FRACTURE TREATMENT AND HEALING

edited by

R. BRUCE HEPPENSTALL, M.D., F.A.C.S.

Associate Professor of Orthopaedic Surgery,
University of Pennsylvania School of Medicine
Chief, Fracture Service,
Hospital of the University of Pennsylvania,
Philadelphia
Chief, Orthopaedic Surgery,
Philadelphia Veterans' Administration Hospital

W. B. SAUNDERS COMPANY   1980
Philadelphia   London   Toronto

W. B. Saunders Company: West Washington Square
Philadelphia, PA   19105

1 St. Anne's Road
Eastbourne, East Sussex BN21, 3UN, England

1 Goldthorne Avenue
Toronto, Ontario M8Z 5T9, Canada

Library of Congress Cataloging in Publication Data

Main entry under title:

Fracture treatment and healing.

1. Fractures.   2. Wounds.   3. Wound healing.
   I. Heppenstall, R. Bruce. [DNLM: 1. Fracture fixation.
   2. Wound healing. WE185 F798]

RD101.F73   617'.15   77–79395

ISBN 0–7216–4638–7

Fracture Healing and Treatment   ISBN 0-7216-4638-7

Last digit is the print number: 9   8   7   6   5   4   3   2   1

To my parents Edna and Al for their support and encouragement and to my wife Carol and children Mark and Darcy for their continued patience and understanding

"I treated him, God healed him."

AMBROISE PARÉ (1510–1590)

Contributors

DANIEL C. BAKER, M.D. Clinical Instructor in Surgery, New York University School of Medicine; Assistant Attending Surgeon, Institute of Reconstructive Plastic Surgery, New York University Medical Center; Assistant Attending Surgeon, Manhattan Eye, Ear, and Throat Hospital; Assistant Attending Surgeon, Head and Neck Service, St. Vincent's Hospital, New York, New York

JONATHAN BLACK, Ph.D. Associate Professor of Research in Orthopaedic Surgery, University of Pennsylvania School of Medicine; Director, Biomaterials Laboratory, Department of Orthopaedic Surgery, University of Pennsylvania, Philadelphia, Pennsylvania

JOHN J. BONICA, M.D., D.Sc., F.F.A.R.C. Professor of Anesthesiology, University of Washington School of Medicine; Director of Pain Clinics, University of Washington Affiliated Hospitals, Seattle, Washington

F. WILLIAM BORA, JR., M.D. Professor of Orthopaedic Surgery, Chief of the Hand Service, University of Pennsylvania School of Medicine; Attending Physician, Hospital of the University of Pennsylvania, Children's Hospital of Philadelphia, and Fitzgerald-Mercy Medical Center, Philadelphia, Pennsylvania

CARL T. BRIGHTON, M.D., Ph.D. Chairman, Department of Orthopaedic Surgery; Paul B. Magnuson Professor of Bone and Joint Surgery, Department of Orthopaedic Surgery, University of Pennsylvania School of Medicine; Chief of Orthopaedic Surgery, Hospital of the University of Pennsylvania; Attending Orthopaedic Surgeon, Children's Hospital of Philadelphia and Philadelphia Veterans' Administration Hospital, Philadelphia, Pennsylvania

STEPHEN H. BUTLER, M.D. Assistant Professor of Anesthesiology, University of Washington School of Medicine; Attending Anesthesiologist, University Hospital, Harborview Medical Center, and Seattle Veterans' Administration Hospital, Seattle, Washington

JOHN MARQUIS CONVERSE, M.D. Lawrence D. Bell Professor of Plastic Surgery, New York University School of Medicine; Director, Institute of Reconstructive Plastic Surgery, New York University Medical Center; Director of Plastic Surgery Service, Bellevue Hospital; Consultant in Plastic Surgery, Manhattan Eye, Ear, and Throat Hospital, and Manhattan Veterans' Administration Hospital, New York, New York

D. A. DeLAURENTIS, M.D. Professor of Surgery, University of Pennsylvania School of Medicine; Director of Surgery, Pennsylvania Hospital, Philadelphia, Pennsylvania

VINCENT DiSTEFANO, M.D. Clinical Assistant Professor of Orthopaedic Surgery, University of Pennsylvania School of Medicine; Team Physician, Philadelphia Eagles Football Club, Philadelphia, Pennsylvania

WILLIAM T. FITTS, M.D. Professor of Surgery, University of Pennsylvania School of Medicine, Philadelphia, Pennsylvania

ZACHARY B. FRIEDENBERG, M.D. Professor of Orthopedic Surgery, University of Pennsylvania School of Medicine; Attending Orthopedic Surgeon, Presbyterian–University of Pennsylvania Medical Center, Philadelphia, Pennsylvania

ROBERT M. GLAZER, M.D. Clinical Assistant Professor of Orthopaedic Surgery, University of Pennsylvania School of Medicine, The Graduate Hospital of Philadelphia, Children's Hospital of Philadelphia, and Philadelphia Veterans' Administration Hospital, Philadelphia, Pennsylvania

EDWIN S. GURDJIAN, M.D. Senior Vice-Chief of Neurosurgery, Grace Hospital, Detroit, Michigan

E. STEPHEN GURDJIAN, M.D., Ph.D. Emeritus Professor of Neurosurgery, Wayne State University School of Medicine, Detroit, Michigan

WILSON C. HAYES, Ph.D. Associate Professor of Orthopaedic Surgery, Harvard Medical School; Director, Orthopaedic Biomechanics Laboratory, Beth Israel Hospital, Boston, Massachusetts

THOMAS K. HUNT, M.D. Professor of Surgery and Ambulatory and Community Medicine, University of California, San Francisco School of Medicine, San Francisco, California

RAE R. JACOBS, M.D. Associate Professor of Surgery, University of Kansas; Chief, Orthopedic Section, Veterans' Administration Medical Center; Chief, Problem Spine Clinic; formerly Director, Emergency Surgical Service, Kansas University Medical Center, Kansas City, Kansas

JEROLD Z. KAPLAN, M.D. Director, Burn Center, Alta Bates Hospital; Assistant Clinical Professor of Surgery, University of California, Davis, California

JOSEPH M. LANE, M.D. Associate Clinical Professor of Orthopedic Surgery, Cornell University Medical School; Chief, Bone Tumor Service, Memorial Hospital for Cancer and Allied Diseases; Chief, Metabolic Bone Disease and Associate Attending Orthopedic Surgeon, Hospital for Special Surgery; Attending Orthopedist, New York Hospital, New York, New York

PETER R. McCOMBS, M.D. Assistant Professor of Surgery, University of Pennsylvania School of Medicine; Associate Surgeon, Pennsylvania Hospital and Northeastern Hospital, Philadelphia, Pennsylvania

JAMES M. MORRIS, M.D. Associate Professor of Orthopaedic Surgery, University of California Medical Center, San Francisco, California

JAMES NIXON, M.D. Clinical Professor of Orthopaedic Surgery, University of Pennsylvania School of Medicine; Chief, Orthopaedic Surgery, The Graduate Hospital of Philadelphia, Philadelphia, Pennsylvania

A. LEE OSTERMAN, M.D. Assistant Professor of Orthopaedic Surgery, University of Pennsylvania School of Medicine; Director of Orthopedic Microsurgery, Hospital of the University of Pennsylvania; Children's Hospital of Philadelphia, The Graduate Hospital of Philadelphia, Philadelphia, Pennsylvania

BASIL A. PRUITT, JR., M.D., Colonel, M.C. Commander and Director, United States Army Institute of Surgical Research, Brooke Army Medical Center, Ft. Sam Houston, Texas

ROBERT B. SALTER, O.C., M.D., M.S., F.R.C.S.(C). Professor and Head of Orthopaedic Surgery, University of Toronto; Senior Orthopaedic Surgeon and Research Project Director, The Hospital for Sick Children, Toronto, Ontario

FREDERICK A. SIMEONE, M.D. Associate Professor, University of Pennsylvania School of Medicine; Chief of Neurosurgery, Pennsylvania Hospital and Presbyterian–University of Pennsylvania Medical Center, Philadelphia, Pennsylvania

WALTON VAN WINKLE, JR., M.D. Emeritus Professor of Surgical Biology, University of Arizona College of Medicine, Tucson, Arizona

Preface

I first entertained the idea for a new fracture text in 1974. At that time no reference text combining basic research and clinical management of the fracture patient was available for the student or the practicing orthopedic surgeon. It is difficult to envision how a practitioner can provide excellence in patient management without a solid understanding of the basic aspects of the healing process. Only within the last decade has research at both a cell and a tissue level provided us with exciting and clinically applicable insights into the healing process. With this in mind, I approached Jack Hanley at the W. B. Saunders Company to discuss the need for a new fracture text. Mr. Hanley agreed that the concept of a text incorporating basic new scientific and clinical findings into the management of patients with fractures would be a useful addition to the medical literature. At times the task appeared almost impossible to combine with a busy clinical practice. My family was always patient and understanding, which provided me with the motivation to continue through many "wee hours" of the morning.

As with any project, many people played key roles in its production. I will be forever grateful to my training chief, Dr. Edgar Lee Ralston, for his guiding hand and stable influence during and following my training years. He also has a specific interest in fractures, and I am sure that much of his enthusiasm has rubbed off on me through the years. During his time as Chairman at the University of Pennsylvania, he always considered the students and residents as part of his family, providing a very friendly and productive working environment.

Following formal training, I was involved in basic research in the wound healing laboratory of Dr. Thomas K. Hunt. This offered an unusual opportunity to apply soft-tissue research techniques to the fracture healing process, with several interesting results. Dr. Hunt has remained a personal friend and has continued to be extremely helpful through the years. The first chapter of this book was written by Dr. Hunt and is an important contribution, as soft tissue plays a vital role in the fracture healing process.

Dr. Carl T. Brighton, the current Chairman at Penn, has continued to play the most vital role in developing my career. During my training period he guided me through several productive research projects, and we have continued this close relationship. It was through his efforts that I was appointed the Chief of the Fracture Service at Penn. He has written a chapter for the book dealing with the exciting new development of stimulating fracture healing through the use of electrical current.

To my many other co-authors I extend my personal gratitude. Mary Jo Larson provided the many medical illustrations and Karl Ott the photography for the book. Marie Tschantz and Frances Hickman provided the secretarial help and many hours of devoted typing. The valuable assistance of Susan Hunter, Ruth Barker, and Constance Burton of the W. B. Saunders Company is greatly appreciated.

I have attempted to integrate the new basic science and clinical aspects of fracture healing into this text, with the goal of providing a useful reference for students, residents, and practicing orthopedic surgeons. I hope this has been accomplished.

R. BRUCE HEPPENSTALL, M.D.

Contents

THOMAS K. HUNT, M.D.

and

WALTON VAN WINKLE, JR., M.D.

Wound —————————————————— *1*
Healing

Repair is a normal reaction to injury and may be the key to prolonged life in a hostile environment. It is the keystone on which surgery is founded. Despite the lessons of surgical history, it seems that most surgeons accept it as an inevitability, a process that will or will not occur, and having occurred will be "normal"—a single immutable sequence. A look at surgical history reveals, however, that a number of our most fundamental advances have coincided with sudden new insights into the reparative mechanisms. Witness Lister's struggle to separate the fact of sepsis from the fact of normal repair. It has been recognized since the time of Hippocrates that union of two cut edges of tissue can occur without inflammation or sepsis. Yet up to a century ago such an event was so unpredictable that surgeons "incorporated" sepsis into their concepts of normal repair; when "laudable pus" appeared, eventual recovery was expected. When cleanliness had become an ideal, and the microbial theory had become a fact, the stage was set for Semmelweis, Lister, and others to achieve a concept so important that it literally made modern surgery possible. They realized that sepsis and repair were separate phenomena. They learned to expect repair without infection.

Refinements in aseptic technique, the introduction of antibiotics, and improvements in surgical technique, now make primary repair by far the rule rather than the exception. Today the argument would seem to have been won—but has it? In fact, we disagree only in quantity with the surgeons of Lister's early days. Sepsis and delayed union of wounds are no longer considered inevitable; we merely expect them part of the time. Scarring is considered controllable in some—but certainly not all—cases. Repair is not simply the surgeon's ally; it is his concern, his lifeline. Unless the surgeon arranges his priorities to aid the forces of repair and to mobilize resistance to infection, he will be, in substance, little more than a surgeon of the last century who somehow has found a modern operating room.

INJURY

When tissue is injured, blood vessels are broken or cut. Platelets bind to the exposed collagen and release their phospholipids, which stimulate the intrinsic coagulation mechanism. Injured tissue cells release thromboplastin, which activates the extrinsic coagulation mechanism. At the same time, the aggregating platelets, and perhaps white cells, release proteolytic enzymes that initiate the cascade of proteolytic enzymes in the complement system. As this enzymatic cascade rapidly amplifies the distress signals of injured tissue, chemotactic substances accumulate and call forth the inflammatory cells, which are first seen sticking to the sensitized endothelial membranes of local vessels. The cells follow the chemical signals to the area of injury and bind their membranes to the various components of injured tissue. The

1

phagocytic cells ingest these altered substances, and the act of phagocytosis "activates" them.

Exactly what calls forth the sudden burst of fibroblast replication near the area of injury is unknown. The evidence suggests that platelets activated by thrombin and macrophages activated by phagocytosis release a substance or substances that can stimulate replication of fibroblasts. No matter what the signal, the evidence is clear that the vast majority of the total fibroblast population originates in the wound itself, probably stemming from cells located in or around local small vessels.

Fibroblasts in cell culture do not necessarily make collagen. It seems necessary to stimulate them to do so. The most prominent stimulators of collagen synthesis in cultured fibroblasts are ascorbic acid and lactate ion, which "activate" enzymes necessary for collagen synthesis. The lactate that accumulates after several hours of hypoxia will also "activate" these enzymes. The hypoxia or the concentrations of ascorbate and lactate necessary to stimulate collagen synthesis in cell culture are actually present in wounded tissue. As the numerous cells that are called into the wound reach the environment of damaged vasculature and limited oxygen supply, anaerobic metabolism inevitably results. The extracellular oxygen tension in this area falls well below 10 mm Hg, a point probably below the critical or lowest optimum level for aerobic metabolism in both fibroblasts and leukocytes. Possibly for this reason, fibroblasts and new epithelial cells start their lives with a prominent capacity for anaerobic metabolism. The by-product of the glycolytic pathway of anaerobic metabolism is lactate. Furthermore, leukocytes and macrophages, when "activated" by the ingestion of altered substances or foreign body, have a prodigious capacity for lactate production in either aerobic or anaerobic conditions. Within a few days, lactate in the extracellular fluid of the central dead space of wounds is in the region of 10 to 15 millimolar.

THE WOUND MODULE

At this relatively adult stage, the wound cells form a rather vague "module of repair"

(Fig. 1–1). In the van of the advancing wound edge is the macrophage. Wound macrophages seem to be chronically activated and are usually found with ingested substances in their digestive vacuoles. Just behind these cells are some maturing but still youthful fibroblasts, apparently the products of nearby cells that are actively dividing. Cells undergoing mitosis are normally found between the first functioning capillary and the first maturing fibroblast of the wound edge. The most distal functioning blood vessel is stationed just behind the first maturing fibroblasts. It sprouts new capillary buds that are destined to complete an arcuate path through the injured tissue, either to unite with a vessel from the other side in primary repair,* to unite with a cut vessel end in a skin graft, or to join another similar bud from a lower or higher pressure point in the granulation tissue of an open or dead space wound.† The new and tender microcirculatory loops find external support in the collagen gel secreted by the immature fibroblasts. Without such support they would inevitably rupture as soon as they were exposed to the pressure of the arterial system. As each new capillary loop becomes functional, more oxygen becomes available to the cells of the wound "module." The fibroblasts, now in a higher oxygen pressure, can synthesize more collagen and can migrate further until they again run out of oxygen. The process continues in a cyclic fashion. As the "module" proceeds, the collagen-synthesizing fibroblasts are left behind to continue their work of constructing and reconstructing the new connective tissue.

---

*"Primary repair" is the term used to describe healing of a wound that is accurately reapproximated and mends with minimal space between its edges. It is sometimes called repair by first intention. Closure of a wound on the fourth or fifth day is often called delayed primary closure.

†Healing of a dead space or open wound is said to occur by second intention. It involves filling of a tissue defect through formation of large amounts of new connective tissue, new vessels, and new epithelium in many cases. The term usually implies an external, open wound, but the repair involved is much the same as in healing of a closed space such as a pneumonectomy space, or a serum or blood collection such as often occurs in fractures.

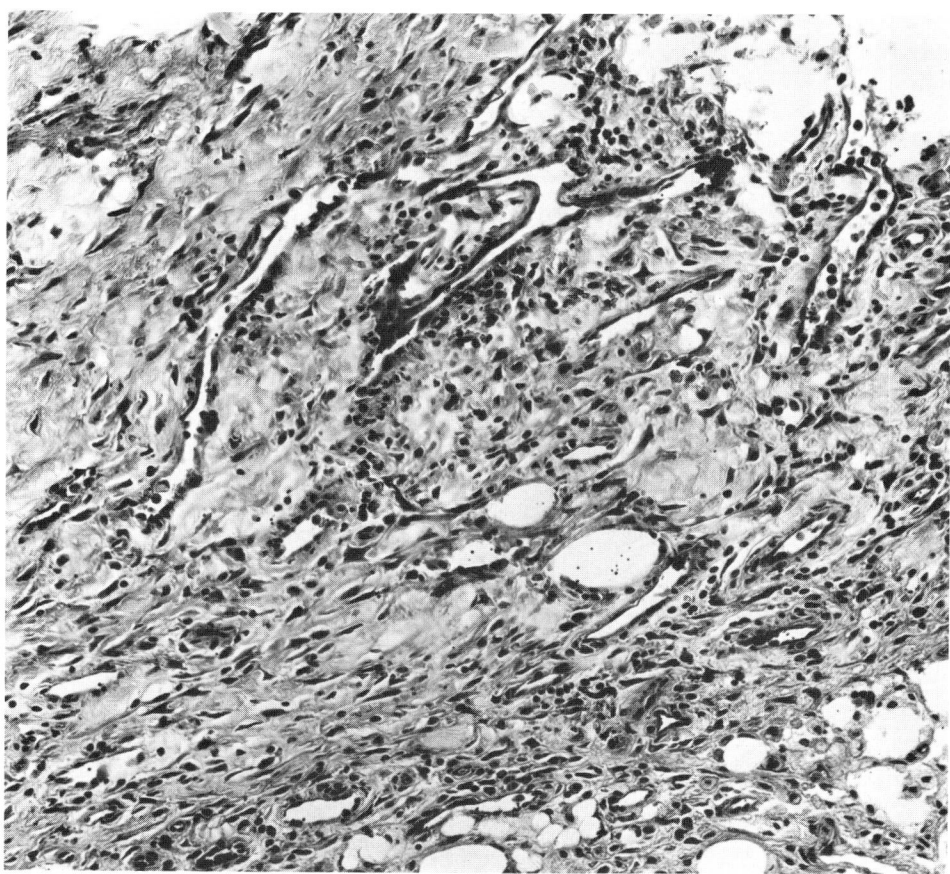

Figure 1-1   Medium-high-power magnification of granulation tissue from a "dead wound" in a rabbit. The central space of the wound is in the upper right corner. All this tissue is new. Small vessels can be seen emptying into the dead space. Macrophages can be seen on the surface, and fibroblasts are scattered about below. Some remodeling of the fibrous tissue into fat is seen in the right lower corner. Reprinted from Fundamentals of Wound Management in Surgery, Chirurgecon, Plainfield, N.J.

The concept of the advancing "module" implies that there are metabolic gradients in the wound that probably influence its form and its motion. One would expect that, if the foregoing description is accurate, there would be a very low oxygen tension at the surface of the macrophage in the wound module. In fact, this is true. Measurements of oxygen gradients show that the P_{O_2}, which is in the region of 50 mm Hg over the arteriolar portion of the capillary, falls to near 0 mm Hg at the surface of the macrophages and in the dead space. The lactate, hydrogen ion, and P_{CO_2} gradients slope in the other direction—that is, high in the dead space and lower near the functioning vessels.

LEUKOCYTES—THE MACROPHAGE

Leukocytes appear in the wound within a few hours. At first, they are mostly polymorphonuclear cells, but by about the fifth day the predominant leukocytes are macrophages. This type of cell remains in the wound until it is healed (Fig. 1–2).

Primary repair occurs uninhibited even by major reductions in the numbers of circulating and tissue neutrophils and lymphocytes in the system. Their role is to inhibit and kill contaminating bacteria. When the macrophage is eliminated from the healing wound, however, even primary repair suffers. Macrophages are wandering mononuclear cells found in tissues and

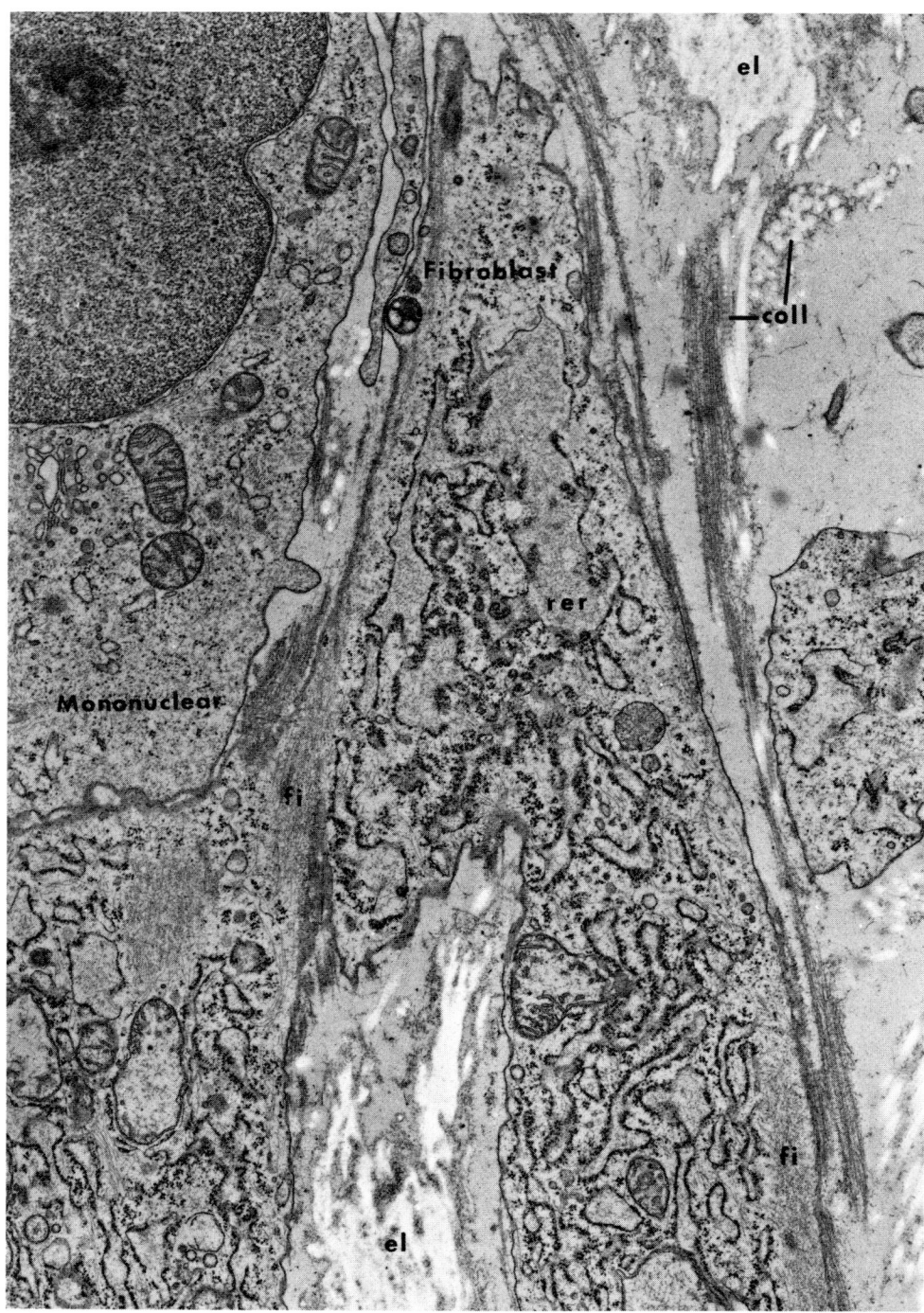

Figure 1–2 Electron microscope view of one field in a wound, demonstrating the intimate relationship between mononuclear cells and fibroblasts. There are a few filaments in the periphery of the fibroblasts, suggesting that there might be some smooth muscle function in the cell. A layer of extracellular collagen (coll) can be seen around the fibroblasts. *el*, elastin; *fi*, fibrin; *rer*, rough endoplasmic reticulum. (Courtesy of Russell Ross, Ph.D., University of Washington Medical School). Magnification × 17,000. Reprinted from Fundamentals of Wound Management in Surgery, Chirurgecon, Plainfield, N.J.

tissue spaces. They are actively phagocytic and can kill organisms in a manner apparently similar to that of polymorphs. They can ingest particles and macromolecules, and excrete the products of digestion into the surrounding environment. Recent laboratory research suggests that local macrophages can play a nutritional role by acting as "the digestive tract of the wound." Probably most important, however, is that macrophages seem to act as director cells. The case is strong that the macrophage is the key cell of the inflammatory response to injury. It (1) debrides injured tissue, (2) processes macromolecules to useful amino acids and sugars, (3) attracts more macrophages, (4) probably signals for fibroblast replication, (5) may signal for neovascularization, and (6) secretes lactate.

In some unknown manner, vitamin A aids the entrance of macrophages into the wound. This important vitamin is vital to the initiation of repair. If macrophage entry is prevented by antiinflammatory steroids, repair can usually be stimulated by giving vitamin A. In this case, the vitamin A administration is followed by increased leukocyte and macrophage entry into the wound.

VASCULAR ENDOTHELIUM

One of the most important and least appreciated aspects of repair is the regeneration of new blood vessels. Neovascularization is seen in injuries, infarcts, areas of inflammation (especially those attended by certain types of macrophagic inflammation), and tumors. The function of angiogenesis or neovascularization in wounds is to nourish tissue that obviously cannot be well nourished unless new vessels can replace and supplement the old, injured system. Present concepts rest on two major facts: First, new vessels originate from existing vessels; and second, whatever their ultimate size or function becomes, all new vessels begin as capillaries (Figs. 1–3, 1–4, 1–5, and 1–6).

The new vasculature is formed, in general, in three ways. The first is by generation of a whole new vascular network where a large tissue defect has to be filled. The second is by union with an unused network as the host bed provides circulation to a skin graft. The third is by joining (or rejoining) of vessels across a primarily closed wound.

It seems most instructive to consider the generation of a new vascular network first.

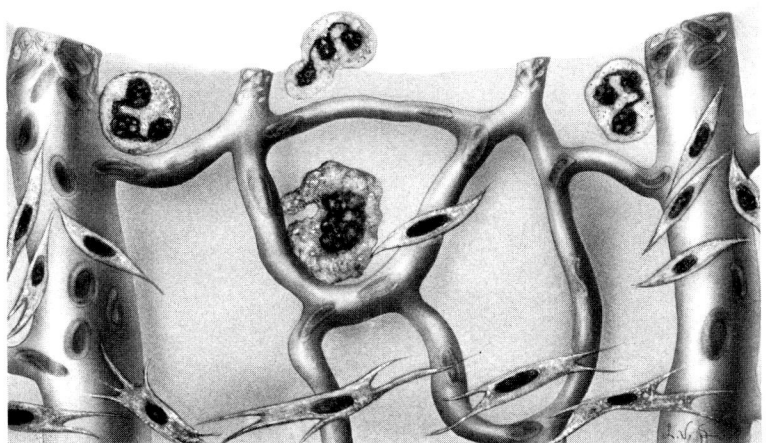

Figure 1–3 Schematic drawing of the wound just after injury. Vessels have become thrombosed with platelet and fibrin clots, and an early inflammatory exudate is appearing. This and the following series reprinted from Fundamentals of Wound Management in Surgery, Chirurgecon, Plainfield, N.J.

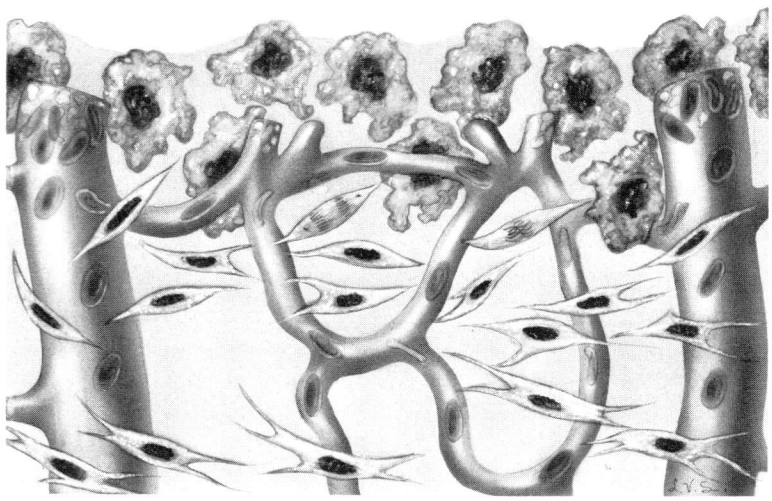

Figure 1-4 This wound, at five to seven days, now shows an inflammatory exudate dominated by mononuclear cells. Fibroblasts have appeared, mostly from their usual origin in perivascular cells. Endothelial capillary buds are present in the center of the preexisting capillary arcade.

The clinical circumstance is healing of a dead space in tissue—a severe fracture, for instance. First, the injured vessels become thrombosed. The wound module is assembled, and from the functioning vessels nearest the wound, sprouts of vascular cells appear from the bases of the existing endothelial cells. Such capillary sprouts are pictured in Figures 1-4, 1-5, and 1-6. These new vessels somehow join with similar sprouts from a lower or higher pressure system to form a functioning capillary loop. Later on, this loop will either participate in formation of a larger vessel or

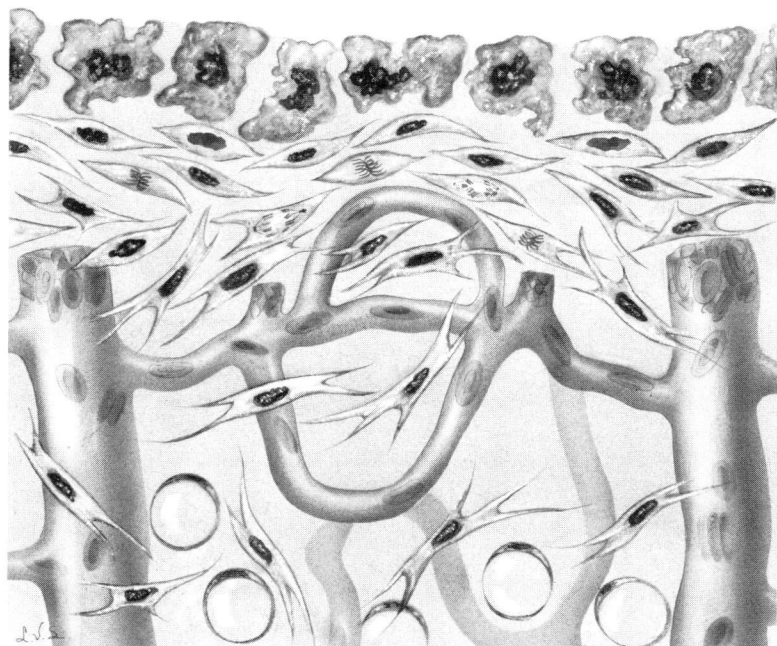

Figure 1-5 At about 10 days the fibroblast response is at its peak. The "wound module" is complete. There is a new functioning capillary loop in the center.

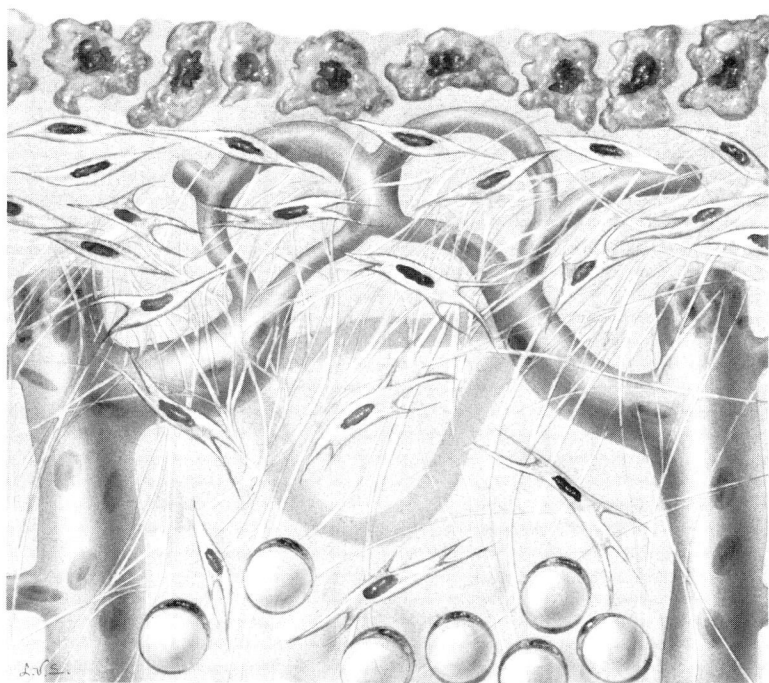

Figure 1–6 The edge of the wound has advanced. More capillary loops have formed and some old loops have dropped out or become "ghost vessels." The supplying artery and vein are becoming larger and larger because they are now supplying an increased volume of tissue. Compare these with Figure 1–19, which shows much the same section in a real wound.

will stop functioning and disappear.

Some vascular sprouts appear to have no lumina. Others appear to be open-ended tubes through which red cells escape. This last type would seem to predominate in primary repair or revascularization of a skin graft. For a while after cannulation has occurred, the new endothelial cells fit loosely and the new vessels are fragile and "leaky." Large particles in blood, colloidal carbon for instance, leak between the cell junctions and are phagocytized by macrophages, perhaps "activating" them. There is no ready explanation for the stimulation for new vessel formation. The molecular signals are entirely unknown, though as noted, macrophages and platelets seem to have the capacity to make the signals. We have seen new veins 2 or 3 mm in diameter traversing the space across totally enclosed wire mesh cylinders. Arteries up to 1 mm or more in diameter have been seen in ear chambers. Vascular studies on healing tissues have shown that arteries up to 3 mm have regained continuity across the base of a pedicle flap. One can only speculate that,

somehow, hypoxia plays a role. The loss of a metabolic stimulant to new circulation would seem to be adequate explanation for lack of flow within vessels, thus explaining the gradual disappearance of unused vessels after healing is complete. Exactly how the stem vessels become larger and larger as more and more tissue has to be traversed and more and more tissue is supplied, is, as yet, an unsolved mystery.

In primary repair, reestablished circulation bridging the wound can be noted by the second or third day. The manner in which reconnection of vessels occurs is not understood. It seems likely, however, that thrombosed vessels may be reopened by the thrombolytic mechanism. Most vessel endothelia contain fibrinolysin, which may open "holes" in the fibrin that initially locks the wound edges together. Pathways for blood cells may form thereafter, just as oft-walked paths in a field become worn by constant use. Such a pathway would be an ideal guide for sprouting endothelial cells.

Vascular regeneration is, as one might expect, a delicate process: Excessive motion can destroy it. Histamine depletion and numerous of the cytoplasmic poisons used in chemotherapy stop it. Vascular regeneration is poor in tissue bearing chronic changes of radiation exposure. Clinically, however, we find that the placement of an autograft or heterograft on viable but wounded and radiation-damaged tissue, followed by administration of oxygen to maintain the arterial PO_2 in the region of 200 mm Hg, is followed by obvious evidence of neovascularization hitherto unseen in the wound in these chronically scarred and wounded tissues.

Vascular regeneration is also poor in steroid-treated patients. Once again, vitamin A seems to restimulate the process, further indication that monocytes have a role in neovascularization. Regeneration is also inhibited in ischemic tissue. As neovascularization goes, so goes the wound.

THE FIBROBLAST

The fibroblast synthesizes and deposits collagen and proteoglycans. There has been controversy about the site of origin of fibroblasts. The basic reason for the controversy has been that the fibroblast, as seen in the actively healing wound, is not seen in normal tissue. Since fibroblasts are rare in tissue, they were once thought to be derived from blood spilled into the injury. Extremely sophisticated experiments with symbiotic animals, however, with radiation inhibition of cells in wounded tissue, give the irrefutable answer that all or almost all fibroblasts found in the wound originate in the injured tissue. Most of the cells appear to rise from perivascular cells. Whatever the signal, the response is extraordinary—especially in connective tissue in which a relatively acellular tissue is converted to one that is almost pure cells within a few days.

The mature fibroblast is pictured in Figure 1–2 and diagrammed in Figure 1–7. It is richly endowed with endoplasmic reticulum, Golgi apparatus, and mitochondria, as are other protein-synthesizing cells. It is mobile and migrates in tissue culture. Its mobility is subject to contact inhibition, leading some to say that the contact of the fibroblasts of one side of a wound with the

fibroblasts of the other is the signal that turns off repair. Unfortunately, this concept does not stand even first examination, since the object of repair is not edge-to-edge fibroblasts. It is edge-to-edge collagen. Contact inhibition may serve as a means of limiting the wound population during the most intense phases of fibroplasia, but any role it has in limiting the totality of repair must be small.

The fibroblast is a hardy cell. It favors a solid surface on which to attach and migrate. It makes collagen best in a slightly acidotic environment with an oxygen tension of over about 10 to 20 mm Hg but below that of air. It needs a reducing environment, usually rich in ascorbate, to produce collagen; and, as outlined earlier, it makes more collagen if that environment contains a high concentration of lactate.

The immature fibroblast is rounded, while the mature one is elongated with long cell processes that aid its mobility. These processes can even guide a fibroblast over or under a nearby fibroblast. Some fibroblasts have a rich supply of myofibrils and appear to be a hybrid "myofibroblast." This cell will contract and relax in response to the usual stimuli. Such cells are found in contracting wounds, where they seem to furnish at least part of the contractile force. They are also seen in large arteries, where they participate in the process of arteriosclerosis.

In view of modern genetic theory, it seems possible that almost any mesenchymal cell could become a fibroblast. Almost every animal organism ever analyzed contains collagen-proteoglycans or chitin-proteoglycans. The genetic code for collagen synthesis would seem to be present in most vertebrate cells; in fact, even some epithelial cells have been induced to produce collagen.

The fibroblast has a full complement of metabolic pathways. It synthesizes collagen, of course, but also synthesizes proteoglycans and elastin. It can synthesize cholesterol and the like. It respires and makes its own adenosine triphosphate. Thus, its requirements probably include most of the B vitamins as well as ascorbate, oxygen, amino acids, and trace metals such as zinc, iron, and copper. Metabolic needs are met by circulating sugars, fats, amino

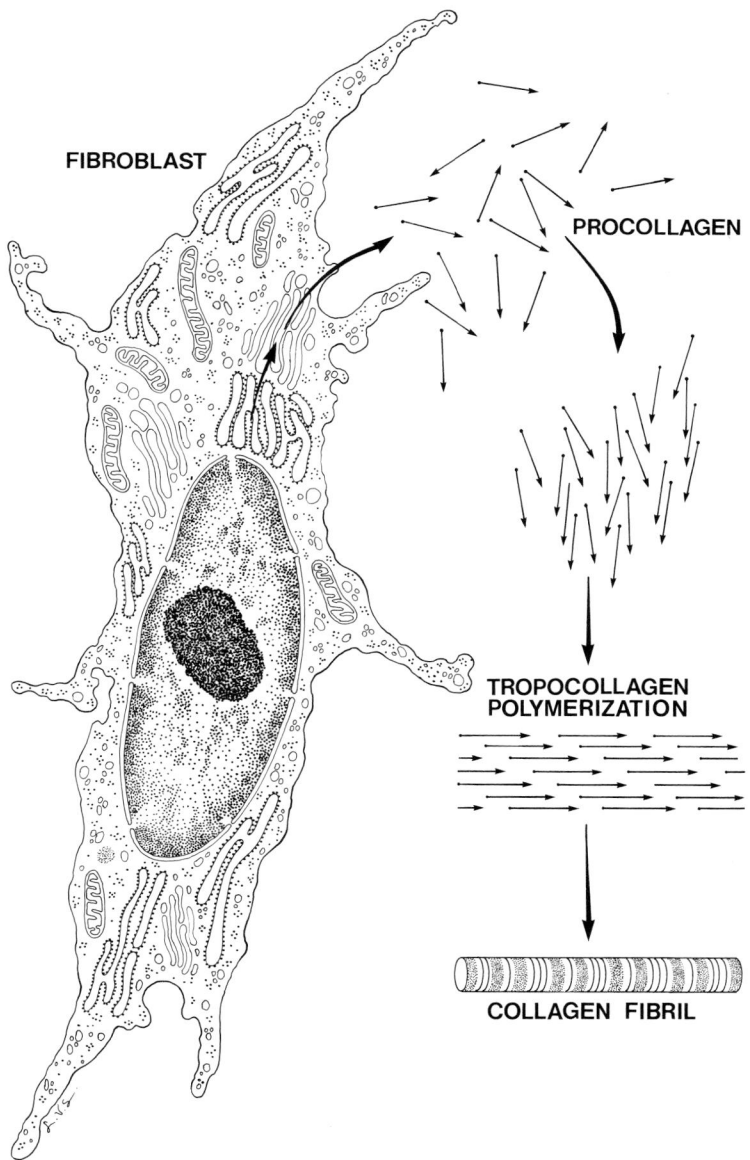

FIBROBLAST

PROCOLLAGEN

TROPOCOLLAGEN POLYMERIZATION

COLLAGEN FIBRIL

Figure 1-7 Schematic diagram of the fibroblast showing the process of collagen synthesis from the endoplasmic reticulum, through the Golgi apparatus, to the extracellular space in the monomer form, and then polymerization of the monomer into collagen fibrils. Reprinted Courtesy of Chirurgecon, Plainfield, N.J.

acids, oxygen, ascorbate, and similar substances. The macrophage may break down local large molecules into reusable amino acids for fibroblast use. Lastly, the fibroblast itself is pinocytic and may supply some of its glucose and amino acid requirement through hydrolysis of more complex molecules.

COLLAGEN

Collagen is the principal structural protein of the body and the major constituent of skin, tendons, ligaments, bones, cartilage, fascia, and the septa of various organs. Of more importance to wound healing, it is the principal component of scar tissue and the

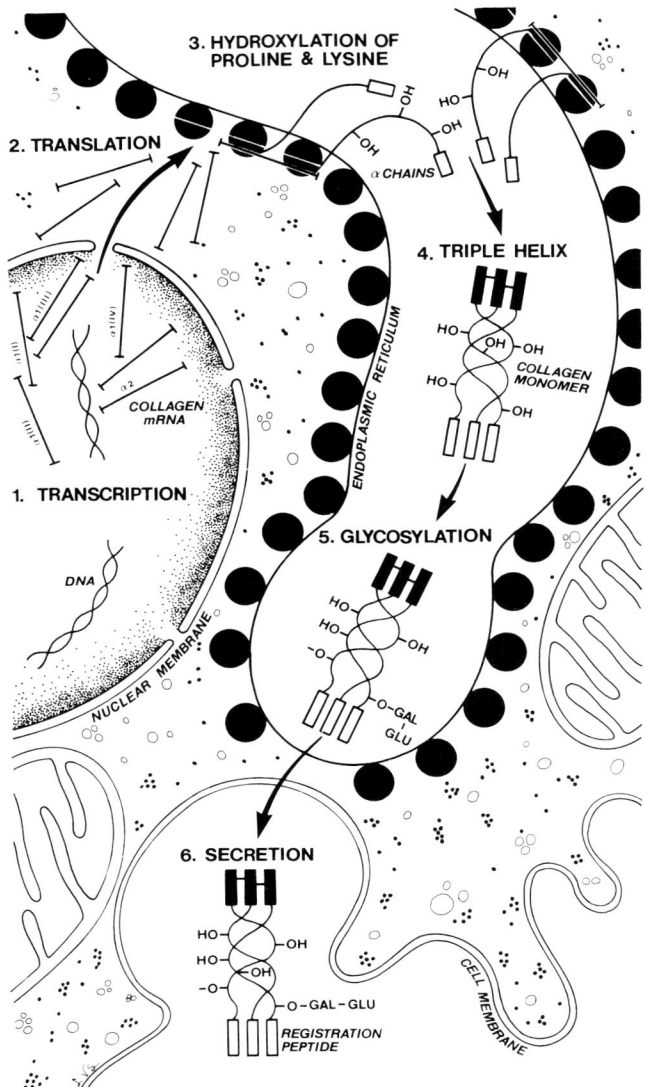

Figure 1-8   Highly diagramatic representation of the steps in collagen synthesis from translation to secretion. The collagen monomer seems to be excreted into the Golgi apparatus, where glycosylation occurs. The molecule is excreted from the cell with the registration peptides still in place. The registration peptides must be cleaved before further polymerization and fibril formation can occur normally. Reprinted Courtesy of Chirurgecon, Plainfield, N.J.

principal product of fibroblasts (Fig. 1–8). It has many chemical and structural properties to distinguish it clearly from other proteins.

When we use the word "collagen" we now mean not a single substance but a group of glycoproteins that have the following attributes in common:

1. They are composed of three separate linear peptide chains of approximately equal length, each containing about 1000 amino acids. These are alpha chains. Each chain is made up of one third glycine, one third proline and hydroxyproline, and one third other amino acids. Glycine occurs in every third position, making a repeating structure of glycine-X-Y. X and Y may be any amino acid, but hydroxyproline and hydroxylysine are usually found in the Y position.

2. Each alpha chain is twisted into a right-handed helix, three of which lie parallel to each other, and the entire structure is then twisted into a left-handed "superhelix." This compound helix is unique to collagen and accounts for its rigidity despite its enormous length of 3000 Å and width of only 15 Å — a ratio of 200 to 1. Its rigidity derives from its ability to cross-link *side to side* with other molecules to form ropelike strands.

Hydroxyproline is almost unique to collagen (it occurs to a small extent in complement). Therefore, the analysis of this amino acid has been a precise means of measuring collagen content.

Four distinct types of collagen are now recognized. All four have the attributes just listed.

Type 1 collagen — found in adult tissues such as dermis, fascia, and bone — is the most common. Two of its three alpha chains, termed alpha-1 chains, are identical. The third, termed alpha-2, is similar but not identical.

Type 2 collagen is found only in cartilage and has three identical alpha-1 chains that differ slightly in amino acid sequence from the alpha-1 chains of type 1 collagen.

Type 3 collagen is found principally in embryonic connective tissue, but is present in small amounts in some adult tissue such as wounds, dermis, and aorta. It also contains three identical chains that differ somewhat from the chains of types 1 and 2 collagen.

A *type 4 collagen* has been identified in certain basement membranes.

Some type 2 collagen is laid down initially in the wound, but as the wound matures it is replaced by type 1 collagen. This is the first hint of an important concept: that collagen composition in wounds changes as time passes. In other words, the original collagen may be removed and replaced before full maturation of the wound can occur. This may be particularly important in bone, in which fracture callus changes from fibrous tissue to cartilagenous tissue to bony tissue. This implies that types 1 and 3 collagen change to type 2 collagen, which changes to type 1 collagen — perhaps three turnovers of collagen before bone can be fully healed.

Collagen Synthesis

Collagen is synthesized in much the same manner as any other protein. There are, however, a few unique steps that make a knowledge of collagen synthesis of great interest to the surgeon and of great potential value in the treatment of healing tissue.

When collagen synthesis is stimulated, the nuclear DNA forms the messenger RNA in a process called transcription (Fig. 1–8). The messenger RNA diffuses into the cytoplasm to control the make-up of the ribosomal network. Transfer RNA attaches specific amino acids to the growing polypeptide chains while they are still attached to the ribosomes. Since no transfer RNA for hydroxyproline or hydroxylysine exists, these two amino acids cannot be directly incorporated into collagen. Instead, proline and lysine are included in the growing chain, and while the chain is still on the ribosome, a significant number of each of these amino acids is hydroxylated through the action of specific enzymes, prolyl hydroxylase or lysyl hydroxylase, with the other substrate being molecular, that is, dissolved, oxygen. The cofactors are ferrous iron, alpha ketoglutarate (a constituent of the Krebs cycle), and a reducing agent such as ascorbic acid. Other substances can take the place of ascorbic acid, but repair proceeds rapidly only with vitamin C. In its absence, prolyl and lysyl hydroxylase, which originate in an inactive monomeric state, will not aggregate into the active enzyme, and oxygen will not be transferred to proline or lysine. Somehow, through a mechanism unknown, lactate participates in the activation (but not the de novo synthesis) of these enzymes; and as already noted, the synthesis of collagen and the activity of prolyl hydroxylase are very much increased in the presence of lactate. Without ascorbate, underhydroxylated collagen is produced, and little of this substance escapes from the cell. That which does escape fails to form characteristic collagen fibers. The condition we recognize as scurvy develops. Wounds fail to heal. Capillaries become fragile because of failure of basement membrane formation. Fractures will not unite, and many other consequences of failure of connective tissue repair occur.

Fibroblasts contain large vacuoles presumably filled with collagen precursor.

The basic chain of collagen can be made with energy derived from anaerobic glycolysis; but without oxygen to hydroxylate proline and lysine, finished collagen production is halted and wound healing cannot take place. As one might expect, a local condition resembling scurvy tends to occur. The mechanism by which ascorbate aids in hydroxylation other than hydroxylase activation is still unclear. It seems that when ascorbate is oxidized in the presence of divalent iron, a high-energy form of oxygen called superoxide ion (O_2^-) results. When more superoxide ion is made available, as when more oxygen is present, collagen synthesis is enhanced. When superoxide ion is produced by photochemical stimulation of riboflavin, collagen synthesis is enhanced as with ascorbate. This may seem rather technical, but the same mechanism becomes important later in the oxidative microbicidal mechanism in leukocytes. The surgeon should remember that adequate oxygen supply is essential to wound well-being in numerous ways.

The collagen resulting from assembly of the alpha chains has special terminal peptides called "registration peptides" that enable the alpha chains to assemble in proper parallel array and at proper distance so that they may assume the superhelical configuration. This molecule (with the registration peptide attached) is transported to the Golgi apparatus where galactose is attached, a step of controversial significance. After glycosylation occurs, the molecule, now called procollagen, is excreted from the cell. Somehow, the microtubule is also important to collagen transport from the cell, because colchicine, which inhibits microtubules, also inhibits collagen transport. When the function of the terminal peptides is over, one or more enzymes termed procollagen peptidases remove them. The resultant molecule is termed tropocollagen. This molecule can polymerize to form the collagen fiber (Fig. 1–9). Deficiency of the enzymes that cleave the registration peptides from procollagen results in a disease of inadequate polymerization found in cattle, called dermatosparaxis, in which skin can be so soft it can be wiped away by the examiner's hand.

Tropocollagen aggregates with other tropocollagen molecules and with partially assembled fibrils, probably by ionic interaction between oppositely charged polar groups in adjacent molecules. These groups occur in clusters along the alpha chains, and somehow the assembly is regulated so that each tropocollagen unit is displaced by one fourth of its length from the adjacent tropocollagen molecule. This "quarter-stagger" arrangement, grouping the polar residues, leads to the characteristic band pattern of collagen seen in transmission electron microscopy. Before and during the assembly of tropocollagen molecules, certain of the lysine residues are acted upon by a specific monamine oxidase, lysyl oxidase. This copper-containing enzyme removes the ε-amino group from the lysine and converts the terminal carbon into an aldehyde, which then reacts with another aldehyde from another lysine, forming an intermolecular cross-link. This link, within each molecule, may not have much significance, but when other lysines from adjacent tropocollagen molecules condense, strong intermolecular covalent bonds are formed. These intermolecular cross-links, which "mature" gradually, are responsible for a major portion of the strength of the collagen fibril.

A disease in cattle and other animals, called lathyrism, is characterized by fragility and weakness of all connective tissues. Bone deformities, skin fragility, and arterial aneurysms are typical. This condition is caused by ingestion of sweet peas of the genus *Lathyris*. The active principle is a compound called β-aminopropionitrile (BAPN), which is a specific inhibitor of lysyl oxidase and thus represses the formation of intermolecular cross-links in both collagen and elastin. Fibril formation proceeds normally, but the fibers have no strength and are soluble in dilute neutral salt solution. Removal of the β-aminopropionitrile allows cross-links to form normally.

Collagen Synthesis in Wound Healing

New collagen can be found in healing wounds as early as the first day. The peak rate of synthesis in a primarily healing wound appears to occur about the fifth to seventh day. The early collagen is highly

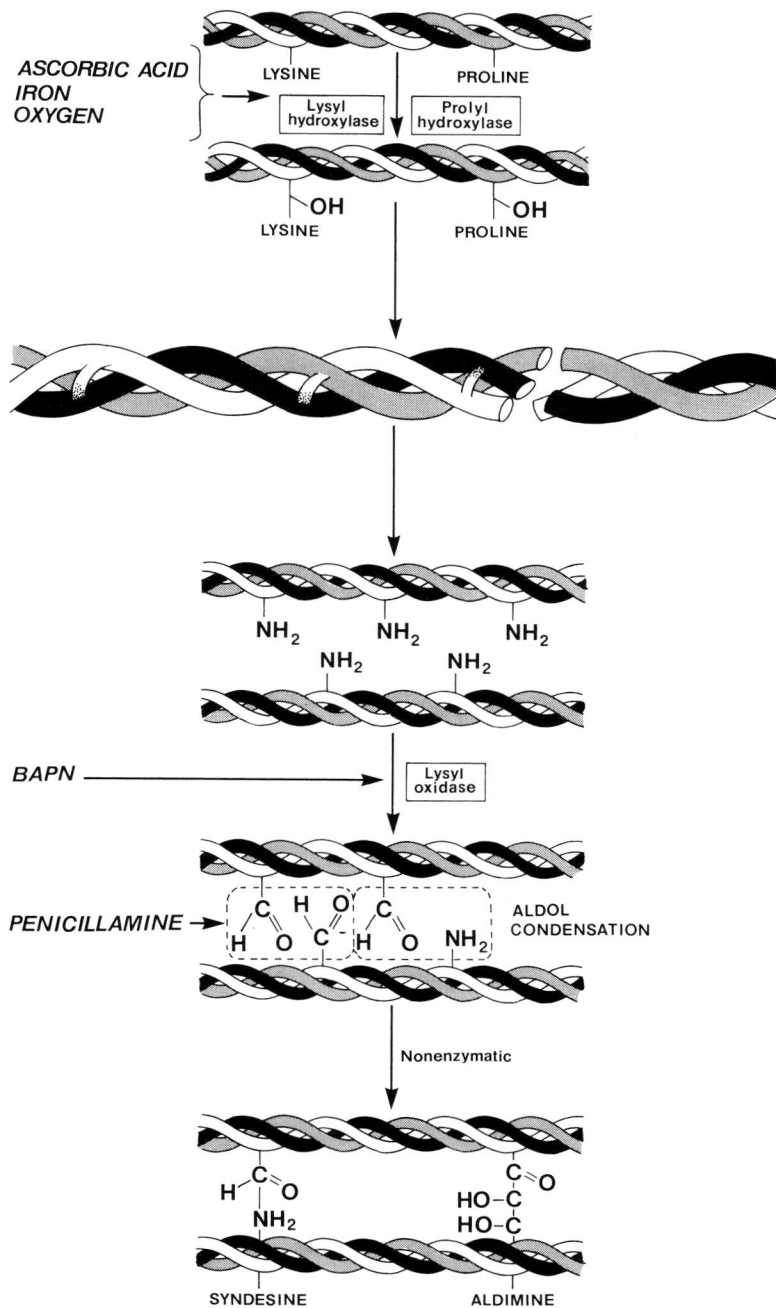

Figure 1-9 A diagram of the extracellular assembly of collagen fibrils. The molecules are aligned to the quarter-stagger arrangement by mechanisms as yet unknown. Covalent cross-links then are formed. Each of the steps noted on the left produces a deficiency or an enzyme inhibitor to fluid. The end result, as shown, is a soft collagen without the usual tensile strength. BAPN, β-aminopropionitrile. Reprinted Courtesy of Chirurgecon, Plainfield, N.J.

disorganized, and views obtained by scanning electron microscopy suggest that collagen exists almost as a gel. The collagen synthesized on the very surface of a wound that is "granulating in" by second intention also exists basically as a gel and can be identified as collagen only through sophisticated immunochemical techniques. The slightly deeper, slightly older collagen appears much more fibrous, mature, and strong.

Collagen synthesis remains rapid for many months after injury, often up to six months or a year. Why, then, does not the wound become hypertrophic and slowly amass collagen until it protrudes from the surrounding tissue? Some scars do continue to amass collagen. Since the vast majority do not, however, one can see that even as collagen is being synthesized it is being lysed and removed in a constant process of collagen turnover.

Collagen Lysis

It might be possible to make an ideal wound if one could use an infinitely sharp knife, protect the wound edge from water loss, and close the wound primarily without sutures within a few seconds of its making. In such a case, little surrounding tissue would have to be debrided by inflammatory cells before the conditions for repair would be suitable. In practice, wounds are not made with infinitely sharp instruments, wounds are exposed and contaminated, and surgeons tend to leave islands of strangulated or coagulated tissue behind them. Before repair can occur, then, the "damaged face of the wound" must be taken down. This process involves collagen lysis as well as removal of noncollagenous tissue. This job is generally left to the macrophage. Polymorphonuclear cells also contribute collagenase. The macrophage can ingest fragments of tissue and can hydrolyze them to amino acids within the digestive vacuole through the action of lysosomal enzymes. In the process of ingestion, macrophages leak these enzymes—which can digest preformed protein, including denatured collagen—into the extracellular fluid. Probably, these enzymes can digest some native

collagen as well, although this point is controversial.

Collagen lysis continues to play a constructive role as normal repair proceeds. At first, newly deposited collagen is essentially a gel, and wound strength is poor. Thus, much of the early-deposited collagen must be broken down, probably ingested, and reduced to amino acids; and these amino acids must be resynthesized into collagen—all in the wound site. This process is essential to maturation of the wound. In order to continue resynthesis, however, amino acids must be brought in from elsewhere, because inevitably some of the original amino acids will be lost to diffusion or to carbohydrate metabolism. Furthermore, some of the by-products of collagen metabolism will inevitably be hydroxyproline and hydroxylysine, neither of which can be resynthesized into collagen and both of which must be replaced from external sources as well as from the pool of unhydroxylated proline and lysine removed from the collagen.

The principal extracellular enzyme involved in collagen lysis is collagenase. This enzyme, at pH7, cleaves native collagen monomer at about a third of its length from one end. The fragments are susceptible to other proteases as well as to ingestion by cells. The intimate details of collagenase are still controversial. It is produced by inflammatory cells, including polymorphonuclear leukocytes. It is also produced by regenerating epidermis and vascular endothelium. Its presence or its activity seems to be enhanced by steroids and inflammatory reactions. Collagen lysis is destructive, and its energy demands are less than those of the constructive process of collagen synthesis. Therefore, lysis continues despite (and may even be accelerated by) starvation, oxygen deficiency, or specific protein deficiency. If collagen synthesis proceeds normally and is not depressed by malnutrition or oxygen deficiency, collagen lysis is offset by synthesis. When the balance is tipped, however, collagen lysis may predominate, and the wound may literally melt away. The reparative process is so delicate that malnutrition or sepsis may shift normal balance to self-destruction.

Balance of Synthesis and Lysis

The most commonly known example of collagen lysis exceeding collagen synthesis in wounds is the well-known proclivity of even apparently healed wounds to break down in a patient who develops scurvy. Here, collagen synthesis and collagen lysis are probably proceeding at a relatively low rate, but in the absence of ascorbic acid, collagen lysis inevitably predominates, and the wound breaks down and falls apart (Fig. 1–10).

The solubility of collagen and its susceptibility to enzymatic destruction are partly dependent on the extent of cross-linking and the stability of the cross-links. Native collagen, in the triple helical configuration, is resistant to the action of such naturally occurring proteolytic enzymes as pepsin, trypsin, or acid proteases. Denatured collagen, however, is susceptible to digestion by most proteolytic enzymes.

Neutral collagenase is a large molecule, and there is some evidence that in wounds its activity is particularly directed toward the already established, highly insoluble collagen. Several studies involving radioactive labeling of old collagen before wounding, or of new collagen after wounding, in rat colon have shown that the old collagen is preferentially destroyed. The end result of this mechanism is that tissue strength suffers until the new collagen can be adequately cross-linked. Every wound passes through a nadir of strength on its way to maturity. Normally, collagenolytic activity is found up to approximately 7 mm away from the wound. Within this region tissue strength diminishes, and sutures placed within this distance of the wound may well cut through. For this reason, it has become customary to close wounds that represent a dehiscence danger with internal retention sutures placed more than 0.5 cm from the wound edge.

The infliction of major trauma not only stimulates collagen lysis in the area of injury but turns on generalized collagen lysis as well. As lean body mass is lost, a disproportional amount of collagen is lost. As the wound becomes larger, and the degree of injury is increased, the ability of each part of the wound to heal diminishes because its content of strong collagen is unduly diminished and also because, for the various reasons already described, collagen synthesis is also diminished.

Although the technical details of collagen lysis in wounds are not available, it is obvious that collagen lysis is an important biological fact. The balance of collagen synthesis and collagen lysis represents the well-being of the wound. Insofar as the surgeon holds this balance in his hands, he also holds the well-being of his patient.

As stated earlier, the peak rate of collagen synthesis in a primarily healing wound occurs at about five to seven days. This corresponds with the most rapid rate of increase in tensile strength. By about the third week, the primarily healing wound has about the greatest mass it will have. This mass is often described as the healing ridge whose absence by the seventh to ninth day may signify the possibility of

Figure 1–10 Tensile strength of the wound is here expressed as a balance between lysis of the old collagen holding the sutures and the new collagen welding the wound edges. Any exaggeration of lysis or deficit of synthesis lowers the nadir of wound tensile strength and increases the time during which the wound is weak. Reprinted courtesy of Lange Publications.

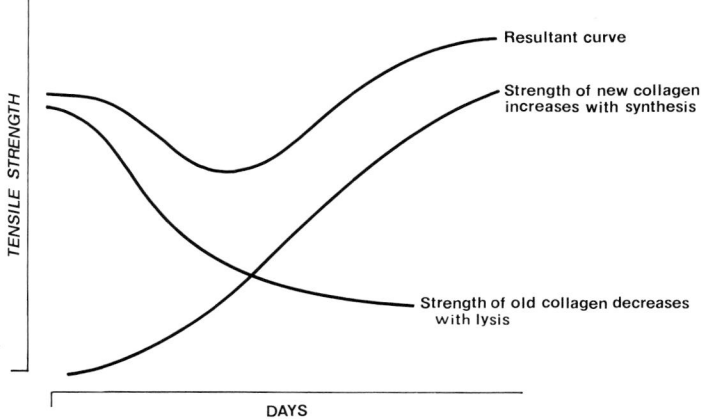

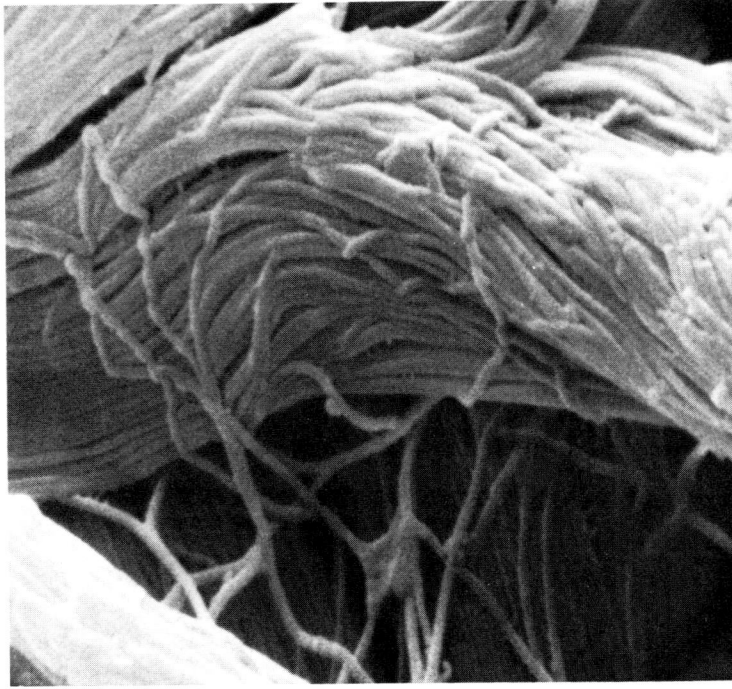

Figure 1-11   Normal skin collagen, probably with some surrounding elastin, magnified approximately 10,000 times. The collagen fiber contains many definable fibrils.

dehiscence of the wound.° This mass, perhaps a simplified counterpart of fracture callus, then recedes, and the tissue softens while its collagen content diminishes. Paradoxically, the strength of the wound increases during this time. The obvious conclusion is that there is remodeling of the structure of the wound and that a more effective structure is being made with less collagen. The major point is that the new structure is not achieved by intelligent *subtraction* of collagen molecules. Instead, it is achieved by intelligent *replacement* of the total collagenous structure. The very close, even gel-like, collagen molecules in the early wound give way to open basketweave tissue structure. Scanning electron microscopic views of normal early and well-remodeled collagen structure from primary wounds in animals are shown in Figures 1-11, 1-12, and 1-13. In this manner, the wound is remodeled and probably remodeled again, and perhaps again, for six months to a year.

Common sense tells us that at some point new collagen must interact with old collagen to form a bond. Either the new collagen physically unites with the ends or sides of old collagen in a sort of "weld" or new collagen fibers interlace with the old, providing a sort of woven junction or "darn." Probably, both possibilities occur. It is very difficult to find cut collagen ends even in an early healing wound, and therefore, we presume that they have united with wound collagen. It is also easy to see, however, as shown in Figure 1-13, that new collagen fibers interlace with old collagen fibers.

If significant inhibitors of collagen synthesis are present in a given case, the surgeon can anticipate wound trouble. If these are coupled with significant enhancers of collagen lysis such as starvation, steroid hormones, and inflammation, they are so potent that, when combined with such factors as arterial hypoxia, hypovolemia, and chemotherapeutic drugs, they greatly impair the likelihood of wound healing and, particularly when infection is present, almost certainly doom the suture line (Table 1-1).

°The converse is also true. A wound that has a healing ridge throughout its length will not dehisce; and sutures, even retention sutures, can safely be removed.

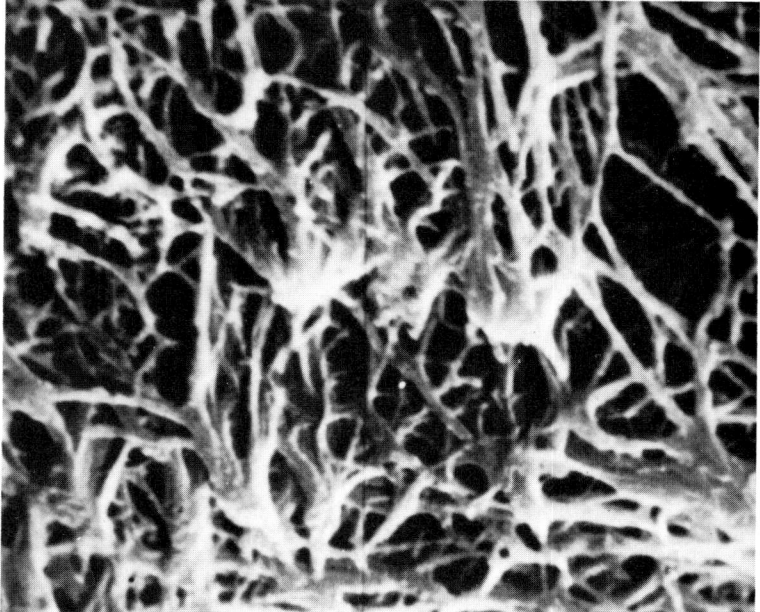

Figure 1–12 Ten-day-old wound collagens by scanning electron microscopy at about 10,000 times' magnification. Note the lack of definition of collagen fibrils and the small fibers as compared to Figure 1–11.

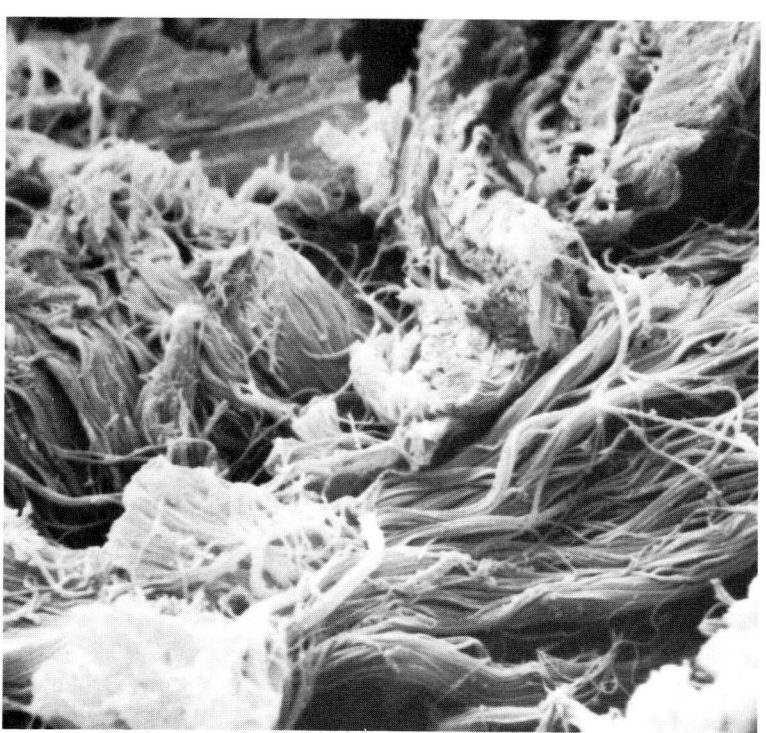

Figure 1–13 Scanning electron micrograph of collagen near a rat colon anastomosis. The most notable feature is the way in which the disorderly new collagen fibrils interlace with more densely packed and orderly older fibers. The new fibers are seen side view in most cases, while the older fibers are seen end view and near the top of the picture.

TABLE 1–1 Factors That Decrease Collagen Synthesis and Increase Collagen Lysis

Synthesis Decreased by
Preoperative
  Starvation (protein depletion)
  Steroids
  Infection
  Associated injuries
  Hypoxia
  Radiation injury
  Uremia
  Diabetes
  Advanced age

Operative
  Tissue injury
  Poor blood supply
  Poor apposition of surrounding tissues
    (pelvic anastomosis)

Postoperative
  Starvation
  Hypovolemia
  Hypoxia
  Drugs (actinomycin, 5-fluorouracil,
    methotrexate, etc.)

Lysis Increased by
Starvation
Severe trauma
Inflammation
Infection
Steroids

° All are active before and after operations.

Normal Collagen Turnover

As collagen in the maturing wound is turned over, its synthesis and deposition probably follow a somewhat different set of rules than on the first synthesis and deposition. The vascular system, which was relatively inadequate the first time around, is now complete. The wound, now having united, is subjected to continuity of stresses and strains as if the tissue were once again normal. The electrical charges produced by these stresses probably result in an alignment of the proteoglycans and collagen fibers. When slight force is applied to it periodically during its maturation phase, the wound is stronger than if it is protected from those forces. Fibroblasts and collagen tend to line up along lines of tension, and in wounds actively resisting tension, such as those surrounding grafts into the abdominal aorta or surrounding fracture or muscle, there is a fibroblastic and collagenous pat-

tern reminiscent of the normal architecture surrounding the original dynamic structure.

PROTEOGLYCANS– GLYCOSAMINOGLYCANS (MUCOPOLYSACCHARIDES)

Among the noncellular components of connective tissue, constituting a substantial portion of what is known as "ground substance," are the glycosaminoglycans. These substances are largely polysaccharides composed of chains of repeating disaccharide units that are in turn composed of glucuronic acid or iduronic acid and a hexosamine. The hexosamine is sulfated in varying degrees, usually at the 4 or 6 position. Glycosaminoglycans rarely exist free in the body, but instead couple to proteins. The combinations are called proteoglycans. The glycosaminoglycans are linked with the carrier protein through an O-glycosidic linkage to a serine or occasionally a threonine residue. There may be several such chains linked to a single protein, and the chain link may vary from about 2000 disaccharides in the case of hyaluronic acid to as few as 10 in the case of keratan sulfate or heparitin sulfate.

Much less is known of the protein core of the proteoglycans. Probably several proteins are involved, all quite large, linear, randomly coiled chains about 4000 Å in length. Thus, proteoglycans are very large molecules and, because of the presence of numerous sulfates and glucuronic groups, are highly charged. The charges tend to repel one another, and the complex molecule occupies considerable space. This space, because of the charge and the steric influences, limits the type and size of molecule that can penetrate. Large negatively charged molecules generally cannot pass through the proteoglycans' domain. Smaller, positively charged molecules may pass through or can even be trapped within the space and bound to the proteoglycans. Thus, the ground substance that contains large amounts of proteoglycans can act as a molecular filter, exactly as does a chromatographic column.

Collagen has groups of charged residues along the alpha chains. These can interact with the charge groups on proteoglycans. The nature, extent, and significance of these interactions is still under investigation. It appears that, however, as we have suspected for years, proteoglycans play a role in collagen fiber formation by binding polymer chains of collagen through electrostatic interactions, orienting and permitting closer proximation of polymer chains, and thus enhancing intermolecular linkages. The fiber orientation and fiber size may be influenced or directed by the characteristics of the proteoglycans. We know that different connective tissues with different architecture contain each a predominance of one or the other type of proteoglycans, and that collagen fiber diameter and orientation are each characteristic for these types of connective tissue. For instance, dermis is composed of large collagen fibers that are coiled about one another in an apparently random fashion. When skin is stretched, however, the majority of fibers orient along the lines of stress. The principal glycosaminoglycan of skin is dermatan sulfate. On the other hand, the collagen fibers of cornea are small and are highly oriented in planes with unidirectional fibers in each plane at approximately right angles to the underlying or overlying fiber bundles. The principal glycosaminoglycan in cornea is keratan sulfate. In corneal scars, however, collagen fibers are randomly arranged and vary greatly in size. The major glycosaminoglycans found in corneal scars are chondroitin sulfate and dermatan sulfate, as in other scars.

Hyaline cartilage presents a special and interesting case of collagen-proteoglycans interaction. The collagen in hyaline cartilage is type 2 and contains a large number of glycosylated hydroxylysine residues. The collagen fibers are small and rarely show a typical banding pattern with the electron microscope. Nearly 50 per cent of the mass of cartilage is proteoglycans. This mixture binds water and releases it slowly under pressure, thus accounting for the elastic and compressive qualities of cartilage. Injury to cartilage is not repaired by the formation of new hyaline cartilage. If repair occurs at all, it is by deposition of fibrocartilage of repair, which contains less proteoglycans and obviously is inferior to the real cartilage. One can imagine the gradual loss of function of the intervertebral disk with wear and the scars of time; scarring in cartilage is very much like scarring in the cornea. There is a loss of normal function as the normal collagen proteoglycans matrix is replaced with one characteristic of scar.

The precise role played by proteoglycans in healing is not understood. Shortly after injury, the hyaluronic acid content of wounds increases rapidly. Some of this comes from the local circulation and seems to be a consequence of microvascular permeability. As healing progresses, the hyaluronic acid decreases and chondroitin sulfates increase. As maturation occurs, the concentration of proteoglycans falls, eventually to a low level. As proteoglycans are lost, water is also lost, and the wound assumes its dense, white appearance owing to the large content of tightly packed collagen fibers. At some point, a small amount of proteoglycans is incorporated into the collagen fiber.

EPITHELIZATION

Since epithelia cover all external surfaces of the body, they are probably the most frequently injured tissues. They have their own style of repair, which usually entails multiplication of the cells at the wound edge, migration across the wound of the resulting new cells, and then maturation of the one or two cell layers into a more (but not quite) normal structure.

Squamous epithelium consists of stratified layers of epithelial cells. The lowermost cells, basal cells, rest on a basement membrane over the connective tissue of the dermis. Above the basal layer are several layers of cells undergoing mitosis or differentiation, known as prickle cells because of the prominent desmosomes, that is, intracellular connections. Above these are well-differentiated cells producing keratin, and on the outermost layers are dead cells that are mostly keratin. Epidermis can be visualized as a modular structure with columns of cells starting at the basal cells and moving slowly outward while differentiating through the prickle cell stage and eventually becoming the dead keratinized residue that constitutes the horny layer of the skin. The outer layers are constantly being desquamated and replaced from below.

When a defect is made in squamous epithelium, the cells at the margin of the wound "flatten" and begin to move toward the area of cell deficit. The migrating cells come from the basal layer. Mitoses appear at the wound edge, and the cells thus produced migrate. Migration is usually started within hours of the making of the defect. There is some tumbling or "leapfrogging" of cells as they move. As the wound becomes covered with flat migrating epithelial cells, those farthest from the margin begin to assume a more cuboidal or rectangular shape and begin to divide. Daughter cells, products of these divisions, pile up, forming once again the characteristic columnar module of the epithelial barrier.

Epithelial cells will migrate only over viable tissue. Thus, the cells often move inward, below the wound debris, blood clot, or eschar. The cells, as one would expect, seek a blood and nutritional supply adequate to function. As the "tongue" of epithelium burrows between the eschar and the living tissue, it releases collagenolytic enzymes that literally cleave through the collagen that connects the viable and nonviable tissues. An eschar produced by exposure therefore impedes epithelization. If the wound is kept moist and is protected from the external environment, but is allowed adequate oxygenation, epithelization will occur on its surface at maximum rate.

Just like the fibroblast, the new epithelial cell is "born" as if its parent recognized the hypoxic nature of wounds. Its enzymes for energy metabolism are primarily glycolytic, but the cell can use oxygen when it becomes available. Epithelial cells can exist but cannot divide or migrate in anoxia. Their rate of division and migration are PO_2-dependent.

The stimulus to repair is a controversial subject. Currently, the most accepted theory is that a "chalone" responsive to catecholamines constantly holds the cells in check. Wounding interrupts this effect, and mitosis results.

Skin sutures create microwounds. Epithelial cells migrate into these wounds just as they do into the major wound. Even dermal appendages will migrate along a suture tract. Occasionally, a plug of keratinizing epithelium will be trapped in the tract when final healing occurs, and small cysts may appear at the side of the mature wound. The epithelized suture tract leaves a scar, which, of course, can be avoided by the use of skin tapes instead of sutures, clips, or staples. Alternatively, the epithelial migration, and hence scarring, can be minimized by removing penetrating fastenings by about the second day and replacing them with tapes.

Epithelization over linear defects, however, is only a minor portion of the wound healing that epithelial cells perform. Superficial injuries—second-degree burns, for instance—epithelize not only from the wound edge but from hair follicles and other deep dermal appendages. Third-degree burns, however, can heal only from the edge of the injury.

The intense cellular activity at the wound edge produces a thickened, active looking hyperplastic zone that disappears after epithelization is complete. Nevertheless, the completed epithelial scar is thin, flat, and devoid of rete pegs. The surface of the scar is often ridged, because epithelization is so often accompanied by contraction. That is, while the covering is becoming complete, the wound is also shrinking, thus throwing the epithelial surface into a set of wrinkles, as discussed in the following section.

Epidermis regenerates faster in hyperbaric oxygen. The underlying blood vessels also regenerate better or are better preserved. Local environment is obviously important to the regenerating squamous cell. Epithelization of second-degree burns is faster under homograft or under microporous tape. The mechanism is not entirely clear, but would seem to involve the conservation of energy that might otherwise be lost to desiccation, heat loss, and the like for more useful metabolic activity. This principle has a number of interesting clinical correlates. For instance, second-degree burns heal more rapidly under intact blisters—a fact proved by many investigators. This does not relieve the surgeon of unroofing milky, white, inflamed, and infected blisters. Infection slows epithelization. Epithelium heals poorly under dressings that are applied wet and removed dry; the clean, moist environment encourages epithelium to grow so the nurse can then tear it off with the dried-on dressing. With this technique one may debride dead tissue, but also one debrides new epithelium that, being only a few cells thick, is easily overlooked.

Squamous cell repair is not totally independent of the underlying wound. The two influence each other by signals that are as yet unknown. Deep repair of inflammation due to a superficial second-degree injury will not occur until epithelization is complete. Or, as epithelium covers granulation tissue, the red, soft tissue loses vessels and shrinks, and its collagen matures. There are many other examples.

WOUND CONTRACTION

Wound contraction is the centripetal movement of full-thickness skin toward the center of the skin defect. It is an active process by which a wound shrinks by "drawing in" surrounding normal skin. The term contraction should not be confused with "contracture," which is the end result of shortening of scar tissue, usually limiting the motion of a joint. For the most part, contraction is a friendly process by which large wounds become small without the necessity for secondary closure or skin graft.

If a rectangular piece of full-thickness skin is excised where the skin is freely movable, the edges of the wound will immediately retract and the wound area may become larger. The retraction is due to the normal skin tension, often recognized in Langer's lines. After three or four days, the area of the wound begins to decrease. Careful examination will show that, although epithelization may have begun, the decrease in area of the wound is due more to the movement of the original wound edges toward the center. The center point of each side of the rectangle will have moved more rapidly than the corners. Eventually, the wound edges will meet, leaving a linear scar in the shape of two Y's, tail-to-tail. Wounds that can heal by contraction often heal to the best cosmetic and functional result in this manner. Whereas almost any wound in an animal can heal by contraction, however, many wounds in the human cannot. For instance, wounds on the anterior

aspect of the lower leg close to the tibia will not close by contraction at all. Wounds of the face will contract, but because the skin is fixed to so many structures nearby, there is a purse string effect and distortion of the features may result; for example, the lower eyelid may be pulled down or the lips may be pulled into a distorted position if a malar wound is allowed to contract. On the other hand, on the back of the neck, even the largest wounds may eventually close with small scars. On the abdomen or the breasts, almost any wound will contract to a size smaller than it began.

Over the years, various theories to explain wound contraction have been advanced. Even today, the last word on this subject has probably not been written. Nevertheless, certain basic facts have been determined: (1) Collagen is not essential for wound contraction. Contraction proceeds normally in the scorbutic animal. (2) The motive force for contraction comes from a cell. Any event that interferes with the viability of cells in the wound edge will inhibit wound contraction. (3) The cells that supply the motive force appear to be a special type of contractile cell having attributes of both the fibroblast and the smooth muscle cell. These cells have been termed "myofibroblasts."

Under light microscopy, the myofibroblasts appear similar to any fibroblast—for that matter, any smooth muscle cell. Under electron microscopy, however, these cells appear to be basically fibroblasts with rough endoplasmic reticulum, but in the periphery of the cytosol, there is contractile protein, actomyosin, in tiny fibrils essentially identical to that found in smooth muscle cells, and microtubules as in normal fibroblasts. These cells have been cultured and have been shown to synthesize and deposit collagen. They have desmosomes and tight intercellular junctions. They become attached to the underlying substrate and respond appropriately to smooth muscle stimulants and relaxants. Therefore, wound contraction can be inhibited by local application of smooth muscle relaxants. It can also be inhibited by antimicrotubular drugs such as vinblastine and colchicine. It appears, therefore, that wound contraction is due to contraction of myofibroblasts and somehow involving the function of microtubules. Certain fibrotic contractures, such as Dupuytren's contracture, also contain myofibroblasts. Strangely, or perhaps fittingly, myofibroblasts are not found in ordinary incised and closed wounds even in areas of skin in which contraction of an open wound would inevitably occur. No one knows what determines whether a mesenchymal cell will differentiate into a myofibroblast or into an ordinary fibroblast. In granulating tissue, cell types vary from pure fibroblasts to fully developed contractile myofibroblasts. Myofibroblasts are also found in high concentrations in wounds of arteries.

Traditionally, a sharp line has been drawn between "contracture" and "contraction." Certainly, scars do shorten, particularly if they often undergo reinjury. With the finding of the myofibroblast in open wounds and contractures, however, the overlapping area between these two concepts requires detailed examination. Why? Because contraction can be inhibited by smooth muscle inhibitors and steroids. If contraction is what causes the early esophageal stricture (it certainly is not the power behind the chronic one), we should learn to be more alert to its early development and prevent it. On the other hand, contracture can often be prevented or treated by local pressure and traction.

Epithelization and wound contraction proceed simultaneously and independently. Neither process seems to affect the other. If a split-thickness skin graft is placed on an excised and contracting wound, contraction may be slowed, but the wound will continue to contract, perhaps even to the same extent as if the graft were not present at all. Clinically, one sees this phenomenon in split-thickness skin grafts that at first lie smooth on a burn wound but later become wrinkled by the contraction of the wound bed. If, however, the wound edges are mechanically splinted so that contraction cannot occur, and if a skin graft is applied immediately, and if the graft and splints remain for at least seven days, contraction will not occur after the splint is removed. A splinted but ungrafted wound will contract rapidly, even after seven days, if the splints are removed. Full-thickness skin grafts, however, either free or as pedicle or rotation flaps, will markedly inhibit contraction if active contraction has not yet commenced.

Lastly, contraction slows with smooth muscle relaxing agents and is literally halted by large doses of antiinflammatory steroids. Epithelization also is stopped by steroids, but is restimulated by vitamin A. Vitamin A does not restimulate steroid-inhibited contraction. Therefore, we have a specific control of the process.

ENDOCRINOLOGY OF REPAIR

Although much has been written on the endocrinology of repair, it seems fair to conclude that few of the usually defined endocrine substances have significant influence.

The major single exception is that cortisol or its congeners impair healing. Small-dose inhibition can be overcome with force feeding, but large-dose inhibition cannot. The effect is most pronounced if steroids are given before or within three days after injury. Poor repair is a common problem in Cushing's syndrome. The effect is within the wound and can be achieved by local steroid administration. The major mechanism appears to be through the exclusion of inflammatory cells, especially macrophages, from the wound. If adequate doses of vitamin A are given topically or systemically, the effect can be mostly, but not entirely, overcome. Clean primary repair often goes to completion, albeit slowly, despite steroid administration. Once the wound is open, however, the effects of steroids become vastly more troublesome.

Sex hormones are also "wound-active." Estrogen does depress collagen synthesis mildly. Progesterone depresses it markedly. The combination of the two, birth control pills, even more markedly retards repair in animals. Progesterone also increases neovascularization and increases oxygen supply, but yet it reduces collagen synthesis. Nevertheless, in most animals, females heal somewhat faster than males, and a pregnant or recently pregnant woman has extraordinary reparative powers.

Anabolic steroids, male hormones, have long been touted as enhancers of repair. They have little practical value except that they have, with vitamin A, the power to counteract steroid retardation of repair.

ACTH, growth hormone, thyroid hormone, all have some influence on repair, but it seems minor in most instances. Some data suggest that aldosterone enhances repair. Insulin, of course, is necessary for repair—if only in the sense that it is required for glucose entry into the fibroblast. Diabetes, on the other hand, inhibits repair in many ways.

A number of substances increase fibroblast replication in culture, including a platelet factor and a human, brain-derived fibroblast growth factor. The clinical significance is uncertain.

PHAGOCYTE FUNCTION

One of the fundamental properties of a well-healing wound is its resistance to infection. Almost all wounds are contaminated, yet few become infected. Nevertheless, a disproportionately large number of human infections begin in injured tissue. Disruption of the epithelial barrier allows entry of a variety of bacteria, yet the wound falls prey to only a small group.

The number of contaminating organisms is important, but the condition of the wound is probably just as important. A wound well made in healthy tissue can resist several orders of magnitude more contaminating organisms than a poorly made wound, especially one in a compromised tissue or host.

Specific or acquired immunity to bacteria account for a significant portion of the wound's resistance to infection. The wound, however, has innate or "natural" defense mechanisms as well. Furthermore, "natural immunity" can be temporarily elevated or depressed. Experience with leukopenic patients illustrates the critical role played by phagocytic leukocytes, and several neutrophil functional deficiency states that increase susceptibility to wound infection have been recognized. At least in the first few days, "natural immune" mechanisms probably are the principal means of defense against bacteria.

As soon as the wound is made, leukocytes of all varieties "marginate," i.e., stick to the endothelium of small vessels. Shortly thereafter, they slip through the "leaky" barrier between endothelial cells, attracted by any of a number of substances ranging from products of macrophages to bacterial metab-olites to complement factors. Although the cells leave the circulation, squeeze through tiny orifices, and migrate long distances through damaged tissue, they arrive in a cleanly incised wound in good functioning order, not detectably changed from their fellows still in circulation. Antiinflammatory steroids suppress chemotaxis and migration.

Having arrived in the wound, the phagocyte must recognize its natural prey. Substances in serum that attach to microorganisms and facilitate recognition and ingestion by phagocytes are referred to as opsonins. Many microorganisms cannot be ingested by phagocytes unless they are first exposed either to serum or specific antibody. The best-characterized opsonic substances are specific IgG antibodies and C3 of the complement system. The alternative properdin system also probably contributes. The opsonic molecules on the microbial surface fix the bacterium to the cell wall through an interaction with receptor molecules on the surface of the phagocyte.

Once the phagocyte fixes the microbe to its surface, its pseudopodia extend around the microbe, eventually engulfing it (Fig. 1–14). In the process, the external cell membrane of the leukocyte invaginates to form the intracellular phagocytic vacuole or phagosome. The energy for this process can be derived totally from anaerobic metabolism, a fact that becomes more important as the process develops.

Enzyme-containing cytoplasmic granules (sometimes called lysosomes) migrate through the cytosol toward the developing phagosome. The granule membranes fuse with the phagosomal membrane, spilling their acid hydrolases, phosphatases, highly cationic esterases, lysozyme, myeloperoxidase, and a variety of other enzymes into the vacuole and onto the microbe. This step is called "degranulation." If phagocytosis of the microbe is incomplete, enzymes may spill into the extracellular wound fluid (Fig. 1–15). Several of the granule proteins and enzymes including lactoferin, lysozyme, and cationic esterases have antimicrobial activity directed against certain organisms either in the phagosomes or in the extracellular fluid.

Granular enzymes soon appear in extracellular wound fluid. Myeloperoxidase and lysozyme are concentrated in human wound

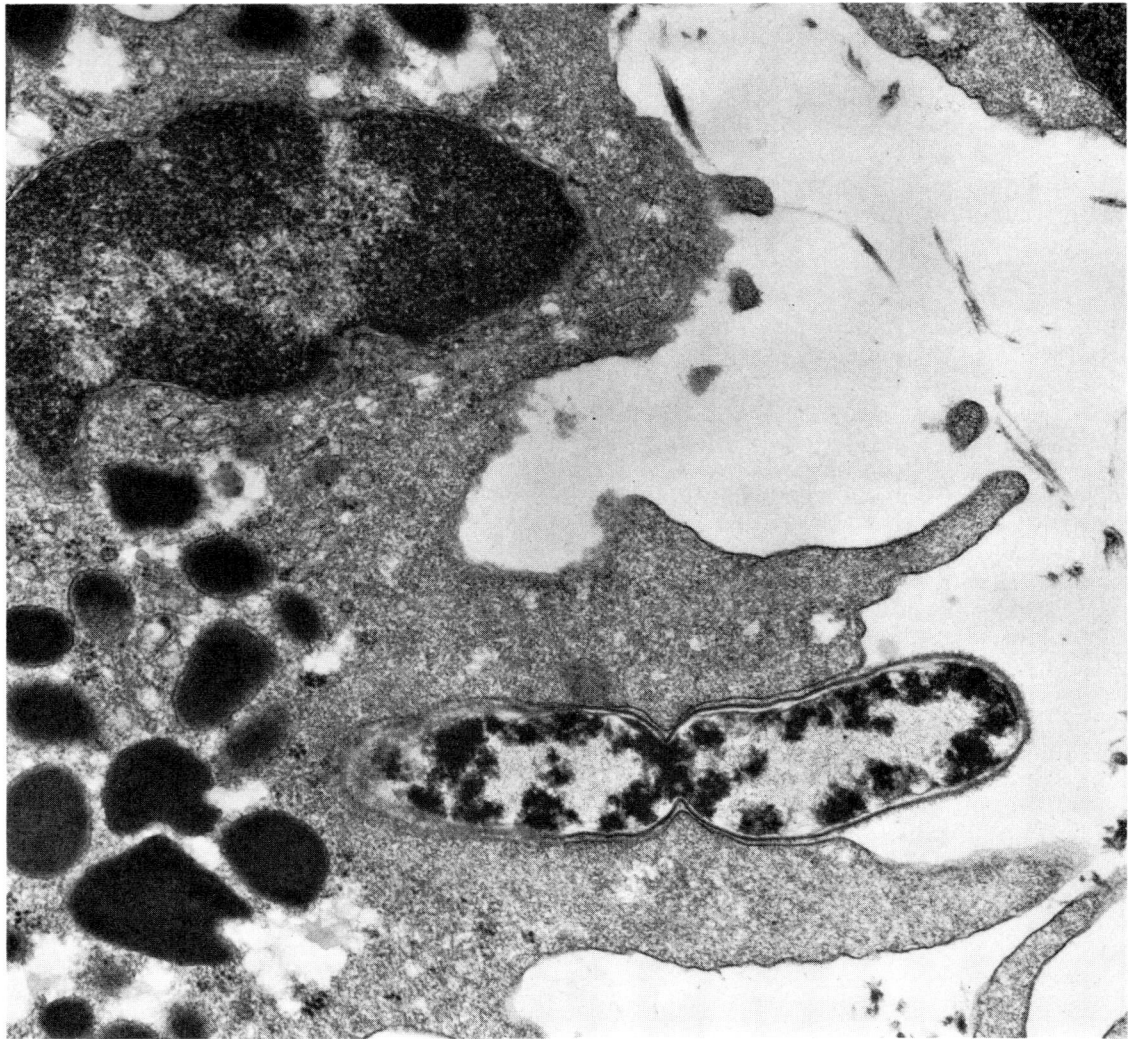

Figure 1–14 A white cell swallowing a bacterium looks like a great jaw as, with big nose pointing up to the right, it surrounds a bacillus in the act of dividing. This is a polymorphonuclear leukocyte caught by the electron microscope in the act of ingesting a bacterium. Opsonization has aided the close approximation of the granulocyte cell membrane to the bacterium. (Courtesy of Dr. Dorothy Bainton.) Reprinted from Fundamentals of Wound Management in Surgery, Chirurgecon, Plainfield, N.J.

fluid by the first postoperative day. Myeloperoxidase, when combined with halide ions and hydrogen peroxide, has potent antimicrobial activity against a broad spectrum of microbes. Lysozyme can hydrolyze the protein capsules of pneumococci. Much of the innate resistance of wounds to infection may be attributable to these enzymes and proteins.

During degranulation, pH values in the phagosome fall as low as 3.0. The change is in part due to the accumulation of lactic acid derived from glycolysis. Lactic acid itself may kill certain organisms such as pneumococcus.

All of the aforementioned systems are effective in the absence of oxygen. Complex mammalian organisms have, however, developed another extremely important system of bacterial killing that selectively uses oxygen (Fig. 1–16). Coincident with ingestion, the normal phagocyte mounts a burst of oxygen consumption as much as 20 times its basal rate. The significance of this

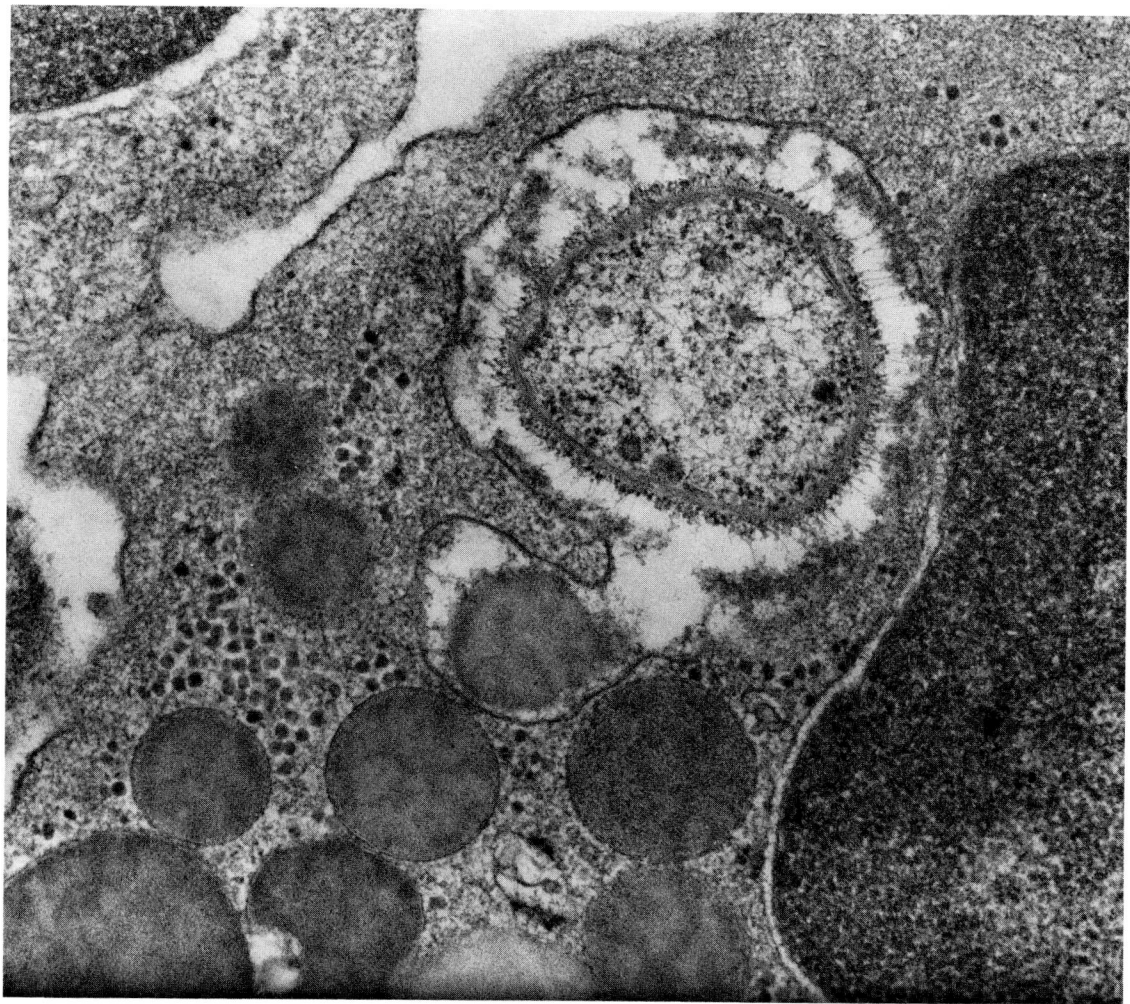

Figure 1-15 Degranulation is shown occurring after ingestion of the bacterium. The phagosome membrane is pulled away from the bacterium, which is now being bathed in the enzymatic contents of the granules. (Courtesy of Dr. Dorothy Bainton.) Reprinted from Fundamentals of Wound Management in Surgery, Chirurgecon, Plainfield, N.J.

phenomenon has only recently been recognized, owing to the discovery of a rare but important heritable disorder called chronic granulomatous disease (CGD). Children with chronic granulomatous disease are unduly susceptible to infections by *Staphylococcus aureus, Serratia marcescens, Candida albicans, Salmonella, Pseudomonas,* and other gram-negative organisms. Note that these organisms are also frequent "wound infectors." Cells from these children cannot mount a respiratory burst because they lack the primary oxygenase and therefore cannot kill efficiently the aforementioned organisms though they in-

gest them normally. The sequence shown in Figure 1-16 has gradually emerged.

In normal phagocytes, some of the oxygen consumed in the respiratory burst is enzymatically reduced by a single electron to form superoxide (O_2^-). Superoxide is an unstable molecule that has demonstrated bactericidal activity against clostridia and other organisms not equipped with superoxide dismutase (which changes superoxide to hydrogen peroxide). Superoxide is rapidly reduced to hydrogen peroxide in the phagosome. Hydrogen peroxide directly kills certain organisms, and in the presence of myeloperoxidase (MPO) and halide ions,

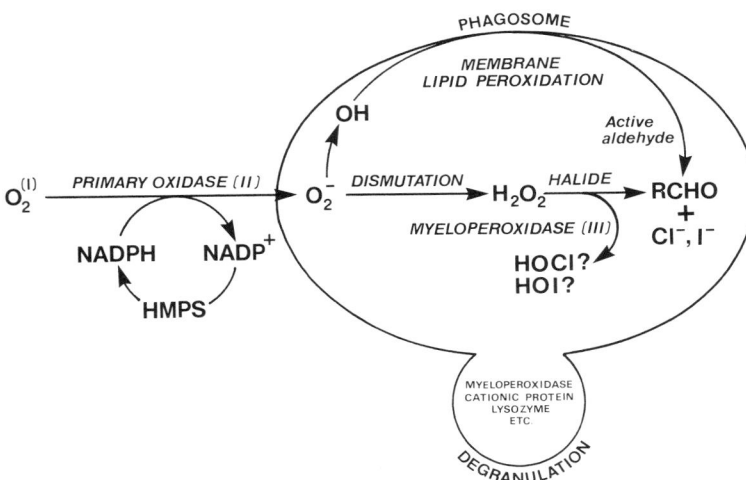

Figure 1–16 Schematic representation of the oxidative microbial killing mechanism. Most of the reduced or active forms of oxygen shown within the phagosome are microbicidal to certain organisms. Note that the absence of oxygen would mimic the absence of the primary oxidase and therefore mimic chronic granulomatous disease. Hexose monophosphate shunt (HMPS) is defective in patients with severe glucose-6-phosphate dehydrogenase deficiency, and these patients are unusually susceptible to infection. Reprinted from Fundamentals of Wound Management in Surgery, Chirurgecon, Plainfield, N.J.

its antimicrobial activity is greatly amplified. Other high-energy derivatives such as hydroxyl radicals and singlet oxygen are formed by normal cells during phagocytosis and may play a role in microbial killing as well.

Normal leukocytes that are maintained in the absence of oxygen exhibit a microbicidal defect resembling that seen in chronic granulomatous disease. The absence of the primary oxygenase is mimicked by the absence of its substrate, oxygen. Obviously, without oxygen, superoxide cannot be made. This may account for the particular sensitivity of wounded tissue to infection by a limited group of microorganisms. The group of organisms that typically causes infections in children with chronic granulomatous disease includes most of the common wound pathogens. Anaerobes make up most of the rest of the wound invaders. While clostridia, bacteroides, and other anaerobes are not affected by the oxidative mechanism, they do grow more rapidly and produce their toxins far better in an anaerobic environment. Thus, the common wound pathogens have one common property—they survive in a hypoxic environment.

Leukocyte oxygen consumption, and presumably peroxide production, is progressively depressed as PO_2 falls into, through, and below the normal range found in wounded tissue. Trauma at a distance from the wound lowers wound space PO_2 and also increases susceptibility to infection. In the test tube, human leukocytes kill certain organisms more than twice as fast in air-equilibrated environments ($PO_2 = 150$ mm Hg) as in nitrogen ($PO_2 < 5$ mm Hg). The major increment is from 5 to 30 mm Hg (Fig. 1–17).

Both white cell and fibroblast function are depressed by hypoxia. Wounds in hypoxic tissue heal poorly *and* become infected. The surgeon can enhance the natural resistance to infection of his wounds by maintaining good blood volume and normal arterial PO_2. In animals, natural resistance can be increased above "normal" by maintaining slight arterial hyperoxia. Although this effect remains to be confirmed in humans, it directs attention to the technique of making wounds. Ischemic tissue, produced by hacking strokes of the knife, resists infection poorly. Tissue desiccated by the cautery or dried by prolonged exposure to air cannot be perfused and is exceedingly infectable. Tissue strangulated by too many, too large, or too tight sutures and contaminated by a minimal number of organisms will become infected. The state

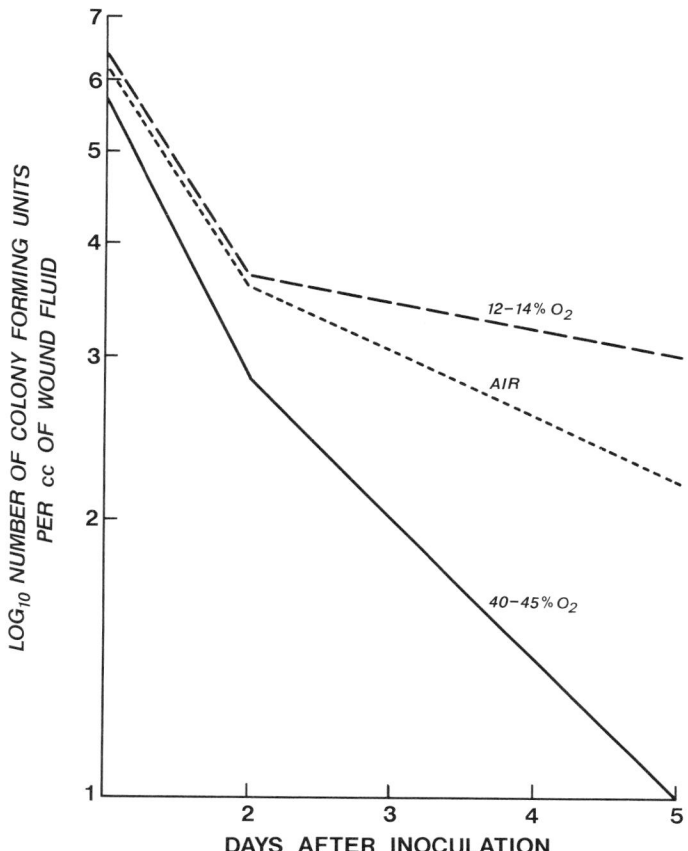

Figure 1-17 Curves resulting when *Staphyloccus* 502-A is incubated with human leukocytes in the test tube in various oxygen environments. Note that there is more than one log difference between points. Days after inoculation is given on the horizontal axis, and $\log_{10}$ number of colony-forming units on the vertical axis. The three lines correspond to 40 to 45 per cent oxygen, air, and 12 to 14 per cent oxygen. Reprinted from Fundamentals of Wound Management in Surgery, Chirurgecon, Plainfield, N.J.

of the microcirculation, as left in the wound by the operating surgeon, determines not only how rapidly the wound will heal—perhaps whether it will heal at all—but also whether it will be able to resist the inevitable bacterial contamination.

Surgeons vs. Granulocytes

Granulocytes and macrophages are scavengers of wound debris and killers of microbes. They "clean up" after the surgeon. Unfortunately, each cell has a limited capacity for phagocytosis. If it expends that capacity to ingest dead fat, for instance, microbicidal capacity is demonstrably diminished. The surgeon has the power to minimize the dead tissue that must be

ingested, and thus he has in his hands a major means of preventing infection.

THE FOREIGN BODY

Certain foreign bodies potentiate infection. Some are less dangerous than others. The degree of potentiation parallels their tendency to incite an inflammatory response. Figure 1-18 shows the oxygen tension of a wound surrounding a relatively well-tolerated foreign body. One can readily see that a microbe caught in the interstices of a porous substance, in a PO_2 of 0 mm Hg, occupies a protected position—even more so if the space it occupies is too small to allow a leukocyte room for

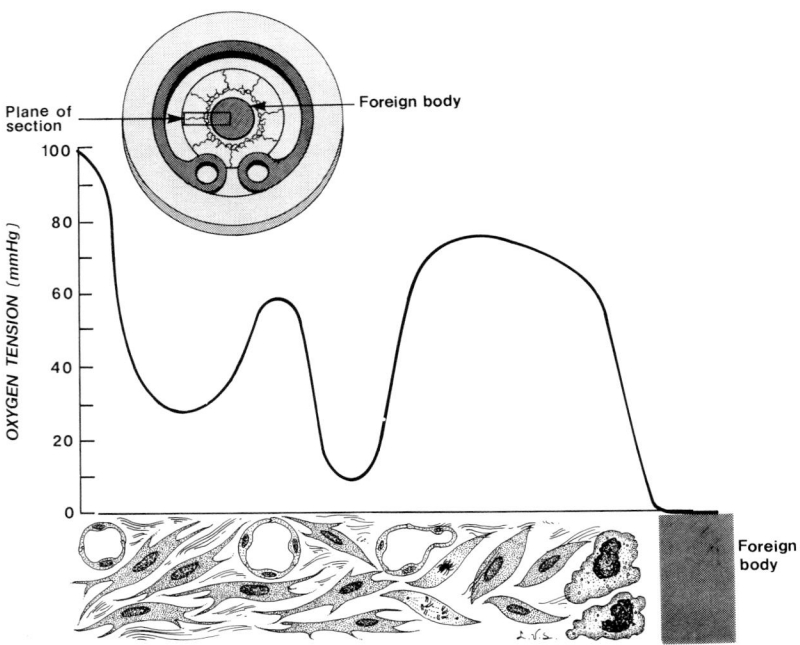

Figure 1–18 Diagrammatic representation of oxygen tension in a well-healed rabbit ear chamber wound containing a well-tolerated foreign body. Despite the fact that this foreign body excites minimal inflammatory response, the PO_2 is essentially zero on its surface. Oxygen tension would start to decrease considerably farther away from a foreign body that excited a greater inflammatory reaction. Courtesy of Dr. Ian Silver. Reprinted from Fundamentals of Wound Management in Surgery, Chirurgecon, Plainfield, N.J.

pursuit. Oxyten tension around a Teflon, Silastic, or nonreactive metal implant remains relatively high, and the smooth surfaces allow no haven for bacteria.

Some foreign bodies cause such an extremely acute inflammation that repair for a short distance around them is inhibited. They become encysted in a fibrous pocket filled with leukocytes. Others cause extensive scar formation. Those foreign bodies that are smooth-surfaced (no pores large enough to accept bacteria) and do not stimulate an inflammatory reaction are well tolerated by tissue and increase infection risk minimally. Catgut and polyfilament sutures are rough surfaced, cause inflammation, and are infectable. Nylon, wire, polypropylene, and polytheylene monofilament sutures are resistant to infection.

CELLULAR INTERACTIONS IN THE WOUND

It seems helpful to visualize repair in terms of a functioning unit of tissue, termed here a "module." The basic concept is that macrophages, fibroblasts, and growing vascular tissue form a unit of interacting cells that support, stimulate, and nourish each other. The function of no one of these components can be understood in the absence of the other. Although the "module" loses some of its identity in primary and delayed primary repair, the concept nevertheless holds there as well. Figure 1–3 is a schematic diagram of tissue in which a wound has been made. The cut microvasculature has become thrombosed and the initial bleeding has stopped. One can now visualize the nutrition of a given point in the wound much as one would the nutrition of an orange seed after the orange has been cut in two through the seed in question and exposed to air. Whereas nutrition previously came from the sphere surrounding the seed, it now comes from a hemisphere. Whereas nutrition could be brought in from sources immediately adjacent prior to cutting and allowing the cut edges to dry, whatever nutrition that can reach the unfortunate seed must now do so by diffusion through damaged tissue. To leave the analogy and return to normal tissue: The vasculature that was once geared to the rather unvarying needs of connective tissue, or fascia, has become thrombosed and is no longer adequate to meet the needs of the exposed tissue; desiccation occurs. Furthermore, in the next few days, the injured area will become suffused with metabolically active white cells and then will become densely populated with metabolically active fibroblasts. Thus, at a time at which a point in connective tissue needs more nutrition than ever before in its life, its nutritional sources are least able to meet the need. Oxygen supply is inadequate and local PO_2 is low. The vasculature responds to hypoxia and the invasion of leukocytes and platelets by sending capillary buds into the wounded area. Now the symbiosis of the ecological unit, the wound module, becomes apparent. The fibroblasts probably cannot migrate into the wounded area until the macrophage gives the signal. The fibroblast is not even actively encouraged to make collagen until a build-up of lactate occurs, and this lactate is probably largely formed by the macrophage. The signal for collagen synthesis cannot be met, however, unless oxygen, amino acids, glucose, trace metals, vitamins, and probably other elements are supplied by the vascular system, and most of these elements cannot diffuse over more than the shortest tissue distances. Hence, the fibroblast cannot respond to its stimulus until the vascular system has regenerated sufficiently to supply it.

On the other hand, the vascular system cannot merely poke a vascular sprout into a space and then pump blood through it unless there is external support to prevent bursting, as one sees in scurvy. Hence, the lead fibroblast must struggle ahead with minimal nutrition until sufficient collagen gel is laid down to support the budding capillary. The capillary cell probably contains a measure of collagenase, since it inevitably must burrow through the collagenous support. Once a cycle of circulation has been established when two capillary buds have met and fused, nutrition suddenly becomes more adequate. The hypoxic fibroblast near the wound edge can now make more collagen and provide a matrix in which the macrophage in the van of the advancing module can once again advance,

and fibroblasts can follow it until the cells once again reach the limits of their supply lines, when they again signal for a new vascular system.

One has the feeling that each fibroblast is "born" into its "permanent" position. It seems to perform its function in that spot while the vascular system advances past it in a "leapfrog" fashion. Meanwhile, the macrophages remain in the van. The new fibroblast is formed from a mitotic figure lying just distal to the most distal functioning capillary loop. It, therefore, is thrust into a hypoxic environment and is activated by it. As the vasculature moves by, the fibroblast is given a more secure environment with greater energy supply, and it secretes more and more collagen into the tissue spaces beside it (see Figs. 1–4 and 1–5). The similarity to the growth and movement of the epithelial plate is apparent.

In uncomplicated repair—the filling of an uninfected dead space, for instance—the fibroblast eventually drops out, perhaps at the end of its life span. The collagen that has been deposited is usually partly removed and replaced by fat. As a result, the empty space made by the surgeon and first filled with tissue fluid is then filled with a few macrophages and early fibroblasts, and then with vessels and collagen. This unit marches across dead space, leaving behind it a kind of subcutaneous tissue of fat and collagen unless, in the process, the new tissue either remains inflamed or performs a mechanical function. In either of these cases, the eventual maturation to fatty tissue does not occur and the area remains collagenous.

The evolution of the vessels is shown in the series of diagrams and in the photomicrograph of a rabbit ear chamber (Fig. 1–19). The advancing edge of granulation tissue is characteristically filled with microvasculature. As this portion of the tissue migrates into the dead space, the older microvasculature drops out, leaving longer and longer and larger and larger stem vessels, giving the effect of a grape arbor that rises from the soil in a stout trunk and arches upward into its small fruit-bearing branches.

In the primarily closed wound, this process is obviously truncated. In the first place, the tissue damage is usually less in the sharply incised wound. If the wound

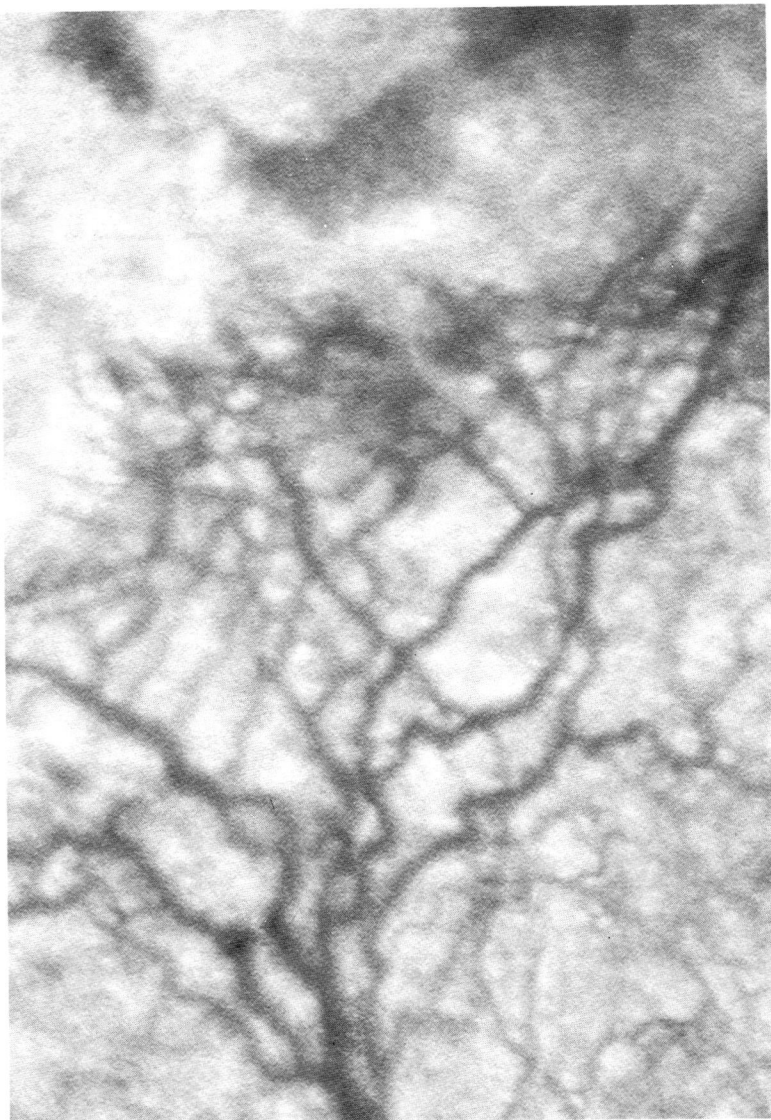

Figure 1–19 Photomicrograph of advancing arterial circulation in a healing ear chamber. The dense vessel that now occupies the junction of the upper and middle thirds of the figure once started at the bottom of the figure. All these vessels have grown anew. As the plexus of small vessels advances, it leaves behind it a few larger feeding vessels. The "ghosts" of several small vessels now no longer used are seen in the right lower corner. The "halo" above the advancing vasculature is the area of new fibroblasts and macrophages. One or two cells can be seen at the upper left. Slide courtesy of Dr. Ian Silver, Professor of Comparative Pathology, Department of Pathology, University of Bristol, England.

edges are reunited well, their nutrition obviously reaches the center point from both sides of the wound. The coagulative process is followed by a fibrinolytic mechanism, and some of the damaged vasculature is probably reopened to flow. Although the mechanism is unknown, it is obviously possible for vessels to reunite across the

wound. With this mechanism available, the macrophage that reaches the center of the wound has little debridement to do. It is exposed to hypoxia for a relatively short period of time. Only a few fibroblasts are needed to give support to already reasonably well-supported microvasculature, and the process proceeds to completion with vastly less machination and vastly less expenditure of energy.

This concept gives an interesting insight into certain clinical situations. Ischemic tissue in the foot of an arteriosclerotic patient may have enough vasculature to support itself, but once wounded may not be able to support repair. Other, perhaps less ischemic, tissue may support primary repair, as in a transmetatarsal amputation, but if that suture line once opens and the underlying tissue is forced to heal by secondary intention, the available energy, that would possibly have been sufficient for primary wound healing cannot support secondary wound healing, and loss of the amputation stump becomes inevitable.

With the two polar situations of the granulating wound and the primarily closed wound in mind, one should have relatively little doubt about how healing by delayed primary closure occurs. The early wound module is formed and by the fourth or fifth day is usually well on its way. When this tissue is then brought together, the macrophagic layer fuses to form one serving both sides, the few ischemic fibroblasts fuse to serve both sides, and the growing capillary buds instead of joining other sprouts from the same side, may find it more convenient to join sprouts from the other side. The microvasculature is thus formed.

The diagrams of the wound module show the gradients of oxygen, lactate, and carbon dioxide occurring in the normally healing dead space wound (Fig. 1–20). On inspection of these gradients, it should become apparent that the advancing edge of the healing wound is in a vulnerable position. Cells have migrated out to the very limits of their ability to survive. If the tenuous oxygen supply is interrupted or depressed, the cells that are at their survival limits may die. At the least, they may be made temporarily inactive because of the extreme shortage of oxygen.

In examination of these gradients, one may find an apparent contradiction. We have stated before that the better the oxygen supply, the better the repair. The converse is also true; the worse the oxygen supply, the slower the repair. If one adds

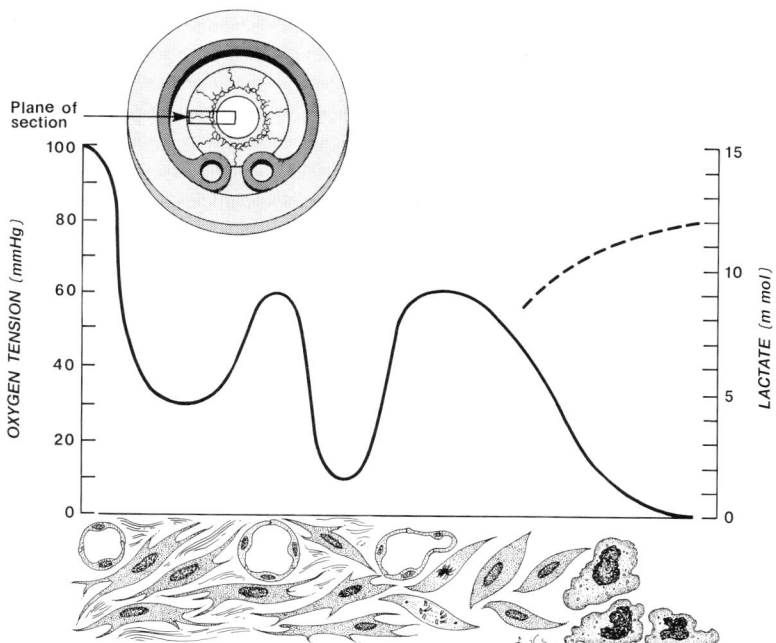

Figure 1–20 Diagram of tissue oxygen tension in a rabbit ear chamber healing wound. The peaks of PO_2 occur over the vessels. Note the long gradiant to almost zero at the edge of the dead space. This demonstrates how the central wound remains hypoxic and acidotic despite the advancing vasculature. The lactate concentration from the dead space to the first capillary is shown on the right. Courtesy of Dr. Ian Silver, Professor of Comparative Pathology, Department of Pathology, University of Bristol, England.

oxygen to this system, however, one would expect the oxygen gradient into the wound space to be shifted upward, the distalmost cells to be better supplied, and the lactate levels in the wound edge to decrease, thus diminishing this stimulus to collagen formation. Conversely, if the oxygen content were to fall, lactate content would rise and the stimulus to collagen synthesis might increase.

The explanation is relatively simple. Fibroblasts and epidermal cells can survive but cannot migrate or divide in the absence of oxygen. In the complete absence of oxygen, even macrophages begin to lose their cell membrane potential, their sodium and potassium pump mechanisms begin to fail, and they together with the fibroblasts begin to leak potassium and eventually die. In the case of the fibroblast, as noted earlier in the section on collagen synthesis, molecular oxygen is required for hydroxylation of lysine and proline. Unless a significant number of proline and lysine molecules are hydroxylated, most collagen cannot leave the cell. Furthermore, in the presence of oxygen, more adenosine triphosphate can be synthesized from a single glucose molecule, and the energy requirements for protein synthesis can be more economically met. Although such a generalization may be dangerous, it would seem that in normal repair, with nondiffusable nutritional substances present in adequate supply, oxygen probably becomes the rate-limiting factor in collagen synthesis in wounds.

If oxygen supply is moderately increased, the PO_2 over the distalmost capillary rises, but the gradient down into the wound space becomes steeper; the oxygen and lactate levels at the surface of the wound edge are essentially unchanged. If hypoxia is maintained in the distal arterioles, lactate levels in the wound remain high. More collagen is made because of the relative surplus of oxygen. This effect is limited, however. Continued arterial PO_2 over about 250 mm Hg becomes toxic.

If, on the other hand, the wound is exposed to arterial hypoxia, lactate levels and the stimulus to collagen synthesis increase. However, collagen synthesis is then limited by oxygen supply. In one experiment, short periods of hypoxia alternating with longer exposures to normal air

actually increased collagen deposition over that in control subjects kept in normal air.

At skin level, squamous epithelium eventually covers the module. Immediately thereafter, energy demands lessen because water loss is decreased, circulation diminishes, and instead of further movement of the module, the macrophages disappear and the new dermis is remodeled to a tighter, denser scar. In most cases, cellularity diminishes sharply. If it does not, a hyperplastic scar is likely to result. One way to ensure continued cellularity is to place the part under motion and tension. Tension "demands" more collagen. Breaking collagen and bursting microvasculature "renew" the wound, and inflammatory cells caught in the microwounds send out their usual signals, which are all too easily heard by the nearby wound cells. Another way is to cause continued inflammation. Then the wound tends not to finish its sequence—that is, it fails to stop healing.

SUMMARY

The wound is a delicately tuned ecosystem in which the meddlings of man, whether intentional or careless, may be disastrous. On the other hand, as ecosystems often do, the wound may need help. The greatest gift a surgeon can give his wounds is his technical skill. If he is gentle, cuts decisively, does not "fuss" with tissue—picking it up and dropping it again and again—if he uses sutures, ligatures, and cautery with restraint, if he does not kill tissue with clamps, retractors, and unnecessary exposure, he and his patients will be rewarded. Next, the surgeon can offer his knowledge of the needs of the wound and supply them.

We are constantly making new demands upon the repair process. We are operating on sicker and older patients, more often invading contaminated tissue. We are doing longer operations and implanting more and more foreign bodies. Under these circumstances, wound problems will arise. It is to be hoped that each surgeon can anticipate these problems and will do what he can to thwart them. The well being of his wound, and his patient, may depend on it.

REFERENCES

Cellular Aspects of Repair

1. Branemark, P. I.: Capillary form and function: The microcirculation of granulation tissue. Bibl. Anat., *D*:9, 1965.
2. Cohen, B. E., and Cohen, I. I.: Vitamin A: Adjuvant and steroid antagonist in the immune response. J. Immunol., *111*:1376, 1973.
3. Harington, J. S.: Fibrogenesis. Environ. Health Persp., 9:271, 1974.
4. Hunt, T. K., Ehrlich, H. P., Garcia, J. A., and Dunphy, J. E.: Effect of vitamin A on reversing the inhibitory effect of cortisone on healing of open wounds in animals and man. Ann. Surg., *170*:633, (Oct.) 1969.
5. Leibovich, S. J., and Ross, R.: The role of macrophages in wound repair. Am. J. Pathol., 78:71, 1975.
6. McLean, A. E. M., Ahmed, K., and Judah, J. D.: Cellular permeability and the reaction to injury. Ann. N.Y. Acad. Sci., *116*:986, 1964.
7. Ross, R., and Odland, G.: Fine structure observations of human skin wounds and fibrinogenesis. *In* Dunphy, J. E., and Van Winkle, W., Jr. (eds.): Repair and Regeneration. New York, McGraw-Hill Book Co., Inc., 1969.
8. Rutherford, R. B., and Ross, R.: Platelet factors stimulate fibroblasts and smooth muscle cells quiescent in serum to proliferate. J. Cell Biol., 69:196, 1976.
9. Sandberg, N.: Time relationship between administration of cortisone and wound healing in rats. Acta Chir. Scand., *127*:446, 1964.
10. Schoefl, G. K.: Studies of Inflammation, III. Growing capillaries: Their structure and permeability. Virchow Arch. Pathol. Anat., 337:99–141, 1963.
11. Spector, W. G., and Lykke, W. J.: The cellular evolution of inflammatory granulomata. J. Pathol. Bacteriol., 92:103, 1966.
12. Weeks, J. R.: Prostaglandins. Ann. Rev. Pharmacol., *12*:317, 1972.

Physiology of Repair

13. Heughan, C., Grislis, G., and Hunt, T. K.: The effect of anemia on wound healing. Ann. Surg., *179*:163, 1974.
14. Hunt, T. K., and Pai, M. P.: Effect of varying ambient oxygen tensions on wound metabolism and collagen synthesis. Surg. Gynecol. Obstet., *135*:561, 1972.
15. Niinikoski, J., Hunt, T. K., and Dunphy, J. E.: Oxygen supply in healing tissue. Am. J. Surg., *123*:247, 1972.
16. Remensnyder, J. P., and Majno, G.: Oxygen gradients in healing wounds. Am. J. Pathol., 52:301, 1968.

Epithelization

17. Im, M. J. C., and Hoopes, J. E.: Energy metabolism in healing skin wounds. J. Surg. Res., *10*:459, 1970.
18. Johnson, F. R., and McMinn, R. M.: The cytology of wound healing of body surfaces in mammals. Biol. Rev., 35:364, 1962.
19. McMinn, R. M. H.: Tissue Repair. London, Academic Press, 1969.

20. Rovee, D. T., Kurowsky, C. A., Labun, J., and Downes, A. M.: Effect of local wound environment on epidermal healing. *In* Mailbach, H. I., and Rovee, D. T. (eds.): Epidermal Wound Healing. Chicago, Year Book Medical Publishers, Inc., 1972.
21. Silver, I. A.: Oxygen tension and epithelization. *In* Maibach, H. I., and Rovee, D. T. (eds.): Epidermal Wound Healing. Chicago, Year Book Medical Publishers, Inc., 1972.

Wound Contraction

22. Higton, D. I. R., and James, D. W.: The force of contraction of full thickness wounds of rabbit skin. Br. J. Surg., *51*:462, 1964.
23. Montandon, D., Gabbiani, G., Ryan, G. B., and Majno, G.: The contractile fibroblast, its relevance in plastic surgery. Plast. Reconstr. Surg., 52:286, 1973.
24. Ryan, G. B., Cliff, W., Jr., Gabbiani, G., Iolé, C., Statkov, P. R., and Majno, G.: Myofibroblasts in human granulation tissue. Hum. Pathol., 5:55, 1974.
25. Stephens, F. O., Dunphy, J. E., and Hunt, T. K.: Effect of delayed administration of corticosteroids on wound contraction. Ann. Surg., *173*:214, 1971.
26. Stone, P. A., and Madden, J. W.: Effect of primary and delayed split skin grafting on wound contraction. Surg. Forum, 25:41, 1974.
27. Van Winkle, W., Jr.: Wound contraction. Surg. Gynecol. Obstet., *125*:131, 1967.

Collagen Structure and Synthesis

28. Barnes, M. J.: Function of ascorbic acid in collagen metabolism. Ann. N.Y. Acad. Sci., *258*:264, 1975.
29. Chung, E., Keele, E. M., and Miller, E. J.: Isolation and characterization of the cyanogen bromide peptides from the α (III) chain of human collagen. Proc. Natl. Acad. Sci., U.S.A., 70: 3521, 1973.
30. Hawley, P. R., Faulk, W. P., Hunt, T. K., and Dunphy, J. E.: Collagenase activity in the gastro-intestinal tract. Br. J. Surg., 57:896, (Dec.) 1970.
31. Hodge, A. J., and Schmitt, F. O.: The charge profile of the tropocollagen macromolecule and the packing arrangement in native type collagen fibrils. Proc. Natl. Acad. Sci., U.S.A., 46: 186, 1960.
32. Ireland, R. L., Kang, A. J., Igarasli, S., and Gross, J.: Isolation of two distinct collagens from chick cartilage. Biochemistry, 9:4993, 1970.
33. Kivirikko, K. I., and Prockop, D. J.: Enzymatic hydroxylation of proline and lysine in protocollagen. Proc. Natl. Acad. Sci. U.S.A., 57:782, 1967.
34. Monson, J. M., and Bornstein, P.: Identification of disulfide-linked procollagen as the biosynthetic precursor of chick-bone collagen. Proc. Natl. Acad. Sci. U.S.A., 70:3521, 1973.
35. Page, R. C., and Benditt, E. P. A.: A molecular defect in lathyritic collagen. Proc. Soc. Exp. Biol. Med., *124*:459, 1967.
36. Tanzer, M. L.: Crosslinking of collagen. Science, *180*:561, 1973.
37. Van Winkle, W., Jr.: The fibroblast in wound healing. Surg. Gynecol. Obstet., *124*:369, 1967.

Phagocytic Function

38. Hohn, D. C.: Leukocyte phagocytic function and dysfunction. Surg. Gynecol. Obstet., *144*:99–104, 1977.
39. Hohn, D. C., and Hunt, T. K.: Oxidative metabolism and microbicidal activity of rabbit phagocytes: Cells from wounds and from peripheral blood. Surg. Forum, *26*:86, 1975.
40. Hohn, D. C., MacKay, R. D., Halliday, B., and Hunt, T. K.: The effect of oxygen tension on the microbicidal function of leukocytes in wounds and in vitro. Surg. Forum, *17*:18–20, 1976.
41. Hunt, T. K., Linsey, M., Grislis, G., Sonne, M., and Jawetz, E.: The effect of differing ambient oxygen tensions on wound infection. Ann. Surg., *181*:35, 1975.
42. Mandell, G. L.: Bactericidal activity of aerobic and anaerobic polymorphonuclear neutrophils. Infect. Immun., 9:337, 1974.

General

43. Bailey, A. J., Sims, T. J., LeLons, M., and Bazin, S.: Collagen polymorphism in experimental granulation tissue. Biochem. Biophys. Res. Commun., *66*:1160, 1975.
44. Bauer, E. A., Eisen, A. Z., and Jeffrey, J. J.: Regulation of vertebrate collagenase activity in vitro and in vivo. J. Invest. Dermatol., 59:50, 1972.
45. Brunius, V.: Wound healing impairment from sutures. Acta Chir. Scand., Suppl. 395, 1968.
46. Chvapil, M.: Zinc and wound healing. *In* Zederfeld, B. (ed.): Symposium on Zinc. Lund, Sweden, A. B. Tika, 1974.

47. Chvapil, M.: Pharmacology of fibrosis: Definitions, limits and perspectives. Life Sci., *16*: 1345, 1975.
48. Ehrlich, H. P., and Hunt, T. K.: Effects of cortisone and vitamin A on wound healing. Ann. Surg., *167*:324, 1968.
49. Hunt, T. K.: Physiology of repair. *In* Wound Healing, 1st International Symposium on Wound Healing, Rotterdam, April 1974. Montreux, Switzerland, Foundation for International Cooperation in the Medical Sciences, 1975.
50. Hunt, T. K., and Hawley, P. R.: Surgical judgment and colonic anastomoses. Dis. Colon Rectum, *12*:167–171, (May-June) 1969.
51. McMinn, R. M. H.: Tissue Repair. New York, Academic Press, 1969.
52. Oegema, T. R., Laidlaw, J., Hascall, V. C., and Dziewiatkowski, D. D.: The effect of proteoglycans on the formation of fibrils from collagen solutions. Arch. Biochem. Biophys., *170*:698, 1975.
53. Pareira, M. D., and Jerkes, K. D.: Prediction of wound disruption by use of the healing ridge. Surg. Gynecol. Obstet., *115*:72, 1962.
54. Peacock, E. E., Jr., and Van Winkle, W., Jr.: Surgery and Biology of Wound Repair. Philadelphia, W. B. Saunders Co., 1970.
55. Silver, I. A.: Local and systemic factors which affect the proliferation of fibroblasts. *In* Pikkarainen, J. (ed.): Biology of the Fibroblast. Sigrid Juselius Foundation Symposium. London, Academic Press, 1974.
56. Viljanto, J.: Biochemical basis of tensile strength in wound healing. Acta Chir. Scand., Suppl. 333, 1964.

R. BRUCE HEPPENSTALL, M.D.

Fracture ———————————————— 2
Healing

The two primary functions of bone are to support the human frame and to provide a source of calcium. Bone also serves as an anchor for the origin and insertion of the surrounding musculature and protects several vital soft tissue structures. Since bone makes up the human skeleton, it is essential to locomotion. Despite its active role in these body functions, bone is a light structure, when one considers that it represents only one tenth of the entire body weight. Bone has a breaking strength comparable to that of medium steel, yet it is a flexible and elastic structure. This elasticity allows bone to be bent or twisted and still return to its original state following removal of the deforming force, provided that force has not exceeded the limits of elasticity. As indicated in Chapter 7, bone is able to resist axial stresses but is limited in its ability to resist rotational forces. One important point to bear in mind with regard to bone is that, like the liver, it is one of the few organs able to undergo spontaneous regeneration rather than just simple repair with restoration of structure. This property is more of a regenerative phenomenon, as the entire anatomical structure is restored to the state that existed prior to injury.

Fracture healing has many similarities to soft tissue healing (as outlined in Chapter 1) but also has some unique features owing to the anatomical structure and characteristics of bone. There has been a lag in investigative studies on the healing of osseous tissue compared with that of soft tissue, because many of the techniques applied to soft tissue studies are not applicable to the anatomical structure of bone. A simple example is the difficulty of isolating intact mitochondria from osseous tissue as opposed to the relative ease of obtaining mitochondria from soft tissue.

BONE STRUCTURE

The gross structure of bone has been divided into two specific types—tubular and flat. Tubular bone provides normal weight-bearing functions and locomotion. Flat bone, such as the skull, serves to protect vital soft tissue structures. Anatomically, tubular bones are formed with a diaphysis and an epiphysis, or secondary ossification center. Diaphyseal bone is made up of a lamellar structure, indicative of mature bone, with collagen fibril bundles which are arranged in layers, strata, or lamellae. Primitive nonlamellar bone is known as fibrous bone, and it occurs in embryonic life, at fracture sites, and at the metaphysis during active new bone formation. The epiphyseal plate is located at the junction of the diaphysis and epiphysis in the area where normal longitudinal growth occurs in tubular bone. In flat bone there is no epiphyseal plate.

The periosteum is a fibrous sheet that surrounds bone. This important anatomical structure plays an active role in the fracture healing process. It is subdivided into an outer fibrous layer and an inner layer known as the cambium layer (Fig. 2–1). Active new bone cell proliferation occurs from the cambium layer during fracture repair. The periosteum has a much greater osteogenic potential in the child than in the adult. This

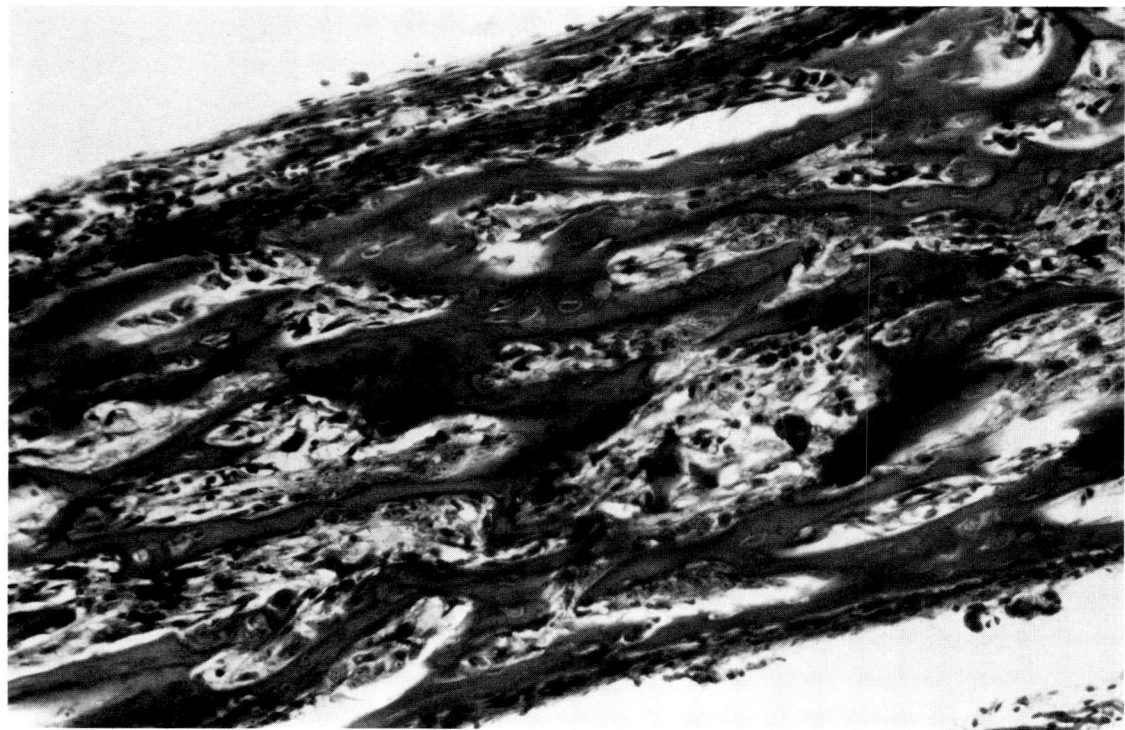

Figure 2-1   Longitudinal section of bone demonstrating the periosteum as an outer fibrous layer and an inner cambium layer.

is important to the fracture healing process since nonunion is very rare in childhood. The inner portion of bone, known as the marrow cavity, is lined with a fibrous sheet called the endosteum, which also is actively involved in the fracture healing process.

The functioning unit of mature bone is known as the haversian system or osteon. This structure consists of a haversian canal in the center, containing one or more blood vessels (capillaries and venules), which is surrounded by lamellae (Fig. 2-2). The surrounding lamellae have lacunae, each of which contains an osteocyte with a cytoplasmic process extending through canaliculi to communicate with the haversian vessels. The size of the osteon is limited by the fact that the haversian canal supplies the nutrition, and Ham has demonstrated that bone cells in general cannot survive farther than 0.1 mm away from a capillary.[42, 43]

BONE FORMATION

Bone formation occurs through two distinct mechanisms, endochondral and membranous. Endochondral bone formation occurs at the epiphyseal plate in long bones and accounts for growth and length. Growth in width of bone develops by subperiosteal appositional bone formation.) Endochondral bone requires the laying down of a pre-formed cartilage model. This cartilage is gradually resorbed and replaced by new bone. It is important to have a thorough knowledge of endochondral bone formation as this sequence of events has been described in fracture healing. An organizational structure, such as the epiphyseal plate, does not develop during fracture healing. However, several of the events, such as the formation of a cartilage model, do occur, and many investigators feel that

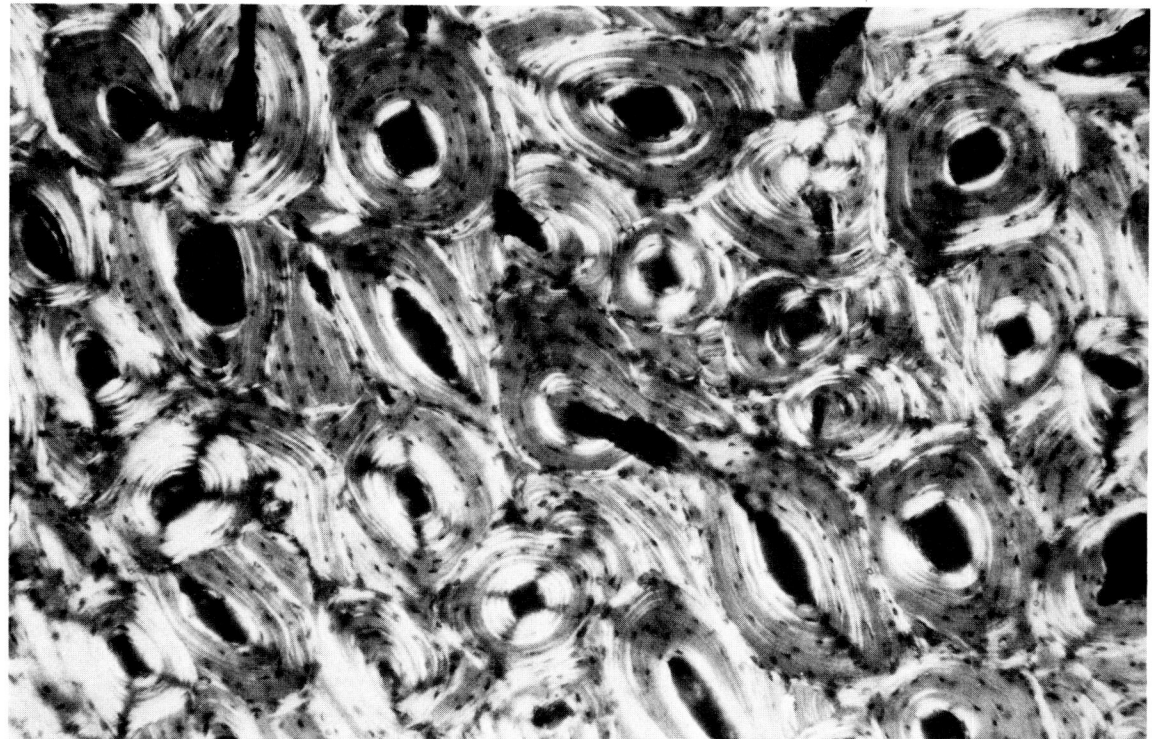

Figure 2-2   Polarized light demonstration of the osteonal structure of bone. Note the surrounding lamellae.

the fracture healing process is similar to events that occur in the epiphyseal plate. In fact, several recent studies have pointed out the similarities in the physiological events that take place at a fracture site and those that take place at the epiphyseal plate.[54] Therefore, it is possible that bone growth and bone repair are governed essentially by the same mechanisms.

Membranous bone formation does not involve a cartilage model. This type of bone forms when mesenchymal cells differentiate directly into osteoblasts, which then lay down osteoid. This is followed by mineralization to form new bone. This type of bone is seen in the calvarium, most facial bones, the clavicle and mandible (both mixed), and subperiosteal bone. The specific type of bone formation has a direct bearing on fracture repair, as skull, for example, generally heals by fibrous union and not by new bone formation.

BONE COMPOSITION

A typical mature lamellar bone has a composition of approximately 8 per cent water and 92 per cent solid material. The solid material portion can be divided into an organic phase of 21 per cent and an inorganic phase of 71 per cent.

Organic Constituents

The organic material, also known as the matrix, supplies form and supporting structure for the deposition and crystallization of inorganic salts. The matrix is composed of approximately 98 per cent collagen, with the remaining 2 per cent or less consisting of ground substance. Bone collagen, as discussed in Chapter 1, is made up of type 1, which consists of two alpha-1 chains and an alpha-2 chain. Type 1 collagen is very similar to skin and tendon collagen. As pointed out in Chapter 1, the hydroxylation of proline and lysine requires oxygen, iron, and ascorbic acid. It is important to bear in mind that very little oxygen is required to hydroxylate all available proline and lysine. Therefore, the hydroxylation process can occur under conditions of relative hypoxia. It is interesting that the number of hydroxylysine residues in humans is the same in both bone and skin collagen. This does not apply to the glycosylation of the hydroxylysine residues, as this process is less frequent in bone collagen than in other types of collagen.

Lane recently demonstrated that in the rat 40 to 60 per cent of collagen synthesis in the callus and pericallus tissues during the second and fourth week postfracture was type 2 collagen. The presence in the fracture callus of type 2 collagen, which had previously been identified in the epiphyseal plate, provided strong biochemical evidence that endochondral bone formation occurs during the fracture healing process.[58] However, if compression plating is employed for the fixation of fractures, very little callus develops, and the collagen formed is then type 1.

Several investigators have felt that the cross-linking pattern in bone collagen may differ from that of other types of collagen. It is true that bone collagen is extremely insoluble compared with other collagens. It has also been demonstrated that animals administered β-aminopropionitrile and made lathyritic have 40 per cent of their bone collagens soluble in neutral salt solution, which consists primarily of the alpha components. Lathyrogens have been demonstrated in the past to prevent covalent cross-linking in collagen. Therefore, it is reasonable to conclude that the insolubility of bone collagen may be due to a high degree of cross-linking, or that the cross-linking is of a different type than that in other collagens. It has also been suggested that the insolubility of bone collagen may be due to keto-aldimine cross-linking as well as other aldimine cross-links which may be reduced during maturation. Collagen degradation occurs by action of the enzyme collagenase. The enzyme cleaves the collagen molecules at a specific site to yield two peptides, which are then susceptible to other proteases under normal physiological conditions. Although the exact regulation of collagenase activity is a very complex subject, it is known that collagenase activity is partially controlled by parathyroid hormone, thyroxin, and steroid metabolism.

The matrix also includes a group of substances that make up less than 2 per cent of its composition and are known as ground substance. They include the glycosaminoglycans (previously known as acid mucopolysaccharides) and proteoglycans. The glycosaminoglycans (GAG) are highly-charged polyanions composed of repeating disaccharide units. These units include a carboxyl or a sulfate group or both, consisting of uronic acid and hexosamine moieties, except for keratan sulfate, which is an exception to this rule.

The GAG structure, which has been evaluated in several studies, includes hyaluronate, chondroitin-4-sulfate, chondroitin-6-sulfate, keratan sulfate, dermatan sulfate, heparan sulfate, and heparin. The difference between these structures is essentially a different repeating disaccharide structure. The GAG structures as a rule do not exist as isolated polysaccharide chains in vivo but are linked covalently to protein and are known as proteoglycans. It has recently been proposed that hyaluronate may not exist as the proteoglycan, in contrast to sulfated GAG, but as individual GAG chains occurring in the extra-cellular matrix. Interestingly, the molecular weight of hyaluronate is several times that of the sulfated GAG chains. Some investigators believe that the glycosaminoglycans and proteoglycans may be involved in the calcification mechanism, although their exact role has not been delineated. It is probable that the interaction of collagen and cartilage proteoglycan plays an important part in cartilage matrix deposition.

Inorganic Constituents

The principal inorganic salt is crystalline in the form of hydroxyapatite, $Ca_{10}(PO_4)_6(OH)_2$. The role played by bone carbonate in relation to calcium carbonate has been extensively debated in the past.[11] Recent theories have focused on the inclusion of carbonate $CO_3^=$ in the interior volume of the apatite structural model. The difficulty of this theory lies in how carbonate is incorporated into the hydroxyapatite structure. It is possible that it may be substituted for phosphate ion, or trapped interstitially, or substituted for the hydroxyl radical. It is also possible that $CO_3^=$ interferes with the formation of hydroxyapatite by replacing $PO_4^=$ or $HPO_4^=$ at the surface of the developing crystallite. Further studies will be required before the exact role of the carbonate ion is definitely established.

The mineral crystals are extremely small, being approximately 25 to 75 Å in diameter and approximately 200 Å in length. This provides a very large surface area. In fact, the surface area of bone mineral is enormous and has been estimated to be approximately 100 square meters per gram. There is a shell of water surrounding the surface crystals (hydration shell), and ions may move freely between the hydration shell and the crystalline surface. Glimcher has demonstrated a definite relationship between bone crystal and collagen structure.[36, 37] The bone crystals appear to align in a specific pattern within the collagen molecule, with the long axis of the crystal aligned parallel to the longitudinal axis of the collagen fiber in a band pattern with the collagen fibril. In other words, bone crystals appear in the hole zone of the collagen fibril, increasing the surface area.[51] As an example, the skeleton of a 150-pound man would equal approximately 100 acres of surface area. Two theories have been advanced regarding the relation of bone crystal and collagen fiber. The first is that a direct physical bond exists between the collagen fibers and the initial apatite crystallites. This theory is based on the results of electron paramagnetic resonance studies. The second theory is that a specific charge exists on the collagen fiber, initiating the formation of crystals, which are held in this position by electrostatic forces.

Cellular Components of Bone

Three principal bone cells are identified during bone formation and remodeling. These are the osteoblast, osteocyte, and osteoclast. A similar series of cells has been demonstrated in cartilage formation, and these are known as the chondroblast, chondrocyte, and chondroclast. In bone, the osteoblast is the cell primarily involved in the formation of the matrix. The osteocyte acts in a dual capacity as a bone-forming and bone-destroying cell. The osteoclast is involved with bone destruction and resorption and also plays a part in the remodeling process.

In an excellent series of investigative studies Bélanger described bone resorption as being mediated by the osteocyte and termed this process osteocytic osteolysis.[9] He felt that the normal day-to-day resorption occurring in bone remodeling was mediated by the osteocyte, whereas pathological resorption was mediated by the osteoclast. The osteocyte produces collagen and is believed to elaborate the proteoglycans and the protein polysaccharides. The osteocyte is found within the haversian system in lamellar bones and in a lacuna communicating with a haversian canal from which it obtains nourishment and oxygen supply. As described by Ham, osteocytes generally occur in compact bone no more than 0.1 mm away from a functioning capillary.[42] The blood supply of compact bone is derived from one or two capillaries or slightly larger vessels that are present in each haversian canal. The haversian canal and the enclosed capillaries lie more or less parallel to the shaft of a long bone.

During fracture repair, osteoblasts appear to originate from cells of the cambium layer of the periosteum and endosteum. Several names have been attached to these cells in the past, including fibroblast, osteoprogenitor, and undifferentiated mesenchymal cell. Many investigators believe that the periosteum contains osteogenic cells and participates in the formation of the external callus (Fig. 2–3).[92, 94] Therefore, it should be preserved, if at all possible, during the surgical management of fractures. However, as will be discussed, the endosteum is ultimately the most important portion of the bone involved in fracture healing.

The osteoclast is a multinuclear cell, which generally is located along the peripheral aspect of the bone substance. Its primary function is bone resorption. The peripheral aspect of an osteoclast presents a ruffled border in association with resorption of the adjacent bone.

It is probable that mesenchymal cells subjected to appropriate mechanical and

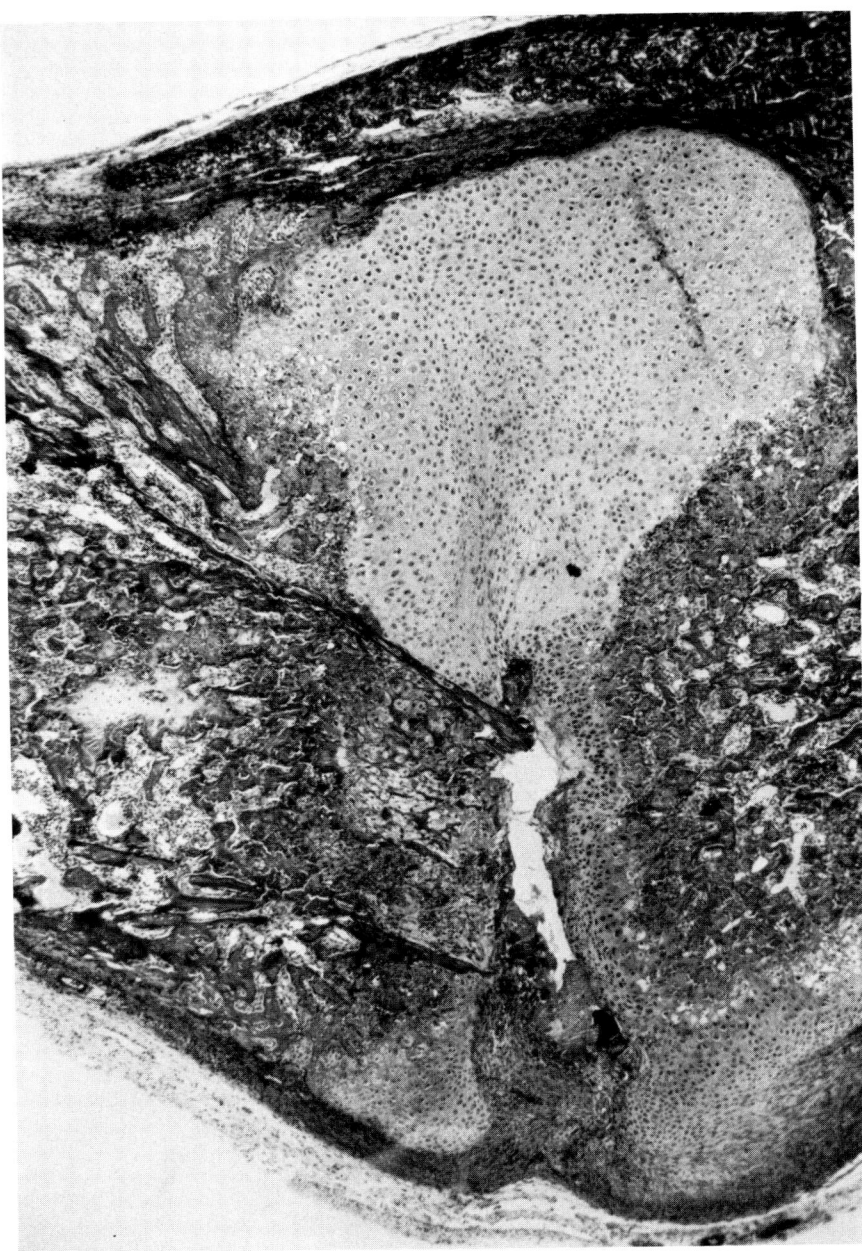

Figure 2–3 The extent of the periosteal collar may be viewed in this fracture at the top of this low power photomicrograph demonstrating the osteogenic potential of the periosteum at the proximal and distal aspects of the fracture and the cartilage cells in the center of the periosteal collar. Development of the abundant periosteal collar is secondary to gross motion at the fracture site.

biophysical stimuli may transform directly into osteoblasts and produce bone. Bassett demonstrated that cells subjected to a combination of compression and low oxygen tensions transformed directly into chondroblasts and formed cartilage.[7] If the cells were then administered an adequate amount of oxygen and placed under tension rather than compression, they differentiated into fibroblasts and produced dense fibrous tissue. One problem in interpreting these results is separating the effects of compression and tension from the effects of varying oxygen tensions on the stimulation of cells to form various linkages. It is a clinical axiom that bone forms in compression and fails in tension.

FRACTURE HEALING

Primary type bone healing is somewhat artificial in that it is possible only with rigid internal fixation and excellent anatomical position. This is not usually the case in the nonoperative treatment of fractures. The goal of primary bone healing is therefore obtained only by primary operative internal fixation. It has been adequately demonstrated by Perren and the Association for the Study of Internal Fixation (AO Group) that fractures treated in this manner reveal evidence of primary bone healing without any sign of fibrous tissue or cartilage during the healing process.[70] There is no evidence of external callus formation with this type of treatment. The destruction of osteons close to the fracture site, initiated by the destruction of local blood supply, stimulates an intensive regeneration of new haversian systems in the area. Osteoclasts form spearheads at the ends of the haversian canals close to the fracture site, and these become enlarged in preparation for the formation of a new system. The osteoclast spearhead (cutting cone) can advance at a rate of 50 to 80 μ per 24 hours up to and through the fracture surface, with the production of enlarged haversian canals, which cross from one fragment to the opposite fragment. Osteoblasts follow immediately to form new osteons which traverse the fracture site. If rigid internal fixation is employed, it will take approximately five to six weeks for new osteons to be constructed. Therefore, the repair is produced by new osteons developing and crossing the fracture site to replace the old osteons that had been deprived of their local blood supply. If a gap exists between the fracture fragments, or if there is not rigid immobilization, this type of healing does not occur. It is replaced by healing that is normally observed in the nonoperative management of fractures, which will be discussed further on. A great deal of credit must be given to the Association for the Study of Internal Fixation for thoroughly evaluating this type of fracture repair, which is further discussed in Chapter 7.

STAGES OF REPAIR

Stage of Impact

Bone will absorb energy until a failure occurs. The greater the rate of application of force or load, the greater the energy bone may absorb. The amount of energy that can be absorbed by bone is inversely proportional to the modulus of rigidity. Also, the amount of energy absorbed by osseous tissue is directly proportional to the volume of bone. A fracture line will follow the path of least resistance. If drill holes have been placed in bone prior to impact, the fracture line will pass through the drill holes because they produce areas of stress concentration. This is extemely important to remember when large compression plates are removed following internal fixation and during fracture healing. The limb must be protected until the osseous tissues around the drill holes have a chance to react to the new stresses and abolish the stress concentration. It usually requires at least four to six weeks for the bone to adapt to the new stress. If compression plates are left on for a prolonged period, osteoporosis may develop beneath them, and this of course will weaken the resistance of bone to impact. This is discussed further in Chapter 7.

Stage of Induction

At the present time, the exact duration of the stage of induction is unknown. This stage may occur at any time from impact to the completion of the stage of inflammation.

Cells in the area of the fracture are induced to form new bone. Although the exact origin of new osteoblasts is still a matter of controversy, it is fair to state that two separate mechanisms appear to operate. In the first mechanism, the periosteal cell, endosteal cell, and osteocyte undergo modulation in order to produce new osteoblasts. The second mechanism involves differentiation of fibroblasts, endothelial cells, muscle cells, and undifferentiated mesenchymal cells. The exact stimulus of modulation and differentiation is unknown at the present time. It is possible that the initial disruption of the blood supply and the production of a state of relative hypoxia with a large oxygen gradient may stimulate formation of an osteoblast linkage, as previously proposed by the author.[47, 48] An acidic pH rapidly develops in the local area, and this may also be a stimulus. Lysosomal enzymes are released following cell disruption. Although each is a possible initial stimulant, it is probable that the stimulation is multifactorial. Urist and his co-workers have published several investigative studies regarding a bone morphogenic stimulating substance (BMP), which is discussed further in Chapter 5.

Stage of Inflammation

This stage begins immediately after the fracture occurs and persists until cartilage or bone formation is initiated. Clinically, the end of this stage is usually associated with a decrease in pain and swelling. This interval varies but usually lasts for three to four days. There is a gross disruption of the vascular supply with attendant hemorrhage and hematoma formation (Fig. 2–4). A state of hypoxia exists with an acidic environment. The bone at the edge of the fracture site, both the periosteal and endosteal surfaces, becomes necrotic. There is a gross disruption of the osteons and the lacunae with the release of lysosomal enzymes. Mast cells, containing vasoactive substances as well as heparin, may be identified now and are thought to play an active role at this stage. As in other areas of inflammation, the macrophage removes metabolic by-products and dead tissue. Recent work suggests that the macrophage may be the activator of fibroblasts in soft tissue repair, and it is conceivable that the same mechanism operates in fracture repair. Osteoclasts begin to mobilize, and osteolytic activity may be seen along the ruffled border of the cell. A further explanation of the inflammatory stage of soft tissue repair can be found in Chapter 1.

Stage of Soft Callus

This is a very active phase in which both an external and an internal soft callus are formed (Fig. 2–5). The external callus plays an important role by helping to immobilize the fracture fragments. Urist and Johnson likened the callus cuff to a bridge span, because it makes it possible to stabilize the fracture and to load the bone long before the process of union is complete. The external callus is achieved by an active proliferation of osteoblasts in the cambium layer of the periosteum. This is evident not only at the

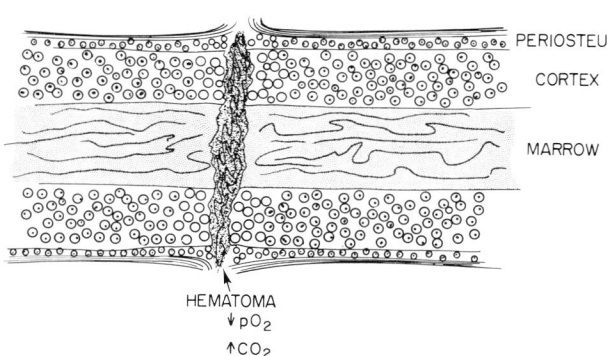

PERIOSTEUM

CORTEX

MARROW

HEMATOMA
$\downarrow pO_2$
$\uparrow CO_2$
$\downarrow pH$

Figure 2–4 A hematoma develops at the fracture site as a result of disruption of the osseous structure and attending vascular supply. The bone at the edges of the fracture site becomes necrotic. This produces empty lacunae at the fracture margins.

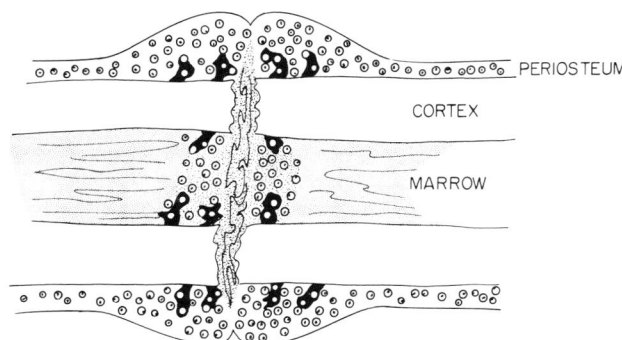

Figure 2–5 The stage of soft callus with a periosteal collar forming to bridge the fracture surface. Note the periosteal reaction that occurs both proximal and distal to the fracture site proper.

fracture site but also along the undersurface of the periosteum away from the fracture site. In effect, this produces a collar of soft tissue callus, with each end approaching the other from each fragment. The fibrous layer of the periosteum is elevated proximal to the fracture site for some distance by the proliferation of the underlying osteoblasts. In the proximal portion of the periosteum the osteoblasts form new bone directly. However, as the fracture site is approached, cartilage cells as well as active osteoblasts are evident. Tonna demonstrated in a series of experiments that cartilage cell formation at the fracture site occurs by means of osteogenic cell progeny transformation.[94] He labeled the cells at the fracture site and found that newly formed cartilage cells were labeled with the same frequency as osteogenic cell progeny. He concluded that osteogenic cells were osteochondrogenic cells which were equally capable of giving rise to osteoblasts, chondroblasts, or chondrocytes. Therefore, these cells can form cartilage or bone, depending on the local environment. As the fracture site is approached, there is an associated gradual ingrowth of new vascularity. However, new cells are increasing at a more rapid rate, and the cellularity outstrips the vascular supply, producing a state of relative hypoxia. This was initially demonstrated by Wray[106, 107] and has been further documented by the author.[47] The importance of the endosteal blood supply has been thoroughly evaluated in several excellent studies by Rhinelander, which will be discussed.[74–79] Suffice it to state that the periosteal circulation initially provides blood supply to the fracture site, but the endosteal circulation eventually plays a major role in the fracture

healing process. The surface of the soft callus is electronegative and remains so throughout this stage, which usually lasts three to four weeks, or until the bony fragments are united by fibrous and/or collagenous tissue. The end of this stage is clinically evident when the osseous fragments are no longer grossly mobile and are at least in a "sticky" phase.

Stage of Hard Callus

At this stage the external and internal callus gradually convert to fiber bone (Fig. 2–6). If internal fixation has not been employed in the treatment of these fractures, endochondral bone formation dominates. If the fragments have been well immobilized with a compression plate, however, membranous bone formation will predominate. This is discussed further in

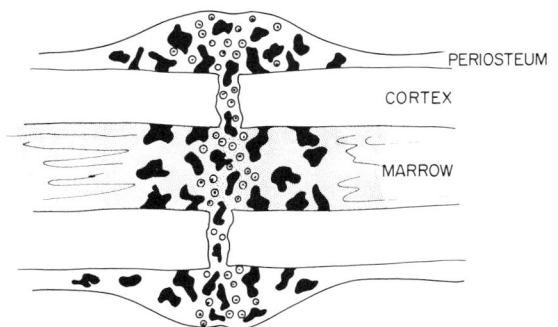

Figure 2–6 The stage of hard-callus formation with the conversion of the internal and external callus to fiber bone. Studies have revealed hypertrophic cells within the callus similar to those seen in the epiphyseal plate prior to calcification.

Chapter 7. In this stage there is a definite increase in vascularity but also an abundant increase in cellularity. Therefore, the cellular structure is still operating under conditions of relative hypoxia. The pH of the matrix now reverts to neutral, but the external and internal surfaces of the callus remain electronegative. There is continued development of the endosteal blood supply throughout this stage, and the osteoclasts are still active in removing the remaining dead bone. This stage begins at three to four weeks and continues until the fragments are firmly united with new bone. The fracture site is now clinically and roentgenographically healed (Figs. 2–7 and 2–8). The average elapsed time in an adult is three to four months for major long bones. As described in Chapter 9, this time is significantly decreased in the pediatric age group.

Stage of Remodeling

In this stage the newly formed fiber bone is gradually converted to lamellar bone. Osteoclasts are active in remodeling the external surface of the bone to decrease the size of callus or "bump." The medullary canal is reconstituted in a similar manner. The local tissue oxygen supply reverts to normal. The surface charge of the fracture site is no longer electronegative. The duration of the remodeling stage is variable: It may last for a few months, but there is evidence in human biopsy studies that it may continue for several years. The capability for remodeling is vastly increased in pediatric patients compared with adults. This effect is believed to be mediated through the epiphyseal plate, but the exact mechanism of its action has not been adequately evaluated. It is not uncommon

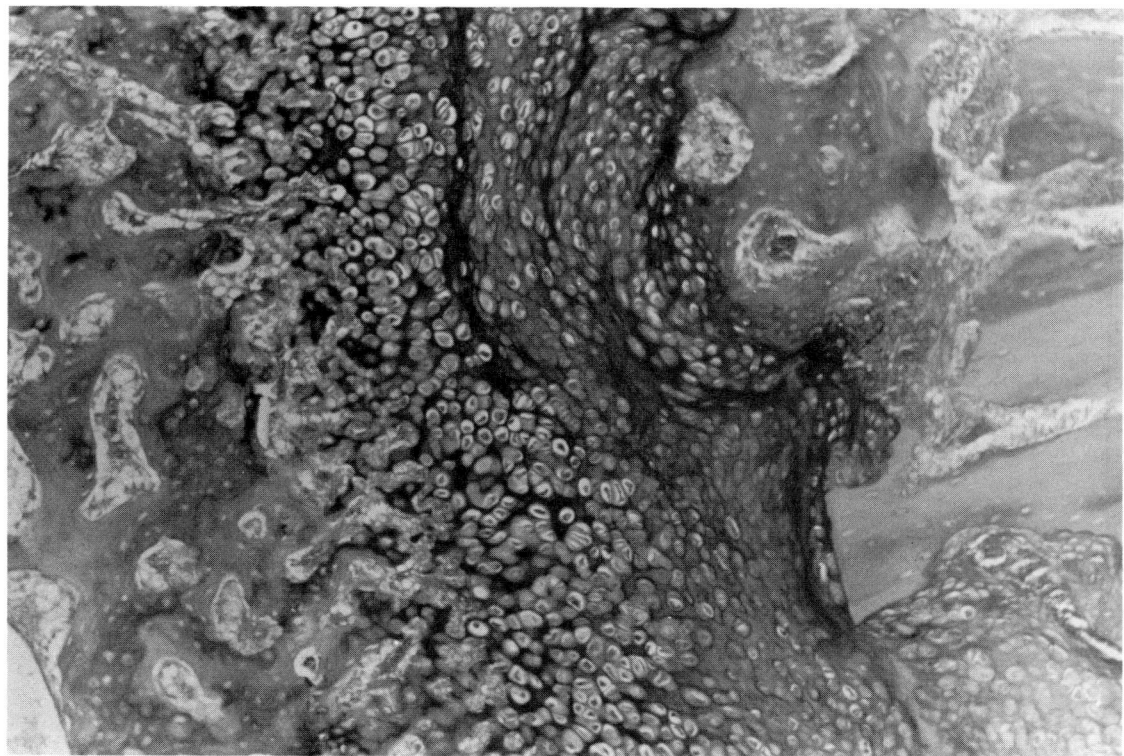

Figure 2–7   A high-power view of the advanced periosteal and endosteal reaction. Note the fracture surface in the midportion on the right. The abundant periosteal new fiber bone and endosteal conversion to fiber bone is evident.

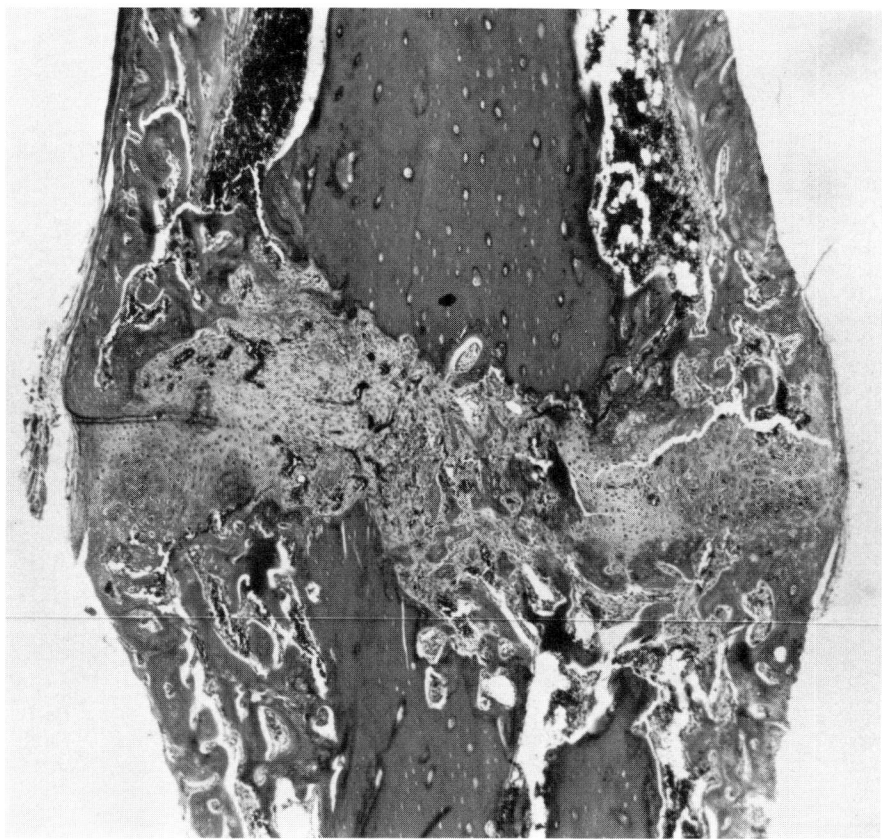

Figure 2–8 This is an obvious nonunion for comparison with Figure 2–7. Note that the periosteal and endosteal callus has not progressed to form new fiber bone. Cartilage and fibrous tissue persist.

in pediatric patients to have a bone heal in an angulated state only to be actively remodeled, and in follow-up one year post-fracture to find that the angulation has been remodeled and the gross anatomical alignment of the bone has been restored. Adult bone lacks this increased ability to actively remodel angulatory deformities at the fracture site, and therefore adult fractures must be properly reduced if alignment is to be maintained (Figs. 2–9, 2–10, and 2–11).

Role of the Hematoma

The exact function of the hematoma at a fracture site has been actively debated in the past. Lexer believed that the fracture hematoma represented an inactive stuffing material between ends of the fracture, without value for union. If the hematoma was increased, then periosteal cells would organize the hematoma extensively. He concluded that if this occurred, the cells produced fibrous tissue instead of bone. On the other hand, Phemister felt that fibrin in the hematoma may stimulate cell regeneration and aid in immobilizing the fracture ends. Through this mechanism, granulation could advance into the hematoma with resorption and perform the same function as in soft tissue repair.

Most investigators now agree that the active role of the hematoma is not as important in the fracture healing process as was once believed.[107, 108] The larger the dead space created by the disruption at the fracture site, then the more extensive the hematoma formation. The real physiological question is the following: Does the hematoma function as an initial stimulus for the differentiation of primitive mesenchymal cells for active repair at the fracture site?

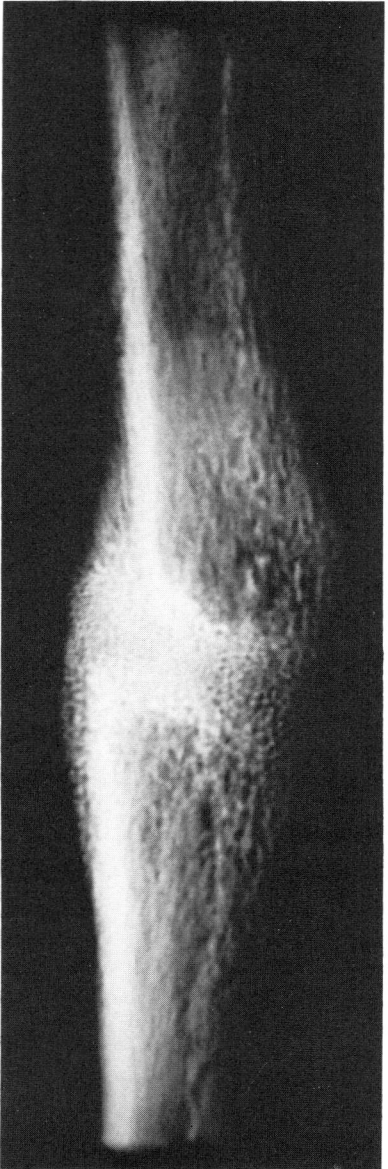

Figure 2-9 A roentgenograph of a healed dog fibula. Note the remodeling that has occurred at the fracture site.

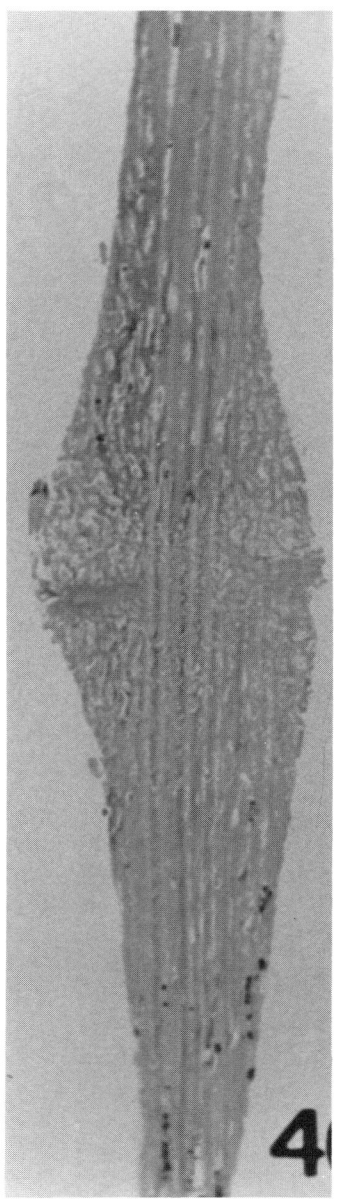

Figure 2-10 A longitudinal section of a healed dog fibula demonstrating the remodeling and reconstitution of the endosteal bone.

Considerable debate continues to surround this point, but the general feeling is that the hematoma itself does not play a significant physiological stimulatory role in the repair of fractures. In fact, the studies of the AO Group demonstrated that the hematoma between the fracture ends is virtually eliminated in rigid anatomical internal fixation, the condition in which primary bone healing occurs.[70]

BLOOD SUPPLY AND FRACTURE HEALING

Our present understanding of the microcirculation in fracture healing was advanced by Trueta's work,[97] but it remained for the classic studies of Rhinelander to outline and document the microcirculatory changes during the fracture healing process.[74-79] These studies represent an excellent example of a scientific approach to the problem, and all personnel involved with skeletal physiology should be thoroughly familiar

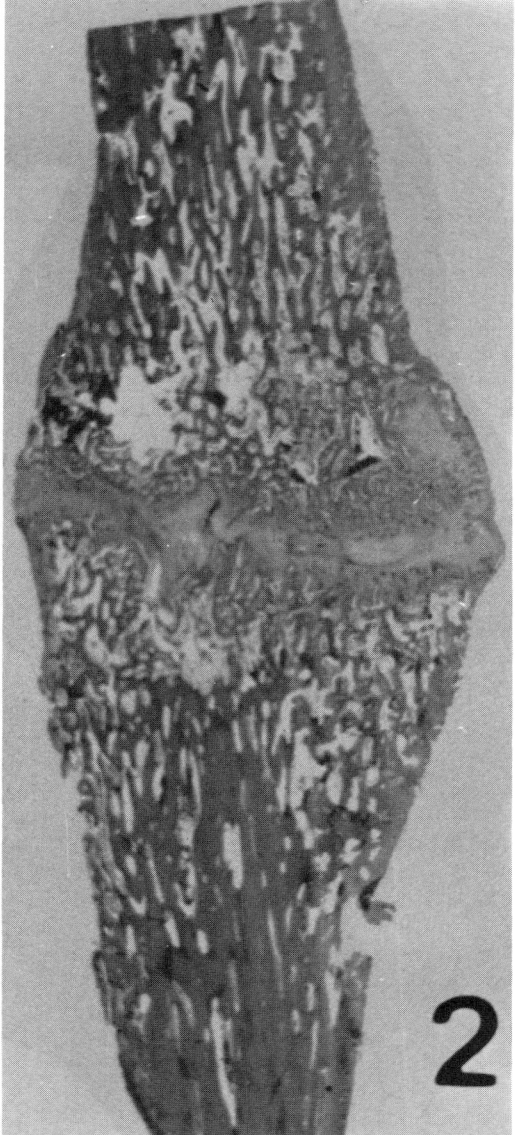

Figure 2–11 Low-power magnification shows that the medullary space has not been reconstituted in this longitudinal section of a dog fibula. Cartilage is still present at the fracture site.

with Rhinelander's work. A brief summary of his findings follows.

Microangiographic techniques revealed that fracture of a contralateral forelimb of a canine ulna produced a physiological stimulation of the circulation of the uninjured forelimb. Rhinelander believed that the difference between the normal stimulated circulation and the normal resting circulation, shown in Figure 2–12, represented an enormous potential for increased vascular function within bone. A classification of the blood vessels comprising the normal circulation was developed on the basis of function rather than anatomical location. An afferent and an efferent vascular system were described. The three primary components of the afferent vascular system were the principal nutrient artery, the metaphyseal arteries, and the periosteal arterioles. The efferent vascular system included the large emissary veins and vena comitans of the nutrient vein, which drain the medullary contents exclusively, the cortical venous channels, and the periosteal capillaries. All these components convey blood toward the exterior. The endosteal circulation supplies the medullary area and the inner two thirds to three quarters of the compactum. The periosteal arterioles supply the outer third or quarter of the compactum only in localized areas that are related to fascial attachments, and these periosteal arterioles become more active when the medullary supply is interrupted.

Brookes felt that the normal centrifugal blood flow could be reversed with interruption of the nutrient blood system so that the periosteal system could convey blood to the compactum.[77] However, Rhinelander was unable to demonstrate a major reversal in direction of flow of blood supplied by the so-called periosteal circulation when the medullary blood supply was interrupted. It is true that a small supply of new blood develops in relation to the soft tissue attachments at the fracture site, and these temporarily provide blood to the external callus (Fig. 2–13). Following canine fractures that were well reduced and stabilized, he was able to demonstrate that the endosteal osseous callus can bridge the fracture gap within three weeks without the intermediate production of fibrocartilage. Arteries derived from the medulla permeated

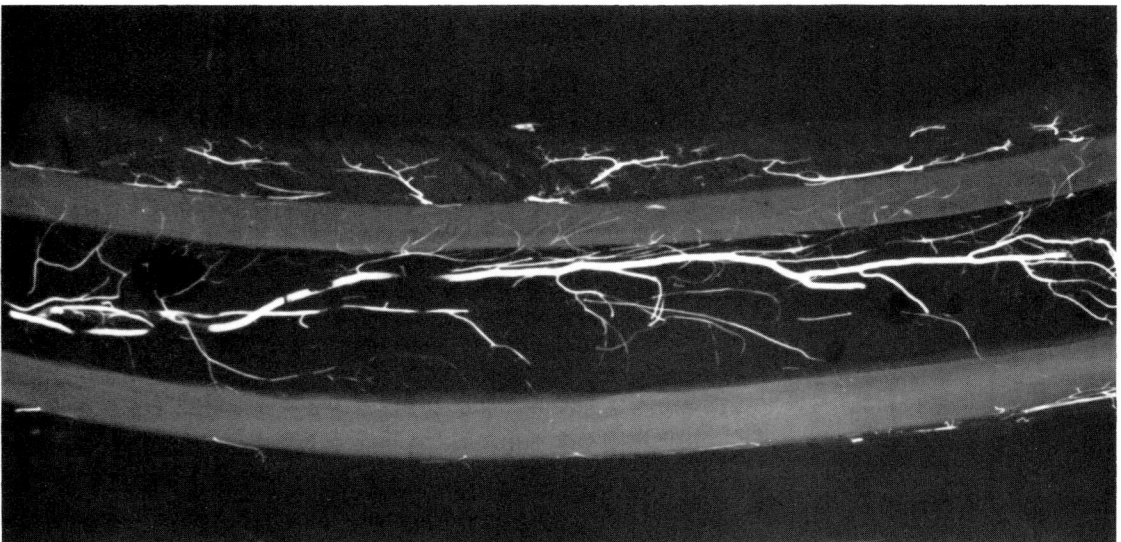

Figure 2–12   Micrograph of the midshaft of a normal dog radius with the circulation in a resting state. Note the prominence of the medullary vessels. (Courtesy of F. W. Rhinelander and *Journal of Bone and Joint Surgery*. The normal microcirculation of diaphyseal cortex and its response to fracture. J. B. J. S. *50A*:784–800, 1968.)

the cortex of both fracture fragments and rendered these fragments extremely porotic, with the result that by six weeks they traversed it completely to afford the major blood supply even to the external callus.

This provided further evidence that blood supply of the cortex was functionally centrifugal in direction of flow.

This sequence of events did not occur when the fracture fragments were widely

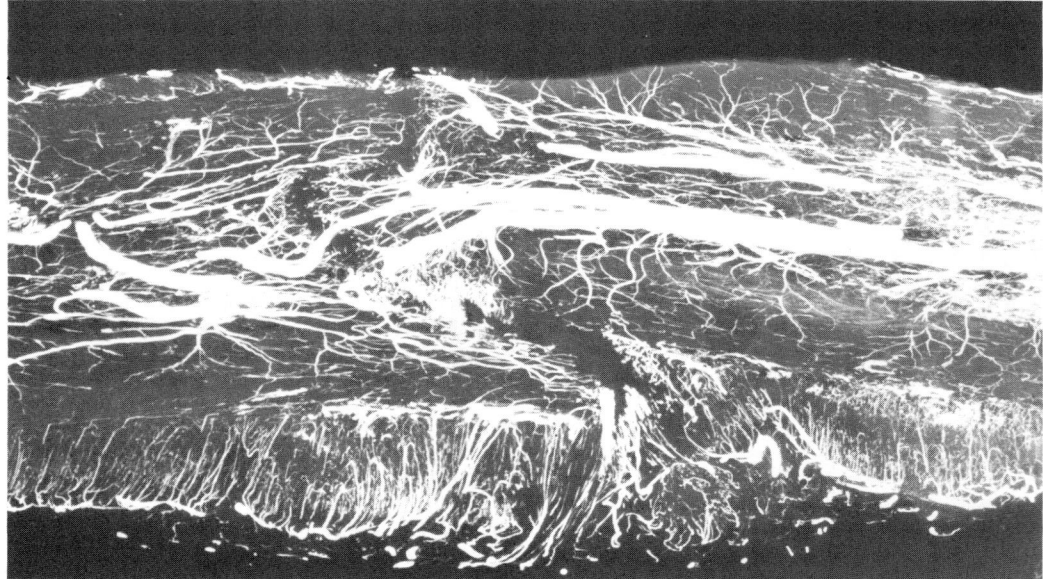

Figure 2–13   Microangiogram of three-week-old displaced radial fracture with reestablishment of the medullary circulation. The extensive periosteal callus shows the characteristic arrangement of blood vessels perpendicular to the cortical surface. (×6) (Courtesy of F. W. Rhinelander and *Journal of Bone and Joint Surgery*. The normal microcirculation of diaphyseal cortex and its response to fracture, J. B. J. S., *50A*:784–800, 1968.)

displaced or comminuted. In displaced fractures the periosteal afferent circulation derived from the overlying soft tissues was initially important in supplying blood to the external callus that attempted to bridge the fracture gap. However, the periosteal bridging callus was never responsible for the primary osseous union. It always contained a zone of fibrocartilage. The medullary circulation was also stimulated following fracture in each main fragment with the production of the endosteal osseous callus. If the fracture fragments were widely displaced or comminuted, then the periosteal afferent circulation persisted for much longer in supplying the chief areas of bone repair. However, Rhinelander was able to demonstrate that the endosteal circulation makes every effort to assume the major function of afferent blood supply as soon as

possible. In short, the endosteal blood supply is ultimately the most important blood supply in the fracture healing process (Figs. 2–14 and 2–15).

SPECIAL TYPES OF REPAIR

Small Osseous Defects

This type of repair has been studied in animals by means of a small drill hole in bone. The periosteum is destroyed at the penetrating site. As in a fracture, the surrounding bone and marrow become necrotic for at least a few millimeters around the hole, and a small hematoma develops in the osseous defect. Polymorphonuclear leukocytes are seen in the hematoma almost immediately, and by 24 hours plasma cells, lymphocytes, and macrophages are evident.

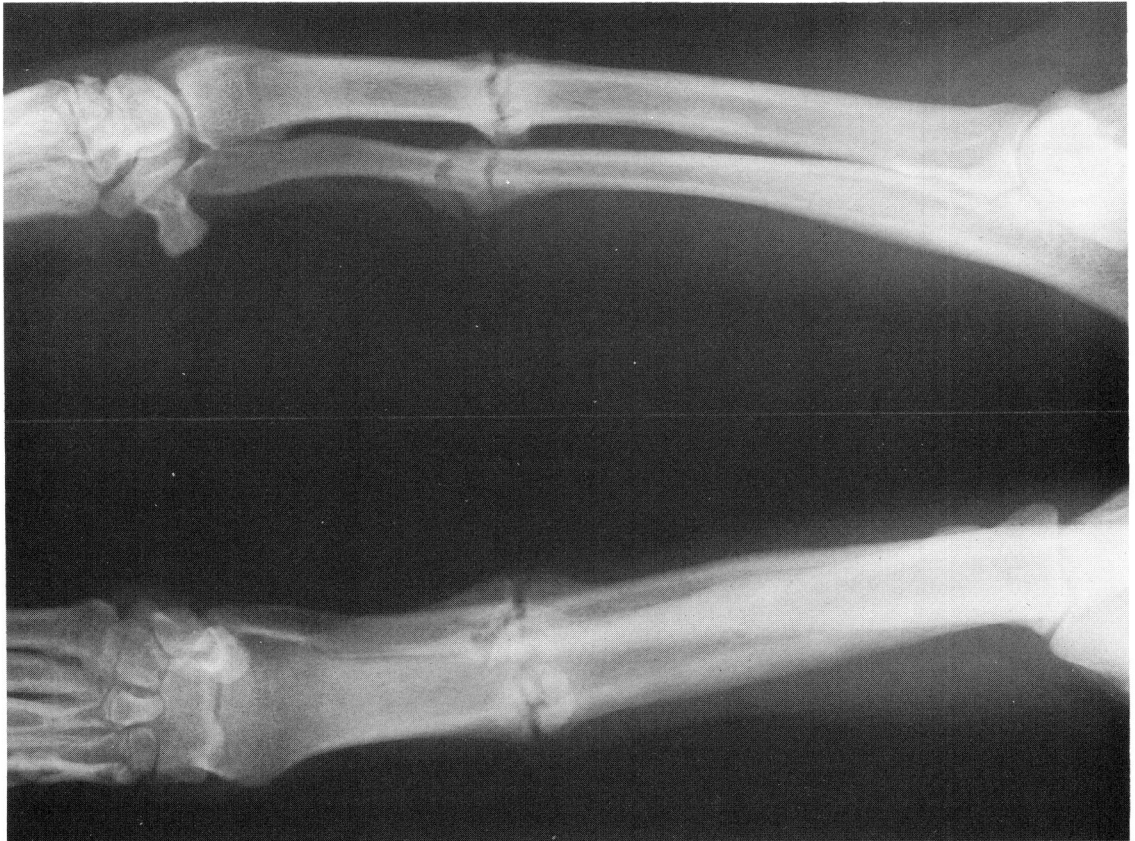

Figure 2–14 Roentgenograph revealing delayed union of six-week-old displaced fractures of both forelimb bones in a dog. (Courtesy of F. W. Rhinelander and *Journal of Bone and Joint Surgery. The normal microcirculation of diaphyseal cortex and its response to fracture, J. B. J. S., 50A:784–800, 1968.)

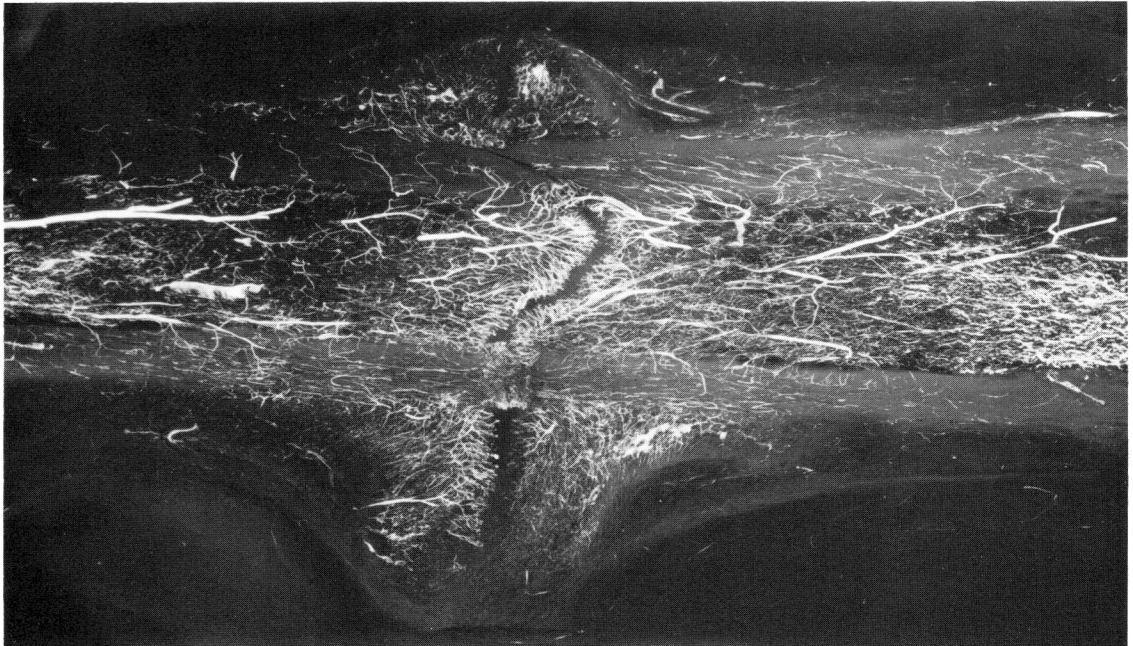

Figure 2–15   Microangiogram of radial fracture shown in Figure 2–14. Note the vascular pattern corresponding to the roentgenographic appearance of delayed union. (×6). (Courtesy of F. W. Rhinelander and *Journal of Bone and Joint Surgery*. The normal microcirculation of diaphyseal cortex and its response to fracture. J. B. J. S., 50A:784–800, 1968.)

Granulation tissue gradually replaces the hematoma. The periosteum reacts as it does to a normal fracture. The cambium layer becomes thickened by the proliferation of new osteoblasts, elevating the fibrous layer. This reaction extends for some distance from the drill site. The osteoblastic cells within the periosteal layer eventually form a bridge across the defect in a peculiar way that resembles the external callus of normal fracture healing. The endosteum responds in a similar manner. The transformation of undifferentiated mesenchymal cells is more rapid with this type of defect. Intramembranous bone formation occurs within the central portion of the defect. In general, the major portion of the trabeculae is oriented at right angles to the osseous shaft. Lamellar bone gradually replaces fiber bone within the osseous defect, and large intertrabecular spaces are gradually abolished. In the early phase of this repair (by three weeks), a mixture of fibrous and lamellar bone bridges the gap. There is no definite evidence of endochondral bone formation in

this defect. Cutting cones gradually replace the reactive bone, with new bone oriented in the same direction as the remainder of the shaft. Remodeling of the excess periosteal and endosteal callus is evident.

Intramedullary Fixation

Several types of intramedullary devices are now available for internal fixation. This technique was introduced by Küntscher in 1940 with a report of the results of intramedullary rod fixation of femoral fractures. This device has its most useful application in the femoral region. Several other devices have been described in the literature over the past two decades and are now available, including the Schneider, Hanson-Street, and Fluted Sampson devices. The femoral medullary cavity must be reamed extensively before any of these is inserted; the effect of such reaming has been studied by Rhinelander with microangiographic techniques. The main intramedullary vascular supply is destroyed during the initial reaming prior to insertion of the rod. The periosteal blood supply then increases its function in an attempt to compensate for the lost endosteal circulation. The deficit is compounded if the periosteum is "stripped" during the insertion of the rod.

Rhinelander demonstrated that the best design for an intramedullary device is a fluted one because it permits control of rotation but at the same time allows regeneration of the endosteal vascular blood supply between the flutes.[78, 79] If a solid intramedullary rod without flutes is employed, the main medullary circulation is destroyed, and an extensive period is required for its regeneration along the border of the device. However, if a fluted rod has been inserted, the endosteal blood supply may regenerate between the flutes. In other words, besides controlling rotation, the fluted design allows for a rapid reconstitution of the endosteal blood supply compared with the nonfluted one.

If there is good solid fixation of the fracture site by the intramedullary device, a small amount of external callus develops, with a decreased amount of endochondral bone formation. However, if a loose-fitting rod is inserted and there is motion at the fracture site, the major portion of the bone deposited between the fragments will be the result of endochondral bone formation. Clinically, it is difficult to decide when a fracture site is completely healed, as a portion of the fracture is obscured by the intramedullary device. Most authors feel that at least one and one half years should elapse before the device is removed.

An important point to bear in mind is that if there is evidence of comminution at the fracture site, a bone graft from the iliac crest should be used along with the internal fixation device. In fact, we have seen many cases presenting with initial comminution that are bone grafted in this manner and the rod removed at a later date. Following removal of the rod, it is not uncommon to see a fracture line in the intramedullary area that was once occupied by the rod. However, there is usually extensive bone formed around this area, bridging the two main fragments. The author takes this to mean that if the fracture had not been bone grafted initially, it probably would not have

healed primarily, even with the internal fixation device. Therefore, it is a good rule of thumb to employ a bone graft as well as internal fixation for open reduction of comminuted femoral fractures.

Compression Plating

As described earlier, the role of a compression plate is to provide rigid internal fixation, reducing motion at the fracture site and allowing excellent apposition of the osseous fragments (Fig. 2–16). As outlined in Chapter 7, several outstanding studies performed by the Association for the Study of Internal Fixation have documented the beneficial effect of compression plates.[70] Primary bone healing is common in this type of repair. The osseous fragments unite with new bone that is osteonal, without endochondral bone formation, and of normal orientation. The bone fragments under the compression plate should be approximated as closely to anatomical as possible. However, the cortices opposite the plate are often poorly approximated owing to the differing configurations of the bone and the compression plate. Every effort should be made to reconcile the two by bending the plate if this is to be prevented. In this connection, it is important to recall that *bone heals under compression and fails under tension.* Therefore, it is not only theoretically sound to obtain good apposition of both cortices, but it is also very practical. A hematoma does not form between the bone fragments if apposition is satisfactory with a compression plate. There is a mild inflammatory reaction in the soft tissues adjacent to the periosteum and in the marrow. New cutting cones originate at the junction of live and dead bone. Osteoclasts lead the cutting cones and migrate directly across the fracture site along an empty haversian canal, resorbing the matrix. They cross the fracture site and enter another apposing empty haversian canal or begin to cut into necrotic bone on the other fragment. This means that a new living osteon is produced immediately behind the cutting cone. The obvious question that arises is, what is the significance of the finding of an external callus? The finding of an external callus means by inference that there has been motion at the fracture site. If

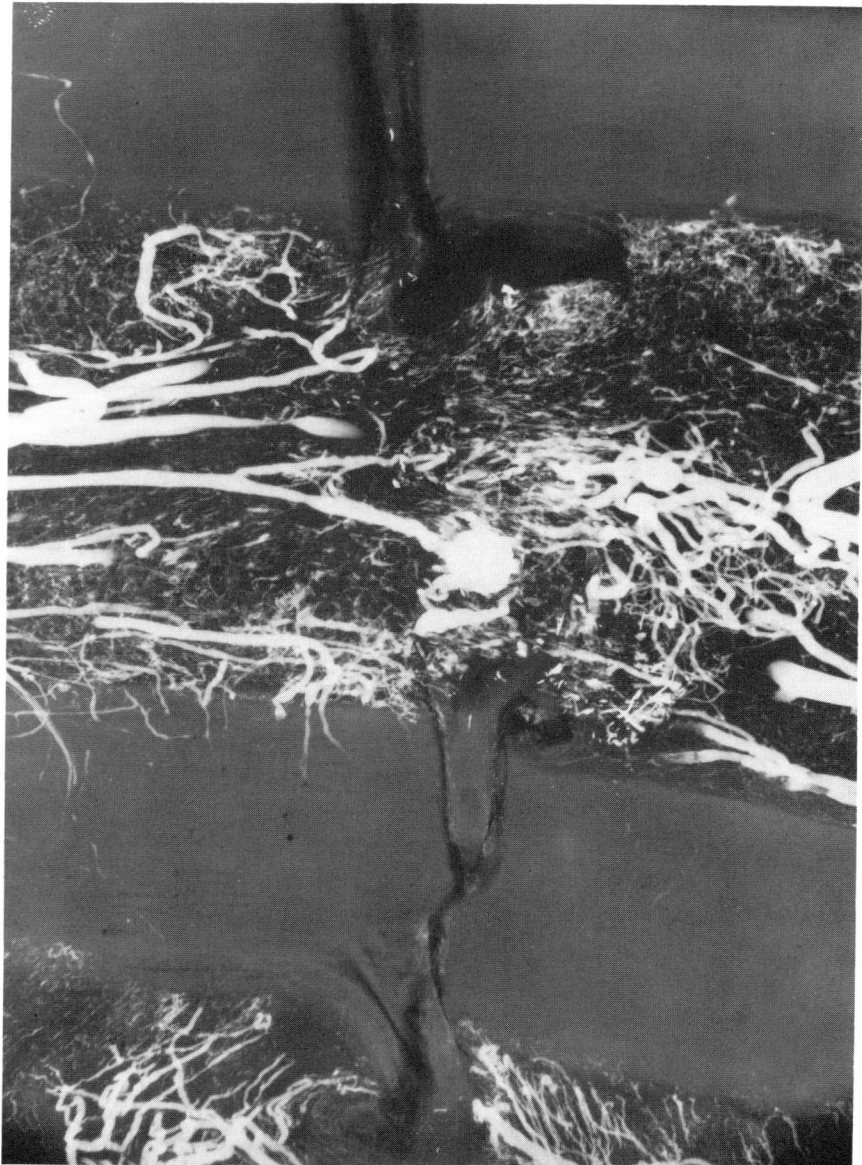

Figure 2–16 Microangiogram of a dog radius one week after transverse osteotomy and secure plate fixation showing reconstitution of the medullary vessels (×25). (Courtesy of F. W. Rhinelander and *Journal of Bone and Joint Surgery*. The normal microcirculation of diaphyseal cortex and its response to fracture. J. B. J. S., 50A:784–800, 1968.

motion at the fracture site can be eliminated, an external callus is not formed, and primary bone healing takes place. With an external callus, endochondral bone formation is present, whereas with compression plating and the consequent absence of an external callus, primary bone healing with-

out intervening cartilage occurs. It is important to remember that a compression plate, if left in place, will continue to absorb the major portion of the stress instead of the stress being absorbed by the osseous tissue underneath the plate. When this occurs, osteoporosis underneath the plate is the ultimate result. If flexible compression plates are employed instead of rigid fixation plates, the severe osteoporosis underneath the plate is not as significant. The design of improved plates and the timing of their removal are the subjects of extensive investigation.

PHYSIOLOGICAL EFFECTS OF OXYGEN ON GROWTH AND REPAIR

In the past, it was felt that adequate blood supply with a high oxygen tension stimulated growth in the epiphyseal plate. Brighton and Heppenstall recently documented the oxygen tensions in various zones of the epiphyseal plate.[16] The result of this study indicates that active bone growth in the metaphyseal area of the epiphyseal plate occurs under conditions of relative hypoxia. It was further noted that a large oxygen gradient existed between the zone of cell columns, the zone of hypertrophic cells, and the metaphyseal area. The oxygen tension in the zone of cell columns averaged 57 mm Hg. In the zone of hypertrophic cells it measured 24.3 mm Hg. In the metaphyseal area where active new bone formation occurs the oxygen tension measured 19.8 mm. Hg. It was postulated that the relative hypoxia in the metaphyseal area might be a stimulus for new bone formation. These studies were then expanded to include fracture repair. Brighton and Krebs, utilizing the same oxygen microelectrode technique, measured the oxygen tensions at a fracture and nonunion site.[18] Once again, the oxygen tensions were noted to be relatively low during active new bone formation in the course of repair. In a separate study utilizing a different oxygen-measuring technique, the author was able to demonstrate that active new bone formation at the site of an osseous defect occurred under conditions of relative hypoxia (Fig. 2–17).[47] An additional finding in the same study was that the oxygen consumption during rapid active new bone formation was not elevated above that of normal bone. This provided evidence that the low oxygen tension was not due to rapid consumption but rather to an increase in cellularity above that of vascularity. In other words, the cells were outstripping their blood supply, in a sequence of events similar to that in soft tissue repair, as outlined in Chapter 1. Kelly and his associates have measured the blood flow to fractures in animals with the use of radioisotope techniques.[59, 68] They were able to demonstrate that the blood flow to a canine fractured tibia reached a maximum

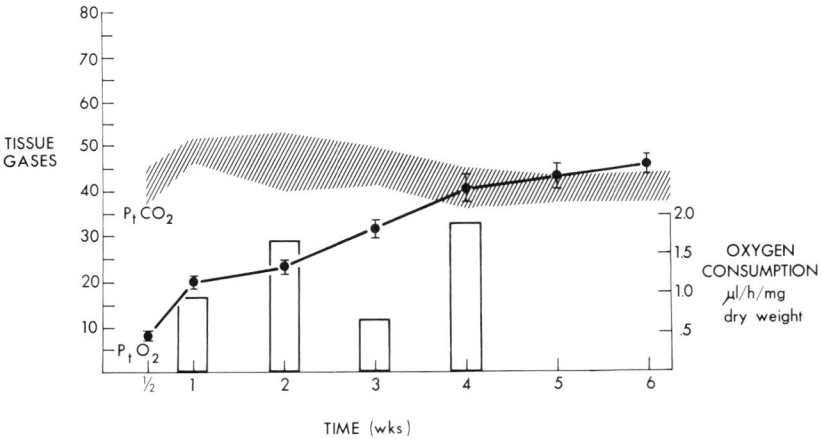

Figure 2–17 The tissue oxygen, carbon dioxide, and oxygen consumption values obtained in healing dog rib defects as a function of time. Of interest was the fact that at three to four weeks, when bone was actively being formed, the oxygen tension remained low and was associated with a slightly elevated carbon dioxide tension and no evidence of an increase in oxygen consumption above that of normal bone. (Courtesy of R. B. Heppenstall et al. and *Clinical Orthopedics and Related Research*. Tissue gas tensions and oxygen consumption in healing bone defects. Clin. Orthop., *106*:357–365, 1975.)

on the tenth day and decreased thereafter but did not return to normal values until 112 days postfracture. Rhinelander has also demonstrated through microangiographic techniques a gradual increase in the vascular supply. If these studies are correlated, it appears that the blood supply is increased at a fracture site, but that cellularity is also increased above vascularity, producing a state of relative hypoxia during active new bone formation.

A further study was performed by the author in an attempt to evaluate the effect of chronic systemic hypoxia on the fracture healing process.[48] It was noted that a sustained chronic systemic hypoxia produced a delay in fracture healing. The author proposed that one cause of delay in fracture healing might be the fact that systemic hypoxia abolished the normally large oxygen gradient at the fracture site, as had been previously demonstrated.

Hyperbaric oxygen studies have produced conflicting results. Some studies have indicated that the fracture healing process may be stimulated by the addition of hyperbaric oxygen treatments.[63] However, a recent study on bone turnover with the use of hyperbaric oxygen reveals that this technique increases the amount of bone resorption above that of bone formation,

with a negative net effect.[28] It is also known that a high concentration of oxygen over a prolonged period is detrimental to cell function.

What then can we accurately state regarding the effect of oxygen on the fracture healing process? Seven facts appear to emerge.

1. All the available proline and lysine that is hydroxylated in tissues can be hydroxylated by a small amount of oxygen, well below the levels measured for normal fracture repair.

2. Fractures normally heal under a state of relative hypoxia by mechanisms similar to those of soft tissue repair.

3. A large oxygen gradient across the reparative surface is probably the initial stimulus for healing.

4. A state of chronic systemic hypoxia definitely delays the fracture healing process.

5. Studies of hyperbaric oxygen have produced conflicting results, but hyperbaric oxygen has been shown to have a detrimental effect on bone turnover by producing increased resorption compared to formation. It is also well documented that a high oxygen concentration for a prolonged period of time is detrimental to cell function.

6. The blood supply to a fracture increases well above normal during the early phases of repair, but a concomitant increase in cellularity produces a state of relative hypoxia during active new bone formation.

7. Bone cells have been demonstrated to follow predominantly an anaerobic pathway (Fig. 2–19).

The unanswered question at present concerns the effect of a mild elevation in local oxygen tension above that normally seen during active repair. Studies are currently in progress.

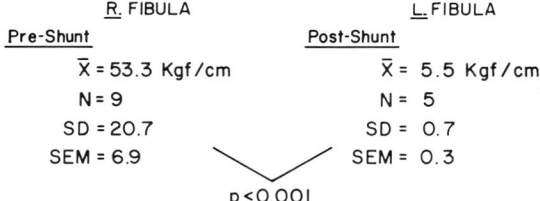

	R. FIBULA		L. FIBULA
Pre-Shunt			Post-Shunt
	$\bar{X}$ = 53.3 Kgf/cm		$\bar{X}$ = 5.5 Kgf/cm
	N = 9		N = 5
	SD = 20.7		SD = 0.7
	SEM = 6.9		SEM = 0.3

$p < 0.001$

$\bar{X}$ = mean
N = number of specimens
SD = standard deviation
SEM = standard error of the mean

Figure 2–18 Modulus of bending of a healing fibula fracture in the dog. The pre-shunt measurements were taken prior to the production of chronic systemic hypoxia. The post-shunt measurements were in dogs with central arteriovenous shunts producing a state of chronic systemic hypoxia. Note the deficit in breaking strength in the post-shunt or chronically hypoxic dogs compared with that in the normal dogs. (Courtesy of R. B. Heppenstall et al. and *Journal of Bone and Joint Surgery*. Fracture healing in the presence of chronic hypoxia. J. B. J. S., 58A:1153–1156, 1976.)

Anemia and Fracture Healing

A review of the literature concerning the effects of anemia on soft tissue healing has produced conflicting opinions. A recent study has provided well-documented evidence that an uncomplicated normovolemic anemia does not alter soft tissue healing. A similar study was performed by the author to evaluate the effect of anemia

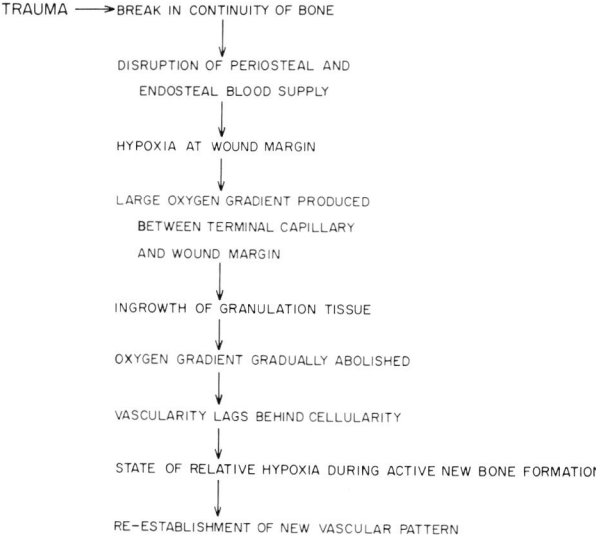

TRAUMA ──→ BREAK IN CONTINUITY OF BONE

    DISRUPTION OF PERIOSTEAL AND
    ENDOSTEAL BLOOD SUPPLY

    HYPOXIA AT WOUND MARGIN

    LARGE OXYGEN GRADIENT PRODUCED
    BETWEEN TERMINAL CAPILLARY
    AND WOUND MARGIN

    INGROWTH OF GRANULATION TISSUE

    OXYGEN GRADIENT GRADUALLY ABOLISHED

    VASCULARITY LAGS BEHIND CELLULARITY

    STATE OF RELATIVE HYPOXIA DURING ACTIVE NEW BONE FORMATION

    RE-ESTABLISHMENT OF NEW VASCULAR PATTERN
    AND REMODELING OF OSSEOUS STRUCTURE

Figure 2–19 A hypothetical sequence of events in relation to oxygen and fracture healing.

on fracture healing (Fig. 2–20).[49] Rothman had earlier demonstrated that an iron deficiency anemia definitely delays the healing process.[83] However, iron deficiency anemia is not the usual clinical situation in fracture healing. The author was able to demonstrate that an uncomplicated normovolemic anemia does not delay fracture healing. If, however, hypovolemia is associated with the anemia, the fracture healing process is definitely delayed. Normally, a hypovolemic anemia is rarely encountered in the course of fracture healing in humans. Therefore, it is not acceptable today to administer blood transfusions when the hemoglobin drops below an arbitrarily selected level (in the past, 8 to 10) in anticipation of stimulat-

ing the fracture healing process. Oxygen delivery to the fracture surface will be normal in the presence of a normovolemic anemia. Since fracture healing is not stimulated by blood transfusion, exposing the patient to the known risks of blood transfusion is not warranted. This rule is probably not valid in managing debilitated patients who have anemia and a fracture. Blood transfusions in this clinical situation may stimulate fracture healing because of the various components present in blood and not because of oxygen delivery.

THEORIES OF CALCIFICATION

A complete discussion of this subject is beyond the scope of this book. A summary of several proposed theories will be outlined.

A significant amount of investigation has been done on the exact mechanism of calcification, and several theories have been formulated on the basis of these experiments. It is fair to state that the exact mechanism of calcification in bone is still unknown. One of the stumbling blocks to developing a theory of calcification is overcoming the fact that calcification can occur in cartilage and osseous tissues without occurring in soft tissue at the same time. This leads the observer to suspect that a

	Hct	Modulus of elasticity	Roentgenogram
Group A	38±2	45 ± 5.2 Kgf/cm	Normal Healing
Group B	30±1	43 ± 4.4 Kgf/cm	Normal Healing
Group C	32±1	16 ± 6.5 Kgf/cm	Delayed Healing

Figure 2–20 Effect of anemia on fracture healing. Group A included fractures of the rabbit fibula at three weeks, blood withdrawn and reinfused. Group B, Normovolemic rabbits. Group C, Hypovolemic Anemia. Note the decreased breaking strength in the hypovolemic state. (Courtesy of R. B. Heppenstall and C. T. Brighton and *Clinical Orthopedics and Related Research*. Fracture healing in the presence of anemia. Clin. Orthop., *123*:253-258, 1977.)

specific mechanism must exist for the calcification of bone. In the past, significant emphasis was placed on hard tissue collagen as a nucleation catalyst. However, recent research has directed attention to the function of mitochondria and matrix vesicles in calcification.[2, 3, 19, 54, 61] It is now recognized that the main inorganic constituent of bone is minute crystals of hydroxyapatite.

One of the earliest theories of calcification was put forth by Robison and revolved around the idea that a local increase in concentration of phosphate ions could be produced by hydrolysis of ester phosphates by a phosphatase.[82] The popularity of this theory has waxed and waned over the past three decades. Some authors have suggested that the protein polysaccharides may play an important role in the calcification process. Chondroitin sulfate may inhibit calcification through a mechanism that limits ion diffusion and binds calcium. It has also been proposed that chondroitin sulfate acts in conjunction with collagen to initiate calcification through the formation of specific nucleation centers.

The theory of crystal nucleation followed by crystal growth has received recent attention and enthusiasm. Glimcher has proposed that hydroxyapatite crystals form within the fibers of the collagen matrix, oriented in a specific way relative to the fiber axis.[36, 37] They appear to be associated with a particular portion of the collagen band pattern (hole zone), which suggests that the collagen matrix may in fact be the nucleation site. It has been demonstrated that fibers with 640 Å periodicity are capable of being calcified.[51] It appears that the other forms of collagen aggregation cannot be calcified, suggesting that the spatial arrangement of a quarter-stagger found in the native form of collagen is required for nucleation to occur.

Another possible mechanism in calcification involves adenosine triphosphate as an energy source. The adenosine triphosphate (ATP) binds calcium in the formation of an ATP–calcium complex. ATPase then hydrolyzes the complex, producing adenosine, sodium acid phosphate, and calcium acid pyrophosphate. The final step involves hydrolysis to form hydroxyapatite. Orthophosphoric acid is also formed, undergoing in turn a reaction with adenosine to regenerate ATP.

A further suggestion is that the specific nucleation site resides in the monosaccharide or disaccharide attached to the hydroxylysine residue of collagen. To carry this a step further, the glycosylation of the hydroxylysine residues may inhibit mineralization through a mechanism of steric hindrance in the hole zones of the polymerized collagen molecule. It is possible that the hole region within the collagen fibril is the nucleation site and that unglycosylated hydroxylysine could be the specific factor in the nucleation process. However, it has been demonstrated that bone treated with β-aminopropionitrile and made lathyritic (which inhibits the cross-linking mechanism) will still calcify. This observation tends to confuse the issue unless we consider the presence of the hydroxyl group of hydroxylysine in the hole region of the collagen fibril to be an important factor.

Current theory, which the author tends to favor, involves the mitochondria and matrix vesicles as key components in the calcification mechanism. This is particularly true in the epiphyseal plate, and it is likely that fracture healing is just an extension of the physiological mechanisms that occur within the growth plate. Ketenjian and Arsenis were able to separate mitochondria from the hypertrophic zone of the growth plate of the calf scapula and costochondral junction. They observed that calcium phosphate ions may be concentrated and stored inside the mitochondria and through a rate-dependent, membrane-regulated phenomenon become transferred to deposition sites along the collagen fibrils.[54] It is possible that the mitochondrial membranes are degraded by lysosomal enzymes, which then set the granules free to become the seeds for growth of extracellular apatite microcrystallites. Lehninger hypothesized that in calcifying tissues, intramitrochondrial deposits of amorphous calcium phosphate were released from the mitochondria and transported as small stable aggregates to other sites, where they served as precursors for the larger and more stable mineral deposits characteristic of calcified tissues.[61] He believed that in this manner the mitochondria played a vital role in the calcification mechanism.

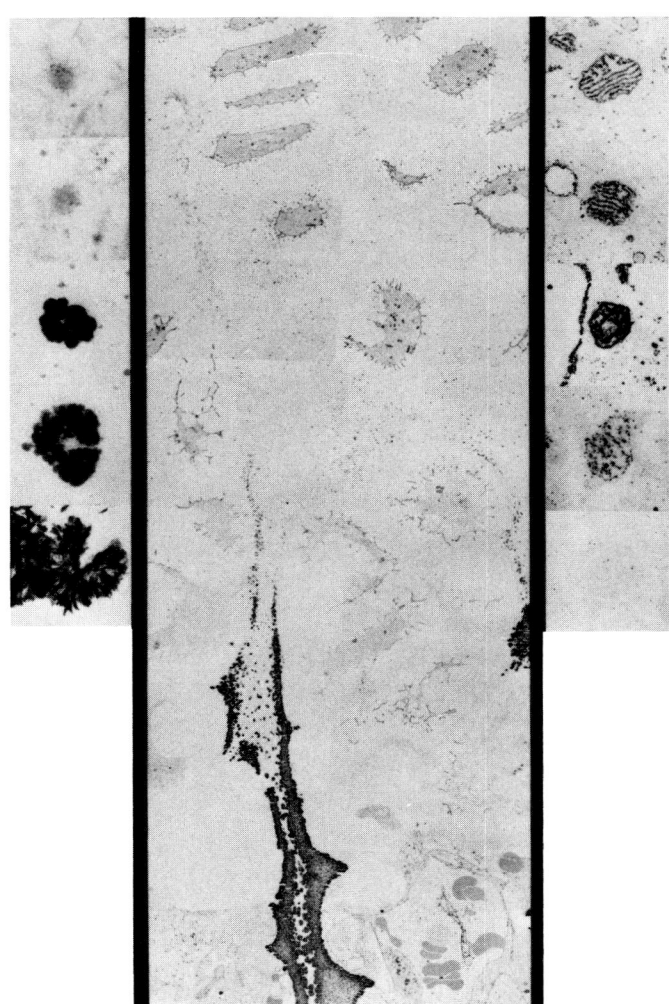

Figure 2–21 Composite electron micrograph of hypertrophic zone of epiphyseal plate. Central portion demonstrates relationship of cartilage cells to calcified matrix. Right hand portion depicts mitochondria calcium at the top of the zone of hypertrophic cells and loss of calcium at bottom of the zone. Left hand portion depicts matrix vesicles taking up calcium as they approach the lower portion of the zone. (Courtesy C. T. Brighton and R. M. Hunt and *Journal of Bone and Joint Surgery.* 1978.)

Brighton and Hunt demonstrated that mitochondria and cell membranes accumulate calcium in the growth plate and concluded that both of these structures may well be involved in the calcification of the growth plate.[19] They noted that the mitochondria and the cell membranes accumulated calcium in the upper zones of the epiphyseal plate, however, at the bottom of the zone of hypertrophic cells the mitochondria tended to lose their calcium as the matrix vesicles began to accumulate calcium (Figs 2–21 and 2–22). It has previously been shown that glycogen storage occurs in the zone of cell columns where the oxygen tension is high and aerobic metabolism occurs. However, the glycogen is utilized in the zone of hypertrophic cells where the oxygen tension is known to be low.[16] Lehninger has demonstrated that the uptake and retention of calcium by mitochondria is an active process requiring energy.[61] Studies by Azzi and Chance have revealed that mitochondria release their calcium when exposed to an anoxic environment.[4] Therefore, it is entirely probable that all of these mechanisms may be involved in the calcification process.

The sequence of events would be as follows. At the upper portion of the growth plate, glycogen is accumulated and aerobic metabolism occurs. As the midportion of the growth plate are approached, mitochondria can be seen to accumulate calcium, as

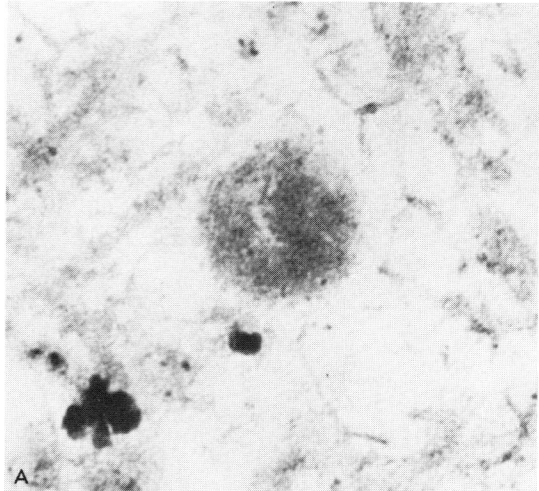

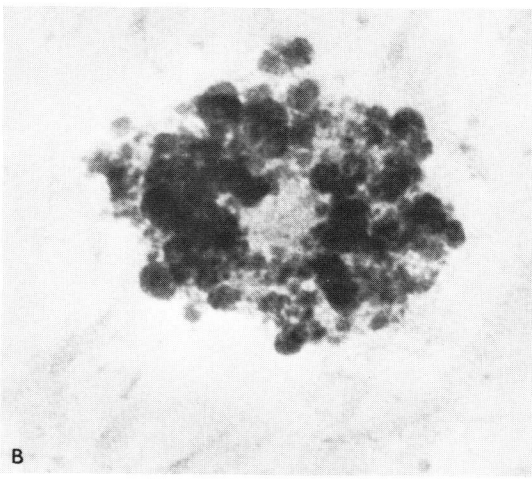

Figure 2–22 A. Electron micrograph of matrix vesicle from top portion of hypertrophic zone. Calcium
stain fails to reveal calcium within the vesicle. B.
Matrix vesicle staining from lower portion of the
hypertrophic zone reveals calcium in the vesicles.

demonstrated by Brighton and Hunt.[19] As
the lower portion of the epiphyseal plate is
approached, particularly the lower half of
the zone of hypertrophic cells, the oxygen
tension is low (as measured previously by
the author), and the glycogen is consumed
as a source of energy. Since there is no other
energy source available for the uptake and
retention of calcium in this region of low
oxygen tensions, the mitochondria lose
their calcium to the extracellular environment. At this level and in the lower portion
of the zone of hypertrophic cells, calcium

begins to appear in the matrix vesicles. It is
true that these studies have been performed
in the growth plate, but if we extrapolate
these theories to fracture healing, the same
physiological mechanism may operate.

The author has demonstrated that the
oxygen tension and the oxygen consumption are low during active new bone formation at the site of an osseous defect.[47]
Ketenjian and Arsensis have shown that all
the components of growth plate cartilage
are found in the callus of a healing fracture.[54] They also demonstrated extracellular
vesicles in the hypertrophic sections of the
fracture callus. Mitochondria tend to accumulate calcium-containing granules in the
callus. A shift of oxidative glycolysis with
cartilage maturation was seen in the callus,
as in the growth plate. Lane has demonstrated a persistence of type 2 cartilage well
into the beginning of the calcification
process.[58] Therefore, it is entirely possible
the same mechanism exists at a fracture site
as in the growth plate to initiate calcification. At the present time, this appears to be
a very attractive hypothesis. However,
there are still several unanswered questions, and a great deal of further investigation into the mechanism of bone formation
is required.

HORMONES IN BONE METABOLISM

Parathyroid Hormone

The parathyroid glands play a primary
role in calcium metabolism. Parathormone
has a direct effect on bone, and its release
increases the serum calcium. It also has a
direct effect on osteoclasts which are normally present in bone. The action of parathormone is believed to take place within
the cell. Osteoclasts contain large quantities
of acid phosphatase and citrate, and it is
possible that a stimulation of both these
substances may be responsible for the
mobilization of calcium from bone. Urinary
hydroxyproline is formed from insoluble
bone collagen and is an indication of
collagen catabolism. Parathormone causes
an increase in hydroxyproline excretion,
which is directly related to the amount of
parathormone released.

The hormone has a stimulatory effect both

on the number and action of the osteoclasts and on osteocytic osteolysis. Bone resorption occurs not only through a mechanism of osteoclast stimulation but also through osteocyte function within the haversian system. Therefore, it may be seen that parathyroid hormone has a direct effect on calcium metabolism. In general it has nine basic functions:

1. It increases plasma calcium concentration and decreases plasma PO_4 concentration.

2. It increases urinary excretion of PO_4 and hydroxyproline-containing peptides and decreases urinary excretion of calcium.

3. It increases the rate of skeletal remodeling and the net rate of bone resorption.

4. It increases the extent of osteocytic osteolysis in bone and increases the number of osteoclasts and osteoblasts.

5. It increases the conversion of 25-hydroxycholicalciferol to 1, 25-dihydroxycholicalciferol in the kidney.

6. It activates adenylcyclase in target cells.

7. It causes an initial increase in calcium entry in target cells.

8. It alters the acid-base balance of the body.

9. It increases gastrointestinal absorption of calcium.

Calcitonin

Copp originally discovered calcitonin and thought it was derived from the thyroid gland.[22] Therefore, it was originally called thyrocalcitonin. It became apparent that calcitonin originates from the C cells of the thyroid, derived embryonically from ultimobranchial origins. This hormone has a direct regulatory function in calcium metabolism. It is believed to act in concert with parathormone to maintain calcium balance.

Its primary function is to decrease the calcium and phosphate plasma concentrations. The effects of calcitonin in bone include the following.: (1) It decreases resorptive activity of osteoclasts and osteocytes; (2) it decreases the rate of activation of osteoprogenitor cells to preosteoclasts and osteoclasts; and (3) it increases modulation of osteoclasts to osteoblasts. When

calcitonin is given prior to parathormone, it initially blocks the effect of parathormone on hydroxyproline excretion, osteocytic osteolysis, and activation of new metabolic units, with the result that eventually parathormone escapes. It does not act at a cellular level as an antiparathormone.

Calcitonin increases the production of both cancellous and compact bone. Although there is still a great deal to learn about the exact mechanism of calcitonin action, we are all indebted to Copp's initial investigative work in isolating and identifying this substance.

Growth Hormone

Recent research has revealed that growth hormone circulates through the liver and acquires a sulfation factor; this metabolite is the growth-stimulating factor and not growth hormone per se. Growth hormone has been demonstrated to increase collagen synthesis in bone and also to increase the ability of tissue to mineralize, as measured by calcium accretion rates. Autoradiographic studies have failed to demonstrate a target cell for growth hormone, and this tends to support the theory that growth hormone operates through its intermediary, known as somatomedin. Animal studies have revealed a decrease in the healing time of fractures with administration of growth hormone. It also may be that its effect on the fracture healing process is due to its direct influence on protein metabolism. Somatomedin increases periosteal bone formation and endosteal bone resorption. It also increases calcium and phosphate absorption in the intestine and renal tubular reabsorption.

Insulin

Insulin appears to increase bone collagen synthesis and may increase excretion of urinary hydroxyproline. The effects of insulin seem to be mediated by protein synthesis. It has been demonstrated that isolated bone cell preparations will increase RNA synthesis after exposure to insulin. A generalized systemic osteoporosis has been noted both in diabetic humans and in alloxan diabetic rats. In humans, the osseous structures of diabetics have reduced numbers of osteoid seams, slower rates of normal osteons, closure, and slower development of resorptive centers. It is also possible that the effect of insulin on bone is related to its effect on carbohydrate metabolism.

Thyroxine

Hypothyroidism leads to a state of generalized growth retardation, and the administration of thyroid hormones produces an acceleration of skeletal and somatic growth. Thyroid hormone itself may have a permissive effect on growth hormone. This is suggested by the fact that growth hormone by itself cannot reverse the linear growth deficit in hypophysectomized–thyroidectomized rats. However, if thyroxin and growth hormone are administered together to hypophysectomized animals, normal linear bone growth will be restored.

Increased bone resorption in humans has been noted in a state of thyrotoxicosis. Another interesting finding is a decrease in the radiodensity in the skeletons of hyperthyroid children. Both triiodothyronine(T_3) and thyroxine(T_4) will increase the differentiation and resorption of cartilage, leading to new bone formation within a fracture callus.

ACTH and Cortical Steroids

It has been demonstrated that low doses of cortisol (0.5 to 2.5 mg per kg) produce direct inhibition of the modulation of osteoclast to osteoblast. If they are administered in higher doses (greater than 5 mg per kg), the rate of osteoprogenitor cell activation falls, so that in spite of secondary increase in parathormone there is a decreased formation of new osteoclasts. The skeleton remodeling rate declines, but net resorption persists. At all doses of administration there is a direct inhibition of osteoblasts.

Soft tissue studies have also shown that administration of steroids will decrease wound healing and may increase susceptibility to infection. This is also true of fracture healing. The net effect is to produce a state of protein catabolism, which definitely retards healing. Steroids have been demonstrated to impair the mobilization

rate of osteogenic precursor cells during fracture healing. It has also been noted that very large doses of cortisone are required to inhibit the initial process of callus formation.

VITAMINS AND BONE METABOLISM

Vitamin A

This vitamin has a direct effect on cartilage cells of the growth plate. Decreased growth may result if it is deficient in the diet, although this is rarely seen today. Severe vitamin A deficiency will produce an apparent overgrowth or thickening of bone. Severe hypervitaminosis A will result in the thinning of cortical bone secondary to the direct effect of lysis. It has been suggested that low doses of vitamin A decrease the fracture healing time and increase cellular proliferation and matrix formation. However, the precise action of vitamin A on bone is poorly documented.

Vitamin C

The role of vitamin C in hydroxylation of proline and lysine has been discussed in Chapter 1. Suffice it to say that collagen formation is dependent upon vitamin C, which is necessary for the hydroxylation of proline. If vitamin C is not plentiful, bone and cartilage matrix will be deficient. Therefore, fracture healing requires the presence of vitamin C for normal collagen formation. If it is not present, normal matrix synthesis will not occur. Vitamin C deficiency is not seen today, and therefore vitamin C supplementation is not necessary to stimulate fracture healing.

Vitamin D

In vitamin D deficiency there is a failure of normal mineralization, a decreased osteoclast count, and diminished bone resorption for the parathormone level. Administration of vitamin D reestablishes the normal calcification front on osteoid surfaces, possibly accounting for the initial decrease in calcium, which requires the presence of parathormone. There is then an increase in the osteoclast count. Vitamin D deficiency also affects the epiphyseal plate. Mitochondrial concentration of calcium is reduced, with fewer matrix calcification vesicles, decreased calcification of cartilaginous matrix, and an absence of chondroclasts to remove calcified cartilage. All of these effects are reversed with vitamin D administration.

The mode of action of vitamin D on bone is as follows: Vitamin D deficiency will cause a decreased rate of entry of calcium into the cells or mitochondria, resulting in a diminished mitochondrial calcium pool and the extracellular calcium pool. It is now known that the active agent of vitamin D is D_3 or cholecalciferol, which was originally thought to be a vitamin but is now considered a hormone. D_3 is converted to 25-hydroxycholecalciferol in the liver and to 1, 25-dihydroxycholecalciferol in the kidney. An increase in parathormone level will stimulate the conversion of 25-hydroxycholecalciferol to 1, 25-dihydroxycholecalciferol. This hormone accelerates the active transcellular transport of calcium and increases the growth and maturation of intestinal mucosal cells.

Vitamin D has been demonstrated to increase citrate production in bone cells by stimulating the conversion of pyruvate first to oxaloacetate and then to citrate in the Krebs cycle. Citrate promotes mobilization of calcium ion from bone by chelating calcium and removing ionized calcium. Many investigators believe that this action of vitamin D plays an important role in the remodeling phase of fracture healing.

It is readily apparent that a great deal is still to be learned in regard to fracture healing in general and to new procedures that may stimulate repair, so that morbidity and recuperation time may be decreased.

REFERENCES

1. Aho, A. J.: Electronmicroscopic and histologic observation on fracture repair in young and old rats. Acta Pathol. Micro-biol. Scand. (Suppl.), *184*:1, 1966.
2. Anderson, H. C.: Matrix vesicles of cartilage and bone. *In* Bourne, G. (ed.): The Biochemistry and Physiology of Bone—Calcification and Physiology. Vol. IV., New York, Academic Press, 1976, pp. 135–157.
3. Ali, S. Y., Sajdera, S. W., and Anderson, H. C.: Isolation and characterization of calcifying matrix vesicles from epiphyseal cartilage. Proc. Natl. Acad. Sci. U.S.A., 67:1513–1520, 1970.
4. Azzi, A., and Chance, B.: The "energized state" of mitochondria; lifetime and ATP equivalence. Biochim. Biophys. Acta, *189*:141–151, 1969.
5. Balogh, K., Jr., and Hajek, J. V.: Oxidative enzymes of intermediary metabolism in healing bone fractures. Am. J. Anat., *116*:429–448, 1965.
6. Bassett, C. A. L., Creighton, D. K., and Stinchfield, F. E.: Contributions of endosteum, cortex and soft tissues to osteogenesis. Surg. Gynecol. Obstet., *112*:145–152, 1961.
7. Bassett, C. A. L., and Herrmann, I.: Influence of oxygen concentration and mechanical factors on differentiation of connective tissue in vitro. Nature, *190*:460–461, 1961.
8. Bassett, C. A. L.: Current concepts in bone formation. J. Bone Joint Surg., *44A*:1217–1244, 1962.
9. Bélanger, L. F.: *In* Bourne, G. (ed.): Biochemistry and Physiology of Bone. Vol. III, 2nd Ed., p. 239–270. New York, Academic Press, 1971.
10. Betts, F., Blumenthal, N. C., Posner, A. S., Becker, G. L., and Lehninger, A. L.: Atomic structure of intracellular amorphous calcium phosphate deposits. Proc. Natl. Acad. Sci. U.S.A., *72*:2088–2090, 1975.
11. Blitz, R. M., and Pellegrino, E. D.: The nature of bone carbonate. Clin. Orthop., *129*:279–292, 1977.
12. Bohr, H. H.: Studies on fracture healing. J. Bone Joint Surg., *37A*:327–337, 1955.
13. Borle, A. B., Nichols, N., and Nichols, G., Jr.: Metabolic studies of bone in vitro. I. Normal Bone. J. Biol. Chem., *235*:1206–1210, 1960.
14. Bridges, J. B., and Pritchard, J. J.: Bone and cartilage induction in rabbit. J. Anat., *92*:28–38, 1958.
15. Brighton, C. T., Heppenstall, R. B., and Labosky, D. A.: An oxygen microelectrode suitable for cartilage and cancellous bone. Clin. Orthop., *80*:161–166, 1971.
16. Brighton, C. T., and Heppenstall, R. B.: Oxygen tension in zones of the epiphyseal plate, the metaphysis and diaphysis. J. Bone Joint Surg., *53A*:719–728, 1971.
17. Brighton, C. T., and Heppenstall, R. B.: Oxygen tension of the epiphyseal plate distal to an arteriovenous fistula. Clin. Orthop., *80*:167–173, 1971.
18. Brighton, C. T., and Krebs, A. G.: Oxygen tension of healing fractures in the rabbit. J. Bone Joint Surg., *54A*:323–332, 1972.
19. Brighton, C. T., and Hunt, R. M.: Mitochondrial calcium and its role in calcification. Histochemical localization of calcium in electron micrographs of the epiphyseal growth plate with K-pyroantimonate. Clin. Orthop., *100*:406–416, 1974.
20. Cohen, J., Maletskos, C. J., Marshall, J. H., and Williams, J. B.: Radioactive calcium tracer studies on bone grafts. J. Bone Joint Surg., *39A*:561–577, 1957.
21. Copp, D. H., and Greenberg, D. M.: Studies on bone fracture healing. 1. Effects of vitamins A and D. J. Nutr., *29*:261–267, 1945.
22. Copp, D. H.: Parathyroid Hormone, Calcitonin and Calcium Homeostasis. Summary. *In* Tal-

mage, R. V., and Bélanger, L. F. (eds.): Para-thyroid Hormone and Thyrocalcitonin (Calci-tonin). New York, Excerpta Medica Founda-tion, 1968.

23. Cuervo, L. A., Pita, J. C., and Howell, D. S.: Ultramicroanalysis of pH, pCO_2 and carbonic anhydrase activity at calcifying sites in car-tilage. Calcif. Tissue Res., 7:220–231, 1971.

24. Deutsch, A., and Gudmundson, C.: Nucleic acids in regenerating rabbit bone. Clin. Orthop., 69:239–244, 1970.

25. Dingle, J. T.: The role of lysosomal enzymes in skeletal tissues. J. Bone Joint Surg., 55B:87–95, 1973.

26. Dixon, T. F., and Perkins, H. R.: Citric acid and bone metabolism. Biochem. J., 52:260–265, 1952.

27. Duthie, R. B., and Barker, A. N.: The histoche-mistry of the preosseous stage of bone repair studied by autoradiography. The effect of corti-sone. J. Bone Joint Surg., 37B:691–710, 1955.

28. Edwards, C. C.: The effect of hyperbaric oxygen and DCAF fluorescein on the rate of bone for-mation in rabbits. Transactions of The Orth-opaedic Research Society Meeting. New Or-leans, 1976, p. 18.

29. Ehrlich, H. P., Grislis, G., and Hunt, T. K.: Metabolic and circulatory contributions to oxy-gen gradients in wounds. Surgery, 72:578–583, 1972.

30. Engstrom, A., and Zetterstrom, R.: Studies on ultrastructure of bone. Exp. Cell Res., 2:268–274, 1951.

31. Engfeldt, B.: Recent observations on bone struc-ture. J. Bone Joint Surg., 40A:698–706, 1958.

32. Enneking, W. F.: The repair of complete fractures of rat tibias. Anat. Rec., 101:515, 1948.

33. Flanagan, B., and Nichols, G., Jr.: Metabolic studies of human bone in vitro. 1. Normal bone. J. Clin. Invest., 44:1788–1794, 1965.

34. Fleish, H., and Newman, W. F.: Mechanism of calcification; role of collagen, polyphosphates, and phosphatase. Am. J. Physiol., 200:1296–1300, 1961.

35. Fleisch, H.: Mechanism of calcification: Inhibi-tory role of pyrophosphate. Nature, 195:911, 1962.

36. Glimcher, M. J.: Molecular biology of mineral-ized tissues with particular reference to bone. Rev. Mod. Physics, 31:359–393, 1959.

37. Glimcher, M. J.: Specificity of molecular structure of organic matrices in mineralization. In Sogn-naes, R. F. (ed.): Calcification in Biological Systems, pp. 421–487. Washington, D.C., The American Association for the Advancement of Science, 1960.

38. Goldhaber, P.: Effect of hyperoxia on bone resorption in tissue culture. Arch. Pathol., 66:635–641, 1958.

39. Goldhaber, P. Some factors affecting bone re-sorption in tissue culture. J. Bone Joint Surg., 43B:180, 1961.

40. Goldhaber, P.: Some current concepts of bone physiology. N. Engl. J. Med., 266:870–877, 924–931, 1962.

41. Ham, A. W.: A histological study of the early phases of bone repair. J. Bone Joint Surg., 12:827, 1930.

42. Ham, A. W.: Some histophysiological problems peculiar to calcified tissues. J. Bone Joint Surg., 34A:701–728, 1952.

43. Ham, A. W., and Harris, W. R.: Repair and transplantation of bone. In Bourne, G. (ed.): Biochemistry and Physiology of Bone. Vol. III, 2nd Ed., pp. 337–397. New York, Academic Press, 1972.

44. Harris, W. H., Heaney, R. P., Towsey, J., et al.: Growth hormone: The effect on skeletal re-newal in the adult dog. I. Morphometric studies. Calcif. Tissue Res., 10:1–13, 1972.

45. Heaney, R. P., Harris, W. H., Cockin, J., and Weinberg, E. H.: Growth hormone: the effect of skeletal renewal in the adult dog. II. Mineral kinetic studies. Calcif. Tissue Res., 10:14–22, 1972.

46. Heppenstall, R. B., Littody, F. N., Fuchs, R., Sheldon, G. F., and Hunt, T. K.: Gas tensions in healing tissues of traumatized patients. Sur-gery, 75:874–880, 1974.

47. Heppenstall, R. B., Grislis, G., and Hunt, T. K.: Tissue gas tensions and oxygen consumption in healing bone defects. Clin. Orthop., 106:357–365, 1975.

48. Heppenstall, R. B., Goodwin, C. W., and Brighton, C. T.: Fracture healing in the pres-ence of chronic hypoxia. J. Bone Joint Surg., 58A:1153–1156, 1976.

49. Heppenstall, R. B., and Brighton, C. T.: Fracture healing in the presence of anemia. Clin. Orthop., 123:253–258, 1977.

50. Holden, C. E. A.: The role of blood supply to soft tissue in the healing of diaphyseal fractures. An experimental study. J. Bone Joint Surg., 54A:993–1000, 1972.

51. Katz, E. P., and Li, S. T.: Structure and function of bone collagen fibrils. J. Mol. Biol., 80:1–15, 1973.

52. Keck, S. W., and Kelly, P. J.: The effect of venous stasis on intraosseous pressure and longitudinal bone growth in the dog. J. Bone Joint Surg., 47A:539–544, 1965.

53. Kelly, P. J.: Anatomy, physiology and pathology of the blood supply of bones. J. Bone Joint Surg., 50A:766–783, 1968.

54. Ketenjian, A. Y., and Arsenis, C.: Morphological and biochemical studies during differentiation and calcification of fracture callus cartilage. Clin. Orthop., 107:266–273, 1975.

55. Koskinen, E. V. S.: The influence of hormonal treatment and orchiectomy, oophorectomy and thyroidectomy on experimental fractures. Acta Orthop. Scand. (Suppl.), 80:1–40, 1965.

56. Kruse, R. L., and Kelly, P. J.: Acceleration of fracture healing distal to a venous tourniquet. J. Bone Joint Surg., 56A:730–739, 1974.

57. Kuhlman, R. E., and Bakowski, M. J.: The biochemical activity of fracture callus in rela-tion to bone production. Clin. Orthop., 107:258–265, 1975.

58. Lane, J., Murphy, L., Irwin, J., and Beller, P.: Collagen and proteoglycan structure and me-tabolism during fracture repair. Transactions of

the Orthopaedic Research Society meeting. Las Vegas, 1977, p. 94.

59. Laurnen, E. L. and Kelly, P. J.: Blood flow, oxygen consumption, carbon dioxide production and blood-calcium and pH changes in tibial fractures in dogs. J. Bone Joint Surg., *51A*:298–308, 1969.

60. LeBlond, C. P., Bélanger, L. F., and Greulich, R. C.: Formation of bones and teeth as visualized by radioautography. Ann. N. Y. Acad. Sci., *60*:631–659, 1955.

61. Lehninger, A. L.: Mitochondria and calcium ion transport. Biochem. J., *119*:129–138, 1970.

62. MacDonald, N. S., Lorick, P. C., and Petriello, L. I.: Healing of bone fractures and simultaneous administration of radioisotopes of sulfur, calcium, and yttrium. Am. J. Physiol., *191*:185–188, 1957.

63. Makley, J. T., Heiple, K. G., Chase, S. W., and Herndon, C. H.: The effect of reduced barometric pressure on fracture healing in rats. J. Bone Joint Surg., *49A*:903–914, 1967.

64. Manabe, S., Shima, I., and Yamauchi, S.: Cytokinetic analysis of osteogenic cells in the healing process after fracture. Acta Orthop. Scand., *46*:161–176, 1975.

65. McLean, F. C., and Urist, M. R.: Bone: An Introduction to the Physiology of Skeletal Tissue. Chicago, University of Chicago Press, 1961.

66. Mela, L., Goodwin, C. W., and Miller, L. D.: In vivo control of mitochondrial enzyme concentrations and activity by oxygen. Am. J. Physiol., *231*:1811–1816, 1976.

67. Mindell, E. R., Rodbard, S., and Kwasman, B. G.: Chondrogenesis in bone repair. Clin. Orthop., *79*:187–196, 1971.

68. Paradis, G. R., and Kelly, P. J.: Blood flow and mineral deposition in canine tibial fractures. J. Bone Joint Surg., *57A*:220–226, 1975.

69. Pearse, H. E., Jr., and Morton, J. J.: The stimulation of bone growth by venous stasis. J. Bone Joint Surg., *12*:97–111, 1930.

70. Perren, S. M., Huggler, A., Russenberger, M., et al.: The reaction of cortical bone to compression. Acta Orthop. Scand. (Suppl. 125), (1969*b*).

71. Penttinen, R.: Biochemical studies on fracture healing in the rat. Acta Chir. Scand. (Suppl.), *432*:7–28, 1972.

72. Pritchard, J. J.: A cytological and histochemical study of bone and cartilage formation in the rat. J. Anat., *86*:259–277, 1952.

73. Prockop, D., Kaplan, A., and Udenfriend, S.: Oxygen-18 studies on the conversion of proline to collagen hydroxyproline. Arch. Biochem. Biophys., *101*:499–503, 1963.

74. Rhinelander, F. W.: Some aspects of the microcirculation of healing bone. Clin. Orthop., *40*:12–16, 1965.

75. Rhinelander, F. W.: The normal microcirculation of diaphyseal cortex and its response to fracture. J. Bone Joint Surg., *50A*:784–800, 1968.

76. Rhinelander, F. W., Phillips, R. S., Steel, W. M., and Beer, J. C.: Microangiography in bone healing. II. Displaced closed fractures. J. Bone Joint Surg., *50A*:643–662, 1968.

77. Rhinelander, F. W., Circulation in bone. *In* Bourne, G. (ed.): The Biochemistry and Physiology of Bone. Vol. II, 2nd Ed. pp. 2–76. New York, Academic Press, 1972.

78. Rhinelander, F. W.: Effects of medullary nailing on the normal blood supply of diaphyseal cortex. AAOS Instructional Course Lectures, pp. 161–187. St. Louis, C. V. Mosby, 1973.

79. Rhinelander, F. W.: Tibial blood supply in relation to fracture healing. Clin. Orthop., *105*:81, 1974.

80. Robinson, R. A., and Watson, M. S.: Crystal–collagen relationships in bone as observed in electron microscope. III. Crystal–collagen morphology as function of age. Ann. N. Y. Acad. Sci., *60*:596–628, 1955.

81. Robinson, R. A.: Crystal–collagen–water relationships in bone matrix. Clin. Orthop., *18*:69–76, 1960.

82. Robison, R.: Possible significance of hexosephosphoric esters in ossification. Biochem. J., *17*:286–293, 1923.

83. Rothman, R. H., Klemek, J. S., and Toton, J. J.: The effect of iron deficiency anemia on fracture healing. Clin. Orthop., *77*:276–283, 1971.

84. Russel, R. G. G., and Fleisch, H.: Pyrophosphate and diphosphonates in skeletal metabolism. Clin. Orthop., *108*:241–263, 1975.

85. Sheldon, H., and Robinson, R. A.: Electron microscope studies of collagen–crystal relationships in bone. IV. Occurrence of crystals within collagen fibrils. J. Biophys. Biochem. Cytol., *3*:1011–1015, 1957.

86. Shim, S. S.: Physiology of blood circulation of bone. J. Bone Joint Surg., *50A*:812–824, 1968.

87. Sissons, H. A., and Hadfield, G. J.: The influence of cortisone on the repair of experimental fractures in the rabbit. Br. J. Surg., *39*:172–178, 1951.

88. Sognnaes, R. F.: Microstructure and histochemical characteristics of mineralized tissues. Ann. N. Y. Acad. Sci., *60*:545–574, 1955.

89. Stern, B., Glimcher, M. J., and Goldhaber, P.: The effect of various oxygen tensions on the synthesis and degradation of bone collagen in tissue culture. Proc. Soc. Exp. Biol. Med., *121*:869–872, 1966.

90. Stinchfield, F. R., Sandaran, B., and Samilson, R.: Effect of anticoagulant therapy on bone repair. J. Bone Joint Surg., *38A*:270–282, 1956.

91. Thompson, R. C., Jr.: Heparin osteoporosis. An experimental model using rats. J. Bone Joint Surg., *55A*:606–612, 1973.

92. Tonna, E. A., and Cronkite, E. P.: Cellular response to fracture studied with tritiated thymidine. J. Bone Joint Surg., *43A*:352–362, 1961.

93. Tonna, E. A.: Fracture callus formation in young and old mice observed with polarized light microscopy. Anat. Rec., *150*:349–362, 1964.

94. Tonna, E. A., and Pentel, L.: Chondrogenic cell formation via osteogenic cell progeny transformation. Lab. Invest., *27*:418–426, 1972.

95. Toole, B. P., and Linsenmager, T. F.: Newer knowledge of skeletogenesis: macromolecular transitions in the extracellular matrix. Clin. Orthop., *129*:258–278, 1977.

96. Trueta, J., and Amato, V. P.: Vascular contribution to osteogenesis. III. Changes in growth and cartilage caused by experimentally induced ischemia. J. Bone Joint Surg., *42B*:571–587, 1960.

97. Trueta, J., and Caladias, A. X.: A study of the blood supply of the long bones. Surg. Gynecol. Obstet., *118*:485–498, 1964.

98. Udupa, K. N., and Prasad, G. C.: Chemical and histochemical studies on the organic constituents in fracture repair in rats. J. Bone Joint Surg., *45B*:770–779, 1963.

99. Urist, M. R., and McLean, F. C.: Calcification in the callus of healing fractures in normal rats. J. Bone Joint Surg., *23*:1–15, 1941.

100. Urist, M. R., Wallace, T. H., and Adams, T.: The function of fibrocartilaginous fracture callus. Observations on transplants labelled with tritiated thymidine. J. Bone Joint Surg., *47B*:304–318, 1965.

101. Urist, M. R.: Biochemistry of calcification. *In*, Bourne, G. (ed.): The Biochemistry and Physiology of Bone. Vol. IV, p. 2–59. New York, Academic Press, 1976.

102. Vaes, G. M., and Nichol, G., Jr.: Oxygen tension and the control of bone cell metabolism. Nature, *193*:379–380, 1962.

103. Vanderhoeft, P. J., Kelly, P. J., Janes, J. M., and Peterson, L. F. A.: Growth and structure of bone distal to an arteriovenous fistula: quantitative analysis of tetracycline-induced transverse growth patterns. J. Bone Joint Surg., *45B*:582–596, 1963.

104. Walker, D. G.: Enzymatic and electron microscopic analysis of isolated osteoclasts. Calcif. Tissue Res., 9:296–309, 1972.

105. Whiteside, L., and Lesker, P. A.: The effects of extraperiosteal and subperiosteal dissection. II. On fracture healing. J. Bone Joint Surg., *60A*: 26–30, 1978.

106. Wray, J. B.: Vascular regeneration in the healing fracture. Angiology, *14*:134–138, 1963.

107. Wray, J. B., and Goodman, H. O.: Post fracture vascular changes and healing process. Arch. Surg., 87:801–804, 1963.

108. Wray, J. B.: The biochemical characteristics of the fracture hematoma in man. Surg. Gynecol. Obstet., *130*:847, 1970.

109. Wuthier, R. E.: A zonal analysis of inorganic and organic constituents of the epiphysis during encochondral calcification. Calcif. Tissue Res., *4*:20, 1969.

CARL T. BRIGHTON, M.D., Ph.D.

Biophysics _____ 3
of
Fracture
Healing

INTRODUCTION

Bone is a peculiar substance, exhibiting certain phenomena that until recently have not been explained by the conventional biological disciplines. Disuse osteoporosis is one such phenomenon: A fully ambulatory healthy adult male, for instance, exhibits tibial cortices that are quite thick as measured in the midshaft region. If this individual is put at bed rest for any reason, as shown in Figure 3–1 in which the lower extremity is in balanced suspension, a very rapid disuse osteoporosis sets in, and the tibial cortices thin measurably. With restitution of weight bearing, the bone very quickly builds back to restore the normal, relatively thick midshaft tibial cortex.

The disuse osteoporosis phenomenon and the rapid return of bone to its original thickness once weight bearing has been resumed are examples of Wolff's law,[50] in which bony structures orient themselves to best resist extrinsic forces (or more simply, form follows function). Wolff's law has been cited as an explanation for disuse osteoporosis for almost 100 years, and yet until recently there was no explanation for its mechanism.

Another example of Wolff's law is seen in the straightening of a malunion of a long bone in a child (Fig. 3–2). With time, growth, and weight bearing, a malunion of up to 25 to 30 degrees of angulation will straighten completely, at least in the infant and young child. This straightening phenomenon of a weight-bearing long bone actually is contrary to the laws of biomechanics, for with repeated weight bearing an angulated structure should in time bend further until fatigue occurs.

But of course the exact opposite happens, and the bone straightens with growth. What is the explanation for this straightening phenomenon? If one considers for a minute, some biological or physical signal must arise from the concave side of the malunion, telling the osteoblasts there to lay down bone, and a corresponding signal must arise from the convex side of the malunion, telling the osteoclasts there to remove bone (Fig. 3–2). What is the nature of this signal? Such a signal has not been found in the biological sciences.

ELECTRICAL POTENTIALS OF BONE

Four research teams began looking at this problem, and all reasoned somewhat in the same manner: If the most important function of bone is physical, namely, to bear load, then perhaps the signal that directs bone formation and resorption is a physical one. In the early 1950's Yasuda and Fukada[24, 52] in Japan, in the late 1950's Bassett and Becker[1] in the United States, and in the early 1960's Shamos and Lavine[47] in the

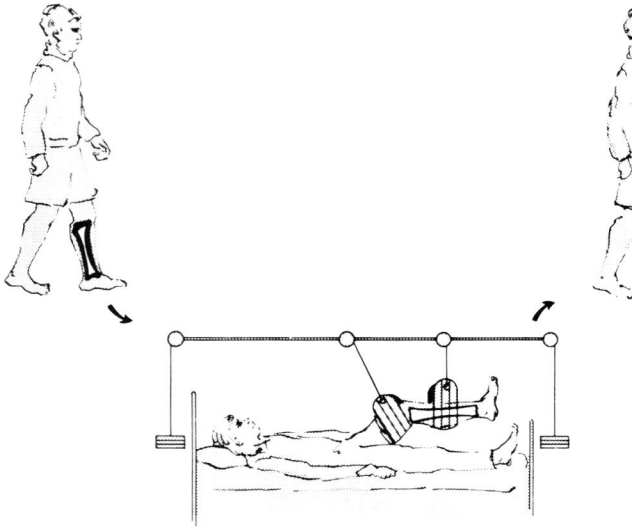

Figure 3-1   The rapid onset of disuse osteoporosis—here highlighted in the tibial cortices—is brought on by non-weight bearing.

United States all began looking for signals in stressed bone. Also in the early 1960's Friedenberg and Brighton[19] began looking for signals in viable nonstressed bone. The signals that were found by these four teams, each working independently and not knowing of the others' existence, were electrical in nature. Two types of electrical signals or potentials were found in bone: (1) stress-generated or strain-related potentials, and (2) bioelectrical or standing potentials.

Stress-Generated Potentials

When bone is stressed one finds that the concave side of the bone, or the area under compression, becomes electronegative, and the convex side of the bone, or the area under tension, becomes electropositive. In a malunion of a long bone in a child (Fig.

3-3), the area of compression where new bone will be formed is electronegative, and the area under tension where bone will be removed is electropositive. These stress-generated potentials arise when the bone is stressed and are not dependent upon cell viability. Areas of compression are electronegative, and areas of tension are electropositive. Research has also shown that the electrical signal arises from the organic component of bone and not from the mineral component. That is to say, even if the bone is completely decalcified these stress-generated signals are obtained.

Bioelectrical Potentials

Bioelectrical potentials are measured from the surface of nonstressed bone (Fig. 3-4). In the intact tibia, the growth plate–

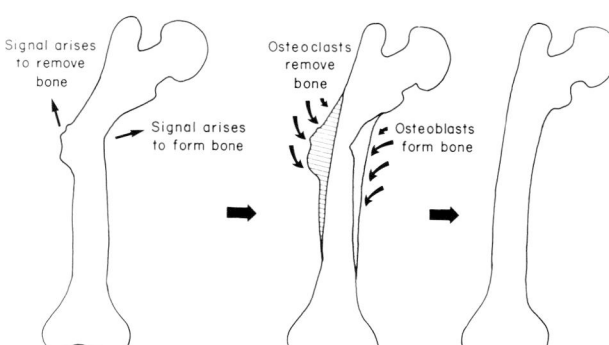

Signal arises to remove bone

Signal arises to form bone

Osteoclasts remove bone

Osteoblasts form bone

Figure 3-2   The straightening phenomenon following malunion in a child's femur. The nature of the signal that directs cell activity was unknown until recently.

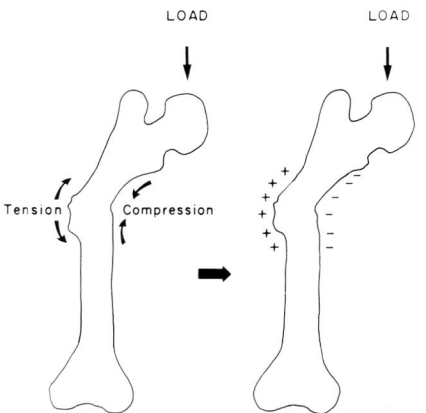

Figure 3–3 Electrical signals arise when bone is stressed. Note that the area under compression is electronegative, and the area under tension is electropositive.

metaphyseal regions are electronegative compared with the diaphyseal or midshaft regions. When a fracture exists in the diaphysis, the entire surface of the tibia becomes electronegative, and a large peak of electronegativity occurs over the fracture site, remaining until the fracture heals. A second peak of electronegativity occurs over the opposite growth plate. This latter finding is fascinating when one considers that a fractured extremity in a child frequently exhibits overgrowth. This overgrowth of course does not take place at the fracture site, but in the growth plate near the end of the bone. The nature of the signal directing

the growth plate to accelerate growth has never been identified. The peak of electronegativity over the growth plate–metaphyseal area that occurs with a midshaft fracture may represent such a signal.

In an attempt to determine the source of the potentials present in nonstressed bone, the following experiments were performed:[21]

1. The vascularity to the lower extremity in the rabbit was interrupted, and yet the electrical potential over the proximal 7 cm of the tibia was not changed. That is to say, the peak of electronegativity of the proximal tibia was not changed significantly 30 minutes after ligation of the vessels.

2. The same was true after the leg in the rabbit was denervated. The peak of electronegativity in the proximal tibia was not changed significantly 30 minutes after denervation of the limb.

3. As soon as a cytotoxic drug (dinitrophenol) was injected into the animal, however, an immediate statistically significant drop in the negative potential occurred. This suggests that the potential, measured from the surface of bone, was indeed due to cell viability.

4. A localized segment of the in situ rabbit tibia was subjected to high-energy ultrasound waves. This resulted in a small segment of bone being killed, with a statistically significant drop in the electrical potential over the nonviable region. In addition, the areas on both sides of the segment that were killed with ultrasound also showed cell injury, and to a lesser

Figure 3–4 The bioelectrical potentials of intact and fractured rabbit tibia.

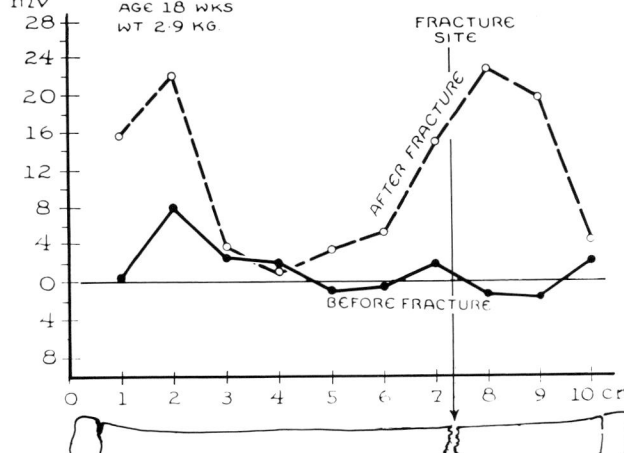

extent cell death. These regions also showed a fall in the potential.

Potentials arising from nonstressed bone are called bioelectrical potentials, meaning that they arise from living bone. Such potentials are not dependent upon stress but upon cell viability. Active areas of growth and repair are electronegative, and less active areas are electrically neutral or electropositive.

ELECTRICITY AND FRACTURE HEALING

Based on the principles that stress potentials are electronegative in areas of compression and that living bone exhibits compression and that living bone exhibits electronegativity over actively growing areas, the next step taken by many laboratories around the world was to implant electricity in bone.[2, 14, 18, 22, 23, 25, 26, 29, 31, 32, 36, 38, 40, 42, 43, 45, 46, 49, 51, 53]

One such model is the intact rabbit femur, in which electrodes are inserted through drill holes into the medullary canal of the bone. The power pack implant has a circuit in it such that as resistance builds up around the electrodes the voltage also increases, and according to Ohm's law the microamperage remains the same. The power packs are programmed to deliver between 5 and 100 microamperes (μA) of constant direct current. The power pack and apparatus are buried under the skin of the rabbit. A constant direct current flowing for 18 days produces abundant new bone formation in the vicinity of the negative electrode or cathode at a current range of 5 to 20 μA. Below 5 μA little or no bone is formed; with greater than 20 μA in the vicinity of the cathode, bone formation gradually gives way to cellular necrosis. Necrosis rather than bone formation occurs around the positive electrode or anode, and the amount of necrosis increases progressively with increasing current magnitudes.

A model in which electricity has been tested for its possible clinical use is that of the healing fractured fibula in the rabbit.[11] The distal fibula in the rabbit is synostotic to the tibia, so that very little motion occurs when a fracture or osteotomy is placed in the upper shaft of the fibula. Electrodes are inserted in various locations in relationship to the fracture site in the fibula. In order to quantitate fracture healing in this model, the fractured fibulae, both control and experimental, are excised at the end of 18 days and are placed in a three-point testing jig. The maximum resistance to bending is obtained for all fractures. Results have demonstrated that in those fractures in which the cathode is inserted directly into the fracture site, the fractured callus on the experimental side is statistically significantly stiffer than the control side. This experiment shows that electricity indeed favorably influences fracture healing.

In the two models just shown, the femoral shaft model in which the electrodes are inserted through drill holes into the medullary canal and the fractured fibula model, bone formation is already occurring whether electricity is present or not. That is to say, in the femoral medullary canal model, bone forms around the drill holes with or without electrical activity, and in the fractured fibula model, the fibulae heal whether electricity is present or not. To be sure, in both instances electricity accelerates bone formation or fracture healing. In both of these models, however, bone healing was already occurring and electricity was simply accelerating bone formation.

OSTEOGENESIS

A third model (Fig. 3–5) answers a much more fundamental biological question: Can electricity induce bone formation in a re-

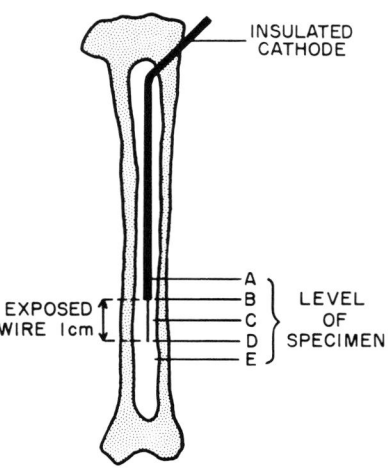

Figure 3–5 An insulated cathode in the medullary canal of the rabbit tibia, with the exposed tip of the cathode located in a nontraumatized area of the bone.

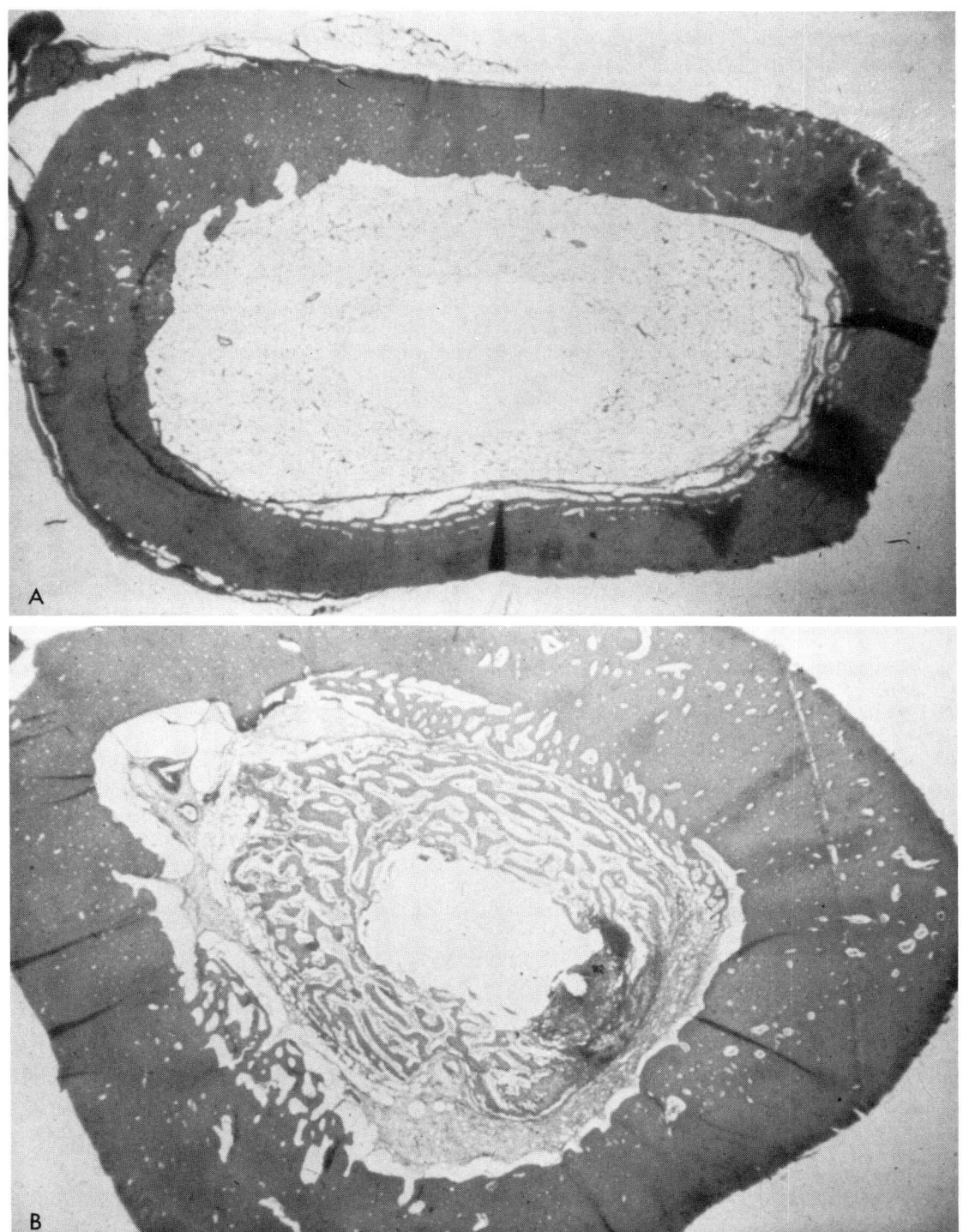

Figure 3–6   *A.* Transverse section of control tibia, showing only normal medullary canal content around the wire (hematoxylin and eosin, × 10). *B.* Transverse section of experimental tibia, showing abundant new bone formation around a 20 microampere cathode (hematoxylin and eosin, × 10).

gion where it is not already occurring? The model is that of the tibia of the rabbit in which an insulated cathode is inserted into a drill hole in the proximal end of the tibia. The cathode is inserted down the medullary canal such that the bare tip of the cathode comes to rest near the distal end of the tibia.[23] Constant direct current of various magnitudes is allowed to flow for 18 days. The bones are then excised, cut transversely at 1/2 cm intervals along the length of the diaphysis, and the amount of new bone present in the medullary canal is determined by point-counting analysis of histological sections. Control sections show little or no bone formation (Fig. 3–6A).

Experimental sections show abundant new bone formation surrounding the cathode in a current range of 5 to 20 μA, with maximum bone formation occurring at 20 μA (Fig. 3–6B). Below 5 μA little or no new bone was formed, and above 20 μA necrosis began to appear in the vicinity of the cathode. Of course, only necrosis occurs in the vicinity of the anode. Thus it is evident that electrical current, given the proper parameters of amperage and voltage, can indeed induce bone formation. Such electrically induced osteogenesis follows a typical dose-response curve: Too little current produces no effect, a given amount of current produces a therapeutic effect, and too much current produces a toxic effect.

To summarize the first two decades of investigation into the electrical properties of bone:

1. Stress-generated potentials arise when the bone is stressed and are not dependent upon cell viability. Areas of compression where bone will form in the in vivo state are electronegative.

2. Live bone exhibits electronegativity over active areas of growth and repair.

3. Exogenous electricity applied to bone, given the proper current and voltage parameters, induces the formation of new bone in the vicinity of the negative electrode or cathode.

Nonunion

Clinical trials based on these principles soon began, utilizing electricity in the treatment of nonunion. The first such trial was initiated in 1970 and utilized constant direct current.[20] The first patient treated with electricity for nonunion, at least in modern times, was a 51-year-old woman with nonunion of the medial malleolus of 14 months' duration (Fig. 3–7A). Under local anesthesia, a 10 μA cathode was inserted across the nonunion site. A constant direct current was allowed to flow for nine weeks, at which time solid bony healing had occurred (Fig. 3–7B).

Encouraged by this initial success, the orthopedic surgery research team at the University of Pennsylvania began a clinical study in 1970 in which stainless steel cathodes were inserted percutaneously under local anesthesia directly into the nonunion site with the aid of roentgenographic localization.[10, 11] A surface anode was applied to the skin, and the power pack was incorporated into a plaster cast. The monitoring leads extended from the cast such that the power pack could be monitored at will (Fig. 3–8). Initially, 10 μA were applied continuously through one cathode for nine weeks in each patient. Later, as experience was gained, the microamperage was increased to 20 for each cathode, the duration of current flow was increased to 12 weeks, and the number of cathodes used in each patient was increased to 4 in the larger bones (see further on).

The patient population of this study is shown in Table 3–1. The average duration of nonunion was 3.0 years. By definition, nonunion was considered present in those fractures in which no progressive signs of healing were demonstrated on roentgenograms over at least a three-month period. Only 22 per cent of the patients had a

TABLE 3–1   Treatment of Nonunion by
Constant Direct Current

Patient Population		
Males:	44	} 72 Patients
Females:	28	
Average patient age	37.7 Years	
Average duration of nonunion	3.0 Years	
Number of closed fractures	44	(61%)
Number of open fractures	28	(39%)
Number with prior infection	16	(22%)
Number with previous surgery	50	(69%)
Average number of prior surgical procedures	2.2	
Number with no previous surgery	22	(31%)

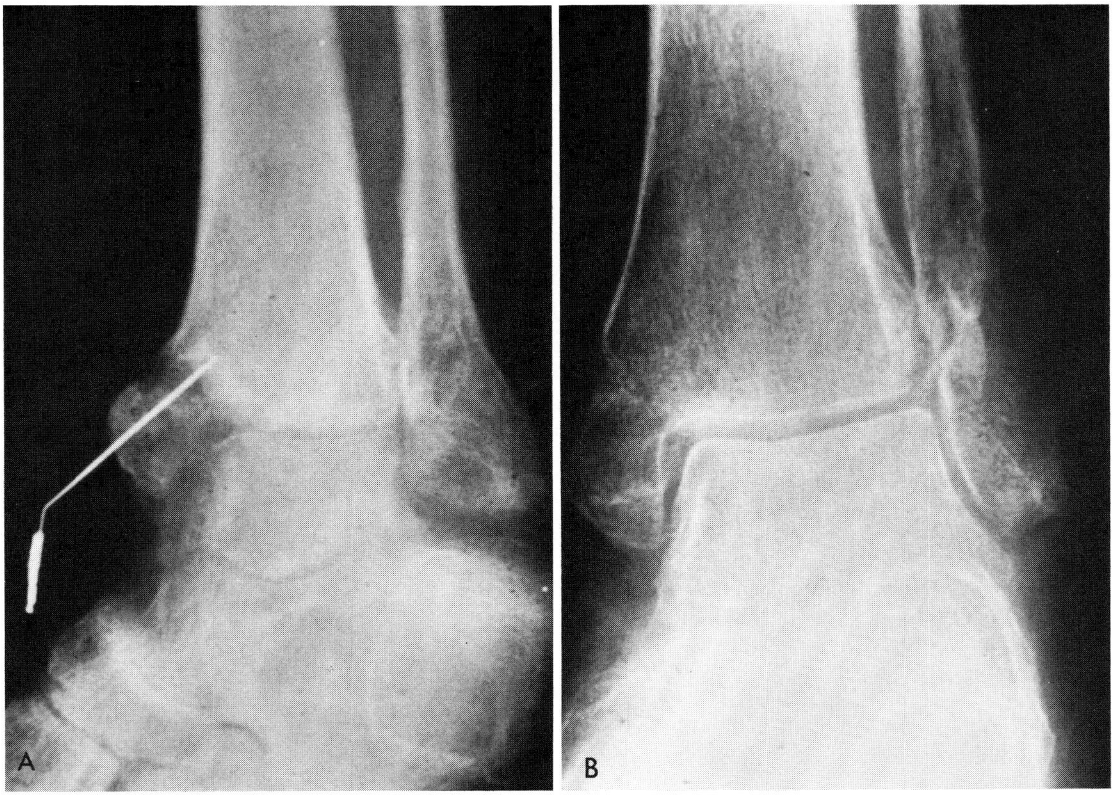

Figure 3-7   *A*. Roentgenogram of ankle showing nonunion of medial malleolus, with a cathode delivering a constant direct current of 10 microamperes crossing the nonunion site. *B*. Roentgenogram of same ankle shown in *A* after discontinuation of current that flowed for nine weeks. The nonunion is healed. (Courtesy of *Journal of Trauma*. J. Trauma, *11*:884, 1971.)

Figure 3-8   Electrical apparatus and electrode placement used in the study described in the test. (Courtesy of *Journal of Bone and Joint Surgery*. J. Bone Joint Surg., 57A:369, 1975.)

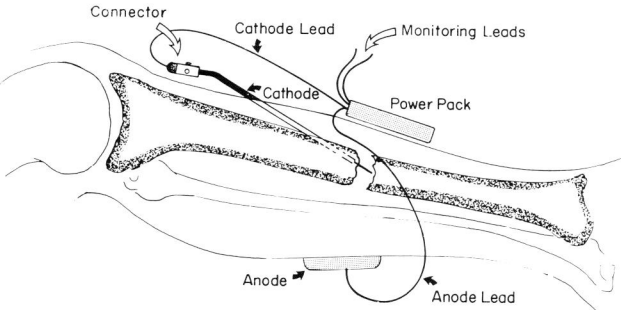

TABLE 3–2   Results of Electrical Treatment

Bone	Number Treated	Number Healed	Number Failed
Tibia	74	59	15
Femur	23	16	7
Clavicle	13	9	4
Ulna	13	10	3
Humerus	12	8	4
Medial malleolus	10	10	0
Radius	5	3	2
Carponavicular	2	1	1
Fibula	1	1	0
	153	117 (76.5%)	36

previous history of infection, while 69 per cent had undergone an average of 2.2 previous surgical procedures. The most common bone involved in nonunion was the tibia, followed by the femur, the clavicle, the medial malleolus, and the remainder of the long bones. The results of treatment of nonunion with direct current in the 72 patients are shown in Table 3–2.

The raw data for all patients show that solid bony union was achieved in 52 out of 72 patients for a rate of 72 per cent. This union rate is comparable to that of most series in which bone grafting is utilized as the primary treatment of nonunion, but it is not as high as that achieved by bone grafting plus internal fixation, particularly compression plating.

More is learned from analyzing the failures in the series, however, than in comparing the success rates of different series. When the failures in the series of 72 patients were analyzed (Table 3–3), it became evident that 11 of the patients had not received adequate electricity. That is, while one 10 μA cathode proved sufficient to heal the small bones, such as the medial malleolus or clavicle, it was not sufficient to heal the large bones, such as the tibia and femur. Once it was realized that the larger

TABLE 3–3   Analysis of Failures of Electrical Treatment

Inadequate Electricity	11
Unknown	4
True Pseudoarthrosis	2
Presence of Chronic Osteomyelitis	2
Electrode Dislodgment	1
	20

bones require more electricity the microamperage per cathode was increased to 20, and the number of cathodes used was increased to 4 for the tibia, femur, and humerus. If the 11 cases of inadequate electricity are eliminated from the series, a truer picture of the present state of the art is obtained (Table 3–4): 52 patients out of 61 were healed for a union rate of 85 per cent. At the present time in the United States, 16 teams in a cooperative study utilizing the techniques described have treated over 300 nonunion patients with constant direct current, and the overall rate of union is 80 to 85 per cent. Since this is about the same success rate as that achieved by bone grafting with internal fixation, it is evident that treating nonunion with electricity is a viable alternative to bone graft surgery. Several typical case studies will now be described.

A 27-year-old male had nonunion of the tibia of two years and five months' duration (Fig. 3–9). The original fracture was open and was treated with open reduction and debridement. No internal fixation device was used. The patient had no history of previous infection of the fracture. Under local anesthesia, four 20 μA cathodes were inserted under roentgenographic control into the nonunion site (Fig. 3–9B). After 12 weeks of constant direct current, during which time the extremity was immobilized in a non–weight-bearing short leg cast, and an additional 12 weeks in a short leg weight-bearing cast, the nonunion healed (Fig. 3–9C).

A 24-year-old male had a nonunion of the femur for one year following a closed fracture that was treated conservatively with skeletal traction and cast immobiliza-

TABLE 3–4   Results of "Adequate" Electrical Treatment

Bone	Number Treated	Number Healed	Number Failed
Tibia	66	59	7
Femur	23	16	7
Clavicle	12	9	3
Ulna	12	10	2
Humerus	11	8	3
Medial malleolus	10	10	0
Radius	5	3	2
Carponavicular	2	1	1
Fibula	1	1	0
	142	117 (82.4%)	25

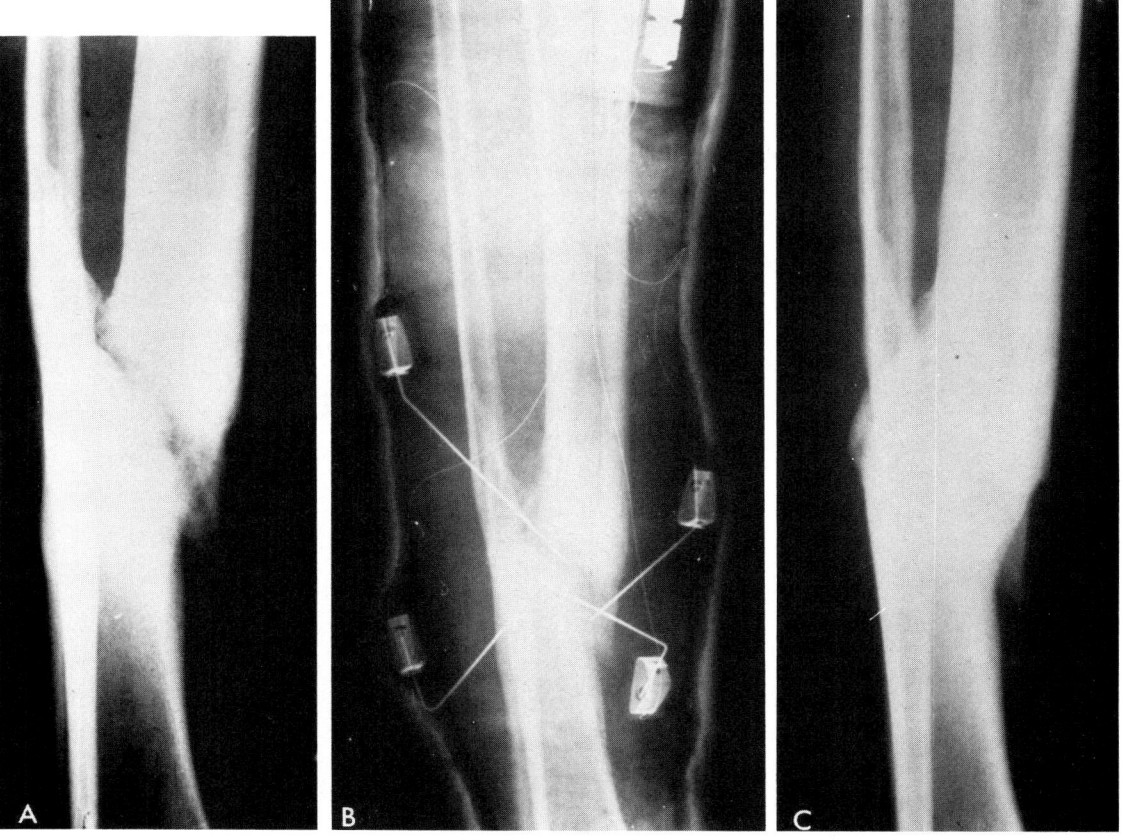

Figure 3–9   A. Nonunion for two years and five months in a 27-year-old male. B. Roentgenogram showing placement of four 20 microampere cathodes into the tibial nonunion site. C. After continuous direct current for 12 weeks and immobilization for an additional 12 weeks, the nonunion is healed. (Courtesy of *Clinical Orthopaedics*. Clin. Orthop., *124*:112, 1977.)

tion (Fig. 3–10A). Three 20 μA cathodes were inserted percutaneously, and after 12 weeks of continuous direct current and long leg cast immobilization for an additional 12 weeks, the nonunion was healed (Fig. 3–10B).

A 40-year-old female had nonunion of the radius of 12 years' duration. She had originally sustained closed fractures of both bones of the forearm which were treated with open reduction and intramedullary rodding of the ulna and compression plating of the radius. Both bones went on to nonunion. Two subsequent bone graft procedures resulted in union of the ulna, but the radius still failed to unite (Fig. 3–11A). Under local anesthesia, a screw at the nonunion site was removed, and one 10 μA cathode was inserted down the empty screw tract (Fig. 3–11B). After 12 weeks of continuous direct current the nonunion was healed (Fig. 3–11C).

The last example is that of a 35-year-old woman with nonunion of the clavicle of 15

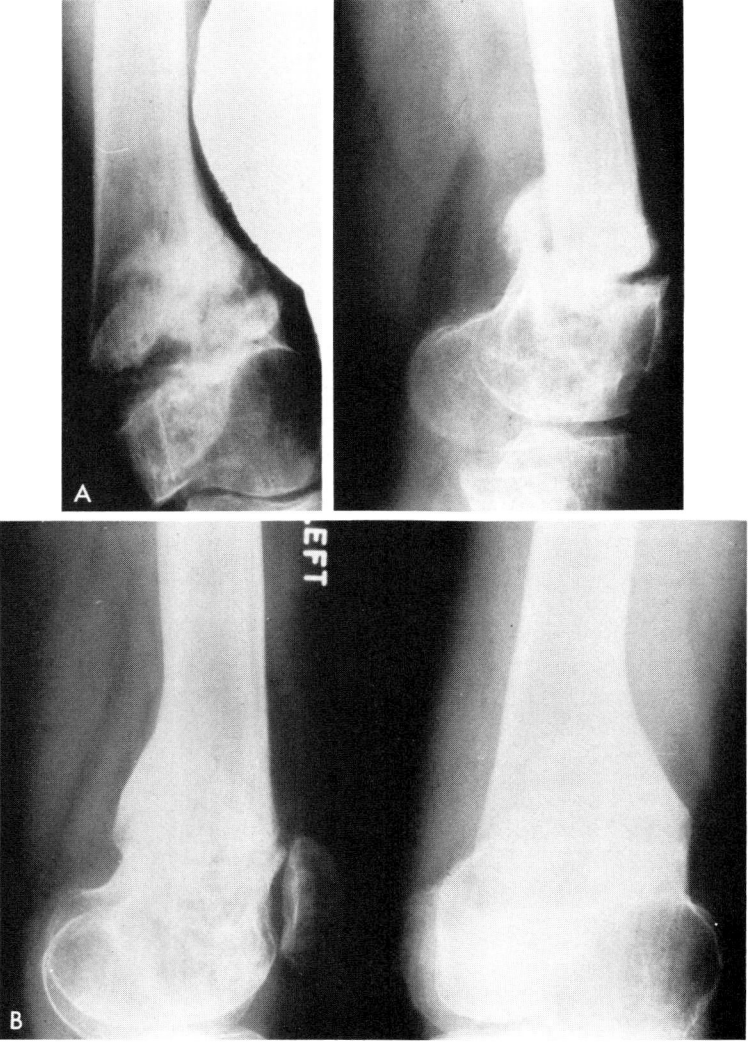

Figure 3–10 A. Nonunion for one year in a 24-year-old male. B. The nonunion is healed after 12 weeks of continuous direct current and an additional 12 weeks of cast immobilization. (Courtesy of *Journal of Bone and Joint Surgery.* J. Bone Joint Surg., 57A:373, 1975.)

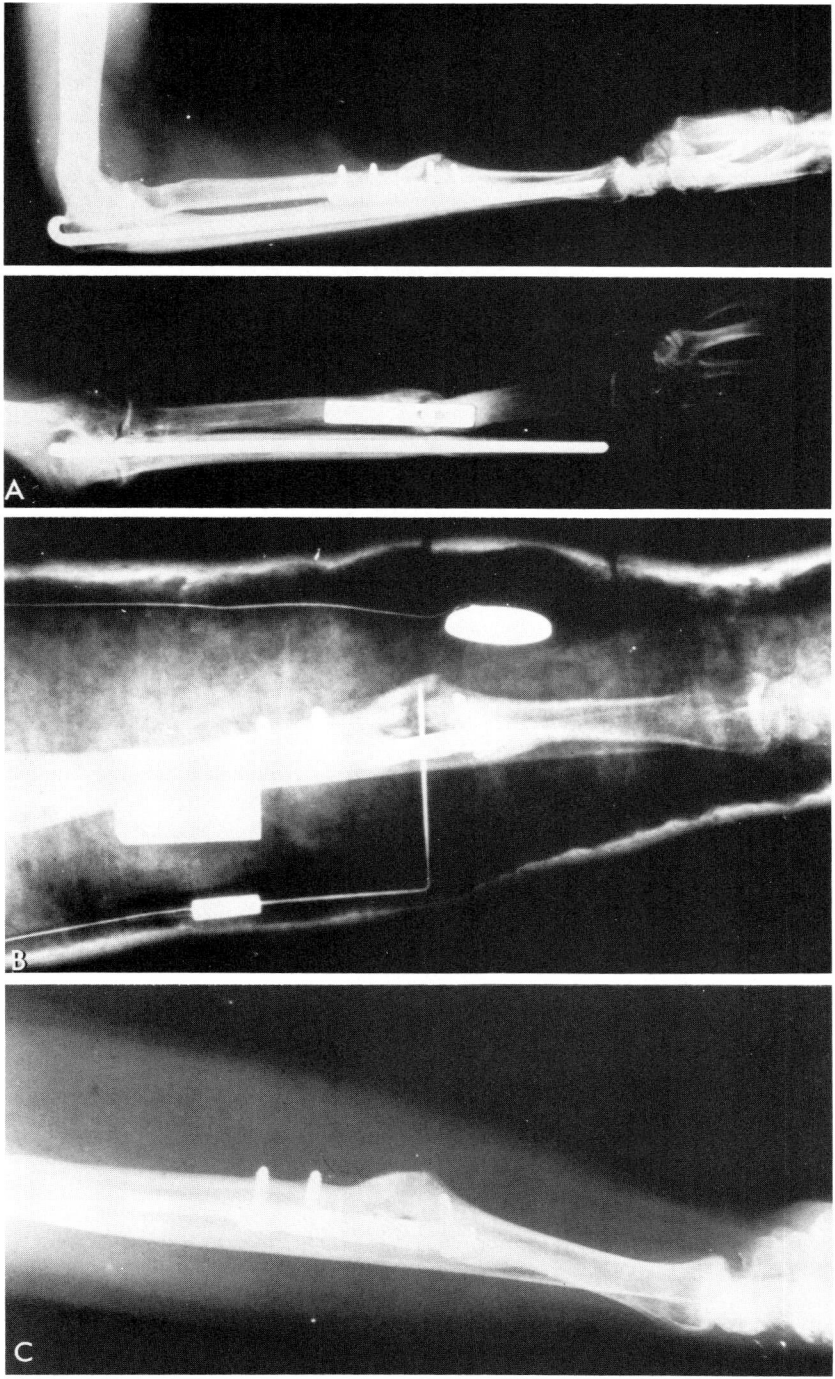

Figure 3–11   A. Nonunion of the radius of 12 years' duration and following compression plating and two bone graft procedures. B. A screw at the nonunion site has been removed and one 10-microampere cathode inserted down the vacant screw hole. The rectangular power pack is incorporated in the plaster cast, and the circular anode is on the skin. C. The nonunion is healed after 12 weeks of continuous direct current. (Courtesy of *Clinical Orthopaedics*. Clin. Orthop., *124*:109, 1977.)

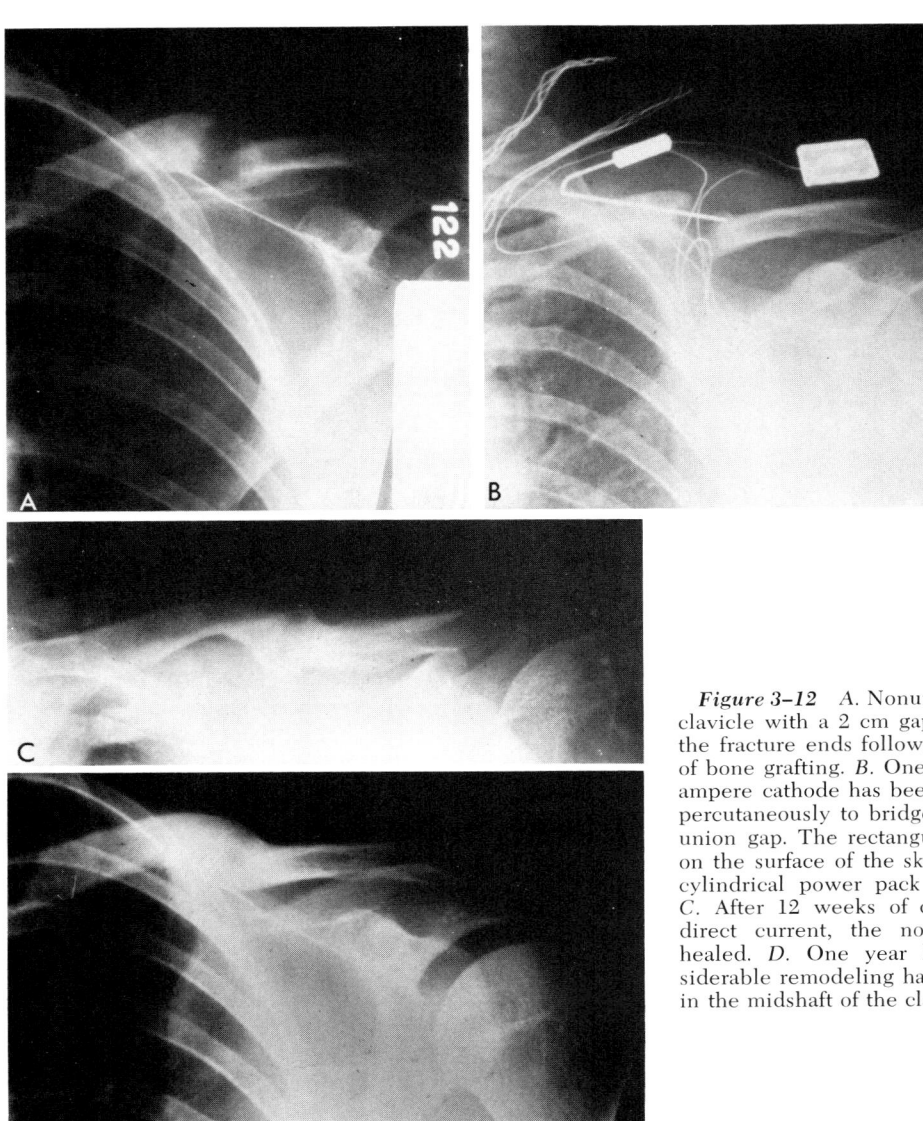

Figure 3–12   A. Nonunion of the clavicle with a 2 cm gap between the fracture ends following failure of bone grafting. *B.* One 20-micro-ampere cathode has been inserted percutaneously to bridge the non-union gap. The rectangular anode on the surface of the skin and the cylindrical power pack are seen. *C.* After 12 weeks of continuous direct current, the nonunion is healed. *D.* One year later, con-siderable remodeling has occurred in the midshaft of the clavicle.

months' duration following an original open reduction and a subsequent bone grafting procedure (Fig. 3–12A). Not only did the nonunion fail to unite, but a resorption process set in such that the graft and the ends of the fracture fragments resorbed, producing a 2 cm gap. Under local anesthesia, one 20 μA cathode was inserted percutaneously across the gap at the nonunion site (Fig. 3–12B). After 12 weeks of constant current, the nonunion healed (Fig. 3–12C). One year later the nonunion has remained healed, and remodeling has occurred (Fig. 3–12D).

Complications with this new technique are about what one would expect. In the series just cited there were six broken wires, six superficial pin tract infections, three cathode dislodgements, and one patient with considerable irritation under an anode. There was one deep postoperative wound infection occurring in a patient who had previously had an osteomyelitis. This infection responded to intensive antibiotic therapy.

Many other investigators have used electricity in one form or another to heal nonunion or congenital pseudarthrosis or to accelerate fracture healing. Continuous direct current,[5, 15, 30, 37, 39, 41] pulsed, asymmetrical direct current,[33, 34] and pulsed electromagnetic fields[3, 4] have all been used with greater or lesser success. The clinical indications for the use of these various forms of electricity in inducing osteogenesis are being evaluated at the present time. Obviously, each form has its advantages and disadvantages. Time and carefully controlled clinical studies will eventually determine the clinical indications for each form.

Mechanisms of Osteogenesis

The mechanism(s) by which electricity in any of its forms induces osteogenesis is unknown. However, all the possible effects of electricity on bone and cartilage cells may be grouped into two broad categories: (1) direct cellular changes, and (2) indirect changes produced in the microenvironment. Direct cellular changes conceivably could include uncoiling or activation of DNA, changes in the surface charge of the cell membrane, and changes in the rate of

ion migration. Indirect changes in the microenvironment conceivably could involve changes in the local tissue oxygen tension, changes in pH, and orientation of collagen due to the electrical current. Because many more data are available on the indirect changes produced by an electrical current, these will be discussed first.

In vitro experiments have shown that oxygen tension is reduced and pH is raised in the vicinity of a cathode according to the following equation:[7]

$$2H_2O + O_2 + 4e^- \rightarrow 4OH^- \tag{1}$$
$$or$$
$$O_2 + 2H^+ + 4e^- \rightarrow 2OH^-$$

Reaction (1) occurs only when the potential is at one volt or less (in the power packs utilized in the laboratory and in the clinical studies discussed previously, the potential average is 0.83 volt). As the potential increases above one volt, oxygen consumption at the cathode gradually gives way to hydrogen production according to the equation:

$$2H_2O + 2e^- \rightarrow H_2 + 2OH^- \tag{2}$$
$$or$$
$$H^+ + e^- \rightarrow \frac{1}{2}H_2$$

In other words, at potentials under one volt oxygen is consumed, and given the proper current, osteogenesis occurs. At potentials over one volt, oxygen consumption at the cathode gives way to hydrogen production, and osteogenesis ceases. That low tissue oxygen tension is conducive to bone formation has been shown (1) by the low P_{O_2} present at the bone-cartilage junction in the growth plate[9] and in newly formed bone and cartilage in fracture calluses;[12, 27] (2) by the maximum bone growth that occurs in vitro in low O_2 environments;[13] and (3) by the fact that growth plate cartilage cells[17, 35] as well as bone cells[6, 16, 48] follow a predominantly anaerobic metabolic pathway.

Since according to equation (1) hydroxyl radicals are produced at the cathode, the local tissue environment becomes more alkaline. That an alkaline environment favors calcification is suggested by the rather high pH (7.70 $\pm$ 0.05) found in the zone of hypertrophic cells of the growth plate.[28]

Collagen may be oriented by an electrical current. When a weak direct current (in the low microamperage range) is passed through a dilute solution of acid-soluble collagen, a band of collagen fibrils is precipitated near the cathode at right angles to the field. Whether or not such orientation of collagen occurs in a fracture callus in the vicinity of a cathode is not known.

Electricity may also have a direct effect on bone and cartilage cells. This is suggested by those studies previously mentioned in which noninvasive methods are used to induce current in bone,[3, 4] and in an in vitro study in which growth plate explants exhibited accelerated growth when subjected to an electrical field of 1500 volts per centimeter.[8] Norton and co-workers[44] demonstrated a change in cyclic AMP content of epiphyseal plate cartilage subjected to an oscillating electrical field of 1500 volts per centimeter. Cyclic AMP is the intracellular or second messenger of the cell. It well may be that the electron or charge or potential is an extracellular or first messenger to bone and cartilage cells.

REFERENCES

1. Bassett, C. A. L., and Becker, R. O.: Generation of electrical potentials by bone in response to mechanical stress. Science, *137*:1063, 1962.
2. Bassett, C. A. L., Pawluk, R. J., and Becker, R. O.: Effects of electrical currents on bone in vivo. Nature, *204*:652, 1964.
3. Bassett, C. A. L., Pawluk, R. J., and Pilla, A. A.: Augmentation of bone repair by inductively coupled electromagnetic fields. Science, *184*:575, 1974.
4. Bassett, C. A. L., Pilla, A. A., and Pawluk, R. J.: A nonoperative salvage of surgically resistant pseudarthrosis and nonunions by pulsing electromagnetic fields: A preliminary report. Clin. Orthop., *124*:128, 1977.
5. Becker, R. O., Spadaro, J. A., and Marino, A. A.: Clinical experiences with low intensity direct current stimulation of bone growth. Clin. Orthop., *124*:75, 1977.
6. Borle, A. B., Nichols, N., and Nichols, G., Jr.: Metabolic studies of bone in vitro. I. Normal bone. J. Biol. Chem., *235*:1206, 1960.
7. Brighton, C. T., Adler, S., Black, J., Itada, N., and Friedenberg, Z. B.: Cathodic oxygen consumption and electrically induced osteogenesis. Clin. Orthop., *107*:277, 1975.
8. Brighton, C. T., Cronkey, J. E., and Osterman, A. L.: In vitro epiphyseal plate growth in various constant electrical fields. J. Bone Joint Surg., *58A*:971, 1976.
9. Brighton, C. T., and Heppenstall, R. B.: Oxygen tension in zones of epiphyseal plate, the metaphysis, and diaphysis. An in vitro and in vivo study in rats and rabbits. J. Bone Joint Surg., *53A*:719, 1971.
10. Brighton, C. T., Friedenberg, Z. B., Mitchell, E. I., and Booth, R. E.: Treatment of nonunion with constant direct current. Clin. Orthop., *124*:106, 1977.
11. Brighton, C. T., Friedenberg, Z. B., Zemsky, L. M., and Pollis, R. P.: Direct-current stimulation of non-union and congenital pseudarthrosis. J. Bone Joint Surg., *57A*:368, 1975.
12. Brighton, C. T., and Krebs, A. G.: Oxygen tension of healing fractures in the rabbit. J. Bone Joint Surg., *54A*:323, 1972.
13. Brighton, C. T., Ray, R. D., Soble, L. W., and Kuettner, K. E.: In vitro epiphyseal-plate growth in various oxygen tensions. J. Bone Joint Surg., *51A*:1383, 1969.
14. Cieszynski, T.: Studies on the regeneration of ossal tissue. II. Treatment of bone fractures in experimental animals with electric energy. Arch. Immunol. Ther. Exp., *11*:199, 1963.
15. Connolly, J. F., Hahn, H., and Jardon, O. M.: The electrical enhancement of periosteal proliferation in normal and delayed fracture healing. Clin. Orthop., *124*:97, 1977.
16. Deiss, W. P., Jr., Holmes, L. B., and Johnston, C. C., Jr.: Bone matrix biosynthesis in vitro. I. Labeling of hexosamine and collagen of normal bone. J. Biol. Chem., *237*:3555, 1962.
17. Eeg-Larsen, N.: An experimental study on growth and glycolysis in the epiphyseal cartilage of rats. Acta Physiol. Scand. (Suppl.), *128*: 1956.
18. Friedenberg, Z. B., Andrews, E. T., Smolenski, B. I., Pearl, B. W., and Brighton, C. T.: Bone reaction to varying amounts of direct current. Surg. Gynecol. Obstet., *131*:894, 1970.
19. Friedenberg, Z. B., and Brighton, C. T.: Bioelectric potentials in bone. J. Bone Joint Surg., *48A*:915, 1966.
20. Friedenberg, Z. B., Harlow, M. C., and Brighton, C. T.: Healing of nonunion of the medial malleolus by means of direct current: a case report. J. Trauma, *11*:883, 1971.
21. Friedenberg, Z. B., Harlow, M. C., Heppenstall, R. B., and Brighton, C. T.: The cellular origin of bioelectric potentials in bone. Calcif. Tissue Res., *13*:53, 1973.
22. Friedenberg, Z. B., Roberts, P. G., Jr., Didizian, N. H., and Brighton, C. T.: Stimulation of fracture healing by direct current in the rabbit fibula. J. Bone Joint Surg., *53A*:1400, 1971.
23. Friedenberg, Z. B., Zemsky, L. M., Pollis, R. P., and Brighton, C. T.: The response of nontraumatized bone to direct current. J. Bone Joint Surg., *56A*:1023, 1974.
24. Fukada, E., and Yasuda, I.: On the piezoelectric effect of bone. J. Physiol. Soc. Jpn., *12*:1158, 1957.
25. Hassler, C. R., Rybicki, E. F., Diegle, R. B., and Clark, L. C.: Studies of enhanced bone healing via electrical stimuli. Clin. Orthop., *124*:9, 1977.
26. Harris, W. H., Moyen, B. J-L., Thrasher, E. L., II, Davis, L. A., Cobden, R. H., Mackenzie, D. A., and Cywinski, J. K.: Differential response to electrical stimulation: A distinction between

induced osteogenesis in intact tibiae and the effect on fresh fracture defects in radii. Clin. Orthop., *124*:31, 1977.

27. Heppenstall, R. B., Grislis, G., and Hunt, T. K.: Tissue gases and oxygen consumption in healing bone defects. Clin. Orthop., *106*:357, 1975.

28. Howell, D. S., Pita, J. C., Marquez, J. F., and Madruga, J. E.: Partition of calcium, phosphate, and protein in the fluid phase aspirated at calcifying sites in epiphyseal cartilage. J. Clin. Invest., *47*:1121, 1968.

29. Ida, H.: Study on dynamic and electric calluses of bone *in vitro*. J. Jpn. Orthop. Surg. Soc., *31*:645, 1957.

30. Inoue, S., Ohashi, T., Imai, R., Ichida, M., and Yasuda, I.: The electrical induction of callus formation and external skeletal fixation using methyl methacrylate for delayed union of open tibial fracture with segmental loss. Clin. Orthop., *124*:92, 1977.

31. Inoue, S., Ohashi, T., Yasuda, I., and Fukada, E.: Electret induced callus formation in the rat. Clin. Orthop., *124*:57, 1977.

32. Jacobs, J. D., and Norton, L. A.: Electrical stimulation of osteogenesis in periodontal defects. Clin. Orthop., *124*:41, 1977.

33. Jorgensen, T. E.: The effect of electric current on the healing time of crural fractures. Acta Orthrop. Scand., *43*:421, 1972.

34. Jorgensen, T. E.: Electrical stimulation of human fracture healing by means of a slow pulsating, asymmetrical direct current. Clin. Orthop., *124*: 124, 1977.

35. Krane, S. M., Parsons, V., and Kunin, A. S.: Studies of the metabolism of epiphyseal cartilage. *In*: Bassett, C. A. L. (ed.): Cartilage Degeneration and Repair. Washington, D.C., National Academy of Science, National Research Council, 1967, p. 43.

36. Lavine, L. S., Lustrin, I., and Shamos, M. H.: Experimental model for studying the effect of electric current on bone in vivo. Nature, *224*: 1112, 1969.

37. Lavine, L. S., Lustrin, I., and Shamos, M. H.: Treatment of congenital pseudarthrosis of the tibia with direct current. Clin. Orthop., *124*:69, 1977.

38. Lavine, L. S., Lustrin, I., Shamos, M. H., and Moss,

M. L.: The influence of electric current on bone regeneration in vivo. Acta Orthop. Scand., *42*: 305, 1971.

39. Lavine, L. S., Lustrin, I., and Shamos, M. H.: Treatment of congenital pseudarthrosis of the tibia with direct current. Clin. Orthop., *124*:69, 1977.

40. Levy, D. D., and Rubin, B.: Inducing bone growth in vivo by pulse stimulation. Clin. Orthop., *88*:218, 1971.

41. Masureik, C., and Eriksson, C.: Preliminary clinical evaluation of the effect of small electrical currents on the healing of jaw fractures. Clin. Orthop., *124*:84, 1977.

42. Minkin, C., Poulton, B. R., and Hoover, W. H.: The effect of direct current on bone. Clin. Orthop., *57*:303, 1968.

43. Noguchi, K.: Study on dynamic callus and electric callus. J. Jpn. Orthop. Surg. Soc., *31*:641, 1957.

44. Norton, L. A., Rodan, G. A., and Bourret, L. A.: Epiphyseal cartilage cAMP changes produced by electrical and mechanical perturbations. Clin. Orthop., *124*:59, 1977.

45. O'Connor, B. T., Charlton, H. M., Currey, J. D., Kirby, D. R. S., and Woods, C.: Effects of electric current on bone in vivo. Nature, *222*:162, 1969.

46. Richez, J., Chamay, A., and Bieler, L.: Bone changes due to pulses of direct microcurrent. Virchows Arch. Pathol. Anat., *357*:11, 1972.

47. Shamos, M. H., Lavine, L. S., and Shamos, M. I.: Piezoelectric effect in bone. Nature, *197*:81, 1963.

48. Vaes, G. M., and Nichols, G., Jr.: Oxygen tension and the control of bone cell metabolism. Nature, *193*:379, 1962.

49. Weigert, M., and Werhahn, C.: The influence of electric potentials on plated bones. Clin. Orthop., *124*:20, 1977.

50. Wolff, J.: Das Gesetz der Transformation der Knochen. Berlin, 1892.

51. Yarington, C. T., Jr., and Jaquiss, G. W.: Electrical control of bone growth in ossicles. Arch. Otolaryngol., *89*:856, 1969.

52. Yasuda, I.: Fundamental aspects of fracture treatment. J. Kyoto Med. Soc., *4*:395, 1953.

53. Yasuda, I.: Electrical callus and callus formation by Electret. Clin. Orthop., *124*:53, 1977.

R. BRUCE HEPPENSTALL, M.D.

4 _____ Delayed Union, Nonunion, and Pseudarthrosis

In the past most standard textbooks and teaching advocated placing an injured part at rest in the expectation that this would stimulate a fracture to heal. It was Hippocrates's belief that a fracture would unite if the bone ends were held together and maintained in this position for an extended period of time. This attitude was shared by Reginald Watson-Jones, who in his classic textbook dealing with fracture healing in the mid-1950's, suggested that the majority of fractures could be managed by closed methods. He also felt that a fracture that was adequately reduced and immobilized for an appropriate length of time would unite in a standard fashion.[79] It was then common practice to maintain patients in plaster casts until there was some roentgenographic evidence of fracture healing. It became apparent, however, that certain fractures would not unite in a standard fashion in spite of adequate reduction and prolonged immobilization.

In the early 1930's materials became available for internal fixation of fractures. These materials were biologically compatible with the body tissues, and this opened an entirely new era in the management of fractures and dislocations. At first, the rationale for using internal fixation was to obtain firm immobilization with the metallic fixation device. With further application of internal fixation, however, it became apparent that it not only provided secure immobilization of the fracture site but also allowed early return of the injured part to functional activity. During the initial stages of the development of internal fixation, it was the practice to supplement the operative procedures with adequate plaster immobilization postoperatively. As further experience was obtained with the use of sturdy metallic internal fixation devices it was realized that the rigid plaster immobilization was not required. In fact, it became apparent that if operative fixation was to be used, rigid fixation with the internal device was necessary and allowed early range of motion of the injured part as well as active contraction of the musculature across the fracture site. The appealing quality of this operative approach to fracture treatment resided in the early return of the injured extremity to active functional use. This had a definite beneficial effect on fracture healing. The risks involved in the management of fractures by the internal fixation technique were those associated with the anesthesia required to perform the operative procedure and also the ever constant possibility of infection inherent in the operative approach.

In several recent studies[63-69] it has been recognized that the return of an injured limb or part to active functional use will in itself stimulate healing of the injured part. This is due to a multitude of factors, including an improved circulatory status, active muscle contraction initiating electrical potentials, the stimulatory effect of active compression of bone ends, and the prevention of significant wasting of the soft-tissue structures surrounding the injured osseous structure as well as of the severe osteoporosis that accompanies disuse. It must be recognized that both the operative and nonoperative methods employed in common practice today should attempt to return the injured part to full functional activity. If internal fixation has been performed and is secure, then external plaster fixation is not necessary and early functional therapy may be instituted. If the conservative nonoperative treatment has been selected, then the use of functional bracing techniques is advocated. Sarmiento, in several recent articles, has demonstrated the superiority of functional bracing for the management of various fractures over rigid immobilization that does not return the injured part to functional activity.[63-69] It is also obvious that some fractures such as those of the proximal third of the femur are best treated by operative methods and not by functional cast bracing because of anatomical location of the fracture and the difficulty of applying an adequate brace.

DELAYED UNION

The fracture healing process requires different time intervals depending on the particular bone involved. In general, the larger bones of the extremities require longer for healing than the smaller osseous structures. Delayed union, by definition, is present when an adequate interval of time has occurred between the initial injury and the average time to union for that particular bone without any roentgenographic or clinical evidence of osseous union. This does not mean that all bones that show evidence of delayed union will necessarily proceed on to nonunion. It does indicate that the particular fractured osseous structure does

not demonstrate early signs of healing at a time when, on average, a fracture in this particular bone would show evidence of healing. This does have direct clinical application, as there are several procedures that may be employed in an attempt to stimulate healing if the treating physician feels that the bone will not unite under the present management. The following factors have been implicated in production of delayed union of various fractures:

Inadequate Reduction

Inadequate reduction is a very important factor in the development of delayed union and nonunion. It is not only common sense but it has been adequately demonstrated that properly reduced fractures heal more rapidly than fractures that are inadequately reduced. A larger amount of callus is required to bridge a large step-off deformity when the fracture is not properly reduced, and a longer time is required to reestablish the blood supply across the fracture site if a stepoff deformity is present. It is possible that soft-tissue interposition may occur with inadequate reduction of the fracture. This also will increase the time required for union across the fracture site.

Soft-Tissue Disruption

Fractures tend to take longer to unite if there has been excessive soft-tissue destruction about the fracture site. The majority of investigators feel that this phenomenon is related to a disruption of the blood supply to the fracture site proper. It is true that the majority of the blood to a healing fracture is supplied through the endosteal vasculature, as demonstrated by Rhinelander and outlined in Chapter 2. A small portion of the blood supply is, however, located in the peripheral zone of the fracture site and is provided by the surrounding soft-tissue structures. If there is significant disruption of the surrounding soft tissues, this outer cortical blood supply is no longer available. Equally important is the fact that the surrounding musculature supplies electrical forces that may well stimulate healing at the fracture site. Disruption of the surrounding musculature eliminates this active electrical potential. It is extremely important to recognize the significance of associated soft-tissue injury in the overall management of fractures; it is no longer acceptable to treat the osseous fragments and ignore the soft-tissue structures. Recent studies by Sarmiento and co-workers have also demonstrated the beneficial effect of the compressive hydraulic action of a snugly applied form-fitting cast that distributes pressures equally throughout the soft tissues and across the fracture area proper. If there is major disruption of the soft tissues, this beneficial compressive effect may not be present.

Inadequate Immobilization

In the past a great deal of importance was attached to the degree of immobilization of fractures. This particular aspect of treatment has received a critical reevaluation. For example, the current therapy advocated for tibial fractures is early active weight bearing with a form-fitting cast, which is felt to have a stimulating effect on the fracture healing process. Active weight bearing with compression of the bone ends appears to produce valuable electrical potentials that are believed to have a direct effect on fracture healing. This is a definitely new concept; in the past it was felt that secure rigid immobilization was required to prevent any disruption of the new vascular supply during the healing process. At present, however, it appears that active compression of the bone ends and contraction of the surrounding musculature are more important than secure immobilization without stress in the treatment of certain fractures. There is no doubt that a small amount of pistoning occurs with this early functional treatment, but this does not seem to have a detrimental effect on the fracture healing process. On the other hand, fractures of certain bones, such as the navicular in the wrist, require adequate immobilization for healing to occur. If mobilization is initiated too soon in these patients or if the initial immobilization is inadequate this may lead to a delay in fracture healing or actual nonunion.

Osseous Distraction

Compression has been advocated in order to stimulate bone healing. Distraction has an adverse effect. If the bone ends are distracted, there is an increased distance between the bone ends, requiring an increased amount of callus to fill the gap, and an increased distance over which the vascular supply must be reestablished. It is also a well-known clinical fact that *bone fails in tension and heals in compression.* Therefore, any distraction of the fracture fragments is to be prevented. This appears to be particularly true in management of fractures of the femur and tibia.

Surgical Management

A decision to manage a fractured bone surgically requires careful evaluation. Some fractures are more properly treated with the conservative closed method, and open surgical fixation is not indicated initially. Surgery performed in treatment of a fracture that would normally heal with conservative closed measures adds the risk of infection and the adverse effect of periosteal stripping of the surrounding soft tissue to the potential adverse effect of the anesthetic required for the operative procedure. The majority of investigators feel that significant stripping of the periosteum and surrounding soft tissue structures to apply an internal fixation device affects fracture healing unfavorably and may lead to delayed union or nonunion. Operative therapy itself may be detrimental to the fracture healing process.

Inadequate Internal Fixation

If open reduction and internal fixation are selected as the treatment of choice for a fracture and adequate internal fixation has not been obtained, this in itself may lead to a delay in the healing process. An example of this type of incorrect therapy is the treatment of a fractured hip with an inadequate internal device. Deforming forces at the fracture site may produce angulation, which may progress to actual disruption. If a fixation device that does not allow for

collapse at the fracture site has been employed, the device itself may penetrate
through the head of the femur.

One of the more serious mistakes in the
application of internal fixation is to use a
rigid metallic device that does not provide
for compression across the fracture site and
actually distracts the fragments. This may in
itself lead to delayed union and possibly
nonunion. Here again it is imperative to
disrupt as little of the soft tissue as possible
during the application of the internal fixation device.

Sacrifice of Osseous Stock

An attempt must be made to preserve all
the bone present at the fracture site during
the operative management of fractures. It is
poor surgical judgment to remove an osseous fragment at the fracture site simply
because it does not have surrounding soft-
tissue attachments. A much more appropriate course is to leave the osseous fragment in position in spite of the loss of soft
tissue. The free fragment, devoid of its
blood supply, will act as a free bone graft—a
much better circumstance than if the fragment were removed and an actual gap left at
the fracture site. This has a more direct
bearing in the management of open fractures. It is good surgical judgment to clean
all the contaminated bone as much as
possible and to leave it in position with
access to the exterior for drainage. The
majority of these wounds can be packed
open with Betadine solutions until the risk
of infection has passed. The wound can
then be secondarily closed, leaving the
osseous fragments in position. This is preferable to excising the contaminated fragments and producing a large osseous defect
that will certainly progress to delayed union
and probably nonunion. The secret in this
particular management is to delay closure to
a later date when there is no longer a
significant risk of infection.

The incidence of delayed union will certainly be reduced if all the foregoing factors
are borne in mind during the active management of patients with fractures. This will
also ultimately reduce the incidence of
nonunion as well.

NONUNION

It has been estimated that there are 2
million cases of long-bone fractures each
year, with 100,000 new cases of nonunion
per year. Nonunion by definition means that
all reparative processes of healing have
stopped, yet bony continuity has not been
restored. All the factors listed in the discussion of delayed union also apply directly to
the production of nonunion. This particular
diagnosis is based on both a clinical and a
roentgenographic evaluation.

Clinically, nonunion is suggested when a
patient has increased pain when he attempts functional use of the involved extremity. If a fracture has gone on to uneventful healing, ambulation or excess stress
do not, as a general rule, elicit pain.
Therefore, the presence of pain at the
fracture site is a definite suggestion of
nonunion. This is not a hard and fast rule,
however, as we have seen the occasional
patient in our nonunion clinic who does not
particularly complain of excessive pain at
the nonunion site. As a rule of thumb,
therefore, pain at the fracture site does
suggest nonunion but the absence of pain
does not definitely rule out nonunion. The
majority of patients with an established
nonunion will have tenderness to direct
palpation at the nonunion site. Again, this is
not a hard and fast rule; the occasional
patient will not have tenderness at the
nonunion site.

The majority of patients with a nonunion
are unable to walk without a significant
antalgic limp. If motion is present at the
fracture site with stress, then the presence
of nonunion is definitely established. A
great deal of motion with stress and very
little pain indicates that a true pseudarthrosis may well be present. Bowing at
the fracture site with attempted ambulation
certainly is diagnostic of a nonunion or a
pseudarthrosis. Persistent edema of the
affected part may be a hint that a nonunion
is present.

ROENTGENOGRAPHIC EVALUATION

Roentgenographically, the presence of a
nonunion is suggested by the following criteria:

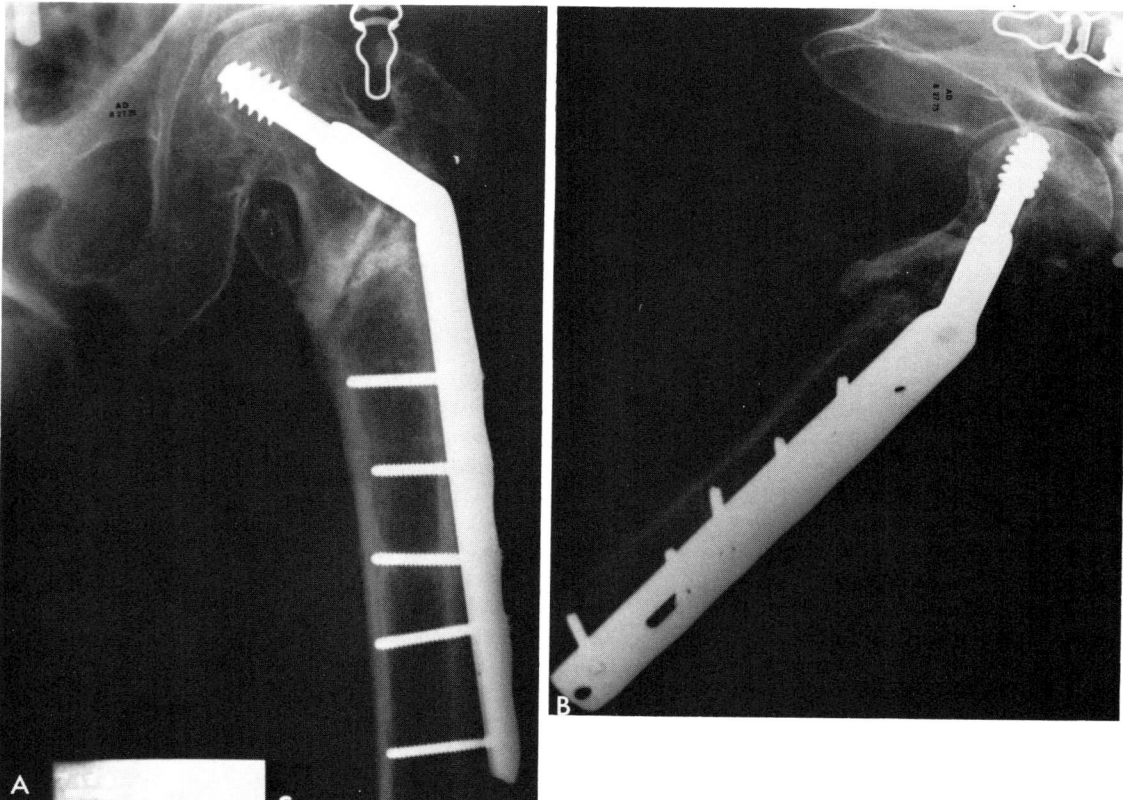

Figure 4-1   A. Anteroposterior view of a left intertrochanteric fracture with nonunion. (Note the sclerotic bone margins.) B. Lateral view of the same hip showing the nonunion site in the intertrochanteric area.

1. Sclerosis of the bone ends at the fracture site has, in the past, been considered very suggestive of nonunion (Fig. 4-1). Because the bone ends are capped, the blood supply is unable to progress across the fracture site to enhance fracture healing. Recently, however, reviewing a large number of nonunions, Brighton found that this sclerotic pattern is present in only approximately 25 per cent of patients.[16] Therefore, although the finding of sclerotic margins at the bone ends is definitely suggestive of nonunion, their absence does not rule out nonunion.

2. Failure to show any progressive change in roentgenographic appearance over a three-month interval has been considered as evidence that nonunion is present.

3. Progressive bowing at the fracture site

in sequential radiographs over a prolonged interval is definitely suggestive of nonunion.

4. An increase in the amount of bone atrophy above and below the fracture site has been associated with nonunions (Fig. 4-2). This osteoporotic pattern has been evident in approximately 25 per cent of nonunions; a combination of osteoporosis and sclerotic margins at the bone ends has been present in approximately 25 per cent.

5. Excess callus formation around the fracture site with a lucent interval through the callus itself has been associated with nonunion. This has been referred to as false callus by some investigators.

6. Remodeling does not occur in cases of nonunion. The presence of remodeling of the osseous structure about the fracture site is a sign that the fracture has achieved some

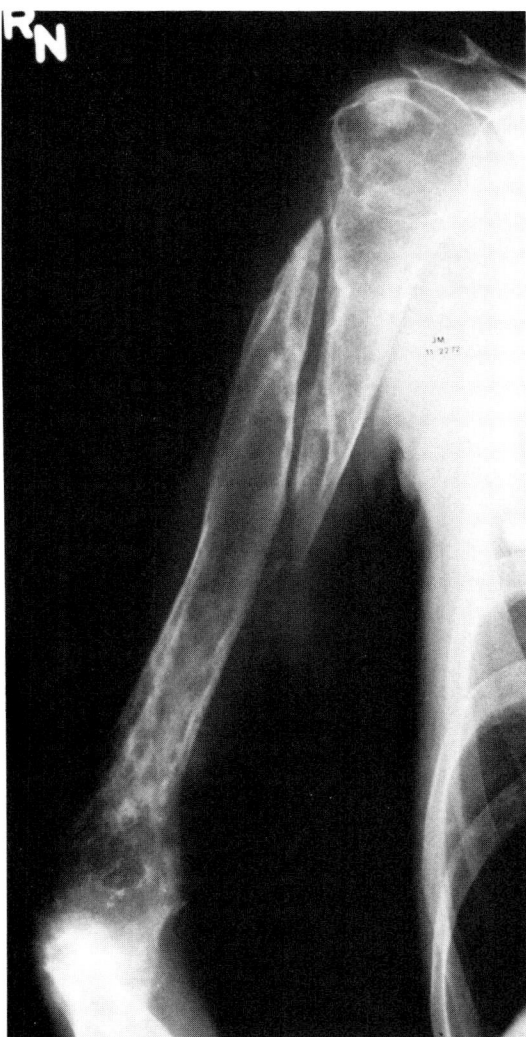

Figure 4-2 Anteroposterior view of the right humerus demonstrating a nonunion with significant osseous atrophy proximal and distal to the nonunion site.

mechanical stability and is progressing on to union. The likelihood that this is a true nonunion is then diminished.

7. Occasionally bone scans are helpful in evaluating the presence of a nonunion or pseudarthrosis. In true nonunion the bone scan remains "hot" directly over the fracture site. This is in contrast to a true pseudarthrosis in which there may be an area of decreased uptake directly in the center of the fracture area surrounded by an area of increased uptake of radioactive material on each side. If this particular pattern is evident, a diagnosis of true pseudarthrosis rather than nonunion should be considered. The bone scan may be helpful diagnostically in differentiating between nonunion and pseudarthrosis, but further documentation will be required in the future.

It is imperative during the evaluation of patients with nonunion to obtain at least four views of the fracture site. In the past, it was routine to obtain an anteroposterior and lateral view of the fracture site only. Patients have, however, presented without evidence of a nonunion in these particular roentgenographic views, only to have one become evident when oblique views are obtained. It is for this reason that four views of the fracture site are essential. These include an anteroposterior, a lateral, and two oblique views of the fracture site proper. With these, few nonunions will be "missed."

INCIDENCE AND MANAGEMENT OF SPECIFIC PROBLEMS

Five specific anatomical areas deserve emphasis in regard to the incidence and management of nonunion.

Type 2 Odontoid Fractures

These fractures have been associated with a high incidence of nonunion, as discussed in Chapter 13. Some authors have felt that this is due to a decrease in blood supply at this particular level. The exact incidence of nonunion varies, but has been reported as from 20 to 64 per cent of cases. For this reason, some authors have advocated primary fusion of C1 to C2 for the management of type 2 odontoid fractures. The author has preferred a conservative program, using a halo brace and then a posterior cervical fusion of C1 to C2 if there is no evidence of any union over a period of four to six months.

Forearm Fractures

The forearm is an area that has been associated with a high incidence of nonunion following conservative management

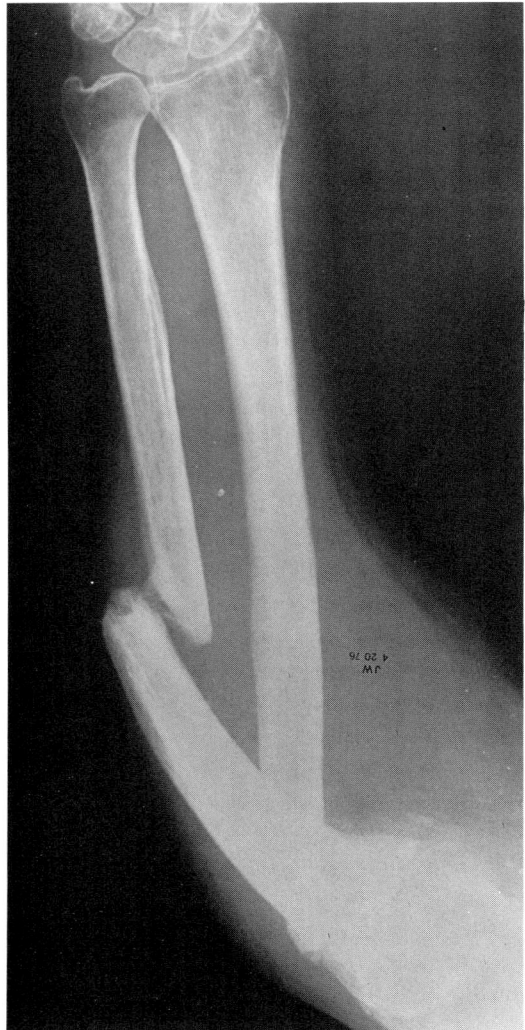

Figure 4–3 A Galeazzi fracture, improperly reduced, resulted in nonunion of the ulna.

(Fig. 4–3). This applies in particular to fractures of both bones of the forearm. The majority of investigators feel that a both-bones-of-the-forearm fracture should be treated initially with compression plating of both the ulna and radius. It has become apparent in recent studies that the incidence of nonunion has been decreased by using internal compression plate fixation rather than conservative management without internal fixation. The improved anatomical reconstruction following an open reduction supplemented with rigid internal fixation appears to enhance the possibility of union of these forearm fractures, particularly the both-bone type. On the other hand, a recent review by Sarmiento of the use of functional bracing techniques for fractures of a single bone of the forearm has suggested that functional bracing may reduce the incidence of nonunion of these fractures.[67] At the present time it appears that the functional bracing technique has a place in the management of single-bone forearm fractures but that further studies will be required to evaluate the effect of this therapy in both-bone forearm fractures. If there is comminution at the fracture site associated with a fracture of both bones of the forearm, the present method of choice is compression plating of both bones and application of a bone graft.

Navicular Bone in Wrist

The navicular bone in the wrist is notorious for delayed union and nonunion of fractures. These fractures are also notorious for being "missed" during the initial physical and roentgenographic evaluation. A repeat roentgenogram 7 to 10 days following an injury may well demonstrate a fracture line that was not evident on the initial postinjury roentgenogram. Fracture of the navicular is one of the few that may require prolonged immobilization for five to seven months if healing is to occur. Once again, it is felt that the reason for the high incidence of nonunion in this particular bone is the lack of blood supply to a fracture through its midportion. Also, this is an intraarticular bone, and some investigators have felt that the presence of synovial fluid is detrimental to healing. The position of the hand in a thumb spica is felt to be very important in an attempt to close the fracture gap. This is discussed further in Chapter 19. Once nonunion has been established, bone grafting is the treatment of choice. A form of the Matti-Russe procedure has been popular in the past for grafting this particular bone.

Subcapital Fractures of Hip

A definite incidence of nonunion is associated with the management of these fractures (Fig. 4–4). This has been felt to be related to the disruption of the blood supply to the femoral head by the fracture. This is also an intraarticular fracture, and the presence of synovial fluid has been felt to be detrimental to healing of this particular fracture as it is to fractures of the navicular. The adequacy of the initial reduction is extremely important in the prevention of nonunion, as outlined in several published reports. Recent large studies have attributed the decrease in incidence of nonunion to an improvement in the type of internal fixation devices as well as to a concentrated effort to obtain adequate reduction prior to insertion of the fixation device (Fig. 4–5). A muscle pedicle graft combined with adequate internal fixation is useful in this type of complication. It is proper to attempt a bone grafting procedure during treatment of the nonunion if the femoral head is viable. A prosthetic replacement can always be performed at a later date if this technique fails.

Fractures of Lower Third of Tibia

In the past it was believed that the distal third of the tibia, long regarded as a specific site for nonunion, failed to unite because of a decrease in blood supply at this particular level (Fig. 4–6). Recent studies, however, have failed to demonstrate any specific increased incidence of nonunion in the distal third of the tibia due to location alone. It is true that nonunion occurs more frequently in these fractures, but this has been attributed to the greater impact associated with many of them and the increased soft-tissue disruption at the fracture site. In reality, it is probably the greater soft-tissue disruption associated with high-velocity or torque injuries that is related to the increased incidence of nonunion.

The author feels very strongly that management of nonunion of the tibia in the presence of a healed fibular fracture must also include resection of a portion of the healed fibula to allow active compression at

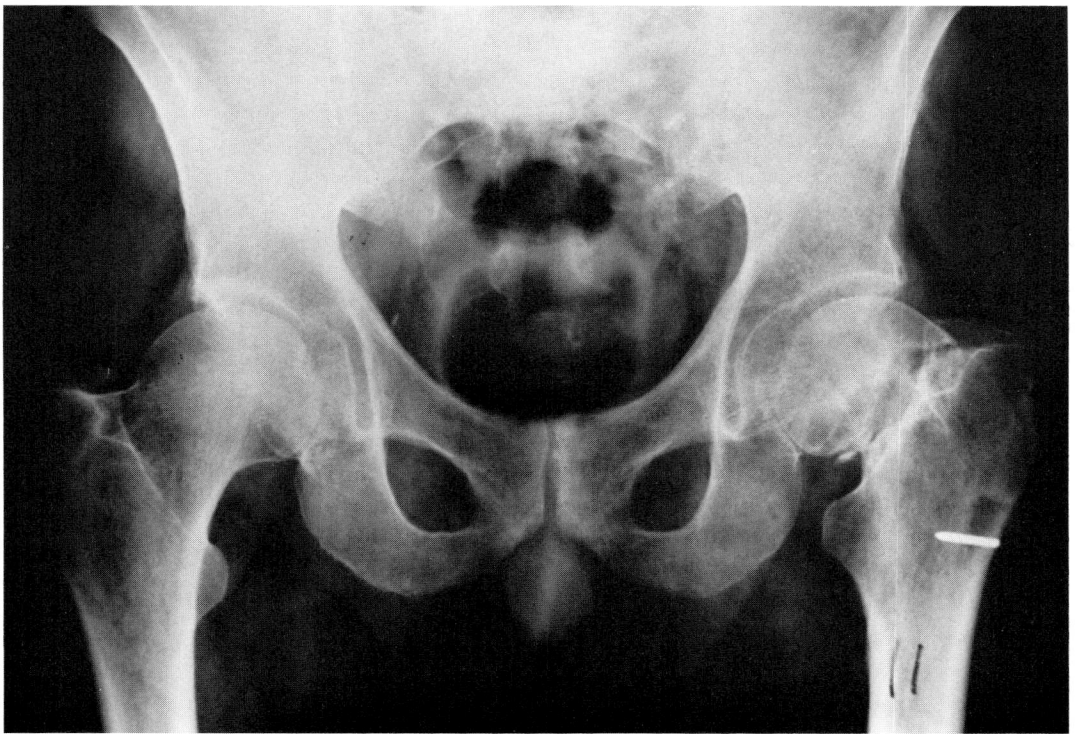

Figure 4–4   Anteroposterior view of the pelvis. There is nonunion of a subcapital fracture on the left.

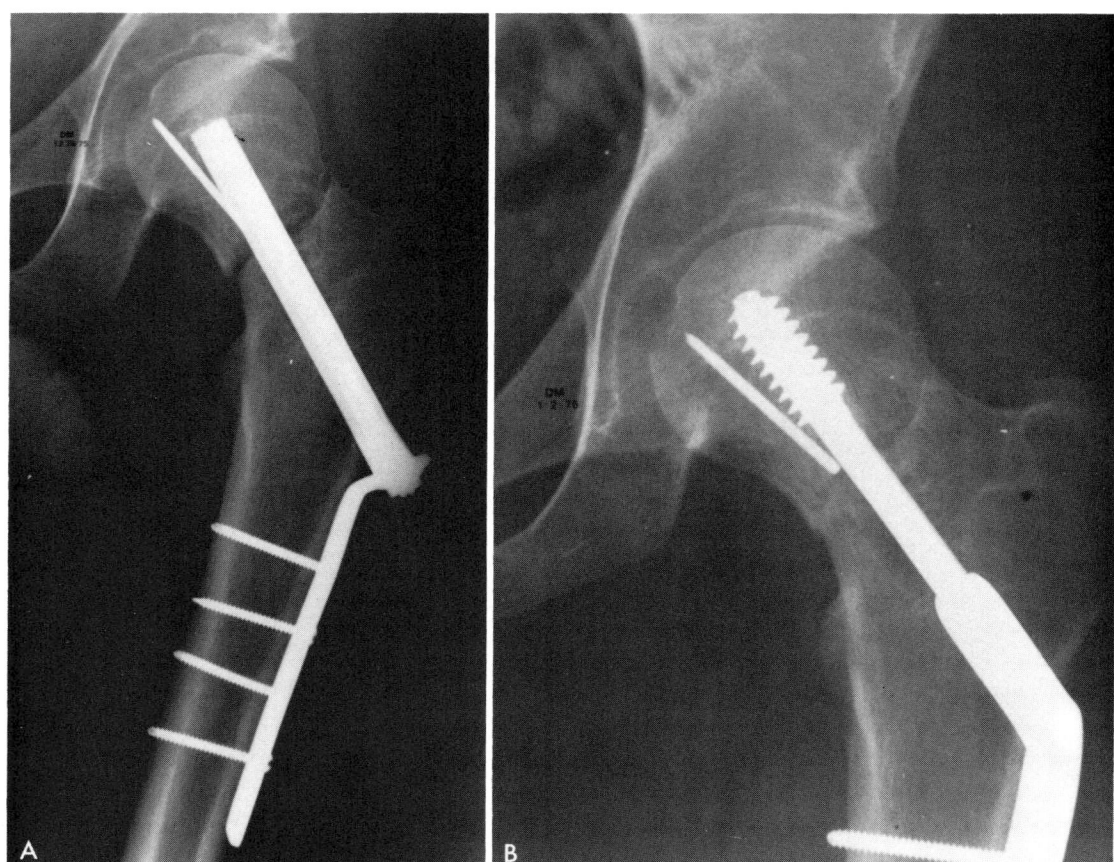

Figure 4–5   *A.* Anteroposterior view of the left hip shows nonunion of a femoral neck fracture treated with a Smith-Peterson nail. There appears to be distraction at the fracture site. *B.* The Smith-Peterson nail and side plate were removed and a compression hip screw and side plate were inserted with active compression at the fracture site. Note the improved position at the fracture site one week postoperatively. This went on to uneventful healing.

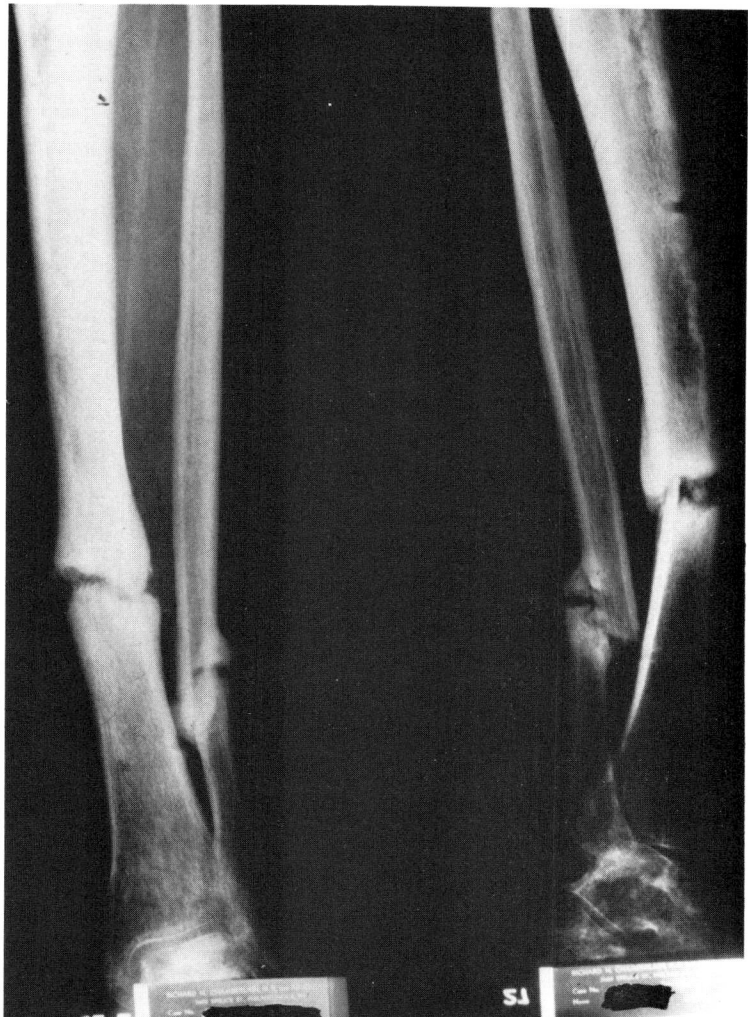

Figure 4–6 Nonunion of a fracture of the distal third of the tibia and fibula. Note the sclerotic margins.

the tibial fracture site to stimulate healing (Fig. 4–7). If a bone grafting procedure has been performed on the tibia without resection or osteotomy of the healed fibula, the fibula itself may act as a strut to keep the tibial bone ends from active compression and thus prevent fracture healing. There have been reports of healing of nonunion of the tibia following resection of a portion of the fibula alone. It is not always necessary to "take down" the entire nonunion site at the time of a bone grafting procedure. It is common practice to leave the central portion of the nonunion intact, to decorticate the involved bone, and to position bone graft along the proximal mid and distal portions of the nonunion site. This does not apply to the management of pseudarthrosis, which is discussed later.

It is interesting to note that fractures of the vertebral body, skull, scapula, and ribs are usually not associated with nonunion.

Infection

Infected open fractures have been associated with a greater incidence of nonunion than closed fractures. It has been estimated that in a large series, in 20 per cent or less of nonunions there may be a prior history of

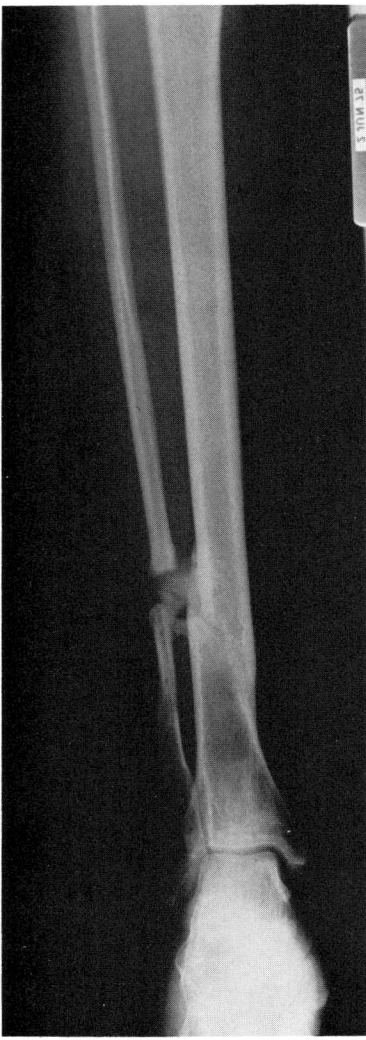

Figure 4–7 Nonunion of the distal third of the tibia treated by resection of the healed fibula and insertion of a bone graft through a posterior Harmon approach. Note that there is solid union of the spiral fracture of the tibia four months postoperatively.

the past, in a patient with a frankly infected nonunion in the presence of a metallic fixation device, removal of the device was advocated in an attempt to control the infection within the bone. Now, however, several studies have evaluated the effect of leaving the metallic appliance in place to provide stability at the fracture site while managing the infection with antibiotics. It is appropriate to provide operative drainage and remove all debris at the fracture site, but the internal fixation device should be left in place if at all possible. It appears that obtaining stability at the fracture site even in the presence of an infection is more beneficial in bringing the infection under control than removing the device and leaving the fracture site unstable as well as infected. This rule of thumb applies unless the patient has recurrent bouts of septicemia that are not controlled by local drainage and debridement. Under these circumstances, the internal fixation device must be removed to avoid toxic manifestations. This is the rare case indeed, however, as the majority of infected nonunions can be managed with the internal fixation device in place.

infection. This association must be borne in mind during the management of patients with open fractures. It is possible that a patient may progress to a nonunion because of a smoldering low-grade infection that is not appreciated clinically. If a surgical procedure is then advocated and metallic internal fixation devices are employed to obtain appropriate fixation, the risk of chronic osteomyelitis will be increased. In

PSEUDARTHROSIS

Pseudarthrosis is a variant of nonunion in which there is formation of dense scar tissue and a false joint with serum loculated in the cicatricial mass. The incidence of true synovial pseudarthrosis is very low—probably less than 5 per cent. There are three anatomical areas that have been associated with pseudarthrosis. These are the clavicle, the humerus, and the tibia. As with an established nonunion, some type of surgical intervention is required to obtain adequate healing, since all true processes of osseous healing have ceased. There are two distinct forms of pseudarthrosis, a congenital form and an acquired form.

Congenital Pseudarthrosis

Congenital pseudarthrosis is a specific type of pseudarthrosis that is present or incipient at birth. The exact etiology of congenital pseudarthrosis has never been firmly established. It is, however, seen in patients with neurofibromatosis. In fact, the tissue obtained from biopsy specimens in the past has been compatible in some cases with neurofibromatosis. The most frequently involved bone structure is the distal half of the tibia and also frequently that of the fibula. Congenital pseudarthrosis has been reported in other areas as well, including the first rib, clavicle, humerus, ulna, and femur.

Congenital pseudarthrosis of the tibia is a very difficult problem to manage. Basically, it presents with four different clinical manifestations. The first type is present at birth and its manifestations are evident. The second type is seen in association with a congenital cyst of bone, which eventually develops a fracture through the cyst. The third type is seen in association with a specific form of congenital bowing when a fracture develops through the bone. Finally, the fourth type occurs following a specific type of insufficiency or stress fracture.

There is a definite pattern to the bowing associated with congenital pseudarthrosis in that there is usually anterior bowing in the distal third of the tibia with evidence of partial or complete absence of the medullary canal at the level of the bowing. Early bone grafting has been advocated in this condition. If bone grafting is delayed, the extremity will frequently be shorter, will fail to develop normally, and will have a deformed and small foot. Several types of bone grafting procedures have been advocated for management of this particular problem. Like any type of operation for pseudarthrosis, it must include complete excision of the dense tissue between the bone and the pseudarthrosis site. McElvenny demonstrated a thick cuff of dense fibrous tissue surrounding the bone at the pseudarthrosis site, and it was his contention that this must be completely excised prior to any bone grafting procedure.[49a] The microscopic picture of this tissue is similar to that described by Aegerter as a type of hamartomatous proliferation of fibrous tissue. The Boyd type of dual onlay graft has been advocated by several authors in the past.[10, 11] Several additional bone grafting procedures are available for this particular problem, but the clinician must always be aware that the incidence of success following bone grafting procedures in a true

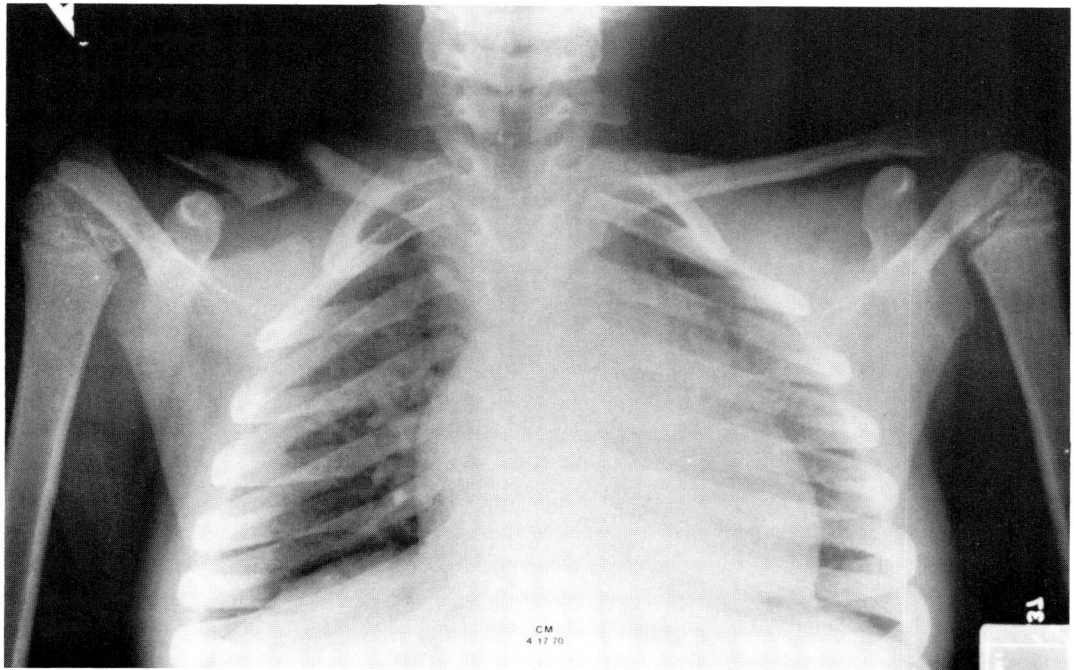

Figure 4–8 Congenital pseudarthrosis of the right clavicle.

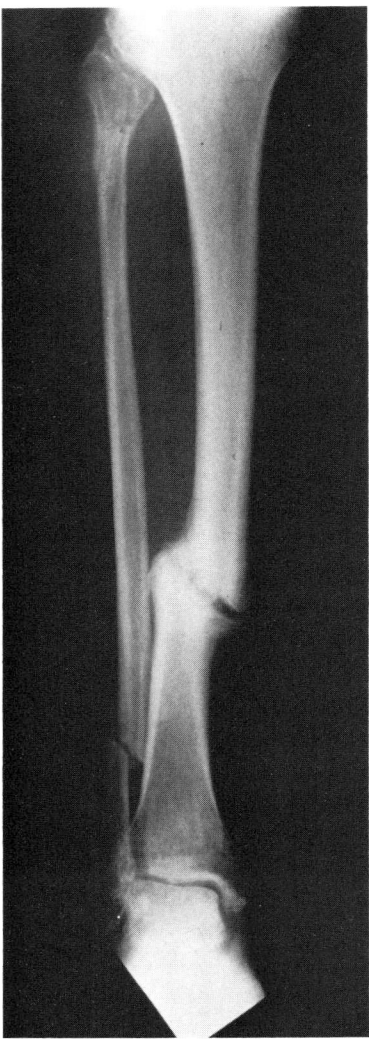

Figure 4-9   A tibial pseudarthrosis. Joint fluid was present, and the pseudarthrosis site had to be excised prior to bone grafting.

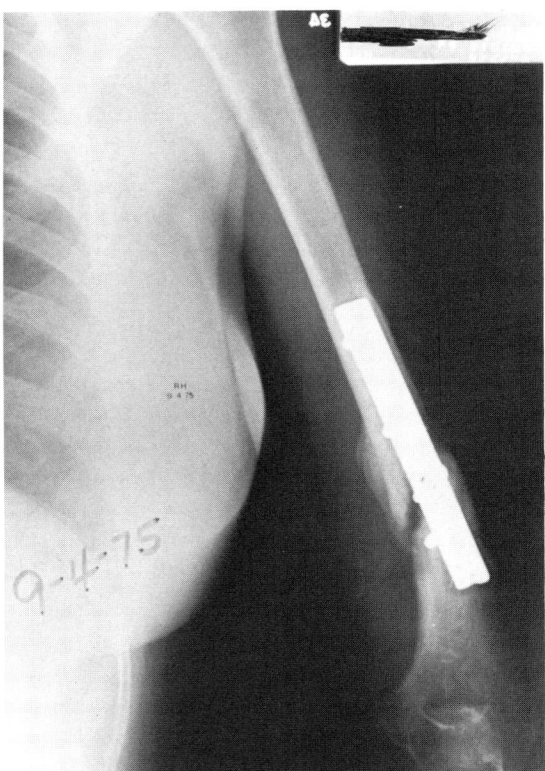

Figure 4-10   Anteroposterior view of a distal humeral fracture that had been initially treated with open reduction and a compression plating procedure. A true pseudarthrosis developed.

congenital pseudarthrosis of the tibia is poor. The parents of these patients must be forewarned that several types of procedures may be required and that ultimately an amputation may be the final result. Recent work with the use of electrical stimulation for this particular problem has had some encouraging results but will require further evaluation before this type of treatment can be advocated.

Congenital pseudarthrosis of the clavicle has also received recent attention (Fig. 4–8). Attempts have been made to correlate this condition with other problems in growth.

The clavicle normally develops from two separate ossification centers, one medial and one lateral. It has been suggested that the pseudarthrosis could be explained by failure of ossification of the precartilaginous bridge that connects the two masses during normal development. The congenital defect frequently will produce an unsightly deformity as well as causing hypermobility of the shoulder girdle. Like other pseudarthroses, this problem will not go on to spontaneous resolution without some type of surgical intervention. Most authors feel that a bone grafting procedure should be carried out before the age of eight years.

Acquired Pseudarthrosis

As with congenital pseudarthrosis, one of the major sites for acquired pseudarthrosis is the distal portion of the tibia (Fig. 4–9). The exact reason why this particular bone shows predilection for both the congenital and acquired types of pseudarthrosis has never been completely understood. Pseudarthrosis in this area is associated with pain, increased instability, and bowing at the site of the defect. In the past, the characteristic roentgenographic picture of acquired pseudarthrosis was that of sclerotic margins at the bone ends and an actual capping or shutting off of the medullary canal associated with a lytic area between the bony fragments. Recent studies,[16] however, have demonstrated that the sclerotic

margins are not always present in this condition. Several cases of pseudarthrosis have been seen in which there were open clear margins at the defect site and what appeared to be a relatively normal medullary canal. Bone scans have been useful in some cases to demonstrate an increased uptake of the radioisotope at both the proximal and distal margins of the pseudarthrosis site with a cold spot directly over the actual pseudarthrosis site. If this picture is present, it definitely suggests a pseudarthrosis. It appears that it is possible to differentiate in this manner between true nonunion and pseudarthrosis. Further correlative studies are required, but this asso-

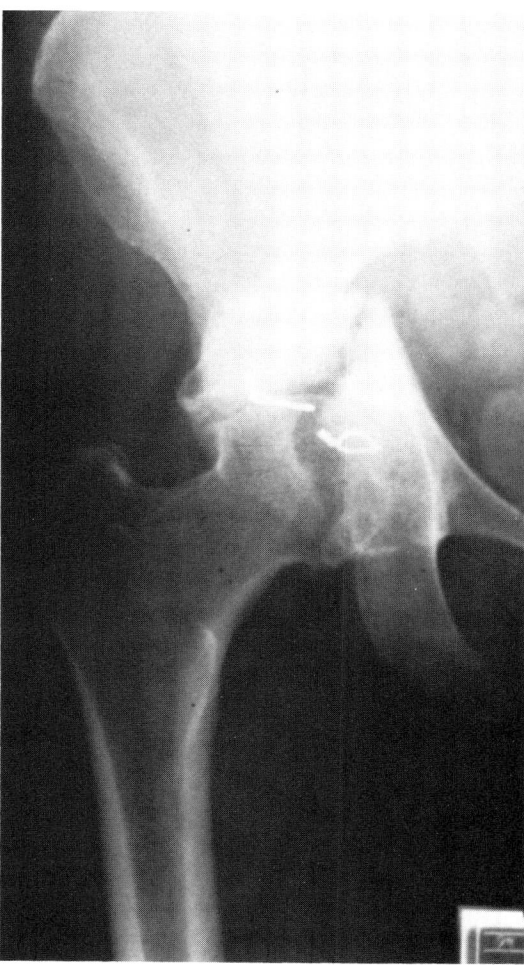

Figure 4–11 A femoral fracture was initially treated with a compression plate. Infection was judged to be a factor in the development of a pseudarthrosis.

Figure 4–12 A pseudarthrosis at the site of a prior entral fracture of the acetabulum.

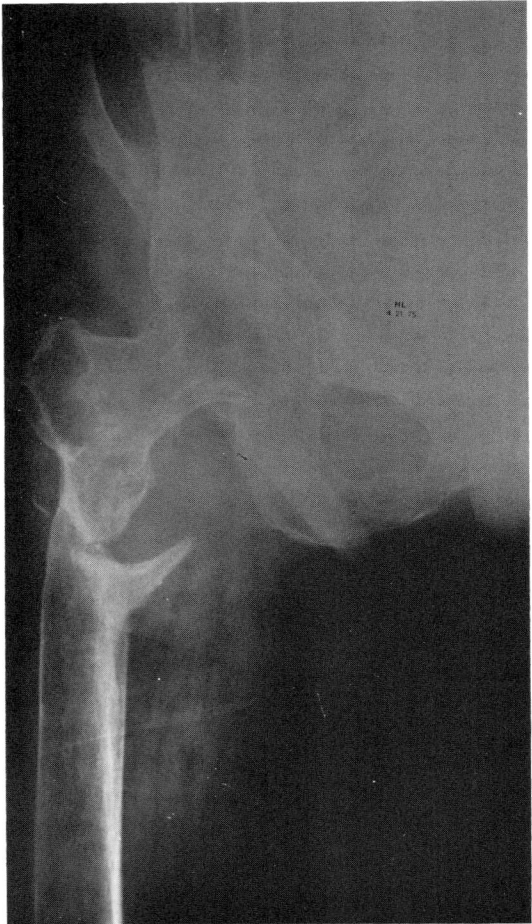

Figure 4–13 An unusual complication of a subtrochanteric fracture. A true pseudarthrosis was present. Note the severe osseous wasting both proximally and distally.

ciation appears to be valid at this particular time.

The tissue between the bone ends in a true pseudarthrosis must be surgically excised and a bone graft must be applied. This differs from the surgical management of a nonunion in that the interposed tissue in the latter does not have to be excised. It is not difficult to differentiate between nonunion and pseudarthrosis at the time of surgical intervention, as joint fluid is present between the fracture fragments in a true pseudarthrosis. At the present time pseudarthrosis has been treated with surgical excision of the intervening soft-tissue structure between the bone ends, resection of

the actual joint margins, and application of rigid internal fixation with a compression plate and a bone grafting procedure (Figs. 4–10 through 4–13).

Recent investigative work with the application of induced electrical potentials combined with resection of the interposing soft tissues has provided encouraging results to date. The beneficial effects are not seen, however, if the interposing soft tissue is not resected before application of the electrical stimulation. This particular form of treatment will have to await further investigative multicenter studies before widespread use of the technique can be justified.

References

1. Albee, F. H.: Principles of the treatment of non-union of fracture. Surg. Gynec. Obstet., 51:289, 1930.
2. Anderson, L. D.: Treatment of ununited fractures of the long bones; compression plate fixation and the effect of different types of internal fixation on fracture healing. J. Bone Joint Surg., 47A:191–208, 1965.
3. Anderson, R.: Delayed union and nonunion; 90% preventable. J. Bone Joint Surg., 25:427–45, 1943.
4. Altner, P. L.: An experimental study on the significance of muscle tissue interposition on fracture healing. Clin. Orthop., 111:269–273, 1975.
5. d'Aubigne, R. M.: Surgical treatment of non-union of long bones. J. Bone Joint Surg., 31A:256, 1949.
6. Bennett, G. E.: Fractures of the humerus with particular reference to nonunion and its treatment. Ann. Surg., 103:994, 1936.
7. Blumenfeld, I.: Pseudarthrosis of the long bones. J. Bone Joint Surg., 29:97, 1947.
8. Bohr, H.: Bone formation and resorption in cases of delayed union and pseudarthrosis. Acta Orthop. Scand., 42:113–121, 1971.
9. Bonfiglio, M., and Voke, E. M.: Aseptic necrosis of the femoral head and non-union of the femoral neck. Effect of treatment by drilling and bone grafting. (Phemister technique.) J. Bone Joint Surg., 50A:48, 1968.
10. Boyd, H. B.: Treatment of difficult and unusual non-unions with special reference to bridging of defects. J. Bone Joint Surg., 25:535–52, 1943.
11. Boyd, H. B.: Causes and treatment of non-union of the shafts of the long bones, with a review of 741 patients. AAOS Instructional Course Lectures. 17:165–83, 1960.
12. Boyd, H. B.: Changing concepts in the treatment of nonunion. Clin. Orthop., 43:37–54, 1965.
13. Brashear, H. R.: Treatment of ununited fractures of the long bones; diagnosis and prevention of nonunion. J. Bone Joint Surg., 47A:174–178, 1965.

14. Brickner, W. M.: Metal bone plating; a factor in nonunion, autoplastic bone grafting to execute osteogenesis in nonunion of fractures. Am. J. Surg., 28:16–20, 1914.

15. Brighton, C. T.: Direct-current stimulation of nonunion and congenital pseudarthrosis; exploration of its clinical application. J. Bone Joint Surg., 57A:368–377, 1975.

16. Brighton, C. T.: Personal communication.

17. Brighton, C. T.: Friedenberg, Z. B., Mitchell, E. I., and Booth, R. E.: Treatment of nonunion with constant direct current. Clin. Orthop., 124:106–123, 1977.

18. deBuren, N.: Causes and treatment of nonunion in fractures of the radius and ulna. J. Bone Joint Surg., 44B:614, 1962.

19. Campbell, W. C.: Transference of the fibula as an adjunct to free bone graft in the tibial deficiency. J. Orthop. Surg., 1:625, 1919.

20. Campbell, W. C.: Malunited fractures. Surg. Gynecol. Obstet., 66:466, 1938.

21. Carrell, W. B.: Transplantation of the fibula in the same leg. J. Bone Joint Surg., 20:627, 1938.

22. Charnley, J.: Surgical treatment of ununited fractures. J. Bone Joint Surg., 42B:3–4, 1960.

23. Christensen, N. O.: Küntscher intramedullary reaming and nail fixation for non-union of fracture of the femur and the tibia. J. Bone Joint Surg., 55B:312–318, 1973.

24. Cleveland, M.: Treatment of non-union in compound fractures with infection. J. Bone Joint Surg., 34A:555–563, 1952.

25. Coleman, H. M., Bateman, J. E., Dale, G. M., and Starr, D. E.: Cancellous bone grafts for infected bone defects; single procedure. Surg. Gynecol. Obstet., 83:392, 1946.

26. Connelly, J. R.: Pedicle coverage in non-union. Plast. Reconstr. Surg., 3:727–39, 1948.

27. Cotton, F. J.: Non-union of fractures of long bones (treatment by bone transplantation). N. Engl. J. Med., 201:895–982, 1929.

28. Coventry, M. B.: Phemister bone graft in ununited fractures of the long bones. Clin. Orthop., 2:194–202, 1953.

29. Crawford, R. R.: A history of the treatment of non-union of fractures in the 19th century in the United States. J. Bone Joint Surg., 55A:1685–1697, 1973.

30. Davis, A. G.: Pin distraction as a cause of nonunion. J. Bone Joint Surg., 25:631–43, 1943.

31. Darrach, W.: Forward dislocation at the inferior radioulnar joint, with fracture of the lower third of the shaft of the radius. Ann. Surg., 56:801, 1912.

32. Farrow, R. C.: Summary of results of bone grafting for war injuries. J. Bone Joint Surg., 30A:31–39, 1948.

33. Freeland, A. E.: Posterior bone grafting for infected ununited fracture of the tibia. J. Bone Joint Surg., 58A:653–657, 1976.

34. French, P. R.: Varus deformity of the elbow following supracondylar fractures of the humerus in children. Lancet, 1:439, 1959.

35. Hanson, L. W., and Eppright, R. H.: Posterior bone grafting of the tibia for nonunion. A review of twenty-four cases. J. Bone Joint Surg., 48A:27, 1966.

36. Harkins, H. N.: Simplified technique of onlay grafts for all fractures in acceptable position. J.A.M.A., 109:1501–1506, 1937.

37. Heiple, K. G.: The pathologic physiology of nonunion. Clin. Orthop., 43:11–21, 1965.

38. Hellstadius, A.: Clinical study of causation of pseudarthrosis of diaphysis of long bones of extremities. Acta Chir. Scand., 73:111–160, 1933.

39. Henderson, M. S.: The treatment of ununited fractures of the tibia by the transplantation of bone. Ann. Surg., 59:486, 1914.

40. Henderson, M. S.: Bone graft in ununited fractures. J. Bone Joint Surg., 20:635, 1938.

41. Hicks, J. H.: Rigid fixation as a treatment for hypertrophic nonunion. Injury, 8:199–205, 1977.

42. Hohl, M.: Treatment of ununited fractures of the long bones; surgical treatment and technique. J. Bone Joint Surg., 47A:179–190, 1965.

43. Jones, K. G., and Barnett, H. C.: Cancellous bone grafting for non-union of the tibia through the posterolateral approach. J. Bone Joint Surg., 37A:1250, 1955.

44. Judet, P. R.: Muscle pedicle bone grafting of long bones by osteoperiosteal decortication. Clin. Orthop., 87:74–80, 1972.

45. Judet, R.: An approach to bony union. Clin. Orthop., 103:95, 1974.

46. Kostwik, J. P.: Treatment of infected ununited femoral shaft fractures. Clin. Orthop., 108:90–94, 1975.

47. Lacey, J. T.: Nonunion of fractures; experimental study. Ann. Surg., 89:813–848, 1929.

48. Loomer, R.: Nonunion in fractures of the humeral shaft. Injury, 74:274–278, 1976.

49. Matti, H.: Technic and results of my operation for pseudoarthrosis. Zbl. Chir., 63:1442, 1936; J. Bone Joint Surg., 19:870, 1937.

49a. McElvenny, R. T.: Congenital pseudo-arthrosis of the tibia. Q. Bull. Northwest. Univ. Med. Sch., 23:413, 1949.

50. McMaster, P. E.: Bone atrophy and absorption; experimental observations. (Nonunion of fibular defects.) J. Bone Joint Surg., 19:74–83, 1937.

51. McMaster, P. E.: Tibiofibular cross-peg grafting. J. Bone Joint Surg., 57A:720–721, 1975.

52. Meyer, S.: The treatment of infected nonunion of fractures of long bones. Study of sixty-four cases with a five to twenty-five year followup. J. Bone Joint Surg., 57A:836–842, 1975.

53. Meyerding, H. W.: Malunion of the radius and ulna preventing closing of the hand and flexion of the wrist. Surg. Clin. North Am., 12:874, 1932.

54. Milch, H.: Cuff resection of the ulna for malunited Colles' fracture. J. Bone Joint Surg., 23:311, 1941.

55. Milch, H.: Tibiofibular synostosis for non-union of the tibia. Surgery, 27:770–79, 1950.

56. Murray, C. R.: Delayed and nonunion in fractures in the adult. Ann. Surg., 93:961, 1931.

57. Murray, G.: End results of bone grafting for non-union. J. Bone Joint Surg., 28:749–56, 1946.

58. Murray, W. R., Lucas, D. B., and Inman, V. T.: Treatment of non-union of fractures of the long bones by the two-plate method. J. Bone Joint Surg., 46A:1027, 1964.

59. Nicoll, E. A.: The treatment of gaps in long bones

by cancellous insert grafts. J. Bone Joint Surg., *38B*:70, 1956.

60. Nilsonne, V.: The distribution of mineral salt in non-union of fractures. Acta Orthop. Scand., *31*:81–89, 1961.

61. Phemister, D. B.: Treatment of ununited fractures by onlay bone grafts without screw or tie fixation and without breaking down of the fibrous union. J. Bone Joint Surg., 29:946, 1947.

62. Phemister, D. B.: Biologic principles in healing of fractures and their bearing on treatment. (Edward D. Churchill Lecture.) Ann. Surg., *133*: 433–46, 1951.

63. Sarmiento, A.: A functional below-the-knee cast for tibial fractures. J. Bone Joint Surg., *49A*:855–875, 1967.

64. Sarmiento, A.: A functional below-the-knee brace for tibial fractures. A report on its use in 135 cases. J. Bone Joint Surg., 52A:295–311, 1970.

65. Sarmiento, A.: Functional bracing of tibial and femoral shaft fractures. Clin. Orthop., 82:2–13, 1972.

66. Sarmiento, A.: Functional bracing of tibial fractures. Clin. Orthop., *105*:202–219, 1974.

67. Sarmiento, A., Cooper, J. S., and Sinclair, W. F.: Forearm fractures and early functional bracing—a preliminary report. J. Bone Joint Surg., *57A*:297–304, 1975.

68. Sarmiento, A., Pratt, G. W., Berry, N. C., and Sinclair, W. F.: Colles' fractures. Functional bracing in supination. J. Bone Joint Surg., *57A*:311–317, 1975.

69. Sarmiento, A., Kinman, P. B., Galvin, E. G., Schmitt, R. H., and Phillips, J. G.: Functional bracing of fractures of the shaft of the humerus. J. Bone Joint Surg., *59A*:596–601, 1977.

70. Segmuller, G.: Diagnostic use of 85 strontium in the preoperative evaluation of nonunion. Acta Orthop. Scand., *41*:150–160, 1970.

71. Solheim, K.: Delayed union and nonunion of fractures: Clinical experience with the A.S.I.F. method. J. Trauma, *13*:121–128, 1973.

72. Sorenson, K. H.: Treatment of delayed union and nonunion of the tibia by fibular resection. Acta Orthop. Scand., *40*:92–104, 1969.

73. Souter, W. A.: Autogenous cancellous strip grafts in the treatment of delayed union of long bone fractures. J. Bone Joint Surg., *51B*:63–75, 1969.

74. Speed, J. S., and Boyd, H. B.: Operative reconstruction of malunited fractures about the ankle joint. J. Bone Joint Surg., *18*:270, 1936.

75. Thompson, A.: The application of rigid-internal fixation to the treatment of nonunion and delayed union using the AO technique. Injury, *8:3*:188–198, 1977.

76. Trueta, J.: Nonunion of fractures. Clin. Orthop., *43*:23–25, 1965.

77. Turner, H.: Probable causes of nonunion. J. Bone Joint Surg., *18*:581–93, 1936.

78. Urist, M. R.: The pathogenesis and treatment of delayed union and nonunion; A survey of 85 ununited fractures of the shaft of the tibia and 100 control cases with similar injuries. J. Bone Joint Surg., *36A*:931–980, 1954.

79. Watson-Jones, R.: Fractures and Joint Injuries. Edinburgh and London, E. & S. Livingstone, Ltd., 1955.

80. Wray, J. B.: Treatment of ununited fractures of the long bones; factors in the pathogenesis of non-union. J. Bone Joint Surg., *47A*:168–173, 1965.

R. BRUCE HEPPENSTALL, M.D.

Bone ——————————————————— 5
Grafting

Bone grafting is a common procedure for the treatment of various delayed unions, nonunions, pseudarthrosis, and osseous defects. It has been estimated that more than 200,000 bone grafts are performed in the United States each year. Although it is so frequently employed, few hard facts are known about the physiological processes that take place at the cell level in bone grafting. Bone was one of the first organs to be transplanted; the first recorded successful bone implant was performed in the year 1688.

Duhamel[27] has been credited with the first scientific approach to the study of osteogenesis. He found that silver wires placed in a subperiosteal location were covered with new bone several weeks after implantation. It was his belief that the new bone was produced from the periosteum. It remained for Ollier,[27] in the mid 1800's, to evaluate further the potential of the periosteum. He concluded from his experiments that transplanted periosteum and bone were viable and under the right circumstances had the ability to be osteogenic. Barth,[27] however, working with replanted bone from the skull, reported that all transplanted bone, marrow, and periosteum died and were replaced by ingrowth from the surrounding tissue.

Of the earliest descriptions of bone transplantation, the most comprehensive and accurate as applied to modern treatment is credited to Axhausen. He performed an excellent set of experiments in 1907 and formulated the principle that the periosteum has great ability to survive and that there is osteogenic activity in autografts.[5]

His view was that periosteum-covered transplants have the potential for clinical application in orthopedic surgery. It is interesting that present-day knowledge of the histological fate of transplanted bone accords very closely with the views originally expressed by Axhausen.

It remained for Phemister to expand the description of the histological changes of bone grafting and to introduce the term "creeping substitution." He felt that the transplanted bone was replaced through a mechanism of invasion of the bone graft by active vascular granulation tissue. The old bone was removed by resorption, and new bone was then actively produced.[59] In 1947 Abbott and co-workers reemphasized the fact that surface cells may survive in the bone graft and participate in active new bone formation.[1]

The role of active viable osteocytes in new bone formation has been further expanded by two recent studies. In 1963 Ray and Sabet were able to demonstrate that bone cells could survive in homografts and isografts. They labeled rat cells with tritiated thymidine. This substance tags cells undergoing DNA synthesis, including marrow cells. The labeled bone was then transplanted into a subcutaneous bed in a host that was not labeled. Ten days later the labeled osteocytes were found scattered throughout the bone graft. This meant that the cells in the bone graft had survived the transplantation.[63]

In a separate experiment reported in 1964, Arora and Laskin used sex chromatin as a cellular label of osteogenesis in bone grafts. They were able to demonstrate that osseous cells within the bone graft survived transplantation. The current feeling in regard to cell survival in bone grafts is that the superficial cells may survive the transplantation but that most of the transplanted bone dies, undergoes resorption, and is replaced by new bone formation. The exact quantity of cells that survive transplantation has never been adequately documented. This quantity, however, also depends on the method employed to obtain the bone graft, the type of bone selected for grafting, and physical factors in the handling of the graft prior to implantation.

HISTOLOGICAL SEQUENCE OF OSSEOUS REPAIR

During the initial stages of osseous repair a similar pattern is noted for both cortical and cancellous transplants. Edema associated with an initial inflammatory response is evident. Most of the bone is necrotic owing to lack of blood supply. It has been adequately documented that bone cells are unable to survive without adequate nutrition, and because of the particular organizational structure of bone, the nourishment that reaches the cells within the graft is limited. The innermost cells can obtain nourishment only through the haversian canal and the canaliculi. Therefore, the only cells that appear to survive are the most peripheral ones that can obtain nutrition from the surrounding tissue. The necrotic tissue in the deep haversian canals and marrow spaces is removed by invading macrophages. An ingrowth of granulation tissue to replace the areas of resorption then occurs. This consists of minute capillaries and primitive mesenchymal tissue. The mesenchymal tissue ingrowth is limited by the forward advance of the fine capillaries, as the cells are unable to survive at any significant distance from the accompanying capillary blood supply. Similar situations exist in both soft-tissue and osseous repair, as outlined in Chapters 1 and 2. This stage continues for at least two weeks, and no particular difference between cortical and cancellous bone grafts is evident at this stage.

In cancellous bone the primitive mesenchymal cells rapidly differentiate into osteogenic cells. The majority of these osteogenic cells are supplied from the host. A seam of osteoid is deposited along the edges of the dead trabeculi by active osteoblast formation. The central portion of the bone is necrotic, and absorption occurs through osteoclastic activity. The gross anatomical architecture of the bone is relatively unchanged as the old necrotic matrix is actively replaced by trabeculi of living bone. The last stage involves replacement of the old marrow spaces by active new marrow cells. Once this occurs the reparative effort is complete.

Cortical bone transplants have a slightly different process of repair. Ingrowth of active vascular granulation tissue occurs, but this phase is much more prolonged than in cancellous bone. The haversian canals are converted into small marrow spaces by osteoclastic resorption of the exposed borders. Invading granulation tissue and primitive mesenchymal tissue fill the large cavities produced in this manner. This process continues until the spaces reach a predetermined size, when the resorption appears to cease and reparative processes predominate as obsteoblasts fill the space with active osteoid tissue. This new bone deposition on the peripheral aspect limits the amount of osteoclasis occurring within the inner necrotic matrix. It is due to this mechanism that the necrotic cortical bone contains many small inner osteons of active new bone formation. Therefore, since the process is not uniform, the peripheral aspect of the bone is actively replaced but replacement of the inner portion is limited.

The physical state of the transplanted bone governs the histological sequence of repair, as evident from the slightly different sequences in cortical and cancellous bone, as previously outlined. Enneking and co-workers have demonstrated that cortical bone grafts are structurally weakened by internal porosity at six weeks and that they remain weak for at least six months. It is only at one year that the graft appears to approach recovery of mechanical strength, and then only approximately 60 per cent of the structure is composed of new bone. Resorption accounts for the early porosity in the grafts. The strength appears to be related to the porosity rather than to the admixture of necrotic and living bone.[37] These studies have recently been expanded by Burchardt and co-workers, who demonstrated that drill holes placed in experimental autologous cortical bone grafts did not appear to accelerate the process of repair in the graft. The drill holes were rapidly filled with cancellous bone, which matured to cortical bone within 12 weeks post-grafting. The holes did not appear to weaken the transplant mechanically at the time of surgery. Microradiography and tetracycline labeling of drilled and undrilled grafts demonstrated similar biological reparative patterns. These authors felt that drilling holes perpendicularly through overlapping portions of an onlay segmental graft and the host bone could possibly lead to early formation of biological pegs to enhance the graft-host union.[15]

SURVIVAL OF BONE GRAFT

Physical Factors

Several physical factors in the handling of the bone graft prior to its implantation in the host site appear to be important. Every effort should be made to place the bone graft into the recipient bed as soon as possible. It has been demonstrated that exposure of a bone graft to the surrounding atmosphere for 30 minutes or more decreases the number of viable cells within the graft. For this reason the graft is not obtained until the recipient bed has been adequately prepared to receive it. Thus the least amount of time elapses between obtaining the graft and placing it in the recipient bed.

Once the bone graft has been obtained, it is important to keep it wrapped in a sponge soaked with the patient's blood. Saline is not an appropriate solution for storage of the bone graft. The blood-soaked sponge appears to have a protective effect on cell survival in the graft and it also eliminates the adverse effect of the high-intensity operating room lights. The lights produce high temperatures as well as bright light, and if the temperature rises above 42° C, damage to the superficial osseous cells may occur. Antibiotic solutions should be avoided, as these also may be detrimental to cell survival.[8]

The thickness of the graft appears to be important. If cancellous bone is obtained, the thickness of the graft should be limited to less than 5 mm. This will provide maximum exposure of superficial osseous cells and allow for rapid ingrowth of peripheral vascular tissue. The bone graft is then placed in close proximity to the host bed, and every attempt is made to eliminate any obvious dead space. It is the author's feeling that if a mixed bone graft is obtained with a cortical surface on one side and a cancellous surface on the opposite side, the orientation of the graft is important to its survival. The cancellous portion should be placed facing the surrounding soft-tissue structures. It must be kept in mind that the graft is replaced by an ingrowth of vascular tissue; if the cancellous surface is exposed to a surrounding bed of vascular soft tissue, this will occur at a more rapid rate than if it is placed into the bone defect site.

Bassett has demonstrated in vitro that compression forces favor specialization of osteoblasts while tension forces favor osteoclasts and fibroblasts. He also demonstrated that a sheet of Silastic placed over the bone graft area between the graft and the surrounding soft tissue would prevent the ingrowth of fresh vascular tissue. Cartilage tended to form in the area instead of the new bone that would have formed without the interposing Silastic membrane.[7-10]

Siffert and Barash found that the best results with bone grafts were obtained when the grafts were inserted into a 7-day-old bed in the rabbit or a 10-day-old bed in the dog. Iliac bone graft appeared to be incorporated more rapidly when the implant was delayed. These authors felt that the large hematoma dead space had been avoided by delaying the transplant and that the conditions for osteogenic stimulation were greatly improved under these circumstances.[68] This observation has been reinforced by several studies involving preparation of the host site two to three weeks prior to actual bone graft procedures. This mechanism is similar to secondary healing in soft tissue.

Origin of Callus Calcium

The origin of callus calcium was extensively investigated by Cohen and associates.[29] They performed radioactive calcium tracer studies in order to evaluate the origin of the calcium. [45]Calcium solutions were injected into dogs, and the single element, calcium, was traced in the grafting procedure in which homogeneous grafts of refrigerated bone were placed in the dogs. The data from this study demonstrated that under the experimental conditions the calcium of the graft entered the blood and was distributed in a manner indistinguishable from that of calcium entering the blood from other sources. There was no evidence of local preferential transfer of calcium to the callus from grafts or from bone stores adjacent to the grafted area. It was the feeling of these investigators that all the data could be used to support the hypothesis that the calcium in the callus was entirely derived from the serum. Dogs receiving nonradioactive grafts and injections of [45]calcium demonstrated that the greater specific activity was observed in the bone, was up to 100 times that of the diffuse component of the host's cortical bone, and was strongly dependent on the relationship between the time of injection and the time of grafting. The calcification of the callus occurred predominantly at about the third week after grafting. Therefore, according to the evidence presented by this study, all the calcium incorporated into the callus came via the circulating blood from skeletal sources situated throughout the body rather than by diffusion from the graft.[29]

Immune Response

A new terminology has evolved for designating transplanted tissues (Table 5–1). In the past it was felt that bone marrow was osteogenic, that autografts were superior to homografts (allografts), and that heterografts (xenografts) failed to survive. The new terminology for transplantation in regard to bone employs the terms "autograft" and "allograft." Autograft refers to tissue from genetically similar individuals of the same species. Allograft refers to tissue from genetically disparate individuals of the same species.

The immune reaction is the result of both a cellular reaction mediated by lymphocytic infiltration and a humorally mediated reaction involving antibodies. In a set of experiments to evaluate the immune response to bone allograft in rats, Muscolo and co-workers found evidence for both a cellular and a humoral immune reaction against the grafts. Complete bone gave a stronger reaction, but marrow-free bone also showed great specific reactivity, suggesting that major histocompatibility antigens were present in bone itself. A gene-dose effect in response was present, since allogeneic grafts gave a stronger reaction than semi-allogeneic grafts. The hypersensitivity-type of humoral immune response was found in grafts in rats regrafted with allogeneic or semi-allogeneic bone. Therefore, it was the impression of these investigators that tissue matching for major transplantation antigen was needed if allogeneic bone grafts were to be used clinically.[55]

Burwell stated that the nucleated cells of bone marrow of fresh homografts (allografts) of cancellous bone were the antigenic component and that the cancellous allograft bone free of bone marrow and blood cells did not elicit in the recipient animal a cytological response associated with incompatability. It was his feeling that marrow-free allografts of cancellous bone that had been decalcified with hydrochloric acid or ethylenediamine tetra-acetic acid and stored by freezing or freeze-drying provided a nonantigenic, sterile, malleable, easily prepared and shaped material that

TABLE 5–1   Bone Graft Terminology

Old	New	Donor
Autograft	Autograft	Same individual
Isograft	Isograft	Identical twin or inbred strain
Homograft	Allograft	Same species (live)
Homoimplant	Alloimplant	Same species (dead)
Heterograft	Xenograft	Different species

acts as an optimal environment for pleurio-potential cells derived from bone marrow of the host to produce living bone.[17-20] Ray and associates performed a series of experiments that demonstrated that fresh autogenous grafts survived in the anterior chamber of the eyes of rats and guinea pigs and that over a period of six weeks new bone was laid down in association with the grafts. In contrast, grafts of fresh adult allograft bone to the anterior chamber of the eye underwent necrosis in the majority of instances and there was a lymphocytic plasma cell–fibroblastic response on the part of the host. Allografts of embryonic bone, however, did survive and grow. In the opinion of these authors, the best substitute for fresh autogenous bone grafts was the organic matrix of bone devoid of its inorganic salt. The presence of the inorganic salt impeded vascular invasion. Ray also felt that the early vascularization was dependent not only on viability of the graft but also on its physical characteristics. Cancellous grafts were vascularized sooner than cortical bone grafts. If cells were grafted that were genetically related to the host, the host connective tissue cells participated in subsequent bone formation, apparently by "induction," which can be demonstrated by 10 days following the transplant. If host and graft are not genetically related, vascular invasion occurs initially, but then the graft is rejected and the blood supply is lost.[62-64]

Friedlander and co-workers performed experiments on the antigenicity of bone to demonstrate that freeze-drying and to a lesser degree deep-freezing of bone allografts markedly reduced or abolished their ability to evoke an immune response in the graft recipient. Their studies revealed that cortical bone was less antigenic than cancellous bone. Fresh allografts of deep-frozen cortical and cancellous bone evoked humoral and cell-mediated immunity, whereas freeze-dried cortical bone allografts failed to sensitize the recipient and were the least antigenic of the allografts examined.[38]

Koskinen and co-workers evaluated the influence of somatotropin, thyrotropin, and cortisone on osteoinduction and osteogenesis of allogeneic bone matrix. Their results indicated that once osteoinduction occurred, growth hormone in combination with thyrotropin acted as a booster, while cortisone was a suppressor of osteogenesis. Growth hormone stimulated formation of protoplasm and increased protein synthesis. It also produced an increase in endosteal mass. Thyrotropin promoted maturation of bone and acted as a booster for the anabolic action of growth hormone.[53]

Goldberg and Lance evaluated the revascularization process and accretion in transplanted bone. They employed azathioprine to produce immunosuppression in rabbits and demonstrated that, with the immunosuppression, rabbits responded to a fresh allograft as if it were an autograft. Revascularization of the autograft proceeded rapidly for four weeks and peaked at six weeks. The new bone formation was maximal at three weeks but continued at a high rate after this time interval. Revascularization in new bone formation in the group treated with immunosuppression was greater than in the untreated group. It was felt that immunosuppression blocked the cell-mediated mechanism involved in immunity.[40] This study was important, as it revealed that the immune response to allografts could be modified with immunosuppressive medication. This has a direct clinical application.

Bank Bone

A bone bank has been developed by the Naval Tissue Laboratory in Bethesda, Maryland, that performs an important service in obtaining adequate bone for grafting and providing appropriate treatment of the bone to reduce the antigenic properties.[42] Several studies have revealed the beneficial effects of banked bone for the treatment of large simple bone cysts in the humerus in children. Recently there has been a definite attempt to perform en-bloc segmental resections of malignant tumors in an attempt to preserve the extremity. The resected bone is then replaced by a large segment of cadaver bone that has been treated by freeze-drying to eliminate any antigenic potential. This bone is also available from the Naval Tissue Bank for replacement of osseous defects in various locations. Compatibility tests can be performed to rule out bone unacceptable for grafting procedures.

The bone that is stored in various bone

banks in the United States is maintained by being frozen, freeze-dried, or freeze-dried and irradiation sterilized. The methods used in hospital bone banks have not changed over the past two decades. Amputations provide the main source for this bone. It is handled under sterile conditions and stripped of its soft tissue. Routine cultures are obtained prior to insertion of the bone into sterile plastic bags to be stored at −70° C. Urist has demonstrated that a delay in collection time of more than 12 hours will activate endogenous proteases. It was his feeling that immediate freeze-drying preserves bone morphogenetic property (BMP) and antigenic substances. Irradiation sterilization with more than 2.0 mrads, however, denatures bone morphogenetic property.[73-78]

Antigen-extracted allogeneic bone (AAA) has been recommended for various operative procedures in patients who are felt to be unacceptable candidates for autologous grafting. Use of this type of bone, however, requires full informed consent procedures as outlined by the National Institutes of Health in guidelines for medical research. The preparation of antigen-extracted allogeneic bone has been fully outlined by Urist.[76]

It is likely that in the future bone banks will play an increasing role in supplying appropriate bone for replacement of segmental and large osseous defects.

Vascular Pedicle Bone Grafts

Vascular pedicle grafts have been employed by plastic surgeons for many years to replace soft-tissue defects. Judet and Patel advocated the use of a muscle pedicle bone graft for the treatment of nonunion of the femoral neck in the hip. It was their feeling that if the bone could be transplanted with its attendant muscular attachments and vascular supply this would encourage new osteogenic potential.[51]

Recently, Doi and co-workers studied vascular pedicle rib grafts by transplanting a segment of the rib with its attendant artery and vein still attached.[34] They demonstrated that osteocytes do not die but remain viable. Creeping substitution did not occur in the pedicle grafts. This study was concerned with fine microvascular anastomosis of the vascular pedicles, but it also demonstrated an important fact: The osseous cells may survive if the blood supply is rapidly reconstituted. These findings have rejuvenated a concept that has an exciting future in regard to bone graft procedures.

Bone Induction

Osteoinduction is a process of differentiation of fibroblast-like migratory mesenchymal cells into osteoprogenitor cells on calcified tissue matrices that are demineralized in the course of resorption or predemineralized in vitro. This process in bone matrix has been thought to be regulated by a hypothetical morphogenetic insoluble polypeptide, specific enzymes, and an enzyme inhibitor. It has been suggested that the potential for bone cell differentiation may be enhanced by transfer of an osteoinductive or bone morphogenetic property inherent in the bone matrix. The morphogenetic property appears to be localized in the organic matrix, and the osseous morphogenetic response is felt to be due to migratory mesenchymal cells. Many facets of the morphogenetic property remain unknown. The critical components, however, appear to be insoluble noncollagenous bone morphogenetic protein (BMP), a proteolytic enzyme (BMPase), and a bone hydrophobic glycopeptide (HGP). The available data suggest that the morphogenetic protein is a low molecular weight noncollagenous polypeptide. Urist and co-workers have performed several studies in evaluating this particular substance.[76, 77]

The generation of structural bone appears to be regulated by the organic matrix. It has been demonstrated that implants of inorganic or denatured bone or nonbiological substances failed to produce bone in a standard muscle pouch. The organic matrix appears to have the ability to stimulate cells that have been preprogramed for differentiation of mesenchymal cells to osteoprogenitor cell populations. Treatment of human bone with sulfhydryl group enzyme inhibitors will elicit a morphogenetic response in extracellular sites in rats.

Chalmers and associates found that bone

decalcified with weak hydrochloric acid acts as a bone-inducing agent in soft tissues in rabbits. They also found that systemic heparin inhibits osteogenic induction by a mechanism similar to that involved in delaying fracture healing.[25, 26]

New and exciting research into the induction of new bone with various chemical substances is currently being performed. Electrical currents are also being vigorously investigated in regard to their effect in inducing bone formation at fracture sites and in areas of large osseous defects. This work is thoroughly discussed in Chapter 3.

DONOR SITES FOR BONE GRAFT

Iliac Bone Graft

Bone graft is commonly obtained from the iliac crest. The iliac crest is relatively subcutaneous and provides ample cancellous bone. Its surface has a natural curve between the anterior superior and posterior superior iliac spines. The anterior gluteal line is an osseous structure extending posteriorly from the anterior superior iliac spine toward the posterior inferior iliac spine. This marks the posterosuperior border of the origin of the gluteus minimus as well as the anteroinferior border of the origin of the gluteus medius. The posterior gluteal line extends downward from just above the posterior superior iliac spine toward the greater sciatic notch. The common posterior border of the origin of the gluteus medius and anterior border of the origin of the gluteus maximus is found in this location. The inferior gluteal line extends from the inferior portion of the anterior superior iliac crest backward toward the greater sciatic notch. Here the inferior border of the origin of the gluteus minimus is found. The insertion of the inguinal ligament is situated directly on the anterior superior iliac spine. The origin of the internal oblique muscle extends backward from the anterior superior iliac spine along the iliac crest for approximately one third of its surface. The middle third of the iliac crest is occupied by the origin of the latissimus dorsi muscle. The remaining third of the iliac crest extending along the posterior superior iliac spine is occupied by the origin of the gluteus maximus.

Just below and similar to the origin of the internal oblique, the insertion of the external oblique extends from the superior iliac spine along the iliac crest for approximately a third of the surface. The gluteus medius muscle origin occupies the main portion between the anterior and posterior gluteal lines. The gluteus minimus is found in a more inferior location extending between the anterior and the inferior gluteal lines. A thorough knowledge of these muscle origins and insertions is important in obtaining a bone graft from the iliac crest. Since the anterior superior iliac spine is in a relatively subcutaneous location, there is easy access to sufficient cancellous bone from the lateral surface of the iliac wing. An incision is made along the anterior iliac crest, extending posteriorly from the anterior superior spine. Here the origin of the internal oblique and the insertion of the external oblique will be found along the anterolateral margin. This interval is identified and an incision down to bone is made just below the insertion of the external oblique muscle. The glutei medius and minimus are then reflected subperiosteally to expose the lateral wing of the ilium. There is an excellent blood supply to the gluteal muscles and they must be carefully reflected subperiosteally from the ilium or a significant amount of bleeding will occur.

Once the gluteal muscles have been reflected, a large osteotome is selected to outline a window in the lateral surface of the ilium from which to obtain the bone graft. It is frequently useful to make longitudinal parallel osteotomy cuts along the lateral surface of the ilium to remove the superficial cortical osseous structure. A curved osteotome is then utilized to reflect the cortical surface in a superior to inferior direction (Fig. 5–1). This will expose sufficient cancellous bone between the inner and outer tables of the ilium. Satisfactory strips of cancellous bone can then be removed with a curved gouge. The gouge is directed into the cancellous bone and the bone is removed by a pronation-supination movement of the operator's wrist. Care must be taken not to violate the inner table of the ilium, or a muscular hernia may result. Care must also be taken not to extend the subperiosteal dissection down to the sciatic notch, where the sciatic nerve may be in-

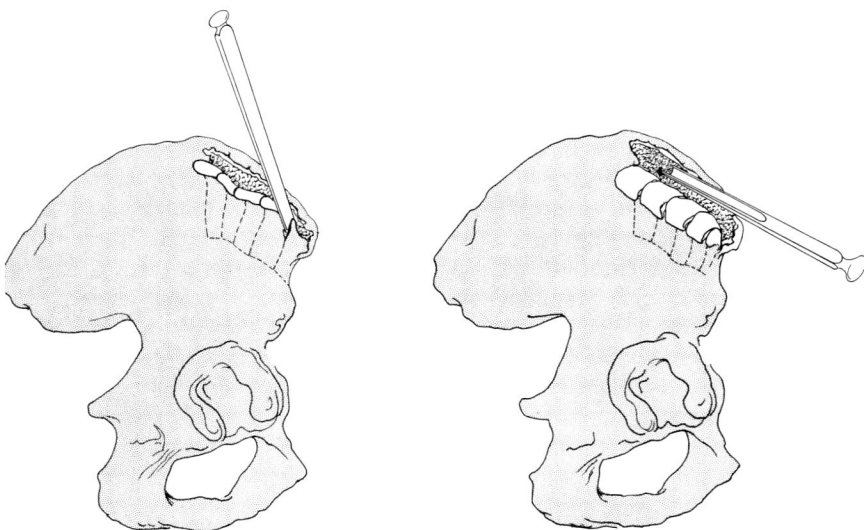

Figure 5–1 Technique of obtaining iliac crest bone graft. The curved gouge is useful in obtaining strips of cancellous bone.

jured. The blood supply in this location is abundant, and it is very difficult to control hemorrhage that occurs inferiorly in the incision.

If additional graft is required, the dissection may be extended toward the posterior superior iliac crest, where the ilium is slightly thicker. Here care must be taken not to violate the sacroiliac joint; failure to observe this caution may cause joint instability at a later date. The hemorrhage from the bone graft site should be controlled with temporary packing with a warm moist sponge. Once the graft has been obtained, the wound is closed in an orderly fashion. It is important to provide for adequate wound drainage, as significant bleeding from the bone graft site can produce a large hematoma in this location. To avoid this, the author finds it very useful to insert a Hemovac drain prior to closure. The gluteal muscles are sutured back to the anterior superior surface of the iliac wing and the subcutaneous tissues and skin are closed in a routine fashion. The Hemovac drain is removed at 24 hours, provided that the drainage has been decreasing.

Tibial Graft

Obtaining bone graft from the tibia should be avoided if at all possible. This method structurally weakens the tibia, and this produces definite stress concentrations that may cause the tibia to fracture with weight bearing. If the iliac crest donor site is not available, however, graft may be taken from the anteromedial surface of the tibia. A slightly curved longitudinal incision is placed over the anteromedial aspect to expose the osseous surface. The periosteum is then reflected, exposing the surface of the bone between the crest and the medial border. The proximal portion of the tibia tends to be wider than the distal portion, and therefore the graft is usually rectangular and wider at the proximal end than at the distal end. Drill holes are placed at each corner of the anticipated graft site area to reduce the stress concentration when the graft is being removed. A power saw can then be employed to remove the graft by cutting the cortex at a slightly oblique angle, which will help to preserve the anterior and medial borders of the tibia. It is important not to overcut the graft beyond the predrilled holes, as this may weaken the donor bone and increase the likelihood of a future fracture. The graft is then pried from its bed with care not to pop it out of the bed onto the floor. Additional cancellous bone may be obtained from the proximal end of the tibia with a curette. The periosteum and the deep portion of the subcutaneous tissues are then closed as a single layer.

It is extremely important to stress to the

patient that this procedure does structurally weaken the donor bone and care must be taken to avoid a fracture at the donor site. It is for this reason that full weight bearing is avoided in the postoperative period. Patients may be allowed protective weight bearing for at least four to six weeks during convalescence.

Fibular Graft

The fibula is a relatively subcutaneous structure and may fairly easily be used for a structurally sound graft. The middle third to half of the fibula may be removed without any untoward effects. Care must be taken not to extend the graft so far distally that it violates the tibiofibular syndesmosis. For this reason, the distal fourth of the fibula must remain intact to provide a stable ankle. The graft may be obtained through a slightly modified Henry approach. The dissection extends down along the anterior

surface of the septum that naturally occurs between the peroneus longus and soleus muscles. The peroneal musculature is reflected anteriorly by subperiosteal dissection. Since the origin of the muscle fibers naturally occurs in an oblique direction, the periosteal stripping is initiated at a distal point and extended proximally. The appropriate length of the graft is then determined, and drill holes are placed through the fibula at the proximal and distal ends of the graft. The author has found a Gigli saw useful for removal of the graft because the graft is not crushed at the proximal and distal ends. Occasionally there is a small amount of bleeding along the posterior surface of the fibula near the middle due to severance of the nutrient artery that enters at this location. This small artery may have to be ligated to control hemorrhage. It is important to bear in mind that the peroneal nerve is located along the proximal end of the fibula; care must be taken to retract this nerve anteriorly to avoid nerve damage. The fibula makes an excellent strut graft, as described later.

BONE GRAFTING TECHNIQUES

Single Onlay Graft

This graft technique was commonly employed prior to the development of the present-day inert metals that provide for stability (Figs. 5–2 and 5–3). It was felt that the cortical onlay graft supplied some stability as well as providing bone for osteogenesis. It was, however, usually supplemented with cancellous bone chips to stimulate osteogenesis. Campbell and Henderson[27] in the early 1900's adopted this technique for the treatment of nonunions.

The surface of the recipient bone is cleared of all scar tissue, and the periosteal surface may be decorticated to provide an adequate osseous surface to receive the graft. An alternative method is to drill small holes along the surface where the onlay graft is to be inserted to encourage ingrowth of new vascular tissue. If the ends of the bone to be united are sclerotic, the medullary cavities should be reamed back to relatively normal marrow. This also will encourage a new blood supply. The large

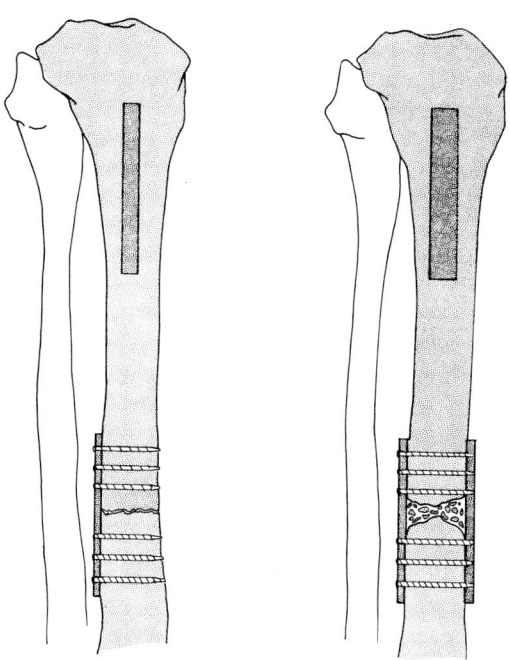

Figure 5–2 Single onlay and dual onlay grafts. The popularity of the single onlay graft has decreased in recent years. In some centers, the dual onlay graft is still popular for the treatment of pseudarthrosis and the management of severely comminuted fractures with bone loss.

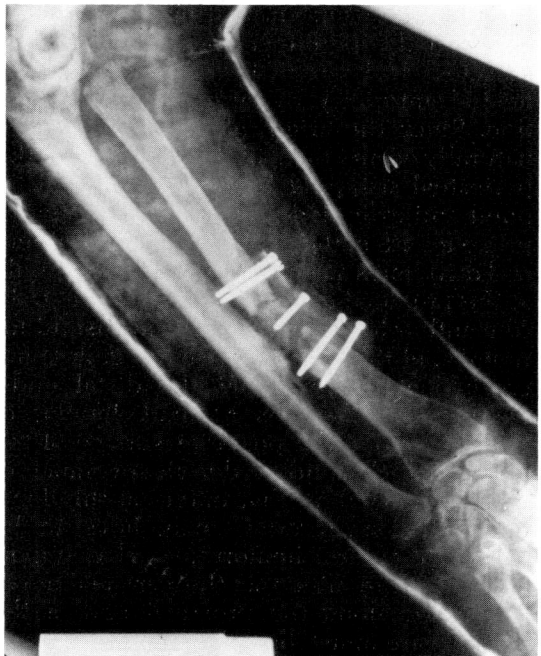

Figure 5-3 An example of a single onlay bone graft used to span a radial fracture with bone loss.

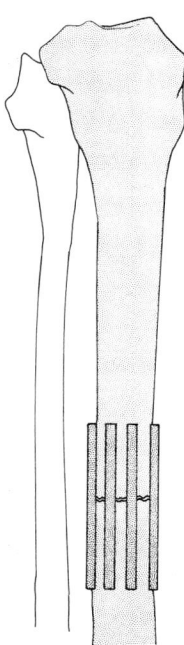

Figure 5-4 Cancellous bone strips may be placed across the fracture site to stimulate osteogenesis.

cortical graft is then obtained from the surface of the tibia or from the fibula. The graft is placed across the site of nonunion or bridging an osseous gap and is held in position until drill holes are fashioned through the graft and into the recipient bone to accept appropriate compression screws. It usually requires two or three screws on each side of the nonunion site or osseous defect to fix the graft. If cortical screws are selected, it is important that they extend through the graft and both cortices of the fragment. This graft is usually supplemented with cancellous bone, which may be obtained from the proximal portion of the tibia if the onlay graft has been obtained from the tibial surface. This type of graft may be employed in addition to a compression plate. It is particularly useful when a defect exists in the recipient bone. The defective area may be filled in with cancellous bone under the cortical onlay graft.

Postoperatively a gutter plaster splint may be applied to protect the site of nonunion or osseous defect. The gutter splint is selected to allow for some swelling in the surrounding soft-tissue structures. If a well-molded

cast is applied and is not bivalved or split, serious swelling may occur under the cast and produce neurovascular compromise.

Phemister described a technique in which osseous bone graft was placed subperiostally across the major bone fragment to provide an osteogenic stimulus (Fig. 5-4). These grafts were not secured with screws but were wedged in beneath the periosteum, spanning the nonunion or osseous defect.[59]

Dual Onlay Grafts

This type of procedure was initially advocated by Boyd in 1941 to be used in the management of congenital pseudarthrosis of the tibia. It was his feeling that the dual onlay grafts provided both some structural stability at the pseudarthrosis site and a stimulus for osteogenesis. The grafts were applied to span the pseudarthrosis site on each side of the bone. They were then held in position by cortical screws that extended through the graft into the recipient bone and into the opposite graft. In this manner the pseudarthrosis was held securely by virtue of the vicelike grip of the cortical onlay grafts. Supplementary cancellous grafts were also used to stimulate osteogenesis. This is a useful technique for bridging an osseous gap between bone ends. In more recent times this type of grafting procedure has been largely supplanted by newly developed compression plates that provide adequate rigid internal fixation in combination with cancellous bone grafts.

Inlay Bone Grafts

This type of bone graft was advocated by Albee for the treatment of fractures and nonunions (Fig. 5–5). Originally suggested for the treatment of fractures of the proximal portion of the tibia, it was then expanded to include other long bones as well.[2, 3] In this method a rectangular bone graft is outlined along the proximal portion of the major osseous fragment. A shorter rectangular graft is then outlined in the distal segment of the bone. The shorter distal graft is removed, and the longer proximal graft is pushed across the nonunion, extending into the trough provided by the prior removal of

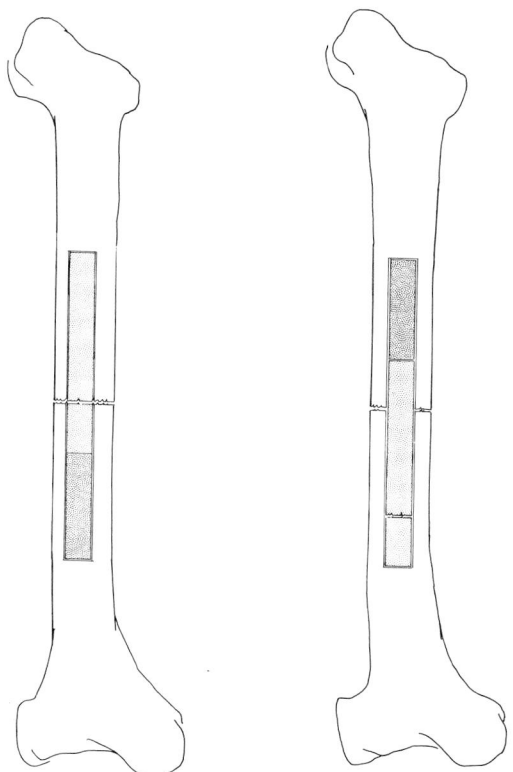

Figure 5–6 Sliding inlay graft. A distal segment of the graft is removed and the large proximal portion is slid into place. The removed distal portion is then placed in the defect in the proximal aspect.

the shorter distal portion. In this manner an inlayed segment of bone spans the fracture site (Fig. 5–6). The removed shorter distal fragment is inserted into the defect created in the proximal portion of the bone by sliding the major portion of the graft in a distal direction. This type of grafting procedure at present has limited application. It may, however, be useful to supplement internal fixation with a compression plate.

Dowel Grafts

This type of bone graft has been employed in the management of nonunion of the navicular in the wrist, depressed tibial plateau fractures, and nonunion of femoral neck fractures (Fig. 5–7). In navicular fractures the two portions of the navicular bone are "hollowed out" and the dowel graft is

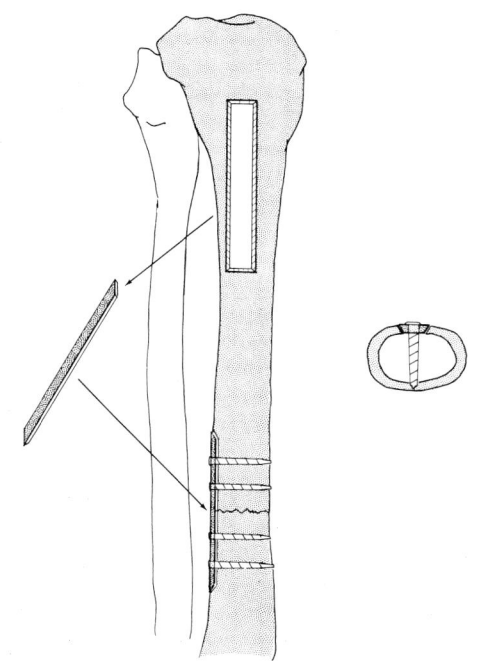

Figure 5–5 Single inlay graft. Note that the edges of the graft are beveled so that they sit into a prepared slot in the recipient bone.

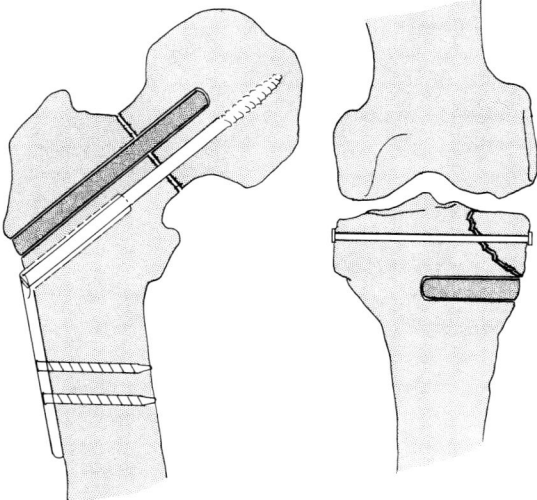

Figure 5-7 The dowel graft. Useful in the management of nonunion of the femoral neck. The graft is inserted across the nonunion site. Supplemental internal fixation is required. This graft is also useful in the management of comminuted depressed tibial plateau fractures. The major portion of the tibial plateau fragment is elevated and secured in position by internal fixation. There is usually an osseous defect under the fragment, and the dowel graft may be inserted in this area for support.

inserted into the osseous substance of both fragments, providing a large cancellous surface of bone to stimulate osteogenesis.

For comminuted depressed tibial plateau fractures, the plateau is elevated and maintained with internal fixation. The dowel graft is then inserted into the defect.

In the past the dowel graft was utilized to supplement internal fixation for the treatment of nonunions of the femoral neck. In this technique a narrow hollow cavity is drilled from the lateral surface of the femur up through the femoral neck into the femoral head. A round long strip of cancellous bone is then obtained and inserted into this defect so that it extends up the femoral neck and across the nonunion site into the femoral head. Dowel grafting does not supply adequate fixation and must be supplemented by additional metallic internal fixation devices. This type of technique has been largely replaced by the muscle pedicle graft, as advocated by Judet.

Muscle Pedicle Grafts

This technique was originally advocated by Judet for the management of femoral neck fractures in young patients, a type of injury in which the incidence of nonunion is significant. A graft is applied so that it extends proximally from a point 3 cm from the tip of the greater trochanter, includes the posterolateral aspect of the intertrochanteric crest along with the insertion of the quadratus femoris muscle, and ends at the level of the lesser trochanter. The graft, usually approximately 1.5 cm in width and 1 cm in depth, is undercut with a curved osteotome and, along with the attached quadratus femoris muscle, is then freed with an osteotome and retracted in the direction of muscle origin along the lateral aspect of the ischial tuberosity. A slot is then produced in the posterior aspect of the femoral neck across the fracture or nonunion site. The muscle pedicle graft is inserted into the prepared slot in the femoral head and is impacted into position and secured with a single screw at each end. It is important to stress that this type of bone graft is employed in conjunction with internal fixation with an appropriate metallic device. It has been demonstrated that a significant amount of the osseous structure survives with a muscle pedicle graft. This has been a very useful technique in the management of nonunions of the femoral neck and also of fractures of the femoral neck in young patients.

Strut Grafts

This type of graft has been useful in management of various spinal conditions. The fibula is usually the donor bone of choice and provides a structurally sound graft that does give some immediate stability. Rib has also been employed with this technique and is extremely useful in the management of severe pathological fractures of the vertebral body. The entire vertebral body may be curetted and removed, and the fibular strut grafts or rib grafts may then be inserted so they span the defect left by the excised vertebra and extend into the vertebrae above and below (Figs. 5-8 and 5-9). The grafts stimulate

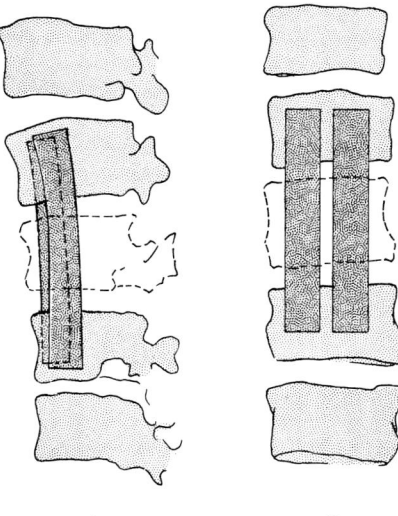

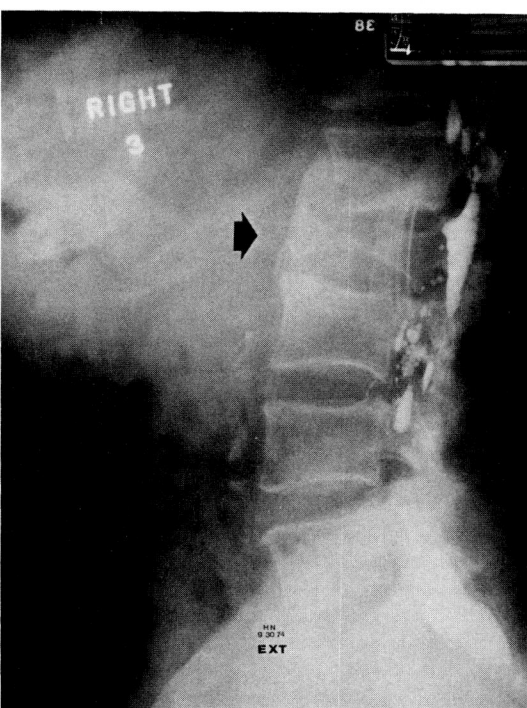

A   B

Figure 5–8 The strut graft. The fibula or rib may be the source of this graft. It is useful in the management of severe fractures of a cervical vertebra with neurological impingement secondary to posterior migration of the vertebral fragment. It is also useful in the management of pathological fractures involving the entire vertebral body. The body may be curetted and excised. The grafts are then wedged in between the bodies above and below, and provide for structural support once incorporation is complete. *A.* Lateral view of the position of the fibular strut graft. The excised vertebral body is represented by the unstippled area. *B.* Anteroposterior view demonstrating the position of the fibular strut graft. This technique is also useful for multiple-level anterior cervical fusions.

Figure 5–9 An example of neural impingement from a burst fracture of the lumbar vertebra in which posterior migration of the vertebral body accounts for the neurological deficit. This was approached anteriorly, the offending portion of the vertebra was excised, and rib strut grafts were inserted. Neurological deficit improved and the patient went on to uneventful spontaneous fusion across the defect site.

osteogenic consolidation and provide structural stability.

The fibular strut graft has also been advocated for the management of multilevel anterior cervical fusions. It may be inserted through a prepared slot along the anterior surface of the vertebral bodies, spanning three or four vertebrae. The graft must then be countersunk into the most proximal and most distal vertebrae within the fusion site. It is important to bear in mind that several structural changes occur within the graft, as outlined by Enneking's work, discussed earlier in this chapter.

Clothespin or H Grafts

The clothespin graft is another type of grafting procedure that has been very useful in the management of disease of the cervical spine. It involves the application of a large rectangular iliac crest full-thickness graft with a slot cut out in both the proximal and the distal portions so that the graft may be wedged in place between the spinous processes. In this manner a large osseous surface is available to stimulate osteogenesis for fusion between the cervical vertebrae. A form of this type of graft has been thoroughly outlined in the illustrations by Fielding in Chapter 13.

Cancellous Bone Graft with Internal Fixation

In modern treatment of various delayed unions, nonunions, and pseudarthroses, this is the technique that is usually selected. In the case of a pseudarthrosis, this involves exposure of the actual bone ends and removal of the interposing joint surface. If a nonunion or delayed union is present, the intervening tissue between the bone ends need not be removed. The surface of the bone is then decorticated to stimulate incorporation of additional bone grafts. A compression plate that provides for adequate stability across the fracture site is then applied to the fracture fragments in a standard fashion. Additional cancellous bone, which is usually obtained from the iliac crest, is useful in supplementing the internal fixation—the strip grafts being placed along the decorticated surface to stimulate osteogenesis. The combination of a compression plate for firm structural stability with a cancellous bone graft to stimulate osteogenesis is the method of choice for treating the majority of nonunions and pseudarthroses.

REFERENCES

1. Abbott, L. C., Schottstaedt, E. R., Saunders, J. B., and Bost, F. C.: The evaluation of cortical and cancellous bone as grafting material. A clinical and experimental study. J. Bone Joint Surg., 29:381–414, 1947.
2. Albee, F. H.: Transplantation of a portion of the tibia into the spine for Pott's disease. J.A.M.A., 57:85, 1911.
3. Albee, F. H.: Evolution of bone graft surgery. Am. J. Surg., 63:421–436, 1944.
4. Arora, B. K., and Laskin, D. M.: Sex chromatin as a cellular label of osteogenesis by bone grafts. J. Bone Joint Surg., 46A:1269, 1964.
5. Axhausen, G.: Histologische Untersuchungen uber Knochen transplantation am Menschen, Dtsch. Z. Chir., 91:388–428, 1907.
6. Axhausen, G.: Die histologischen und klinischen Gesetze der Freien Ostoplastik auf Grund von Tierversuchen. Arch. Klin. Chir., 88:23, 1909.
7. Bassett, C. A. L.: Current concepts of bone formation. J. Bone Joint Surg., 44A:1217–1244, 1962.
8. Bassett, C. A. L.: Clinical implications of cell function in bone grafting. Clin. Orthop., 87:49–59, 1972.
9. Bassett, C. A. L., and Ruedi-Lindesker, A.: Bibliography of bone transplantation. Transplantation, 2:668–679, 1964.
10. Bassett, C. A. L., Creighton, D. K., and Stinchfeld, F. E.: Contributions of endosteum, cortex and soft tissues to osteogenesis. Surg. Gynecol. Obstet., 112:145–152, 1961.
11. Bishop, W. A., Jr., Stauffer, R. C., and Swenson, A. L.: Bone grafts. An end-result study of the healing time. J. Bone Joint Surg., 29:961, 1947.
12. Bohr, H., Ravan, H. O., and Werner, H.: The osteogenic effect of bone transplants in rabbits. J. Bone Joint Surg., 50B:866–973, 1968.
13. Bonfiglio, M., and Jeter, W. S.: Immunological responses to bone. Clin. Orthop., 87:19–27, 1972.
14. Brooks, D. B., Heiple, K. G., Herndon, C. H., and Powell, A. E.: Immunological factors in homogenous bone transplantation. Part IV. The effects of various methods of preparation and irradiation on antigenicity. J. Bone Joint Surg., 45A:1617–1626, 1963.
15. Burchardt, H., Glowczewskie, F. P., and Enneking, W. F.: Allogeneic segmental fibular transplants in azathioprine-immunosuppressed dogs. J. Bone Joint Surg., 59A:881–894, 1977.
16. Buring, K., and Urist, M. R.: Transfilter bone induction. Clin. Orthop., 54:235–242, 1967.
17. Burwell, R. G.: Studies in the transplantation of bone. Part VII. The fresh composite homograft-autograft or cancellous bone: An analysis of factors leading to osteogenesis in marrow transplants and in marrow-containing bone grafts. J. Bone Joint Surg., 46B:110–140, 1964.
18. Burwell, R. G.: Studies in the transplantation of bone. J. Bone Joint Surg., 48B:532–566, 1966.
19. Burwell, R. G.: In Recent Advances in Orthopaedics. A. G. Apley (ed.): London, Churchill, 1969, p. 115.
20. Burwell, R. G., Gowland, G., and Dexter, F.: Studies in the transplantation of bone. Part IV. Further observations concerning the antigenicity of homologous cortical and cancellous bone. J. Bone Joint Surg., 45B:597–608, 1963.
21. Campbell, C. J., Brower, T., MacFadden, D. G., Payne, E. B., and Doherty, J.: An experimental study of the fate of bone grafts. J. Bone Joint Surg., 35A:332–346, 1953.
22. Campbell, W. C.: The antogenous bone graft. J. Bone Joint Surg., 21:694, 1939.
23. Carnesale, P. L., and Spankus, J. D.: A clinical comparative study of autogenous and homogenous bone grafts. J. Bone Joint Surg., 41A:887, 1959.
24. Chalmers, J.: Transplantation immunity in bone homografting. J. Bone Joint Surg., 41B:160–179, 1959.
25. Chalmers, J., and Ray, R. D.: The growth of transplanted foetal bones in different immunological environments. J. Bone Joint Surg., 44B:149–164, 1962.
26. Chalmers, J., and Rush, J.: Observations on the induction of bone in soft tissues. J. Bone Joint Surg., 57B:36–45, 1975.
27. Chase, S. W., and Herndon, C. H.: The fate of autogenous and homogenous bone grafts: A historical review. J. Bone Joint Surg., 37A:809–841, 1955.
28. Cobey, M. L.: A national bone bank survey. Clin. Orthop., 110:333, 1975.
29. Cohen, J., Maletskos, C. J., Marshall, J. H., and Williams, J. B.: Radioactive calcium tracer studies in bone grafts. J. Bone Joint Surg., 39A:561–577, 1957.
30. Curtiss, P. H., Jr., and Herndon, C. H.: Immunological factors in homogenous-bone transplantation. 1. Serological studies. J. Bone Joint Surg., 38A:103–110, 1956.
31. Curtiss, P. H., Chase, S. W., and Herndon, C. H.: Immunological factors in homogenous-bone

transplantation. II. Histological studies. J. Bone Joint Surg., 38A:324–328, 1956.

32. DeBruyn, P. P., and Kabisch, W. T.: Bone formation by fresh and frozen, autogenous and homogenous transplants of bone, bone marrow and periosteum. Amer. J. Anat., 96:375–417, 1955.

33. Deleu, J., and Trueta, J.: Vascularization of bone grafts in the anterior chamber of the eye. J. Bone Joint Surg., 47B:319–329, 1965.

34. Doi, K., Tominaga, S., and Shibata, T.: Bone grafts with microvascular anastomoses of vascular pedicles. An experimental study in dogs. J. Bone Joint Surg., 59A:809–815, 1977.

35. Enneking, W. F.: Histological investigation of bone transplants in immunologically prepared animals. J. Bone Joint Surg., 39A:607–615, 1957.

36. Enneking, W. F., and Morris, J. L.: Human autologous cortical bone transplants. Clin. Orthop., 87:28–35, 1972.

37. Enneking, W. F., Burchardt, H., Puhl, J., and Piotrowski, G.: Physical and biologic aspects of repair in dog cortical bone transplants. J. Bone Joint Surg., 57A:237–252, 1975.

38. Friedlaender, G. E., Strong, D. M., and Sell, K. W.: Studies on the antigenicity of bone. I. Freeze-dried and deep-frozen bone allografts in rabbits. J. Bone Joint Surg., 58A:854–858, 1976.

39. Gallie, W. E.: The transplantation of bone. Br. Med. J., 2:840–844, 1931.

40. Goldberg, V. M., and Lance, E. M.: Revascularization and accretion in transplantation. Quantitative studies of the role of the allograft barrier. J. Bone Surg., 54A:807, 1972.

41. Goldhaber, P.: Osteogenic induction across millipore filters in vivo. Science, 133:2065–2067, 1961.

42. Grishaw, R. B., Perry, V. P., and Wheeler, T. E.: U. S. Navy tissue bank. J.A.M.A., 183:99, 1963.

43. Ham, A. W., and Harris, W. R.: Repair and transplantation of bone. In Biochemistry and Physiology of Bone. Vol. III. ed. by G. Bourne. New York, Academic Press 1972, pp. 337–399.

44. Harkins, H. N., and Phemister, D. B.: Simplified technic of onlay grafts. J.A.M.A., 109:1501, 1937.

45. Harris, W. H., Haywood, E. A., La Vorgna, J., and Hamblem, D. L.: Spatial and temporal variations in cortical bone formation in dogs. J. Bone Joint Surg., 50A:1118–1128, 1968.

46. Heiple, K. G., Chase, S. W., and Herndon, C. H.: A comparative study of the healing process following different types of bone transplantation. J. Bone Joint Surg., 45A:1593–1616, 1963.

47. Henry, M. O.: Homografts in orthopaedic surgery. J. Bone Joint Surg., 30A:70, 1948.

48. Holmstrand, K.: Biophysical investigations of bone transplants and bone implants. Acta Orthop. Scand., Suppl. 26:1–50, 1957.

49. Horwitz, T.: The behaviour of bone grafts. Surg. Gynecol. Obstet., 89:310, 1949.

50. Johnson, J. T. H., and Southwick, W. O.: Growth following transepiphyseal bone grafts. J. Bone Joint Surg., 42A:1381–1412, 1960.

51. Judet, P. R., and Patel, A.: Muscle pedicle bone grafting of long bones by osteoperiosteal decortication. Clin. Orthop., 87:74–80, 1972.

52. Kingina, M. J., and Hampe, J. F.: The behavior of blood vessels after experimental transplantation of bone. J. Bone Joint Surg., 46B:141–150, 1964.

53. Koskinen, E. V. S., Ryoppy, S. A., and Lindholm, S.: Osteoinduction and osteogenesis in implants of allogeneic bone matrix. Influence of somatotropin, thyrotropin and cortisone. Clin. Orthop., 87:116–130, 1972.

54. Lloyd-Roberts, G. C.: Experiences with boiled cadaveric bone. J. Bone Joint Surg., 34B:428–432, 1952.

55. Muscolo, D. L., Kawar, S., and Ray, R. D.: Cellular and humoral immune response analysis of bone-allografted rats. J. Bone Joint Surg., 58A:826–832, 1976.

56. Nisbet, N. W.: Immunology of bone transplantation. Clin. Orthop., 47:199–228, 1966.

57. Ottolenghi, C. E.: Massive osteoarticular bone graft; transplant of the whole femur. J. Bone Joint Surg., 48B:646, 1966.

58. Pappas, A. M., and Beisaw, N. E.: Bone transplantation; correlations of physical and histologic aspects of graft incorporation. Clin. Orthop., 61:79–91, 1968.

59. Phemister, D. B.: The fate of transplanted bone and regenerative power of its various constituents. Surg. Gynecol. Obstet., 19:303–333, 1914.

60. Post, R. H., Heiple, K. G., Chase, S. W., and Herndon, C. H.: Bone grafts in diffusion chambers. Clin. Orthop., 44:265–270, 1966.

61. Puranen, J.: Reorganization of fresh and preserved bone transplants; an experimental study in rabbits using tetracycline labelling. Acta Orthop. Scand., Suppl. 92:9–75, 1966.

62. Ray, R. D.: Vascularization of bone grafts and implants. Clin. Orthop., 87:43–49, 1972.

63. Ray, R. D., and Sabet, T. Y.: Bone grafts: cellular survival versus induction. J. Bone Joint Surg., 45A:337, 1963.

64. Ray, R. D., Degge, J., Gloyd, P., and Mooney, G.: Bone regeneration; an experimental study of bone-grafting materials. J. Bone Joint Surg., 34A:639–647, 1952.

65. Sako, K., and Marchetta, F. C.: Delayed autogenous bone and callus transplants and prepared host beds. An experimental study. Arch. Surg., 92:771–777, 1966.

66. Scuderi, C.: Restoration of long bone defects with massive bone grafts. J.A.M.A., 137:1116, 1948.

67. Siffert, R. S.: Experimental bone transplants. J. Bone Joint Surg., 37A:742–758, 1955.

68. Siffert, R. S., and Barash, E. S.: Delayed bone transplantation: An experimental study of early host-transplant relationships. J. Bone Joint Surg., 43A:407–418, 1961.

69. Simmons, D. J., Ellsasser J. C., Cummins, H., and Lesker, P.: The bone inductive potential of a composite bone allograft marrow autograft in rabbits. Clin. Orthop., 97:237, 1973.

70. Stringa, G.: L Studies of the vascularization of bone grafts. J. Bone Joint Surg., 39B:395–420, 1957.

71. Sudmann, E.: Vital microscopy of bone remodelling in rabbit ear chambers. Acta Orthop. Scand., Suppl. 160, 1975.

72. Turner, T. C., Bassett, C. A. L., Pate, J. W., and Sawyer, P. N.: An experimental comparison of freeze-dried and frozen cortical bone-graft healing. J. Bone Joint Surg., 37A:1197–1205, 1955.

73. Urist, M. R.: Bone; Transplants, Implants, Derivatives and Substitutes—A Survey of Research of the Past Decade. AAOS Instructional Course Lectures, Vol. XVIII, p. 184. St. Louis, C. V. Mosby, 1960.
74. Urist, M. R.: Osteoinduction in undemineralized bone implants modified by chemical inhibitors of endogenous matrix enzymes. Clin. Orthop., 87:132, 1972.
75. Urist, M. R.: Practical application of basic research on bone graft physiology. AAOS Instructional Course Lectures, Vol. XXV, pp. 1–26. St. Louis, Mosby, 1976.
76. Urist, M. R., Mikulski, A. J., and Boyd, S. D.: A chemosterilized antigen extracted bone morphogenetic alloimplant. Arch. Surg., *110*:416, 1975.
77. Urist, M. R., Earnest, F., Kimball, K. M., Di Julio, T. P., and Iwata, H.: Bone morphogenesis in implants of residues of radioisotope labelled bone matrix. Calcif. Tissue Res., *15*:269, 1974.
78. Urist, M. R., Silverman, B. G., Buring, K., Dubuc, F. L., and Rosenberg, J. M.: The bone induction principle. Clin. Orthop., *53*:243, 1967.
79. Williams, R. G.: Comparison of living autogenous and homogenous grafts of cancellous bone heterotopically placed in rabbits. Anat. Rec., *143*:93–196, 1962.
80. Yu, W. Y., Siu, C. M., Shim, S. S., Hawthorne, H. M., and Dunbar, S.: Mechanical properties and mineral content of avascular and revascularizing cortical bone. J. Bone Joint Surg., *57A*:692–695, 1975.

JONATHAN BLACK, Ph.D.

Biomaterials _____ 6
for
Internal
Fixation

The central problem of internal fixation of a fracture is to restore the structural integrity of the damaged bone. This may be achieved by a number of approaches, varying from cerclage at one extreme to segmental or partial prosthetic replacement at the other extreme. The design of an internal fixation device is dependent upon a large number of considerations including the site and type of fracture, the possible operative approaches, the desired or feasible postoperative care program, and the like. The mechanical and functional aspects of this process are discussed in Chapter 7.

A common factor that underlies all these considerations is the performance of the material from which the device is to be made. Materials' selection is not arbitrary; it must occur early in the design process and it has a profound effect on the design, fabrication, surgical implantation technique, and performance in vivo. An immediate corollary to this statement is that, necessarily, materials are *not* interchangeable in any one design. A change in the material from which a device is fabricated can produce as profound a change in performance as a change in mechanical design. In this chapter, I deal with four topics related to materials for use in internal fixation: (1) the general requirements for a material to be used in internal fixation applications, (2) the

properties of specific materials in use for internal fixation devices, (3) the selection of materials for particular devices, and (4) the materials-associated complications that may arise in the use of internal fixation devices.

REQUIREMENTS FOR FIXATION MATERIALS

The general requirements for materials for internal fixation devices may be summarized as follows:

1. The materials must reflect a suitable combination of properties that permit the design and fabrication of devices that perform satisfactorily in clinical use.

2. The materials must sustain the forces placed upon them in a particular application without deformation or fracture that would lead to loss of function or reduction.

3. The materials must not be degraded by the biological environment sufficiently either to impair their mechanical function or to release degradation products that are harmful locally or systemically.

Thus we can see that characterization of materials requires knowledge of their static and dynamic mechanical properties, their chemical and biological interactions in vivo and their other properties that may be dictated by clinical requirements.

113

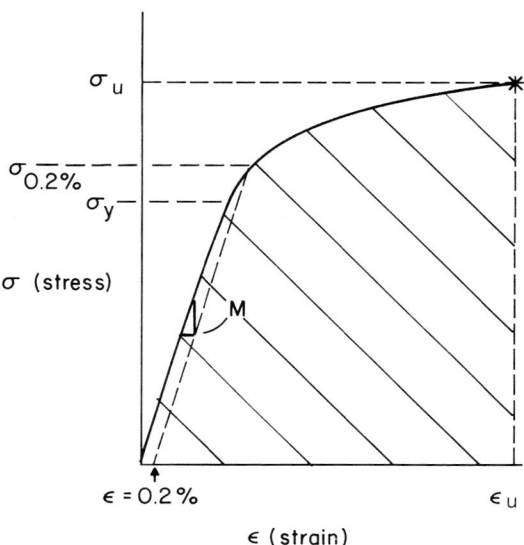

Figure 6–1 Idealized stress-strain curve summarizing the static and low-cycle properties of materials. *Stress*, the vertical coordinate, is the applied load divided by the cross-sectional area of the material. *Strain*, the horizontal coordinate, is the resulting elongation per unit length.

σ_y, the *yield stress*, the greatest stress that can be applied without permanent deformation after removal of stress; $\sigma_{0.2}\%$, the *0.2 per cent stress* that causes a permanent strain of 0.2 per cent after removal; σ_u, the *ultimate stress* that produces material failure by fracture; ϵ_u, the *ultimate strain* or *strain to failure*; M, the *modulus*, the ratio of *stress* divided by *strain* in the linear portion of the curve and a measure of the intrinsic *stiffness* of the material. An additional parameter of interest, shown as the cross-hatched area, is the *work to fracture* per unit volume of the material, or the amount of energy that must be absorbed per unit volume before fracture takes place, a measure of *toughness*.

PROPERTIES OF MATERIALS

Mechanical Properties

Short-Term Behavior of Materials. The static and low-cycle properties of materials can be summarized in a *stress-strain* diagram (Fig. 6–1). Data for such a graph are obtained by standard materials testing methods, usually in tension. *Stress*, the vertical coordinate, is the applied load divided by the cross-sectional area of the material. *Strain*, the horizontal coordinate, is the resulting elongation divided by the length of the specimen to yield elongation per unit length.

Other parameters of interest are:

σ_y: the *yield stress*. This is the greatest stress that can be applied without permanent deformation after the removal of stress.

$\sigma_{0.2}\%$: the *0.2 per cent offset stress*. This yield stress, the stress that causes a permanent strain of 0.2 per cent after removal, is often used as an indication of the point of yielding for materials with a poorly defined yield point.

σ_u: the *ultimate stress*. The stress that produces material failure by fracture, is sometimes called the UTS (in tension) for *ultimate tensile stress*.

ϵ_u: the *ultimate strain* or *strain to failure*. Occasionally this is also called the *ductility*.

M: the *modulus*. The ratio of *stress* divided by *strain* in the linear portion of the curve (stress less than σ_y) is called the modulus. If measured in tension, it is called the *tensile modulus* or *Young's modulus*. This is a measure of the intrinsic *stiffness* of the material. An additional parameter of interest is the area under the stress-strain curve, shown in Figure 6–1 as the cross-hatched area. This area is the *work to fracture* per unit volume of the material. It is the amount of energy that must be absorbed per unit volume before fracture takes place. Thus, it is a measure of *toughness*; this term is sometimes used interchangeably with work of fracture.

These parameters define the short-term behavior of a material.

Long-Term Behavior of Materials. Fixation devices, however, remain in place for periods of months and years and are subjected to a variety of repeated loads. There are three other types of mechanical behavior that help to describe the response of materials to such conditions: fatigue, creep, and stress relaxation.

Fatigue. When a material is repeatedly loaded and unloaded, it may eventually break, although none of the loads produces a stress above the ultimate stress. This failure is termed *fatigue failure*. Generally, the greater the peak stress produced in a given cycle of loading and unloading, the fewer cycles can be sustained before failure. This relationship, termed the *S–N curve*, is shown in Figure 6–2 in a form characteristic of metals. Combinations of stress (S) and number of cycles (N) that fall

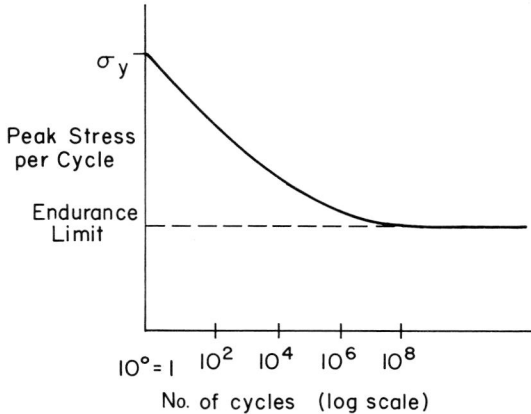

Figure 6-2 Idealized S-N curve for metals. The higher the peak stress produced in a given cycle of loading and unloading, the fewer cycles can be sustained before failure. Combination of stress (S) and number of cycles (N) that fall above this curve predict failure of the material by fracture. The region to the left (high S, low N) represents failure at stresses above the yield stress after a small number of cycles; that to the right (low S, high N) reflects repeated deformation, primarily due to stress below the yield stress. Many materials display an endurance limit, a level of stress below which fatigue failure will not occur, no matter how many cycles of loading and unloading are experienced.

above this curve predict failure of the material by fracture. The region to the left (high S, low N) represents failure at stresses above the yield stress after a small number of cycles. This would be the environment for a device implanted in an unstable fashion or in a patient who was too active during the early stages of fracture healing. The region to the right (low S, high N) represents the environment that is more usual for fracture fixation applications and reflects repeated deformation, primarily due to stress below the yield stress. The usual assumption made is that fixation hardware in the lower limbs will experience 2×10^6 cycles per year. For many materials, there is a level of stress below which fatigue failure will not occur, no matter how many cycles of loading and unloading are experienced. This is called the *endurance limit.* In the absence of an endurance limit, designers try to keep maximum stress below that required to cause failure in 5×10^7 cycles, approximately 25 years of normal use.

Creep. In the presence of sustained loads, even at stresses below the normal yield point, materials may undergo a slow deformation. This process is termed *creep.* Creep rates at body temperature are generally quite low, and periods of months or years would be required for currently used rigid implant materials (except for a few polymers) to undergo rupture or fracture as a result of creep.

Stress Relaxation. In a response to stress similar to creep, materials that are placed under load by a system that has fixed dimensions can accommodate themselves so as to relieve the applied stress. This reduction in stress with time under constant strain conditions is termed *stress relaxation.*

Both creep and stress relaxation phenomena tend to make materials unsuitable for fracture fixation because they release frictional forces that must be maintained to maintain reduction.

Additional factors of importance in selected fracture fixation applications include *hardness, wear behavior, fabricability,* and *cost.*

Nonmechanical Properties

In addition to the mechanical requisites, materials used for internal fixation devices must meet the general requirements of implant materials. They must either be nondegradable or undergo degradation in a fashion that does not interfere with their intended clinical function. Similarly, the materials to be used must not evoke an unwanted biological response, either locally or systemically. These requirements have acted to restrict the choice of materials for internal fixation. Those described in the next section have been found by experience to be generally acceptable, but it must be emphasized that no material used for internal fixation either is sufficiently stable or has sufficiently well-known behavior that it can be considered, a priori, as a permanent implant. Much of this uncertainty stems from the need to use multipart devices in many fracture fixation applications. The properties of the individual parts may vary, even though those parts are nominally made from the same material. Variations in manufacturing processes and interactions between parts, such as fretting and corrosion, further complicate the situation. Thus, it is well to continue to consider devices for fracture fixation as temporary implants and to remove them whenever the clinical course and the patient's condition make such removal reasonable in the surgeon's judgment.

Specific Implant Materials

Metals in Current Use. Metals are widely used in devices for fracture fixation—for the same reasons that have led to their use in other applications: (1) They exhibit high tensile and compressive moduli coupled with reasonable elastic ranges such that structures may bear considerable loads without permanent deformation. (2) When loads exceed the yield point, increasing yield stresses cause sufficient plastic deformation that the devices may be observed to bend or take a permanent set before catastrophic failure, permitting replacement before their function is totally lost. (3) Metals may be fabricated into parts by a variety of conventional techniques and, in many cases, may then be hardened to improve their performance. (4) With reasonable care in preparation and use, metals provide good to excellent resistance to environments, including those encountered in sterilization and implantation.

There are six metallic alloys in common use in orthopedics today. Their chemical composition is given in Table 6–1. Note that the various trade names used by manufacturers describe essentially the same materials. This is the result of the activities of standards organizations such as the American Society for Testing and Materials (ASTM), the American National Standards Institute (ANSI), the British Standards Institution (BSI), and others. References to relevant specifications and a short list of manufacturers' trade names are included in Table 6–1.

These metal alloys divide, by composition, into three groups. The two stainless steel alloys, one of which is generally fabricated into devices by casting and the other by forging, are derived from the very common 18–8 alloy (18 per cent chromium, 8 per cent nickel) used in tableware, countertops, and building trim. The increase in the nickel content and the decrease in the carbon content to 0.03 per cent maximum in the 316L type were vitally necessary to provide the improved corrosion resistance required in implant applications. Inclusion of impurities decreases corrosion resistance and ductility. Therefore, many manufacturers remelt the base alloy in vacuum once or twice, thus further purifying it without markedly changing its composition. This material is often referred to as "vacuum remelt," and the letters VM are added to the symbol or name of the alloy. It should be noted that parts made by casting may have higher impurity levels than those made by forging, since there is the possibility of contamination during processing. These alloys are in wide use, constituting between them about 60 per cent of the implants used in the United States, as judged by retrieval studies.

The forged alloy is more commonly used in fracture fixation devices, greatly dominating this field. Although forging is generally a more expensive process than casting, it can be used to impart a "fiber texture" to the finished part. This means that, by selective directional deformation during the various stages of forging, the grains of the metal are elongated into fibrous or spindle shapes. The forming process is so designed that the long axes of these deformed grains lie parallel to the expected deforming forces. For instance, in a long bone fracture fixation plate, it would be desired that the grain axis lie along the length of the plate. In such a device, by controlling the crack initiation process, the elongated-fiber textures provide greater resistance to breakage than the equi-axised grains in cast materials of the same composition that have been heat treated to the same final condition.

The two chromium-cobalt alloys are termed "super alloys" rather than steels, since they are based on cobalt rather than iron, as are steel alloys. The name Vitallium, actually a trade name, has been widely applied to these alloys and leads to the incorrect assumption that they are identical. In fact, they differ in composition. The casting alloy contains a nominal 6 per cent molybdenum, less nickel, and more chromium than the molybdenum-free wrought alloy. Although a variety of trade names are used, as shown in Table 6–1, with respect to adherence to specifications, these two alloy systems describe all the materials in use.

TABLE 6–1   Composition of Surgical Implant Alloys*

Composition (per cent weight)	Stainless Steel ASTM F55 or F56 Wrought Type B	Co-Cr ASTM F75 Cast	Co-Cr ASTM F90 (Vitallium) Wrought
Tungsten	– – – –	– – – –	14–16
Cobalt	– – – –	Bal (57.4–65)	Bal (46–53)
Chromium	17–20	27–30	19–21
Nickel	10–14	2.5 max	9–11
Molybdenum	2–4	5–7	– – – –
Iron	Bal (59–70)	0.75 max	3.0 max
Carbon	0.03 max	0.35 max	0.05–0.15
Manganese	2.00 max	1.0 max	2.0 max
Phosphorus	0.03 max	– – – –	– – – –
Sulfur	0.03 max	– – – –	– – – –
Silicon	0.75 max	1.00 max	1.00 max

Composition (per cent weight)	Stainless Steel ASTM A296 Cast	Titanium (Pure) ASTM F67 Grade 4, Flat Product Cast/Wrought	Titanium 6A1-4V Alloy ASTM F136 Cast/Wrought
Cobalt	– – – –	– – – –	– – – –
Chromium	16–18	– – – –	– – – –
Nickel	10–14	– – – –	– – – –
Molybdenum	2–3	– – – –	– – – –
Iron	Bal (62–72)	0.5 max	0.25 max
Aluminum	– – – –	– – – –	5.5–6.5
Vanadium	– – – –	– – – –	3.5–4.5
Titanium	– – – –	Bal (99+)	Bal (88.5–92)
Carbon	0.06 max	0.10 max	0.08 max
Manganese	2.00 max	– – – –	– – – –
Phosphorus	0.045 max	– – – –	– – – –
Sulfur	0.030 max	– – – –	– – – –
Silicon	1.0 max	– – – –	– – – –
Oxygen	– – – –	0.45 max	0.13 max
Nitrogen	– – – –	0.07 max	0.05 max
Hydrogen	– – – –	0.015 max	0.015 max

Trade Name	Type	Manufacturer
Alivium	Co-Cr	Zimmer, Orthopaedic Ltd., London, England
CoCroMo	Co-Cr	Orthopaedic Equipment Co., Bourbon, Indiana
Francobal	Co-Cr	s.a. Benoist Girard & Cie, Heronville, France
Orthochrome	Co-Cr	DePuy, Warsaw, Indiana
Protosul-2	Co-Cr	Protek & Sulzer, Zurich, Switzerland
Tivanium	Ti-6A1-4V	Zimmer USA, Warsaw, Indiana
Vinertia	Co-Cr	Deloro Surgical Ltd., Stratton St., Margaret, England
Vitallium	Co-Cr	Howmedica, Rutherford, New Jersey
Zimaloy	Co-Cr	Zimmer USA, Warsaw, Indiana

*Adapted from J. H. Dumbleton and J. Black: *An Introduction to Orthopaedic Materials* with permission of Charles C Thomas, Publisher, Springfield, Ill.

The final two materials are essentially pure titanium and alloyed titanium referred to as Ti–6Al–4V because it contains a nominal 6 per cent of aluminum and 4 per cent of vanadium.

There is little to choose between these six alloys on the basis of chemistry and corro-sion resistance. With the possible exception of the cast stainless steel, which is a recently introduced alloy, all have been proved to have good tissue acceptance and good to excellent corrosion resistance in vivo. The cast stainless steel alloy is still in evaluation. Both the stainless steel and the cobalt-chromium alloys exhibit uniform attack as well as pitting and crevice corrosion, and are subject to galvanic corrosion in mixed metal devices. It seems fairly certain that the stainless steel is more subject to corrosion than the cobalt-chromium alloys, since it is a passivated material, and there is evidence that the passive layer is metastable; thus, physical damage to surfaces of stainless steel implants at or after implantation may result in accelerated corrosion. The mechanism of corrosion resistance of the cobalt-chromium alloys is less well understood. They do not exhibit the uniform passive surface layer of chromium oxide of the type found on stainless steels but seem to have a mixed oxide protective film.

It has also been suggested that the components of these alloys display mutually protective behavior. That is, each component of the alloy has a characteristic potential, depending upon its chemical composition, and this potential may act on another component, conferring cathodic protection upon this second component. The net result is the generation of a "mixed potential," that is, a potential intermediate between those of the components and one at which the alloy is in an immune state.

The titanium alloys are quite corrosion resistant, at least with respect to uniform attack, since they possess a natural surface coating of titanium dioxide formed in response to air exposure. This natural coating, similar to the mineral rutile, is highly insoluble and resistant to corrosive attack. There is, however, some question as to their fatigue corrosion resistance in vivo.

Materials that have passivating layers tend to be prone to stress corrosion or what is sometimes called *fatigue corrosion.* The effect is due to mechanical disruption of the passive film. There is then a competitive interaction between corrosion and passivation during the repassivating interval. Thus, each strain that disrupts the passive film results in a small amount of additional corrosion. Since this is concentrated in areas of severe strain rather than being distributed uniformly, local cracking and formation of stress raisers may result. This will markedly reduce the fatigue life of the material. Future experience will no doubt contribute to understanding in this area.

Titanium and titanium-base alloys are, however, very well accepted by tissues—to the extent that some European practitioners use titanium as the material of choice for implants in operative sites thought to be infected.

The mechanical properties more closely govern the performance of a device and its initial design than the chemical composition. In Table 6–2 the more important mechanical parameters are summarized for these six alloys. The stainless steel alloys have lower yield and ultimate strengths than the cobalt-chromium alloys, but exhibit rather better ductility. The titanium alloys are rather less ductile than either of the two other types. Although they have greater yield strength their strain to failure levels are disappointingly low, thus qualifying them as relatively brittle materials. Ti–6A1–4V, however, has an endurance limit that is significantly above that for either wrought stainless steel or wrought cobalt-chromium.

New Metallic Materials. One of the motives for developing new metallic materials has been the desire to obtain the good ductility of stainless steel along with the greater corrosion resistance of the cobalt-chromium alloys in use. Additionally, the reduction in the volume of fixation devices that becomes possible as the yield strength increases is extremely desirable.

A promising material is the MP35N alloy. This is an alloy of cobalt, nickel, chromium, and molybdenum. Its designation results from the fact that it contains nominally 35 per cent nickel. Unlike the alloys in use today, it is deliberately made in a multiphase state.

A *phase* is defined as a portion of a material that, despite variations in chemical composition, maintains the same physical structure. Multiphase materials are generally avoided in corrosive environment applications such as surgical implantation. These phases are often inadvertently "frozen in" during processing and may not be in chemical equilibrium with each other. The lack of chemical equilibrium is then expressed as localized galvanic corrosion.

MP35N is primarily a three-phase material. It is a peculiarity of this material that these phases appear to be very nearly in chemical equilibrium, and as a result, early

TABLE 6–2 Mechanical Properties of Surgical Implant Alloys*

Properties	Stainless Steel ASTM F55 Type B Wrought	Co-Cr ASTM F75 Cast	Co-Cr ASTM F90 Wrought
Hardness	Rb 85 to 95	Rc 25 to 34	Rb 98
"(CW)†	Rc 30	– – – – –	Rc 65
UTS	70,000 psi min	95,000 min	130,000 min
"(CW)	125,000	– – – – –	250,000
0.2% YS:	25,000 min	65,000 min	55,000 min
"(CW)	100,000	– – – – –	190,000
Endurance Limit:‡ (N > 10^6 cycles)	35,000	35,000 to 40,000	55,000
Max Strain:	40% min	8% min	50% min
"(CW)	12%	– – – – –	10%
Modulus: E	29×10^6 psi	36×10^6	35×10^6

Properties	Stainless Steel ASTM A296 Cast	Titanium (Pure) ASTM F67 Type 4 Cast/Wrought	Titanium 6A1-4V Alloy Annealed Cast/Wrought
Hardness	Rb 70 to 85	Rb 100	Depends on surface treatment
UTS:	70,000 psi min	80,000 min	125,000 to 130,000
0.2% YS:	30,000 min	70,000 min	115,000 to 120,000
Endurance Limit:‡ (N > 10^6 cycles)	– – – – –	35,000	77,000
Max Strain:	30% min	18% min	10% min
Modulus: E	28×10^6 psi	15×10^6	16×10^6

*Courtesy of J. H. Dumbleton, J. Black, and Charles C Thomas, Publisher, Springfield, Illinois. *An Introduction to Orthopaedic Materials*, 1975.

†CW = maximum cold work.

‡Data from H. J. Grover: Values for plane bending (SS, Ti–alloys) and rotating bending (Co-Cr alloys) J. Metals, *1*:413, 1966.

studies of its corrosion rate and biocompatibility rank it as very similar to the present wrought cobalt-chromium alloy. Its mechanical properties are outstanding, with a yield strength of 60,000 psi when fully annealed but with an elongation of 70 per cent. Work hardening and heat treatment can produce yield strengths of up to 300,000 psi while retaining 10 per cent elongation. Thus, it appears to combine many of the good properties of stainless steel and cobalt chromium alloys.

Another interesting material more closely resembles stainless steel. Actually a group of alloys, called TRIP (transformation induced plasticity) steels, these materials exhibit strength, ductility, and toughness that is superior to that of 316L stainless steel. The unique properties of this group of alloys are due to a partial change in structure induced by cold working. Thus, these are actually two-phase materials. The

most promising is an alloy, based on iron as all steels are, containing 9 per cent chromium, 8 per cent nickel, 4 per cent molybdenum, and 0.3 per cent carbon. This TRIP alloy exhibits yield strengths up to 300,000 psi while retaining as much as 15 to 20 per cent elongation.

TRIP steels are still in the research stage. Questions remain to be answered about their corrosion resistance, fatigue life, and compatibility. The unique ductility-strength behavior of this system, however, is a strong recommendation for its further investigation.

A third alloy has attracted attention for reasons other than strength. Known as Nitinol this is an alloy of nickel containing 45 per cent titanium.* It is highly corrosion resistant and displays good ductility but

---

*National Bureau of Standards, Washington, D.C.

relatively poor strength. In the annealed condition it has a yield strength of between 15,000 and 20,000 psi with an elongation of 60 per cent. Cold working produces strengths up to 50,000 psi, still inferior to other titanium alloys, with a corresponding reduction of elongation to 10 to 12 per cent.

This material, however, displays an interesting mechanical "memory." The 45 per cent titanium alloy may be deformed at room temperature and, when heated above 60°C, rapidly reverts to its original undeformed shape. The temperature at which this reversion takes place, which is actually a transformation from one phase structure to another, is controllable by alloy additions. In particular, addition of small amounts of cobalt during alloy production lowers the transformation temperature. Corrosion rate data and compatibility test results are becoming available and are encouraging. Applications of this type of alloy may have important ramifications in the implant field; one such, incorporating a shape change at body temperature, has been considered for use in internal fixation devices.

Materials Selection

Materials and the Design Process

The actual choice of materials lies with the designer, and the function of his design reflects both the properties and the processing of the material. The surgeon cannot make an independent decision concerning material choice, and therefore he should keep in mind some general observations.

1. These metals do have different properties. Thus, changing the metal that a device is made from may be expected to have an effect upon the performance of the device. Just because a surgeon experiences only a very small amount of cutting out of the trifin portion of stainless steel Jewett hip nails he uses to treat a particular class of femoral neck fractures, he cannot necessarily expect this experience to be unchanged if he begins to use nails of the identical design but of another material.

2. Materials' properties depend to a certain extent upon levels of impurities and processing during device manufacture. The surgeon should be alert to changes in processing of devices that he is accustomed to work with. The results of these changes may well be totally desirable, but the clinician's awareness will protect the patient by providing early warning of any possible adverse effects.

3. No one of these metals is inherently superior to any other nor to possible new materials to be developed. Each has its weaknesses and strengths. All factors should be considered by the designer. Thus, successful experience with a particular alloy in one type or design of device should not necessarily influence the surgeon in the choice of material in a new device. This point is important, since the most common devices, particularly in the area of fracture fixation, are often available in identical designs in different metals.

4. Unsatisfactory experience in a particular patient with one metal suggests that a change of alloy is one clinical alternative. If a patient has broken two fracture fixation devices of a particular alloy, for example, and the surgeon decides to continue with a device of the same design, he might well inquire of the availability of the device in a more fatigue- or corrosion-resistant alloy.

The concern expressed here for the effect of materials' properties on performance of devices should be reflected in the handling of these devices by the operating room staff and the surgeon. The manufacturer takes some care in processing implants and in producing those properties that he wishes to be present in the materials upon implantation. Protective coverings and housings are usually supplied to protect critical portions of implants, and manufacturers' instructions in their use should be followed (they should be left in place while the implant is being handled). Care should be taken not to mark, scratch, or otherwise damage implants.

Notes Regarding Specific Applications. A subject of some debate among orthopedic engineers is that of "contouring" or, more specifically, bending of fracture fixation hardware at the operating table to bring it into better conformation with the local bony anatomy. On the positive side, it is true that such deformation will probably result in better fixation, and the resulting work hardening raises the yield point, thus effectively extending the range of elastic deformation. On the negative side, however, the following points must be made: (1) The increased elastic deformation is obtained at the cost of a reduction in toughness. (2) Work hardening of a local area may cause an electrochemical change that can initiate a differential corrosion. (3) The use of the more common designs of bending irons, which are flat plates with slots to accept the fracture fixation device, may result in nicking or marking of the fixation device. These mechanical defects serve as stress raisers and may decrease the resistance to plastic deformation and fatigue fracture.

Clearly, the positive and negative points must be weighed. In balance, some contouring is probably permissible, given that the resulting bends are of a large radius (not sharp) and that no damage by the bending irons is observed.

A similar and older controversy surrounds the use of different alloys in a single location, for instance, the use of cobalt-chromium screws to attach the side plate of a stainless steel Jewett hip nail or the use of stainless steel cerclage wire in conjunction with a cobalt-chromium intramedullary rod.

Despite the generally good electrochemical behavior of these alloys, it is undesirable to use them in combination. Such combinations often lead to corrosive attack of one of the alloys involved. This comment may seem to be in conflict with that made previously on the possible mechanism of protection from corrosion in the cobalt-chromium alloys. A multipart device introduces factors that are not present in a multicomponent alloy. Motion between parts of the device may result in fretting, local loss of the passive layer, and enhanced corrosion. Low oxygen concentration in the "cracks" between parts of the device owing to diffusion limitations may result in another form of enhanced corrosion, termed crevice corrosion. While these factors are present in any multicomponent device, it seems possible that the use of different materials in the same device will exacerbate the difficulties encountered.

Processing variables can also affect the electrochemical behavior of metallic parts. Since different parts, such as wire, screws, and plates, are made by different combinations of processes, manufacturers routinely treat hardware components that are intended for use together to minimize these differences. The approach to this problem may, however, vary from one manufacturer to another. Thus, in addition to keeping alloys separate, it is probably desirable to obtain components for a given system from a single manufacturer.

The need to unite bone fragments in areas of severe stress combined with the clinical preference for union with displacement over failure of fixation has led to the wide use of wrought stainless steel in internal fixation devices. Cobalt-chromium alloys, although somewhat stronger, enjoy no real advantage in fatigue resistance, having similar endurance limits. This, combined with less ductility and greater difficulty of fabrication, has made them less popular. The titanium-6 aluminum-4 vanadium alloy is arousing increasing interest for fracture fixation applications. Despite being a relatively brittle material, it has fatigue properties that are superior to those of the other two alloy systems. To date, it has been used sparingly in fracture fixation devices. The Jewett hip nail and the Schneider intramedullary rod designs are available in Ti-6Al-4V variants. More recently, other device designs, such as fluted intramedullary rods that take advantage of the alloy properties, are appearing. This use of this alloy is more widespread in Europe, with American adoption moving at a slow pace.

Ceramics have found no general clinical role in fracture fixation, but polymers have achieved some limited applications. Replication of conventional designs, such as plate and screw combinations, is unsatisfactory, because of the creep and stress relaxation behavior of the available compatible materials. The necessary frictional forces that provide stability of reduction are lost too rapidly to permit satisfactory union. Limited testing of polymers in intramedullary rod designs and fiber-reinforced polymers in plate applications is under way, however. Initial animal studies in both of these areas show considerable promise.

Polymethylmethacrylate (PMMA) cement, usually used in support of partial and total joint replacement components, is now being used in conjunction with metallic components in the treatment of pathological fractures. The combination of screw-attached web, mesh, or straps with cement encasement can bring about stable fixation after excision of large amounts of bone. Although such cement and metal–filled defects will obviously not heal, such treatment can provide mobility for patients with pathological fractures. Ti–6A1–4V appears to be the material of choice for use in conjunction with polymethylmethacrylate in such applications.

MATERIALS-ASSOCIATED COMPLICATIONS

Local Effects

When fixation devices are overloaded and fail, either through fracture associated with a single event or through progressive fatigue failure, the failure is not usually related to the materials. That is, the failure is most often one of a properly constructed device that is unsuitable because it is an inappropriate device for the fixation requirements, is inadequately inserted, or is subjected to inappropriate postoperative therapy. Even the best-constructed internal fixation device cannot continue to function in the absence of adequate reduction (with load sharing) and progressive healing of the bony defect. Failures of this sort are usually termed *mechanical*.

Fracture of devices may be initiated or accelerated by defects in the device itself. These include inclusions and segregation defects in cast devices, surface defects in wrought devices, and surface damage introduced during insertion. This class of defects leads to failures that are properly termed *material* failures, in the sense that the device would have performed satisfactorily in their absence. Failures from these causes are avoidable through careful control of manufacturing processes and careful handling of implants in the hospital and operating room.

There are additional local conditions associated with materials that can lead to unsatisfactory function of fixation devices in the absence of device fracture. The most important of these is apparently related to corrosion of the fixation devices.

A small group in any large series of patients with fractures fixed with multipart devices will present with evidence of local infection at a time six months or longer after initial surgery. The local evidence (pain, inflammation, edema, aspiratable fluid, or in some cases, drainage) usually cannot be confirmed by systemic studies, and attempts to culture microorganisms from the site are unsuccessful. This presentation is often called a "sterile abscess."

On surgical exploration, these patients are found to have marked discoloration in the tissue planes adjacent to the device and to have a quantity of gray or black fluid in the operative site. Removal of the device brings prompt relief of pain (24 to 48 hours).

Cases of this sort appear to be ones in which there is an active corrosion process going on and a local inflammatory response to the products of corrosion. Since tests of the device components often reveal significant differences in electrochemical potential, they may or may not be associated with antigenic response to components of the metallic alloys involved. In case reports in which antigenic activity is documented by positive cutaneous or intradermal tests, the clinical signs previously mentioned are accompanied by some remote antigenic response, such as dermatitis or hives.

In cases of this sort, in which tissue response to the components of the alloy is suspected and there is a continuing need for internal fixation, the use of a device constructed of a different material is indicated.

There is additional local response that is often mistakenly thought to be material-related. The use of rigid fixation devices is often associated with osteoporotic remodeling in the immediate vicinity of the implant. This is usually interpreted as a Wolff's law dynamic remodeling response to the distribution of load between the implant and the underlying bone. Often, one speaks of the bone being "protected" or "bypassed." Such a finding is common upon removal of screw-plate devices.

Much emphasis is placed upon *modulus* of the material used in the device. In fact, if osteoporosis is a response to the load-sharing situation, then it depends upon the stiffness of the device and the rigidity of its attachment to the fracture fragments. The modulus of the material is only *one component* of these calculations; different designs and different applications can yield the same mechanical stiffness with materials of widely differing moduli. Thus it is inappropriate to associate these remodeling effects with materials' properties. They should more properly be associated with the over-all biomechanics of fixation.

Systemic Effects

The materials used for fabrication of internal fixation devices are the same as those used in partial and total joint replacements. Thus, the concerns that may be voiced over the possible systemic effects of fixation devices are part of the larger concern over the long-term prognosis for artificial implants.

Theories have been proposed and animal studies performed that suggest roles for corrosion and wear products in production of allergic response, depression of bacterial resistance, interference with various enzyme systems, and carcinogenesis, both locally and at remote sites. Of these proposed effects, only the allergenic has been documented with reports of isolated cases of systemic response to cobalt, chromium, and nickel.

The other possible effects remain conjectural. It has been suggested that the great volume of devices used in internal fixation and the lack of reports of systemic effects argue against their presence. It is more probable that the absence of reports stems from the similarity of the proposed effects to those induced by other causes, coupled with the absence of controlled, prospective studies with matched control groups of individuals who have not received internal fixation devices.

Most of the proposed effects depend upon long induction time, however, either for accumulation of corrosion products or for biological transformation to take place. Thus, the uncertainty concerning systemic response to materials used in internal fixation devices should be recognized as an additional reason to consider such devices temporary and to seek their removal at appropriate times after insertion.

Acknowledgment: Portions of this chapter are adapted from

J. H. Dumbleton and J. Black: *An Introduction to Orthopaedic Materials* Chapter 8. Charles C Thomas, Springfield, Ill., 1975. The author is grateful to Dr. Dumbleton for his permission to use this material and for his careful reading of this manuscript.

WILSON C. HAYES, Ph.D.

7 _____ *Biomechanics of Fracture Treatment*

Bone tissue exhibits two remarkable properties that distinguish it from other structural materials. Bone may alter its local mechanical properties in response to changes in functional demand. For instance, bone density changes are commonly observed after periods of disuse or chronically increased function. Bone tissue also exhibits the remarkable capacity to heal itself through a repair process resulting not in a scar but in an actual reconstitution of the injured tissue.[47] This process is the result of a delicate interplay of complex biological and mechanical processes.

Fractures are part of the injury pattern associated with high-speed transportation, industrial accidents, and leisure activities. As measured by days of disability per year, such fractures are among the most serious types of disabling accidental injury. Yet, despite the obvious medical and economic relevance of fracture prevention and optimal management, many aspects of the biomechanics of fracture healing and treatment are only partially understood.

This chapter is an attempt to bring together information on three aspects of the biomechanics of fracture healing and treatment. The first is related to the return of stiffness and strength in healing bone. Bones are structural members whose mechanical functions are to support the body, to protect vital organs, and to permit the skeletal motions necessary for survival. Since these are structural functions, it seems natural that fracture healing should be evaluated by the return of prefracture stiffness and strength. Instead, however, clinical assessments of the extent of fracture healing are made primarily by radiographic criteria. Little is known about the temporal sequence of the return of stiffness and strength to healing bone.

Therefore, one purpose of this chapter will be to summarize the available data on the biomechanical stages of fracture repair and the mechanical factors that influence the process. Such data have been generated primarily from animal models, but wide variations in experimental design, treatment modalities, and normal biological variability have made it difficult to compare results and to draw clinically relevant conclusions. The hope here is that by bringing these data together, comparisons can be made more easily.

A second aspect of the biomechanics of fracture treatment is the optimizing of fracture management. All fracture treatment is an attempt to provide those environmental conditions that allow the healing process to occur as quickly as possible. However, the physiology of bone and of fracture healing poses a unique set of mechanical demands that usually involve trade-offs between conflicting requirements. Plaster immobilization is designed to prevent fracture fragment mobility, and yet there is evidence that some fragment motion may be tolerated and may even be beneficial to the healing bone. The purpose of internal fixation by compression is to provide rigid immobilization during the early stages of fracture healing. During the late stage of the repair process, however, this rigid immobilization may lead to a reduction in bone stresses sufficient to cause a disuse osteoporosis which can lead to refracture upon removal of the plate. When more than mechanical factors are considered, these trade-offs become even more complex.

A second purpose of this chapter, then, is to summarize available information on attempts to optimize the mechanics of fracture management. These include in vitro mechanical comparisons of internal fixation methods, studies of stresses in walking casts and functional bracing, the mechanics of surgical screws and their insertion, and theoretical analyses of plate fixation.

The third aspect of the biomechanics of fracture treatment is the application of mechanical testing techniques to the evaluation of fracture healing in human patients. Currently, to determine the progress of fracture healing, the clinician uses a manual examination for stability, radiographic criteria, the empirical passage of time, and the patient's evaluation of symptomatic pain. Only the first of these can be thought of as a test of the mechanical integrity of the healing fracture, and it obviously is only qualitative. Efforts are underway at a number of laboratories to improve the precision of the biomechanical evaluation of healing fractures. None of the techniques can yet be thought of as a clinical tool for the noninvasive assessment of the mechanical integrity of healing fractures. Considerable progress has been made, however, and this chapter will summarize the techniques under development.

The chapter is organized into four sections. The first is an introduction to some of the mechanical concepts involved. The second summarizes the major findings on the biomechanics of fracture healing using animal models. The third section deals with in vitro and theoretical studies directed toward improved fracture management, and the fourth summarizes developing techniques for the clinical assessment of the mechanical integrity of healing fractures.

MECHANICAL CONCEPTS

In normal daily activities a complex pattern of forces is imposed on the bones of the skeletal system. These forces arise from direct contact occurring at the articular surfaces of joints and the ligaments surrounding joints, and from muscles acting through the insertion of tendons on the bone. The application of these forces causes microscopic deformations of the bone. The nature and magnitude of these deformations are dependent upon: (1) the pattern and magnitude of the imposed loads; (2) the bone structural geometry (i.e., length and curvature); (3) the local cross-sectional geometry; and (4) the material properties of the bone tissue. The mechanical response of a bone under these conditions can be described by quantitatively assessing the relationships between applied loads and the resulting microscopic deformations. These relationships reveal the structural behavior of the whole bone.

The local deformations at any point in the bone are referred to as *strains*, and the local force intensities are the *stresses* at that point. The relationships between stresses and strains at a particular point in the bone are governed by the local material properties of the bone tissue. If the whole bone is loaded with very high forces, the stresses and strains in one region may exceed the ultimate stresses or strains that can be tolerated by the tissue. Local mechanical failure will occur at that point, causing bone fracture.

The two most important parameters for the mechanical behavior of bone tissue are its modulus and its strength. The *modulus* is a measure of the amount of deformation experienced by the tissue when subjected to loads. Low-modulus materials deform more than high-modulus materials when subjected to the same loads. *Strength* is related to the amount of load required to cause failure of the material. Usually the failure load is normalized to account for differences in cross-sectional area.

The case of tensile loading provides a simple instructive example of how the failure load is normalized to account for differences in cross-sectional geometry. Two rods subjected to pure tension are shown in Figure 7-1. Their corresponding load-deflection curves are also shown. Both rods are made of the same material, and yet the first fails at a load level that is half that of the second rod. This is simply because

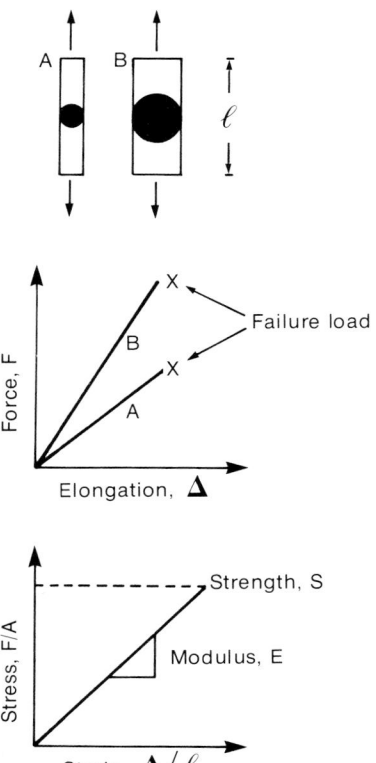

Figure 7–1 Simple tensile test of two rods of the same material showing the effect of cross-sectional area on failure load. To account for this effect, the failure load is divided by cross-sectional area to compute tensile strength. The upper graph corresponds to *structural parameters*, and the lower graph provides *material parameters*.

the stronger rod has a cross-sectional area twice that of the weaker rod. To account for these differences and to provide a parameter that effectively describes the behavior of the material, the failure load is divided by the cross-sectional area, yielding a parameter referred to as *strength*. This parameter has the same units as stress (newtons per meter squared), and thus we may define strength as that stress at which failure occurs. In the case of tension loading, the parameter is referred to as the *ultimate tensile strength*. For bending loads, the strength parameter is called the *flexural strength*, for torsion the torsional strength.

It is important to note that two parameters have been used to describe the ultimate load-bearing capacity of the material. The first is the ultimate failure load, which is simply the maximum force that the specimen can sustain before failure, and it is commonly referred to as a *structural parameter*. The second is the ultimate strength, which by normalizing the results to account for differences in cross-sectional geometry, provides a property descriptive of the material. It is therefore referred to as

a *material parameter*. Material parameters are commonly displayed by plotting a curve of stress (force divided by area) against strain (elongation divided by original length) as shown in the lower portion of Figure 7–1. This plot provides a single curve representing the mechanical properties (strength and modulus) of the material making up the two rods. The two graphs shown in Figure 7–1 represent two different methods for describing the load-bearing capacity of structural components, and thus it is important to distinguish between structural and material parameters. The discussions in this chapter will emphasize this point.

Similar approaches can be used to investigate the mechanical behavior of whole bones. In this case the analysis is more complex, since the mechanical behavior is governed by the tissue mechanical properties, by local geometrical factors, such as cross-sectional area, by global geometrical factors, such as bone length and curvature, and by the imposed loads. Still, the mechanical behavior is characterized using an approach similar to that taken with small specimens. The whole bone is subjected to well-defined loads which are gradually increased until failure occurs. The failure load provides a structural parameter that includes effects due to material properties and to local and global geometry. Removing these geometrical factors results in an assessment of tissue strength, a material parameter. Again, the particular parameters used to characterize the mechanical behavior depend on the loading configuration chosen for the test, with tension, bending, and torsion being most commonly used. Such tests can be employed with whole bones to characterize the modulus, the ultimate failure load, and the tissue strength if appropriate analyses are applied. However, with whole bones these experiments and their interpretation are considerably more complex than with small specimens, since it is far more difficult to control the loads applied and to monitor the resulting deformations. With healing bones or with composite systems including both bone and an internal fixation device, even greater complexities arise.

The difference between material and structural parameters is of considerable importance in determining the strength and stiffness of healing fractures and in assessing the mechanical performance of an internal fixation device. As suggested earlier, the mechanical response of the whole system is governed not only by local tissue mechanical properties but also by local and global geometrical factors. Both sets of factors may be changing markedly during fracture healing. For instance, two healing fractures may exhibit similar values for ultimate load when tested in bending. In one case the results may be strongly related to increasing tissue stiffness and strength at the fracture site. In the second case they may be due to the presence of an abundant callus with a large increase in cross-sectional area. Thus, while the functional capacity of the two fractures may be similar (as measured by a structural parameter, such as ultimate bending load), the mechanical properties of the healing tissues may be quite different. While the ultimate load may be the most relevant parameter for determining the capacity of a healing fracture to withstand load, material and geometrical factors must also be taken into account in order to better understand the mechanics of fracture healing and to optimize fracture management. In much of the research summarized in the following sections this distinction has not always been made.

BIOMECHANICS OF FRACTURE HEALING

In early attempts to monitor the return of prefracture stiffness and strength, the strength of a healing fracture was measured by simply bending the healing bone and noting the failure load.[22, 37, 38, 44, 46, 81] A common finding of these studies was that experimental variability was too great to allow meaningful comparisons of fracture management methods or to assess the effects of systemic or dietary factors. Much of this variability was due to poor control over the mechanical testing conditions. In order to reduce this variability, some attempts were made to normalize the measured failure loads to account for differences in the cross-sectional areas of the healing fractures. In many cases this did not significantly reduce scatter, again owing to poorly controlled measurement methods and the wide variability exhibited by experimental animals.

Recently, through careful control of both animal models and mechanical testing conditions, this situation has improved to the point that several distinct biomechanical stages have been identified for the repair process. In addition, more data are available on some of the factors that influence fracture repair as judged mechanically. These include functional use, surgical intervention, and electrical stimulation. A number of studies have also considered the differences in the mechanics of the repair process when internal fixation devices are used. Some controlled comparative data are also available on the return of prefracture stiffness and strength using different methods of internal fixation.

BIOMECHANICAL STAGES OF FRACTURE REPAIR

Existing classification schemes for the stages in fracture healing are based on radiographic criteria, histological appearance, biochemical observation, and clinical judgment. To provide a classification in which the stages of fracture repair are based on objective measurements of the mechanical properties of the healing bone, White and co-workers[74] designed experiments to correlate radiological and histological information on fracture healing with torsional strength and other biomechanical parameters. By analysis of roentgenograms and the torque-angle curves made after failure at healing fracture sites in rabbits, they identified four clearly delineated biomechanical stages of fracture repair.

The changing patterns of the torque angle graphs of six representative bones from this investigation are shown in Figure 7–2. The earliest evidence of returning strength was seen after 21 to 24 days of healing. In bones with a healing time of 21 to 26 days, the soft tissue exhibits a rubbery type of behavior characterized by low torque values and a large angular deformation. In a later phase of healing, after 49 to 56 days, the bone has a hard tissue type of behavior, characterized by high torque values and small angular deformations associated with a high degree of stiffness. The soft tissue and hard tissue phases are sharply demarcated at approximately 26 to 27 days by an abrupt change in the torque-angle curves. This sharp transition from a rubbery quality to a much stiffer, hard tissue type of behavior is sometimes evident clinically and is characterized by "stickiness" at the fracture site.

In those healing tibial fractures tested in torsional loading, failure occurred in one of three ways: (1) purely through the experimental fracture (healing osteotomy site); (2) partially through the healing experimental fracture and partially through the intact bone; and (3) entirely through the intact bone without involving the healing experimental fracture. Based on these characteristics of healing bone tested to failure, the authors established the following four biomechanical phases of fracture repair.

Stage 1: The bone fails through the original experimental fracture site with a low-stiffness, rubbery pattern, as illustrated in Figure 7–2.

Stage 2: The bone fails through the original experimental fracture site with a high-stiffness, hard tissue pattern.

Stage 3: The bone fails partially through the original experimental fracture site and partially through the previously intact bone with a high-stiffness, hard tissue pattern like the 49-day torque-angle curve shown in Figure 7–2.

Stage 4: The site of failure is not related to the original experimental fracture, and occurs with a high-stiffness pattern similar to the 56-day curve illustrated in Figure 7–2.

The authors reasoned that these stages should correlate with the quantitative measurements of strength. The bones were therefore grouped into the four biomechanical stages on the basis of the test data, and the average maximum torque and average

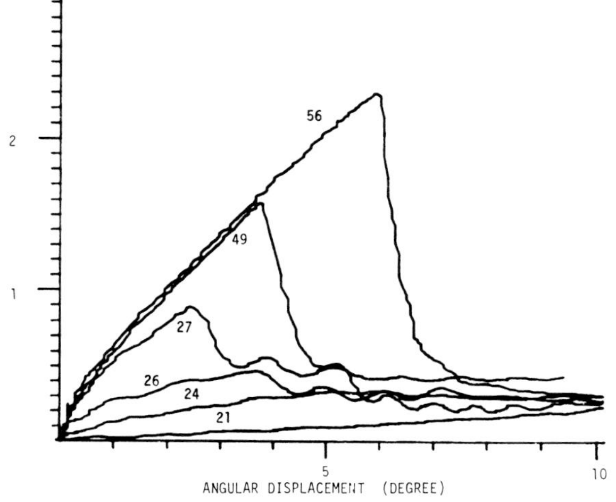

Figure 7–2 A composite torque-angle graph of six bones representative of the entire healing period. The numbers indicate days of healing time. As healing progresses, there is an increase in the strength of union shown by the changes in the torque-angle graphs. (Courtesy of A. A. White, M. M. Panjabi, W. D. Southwick and *The Journal of Bone and Joint Surgery.* J. Bone Joint Surg., 59A:188, 1977.)

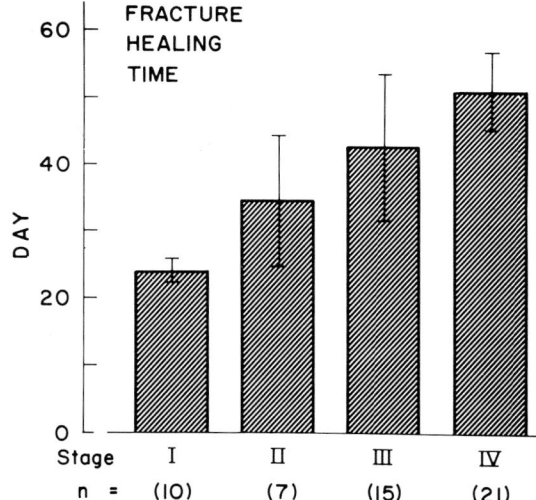

Figure 7–3 Histogram showing average healing times and standard deviations for the four biomechanical stages of fracture healing. (Courtesy of A. A. White, M. M. Panjabi, W. D. Southwick and *The Journal of Bone and Joint Surgery.* J. Bone Joint Surg., 59A:188, 1977.)

energy absorption to failure for each group were determined. Although there was considerable variation in the data, a distinct trend was evident in the progressive increase in strength from stage 1 to stage 4. When the average times after fracture for the bones in each of the four stages were compared, the same progression was evident (Fig. 7–3). As demonstrated by the histogram, the four stages correlated closely with strength and healing time.

A later study,[54] designed to focus specifically on the temporal changes in the physical properties of healing fractures, used the same experimental model. It should be noted that the original purpose of these studies was to determine the effect of superimposed cyclical loads on the rate of fracture repair. The original hypothesis was that cyclical loading would accelerate fracture repair by a stress-related adaptive process.[75] No significant differences were found in comparison with fractures treated with constant compression. Therefore, the results in all healed bones were grouped for

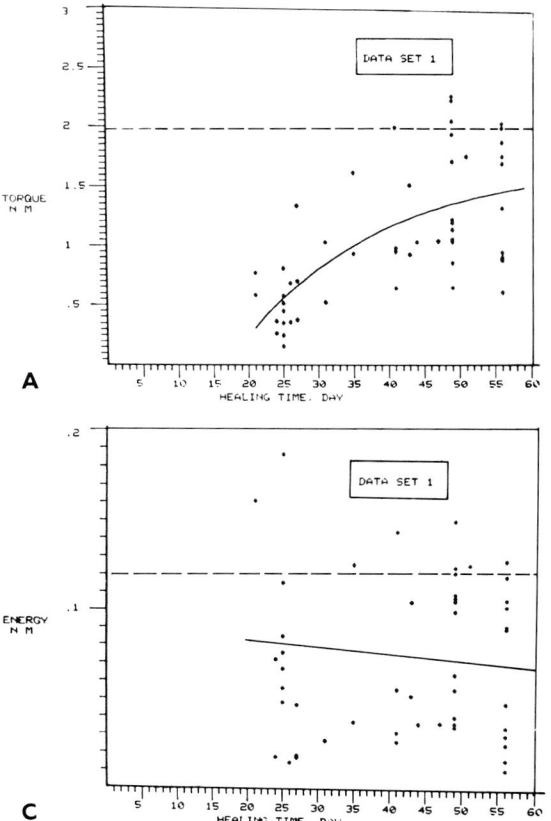

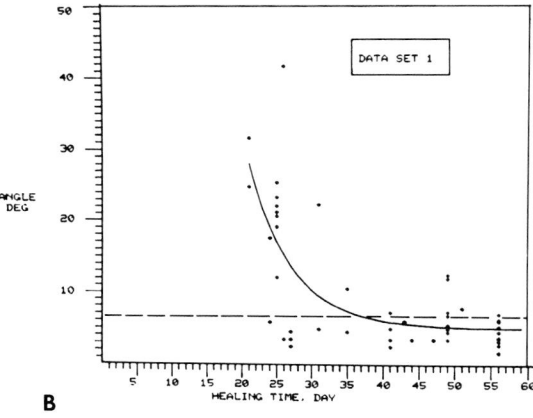

Figure 7–4 Temporal changes in the physical properties of healing fractures. *A.* Maximum torque as a function of healing time. *B.* Angular deformation at maximum torque as a function of healing time. *C.* Average torsional stiffness at maximum torque as a function of healing time. (Courtesy of M. M. Panjabi, A. A. White, W. D. Southwick and *The Journal of Biomechanics.* J. Biomech., *10*:689, 1977.)

the study of temporal changes in physical properties.

The data for maximum torque as a function of healing time are plotted in Figure 7–4A, with the dashed line representing the average values of intact sham bone. Maximum torque is seen to increase from a value of approximately 25 per cent of the intact bone at three weeks to a value of approximately 75 per cent at nine weeks. Exponential curves computed by a least squares procedure are also shown. The angular deformations at maximum torque as a function of healing time are shown in Figure 7–4B. At three weeks the fracture exhibits large angular deformations prior to failure; this is reduced to a value slightly less than that of the intact bone by nine weeks. This result could be expected to be related to the large increases in the cross-sectional area of the healing fracture callus. Finally, the average torsional stiffness at maximum torque as a function of healing time is shown in Figure 7–4C. Examination of these data suggests that the mechanical parameters used to assess fracture healing progress at different rates. It should also be noted, however, that the data obtained in these studies represent structural parameters that include the effects of changes in both the material properties and the geometry of the healing bones. Perhaps modeling the testing procedure analytically in order to account for the geometrical changes will allow a more careful examination of the temporal changes in the mechanical properties of the osseous tissues involved in fracture healing.

BIOCHEMICAL AND RADIOGRAPHIC CORRELATIONS

Since the radiographic appearance of fracture callus is an important clinical variable used to assess fracture healing, the correlation of biochemical and mechanical characteristics of callus with radiographic appearance is important. Whiteside and co-workers[76] investigated the physical changes associated with different radiographic stages of fracture healing and correlated them with changes in the biochemical composition of the fracture callus.

Transverse midshaft osteotomies were made on both tibiae of 36 adult New Zealand white rabbits. The osteotomies were fixed with intramedullary pins, and the rabbits were allowed full activity in their cages. Groups of six animals were sacrificed at one, two, three, four, six, and eight weeks. Roentgenograms were made of the tibiae, and the stage of healing was graded as follows: (1) no visible callus, (2) early callus, (3) abundant callus but not bridged, (4) fully bridging callus, and (5) mature callus. At sacrifice, the fractures were loaded to failure in tension at a constant strain rate, and the failure load, tensile strength, ultimate strain, and energy to failure were determined. The callus was removed and lyophilized, and hydroxyproline, hexosamine, and calcium content was determined and expressed as mg per gm dry weight.

The callus showed a progressive increase in load to failure and tensile strength through the radiographic stages of healing. Energy to failure increased through stages 1 to 3, but decreased significantly (P <0.01) at stage 4, when early bridging callus was detectable radiographically. This decrease in energy resulted from the decrease in the strain to failure. Hexosamine content increased through the first three stages of healing, but dropped sharply at the fourth stage. Calcium increased progressively through the first four stages and leveled off during callus maturation. The concomitant gain in calcium and loss of hexosamine in the fourth stage of healing was associated with a decrease in deformation and energy to failure. Hydroxyproline increased slightly through the first three stages of healing and showed a tendency to decrease in the last two stages. Changes in hydroxyproline content could not be correlated with any of the mechanical changes in the callus.

When all the specimens were grouped, there was a strong positive correlation between hexosamine level and total strain to failure (r=0.90). During the third and fourth stages of healing (and only during these stages) there was a positive correlation (r=0.81) between hexosamine content and energy to failure. There was a strong negative correlation between calcium level and deformation to failure (r=0.90). In the third and fourth stages there was a strong negative correlation between calcium content and energy to failure (r=0.86).

The most striking observation in this

study was the brittleness of the callus in the early bridging stage of healing. Although the callus gained in tensile strength during this stage, it lost a proportionately greater degree of deformability, and thus suffered a decrease in total energy to failure. The loss in deformability appeared to be associated with a reduction in the mucopolysaccharide content of the callus. Throughout the healing period, deformation to failure was negatively correlated with calcium content. However, this did not seem to be damaging except in the early bridging state (stage 4) of the healing, when a marked loss of mucopolysaccharide occurred. These two factors appeared to work in concert in the early bridging callus phase to cause a decrease in the fracture toughness (energy to failure) of the callus.

According to this investigation, the final stage of healing is not associated with any detectable changes in the biochemical characteristics of the fracture callus. However, the most marked changes in mechanical properties occurred during this stage. It seems likely that these alterations are brought about by internal remodeling in order to optimize the structural characteristics of the system.

FACTORS INFLUENCING HEALING

Function Versus Immobilization

There has been relatively little experimental work correlating functional loading with temporal progression of fracture healing. The experiments of White and coworkers failed to show significant differences due to superimposed cyclical loads on healing fractures. Sarmiento and associates[67] assessed the influence of function on fracture healing in the rat, using differences in the fracture callus of immobilized and functional animals based on radiographic, histological, and biomechanical criteria. A standard experimental fracture was created in the rat femur and stabilized with a loose-fitting intramedullary pin. For the immobilized group, spica casts were fashioned to restrict the joints above and below the fracture site. The animals were sacrificed at regular intervals, and the healing callus in the functional and immobilized

groups subjected to histological and biomechanical evaluation.

Three-point bending tests were performed to determine the strength of the healing fracture and the modulus of elasticity of the callus. Approximate calculations were made of the bending stresses that developed at the fracture site, using simple beam approximations. The area moment of inertia used in these calculations was approximated by assuming the cross section at the healing fracture to be an ellipse.

Radiographic and histological findings were consistent and demonstrated more abundant fracture callus in the functional group at the end of the second week. At three weeks the differences in the size of the fracture callus were still present but less striking. The presence of a radiographic fracture line persisted in the functional group well into the third and fourth weeks of fracture healing. This was not the finding in the immobilized group, in which the fracture line had uniformly disappeared by the end of the fourth week.

Although the appearance of the fracture line on roentgenograms suggests clinically that healing is not complete, its disappear-

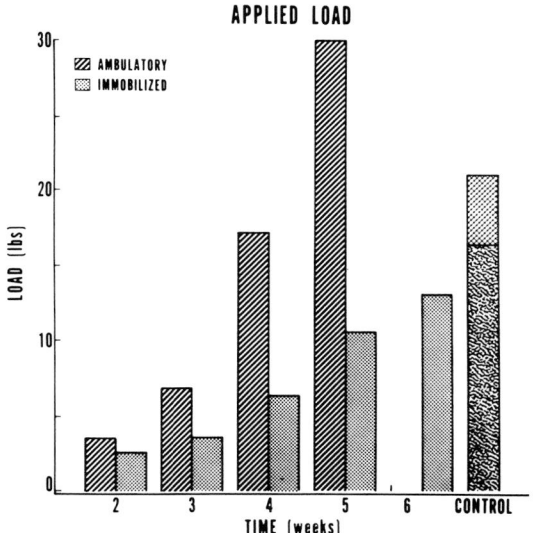

Figure 7-5 Average maximum failure loads in three-point bending as a function of healing time for healing rat femora treated with ambulation and immobilization. (Data from A. Sarmiento, J. F. Schaeffer, L. Beckerman, et al., and *The Journal of Bone and Joint Surgery.* J. Bone Joint Surg., 59A:369, 1977.)

ance in this study did not necessarily indicate completed fracture healing based on biomechanical criteria. The load-displacement curves in three-point bending revealed increasing failure loads as healing progressed. Similarly, the displacement occurring at the fracture site prior to failure decreased with healing time. A comparison of the average maximum loads as a function of healing time for functional and immobilized animals reveals significant differences, as shown in Figure 7–5. At two weeks, the average maximum load for those fractures in the immobilized group is about 25 per cent less than that sustained by the functional group. By three weeks, the average difference is approximately 50 per cent. Using simple beam theory and the assumption of elliptical cross sections, the calculated maximum bending stresses do not show significant differences at the second and third week, but do so at four and five weeks. Calculations of the modulus of elasticity of the healing callus also reveal that the modulus increased with healing time in both groups, but no significant differences were noted between groups.

In discussing their results, the authors noted that their finding of an increased amount of cartilage in response to increased motion in the functional group was compatible with a number of previous experiments.[26, 43, 49, 82] While the formation of cartilage at the fracture site is considered detrimental by some, in this experiment it was rapidly replaced through the process of vascularization and enchondral ossification in the functional group. This increased periosteal osteogenesis in the ambulatory animals was considered an important factor in fracture healing. This increase was assumed to represent the response of the fracture callus to the mechanical forces imposed upon it. In addition, the presence of a number of vascular connections between the appositional new bone and the original cortex, which was not noted in the immobilized group, was felt to indicate a pattern of increased circulation based on the activity of the involved extremity.

The experimental results also suggest caution in the use of radiographic criteria to judge the rate of fracture healing. Functional specimens in which the fracture line persisted on roentgenograms were stronger mechanically than the immobilized group, in which the fracture line had already been lost radiographically. In the latter, excess periosteal callus, delayed union, and non-union appeared on roentgenograms to be similar to the healing callus of the functionally loaded limb, but the material properties were found to be radically different.

In this comparison of functional and immobilized fracture healing, the material properties of the healing tissues (Young's modulus) were not found to be significantly different at any time during the healing process. Marked differences were observed in the structural properties, such as flexural rigidity, and in the maximum load to failure. These findings are consistent with the concept that the geometrical arrangement of the material at the fracture site is responsible for some of the differences in the structural properties of the healing bone. In addition, a marked increase in the modulus of elasticity between the third and fourth weeks in both groups was assumed to represent that phase of fracture healing in which rapid mineralization of the fracture callus occurs. Similar results were noted by White and co-workers.[75] This rapid increase in the stiffness of the fracture callus is of considerable importance in fracture healing. Without sufficient stiffness provided by either a stiff material in the callus or a large callus with a high area moment of inertia, the healing fracture cannot withstand the constant loading that occurs in weight-bearing ambulation.

These findings are in agreement with a number of previous investigations.[57] From their histological investigations, the authors noted that periosteal callus not only develops a large peripheral bulk, but that its best mechanically developed materials lie in those regions most distant from the centroid of the fracture cross-section. Newly formed fibrocartilage develops near the center of the callus and pushes the older, more developed hyaline cartilage outward. Since osseous tissues are continuously being formed between the cartilage and the osseous layers, the earliest remodeling of osseous tissues takes place in the most peripheral portion of the periosteal callus. Therefore, the materials in the callus best suited to resist stresses have been advantageously placed farther from the centroid of the cross-section and provide maximum resistance to bending and torsional loads.

In summary, this experiment represents an important contribution to the understanding of the effects of functional activities on the mechanical properties of healing fractures. Those fractures subjected to functional loading exhibited increased maximum loads at failure. This suggests that functional loading along with maintenance of a normal muscle mass and vascular supply provides a more suitable environment for the development of a strong union compared with total immobilization of the limb. Although the fractures in both the immobilized and the functional groups healed, those fractures in the immobilized group never reached prefracture mechanical strength within the time period of the study. This indicates a decreased functional capability of the fractured bone when complete immobilization is used. In addition, the amount of fracture callus produced was a function of the mobility of the fracture fragments, and continued mechanical stimulation appeared to accelerate the ossification process. The more rapid ossification of a more abundant callus resulted in significant increases in the structural stiffness and strength of the healing fracture.

Sciatic Denervation

Altered fracture healing has been reported in many neurological conditions, and clinicians have observed both increased and decreased rates of healing in neurologically injured patients. Despite these clinical observations, relatively little experimental effort has been directed to this phenomenon. Frymoyer and Pope[29] studied the biomechanics of fracture healing in peripherally denervated animals. Relatively stable fractures of the rat fibula were created. In experimental animals the sciatic nerve was excised.

Biomechanical testing was conducted using a tensile testing device of special design. After failure, the area of the callus at the fracture site was determined using a reflected light microscope. These area measurements were used to calculate the ultimate tensile strength of the healing fractures as a function of healing time. Owing to the large variability in the experimental results, special statistical techniques were used to test the differences between the two groups at 15 and 30 days. At these times there were highly significant differences in fracture strength, elastic modulus, and energy absorbed to failure, with the neurologically injured groups showing higher values in all cases. The data showed that increased healing of fibula fractures occurred in sciatically denervated rats 15 to 20 days following combined fracture and sciatic denervation. Considerable data scatter was observed in both the biomechanical results and the histological evaluations.

The authors proposed a number of mechanisms to explain their observations of enhanced healing in denervated fractures: (1) a neurohumeral mechanism; (2) alterations in fracture motions; (3) altered vascular supply; or (4) altered electrical fields. Lindholm[43] has observed that the fractured rat tibia manipulated daily healed with more exuberant callus and increased cartilage formation than nonmanipulated fractures. Similar observations were noted by Sarmiento and co-workers[67] in rat femoral fractures under conditions of functional weight bearing. In the peripherally denervated animal, a flaccid paralysis may permit greater motion between the fracture fragments than in the nonparalyzed animal. In the rat model, this would seem to be less likely because the synostosis of the proximal and distal portions of the fibula imparts considerable stability to the fracture. Another possibility is that changes in vascular supply may play a role.

Surgical Intervention

Piekarski and colleagues[57] tested the effects of delayed intramedullary internal fixation on fracture healing and explored the hypothesis that a "second injury" phenomenon in callus renders more efficient healing. For the experimental model, osteotomies of the radius were created in adult rabbits. Splinting was not required, since the rabbit radius is tightly bound to the ulna by the interosseous membrane. Three experimental groups consisted of animals with: (a) no intramedullary fixation; (b) intramedullary fixation at the time of fracture using a Kirschner wire; and (c) delayed intramedullary fixation one week after the fracture.

The maximum tensile failure loads as a function of healing time are shown in Figure 7–6A. The group with no intrame-

dullary fixation attained greatest strength at five and six weeks, but the differences are not significant (P >0.3) when compared with the groups with intramedullary fixation. The cross-sectional area data further showed that the delayed internal fixation group developed the largest callus cross

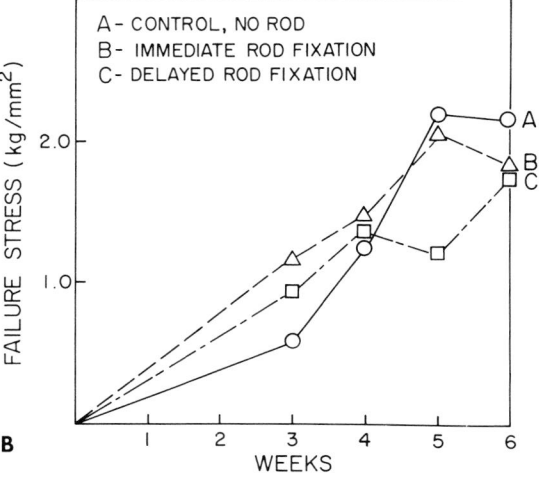

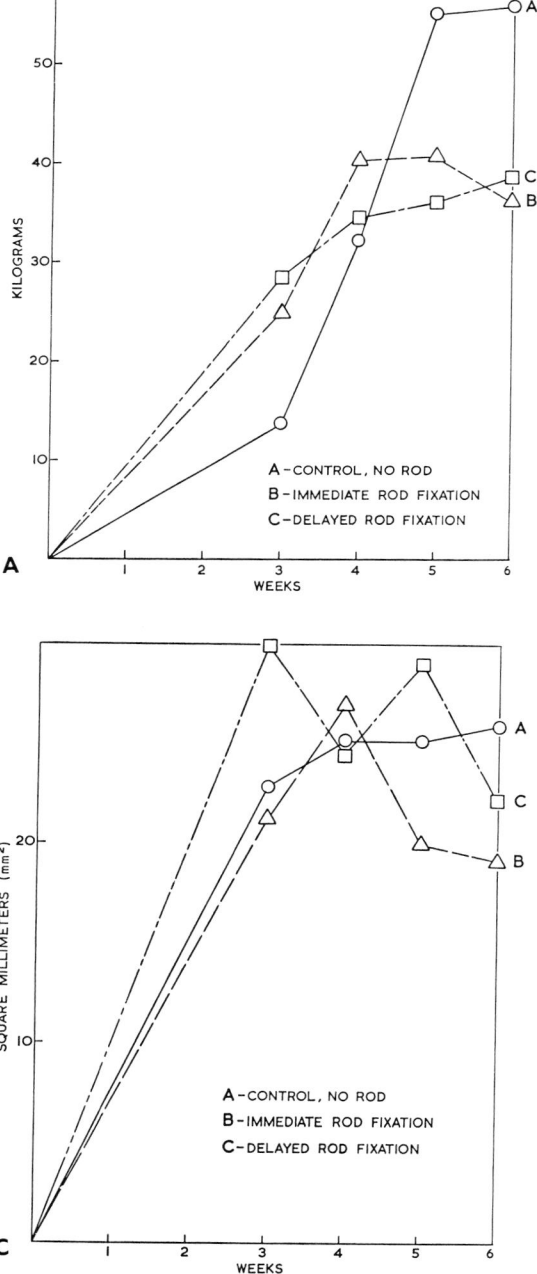

Figure 7–6 The effect of delayed internal fixation with intramedullary rods on fracture healing. *A.* Fracture load. *B.* Fracture strength. *C.* Porosity of callus. (Courtesy of Peikarski, K., Wiley, A. M., and Bartels, J. E. and *Acta Orthopaedica Scandinavica. Acta Orthop. Scand., 40:543, 1969.*)

section in the early stages (up to three weeks) and then tapered off until, at six weeks, both intramedullary fixation groups had smaller cross sections than the group with untreated fractures. Similar results were noted for total callus volume. The findings thus indicate a stimulation of callus production in fractures treated by delayed internal fixation. This effect was greatest shortly after the insertion of the intramedullary rod and diminished thereafter, owing to more intensive remodeling and resorption of the callus in fractures treated with intramedullary fixation.

When the average failure loads of Figure 7–6A are divided by the reported average cross-sectional area values, a failure strength is obtained (Fig. 7–6B). This value gives an indication of the specific local mechanical properties of the healing tissue. The average failure strengths of the three groups are clustered more closely than the failure loads, indicating that the callus tissue strengths are similar for all three methods of treatment. These results can be explained in part by measurements of the porosity of the callus (Fig. 7–6C). At three weeks the delayed internal fixation group exhibits a highly significant increase in callus porosity when compared with controls having no fixation. Thereafter, the porosity of both the controls and the immediate fixation groups decreases almost linearly, while the porosity of the delayed internal fixation group decreases less rapidly. This porosity effect, in combination with the more rapid reduction in the external dimensions of the callus in the intramedullary fixation groups, results in the reduced failure loads and tissue strengths observed in these groups compared with controls with no internal fixation.

The experiment indicates that a relatively immobilized fracture treated by internal fixation with intramedullary rods results in more exuberant callus production in the early stages of fracture healing. This factor imparts increased strength to the healing bone during this period. However, in the later stages of fracture healing, internal fixation under these conditions also results in more rapid reductions in the external dimensions of the callus and in less rapid reductions in the porosity of the callus. The effect of these factors is to reduce the load-carrying capacity of the healing frac-

ture and of the healing tissue in comparison with controls without fixation.

While this experiment may be questioned for the use of formalin-preserved bones and unphysiological mechanical test methods, it remains one of the few temporal studies of the structural capacity of healing fractures to consider both the geometrical factors involved in callus production and the differences in porosity involved in remodeling of the callus.

Henry and co-workers[34] also used the osteotomized rabbit radius as an experimental model in a study of the effects of surgical interference on the mechanical properties of healing fractures. Three experimental groups were used, including a control group in which no implant was inserted. A second group had intramedullary wires passed into each fragment from the fracture site, with no periosteal stripping beyond that necessarily associated with the osteotomy. The third group had plates and screws applied with stripping of the periosteum. In order to eliminate variations in the degree of fixation none of the implant devices crossed the fracture site.

Figure 7–7 shows the results at five weeks' healing time for the three experimental groups. The strength ratio (fractured/intact) is plotted against the stiffness ratio (fractured/intact). There is no significant difference between the three groups (no implant, intramedullary wire, plate and screws). Thus, at least at five weeks, the different modes of treatment and their

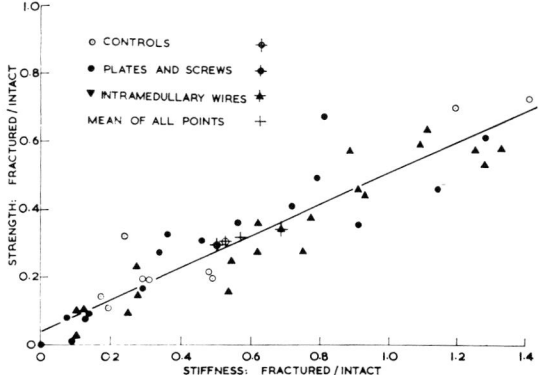

Figure 7–7 Variation of strength ratio with stiffness ratio for fractures tested after 5 weeks. The slope of the line indicates that the stiffness of the fracture returns to normal more rapidly than does the strength.

relative disturbance of the blood supply appear to have no observable effect on the return of strength and stiffness. In addition, although both strength and stiffness ratios vary widely, the slope of the line in Figure 7–7 is 0.48, meaning that when the stiffness ratio returns to a normal value of 1.0, the corresponding strength ratio is only about 0.5.

The statistical significance of the correlation (r=0.92) indicates that for every pair of bones represented, the stiffness had approached that of the intact bone more nearly than had the strength. Similar results were noted when the stiffness and strength ratios were plotted as a function of healing time. In spite of the large scatter observed, which made it impossible to differentiate between the experimental groups, the increase in the stiffness ratio was consistently more rapid than in the strength ratio. This observation led Henry and co-workers[34] to suggest the hypothesis that fracture healing is a self-regulating mechanism governed by signals dependent on deformations occurring in the healing bone. The authors also noted that there were not two clearly separate groups within any one type of fracture, i.e., those in which union had failed and those in which union had succeeded. On the contrary, there was a continuous scatter in the mechanical test results over the entire range of the healing outcomes. Therefore, they concluded that healing had occurred at widely differing rates throughout a spectrum of rapid progression to union on the one hand and to nonunion on the other. These results emphasized the arbitrary nature of the terms "nonunion" and "time to union."

Electrical Stimulation

Accelerating the healing of fractures by artificial stimulation of osteogenesis is an exciting prospect. A variety of experimental techniques, both physical and chemical, local and systemic, have been considered as potential means for stimulating the formation of bone. The concept of stimulating bone formation electrically is suggested by the presence of physiological electrical currents in living bone. These currents are thought to represent part of a control system that affects the remodeling of bone as well as the healing of fractures. A number of experimental approaches for electrical stimulation of bone healing are possible.[20] Each has advantages and limitations, especially from a future clinical standpoint. Direct application of continuous or pulsed currents appears to offer the best possibility for practical utilization, pending development of techniques for stimulation by electrostatic or magnetic fields. The direct application of electrical current to stimulate fracture healing is dealt with in Chapter 3, and only the biomechanical assessments of this approach will be reviewed here.

In an early study, Friedenberg and Brighton[25] demonstrated that live, non-stressed bone exhibited a low-magnitude steady-state potential that is electronegative in the metaphyseal regions and approaches isopolarity in the midshaft. In the presence of a fracture, the entire shaft becomes electronegative, the metaphyseal electronegativity becomes even higher, and a secondary increase in electronegativity appears over the fracture site. With healing of the fracture, the pattern of electropolarity returns to normal. In subsequent studies the effects of applying direct current to bone were evaluated.[24, 27] Battery implants, designed to deliver a constant current to bone in spite of increasing tissue resistance, were employed to provide current sources between 1 and 100 μA. The optimal current for new bone formation in the rabbit femur was from 5 to 20 μA, and such new bone formation occurred at the cathode. Varying amounts of bone destruction occurred at the anode at every magnitude of current evaluated.

In order to determine if direct current of proper amperage and electrode placement can stimulate fracture healing, Friedenberg and co-workers[28] designed a series of experiments in which a galvanic current of 10 μA was applied to the rabbit fibula in several locations relative to a fracture (Fig. 7–8). At sacrifice the fibula was resected, and the degree of fracture healing was rated using roentgenographic criteria. The fibulae were then fixed in buffered formula for up to 10 days, and the maximum resistance to three-point bending was measured with an Instron testing machine.

The degree of fracture healing as determined by maximum resistance to bending is shown in Table 7–1. Statistically signifi-

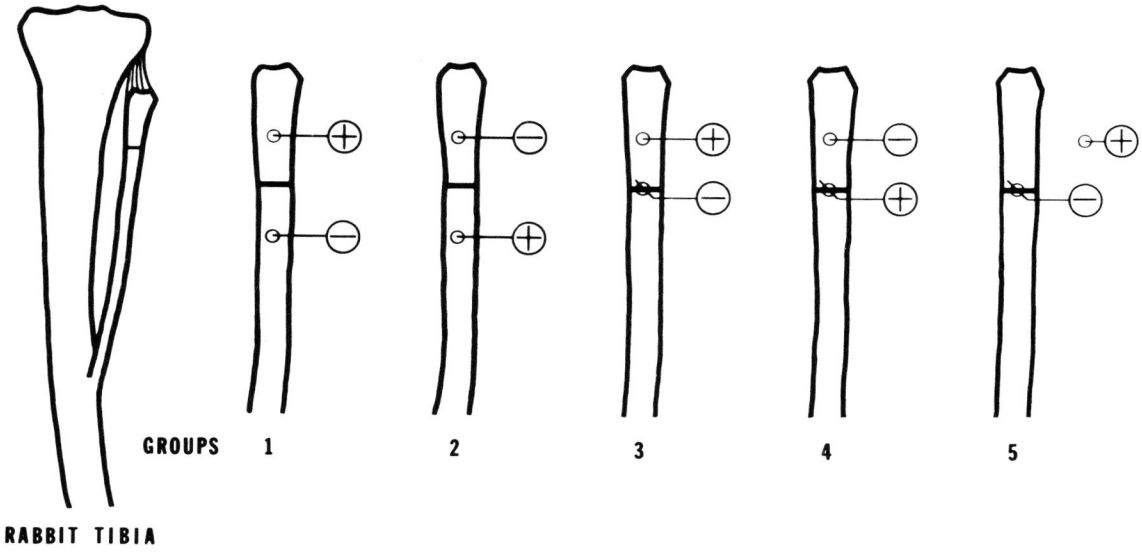

GROUPS   1   2   3   4   5

RABBIT TIBIA
AND FIBULA

Figure 7–8 Electrode placements used in the stimulation of fracture healing by direct current in the rabbit fibula. In groups 3 and 5 the cathode is inserted directly into the fracture site.

cantly greater resistance to bending is found in the experimental groups when compared with control fractures for groups 3 ($P<0.01$) and 4 ($P<0.05$). In group 3, the anode was placed proximally in the medullary cavity, and the cathode was placed in a drill hole crossing the fracture site. Group 5 was identical to group 3, except that the proximal lead or anode was anchored subcutaneously 5 mm from the fracture site. These results show that a cathode implanted at the fracture site is an effective source of stimulation. In the remaining experimental groups the stimulating effect of the cathode was confined to bone at a distance from the fracture and did not influence fracture healing. Group 5 was included to determine if the destructive reaction to the anode could be placed at a distance from the fracture in the soft tissue and still retain the stimulating current effectiveness. This was shown to be successful.

The biomechanical assessment method demonstrated significantly enhanced fracture healing response using two electrode placements with the cathode at the fracture

TABLE 7–1   Maximum Resistance to Binding (Paired t Test of Matched Slopes) *

Group	N	Mean Control	Mean Experimental	Change (Per cent)	SDD	SED	p
I	8	.61	.47	−22.9	.43	.15	0.2
II	6	.50	.31	−38.0	.25	.10	0.1
III	7	.37	.61	+64.8	.27	.10	0.01
IV	8	.58	.27	−53.4	.32	.11	0.5
V	10	.31	.61	+96.7	.21	.07	0.05†

*Maximum resistance to bending of paired fibulae (direct current side versus sham operated side) in the five different electrode placement groups. In groups III and V the cathode was at the fracture site.
† = significant at 99.9 per cent confidence level.
N = degrees of freedom.
SDD = standard deviation of difference between ratings of paired experimental and control tibiae.
SED = standard error of difference between paired ratings.

site. A number of questions remain unanswered, however. The load-deflection curves measured in three-point bending provide an indication of the bending resistance or flexural rigidity of the healing bone. The flexural rigidity in turn includes contributions from the changes both in the material properties of the fracture callus and in the cross-sectional geometry due to the periosteal proliferation of bone.

While a flexural test provides the best indication of clinical stability, it does not allow the separation of changes in mechanical properties from changes in cross-sectional geometry. The use of three-point bending with localized loading at the fracture site may also be questioned. The authors were required to interpret their results on the basis of a somewhat arbitrary discontinuity in the midrange of the load-deflection curve. Despite these shortcomings in biomechanical evaluation, the evidence strongly suggests that a cathodal current of 10 μA intensity placed within the fracture site stimulates fracture healing. As a result, an extensive study of clinical applications to nonunions and congenital pseudarthroses is currently underway in several centers.

While the early clinical trials with the use of continuous direct current for nonunion and congenital pseudarthrosis are encouraging, the mechanisms involved are poorly understood, and relatively little is known concerning the biomechanics of fracture healing using electrical stimulation. For instance, it is not known if the increased rigidities noted in both experimental and clinical trials are due to differences in the specific mechanical properties of the fracture callus, to changes in the amounts of bone formed, or to differences in the sites of the proliferative reaction. In this regard, from a biomechanical standpoint it would be clearly advantageous to induce bone formation as far from the centroid of the bone cross section as is practical, in order to maximize the section properties and the associated torsional and flexural rigidities. To this author's knowledge, no work has been done toward optimizing the location of the osteogenic response based on biomechanical criteria. Also, in common with other biomechanical assessments of fracture treatment techniques, little is known about

the temporal factors involved in fracture repair using electrical stimulation.

INTERNAL FIXATION

The aim of fracture treatment is to reestablish the proper anatomical relationships between bone fragments and to support the region until bony union can occur. Whenever possible, reduction is maintained by the application of external forces, as with traction or casting. In many instances the fragments cannot be adequately controlled, and surgical intervention with open reduction and internal fixation is necessary.

In the absence of internal fixation, fracture healing is accomplished by the formation of fracture callus on the surfaces of living bone adjacent to the defect. Callus grows centripitally until a bony bridge is established. When rigid internal fixation is employed, callus is absent, suggesting that some measure of biomechanical stimulus is necessary for its formation. Further, functional cast bracing is thought by some to facilitate healing through the controlled application of stress at the fracture site. Another possible disadvantage of rigid fixation has been described as a loss of bone density and disuse osteoporosis when the bone is protected from stress by internal fixation devices.

Perhaps because fractures can be stabilized in experimental animals more easily with internal fixation devices than with external immobilization, most experimental work has emphasized the biomechanical evaluation of fractures treated with internal fixation devices. Animal models have been used to study the biomechanics of compression plate fixation, plate-induced osteopenia, the stress-concentrating effects and healing of screw holes, and intramedullary rodding with low-modulus materials. In addition, a number of comparative studies of different treatment modalities have been conducted.

Compression Plate Fixation

Rigid internal fixation depends on the production of local areas of compression between implant and bone or between the fractured bone ends. Wherever "pressure

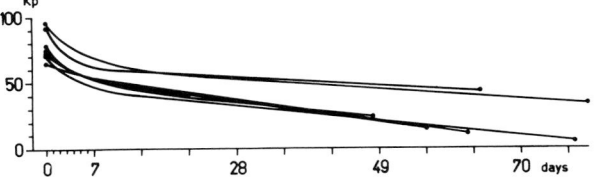

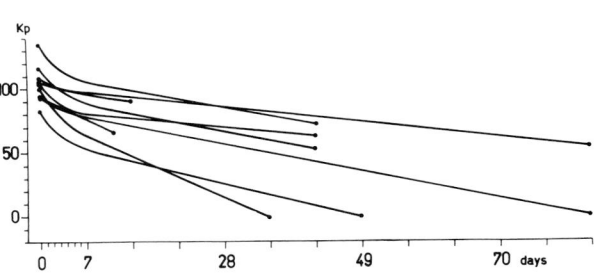

Figure 7–9 Strain gauge plate tension as a function of healing time. *A.* Intact bone. *B.* Osteotomized bone. The rate of change of plate tension is similar with or without osteotomy. (Courtesy of S. M. Perran, A. Haggler, M. Russenberger, et al., and *Acta Orthopaedica Scandinavica.* Acta Orthop. Scand., *125*:19, 1969.)

necrosis" and bone resorption occur, there can be a loss of fixation stability. It is vital, therefore, to understand the reaction of bone to different levels of compressive stress. In order to better understand the reaction of living cortical bone to compression plate fixation, Perren and co-workers[56] designed four-hole compression plates with built-in strain gauges. The gauge plate, a modification of the standard AO design, gave either continuous or intermittent recordings of plate tension with the results unaffected by bending moments or temperature variations. Two- to four-year-old sheep were used as experimental animals. In six sheep the plates were applied to both intact and osteotomized bone, and recordings of plate tension were made at weekly intervals.

Plate tension for the intact bone group is shown in Figure 7–9A. There is a gradual decrease in plate tension over 12 weeks after a somewhat steeper decrease in the first few days following plate application. The plate tension recordings from the osteotomized bone are shown in Figure 7–9B. The same initial decrease in plate tension as in the intact bone is seen. The results demonstrate that after application of longitudinal compression to bone using rigid internal fixation, there is no sudden drop in plate tension. This holds for intact as well as for osteotomized bone under compressive loads of 60 to 140 kiloponds.

The results indicate that there is no pressure necrosis in these animals, since if a layer of bone of 10 to 20 μ thickness were to be resorbed the compressive load would fall to zero. From these results it is reasonable to conclude that rigid fixation can be maintained throughout the healing period.

The histological results (Fig. 7–10) confirm the roentgenographic findings of primary bone healing. In spite of full weight bearing immediately after application of the plate, the osteotomy is bridged by direct haversian remodeling. The histological pattern also suggests a mechanism for the observed slow decrease in plate tension. It is postulated that the intense haversian remodeling of the compressed tibia results in a reduction in the bone modulus. This is reflected in the gradual decrease in plate tensile force. The experiment shows that a static preload of from 60 to 140 kiloponds on a cortical bone segment does not induce pressure necrosis of the bone fragments. An osteotomy does not appreciably alter the bony response to static pressure as long as it is rigidly fixed.

Plate-Induced Osteopenia

The development of disuse osteoporosis leading to refracture after plate removal came into question primarily because of the use of dual plates in treatment of femoral shaft fractures. This practice has since been discontinued, with much improved results.[52] However, the fact remains that bone

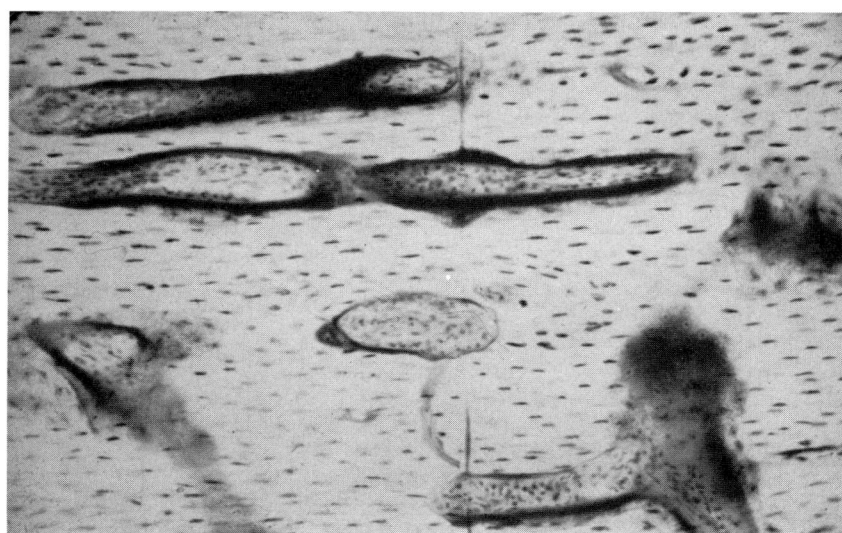

Figure 7–10 Histological characteristics of primary bone healing directly beneath the plate after 12 weeks of fracture healing. There is evidence of direct haversian remodeling and no resorption of the compressed surfaces.

is subjected to lower stress levels owing to the presence of the plate in the late stages of healing, and this may lead to cortical disorganization. These factors have been studied using animal models, theoretical analyses, and biomechanical evaluations.

Using a canine model, Uhthoff and Dubuc[73] observed gradual cortical thinning in roentgenograms taken 2, 7, 20, and 24 weeks following osteotomy and fixation with compression plates. Histological evidence suggested that the thinning process was caused by periosteal resorption and was accompanied by increased porosity at about 10 weeks after surgery. Removal of the plate in two dogs on one side after three months and sacrifice after six months allowed a study of the effects of plate removal. As long as the plate was present, woven bone was laid down in a disorganized fashion, and the bone was incompletely mineralized. Only after removal of the plate did the bone become axially oriented. These observations suggest that plate-induced osteopenia is almost completely reversible three months after plate removal.

Quantitative histological evaluations of the extent of healing in osteotomies of the canine radius treated with two compression plates of differing stiffness were provided by Akeson and co-workers.[2] At 16 weeks all osteotomies had healed, and biomechanical tests showed that radii from the two sides had equivalent strength. The methods of Harris and Weinberg[31] were used to measure cortical porosity. The results showed significantly less cortical porosity on the side having the plate of reduced stiffness compared with the side having a stiff stainless plate.

Similar experiments using stainless steel and plastic plates in dogs were reported by Tonino and associates.[72] In control experiments the authors measured bone mineral mass and mechanical properties in bending for paired canine femora and verified the symmetry of the observed parameters. Plates were then applied to intact canine femora, and the dogs were sacrificed at 10, 12, 14, 16, and 18 weeks. All results were combined, and the data were not presented as a function of healing time. However, significant decreases were noted for the stainless–steel-plated bones in measurements of bone mineral mass and in mechanical properties. Microradiography showed that this was due to massive endosteal resorption.

Thus the experimental evidence suggests that cortical disorganization and disuse osteoporosis occur during the latter stages of bone healing, especially if the plate is left on the bone after cortical continuity is reestablished. These findings are supported by clinical studies reporting refractured bone following the use of dual plates for femoral shaft fractures. Presumably this effect is caused by a reduction in the normal mechanical stimuli in the late stages of healing owing to the presence of the internal fixation device. To explore this phenomenon, Cochran[21] applied strain gauges in vitro around canine femoral diaphyses to which compression plates were applied. He reported reduction in surface strains by as much as 84 per cent with the application of compression plates, thus confirming that mechanical stimuli are indeed decreased.

Woo and co-workers[78] used the torsional testing methods of Burstein and Frankel[17] to test the mechanical properties of fractures treated with compression plates of two different stiffnesses. Six adult mongrel dogs were used and the strength of bilateral osteotomies compared when treated with an ASIF stainless steel plate and with a composite plate of graphite–fiber-reinforced polymethyl methacrylate (GFMM). After four months, fractures treated by both methods were healed, and their mechanical properties (based on measurements of fracture torque, ultimate deformation, fracture energy, and maximum shear stress) were indistinguishable. It should be noted that no attempts were made to determine the development of these properties as a function of healing time. In fact, in four months the fracture sites were healed and usually failed at sites other than the original osteotomy site. Akeson and associates[2] later compared these data with torsion tests on additional radii (without osteotomies but with tapped screw holes), and showed that the maximum shear stress to develop at failure was significantly less for the plated radii. Since the size of the animals in both series was not comparable, comparisons of parameters other than maximum shear strength could not be made.

Woo and colleagues[79] also used strength measurements to compare the extent of plate-induced osteopenia using compression plates of two different stiffnesses. Six adult mongrel dogs were used in a paired experiment. Osteotomies allowed to heal to 9 and 12 months resulted in significantly increased amounts of bone atrophy on the more rigidly plated side. Strength measurements of small bending specimens from the four quadrants of both diaphyses showed that material properties of the healing tissues (as measured by the bending strength and flexural modulus) were similar, but that the structural properties (as measured by the maximum bending load and maximum energy to failure) were significantly different. These differences were attributed to cortical thinning beneath the more rigid plate rather than to changes in the mechanical properties of the tissues themselves. Again, in this experiment no attempt was made to determine the healing rate, and only the late stage of fracture healing was investigated.

These observations of plate-induced osteopenia after rigid internal fixation with compression plates were made during fracture repair. In order to better understand the reaction of intact bone to plate fixation, Slätis and co-workers[70a] studied the successive morphological changes in intact bone after application of a rigid plate with and without compression. Adult rabbit tibiae were instrumented with a stainless steel four-hole dynamic compression plate (DCP-ASIF). In the right tibia, compression was applied, and in the left tibia it was not. The animals were killed at 1 and 3 days, and at 1, 3, 6, 12, 18, 24, and 36 weeks after operation. After sacrifice, transverse sections of the plated area of bone were analyzed by a point-counting technique.[31] Planimetry gave data on the entire cross-sectional area of bone and on the percentage area occupied by the medullary canal.

The morphometric measurements of the porotic changes in cortical bone were divided into four subgroups according to the time of observation after operation. The subgroups were 1 to 3 weeks, 6 to 12 weeks, 18 to 24 weeks, and 36 weeks (Fig. 7–11). During the first three weeks, the proportion of the cross section represented by haversian canals remained unchanged in both the compressed and the noncompressed plated bones (7.3 ± 0.64 per cent and 7.4 ± 0.69 per cent, respectively). The data for 6 to 12 weeks showed that resorption areas occupied 16 ± 3.6 per cent of the cortex in the compressed bones and 14.2 ± 3.5 per cent in the noncompressed bones. Thereafter, resorption progressed more rapidly in the compressed bone, so that by 18 to 24 weeks after operation, porotic areas in the com-

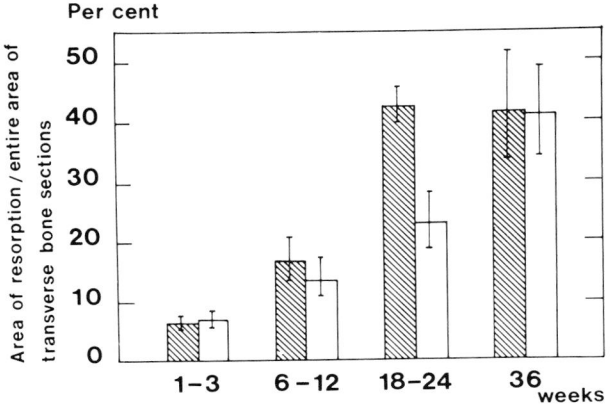

Figure 7–11 Areas of cortical bone resorption expressed as percentages of the total cross-sectional area of cortical bone. Hatched columns indicate the changes after plating with compression. White columns indicate the changes after fixation without compression. (Courtesy of P. Slätis, E. Karaharju, T. Holmström, et al. and *The Journal of Bone and Joint Surgery.* J. Bone Joint Surg., *60A:516–522,* 1968.)

pressed and noncompressed bones were 42.4 ± 2.9 per cent and 22.9 ± 4.9 per cent of the cortical area, respectively (P <0.001). At 36 weeks, however, the two groups showed porotic changes of the same magnitude (40.6 ± 10.0 per cent and 41.2 ± 8.8 per cent, respectively).

The histologically demonstrated formation of subperiosteal new bone and resorption of subendosteal cortical bone could be quantified planimetrically from the enlarged micrographs of transverse sections of the midshaft. Because the changes were of the same magnitude regardless of whether or not compression had been used, the data of both groups were combined (Table 7–2). The increase in the total area of the transverse sections and the increase in the area occupied by the medullary canal both reached a high level of significance (P <0.001) at 36 weeks postoperatively, when compared with the values of 1 to 3 weeks.

Thus, after rigid plating the shaft of the bone is transformed into a tube with a thinner wall and a greatly increased diameter, in which the medullary canal occupies greater area than it did initially. Overall, the area of cortical bone actually increased during the observation time. In this study, no attempts were made to compute other cross-sectional properties (i.e., area moment of inertia), although it would have been extremely interesting to do so. The hypothesis to be investigated with such calculations is whether the bone remodels to produce section properties that are constant, or whether these properties change under the application of a rigid plate.

In summary, after rigid plate fixation of experimental fractures the essential feature of repair is end-to-end consolidation of the fractured bone with minimal formation of ensheathing subperiosteal callus. This primary bone healing is accomplished by

TABLE 7–2 Planimetry of Transverse Sections from the Mid-diaphyseal Bones Plated with and without Compression [*]

Time After Operation (Weeks)	Number of Bones [†]	Total Area of Cross Section (mm² ± SEM)	Area of Medullary Canal (mm² ± SEM)	Area of Cortical Bone (mm² ± SEM)	Intramedullary Area/Total Cross Section (Per cent)
1 to 3	36	40.5 ± 1.7	15.9 ± 1.3	24.5 ± 0.6	39.3
6 to 12	12	47.9 ± 1.6	20.5 ± 0.9	27.5 ± 1.2	42.8
18 to 24	12	55.0 ± 2.9	25.4 ± 1.9	29.6 ± 3.1	46.2
36	6	60.3 ± 1.8	28.6 ± 1.2	31.9 ± 1.8	47.4

[*] From Slätis, P., Karaharju, E., Holmström, T., et al.: J. Bone Joint Surg., *60A:516–522*, 1968.
[†] Right and left tibiae of 33 rabbits.

widening of the haversian canals, formation of resorption cavities, and subsequent formation of new bone across the fracture gap. However, along with this primary healing, rigid metallic implants also induce changes in the underlying cortical bone at a distance from the fracture area. These include widening of the haversian canals, so that the dense lamellar bone becomes more porous. The resulting transformation of cortical bone to more porous bone may contribute to the refractures that sometimes occur after removal of these implants.

Screw Holes

It has been observed clinically that when refractures occur, they usually do so through one of the screw holes during the first few months after removal of the bone screws. Mechanical testing has demonstrated that a fresh screw hole in bone concentrates the stress, making the bone weaker under bending and torsional loads. This weakening is of approximately the same magnitude for any hole that involves less than 30 per cent of the bone diameter. Brooks and co-workers[13] showed that the stress concentration factor under torsional loading for holes either 2.8 mm or 3.6 mm in diameter in the midshafts of the canine femur is about 1.6. This indicates that the stresses around the hole are 1.6 times greater than those over the remainder of the bone. These authors also showed that the hole influences the localization of the resultant fracture, since in over 90 per cent of their experiments the fracture passed through the hole.

To investigate the recovery of bone strength after removal of a bone screw, Burstein and colleagues[18] designed experiments to determine (1) if faster osseous healing occurs when holes are redrilled immediately after screw removal; and (2) the rate of recovery of strength after removal of the screw. In the canine models used in the redrilling experiment, almost every hole was completely filled with a plug of dense woven bone, even by four weeks. Histological evaluation showed that there was no apparent difference in the healing of the screw holes when the fibrous core was removed by redrilling. In addition, the healing pattern in fresh drill holes with no enclosed fibrous tissue was the same as that in the redrilled holes. However, in spite of the histological evidence of healing and the filling of the screw holes, roentgenograms of the specimens showed radiolucent defects similar to those seen clinically months after removal of the screws. In the canine specimens, the radiolucent area did not contain fibrous tissue, but rather bone with reduced radiodensity. These data indicate that there is no apparent advantage to redrilling the original screw hole with a larger sized drill to remove any fibrous tissue, since this does not accelerate the filling of the hole with new bone.

A second group of dogs was used for biomechanical evaluation. One 2.8-mm screw was inserted in the midshaft of each femur and left in place until removal at 90 days. In this procedure, one screw hole in each pair of femora was redrilled with a 3.6-mm drill, and the dogs were sacrificed at either 4 or 12 weeks after the second operation. The femora were then tested in the torsional loading machine.[18] The maximum torque, the maximum angle of deflection at fracture, and the maximum energy absorption at failure were determined for each specimen. A paired comparison of these parameters demonstrated no discernible benefit produced by redrilling the screw holes. The results at the four weeks' interval even suggested that the redrilled specimens were weakened compared with their non-redrilled counterparts. The specimens were comparable in strength at 12 weeks. In direct contrast to the findings of previous investigations with fresh screw holes,[13] the presence of screw holes in this experiment had no significant effect on the localization of fracture lines.

In a related experiment the authors investigated the time sequence over which the recovery of strength occurred in a drilled bone after removal of the screw. In this experiment, rabbits were used because of the number of animals needed for statistical significance. One femur of each rabbit was used as the experimental bone, with a sham operation performed on the opposite femur. Three different stress concentrations were studied: (1) holes resulting from the insertion of a self-tapping screw with immediate screw removal; (2) screw in place; and (3) drill hole with soft Silastic plug. The two latter configurations were used to study the stress concentration effects of a hole when the concentration could not be alleviated by the growth of bone into the hole.

The animals were sacrificed at 1, 2, 4, or 8 weeks, and the bones were subjected to torsional loading at high strain rates. The torque ratios for all three types of stress concentrations as a function of recovery time are presented in Figure 7-12. By the eighth week, the torque ratios showed no significant difference from ~100. At zero time, the presence of a screw hole alone reduced the maximum torque ratio to approximately 50 per cent. The presence of the screw in situ increased the torque ratio to approximately 70 per cent at this time. In order to determine whether the bone incorporates the retained screw into structure, some screws were removed from five of the eight-week animals prior to testing. In this case, the torque ratio dropped to a value approximately the same as that obtained at

two weeks with the screw in place. This was significantly less than the torque ratio for both the screw-in-place and the filled hole at eight weeks.

The authors concluded from these experiments that the stress concentration induced by all types of holes studied (i.e., either filled or unfilled) is adaptively reduced by about eight weeks. If a screw is removed after this adaptation has occurred, the bone is again significantly weakened. In addition, since holes filled with a soft Silastic plug do not act as stress concentrators after adaptation, bones must develop a system for transmitting the forces around the hole. The experimental findings suggest that the bone responds to eliminate the stress-concentrating effect no matter what the nature of the inclusion.

To the extent that these observations are applicable to the clinical situation in humans, this study suggests that refracture after an adaptation period may not be

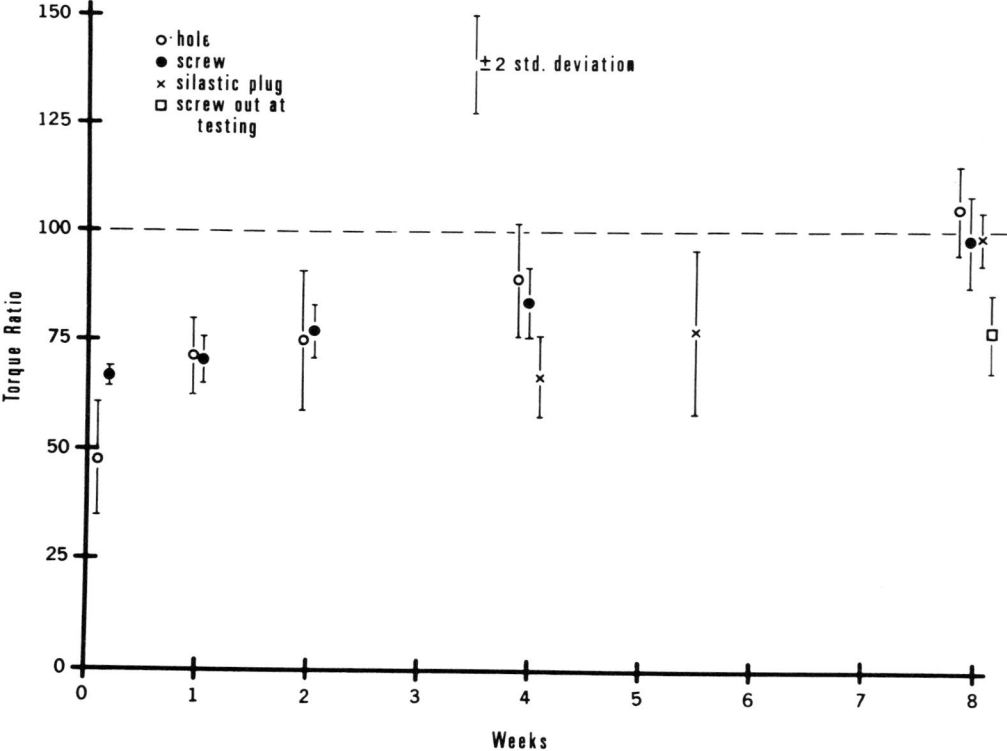

Figure 7–12   Recovery of strength for bones with screw holes expressed by torque ratios (bone with stress concentration/contralateral control) for an eight-week healing period. (Courtesy of A. H. Burstein, J. Currey, V. H. Franke, et al., and *The Journal of Bone and Joint Surgery. J. Bone Joint Surg., 54A:1143, 1972.)

related to the presence of an old screw hole, but instead may be no more than a chance occurrence. The other factor to be considered is that when bone heals, a greater bone mass is formed in the region of the fracture, thus altering the cross-sectional geometry of the bone. As a result, regions of reduced cross-sectional area are created both distal and proximal to the fracture site. After fracture healing has occurred, these areas are potentially weaker than the rest of the bone, and fracture could occur through these regions before failing through the fracture site.

Intramedullary Rods

Brown and Mayor[14] examined the effects of function on the healing of experimental fractures using intramedullary rods of different elastic moduli. The specific question addressed was whether, in conjunction with temporary external support to control alignment, polymeric intramedullary fixation devices could provide sufficient stabilization to facilitate healing without affecting remodeling. A larger study considered the biomechanics of the healing response as a function of healing time. Recently, results have been reported for a group of midshaft tibia fractures in rabbits followed for ~16 weeks after injury.

All of the rods were round in cross section, the same size (70 × 3.2 mm), and had the same surface finish. Four materials were used, including stainless steel and titanium (with elastic moduli of 200 and 110 GPa, respectively), and Delrin and nylon (with elastic moduli of 3 and 2 GPa, respectively). This selection provided a range of stiffness relative to that of bone of

TABLE 7-3 Strength and Energy Absorption for Rabbit Tibial Fractures Treated with Metallic and Polymeric Intramedullary Rods*

	Plastic Rods†	Metal Rods†	P
Strength	90 ± 11	69 ± 22	P < .001
Energy Absorption	72 ± 17	53 ± 30	P < .02

*Courtesy of S. A. Brown, M. B. Mayor, and *The Journal of Biomedical Materials Research.* J. Biomed. Mater. Res., *12*:67, 1978.
†Means ± standard deviations.

10 ×, 6 ×, 0.1 ×, and 0.03 ×. After 16 weeks the mechanical properties of the tibiae were determined in torsion with the intramedullary rods in situ.

Means and standard deviations for strength and energy absorption of the metal-rodded fractures and the plastic-rodded fractures are shown in Table 7-3. The average strengths of the plastic-rodded fractures are 30 per cent greater than those with metal rods; the energy absorption is 36 per cent greater. The results of torsional strength testing of these fractures, broken down by individual materials and animals, are shown in Figure 7-13. The results are ordered from left to right according to implant modulus, and are arranged chronologically within each material. The following differences are statistically significant: (1) nylon versus 316L (P < 0.05); (2) nylon versus titanium (P < 0.001); and (3) Delrin versus titanium (P < 0.001). The differences in nylon versus Delrin, Delrin versus stainless steel, and stainless steel versus titanium are not statistically significant.

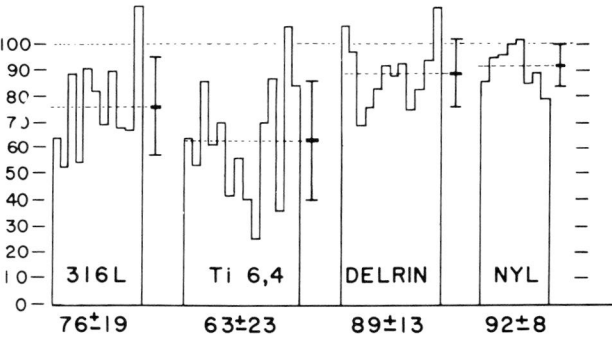

Figure 7–13 Torsional strength at 16 weeks of rabbit tibial fractures treated with metallic and polymeric rods. Results are expressed as a percentage of contralateral control with means and standard deviations shown. (Courtesy of S. A. Brown, M. B. Mayor, and *The Journal of Biochemical Materials Research.* J. Biomed. Mater. Res., *12*:67, 1978.)

Radiographic and histological comparison between fractures stabilized with metallic rods and those stabilized with polymeric rods demonstrated a number of consistent differences in the remodeling phases of healing. With metallic rods, bony caps were seen radiologically by nine weeks after surgery. After sacrifice and mechanical testing, entire sleeves of bone were seen around the rods. The formation and structure of the bony caps would suggest that the load was being transferred from metaphyseal bone to the metal rod in each end. The lack of remodeling and loss of cortical bone density in the diaphysis were probably manifestations of stress protection of the bone. The results further suggest that the rigid metal rods inhibited fracture remodeling. In contrast, the polymeric rods were at least an order of magnitude more flexible than bone and furnished no stress protection after a bony bridge had been established. Thus the biological response of remodeling was not inhibited by the plastic rods, resulting in 50 per cent of the fractures having strengths within ~10 per cent of control by~16 weeks.

This study suggests that fractures stabilized with flexible polymeric intramedullary rods remodel more effectively than those supported by metallic devices.

COMPARATIVE STUDIES OF HEALING WITH INTERNAL FIXATION

In a comparative biomechanical evaluation of fracture healing in the dog, Braden and co-workers[9] reported comparisons of torsional ultimate strength and stiffness for femoral midshaft fractures treated with intramedullary pins, with intramedullary pins and half Kirschner splint, and with compression plates. The half Kirschner devices were removed at the fourth postoperative week, the intramedullary pins at the sixth week, and the compression plates at the tenth week. All tests were conducted after sacrifice at ten weeks. The percentage recovery of strength and stiffness was calculated by normalizing the data with respect to the contralateral normal femur. At ten weeks, the group treated with intramedullary and half Kirschner rods were strongest, having recovered 80.2 per cent of their

original strength. The intramedullary pin group and the compression plate group recovered 61.9 and 36.0 per cent of their strength, respectively. The authors interpreted these results as showing that healing bone is weaker when plate fixation is used than when intramedullary pins or intramedullary pins and Kirschner rods are used.

Although the experiment was an attempt to compare the functional capacities of healing fractures based on strength data, this interpretation of the results may be criticized on a number of grounds. First, it is questionable whether the experimental groups were strictly comparable, since the two intramedullary groups were tested at six weeks and four weeks after removal of the fixation device, and the compression plate group was tested immediately after plate removal. Later data from the same group[12] showed that plated fractures also undergo a rapid increase in strength after removal of the fixation device. Thus a more representative comparison would result from testing immediately after removal of the fixation device in all three groups. Second, the mechanical testing methods subjected the test specimens to extremely uncertain stress fields, resulting in very different failure modes for the three experimental groups and for the contralateral controls.

Mosley, Heiple, and Burstein[51] recently conducted a more controlled experimental investigation into the effects of different types of internal fixation devices on the mechanical properties of healing fractures. Transverse fractures were produced in the femur of adult mongrel dogs by first scoring the midshaft with a Gigli saw and then striking the opposite cortex. Four fixation devices were used: (a) fracture clamps of special design, (b) Kirschner nails, (c) normal bone plates, and (d) compression plates of approximately twice the thickness of the normal plate. In the plated fractures no attempts were made to bend the plate to conform to the curvature of the bone, and no special attempts were made to apply interfragmentary compression.

Figure 7–14 shows the recovery of torsional strength and stiffness as a function of healing time in the four experimental groups. In Figure 7–14A, the average torque ratios (fracture/control) show that the

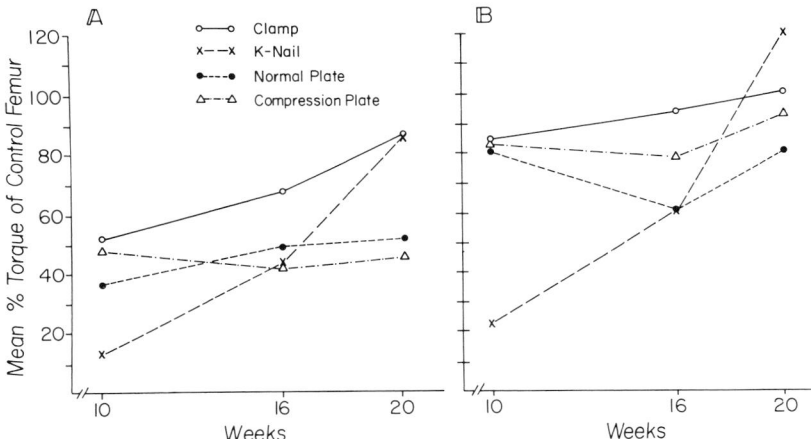

Figure 7–14 Recovery of torsional strength and stiffness as a function of healing time for four methods of internal fixation. *A*, Per cent torque recovery. *B*, Per cent stiffness recovery. (Courtesy of Mosley, Heiple, and Burstein, 1978)

clamp resulted in the highest load-carrying capacity, varying from approximately 50 per cent at 10 weeks to 85 per cent at 20 weeks. The K nail began at about 15 per cent of controls and then increased rapidly in strength to 85 per cent of controls at 20 weeks. Both plated groups remained in the 35 to 50 per cent range throughout the healing period. Statistical analysis of the results indicates that differences between the compression and the normal plate at various times are not significant. Figure 7–14*B* shows the percentage stiffness recovery as a function of healing time for the experimental groups. From 10 to 16 weeks, the clamp and the K nail showed increases in stiffness, the normal plate exhibited a decrease in stiffness, and the compression plate showed no change. From 16 to 20 weeks, clamp and plate recovered stiffness at about the same rate, but the K nail resulted in a sharp increase in the stiffness relative to its previous level. Statistical analysis of these results shows significant differences between the experimental groups when the results are adjusted for the time variation. The K nail over the course of the experiment resulted in an average 57 per cent recovery of stiffness, the normal plate 74 per cent, the compression plate 83 per cent, and the clamp 91 per cent. Analysis and interpretation of this experiment are still underway at the time of this writing. However, this appears to be the only study to date in which sufficient control has been exercised over the experimental variables to demonstrate statistically significant differences between fracture fixation methods.

BIOMECHANICS OF FRACTURE MANAGEMENT

It is evident from the previous section that there are formidable difficulties associated with the use of animal models to study the biomechanics of fracture healing. This is particularly true when plaster immobilization or functional bracing is studied, since these treatment modalities are difficult to control in experimental animals, and the resulting exuberant fracture callus is difficult to test biomechanically.

In response to this situation, investigators have used in vitro methods to explore the biomechanics of fracture treatment. In this case the biological response is not modeled, and primary emphasis is placed on the strength and rigidity of the fracture fixation device immediately after application to bone in vitro. As in the previous section, the major emphasis of research has been on methods of internal fixation, since these are easily studied in vitro and many of the systems are rather similar to other engineering fixation devices. Plaster casting and functional bracing have received relatively little attention, since these methods depend largely on soft tissue responses and soft tissues are not easily modeled in vitro.

This section will cover research efforts on the biomechanics of fracture treatment using plaster casts and functional bracing. The extensive experimental and theoretical studies of internal fixation methods will then be reviewed. These include experimental investigations of the strength and rigidity of plate and intramedullary rod fixations, the mechanics of surgical screws, and an extensive series of comparative studies of different methods of internal fixation.

EXTERNAL IMMOBILIZATION

Functional Bracing

Braces that permit weight-bearing ambulation and early mobilization of joints of patients with fractures of the tibia were developed by Sarmiento.[64-66] Treatment by this technique has demonstrated that rigid immobilization of joints is not a prerequisite for fracture healing. Furthermore, for most fractures of the tibia the initial shortening remains unchanged, despite the fact that weight-bearing ambulation is introduced relatively soon after the initial insult.

When the first below-the-knee functional cast for tibial fractures was developed, it was thought that maintenance of the length of the fractured extremity was the result of direct transmission of ground reaction forces to the patellar tendon and proximal tibia. Clinical observations, however, cast doubt on the validity of this explanation, since patients failed to experience pressure over these areas during ambulation. Patients instead consistently reported that the soft tissues of the calf were primarily responsible for the concentration of forces, even though pressures were felt throughout the distal extremity.

In order to clarify this matter, braces were instrumented with pressure transducers which demonstrated greater pressure readings over the gastrosoleus mass and significantly reduced readings over the bony prominences of the proximal tibia. However, these differences may have been due to the greater reliability of pressure measurements made over soft tissues, where a

hydrostatic effect is to be expected. These studies also revealed that the ground reaction force carried by the plastic brace was about 15 per cent, indicating that the limb itself carried over 80 per cent of the ground reaction forces. These findings gave credence to the belief that the soft tissues play a major role in stabilizing tibial fractures and in preventing shortening of the extremity.

In further studies, patients with oblique fractures of the tibia and fibula were anesthetized, and their fracture fragments were visualized under fluoroscopy. Intermittent vertical loading of 25 lb showed overriding of the fragments by as much as 21 mm in one case. Tests were repeated after the application of a plastic brace extending from below the knee to just above the ankle joint. A similar phenomenon was observed with overriding of the fragments, but the excursion was reduced to 2 mm, 75 per cent less than that observed prior to application of the brace.

The documented fact that the below knee brace is responsible for only 15 per cent of the load bearing of the braced extremity led Sarmiento and co-workers[63] to postulate that a combination of factors result in fracture stability with functional bracing. They assumed that: (1) a hydrostatic environment prevents shortening, because of the incompressibility of the soft tissues and the musculature of the leg; (2) the elastic properties of the muscular and ligamentous structures attached to and surrounding the fractured bones allow significant displacements but prevent permanent plastic deformation; and (3) the interosseous membrane provides a final limiting factor on fracture fragment motion.

The anatomy of the lower extremity between the knee and the ankle supports the hypothesis that hydrostatic mechanisms add stability to the fracture fragments. To study this hypothesis, unstable fractures of the tibia and fibula were created in freshly amputated above-the-knee specimens. Portions of the musculature in the vicinity of the fracture were removed and filled with transparent gelatin of a homogeneous consistency. Specimens were then enclosed in a transparent below-knee functional brace and placed in a compression apparatus to permit intermittent loading of 150 lb peak value. Initially, the limb shortened by approximately 1/8 inch. This value did not increase after repeated cyclical loading.

Fractures were also produced in fresh anatomical specimens. The limbs were then loaded, and the deformities were observed with and without the support of the brace. Reduction of the fracture and application of the brace restored the limb to its original length within a millimeter. Axial loading of 60 lb in the brace caused shortening of slightly more than 1 mm and negligible angulation. Loading of 50 lb after the brace had been removed caused shortening of more than 6 mm and an angulation increase of approximately 8 degrees. Stripping of the interosseous membrane resulted in increased shortening which exceeded 35 mm, indicating that the membrane plays an important role in the prevention of shortening.

Stresses in Orthopedic Walking Casts

Immobilization by plaster cast is probably the most common mode of fracture treatment, but little is known about the effectiveness of immobilization with this method. The role of soft tissues in fracture fragment immobilization has not been extensively investigated, and few papers have dealt with the question of stresses in orthopedic casts.

Schenck and co-workers[69a] described an experimental program to evaluate and improve various cast immobilization techniques. Experiments were conducted to determine the mechanical properties of molded plaster bandage material and to determine the stresses in a completed cast when it is subjected to normal and abnormal use. The experiments were divided into two general categories: (1) material tests, to determine the mechanical properties of the plaster bandage, and (2) volunteer experiments to measure the stresses developed in lower leg casts in normal and abnormal use.

For the mechanical tests of plaster cast material, ultimate compressive strength averaged 1830 psi and tensile strength averaged 740 psi. To determine the ultimate strength in compression as a function of moisture content, mechanical properties tests were conducted as a function of drying time. Plots of the ultimate strength of test cubes against moisture content revealed that maximum ultimate strength was not developed until at least 60 hours of drying time.

To determine the stresses developed in a lower leg walking cast during normal and abnormal activity, experiments were performed on 16 healthy volunteer subjects. Casts were applied using generally accepted techniques, with the subjects instructed not to apply stresses to the cast during the drying period. Clinical experience suggested that cast failure occurs most often in an anteroposterior plane lying just below the ankle and making an angle of about 45 degrees with the tibia. In all experiments, gauges were placed at the anterior and posterior regions of the ankle, with one gauge parallel and one gauge perpendicular to the tibia at each location. Six gauges were monitored in each experiment as the subjects were observed in the following postures: (1) gentle plantar flexion, (2) weight evenly distributed between cast and free leg, (3) entire weight on cast, (4) marking time in place, (5) treadmill walking at various speeds, (6) jumping on cast, (7) vigorous plantar flexion, and (8) vigorous dorsiflexion. Cast stresses were calculated using standard strength of materials relations and the experimental values for modulus of elasticity and Poisson's ratio.

The stress distributions from cast to cast and from activity to activity varied greatly. During the plantar flexion activity, longitudinal strains at the ankle were always tensile anteriorly and compressive posteriorly. In other activities, corresponding points of different casts exhibited totally different stress patterns for each activity. Although there was great variation from cast to cast, the strain pattern in each cast from cycle to cycle (i.e., for each step in a walking activity) was quite uniform. During walking, the anterior ankle section of some casts was always in tension longitudinally, while in others the same section was always in compression. In still other casts, the sections alternated from tension to compression during each step. This inconsistency was typical of all activities except flexion.

The authors attributed these large variations in strain patterns to: (1) anatomical differences, such as leg configuration, muscle strength, and gait pattern; and (2) structural differences, such as walking heel position, cast dimensions, and least important, cast thickness. Stress calculations showed that normal walking resulted in maximum stresses on the order of 295 psi compression. Considerably higher stresses were noted with jumping, with a maximum measurable stress of 585 psi in tension. In all casts, the largest stresses occurred during vigorous plantar flexion. Maximum stresses of 625 psi in compression and 415 psi in tension were measured. Vigorous dorsiflexion produced stresses somewhat lower than those that developed in jumping.

For all activities in all casts the maximum stresses measured, whether tensile or compressive, were developed longitudinally in the anterior and posterior regions of the cast just below the ankle. These results were supported by simple beam analyses of the structure. Because the highest stresses were developed in plantar flexion, it may be concluded that muscle activity induces the largest bending moments in these casts. Even in the seemingly more abusive jumping tests, the load was more directly transmitted to the walking heel of the casts, and the resultant moments were of lower magnitude. Of the 16 casts tested, 7 failed and 4 others developed surface cracks in the ankle region. All failures occurred in the anteroposterior plane, three during jumping and four during vigorous plantar flexion.

From this study it is apparent that the stresses developed in the lower leg walking cast are sufficient to cause failure if the cast has not undergone an adequate drying time before use. After 24 hours, the usual recommended drying period, the cast has reached only about one third of its ultimate strength. A drying period of at least 48 to 60 hours is recommended for plaster walking casts to develop adequate strength. If it is deemed necessary to apply a cast that is thicker than 1/4 inch at the ankle, added drying time should be allowed. In addition, more plaster is necessary in the ankle region of the plaster cast than at the extremities. A thickness of approximately 1/4 inch in the heel-ankle region of the cast is sufficient if the cast is thoroughly cured. Less plaster is necessary in the calf region, with the added advantage of increased drying rate and lighter weight. Reduction in length of the sole plate would also decrease the moment caused by plantar flexion, but the resulting cast would be uncomfortable for the patient.

Because tensile stresses are the most undesirable in a walking cast (the ultimate strength in tension is only about one third of the ultimate strength in compression), the walking heel should be positioned on the cast to induce direct compression of the plaster material. Since drying of the cast in the region under the foot is greatly inhibited by the excess plaster needed to attach the rubber walking heel, the authors suggested that the walking heel should be redesigned to require less plaster and to facilitate drying.

INTERNAL FIXATION

Intramedullary Rod Fixation

Intramedullary nailing is a common method in the treatment of fractures of the long bones. A number of different designs may be used, including a V-shaped nail, a flexible round nail, a diamond cross section nail, and a square cross section rod with grooves.[3] However, there are still complications with this method, and many of these are due to mechanical factors. Typical mechanical failures include rod migration, plastic deformation of the rod, and fatigue fracture. Delayed union or nonunion after intramedullary nailing are also often the result of mechanical factors. Allen and co-workers[3] recently pointed out some of the deficienices with existing intramedullary nailing systems for the fixation of femoral fractures. These include excessive flexibility, poor torsional load transmission characteristics, relatively poor fixation of the nail in the intramedullary canal, and increased incidence of nonunion, malunion, and implant failure when proper reaming techniques are not observed.

In previous studies of the biomechanical characteristics of the commonly used intramedullary nails,[4] these authors identified three mechanical characteristics that are relevant to the performance of intramedullary rods: bending strength, bending rigidity, and torsional rigidity. Since fatigue failure in bending is the usual mode of failure, and since fatigue strength is usually some fraction of the static bending strength (usually about one half), the fatigue resistance was evaluated from the foregoing static measurements.

In an attempt to eliminate some of the deficiencies of intramedullary fixation systems, Allen and co-workers[3] designed a fluted femoral intramedullary rod, using a circular cross section for maximum bending strength and rigidity, a closed cross section to gain torsional strength and rigidity, external fluting to enable the rod to couple to the bone above and below the fracture, and both straight and precurved rods for maximum versatility. The bending strength and bending rigidity were determined using a four-point bending test and compared with Schneider, Küntscher, and Hansen-Street nails. Torsional rigidity was determined in a torsional testing machine with the various rods held in specially machined grips. In addition, the authors tested the intramedullary grip of these fluted rods, comparing it with the grips of three commonly used nails.

These tests were done using 2.5-cm reamed segments of cadaver femora held stationary in the Burstein torsion-testing apparatus. The torsional gripping capacity of these nails on the intramedullary surface

TABLE 7–4   Comparative Torque Capabilities of Intramedullary Rods in Reamed 2.5-Centimeter Segments of Femur

Type of Nail	Average Break-away Torque ($\eta=3$) (kg-cm)
Küntscher (13mm)	110
Two nested Küntscher nails (9 mm/10 mm)	115
Hansen-Street (13 × 11 mm)	160
Schneider (13 mm)	160
Fluted (13 mm)	230
Average torque required to fracture the femoral shaft	700

of the femoral segments was then measured as breakaway torques (Table 7–4). The results of mechanical testing showed that the fluted rods were stronger than the other rods tested, but they still were not as strong (or as rigid) in bending as the femora in which they were placed. Thus an intact bone that would require a 13-mm fluted rod for proper fit would have a bending strength of approximately 450 newton meters, which is three times that of the rod. The bending stiffness of the bone was also 25 per cent greater than that of the rod.

The torsional rigidity (Fig. 7–15) of these nails is greatly influenced by both size and

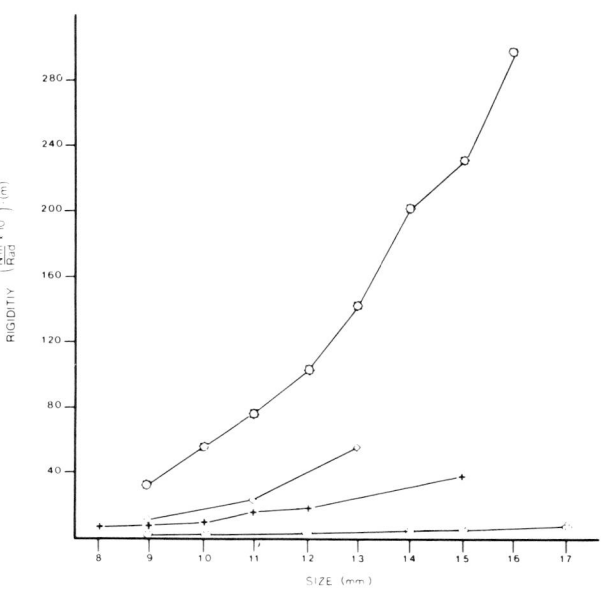

Figure 7–15 Torsional rigidity of intramedullary devices. The four rods tested were the fluted, Schneider, Küntscher, and Hansen-Street. Each is indicated by a symbol approximating the cross-sectional appearance: fluted, cross, cloverleaf, and diamond, respectively. The rigidity of the fluted rod is apparent. (Courtesy of W. C. Allen, K. G. Heiple, A. H. Burstein, and *The Journal of Bone and Joint Surgery.* J. Bone Joint Surg., 60A:506, 1978.)

cross-sectional geometry. The differences between the various configurations are striking, with the open-section cloverleaf design having the least rigidity in this test, and the diamond-shaped rod performing better in this loading configuration than in bending. The rigidity of the fluted rod is apparent, but even more important is its ability to transfer this rigidity to the bone-rod system by virtue of the multiple flutes.

The average breakaway torque for three tests was 230 kg-cm for the fluted rod, 160 kg-cm for both Hansen-Street and Schneider nails, and ~110 kg-cm for the 13-mm Küntscher nail. These values compare with an average torque required to fracture the femoral shaft of 700 kg-cm. The rigidity of fixation achieved by this device is approached clinically only by dual compression plating. With the intramedullary rod, however, the excessive periosteal stripping required for dual plating is not necessary. Moreover, the authors reported no evidence of the excessive bone atrophy that may accompany dual plating, perhaps because the axial stress in the bone caused by weight bearing is not affected by the intramedullary rod.

Compression Plate Fixation

Interfragmentary relative motion has been shown by a number of workers to influence the healing pattern of cortical bone,[6, 34, 56] and this has led to a number of studies of fixation rigidity with plates. Lindahl[40–42] conducted gross studies of the rigidity of immobilization of both transverse and oblique fractures with various internal fixation methods. Using both bending and torsional loads, he concluded that there were marked reductions in both flexural and torsional rigidity with all types of fixation devices in comparison to intact bone. Plates, however, were shown to provide the maximum rigidity of all the devices tested, although no attempts were made to explore the use of interfragmentary compression to increase rigidity.

To test the assumption that the addition of interfragmentary compression to plate fixation results in increased rigidity, Hayes and Perren[32] measured the torsional rigidity of composite plate-bone systems. The proximal and distal ends of moist sheep tibiae

were embedded in rapid-hardening plastic steel and fixed to a test frame. Torques in the range of 0 to 50 kp-cm were applied to the proximal end, and deformations were measured with a dial gauge. After testing the intact bone, an osteotomy was performed at the midshaft. Fixation was accomplished using an eight-hole AO self-compressing Dynamic Compression Plate (DCP).[5] Several methods of compression application as well as the case of no compression were investigated.

The formula for simple torsion of a cylinder, $\phi/l = T/GJ$, was used to calculate torsional rigidity of the plate-bone system. In this formula, ϕ/l is the angle of twist per unit of length, T is the applied torque, and GJ is the torsional rigidity. The torsional rigidities in 10^4 kp cm² expressed as means ± 1 SD were: (1) eight-screw compression, 2.23 ± 0.439; (2) compression, inner and outer screws, 1.67 ± 0.501; (3) compression, outer four screws, 0.82 ± 0.127; and (4) no compression, 1.41 ± 0.251. These compared with a torsional rigidity of 3.71 ± 0.875 found for intact bone.

Statistical analysis of the data revealed that there was a highly significant ($P < 0.001$) reduction in torsional rigidity when compression was not utilized or when compression was applied with only the outer four screws. The authors concluded that the addition of properly applied interfragmentary compression to plate fixation significantly increased the overall torsional rigidity of osteotomized long bones. The results also emphasized the importance of using screws close to the fracture or osteotomy site in order to increase the length over which the bone and plate act as a composite system. If only the outer four screws are used the plate and bone do not act as a single unit, and the torsional rigidity becomes that of the plate acting alone.

These results on the use of longitudinal interfragmentary compression in plate fixation were then extended to the case of rigidity in bending.[32] Moist human tibial and femoral preparations were tested in four-point bending. Uniform bending moments of from 0 to 130 kp-cm were applied in the central test section, and deflections at midspan were measured with a dial gauge. Flexural rigidities were compared, using the slopes of plots of bending force versus

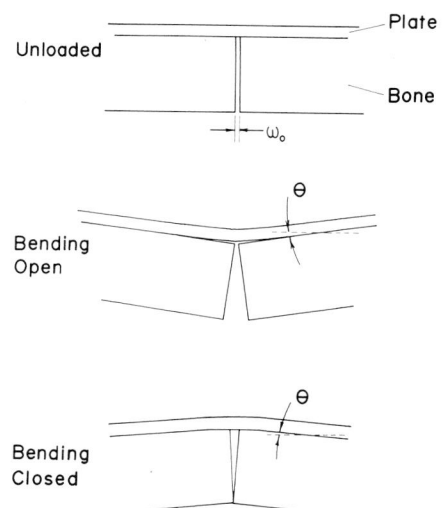

Figure 7-16 Loading configurations for flexural testing of bone-plate systems.

midspan deflection. In such a plot an increased slope indicates an increased flexural rigidity. After the intact bone was tested an osteotomy was performed at midshaft. Fixation was again accomplished using an eight-hole AO self-compressing Dynamic Compression Plate. Two bending configurations were investigated, one in which the bending forces tended to open the osteotomy site (bending open) and one in which the bending forces tended to close the osteotomy site (bending closed) (Fig. 7-16).

In both femoral and tibial preparations, the rigidity of the plate-bone system with compression was compared with the rigidity of the system without compression. The rigidity of the tibial preparations was also measured after a slight bend was introduced in the plate prior to tightening the screws and applying compression (overbent plate). The bend was made concave to the bone and directly above the osteotomy. A plot of bending force versus midspan deflection for one femoral preparation (Fig. 7-17) shows the generally observed sharp transition between two regimes of rigidity in each test. The regime of increased rigidity presumably reflects the stiffness of the plate and bone working together as a composite system, whereas the regime of reduced rigidity reflects the stiffness of the plate acting alone to resist bending. Because of

this transitional behavior, the data were analyzed by fitting separate straight lines through the initial and final portions of plots of bending force versus midspan deflection. When there was no break in the curve, as in some of the tests in the bending closed configuration, the initial and final slopes were taken to be the same.

Two comparisons of average initial and final slopes were made for each of the loading configurations: (1) compression versus no compression, and (2) straight plate with compression versus overbent plate with compression. In the comparison of compression with no compression for the femoral preparations, the use of compression resulted in highly significant increases in initial slope in both the bending closed and the bending open configurations. Differences in final slope were not significant. For the tibial preparations the use of compression did not yield significant increases in initial or final slope in either configuration. In the comparison of the straight plate versus the overbent plate, the use of the overbent plate yielded highly significant increases in initial and final slopes in both the bending open and the bending closed configurations.

The authors concluded that although the use of compression alone is not certain to increase flexural rigidity, the use of an overbent plate with compression provides significant increases in flexural rigidity. The

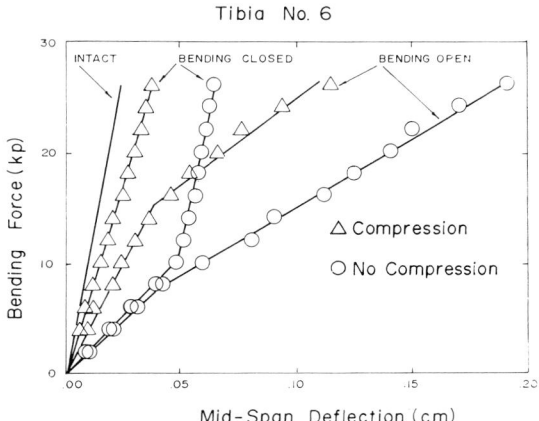

Figure 7-17 Bending force versus midspan deflection for flexural testing of bone-plate systems. The results show that plates should be applied so that the forces acting on the bone tend to close the fracture site.

generally increased rigidity of the bending closed configuration also suggests that, when possible, plates should be applied so that the acting forces tend to close the fracture or osteotomy site. In the case of curved long bones, this means that the plate should generally be applied on the convex surface such that the plate is loaded in tension and the bone in compression.

In an attempt to provide an adequate structural design for plate fixation in the horse, Bynum and co-workers[19] conducted multiple loading tests on commercially available plates installed on whole equine metacarpals. The modes of loading were compression, torsion, and flexure of systems corresponding to the bending open and bending closed modes of the study just reported. In addition, a flexural loading mode corresponding to lateral bending was investigated. All plates were fixed to the dorsal surfaces of the bone. The lowest capacity resulted with flexural loads applied on the dorsal surface of the bone corresponding to the bending open configuration. The maximum capacity occurred with a flexural load applied to the palmar surface (bending closed), such that the plate was loaded in tension and the bone in compression. The capacity of the installed plates with respect to the unfractured strength of the whole bone was between 16 and 67 per cent.

Although only a few specimens were tested and statistical analysis of the results was not possible, this investigation emphasizes that the relative strength of a plated bone compared with the strength of an unfractured bone is highly dependent upon the type of fracture and the mode of loading. Thus, while internal fixation methods may appear adequate under ideal loading conditions, they may be inadequate under many other possible loading conditions. This inefficiency may be tolerable in human orthopedics, because the patient can take extreme care to avoid imposing undesirable loads on an injured extremity. However, the inefficiency of the design in a variety of possible loading modes is most likely responsible for the limited success thus far achieved in internal fixation in the horse.

Ray and associates[59] continued the evaluation of the structural integrity of fractured equine metacarpals treated with internal fixation plates by conducting parametric

studies of the effects of varying plate lengths, widths, and screw diameter. All tests were conducted in flexure and were normalized with respect to the strengths of intact bones of animals of the same age. The results were reported as load factors calculated by dividing the failure loads by the cross-sectional properties of the bone, but without including the load-carrying capacity of the plate itself. A full-factorial experiment was designed and included four plate lengths (3, 4, 5, and 6 inch), three plate widths (0.5, 0.75, and 1 inch) and three sizes of bone screw. All tests were conducted with the plate on the tensile side of the bone corresponding to the bending closed configuration. In all, 27 experiments were carried out corresponding to the $3 \times 3 \times 3$ factorial design.

Figure 7-18 illustrates one of the most significant findings — the effect produced by an increase in length. It can be seen that, regardless of the width of the plate or the size of the bone screw employed, the 6-inch long plate demonstrates approximately twice the capacity of the 3-inch long plate. This increase presumably results because the longer plate can better distribute the stresses over a greater length of bone. The net effect of distributing the load between plate and bone over a greater portion of the bone surface produces a corresponding increase in the capacity of the structure.

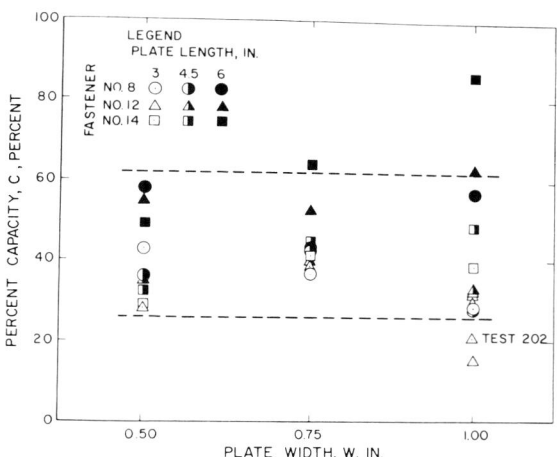

Figure 7-18 Influence of plate length on the capacity of bone-plate systems. Results were normalized with respect to contralateral, unplated control. (Courtesy of D. R. Ray, W. B. Ledbetter, D. Bynum, et al., and *The Journal of Biomechanics.* J. Biomech., 4:163, 1971.)

The data also show that for a particular size of fixation plate, increasing the screw size produced no substantial increase in the capacity of the composite structure. In addition, increasing the plate width from 0.5 to 1 inch produced no significant increase in the overall capacity.

Figure 7-18 also shows that the structural capacity of the plate-bone system is not likely to be greater than approximately 60 per cent of the intact bone. This represents the maximum support that can normally be expected, using the largest feasible plate under the described loading conditions. When combined loading conditions occur, as reflected in the earlier studies, the capacity of the composite structure can be substantially reduced. The authors tentatively concluded that the use of single fixation plates would not provide adequate structural support for internal fixation in large animals, such as the horse.

Minns and co-workers[50] conducted a comprehensive theoretical study of internal fixation of the human tibia that confirmed a number of the findings described earlier and extended the results to more physiological loading regimes. Based on gait analysis data by Paul[55] and previous studies of the geometrical properties of the tibia, a theoretical study was conducted on the variation in the stresses around and along the shaft of the tibia subjected to the loads expected during the gait cycle. These loads were then generated in the laboratory using a loading rig of special design and the performance of various plating configurations was compared. Deflection measurements were recorded when plated, fractured human tibiae were subjected to static loads at four positions in the walking cycle (3, 9, 41, and 52 per cent). The theoretical calculations suggested that the position of maximum tensile stress is the anterolateral surface of the tibia.

The authors further hypothesized that a plate placed in an area of predominantly tensile stress would be mechanically more stable than one placed in an area of compression (anteromedially). The experimental studies were designed to test this hypothesis by comparing the flexural and torsional rigidities of plated transverse osteotomies of the human tibia. In addition, two commercially available plates were tested. One was a thin type, Venables 5-inch, 8-hole plate, and one was a thick Mueller 5¼-inch, 8-hole plate. Results were normalized by comparing the deflections of each intact tibia under the applied physiological loads with the deflections of the same tibia when plated. In one set of tests the fractured tibiae were plated with and without the use of longitudinal interfragmentary compression.

The results were presented as the ratio of deflections of the intact tibia to deflections of the plated fractured tibia under the same load. Values above unity thus indicate a stiffer combination than the intact tibia. The ratio of bending deflections under physiological loading for the tibiae plated with compression after being osteotomized are shown in Figure 7-19. When placed laterally, the plate and bone produce a stiffer composite structure than when placed medially. The thicker Mueller plate, as expected, was stiffer in combination with the bone than the thinner Venables plate. The reason for this higher ratio is that at 41 per cent of the gait cycle the bending moments are resisted by the width of the plate. The plates applied without compression gave lower ratios than with compression, but the general trend of improved bending stiffness with lateral plating was still evident.

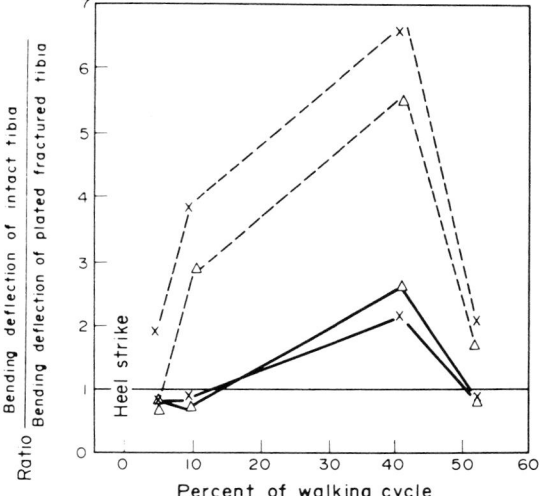

Figure 7-19   Bending behavior of tibiae with eight-hole plates with compression. (X) Muller plate, (∆) Venables plate. Plated surface. (— — —) anterolateral, (————) anteromedial. (Courtesy of R. J. Minns, G. R. Bremble, J. Campbell and *The Journal of Biomechanics*. J. Biomech., 10:569, 1977.)

In general, either with or without compression, the stiffness and bending of the plated fractured tibiae were always lower than the intact tibia at 4 per cent of the loading cycle. The greatest increase in bending stiffness was at 41 per cent of the gait cycle because the bending forces tended to act in the plane of the plate width, a direction in which its bending rigidity is maximal.

Similar results were noted for torsional deflections, suggesting that plates on the anterolateral surface produce less deflection of the bone-plate composite than plates on the medial surface. This was attributed partly to the fact that the medial surface is closer to the longitudinal axis of the tibia than the lateral surface. The thicker Mueller plate again resisted torsion better than the Venables plate. In conclusion, plates applied to the anterolateral surface of fractured tibiae exhibited more resistance to physiological load than those applied anteromedially. The thicker plate resisted bending and torsion better than the thinner plate, and plates applied with compression produced a more rigid bone-plate configuration than plates that were applied without compression.

Mathematical Analysis of Plate Fixation

Until recently, studies concerning the mechanics of plate fixation have been limited to the experimental studies described earlier. While these studies provide important information, they have limitations. It is difficult and expensive to alter experimentally the many parameters influencing the mechanical behavior of musculoskeletal components in order to study the response. These limitations can be overcome by combining experimental studies with mathematical analyses based on theoretical mechanics. One approach that has become increasingly popular is the finite element method. It is ideal for the analysis of musculoskeletal structures, since it can incorporate geometrical and material properties complexities and can be used to investigate a wide variety of loading conditions. A number of authors have used this approach to optimize internal fixation methods and to shed light on the relationships between internal stresses and bone remodeling responses.

Rybicki and co-workers[62] developed a finite element model of an equine third metacarpal-compression plate composite system. A transverse midshaft osteotomy was modeled, and the plate-bone system was subjected mathematically to axial loads in both tension and compression which were applied to the bone ends at some distance from the plate. The fracture site was free to open, simulating an unhealed condition. As expected, the results demonstrated that tensile loading tended to open the fracture site, resulting in bending and stretching of the plate, with the entire load supported by the plate. Conversely, compressive loading tended to close the fracture site, and reduced the deflections of the system by a factor of 100 over that predicted under tensile loadings. In this case the analysis predicted that 18 per cent of the applied load was supported by the plate, with the remainder carried across the fracture site by the bone.

These results for a simple transverse fracture were extended to the more complex case of an oblique fracture by Rybicki and Simonen.[60] The purpose of this theoretical study was to examine the influence of plate tension, bone screws, and axial forces on the stress distributions at the fracture site. The contact stress distribution for a bone containing an oblique fracture subjected to a uniform end compression is shown in Figure 7–20. The forces applied by the bone screws and an initial tensile force of 75 lb in the plate are also shown. An applied force of 400 lb represents a 200 lb human in a one-legged stance. As expected, an axial load increases both the contact stresses and the area of contact at the fracture site when compared with the effects of plate tension alone or with combined plate tension and screw forces. By comparison, plate tension alone results in a highly concentrated contact stress directly beneath the plate and a distraction of the fracture fragments. The application of a single screw perpendicular to the long axis of the bone gradually increases this contact area and reduces the stress concentration.

It is of interest to note that the beneficial effect of screw tightening is limited to approximately 50 per cent of the pull-out strengths of screws. Above this value, addi-

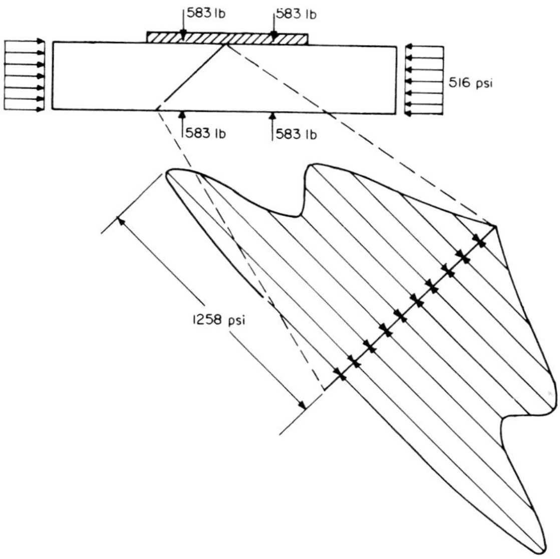

Figure 7–20 Contact stress distribution for an obliquely fractured long bone which has been plated and subjected to uniform axial compression. (Courtesy of E. F. Rybicki, F. A. Simonen and *The Journal of Biomechanics*. J. Biomech., 10:141, 1977.)

tional screw tightening actually reduces the contact area and increases the concentration of the contact stress. Screws applied more perpendicularly to the oblique fracture actually reduce the contact area.

These theoretical investigations emphasize a fundamental feature of compression plate fixation. Since the plate is applied asymmetrically to one surface of the bone, the application of a compression plate induces both bending and compressive stresses in the bone-plate system. The induced bending moment may be large enough to cause distraction (separation) of the fracture surfaces opposite the plate. In addition, highly concentrated contact stresses may occur in the bone directly beneath the plate. The bending effect may dominate, since the fractured bone is unable to support tensile loads.

These factors were demonstrated by Askew and colleagues[8] using photoelastic models and mathematical analyses. Their results indicated that with straight plates applied to straight bones, only a small fraction of the cross-sectional area of the fracture surface (8 to 20 per cent) is in contact. The resulting effect in the compact bone is the creation of high-compression stresses, reaching 5.8×10^7 newton/meter^2 under the action of a bending moment of 10 newton meters and an axial plate load of 534 newtons. To offset this bending effect, Askew and co-workers suggested prebend-

ing the plate prior to installation so as to impact an opposing moment and to close the fracture fragments.

Similar conclusions were reached by Plant and Bartel[58] from a finite element analysis of a bone-plate system. Their results indicated that the application of plate compression resulted in contact of only 25 to 50 per cent of the fracture surface. When the elastic modulus of the plate was reduced to a value equal to bone, the contact area of the fracture surface was reduced to less than 25 per cent. The results in this model support the basic premise of Askew and colleagues[8] that application of tension in the fixation plate induces bending moments that may lead to fracture surface distraction. These effects are exaggerated by the use of plates of reduced modulus.

Since a number of investigators have noticed a tendency for a gap in the cortex to form opposite the plate when straight plates are applied to bone, we have investigated the mechanical consequences of the use of prebent plates.[33] A finite element analysis of an idealized bone-plate system was the model. The results of the analyses show that since the tensile force in the plate is offset from the bone axis, a bending moment is introduced. The contact stresses at the osteotomy site are thus nonuniform, being highly compressive beneath the plate and becoming less compressive across the cortex (Fig. 7–21). Parametric studies of plate

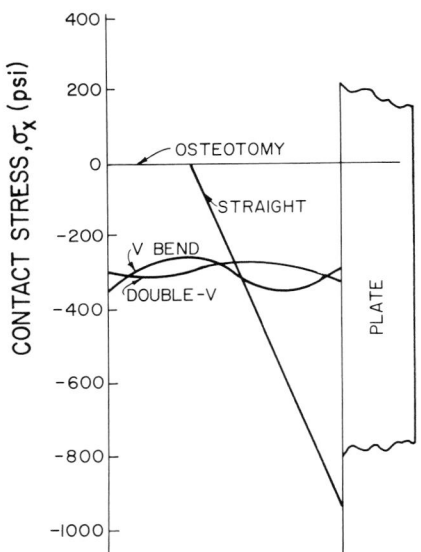

Figure 7–21 Contact stresses at an osteotomy site for straight and prebent plates. For straight plates, the stresses are highly compressive directly beneath the plate. Prebending the plate results in a more nearly uniform distribution of contact stress.

modulus and thickness showed that with straight plates such gaps can be avoided only by the use of plates of unrealistically high values of thickness and modulus. Because of their reduced stiffness, plates of low modulus actually increase the bending moment, and thus increase the tendency for gaps to form in the opposite cortex. These results again confirm the findings of other workers.

The use of prebent plate results in more nearly uniform compressive contact stresses across the osteotomy site (Fig. 7–22). Two bent configurations were analyzed: (1) a V-bend directly over the osteotomy, and (2) a double V-bend on both sides of the osteotomy. One surprising result is that plate bend angles of less than 0.2 degrees are required to induce these nearly uniform contact stresses. This suggests that ex-

tremely small bending angles are required surgically, and that these values are less than the local variations in surface contour. The results also emphasize the large stress variations that may occur owing to differences in the contour of plate and bone.

Woo and co-workers[80] also used finite element methods to evaluate the effects of internal fixation plates on long bone remodeling. The models were designed to explain the differences in plate-induced osteopenia observed with the in vivo use of plates having large differences in bending stiffness. A one-dimensional finite element model of the human femur was constructed after it was verified that such simplified models accurately represent the characteristic behavior of plate-bone systems at locations far distant from screw holes.[70] Two fixation plate materials were considered in the models: a graphite–fiber-reinforced plate and a Vitallium plate. Both plates were of the same length and cross-sectional dimensions, and the geometrical placement of screw holes was the same. The only difference was an order of magnitude reduction in the elastic modulus of the GFMM plate.

The results of bending stress distribution for the unplated models were similar to those reported by Rybecki and associates.[61] After the inclusion of a compression plate in the model, significant bone stress reductions were evident; these were more pronounced with the more rigid Vitallium plate. For the typical load case, the stress distributions along both the medial and lateral cortices of the plated femur differed significantly from those of the unplated femur. However, the bone stresses beneath the GFMM plate were not as low as the bone stresses beneath the more rigid Vitallium plate. The Vitallium-plated bone stresses were only 7 per cent of those of the unplated femur, compared with 53 per cent of the GFMM-plated femur in the lateral

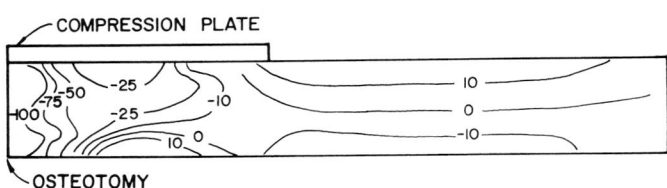

Figure 7–22 Stress contours in the bone with the use of a prebent plate. For a perfectly straight bone, plate bend angles of less than 0.2 degrees result in this nearly uniform contact stress distribution.

cortex directly beneath the plate. In addition, these stress reductions occurred in the same area as the plate-induced osteopenia observed in canine femora.[2] The authors postulated that the reductions in thickness observed in the experimental animals were due to differences in the stresses applied to bone using the two systems.

These predictions of plate-induced osteopenia have led several authors to make in vitro experimental investigations of the strains induced in cortical bone by the application of compression plates. Cochran[21] applied three longitudinally oriented strain gauges to the middiaphyses of dog femora. A four-hole AO plate was then attached over the anterolateral gauge and the strain response to axial loads measured with and without the plate. The application of a single anterolateral plate resulted in an 84 per cent reduction in bone strain beneath the plate, a 22 per cent reduction in strain over the medial surface, and a 27 per cent reduction over the posterior surface. With an additional anteromedial plate, the strain values were reduced more uniformly around the diaphysis: 72 per cent anterolaterally, 32 per cent medially, and 41 per cent posteriorly. The addition of two oblique osteotomies (to simulate a butterfly fragment) did not substantially alter these results.

Similar observations were made by Schatzker and co-workers.[69] Canine femora were instrumented with four-hole semitubular plates and with four-hole AO Dynamic Compression Plates. Plates were applied to the lateral surface, and the bone strains were monitored with strain gauge rosettes. When instrumented with AO semitubular plates, the lateral cortex showed an average decrease in tensile strain of 64 per cent. The medial cortex exhibited a decrease in compressive strain of 20 per cent when compared with strains in the intact bone. These strain reductions did not depend on the presence of an osteotomy.

Even more pronounced strain reductions were observed with AO Dynamic Compression Plates, with the lateral cortex showing a decrease in tensile strain of 77 per cent, and the medial cortex a decrease in compressive strain of 34 per cent. These results demonstrate that internal fixation of bones with plates produces a significant decrease in the mechanical deformations of

compact bone. Thus, although rigid internal fixation initially provides conditions conducive to primary bone healing, protection from mechanical stimuli during the latter stages of healing can encourage atrophic changes that decrease bone strength.

Surgical Screws

The most commonly used orthopedic implant is the surgical screw. Its function is to clamp together the bone and bone plate or to fix bone fragments. This is achieved by the generation of a tensile stress along the length of the screw which is derived from the torsional moment introduced during this screwing process. There are a variety of surgical screws in use, and it appears that certain aspects of their design have not been extensively studied. There also seems to be a difference of opinion about the size of the screw that should be used and some question about the relative advantages of using pretapped screw holes. The relationship of drill size to core diameter of the screw is also of interest. Finally, a screw may fail during insertion, during use, or during removal from the patient. Obviously, the force applied to a screw during its insertion should be below the yield stress of the screw; a number of authors have advocated the use of a torque-limiting screwdriver for surgical use.

Hughes and Jordan[34b] outlined some of the factors governing the use of surgical screws. To drive a screw into a pilot hole it is necessary to apply a clockwise turning force to the screw head. When the leading end of the screw meets some resistance, as when cutting a thread, a shear stress develops along the length of the screw. The insertion of a screw also involves the application of an axial compression force to the screw. If this load is applied axially, then the stress induced in the screw will be pure compressive stress. In practice, the load can be applied at an angle to the screw axis, thus introducing bending stresses in the screw. These can be particularly high at the start of insertion when most of the screw length is unsupported.

When the countersink of a screw meets the countersunk surface of a bone plate or the bone itself, continued turning of the screw pulls the bone plate and the underlying bone together. The magnitude of the clamping force depends on the tensile stresses induced in the screw. Thus the tensile stress in the screw is derived from the torque applied to the screw head. The efficiency of this system may be determined by the ease with which the applied torque is converted into screw tension. The useful torque may be defined as the torque available for conversion into screw tension. The situation may be simply represented by equating the total applied torque to the sum of the torques required to: (1) cut threads, (2) overcome thread friction, (3) overcome friction at the countersink interface, and (4) produce useful torque resulting in tensile forces in the screw.

In practice, the various stresses, including the effects of bending at insertion, compression from the screwdriver, tension required to clamp the plate to the bone, and torsional shear, can combine to result in fracture of the screw. In particular, if a screw is subjected to torsional shear stresses followed by tensile stresses, the tensile stresses required to cause fracture will be lower than the tensile strength owing to the effects of the combined stresses. Thus for a very high tensile stress the application of a small shear stress can be sufficient to cause failure. Conversely, when a high shear stress is present a small tensile stress is sufficient to cause fracture. In the latter event, failure may occur before a sufficient clamping force has been generated.

On the basis of this discussion, one of the most important considerations in testing programs designed for screw evaluation is to determine the factors contributing to the torque required to produce a given level of tension in a screw. These factors can then be used during insertion to insure that the highest practicable tensile stress is obtained with the minimum shear stress. Thus work must be undertaken that deals not only with the conventional mechanical properties of the screw themselves, but also with the mechanics of screw insertion. This is necessary because in clinical applications of bone screws the two factors are interdependent. One final aspect of surgical screw performance is the holding force or stripping strength of a screw. Tensile stresses in a screw result in corresponding opposing shear stresses in the threaded

length of the screw, and these can be utilized only if the bone can sustain these shear stresses. Thus the holding power of a screw (i.e., the axial tensile load that will extract it intact from the bone) is very largely dependent upon the strength of the bone. It can also be shown that when a screw is inserted into a pilot hole, the size of that hole has a strong effect on the holding power of the screw.

Ansell and Scales[7] studied insertion torque and pull-out force for non–self-tapping and self-tapping screws in human cortical bone. They found that it is possible with certain screwdrivers to apply a torque of such a magnitude as to exceed the torsional yield stress of surgical screws having a core diameter of less than 0.120 inch. Of the five groups of screws tested, the most suitable was one with an external diameter of 4 mm and a core size of 0.119 inches. When 9/64-inch diameter screws were compared with 4-mm screws, it was found that a 13 per cent increase in the core diameter resulted in a 44 per cent increase in the torsional yield stress. While the experiments indicated that self-tapping screws yield lower insertion torques and increased pull-out forces, the authors concluded that screws should be inserted into pretapped holes using a torque-limiting device if the failure of screws at insertion is to be prevented. They also found that a 0.125-inch diameter drill is the most suitable size to use with a 4-mm (5/32-inch) screw having a nominal core diameter of 0.118 inches. If the bone is exceptionally hard, then a drill of 0.1285 inches (number 30) can be used.

Bynum and co-workers[19] studied the holding characteristics of five types of screws at five stations along the long axis of the equine metacarpus. The screw types tested were two sizes of sheet metal screws with various interference fits, commercial self-tapping orthopedic screws, and two sizes of machine screws inserted in pretapped holes. Interference was defined as the difference between the major diameter of the screw and the drill diameter, divided by the difference between the major and minor diameters of the screw. Thus the smaller the initial hole, the greater the interference. By increasing the interference, the stress between the screw thread and the surrounding bone was increased. The results were reported both as ultimate push-out force and as ultimate shear stress in order to account for differences in cortical thickness and bone diameters.

The ultimate push-out force was found to be maximal at the midlength of the bone and minimal at the distal end. With sheet metal screws, the ultimate shear stress at midlength ranged from 3.5 to 4.6 ksi for number 10 screws, and from 3.5 to 5.8 ksi for number 14 screws. These results depended upon the interference, with 35 per cent interference resulting in maximum push-out forces for the number 10 screw and 50 per cent interference for the number 14 screw. The average ultimate shear stress at the midlength of the bone was about the same for sheet metal screws as for machine screws in pretapped bone holes. The ultimate shear stress obtained with self-tapping surgical screws was about 50 per cent greater than that for machine screws in tapped bone holes.

Failure mechanisms also depended markedly on screw diameter and on ultimate push-out force. The failure mechanism was thread shear for low push-out forces, bone splitting for intermediate push-out forces, and bone fragmentation for large push-out forces. The propensity of the bone to shatter also increased with increasing fastener size. Since multiple comminuted fractures are difficult to repair surgically, the results indicate that maximum holding force may not be a suitable design criterion for surgical screws. Stated in a different way, this suggests that surgical screws should be designed to encourage failure by the thread shear mode rather than by bone fragmentation.

On the basis of the theoretical considerations outlined at the beginning of this section, Hughes and Jordan[34b] studied the tensile and torsional strength of surgical screws and some effects of the manner of insertion on their performance. To study tensile and torsional strength, cortical bone screws of stainless steel, titanium, and cast Co-Cro-Mo alloy of 2.75-mm, 3.5-mm, and 4-mm major diameter were inserted into pretapped holes in Delrin blocks. Delrin was shown to be a good substitute for bone by Ansell and Scales.[7]

The screws were inserted to a depth sufficient to insure that the holding strength of the screw would exceed its breaking strength. Tensile and torsional loads sufficient to cause failure were then applied to the screw heads. It can be shown theoretically that for cylindrical specimens, the maximum torsional shear strength of a screw is proportional to the core diameter cubed, while the tensile strength is related to the diameter squared. The results were therefore presented as plots of tensile strength versus (core diameter)^2 for each screw material. The relationship was found to deviate somewhat from linearity, because the core diameter underestimates the true stressed area of a helical thread form. For the screws tested, the descending order of strength is: stainless steel, cast Co-Cro-Mo, and titanium. Similarly, when torsional strength was plotted against (core diameter)^3 the relationship was approximately linear, with the screw materials in the same descending order of strength.

The results clearly demonstrate that both the tensile and the torsional strength of surgical screws are critically dependent on the core diameter. Considerable increase in strength can be obtained by an increase in core diameter to 3.4 mm. This would provide a torsional strength for a stainless steel screw of about 80 inch-pounds and for a titanium screw of about 56 inch-pounds. These values compare with 54 and 38 inch-pounds as the maximum torsional strength of currently available 4-mm screws of these materials. An alternative means of strengthening the weaker titanium screws would be to change their composition to a titanium alloy. Results of a small number of tests indicated that 4-mm screws of the titanium alloy were comparable to 4-mm stainless steel screws.

Under combinations of torsion and tension, it is likely that there would be some divergence from these values. Since torsion is the most easily measurable component during screw insertion (by using a torque-limiting screwdriver), the maximum torsional moment for 4-mm screws should not exceed approximately 50 per cent of the ultimate torsional strength for Co-Cro-Mo (21 inch-pounds), 60 per cent for titanium (20 inch-pounds), and 70 per cent (33.5 inch-pounds) for stainless steel. However, since frictional forces at the countersink interface may absorb up to 40 per cent of the total torsional input, Hughes and Jordan suggested a figure of 65 per cent of the ultimate strength as a good overall value incorporating a reasonable margin of safety.

The results emphasize that for maximum efficiency and least risk of premature screw failure, screw tensile stresses should be generated with the lowest possible shear stresses in the screw. In the most adverse circumstance (without lubrication and without pretapping of the bone) only about 5 per cent of the applied torque can be usefully employed to induce screw tension. The important factors in improving this situation are: (1) the use of a pilot hole with the largest practical diameter; (2) the use of a pretapped hole; and (3) the use of saline as a lubricant to reduce friction at the countersink faces. Under these circumstances, about 65 per cent of the applied torque can be usefully employed to induce screw tension. Practical observations by these authors also lead to the conclusion that the poorest screwhead design is the single slot, and the best is probably the recessed hexagon.

Hughes and Jordan further described the strength of surgical screws under combined tensile and shear stresses by a critical resolved shear stress necessary to induce failure. Expressed in arbitrary units, the relative strengths of commercially available bone screws are approximately: (1) stainless steel, 100; (2) cast Co-Cro-Mo, 80; (3) titanium, 65; and (4) titanium alloy, 100. The holding power of a screw is also independent of the mechanical properties of the screw and dependent on the shear strength of the bone into which the screw is inserted. For a given bone strength, the optimal pilot hole size for maximum holding power depends solely on the major diameter of the screw. The experiments indicated that the pilot hole diameter for 4-mm screws should be made with a 3.45-mm drill, which is larger than that usually recommended. Where increased holding power is required, as in cancellous or diseased bone, a larger major diameter of the screw should be considered.

Nunamaker and Perren[53] provided further estimates of the effect of core diameter on the holding power of surgical screws. An entire range of screw sizes and types were inserted in bovine cancellous bone to measure the torque of insertion, screwdriver pressure, axial compression generated by the screw, screw breaking strength, and efficacy of various head types. The results indicated that the core diameter of the screw should be as large as conditions allow, since the torque required to break a screw is largely determined by the core diameter. In this direct comparison of the screws made of the same material, the ratio of breaking torques was equal to the ratio of the cubes of their respective core diameters. This finding supports the similar observation of Hughes and Jordan.[34b] The experiments in bovine cancellous bone showed that larger screws hold better and should be used whenever possible, especially in soft bone. Since the stress-concentrating effects of a screw hole in cancellous bone would not be expected to be as severe as in cortical bone, the results suggest the use of the largest possible screw diameter in cancellous bone for optimal fixation.

The foregoing studies are in vitro tests of the holding power of surgical screws. However, holding power is inseparably a function of the bone adjacent to the screw. The holding power can be expected to be a function not only of screw design but also of the changes induced in bone by the trauma of insertion, and by the resorption and remodeling of the bone during healing. To investigate these factors, Schatzker and co-workers[68] tested the holding power of surgical screws after implantation in mongrel dogs for periods of 2, 4, 6, and 12 weeks. Three non–self-tapping and one self-tapping screw were used, with outer diameters varying from 3.5 to 4.5 mm (core diameters ranged from 2.0 to 3.0 mm). Both stainless steel and cobalt chrome screws were investigated.

The push-out force was weakly dependent on the thickness of the cortex. The rather substantial data scatter was attributed to uncontrolled variations in insertion and testing techniques as well as to variations in the in vivo healing and remodeling responses. The mean values of the holding power of the four screw types, when plotted as a function of time, increased at six weeks to between 150 and 190 per cent of the initial values, and at 12 weeks to between 100 and 125 per cent of initial values. Statistical analyses also showed a significant difference (P<0.05) in mean values between the stainless steel AO 4.5-mm diameter non–self-tapping screw (the largest in the series) and each of the other screw types at zero, two, and six weeks. The 4- and 12-week values showed no differences. No differences were observed between the two cobalt chrome screws (only one of which was self-tapping). At no time during the phase of maximal bony reaction did bone death or remodeling weaken the holding power below initial values.

Histological investigations revealed that the amount of new bone formation was directly related to the ratio of the pilot hole diameter to the core diameter. When large pilot holes were used, more new bone formation was found near the inner core of the screw. Consistently, at two, four, and six weeks, cortical bone was found to be devoid of nuclear material in the lacunae for an average distance of 1 mm from the margins of the drill hole. The self-tapping and non–self-tapping screws gave rise to similar proliferative reactions, which resulted in the formation of bone without a fibrous layer interposed between thread and cortex.

The results of this experiment indicate that with normal care on insertion, for the four screw types tested, the tissue reaction to a minimally loaded screw is not deleterious to its holding power during the initial 12-week period. The largest screw tested, the 4.5-mm non–self-tapping stainless steel screw of the AO type, provided the greatest holding power over the testing period.

COMPARATIVE STUDIES

In order to provide comparisons of the structural performance of different methods of internal fixation, a number of in vitro studies have been conducted. Hubbard[34a] measured the failure torques of intact fresh human femora. Each fractured specimen was reconstructed using a Küntscher rod and then retested. The rod was removed and the femur again reconstructed by application of two compression plates. Following that procedure the Küntscher rod

was reinserted with PMMA fixation in the distal metaphyseal region. Hubbard[34a] recorded failure torques of only 2 per cent of the control value after the first test, because the Küntscher rod without PMMA did not adequately grip the distal segment. The second test showed that compression plates failed at 7 per cent of the control value, primarily as a result of poor plate fixation and the two previous test fractures. The third series, after fixation by Küntscher rod and PMMA, produced the best results at 31 per cent of the control value.

Laurence, Freeman, and Swenson[36] reported engineering considerations in the internal fixation of fracture of the tibial shaft. First, measurements and calculations provided estimates of the bending and torsional loads that might be applied to fixation devices during non–weight-bearing mobilization and during restrictive weight bearing. Second, experiments were conducted in which intact and drilled tibiae were fractured by bending or torsion in order to provide a standard of comparison for the strengths of fixation devices. Third, tests in bending and in torsion for various plates and intramedullary nails were conducted. These tests, including measurements of the tensile loads acting on screws while the device was transmitting bending loads, were designed to provide a better understanding of the functioning of intramedullary nails and onlay plates. Tests were conducted so that bending loads tended to open the fracture site, a load that tests the bending properties of the plate alone.

These authors estimated that the greatest bending moment applied to a plated or nailed fracture of the tibia during restricted weight bearing in men is up to about 79 newton meters. The maximum twisting moment was estimated to be about 29 newton meters. Twenty-two human tibiae were loaded in three-point bending and failed at bending moments of from 57.9 to 294 newton meters (mean ± 1 S D, 152.4 ± 62.7) if they had not previously been drilled. Tibiae that had 3-mm drill holes through both cortices broke at from 32.4 to 144 newton meters (96.8 ± 46.7). Tibiae loaded at torsion broke at twisting moments of from 27.5 to 89.2 newton meters (56.85 ± 21.0) when not drilled, and from 23.6 to 77.5 newton meters (54.8 ± 18.0) when drilled.

In bending, the rankings of the internal fixation devices tested were similar to those reported by other workers. As expected, two plates were stiffer and stronger than any single plate and were as strong as the weaker of the drilled tibiae. In torsion, as in bending, two-plate preparations were appreciably stronger than a single plate. It is of interest that the two-plate preparations tested in torsion failed by fracture of the bone through screw holes at twisting moments similar to those needed to break drilled tibia. The torsional stiffness and strength of the intramedullary nails tested were found to be unsatisfactory. Of the three available metallic materials tested (stainless steel, cobalt chrome, and titanium), all provide mechanical properties so similar that the choice between them can be made on other grounds.

With the use of a special transducer, the highest tensile load applied to a screw during bending tests was about half of that necessary to pull a screw out of a thin-walled tibia. Screws beyond four for a single plate were found to be mechanically redundant at the moment of implantation, but may be necessary as insurance against subsequent deterioration in strength. The authors emphasized that if at all possible every hole in the plate should be occupied by a firmly held screw, since empty screw holes can act as stress concentrators. In conclusion, these authors found that only the strongest implants tested were strong enough to withstand the bending and twisting moments to be expected in restricted weight bearing. Significantly, in two-plate preparations an additional danger is introduced, because these moments are close to those required to fracture a drilled tibia. As a result, failure for two-plate preparations can be expected to occur by bone fracture rather than by excessive deformation of the internal fixation device.

Mensch and co-workers[48] compared the torsional response of three groups of internal fixation devices. All results were normalized by comparing the torsional response of reconstructed femora with that of their intact contralateral bones. The experiment was conducted with paired fresh human femora collected at autopsy within eight hours of death. In order to simulate the most severe pathological conditions in

which there is great gross destruction of bone, a model was developed in which a segment of 20 per cent of the mid-diaphysis was resected from one of each pair. The opposite femur remained intact and was tested as a control. Continuity in the resected specimen was reestablished by the application of internal fixation devices with and without PMMA.

Three types of internal fixation devices were used: intramedullary rods, titanium mesh, and bone plates. Three stainless steel intramedullary devices were evaluated: Küntscher cloverleaf nails, Schneider self-broaching rods, and multiple 2.8-mm Steinmann pins. For the titanium mesh group, 0.89-mm titanium mesh was cut into 3.8 × 15.2 cm strips, and each strip was bent to conform to the outer cortex of the femur. Configurations of one, two, and three strips were used. Prior to application of the mesh, PMMA was inserted into the medullary canal as well as on the cortex adjacent to the mesh.

For the bone plate group, stainless steel compression plates were applied in two configurations: (1) single plates were screwed to the lateral aspect of the femur, and (2) lateral and anterior plates were applied. In order to judge whether cement enhanced the strength of these bone-plate configurations, specimens were also prepared by packing cement within the segmental defect and into the medullary canals. In order to achieve dynamic torsional loading of the test specimens, a special apparatus similar to that of Burstein and Frankel[17] was designed. Both the applied torque and the torsional rotation were monitored, and torque versus rotation curves were displayed on a storage oscilloscope.

A summary of the torque ratios is shown in Figure 7–23. The combination of two bone plates and cement exhibits the highest relative average fracture torque (73 per cent of control). One bone plate and cement, a less complicated configuration, is nearly as strong (on average, 72 per cent of control, although with greater variability). Cement added to a single bone plate appears advantageous, since the femora fixed without cement fail at a lower torque (on average, 40 per cent of control). Of the titanium mesh tests, the three strips-and-cement configu-

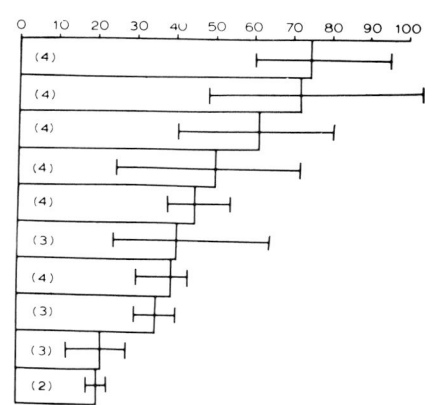

PERCENT OF CONTROL FAILURE TORQUE

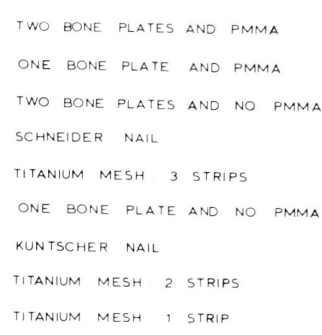

Figure 7–23 Experimental stabilization of segmental defects in the human femur. Torque capacity as a percentage of contralateral control. Numbers of specimens are shown in parentheses. (Courtesy of J. S. Mensch, K. L. Markolf, S. B. Roberts, et al., and *The Journal of Bone and Joint Surgery.* J. Bone Joint Surg., 58A:185, 1976.)

TWO BONE PLATES AND PMMA
ONE BONE PLATE AND PMMA
TWO BONE PLATES AND NO PMMA
SCHNEIDER NAIL
TITANIUM MESH 3 STRIPS
ONE BONE PLATE AND NO PMMA
KUNTSCHER NAIL
TITANIUM MESH 2 STRIPS
TITANIUM MESH 1 STRIP
MUTIPLE STEINMANN PINS

ration gives the best results. Of the configurations with intramedullary devices, the Schneider and Küntscher nails produce average torsional failure loads twice those of the Steinmann pin group. This is not unexpected, in view of the fact that the torsional rigidity of the multiple pin bundles is relatively low.

These results indicate that under the severe test conditions represented by the 20 per cent resection model, bone-plate is the strongest configuration for withstanding torsional loading. The torsional strength of femora fixed with single and double bone plates with and without cement averages 63 per cent of control values. As a group, the specimens reconstructed with plates are significantly stronger than specimens fixed with intramedullary nails or with titanium mesh strips. The torsional strengths of the plated femora are limited in all cases by the stress concentration effects at the holes drilled in the bone for screw fixation.

Femora fixed with Küntscher and Schneider nails average 45 per cent of control strength and are significantly stronger than femora fixed with titanium mesh strips. The torsional strength of femora fixed with intramedullary nails anchored in cement is limited by failure of the acrylic and bone adjacent to the resected section. The use of titanium mesh applied with screws and cement in one- and two-strip configurations is the least effective of the three categories tested, averaging only 28 per cent of control values. The two specimens fixed with multiple Steinmann

pins and cement fail at an average of 19 per cent of normal. As a group, this is the weakest configuration. The use of multiple Steinmann pins packed with PMMA in the intramedullary cavity should therefore be discouraged because of severe twisting and fragmentation of the surrounding acrylic at low levels of torque.

It should be emphasized that these results apply only to torsional loading. Different rankings of fixation methods may occur under other loading conditions. However, under the severe test conditions represented by the 20 per cent resection model, this study emphasizes the mechanical superiority of plate fixation with and without PMMA reinforcement over intramedullary fixation and titanium mesh fixation.

CLINICAL ASSESSMENT OF FRACTURE HEALING

Currently, to evaluate the progress of fracture healing the clinician utilizes a manual examination for stability, radiographic evidence of healing, the empirical passage of time, and the patient's evaluation of symptomatic pain.[71] For bones deeply underlying muscular and subcutaneous tissue, manual tests of stability are of questionable value. Similarly, radiographic evidence may be open to interpretation, since in many fractures the bone is functionally normal before a roentgenogram indicates obliteration of the fracture line. Since the rate of union is also variable, the elapsed time since fracture does not afford a precise prediction of union in individual cases. And finally, tenderness over the fracture site may be difficult to determine. As a result of these uncertainties, many fractures are subjected to immobilization for a longer time than necessary. Conversely, conventional methods do not indicate precisely when the healing process has failed. Diagnosis of a malunion or a nonunion and the need for surgical intervention may thus be unduly postponed.

Because of these limitations, various investigators have attempted to devise objective methods for nondestructively estimating the ability of a healing fracture to withstand functional demands. A number of different techniques have been explored, but because of the variability of bone response, few have been brought to clinical trial and none has gained widespread clinical acceptance. However, because of the potential usefulness of a means to precisely dictate time for cast removal or to predict occurrence of nonunion, efforts continue to be made in a number of laboratories to develop a noninvasive method for assessing fracture healing. In this section, some of the techniques will be explored briefly, and two methods that have been brought to clinical trial will be dealt with in more detail.

ULTRASOUND

Floriani and co-workers[23] measured the speed of propagation of ultrasound in guinea pig femora six months after osteotomy and reported a significant decrease in sonic velocity in nonunion (67 per cent of normal) and in incomplete union (81 per cent of normal). This work was extended by Abendschein and Hyatt,[1] but their attempt was not totally successful because there was no clear distinction between the delay of the wave in freshly fractured, solidly united bones and fractures with disjointed fragments. Thus when the speed of ultrasound propagation through an intact bone is compared with that of a bone that has been transversely sectioned, there is no difference if the sectioned ends are closely approximated. If the sectioned ends are separated by a material of reduced sonic

velocity, such as soft tissue, the propagation rate is decreased to an extent determined by the thickness of the soft tissue. Another intrinsic limitation of the ultrasound propagation technique is the requirement that the wavelength of the propagated sound be negligible in comparison with the dimensions of the bone. This results in a requirement for sound frequencies higher than 3 mHz. At these frequencies, the attenuation of ultrasound becomes so great that it is nearly impossible to measure propagation velocities. At frequencies below 1 mHz, the wavelength becomes long enough to violate the basic theoretical assumptions required to calculate mechanical properties from sonic velocity measurements.

In spite of these limitations, Gerlanc and colleagues[30] published data showing empirically derived correlations between ultrasound propagation velocities and degree of fracture healing. A number of other workers are also exploring the use of sound propagation as a possible means of evaluating fracture healing. Brown and Mayor[15] are using ultrasound attenuation measurements to assess callus formation during the early stages of fracture healing.

STRESS WAVE PROPAGATION

Another approach has been to use changes in the characteristics of a propagating flexural wave when a discontinuity, such as a fracture, is introduced in a long bone. Lewis and associates conducted limited clinical trials of this method and compared the results with identical tests involving the corresponding uninjured limb. The stress wave was generated by applying a dynamic load with a small amplitude force (10 newtons) produced by the impact of a spring-loaded 1/8 inch-diameter steel ball on a bony prominence at the proximal tibia. The transmitted wave was recorded by means of an accelerometer applied externally to the distal tibia. The output exhibited acceleration amplitudes on the order of 0.2 g with frequencies in the range of 3 kHz, corresponding to noninjurious strain levels. The results were also compared with the healing state as judged radiographically. A set of data taken from a patient with a fractured tibia and fibula is

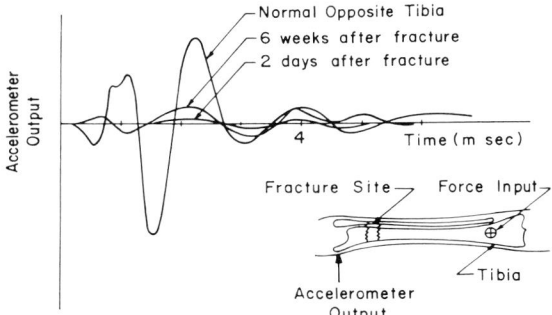

Figure 7–24 Stress wave propagation used to evaluate healing of clinical fractures of tibia and fibula. (Courtesy of J. L. Lewis and *The Journal of Biomechanics.* J. Biomech., 8:17, 1975.)

shown in Figure 7–24. While the data scatter is considerable with this method, it is not so great as to alter the major signal shape. The two main aspects of the signal altered by the healing are: (1) the amplitude increases with healing, and (2) the high-frequency content increases with healing. To date, sufficiently satisfactory reproducibility of the results has not been obtained owing to difficulties in the proper control of the boundary conditions at both loading and recording ends. Nevertheless, the data suggest potential clinical applicability. Toward this end, fundamental investigations of the process of wave propagation in intact and discontinuous long bones have been undertaken.[39, 77]

In order to avoid some of the limitations presented by the uncertain boundary conditions in the foregoing method, Sonstegard and Matthews[71] explored the use of stress wave disturbances imposed on the bone

BASIC APPROACH

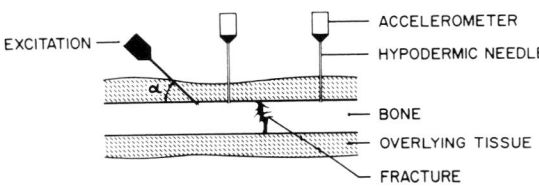

Figure 7–25 Measurement technique for the sonic diagnosis of fracture healing. An excitation and two sensing needles are used in intimate contact with the bone surface. (Courtesy of D. A. Sonstegard and L. S. Matthews and *The Journal of Biomechanics.* J. Biomech., 9:689–694, 1976.)

through direct coupling. The guiding criterion in the design of their sonic diagnosis techniques was the mitigation of surrounding tissue influences. Thus direct attachment to bone at excitation and sensing locations was desired. A three-needle configuration (Fig. 7–25) is shown, with one needle attachment providing the source of excitation. Standard hypodermic needles are used; light tapping of the needle base yields tip penetration through the periosteum and into the adjacent cortical surface. Two additional needles are placed perpendicular to the longitudinal bone axis at a predetermined separation distance spanning the fracture. The first of these needles provides a control measure of the incoming excitation, and the second measures the disturbance after it has traversed the fracture site. A suitable input signal is provided by simply tapping the excitation needle. Unidirectional piezoelectric accelerometers are attached in a vertical orientation to the measurement site.

The parameters used to characterize the pre- and postfracture wave fronts are the propagation velocity and the amplitude and slope ratios of the incoming and transmitted waves. No attempt has been made to relate the parameters to the stiffness or strength of the fracture. Results from laboratory animal experimentation and subsequent limited clinical trials indicate that this approach holds some potential for the clinical and experimental diagnosis of fracture healing. It circumvents some of the limitations of the methods previously described, in that the influences of adjacent bone and soft tissues are effectively removed from the measurement system. The approach is limited, however, by the requirement that the needles be inserted directly into the bone.

RESONANT VIBRATION

In order to develop a noninvasive measure of bone integrity, Markey and Jurist[45] explored the use of steady-state resonant vibration measurements of long bones. One difficulty with this index is that in vibrating systems, resonant frequencies depend on the ratio of stiffness to mass. A bone with a reduced load-carrying capacity may have both a reduced stiffness and a reduced mass and yet display normal resonant fre-

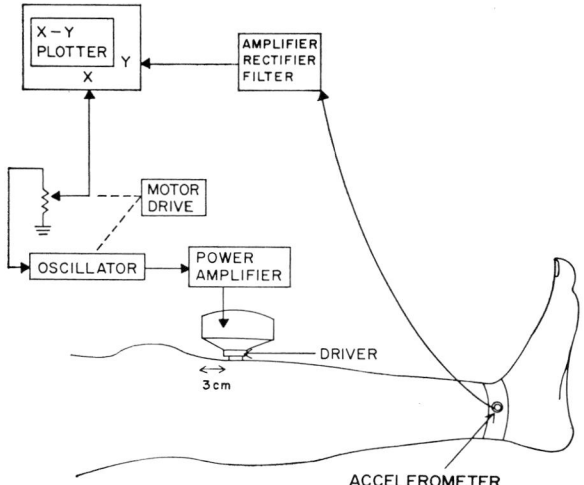

Figure 7-26 Tibial resonant frequency apparatus for the diagnosis of fracture healing. (Courtesy of E. Markey, J. Jurist, and *The Wisconsin Medical Journal,* Wisc. Med. J., 73:62, 1974.)

quency characteristics. The resonant frequency of a long bone is related to its flexural rigidity as well as to the speed of sound in the bone tissue. The apparatus used by Jurist to measure tibial resonant frequency in vivo is shown in Figure 7–26. The resonant frequency is obtained from a recording of the acceleration response as a function of frequency. The bone is driven by a mechanical oscillator about 3 cm distal to the tibial tubercle, with the driver axis aligned in an anteroposterior direction perpendicular to the long axis of the bone. The response of the tibia is monitored by means of a small piezoelectric accelerometer strapped to the medial malleolus.

The original hypothesis developed by these workers was that the tibial resonant frequency would increase progressively with healing, and at the same time the amplitude of the resonant peak would increase. Figure 7–27 shows the evolution of the tibial response spectrum of a normally healing fracture.[45] Note the increase in both frequency and amplitude. Note also that the vertical scale of the recording made 97 days after fracture is compressed by a factor of 20, relative to the other two tracings. Simple conceptual models were developed which suggested that the square of the ratio of the resonant frequency of the fractured tibia to that of its contralateral control provides an index of the strength of union relative to that of the intact bone. The use of this ratio

eliminates geometrical variations between individuals.

To test the hypothesized squared relationship, defects were created in the fe-

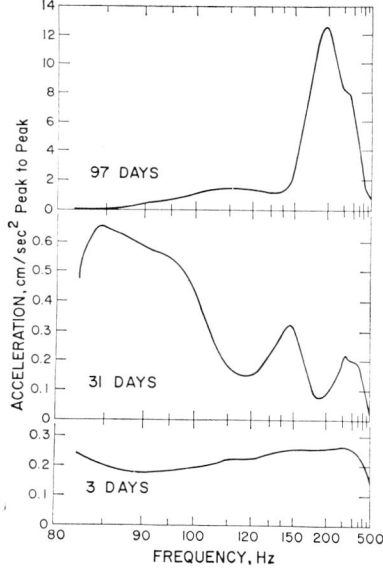

Figure 7-27 Tibial response spectra for a normally healing fracture. Note the flat response obtained three days following fracture. By one month, a low amplitude peak was obtained at 84 Hz. By three months, the resonant frequency had increased to 191 Hz, and the amplitude had increased by a factor of about 20. (Courtesy of E. Markey, J. Jurist, and *The Wisconsin Medical Journal.* Wisc. Med. J., 73:62, 1974.)

moral cortex of dogs. In some dogs the femora were excised for testing immediately, and the others were sacrificed three to eight weeks postoperatively. The resonant frequency was determined, and then the femora were tested to failure in three-point bending. Significant correlations were found between the failure load and the resonance frequency (r=0.428) and between resonant frequency and flexural rigidity (r=0.456). Plots of the ratios of bending strength (defective/intact) against the resonance frequency ratio provided highly significant correlations, supporting the squared relationship between the strength ratio and the frequency ratio (r=0.932).

In addition, both the relative strength and the relative resonant frequency were found to be associated with healing time, with correlation coefficients averaging about 0.55. These weak correlations were assumed to be due to variations in size of the dog femora, depths of the artificial defects, and differences in individual healing rates. It should be noted that this conclusion – the strength of healing bones is proportional to the square of the resonant frequency – is based on the assumption that a partially healed fracture can be simulated by a healing partial osteotomy. This simulation is unrealistic in the early stages of fracture healing, but is presumably more realistic in the later stages.

With this background, Markey and Jurist[45] used the tibial resonant frequency meas-

urement method on 19 patients with uncomplicated fractures on 58 separate occasions to derive a normal healing curve (Fig. 7–28). This was accomplished by plotting squares of the ratios of the resonant frequencies of the fractured tibiae to their controls as a function of time since fracture. The development of a normal healing curve allowed a comparison of longitudinal measurements on individual patients to be compared with the normal healing response. Patients who went on to develop nonunion exhibited frequency response curves that followed the normal healing curve but then fell markedly below it. This suggests that fracture healing may initially be normal, and only in the later stages become abnormal (Fig. 7–28).

In summary, the technique of resonant frequency measurement appears to have merit in the in vivo evaluation of fracture healing and is certainly the best developed method in terms of clinical applicability. It has value in the study of both normal and pathological fracture healing and may prove useful as a predictive tool for estimating individual healing rates. In some cases, this could allow earlier removal of immobilization devices. This approach represents an objective yet noninvasive method of evaluating fracture healing and provides supportive data to roentgenographic and clinical examination. It is not without difficulties, however, and questions concerning repeatability and the effects of soft tissues and edema require further study. In addition,

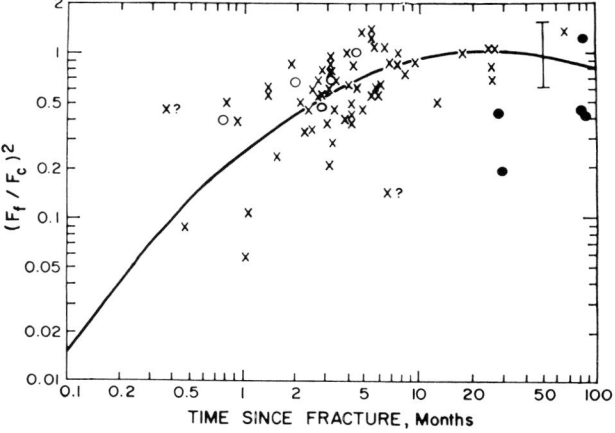

Figure 7–28 Normal healing curve for tibial fractures monitored by the resonant frequency technique. The ordinate represents the square of the resonant frequency ratio (fracture/control). The open figures represent a 14-year-old boy; the closed circles, those with delayed or nonunion; and the crosses, all other adults.

this method has been applied primarily to the ulna and tibia, and much work remains to extend its applicability to other bones. Resonant frequency measurements remain, however, the most advanced tool for the noninvasive assessment of the mechanical integrity of healing fractures.

SUMMARY

Trauma associated with high-speed transportation, industrial accidents, and leisure activities often involves fractures of the long bones. Despite the obvious medical, economic, and scientific relevance of information relating to the healing of such fractures, many aspects of the healing process are poorly understood. In particular, rational methods for comparing therapeutic approaches in fracture management have not been advanced. This chapter has been an attempt to bring together information on three aspects of the biomechanics of fracture healing and treatment. The first is related to the return of stiffness and strength in healing fractures. Available data on the biomechanical stages of fracture repair and the mechanical factors that influence this process have been summarized. While many data have been generated, wide variations in experimental design, treatment modalities, and normal biological response have made it difficult to compare results and draw clinically relevant conclusions.

The optimization of fracture management techniques has also been reviewed. Fracture healing poses a unique set of mechanical demands that involve trade-offs between conflicting requirements. In the face of these conflicting demands, attempts have been made to optimize the mechanics of fracture management. These have included in vitro mechanical comparisons of internal fixation methods and studies of stresses in walking casts and functional bracing. Studies are relatively advanced and have led to a good understanding of the mechanics of surgical screws and their insertion and of plate fixation. Less research has been done on methods of external immobilization, such as plaster casts and functional bracing.

The use of mechanical testing techniques in the evaluation of fracture healing in human patients has also been reviewed. Although none of the techniques currently under investigation can be yet thought of as a clinical tool for the noninvasive assessment of fracture healing, considerable progress has been made. In particular, resonant frequency measurements show promise for the clinical diagnosis of the return of stiffness and strength to healing fractures.

REFERENCES

1. Abendschein, N., and Hyatt, G. N.: Ultrasonics and selected physical properties of bone. Clin. Orthop. Rel. Res., 69:294–301, 1969.
2. Akeson, W. H., Woo, S. L-Y., Coutts, R. D., Matthews, J. V., Gonsalves, M., and Amiel, D.: Quantitative histological evaluation of early fracture healing of cortical bones immobilized by stainless steel and composite plates. Calcif. Tiss. Res., 19:27–37, 1975.
3. Allen, W. C., Heiple, K. G., and Burstein, A. H.: A fluted femoral intramedullary rod. J. Bone Joint Surg., 60A:506–515, 1978.
4. Allen, W. C., Piotrowski, G., Burstein, A. H., and Frankel, V. H.: Biomechanical principles of intramedullary fixation. Clin. Orthop. Rel. Res., 60:13–20, 1968.
5. Allgöwer, M., Ehrsam, R., Ganz, R., Matter, P., and Perren, S. M.: Clinical experience with a new compression plate "DCP." Acta Orthop. Scand. (Suppl.), 125:45–61, 1969.
6. Anderson, L. D.: Compression plate fixation and the effects of different types of internal fixation on fracture healing. J. Bone Joint Surg., 47A: 191–208, 1965.
7. Ansell, R. H., and Scales, J. T.: A study of some factors which affect the strength of screws and their insertion and holding power in bone. J. Biomech., 1:279–302, 1968.
8. Askew, M. J., Mow, V. C., Wirth, C. R., et al.: Analysis of the intraosseous stress field due to compression plating. J. Biomech., 8:203, 1975.
9. Braden, T. D., Brinken, W. O., Little, R. W., et al.: Comparative biomechanical evaluation of bone healing in the dog. J. Am. Vet. Med. Assoc., 163:65–69.
10. Brighton, C. T.: Biophysics of fracture healing. *In* Heppenstall, R. B. (ed.): Fracture Healing and Treatment. Vol. I. Philadelphia, W. B. Saunders, 1979.
11. Brighton, C. T., Friedenberg, Z. B., Zemsky, L. M., and Pollis, P. R.: Direct current stimulation of non-union and congenital pseudarthrosis. J. Bone Joint Surg., 57A:368–377, 1975.
12. Brinker, W. O., Flo, G. L., Braden, T., Noser, G., and Merkley, D.: Removal of bone plates in small animals., J. Vet. Med., 11:577–586, 1975.
13. Brooks, D. B., Burstein, A. H., and Frankel, V. H.: The biomechanics of torsional fractures: The stress concentration of drill holes. J. Bone Joint Surg., 58A:507–514, 1970.

14. Brown, S. A., and Mayor, M. B.: The biocompatibility of materials for internal fixation of fractures. J. Biomed. Mater. Res., *12*:67–82, 1978.

15. Brown, S. A., and Mayor, M. B.: Ultrasonic assessment of early callus formation. Biomed. Eng., *11*:124–136, 1976.

16. Brown, S. A., Vandergrift, J. A., Kennedy, F. E., and Mayor, M. B.: Biomechanical compatibility in fracture fixation. Transactions of the 9th International Biomaterials Symposium, p. 79. New Orleans, 1976.

17. Burstein, A. H., and Frankel, V. H.: Technical note: a standard test for laboratory animal bone. J. Biomech., *4*:155–158, 1971.

18. Burstein, A. H., Currey, J., Frankel, V. H., Heiple, K. G., Lunseth, P., and Vessely, J. C.: Bone strength: the effect of screw holes. J. Bone Joint Surg., *54A*:1143–1156, 1972.

19. Bynum, D., Jr., Ray, D. R., Boyd, C. L., and Ledbetter, W. B.: Capacity of installed commercial bone fixation plates. Am. J. Vet. Res., *32*:783–791, 1971.

20. Cochran, G. V. B.: Experimental methods for stimulation of bone healing by means of electrical therapy. Bull. N. Y. Acad. Med., *48*:899–911, 1972.

21. Cochran, G. V. B.: Effects of internal fixation plates on mechanical deformation of bone. Surg. Forum, *20*:469, 1969.

22. Copp, D. H., and Greenberg, D. M.: Studies on bone fracture healing. J. Nutr., *29*:261–267, 1945.

23. Floriani, L. P., Debevoise, N. T., and Hyatt, G. W.: Mechanical properties of healing bone by the use of ultrasound. Surg. Forum, *18*:468–470, 1967.

24. Friedenberg, Z. B., Andrews, E. T., Smolenski, B. I., Pearl, B.W., and Brighton, C. T.: Bone reaction to varying amounts of direct current. Surg. Gynecol. Obstet., *131*:894–899, 1970.

25. Friedenberg, Z. B., and Brighton, C. T.: Bioelectric potentials in bone. J. Bone Joint Surg., *48A*:915, 1966.

26. Friedenberg, Z. B., and French, G.: The effects of known compression forces on fracture healing. Surg. Gynecol. Obstet., *94*:743–748, 1952.

27. Friedenberg, Z. B., and Kohanim, M.: The effect of direct current on bone. Surg. Gynecol. Obstet., *127*:97–102, 1968.

28. Friedenberg, Z. B., Roberts, P. G., Jr., Didizian, N. H., and Brighton, C. T.: Stimulation of fracture healing by direct current in the rabbit fibula. J. Bone Joint Surg., *53A*:1400–1408, 1971.

29. Frymoyer, J. W., and Pope, M. H.: Fracture healing in the sciatically denervated rat. J. Trauma, *17*:355–361, 1977.

30. Gerlanc, M., Haddad, D., Hyatt, G., Langloh, J., and St. Hilaire, P.: Ultrasonic study of normal and fractured bones. Clin. Orthop. Rel. Res., *111*:175–180, 1975.

31. Harris, W. H., and Weinberg, E. H.: Microscopic methods for measuring cortical bone volume. Calcif. Tiss. Res., 8:150–156, 1972.

32. Hayes, W. C., and Perren, S. M.: Plate-bone friction in the compression fixation of fractures. Clin. Orthop. Rel. Res., 89:236–240, 1972.

33. Hayes, W. C., Grens, W. B., Murch, S. A., and Nunamaker, D. M.: Effects of plate modulus, thickness and pre-bending on the mechanics of compression plate fixation. Transactions of the 24th Annual Orthopaedic Research Society, Dallas, February, 1978.

34. Henry, A. N., Freeman, M. A. R., and Swanson, S. A. V.: Studies on the mechanical properties of healing experimental fractures, Proc. R. Soc. Med., *61*:40–44, 1968.

34a. Hubbard, M. J. S.: The fixation of experimental femoral shaft torque fractures. Acta Orthop. Scand., *22*:55–61, 1973.

34b. Hughes, A. N., and Jordan, B. A.: The mechanical properties of surgical screws and some aspects of insertion practice. Injury, *4*:25–32, 1972.

35. Hutzschenreuter, P., Perren, S. M., Steinmann, S., Geret, V., and Kiebl, M.: Some effects of rigidity of internal fixation on the healing pattern of osteotomies. Injury, *1*:77–81, 1969.

36. Laurence, M., Freeman, M. A. R., and Swanson, S. A. V.: Engineering considerations in the internal fixation of fractures of the tibial shaft. J. Bone Joint Surg., *51B*:754–768, 1969.

37. Laurin, C. A., Sison, V., and Roque, N.: Mechanical investigation of experimental fractures. Can. J. Surg., *6*:218–228, 1963.

38. Lettin, A. W. F.: The effects of axial compression on the healing of experimental fractures of the rabbit tibia. Proc. R. Soc. Med., *58*:882–886, 1965.

39. Lewis, J. L.: A dynamic model of a healing fractured long bone. J. Biomech., *8*:17–25, 1975.

40. Lindahl, O.: The rigidity of fracture immobilization with plates. Acta Orthop. Scand., *38*:101–114, 1967.

41. Lindahl, O.: Rigidity of immobilization of oblique fractures. Acta Orthop. Scand., *35*:39–50, 1964.

42. Lindahl, O.: Rigidity of immobilization of transverse fractures. Acta Orthop. Scand., *32*:237–246, 1962.

43. Lindholm, R. V., Lindholm, T. S., Toikkanen, S., et al.: Effect of forced interfragmental movements on the healing of tibial fractures in rats. Acta Orthop. Scand., *40*:721–728, 1969.

44. Lindsay, M. K., and Howes, E. L.: The breaking strength of healing fractures. J. Bone Joint Surg., *13*:491–501, 1931.

45. Markey, E., and Jurist, J.: Tibial resonant frequency measurements as an index of the strength of fracture union. Wis. Med. J., *73*:62–65, 1974.

46. McKeown, R. M., Lindsay, M. K., Harvey, S. C., and Howes, E. L.: The breaking strength of healing fractured fibulae of rats. Arch. Surg., *24*:458–481, 1932.

47. McKibbin, B.: The biology of fracture healing in long bones. J. Bone Joint Surg., *60B*:150–162, 1978.

48. Mensch, J. S., Markolf, K. L., Roberts, S. B., and Finerman, G. M.: Experimental stabilization of segmental defects in the human femur. J. Bone Joint Surg., *58A*:185–190, 1976.

49. Mindell, E. R., Rodbard, S., and Kuasman, B. G.: Chondrogenesis in bone repair: a study of healing fracture callus in the rat. Clin. Orthop. Rel. Res., 79:187–196, 1971.

50. Minns, R. J., Bremble, G. R., and Campbell, J.: A biomechanical study of internal fixation of the tibial shaft. J. Biomech., 10:569–579, 1977.

51. Mosley, C. K., Heiple, K. H. and Burstein, A. H.: Personal communication, 1978.

52. Muller, M. E., Allgower, M., and Willenegger, H.: Manual of Internal Fixation. Berlin, Springer-Verlag, 1970.

53. Nunamaker, D. M., and Perren, S. M.: Force measurements in screw fixation. J. Biomech., 9:669–675, 1976.

54. Panjabi, M. M., White, A. A., and Southwick, W. O.: Temporal changes in the physical properties of healing fractures in rabbits. J. Biomech., 10:689–699, 1977.

55. Paul, J. P.: Bioengineering studies of the forces transmitted by joints. In Kenedi, R. M. (ed.): Biomechanics and Related Bioengineering Topics. London, Pergamon Press, 1965.

56. Perren, S. M., Huggler, A., Russenbergon, M., et al.: Cortical bone healing. Acta Orthop. Scand. (Suppl.), 125:19–29, 1969.

57. Piekarski, K., Wiley, A. M., and Bartels, J. E.: The effect of delayed internal fixation on fracture healing. Acta Orthop. Scand., 40:543–551, 1969.

58. Plant, R. E., and Bartel, D. L.: Finite element analysis of a bone-plate-screw system. Paper presented at Annual Meeting of American Society of Engineers. New York, November, 1974.

59. Ray, D. R., Ledbetter, W. B., Bynum, D., and Boyd, C. L.: A parametric analysis of bone fixation plates on fractured equine third metacarpal. J. Biomech., 4:163–174, 1971.

60. Rybicki, E. F., and Simonen, F. A.: Mechanics of oblique fracture fixation using a finite element model. J. Biomech., 10:141–148, 1977.

61. Rybicki, E. F., Simonen, F. A., and Weiss, E. B.: On the mathematical analysis of stress in the human femur. J. Biomech., 5:203–215, 1972.

62. Rybicki, E. F., Simonen, F., Mills, E. J., et al.: Mathematical and experimental studies on the mechanics of plated transverse fractures. J. Biomech., 7:377–384, 1974.

63. Sarmiento, A.: Functional bracing of tibial fractures. Clin. Orthop. Rel. Res., 105:202–219, 1974.

64. Sarmiento, A.: Functional bracing of tibial and femoral shaft fractures. Clin. Orthop. Rel. Res., 82:2–13, 1972.

65. Sarmiento, A.: A functional below-the-knee brace for tibial fractures. A report on its use in one hundred thirty-five cases. J. Bone Joint Surg., 52A:295–311, 1970.

66. Sarmiento, A.: A functional below-the-knee cast for tibial fractures. J. Bone Joint Surg., 49A:855–875, 1967.

67. Sarmiento, A., Schaeffer, J. F., Beckerman, L., Latta, L. L., and Enis, J. E.: Fracture healing in rat femora as affected by functional weightbearing. J. Bone Joint Surg., 59A:369–375, 1977.

68. Schatzker, J., Sanderson, R., and Murnaghan, J. P.: The holding power of orthopaedic screws in vivo. Clin. Orthop. Rel. Res., 108:115–126, 1975.

69. Schatzker, J., Sumner-Smith, G., Clark, R., and McBroom, R.: Strain gage analysis of bone

69a. Schenck, T., Somerset, J. H., and Porter, R. E.: Stresses in orthopedic walking casts. J. Biomech., 2:227–239, 1969.

70. Simon, B. R., Woo, S. L.-Y., Stanley, G. M., Olmstead, S. R., McCarty, M. P., Jemmott, G. F., and Akeson, W. H.: Evaluation of one-, two-, and three-dimensional finite element and experimental models of internal fixation plates. J. Biomech., 10:79–86, 1977.

70a. Slätis, P., Karaharjn, E., Holmström, T., Ahonen, J., and Paavolainen, P.: Structural changes in intact tubular bone after application of rigid plates with and without compression. J. Bone Joint Surg., 60A:516–522, 1968.

71. Sonstegard, D. A., and Matthews, L. S.: Sonic diagnosis of bone fracture healing—A preliminary study. J. Biomech., 9:698–694, 1976.

72. Tonino, A. J., Davison, C. L., Klopper, P. J., and Lineau, L. A.: Protection from stress in bone and its effects. J. Bone Joint Surg., 58B:107–113, 1976.

73. Uhthoff, H. K., and Dubuc, F. L.: Bone structure changes in the dog under rigid internal fixation. Clin. Orthop. Rel. Res., 81:165–170, 1971.

74. White, A. A., Panjabi, M. M., and Southwick, W. O.: The four biomechanical stages of fracture repair. J. Bone Joint Surg., 59A:188–192, 1977.

75. White, A. A., Panjabi, M. M., and Southwick, W. O.: The effects of compression and cyclic loading on fracture healing—A quantitative biomechanical study. J. Biomech., 10:233–239, 1977.

76. Whiteside, L. A., Lesker, P. A., and Sweeney, R. E.: The relationship between the biochemical and mechanical characteristics of callus during radiographically determined stages of fracture healing. Transactions of the 24th Annual Orthopedic Research Society, Dallas, February 1978.

77. Wong, A. T. C., Goldsmith, W., and Sackman, J. L.: Flexural wave propagation in discontinuous model and in vitro tibiae. J. Biomech., 9:813–825, 1976.

78. Woo, S. L.-Y., Akeson, W. H., Levenetzy, B., Coutts, R. D., Matthews, J. V., and Amiel, D.: Potential application of graphite fiber and methyl methacrylate resin composites as internal fixation plates. J. Biomed. Mater. Res., 8:321–338, 1974.

79. Woo, S. L.-Y., Akeson, W. H., Coutts, R. D., Rutherford, L., Doty, D., Jemmott, G. F., and Amiel, D.: A comparison of cortical bone atrophy secondary to fixation with plates with large differences in bending stiffness. J. Bone Joint Surg., 58A:190–195, 1976.

80. Woo, S. L.-Y., Simon, B. R., Akeson, W. H., and McCarty, M. P.: An interdisciplinary approach to evaluate the effect of internal fixation plate on long bone remodeling. J. Biomech., 10:87–95, 1977.

81. Wray, J. B., and Goodman, H. O.: Postfracture vascular changes and healing process. Arch. Surg., 87:801–804, 1963.

82. Yamagiski, M., and Yoshimura, Y.: The biomechanics of fracture healing. J. Bone Joint Surg., 37A:1035–1068, 1955.

STEPHEN H. BUTLER, M.D.,
and
JOHN J. BONICA, M.D.

Regional Anesthesia for Fractures and Dislocations ———— 8

Regional anesthesia is a most useful adjunct in the treatment of fractures and dislocations. To perform these procedures one must be familiar with the techniques of nerve blockade, with anatomy, with the pharmacology of the local anesthetics and vasopressors, with the complications of the techniques, and with the treatment of these complications. Experience must be gained under the supervision of skilled teachers before regional anesthesia is attempted. The following discussion of the uses, advantages, and disadvantages of some of the block procedures includes only sparse explanations. Explicit directions for performing them can be found in standard textbooks.[1-4] The surgeon, especially the one who now or in the future may have little professional help with anesthesia, might well seek out instruction in these techniques to aid himself and his patients.

As for other such procedures, it is advisable to prepare patients for regional anesthesia with a preoperative discussion of the technique and its advantages. Preoperative sedation may be indicated as well in patients anxious about the procedure. Intravenous sedation is a useful adjunct, but must be used with care in emergency surgery on the patient with a full stomach.

ADVANTAGES OF REGIONAL ANESTHESIA

The first obvious advantage of regional anesthesia is that it may be used in a patient with a full stomach or with head or facial injuries in whom general anesthesia is prone to complications and should be postponed or avoided. Vomiting or regurgitation and aspiration in an unconscious patient under general anesthesia are potentially lethal complications to be avoided at all costs. Stomach emptying time is delayed following trauma and preoperative medication, and this problem should be considered in emergency surgery.

For limb surgery, regional anesthesia imposes none of the trespasses on the cardiovascular and respiratory systems inherent in general anesthesia. This is important in the old and debilitated and in those with chronic or acute cardiac or respiratory disease when immediate surgery is indicated. In patients with severe pain from

173

extensive injury, regional anesthesia produces a specific block of nociceptive ("pain") pathways and thus provides prompt and complete relief. Moreover, the anesthetic interrupts the efferent limb of the abnormal reflex responses to trauma that often cause vasoconstriction of the splanchnic region and consequent production of myocardial depressant factors and other toxic substances that aggravate the shock. These injured patients and others who are in shock tolerate regional anesthesia well and often improve as soon as complete pain relief is achieved with the block.

By using one of the newer long-acting agents such as bupivacaine or a continuous epidural technique for the lower extremity, the anesthesia may be tailored to outlast the duration of surgery or manipulation or both. This leaves an awake, comfortable patient without the hangover of general anesthesia, obviating the need for immediate postoperative narcotic with its depressant effects. It also makes this a method of choice for providing outpatient anesthesia for minor procedures. By providing this kind of relief, regional anesthesia decreases the incidence of respiratory complications such as atelectasis and pneumonia.

Regional anesthesia can be tailored to provide complete muscle relaxation to facilitate reduction of fractures and dislocations. A comparable degree of relaxation can otherwise be achieved only with deep general anesthesia or large doses of muscle relaxant. These produce widespread relaxation that outlasts the operation, a significant disadvantage.

When the services of an anesthesiologist or nurse anesthetist are not available, certain regional anesthetic techniques can be performed by the surgeon, given a patient with cardiorespiratory stability. The surgeon can then proceed with operations that would be impossible without anesthesia. This is especially true for outpatient or office procedures.

Regional anesthesia is not expensive. Little equipment is necessary, and that can be easily transported. Thus it is readily adaptable to various situations and can be employed without a formal operating room environment.

It deserves reemphasis that all these advantages can be gained only if the anesthesiologist or surgeon learns the procedures well. This requires, in sequence, acquiring a knowledge of the pertinent anatomy and of the pharmacology of local anesthetics, watching the procedure being done by a skillful operator, performing the block under the direct supervision of such a person, and maintaining the skill by doing the procedure frequently. Another essential requisite is full knowledge of possible complications, how they are prevented, and if they occur, how to treat them properly. *None of these procedures that require the injection of more than 50 mg of lidocaine (Xylocaine) or an equivalent amount of drug should be started without having resuscitation equipment available for immediate use.* This should include an oxygen source, an "ambu" bag and mask or alternate means to facilitate positive pressure ventilation, intravenous diazepam, and a source of suction. Patients for these blocks should have an intravenous route established prior to commencement of the block.

DISADVANTAGES OF REGIONAL ANESTHESIA

It takes time to perform blocks, and there is also a latent period before onset of analgesia and muscle relaxation. With skill, however, the time necessary to provide anesthesia can be considerably reduced.

Most regional anesthesia with the exception of intravenous blocks makes immediate postoperative evaluation of neurological function impossible. For this reason it may be contraindicated.

Many patients dislike the necessary needle punctures or being awake during surgery or both. Most, however, will accept regional anesthesia if they are assured they will experience little discomfort and will be given sedation to provide amnesia. Nevertheless, there are always patients who will refuse this form of anesthesia despite adequate explanation.

It must be recognized that regional anesthesia is an all-or-none phenomenon. Failure to produce complete anesthesia occurs even in the most skilled hands. This requires supplemental injection of the missed nerves, repetition of the entire primary block procedure, or complementation with a general anesthetic.

Patient cooperation, other than being reasonably immobile through the block procedure, is not necessary to perform regional anesthesia. Children and stuporous patients needing immediate care can be easily anesthetized with any of the procedures outlined, with certain modifications. For instance, insulated needles and a source of current enable the operator to elicit motor responses from individual nerves ("motor paresthesiae") for accurate needle placement when patient cooperation is lacking. This is just one of the modifications to allow us to use regional anesthesia in other than the calm, awake, cooperative, intelligent patient.

REGIONAL ANESTHESIA FOR THE UPPER EXTREMITY

Brachial Plexus Block

The brachial plexus is contained in an envelope or sheath of prevertebral fascia stretching from the vertebral bodies to the midpoint of the arm. Deposit of an adequate volume of local anesthetic drug into this fascial sleeve at any point will interrupt nervous impulses through the plexus. Two absolute requisites for successful blockade are sufficient knowledge of the location of this sleeve and its contents and an indication that the needle for injecting the drug is indeed within the sheath. Needle placement is guided by eliciting sensory paresthesiae, by "popping" through the fascial sleeve, by gauging proximity to arteries in or near the sheath, by laying down a wall of local anesthetic so that a good proportion will be deposited in the fascia as the needle passes through. Any or all of these techniques can be used by the practitioner.

Interscalene Approach. This is the most cephalad approach to the brachial plexus. Its advantage is that, for surgery on or manipulation of the shoulder, it invariably produces a blockade of part or all of the cervical plexus that traverses the prevertebral fascial sheath as well. Its disadvantage is that, without large volumes and high dosages of local anesthetic, the dermatome of T1 may be inadequately blocked (Fig. 8–1). For surgery involving this area, another approach to the plexus may be more

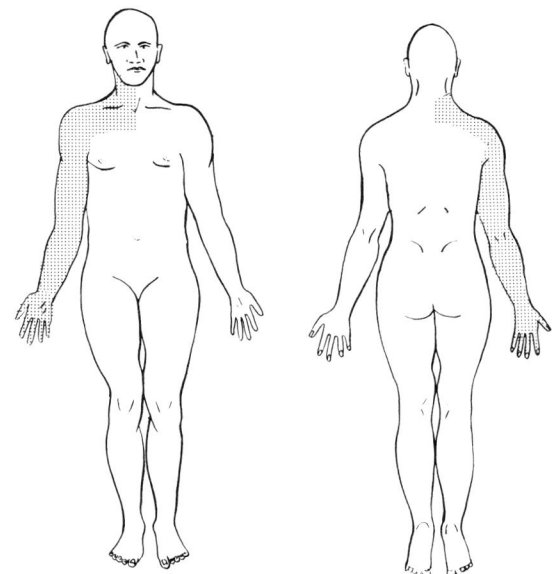

Figure 8–1 The area of anesthesia provided by an interscalene brachial plexus block.

reliable. Another disadvantage is that the ipsilateral phrenic nerve is often involved, which may have to be considered in the patient with compromised respiratory function. There is also the possibility that the needle will enter a dural sleeve and local anesthetic will be injected into the subarachnoid space, producing a widespread "spinal" block with severe cardiorespiratory complications.

To perform the block, the needle is inserted perpendicular to the trunks of the brachial plexus at the level of C6 in the groove between the anterior and the middle scalene muscles. When a paresthesia is obtained, a suitable volume of local anesthetic solution is injected in accordance with the required extent of analgesia.[5]

Supraclavicular Approach. This is the approach most commonly used for hand and arm surgery when pain, vascular compromise, neurological compromise, or a combination of them prevents arm movement prior to nerve blockade. The block provides excellent analgesia for surgery or manipulation of arm, forearm, and hand (Fig. 8–2). It can be used for shoulder work, provided that the skin over the joint is anesthetized by subcutaneous infiltration over the clavical and acromion process to block the

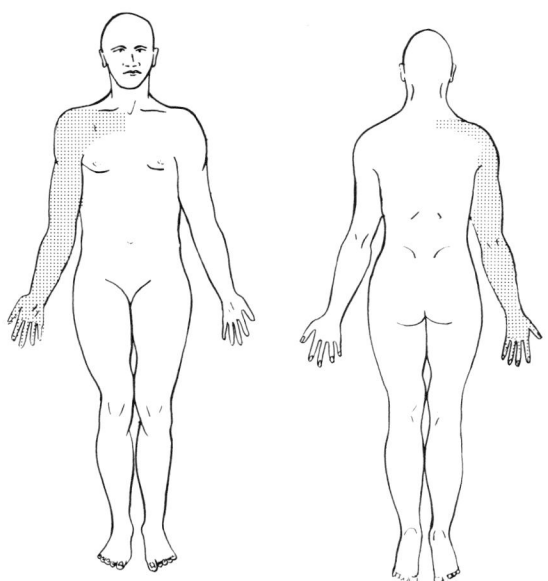

Figure 8–2 The distribution of anesthesia for a supraclavicular block.

appropriate branches of the superficial cervical plexus. There are good landmarks for the block, but in unskilled hands it is attended by a significant incidence of pleural puncture and pneumothorax.

Descriptions of the approach vary, but it involves inserting the needle just above the clavical in the groove between the anterior and medial scalene muscles just posterior to the subclavian-brachial artery. The needle is advanced caudad, mesiad, and dorsad, toward the first rib in a search for paresthesiae. When they are encountered, the local anesthetic is injected (Fig. 8–3).[3, 4]

Axillary Approach. The axillary block provides good analgesia for surgery on and manipulation of the arm, forearm, and hand. It does not provide analgesia for shoulder work (Fig. 8–4). There may be problems with blockade of the musculocutaneous nerve if the block is not done carefully, and some practitioners avoid its use for cases in which surgery or manipulation involves an area supplied by this nerve, i.e., the lateral arm and forearm. A relative disadvantage is the slightly longer period of latency between injection and onset of analgesia than with supraclavicular blockade. This block does avoid the danger of pneumothorax inherent in the supraclavicular approach

and lends itself to easy blockade of the intercostobrachial nerve, a branch of T2 supplying the inner aspect of the arm. This is questionably necessary when an arm tourniquet is used. As this technique is the simplest and safest approach to the brachial plexus, it is the technique recommended by the authors for those people who wish to begin regional anesthesia of the upper extremity.

To begin this block, the patient should be in the supine position with the arm to be blocked abducted and externally rotated. A skin wheal with local anesthetic is raised superficial to the pulse of the axillary artery at the level of insertion of the pectoralis major and latissimus dorsi muscles. Generous skin infiltration and subcutaneous infiltration in this area will provide blockade of the intercostobrachial nerve. The needle for performing plexus block is then inserted through the skin wheal toward the pulse of the artery. Some physicians rely on the "pop" of the needle through the sheath, some on the presence of one or more paresthesiae, some on the arterial pulsation transmitted to the needle for the end point before injecting a volume of local anesthetic. The most reliable test is to elicit a paresthesia (Fig. 8–5). Most commonly that will be in the distribution of the median or ulnar nerve, as these are superficial to the artery at this point.

When the paresthesia has been obtained, compression of the arm distal to the needle by using a simple tourniquet or the pressure of the hand is needed before injection of the local anesthetic to prevent it from spreading distally in the fascial sheath. At this point a volume of 30–40 ml of local anesthetic solution is injected, with care being taken not to dislodge the needle from its position adjacent to the nerves. After injection of the volume of local anesthetic and before compression distal to the injection has been released, the arm is brought back to the anatomical position. This allows spread of the local anesthetic solution past the head of the humerus to bathe the brachial plexus more proximal than the point of injection in the axilla. This insures that adequate blockade of the radial and musculocutaneous nerve distributions occurs. Some practitioners who wish to insure radial nerve blockade will advance the needle through

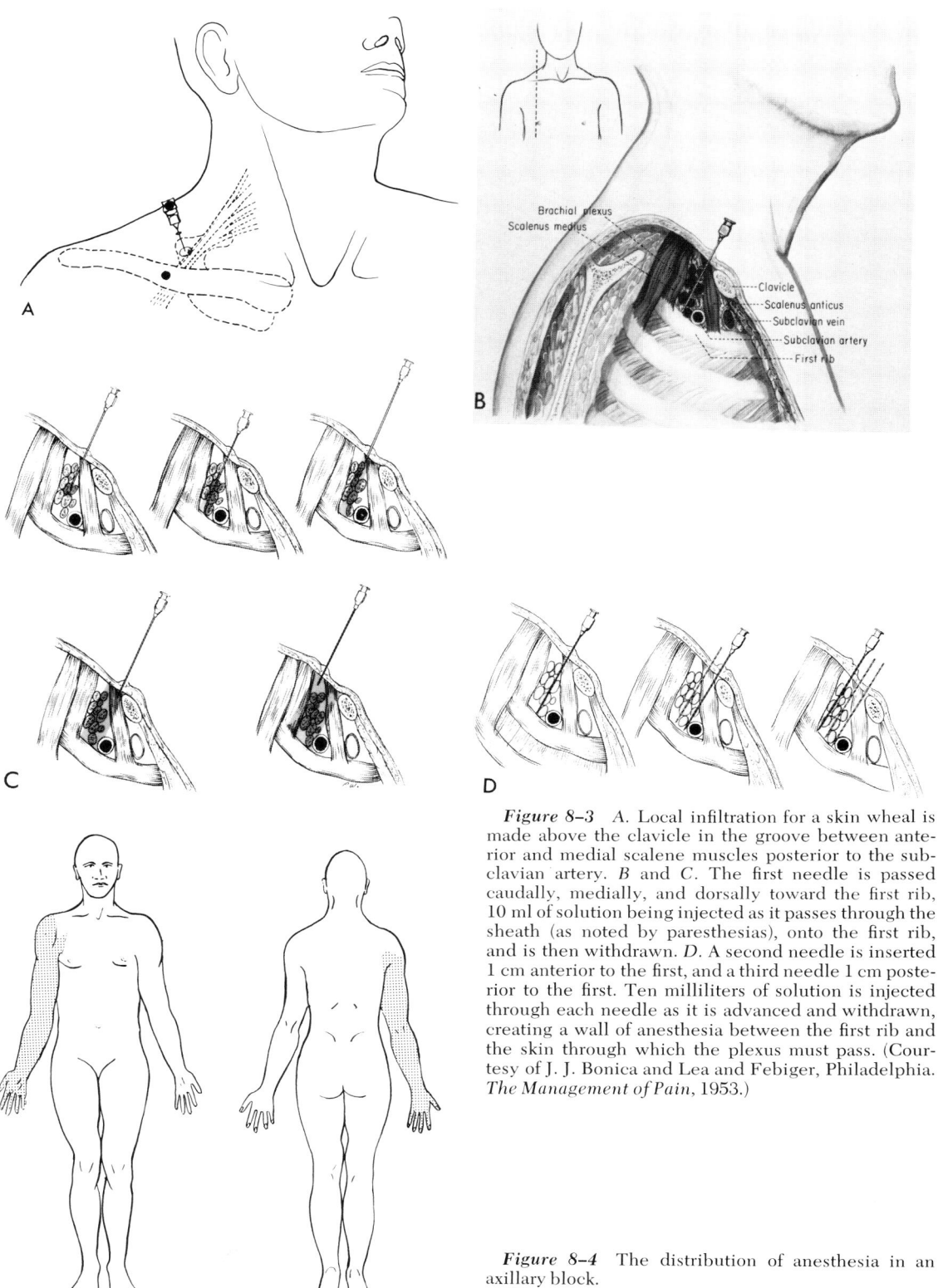

Figure 8–3 *A.* Local infiltration for a skin wheal is made above the clavicle in the groove between anterior and medial scalene muscles posterior to the subclavian artery. *B* and *C.* The first needle is passed caudally, medially, and dorsally toward the first rib, 10 ml of solution being injected as it passes through the sheath (as noted by paresthesias), onto the first rib, and is then withdrawn. *D.* A second needle is inserted 1 cm anterior to the first, and a third needle 1 cm posterior to the first. Ten milliliters of solution is injected through each needle as it is advanced and withdrawn, creating a wall of anesthesia between the first rib and the skin through which the plexus must pass. (Courtesy of J. J. Bonica and Lea and Febiger, Philadelphia. *The Management of Pain*, 1953.)

Figure 8–4 The distribution of anesthesia in an axillary block.

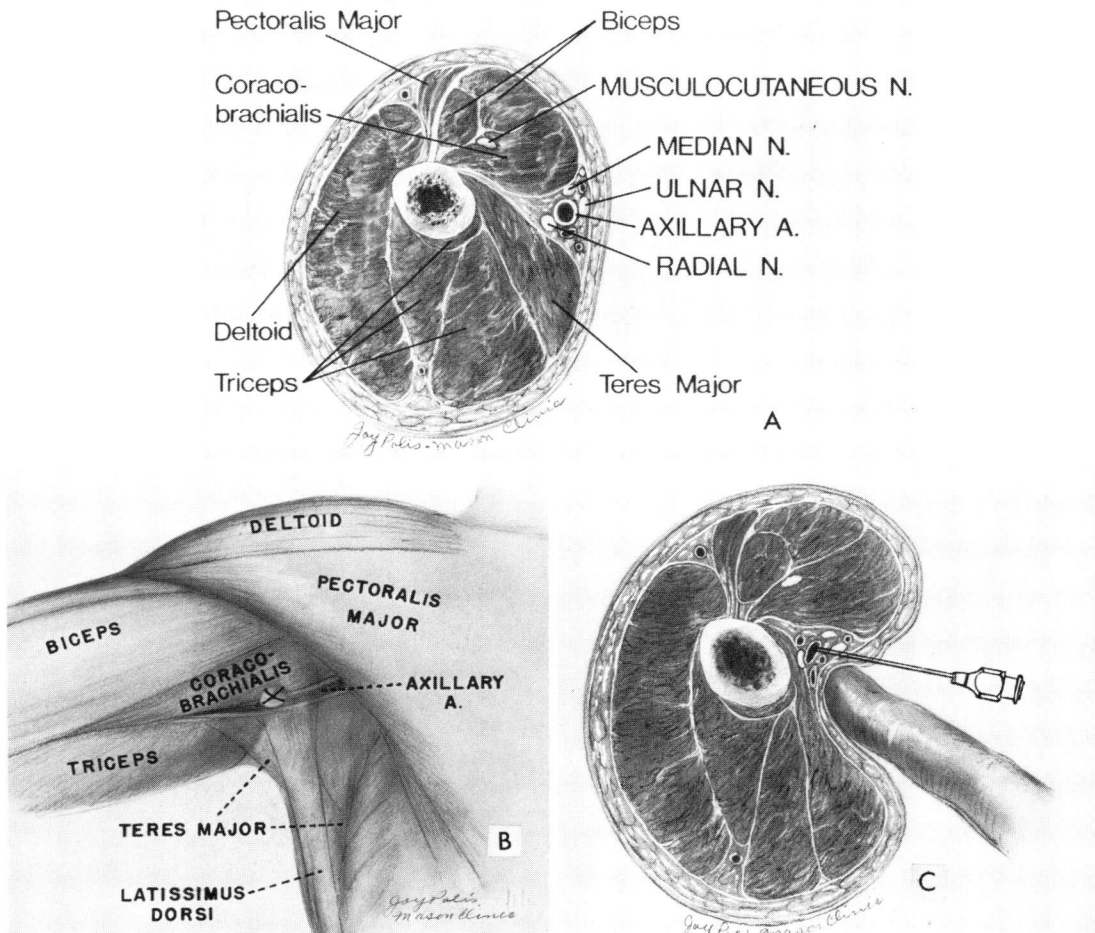

Figure 8–5   *A.* A cross section of the arm through the axilla. Note that the median, radial, and ulnar nerves are grouped around the axillary artery, but that the musculocutaneous nerve is outside the sheath between the coracobrachialis and biceps. *B.* The site of the skin wheal in the axilla over the axillary artery pulse where the latissimus dorsi meets the coracobrachialis. A generous subcutaneous infiltration at this point will block the intercostobrachial nerve to give a complete upper arm block. *C.* The palpating finger over the axillary artery compresses the neurovascular bundle against the humerus. The needle is advanced toward the artery and at this point should produce an ulnar or median nerve paresthesia. The volume of drug needed for block can then be injected, or 10 ml can be injected, with further paresthesias being sought and additional injections made. (Courtesy of D. C. Moore and Charles C Thomas, Publisher, Springfield, Illinois. *Regional Block.* 4th edition, 1969.)

the axillary artery to elicit a radial nerve paresthesia prior to injection of the local anesthetic. This will insure more rapid onset of radial nerve blockade but is not necessary.[3, 4]

Elbow Block

This is a suitable technique for surgery on or manipulation of the wrist or hand when an upper arm tourniquet will not be necessary. It avoids many of the complications of the brachial plexus block at various levels, including subarachnoid injection and pneumothorax. A smaller total dose of local anesthetic is necessary, which can be an advantage in poor-risk individuals. These nerves may also be blocked individually to supplement an incomplete brachial plexus block.

The elbow block is a three-needle technique. The ulnar nerve can be found in the groove between the medial epicondyle and the olecranon, and infiltration of 5 ml of local anesthetic with or without a paresthesia in that area will provide good ulnar nerve block. The median nerve lies just medial to the brachial artery in the antecubital fossa at the level of the elbow crease. It can be blocked by deposition of 5 ml of local anesthetic following an appropriate paresthesia or by fanwise injection of 10 ml of local anesthetic solution through this area without the elicitation of a paresthesia. The radial nerve is found in the antecubital fossa by following the elbow crease 1 cm lateral to the biceps tendon and inserting a needle at this point. After a paresthesia has been elicited, 5–10 ml of local anesthetic will adequately block the radial nerve at this point (Fig. 8–6).[1, 3, 4]

Wrist Block

This is useful for minor procedures on the hand and fingers in which an arm or forearm tourniquet is not needed. It avoids the complications of brachial plexus block and leaves the patient in full control of the limb postoperatively.

The ulnar nerve can be found just lateral to the tendon of the flexor carpi ulnaris muscle. Insertion of the needle at this point and infiltration of 3–5 ml of local anesthetic following an appropriate paresthesia will adequately block the nerve. The median nerve is found between the tendons of palmaris longus and flexor carpi radialis. Insertion of the needle through a skin wheal at this point and deposition of 5–10 ml of local anesthetic following elicitation of an appropriate paresthesia will block this nerve. The terminal fibers of the radial nerve here can be blocked adequately by a subcutaneous wheal of local anesthetic solution from dorsal to volar surface over the lateral border of the wrist (Fig. 8–7).[1, 3, 4]

Intravenous Block

This is technically the easiest form of regional anesthesia and is more suited to the arm than the leg, as in the leg fairly substantial volumes of local anesthetic are needed to perform the block adequately. The requisite skills are ability to put on a tourniquet and to start an intravenous line. A suitable vein is found as close to the operative site or fracture as possible, and a needle (preferably a small-bore plastic cannula) is fixed in the vein at that site. A double cuffed pneumatic tourniquet is applied to the upper arm following this. The arm is then exsanguinated by compression with an Esmarch bandage or a pneumatic splint, and while pressure is applied in this way the proximal of the two cuffs is inflated above arterial pressure. With removal of the compression, 25–30 ml of a dilute solution of local anesthetic (i.e., 0.75 per cent lidocaine) is administered through the intravenous cannula to fill the venous compartment of the arm. Within 10 minutes adequate anesthesia for surgery or fracture reduction will be obtained. At this time the intravenous cannula is withdrawn, the distal arm cuff is inflated to above arterial pressure, and the proximal arm cuff is deflated. This switch in tourniquets transfers the pressure of the tourniquet to an anesthetic area and thus will be well tolerated by an awake patient. This technique gives adequate anesthesia for surgery of the elbow and more distal structures. There is some argument against its use for fractures and dislocations, as exsanguination of the arm is necessary before inflating the tourniquet and injecting the volume of local anesthetic. This maneuver is usually done with the aid of an Esmarch bandage. In the case of fractures and dislocations, a pneumatic splint can be substituted for this purpose so the procedure is painless and there is less risk of damaging vessels and nerves.

As stated, anesthesia begins within 10 minutes of injection of the local anesthetic solution. It covers structures distal to the cuff and lasts up to two hours with the agents commonly used, but is gone within 10 minutes of cuff deflation, allowing evaluation of the limb's neurological status soon after surgery is completed.[3, 4]

REGIONAL ANESTHESIA FOR THE LOWER EXTREMITY

Regional anesthesia is well suited to providing excellent analgesia and muscle

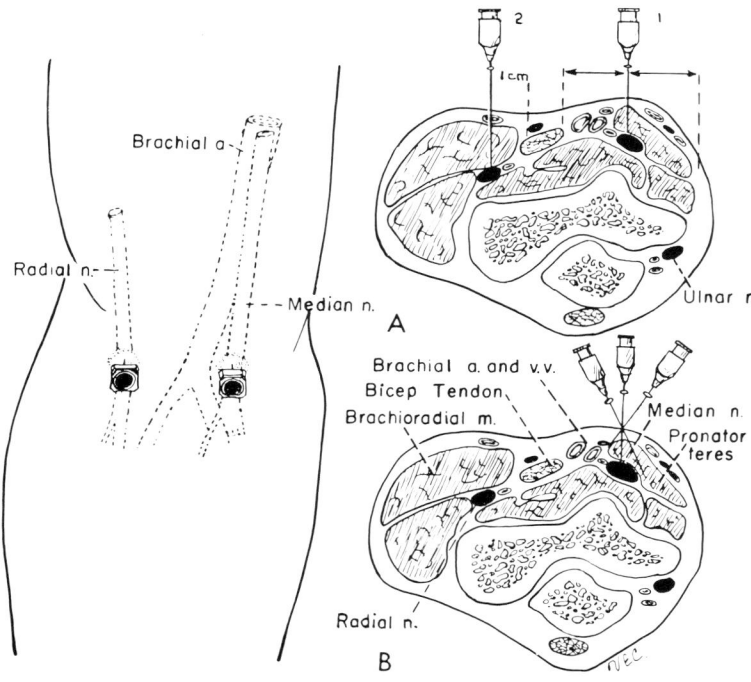

Figure 8–6 Techniques for blocking the median, radial, and ulnar nerves at the elbow. *A.* A single injection technique for blockade of the radial (2) and median (1) nerves when paresthesias are elicited. Note that the needle for radial nerve block is 1 cm lateral to the biceps tendon and the needle for the median nerve block is midway between the medial epicondyle and the biceps tendon. The ulnar nerve is easily blocked as it passes superficially behind the medial epicondyle. *B.* Fanwise injections are used when no paresthesia is elicited. This technique can be done for the median nerve as is shown here, and also for the radial nerve. (Courtesy of J. J. Bonica and Lea and Febiger, Philadelphia. *The Management of Pain,* 1953.)

Figure 8–7 *A.* Sites of injection for ulnar and median nerves and the subcutaneous bracelet on the volar aspect of the wrist to anesthetize the cutaneous nerves. *B.* A cross section of the wrist to show sites of injection for the median and ulnar nerves. Note that the needle for the median nerve is between the palmaris longus tendon and the flexor carpi radialis tendon. That for the ulnar nerve is just lateral to the flexor carpi ulnaris tendon. *C.* The bracelet injection for subcutaneous block of cutaneous nerves on the dorsal aspect of the wrist plus the sites for metacarpal block of the third finger. (Courtesy of J. J. Bonica and *Postgraduate Medicine.* Regional anesthesia for surgery of the extremities. Postgrad. Med., 28:324–332, 1960.)

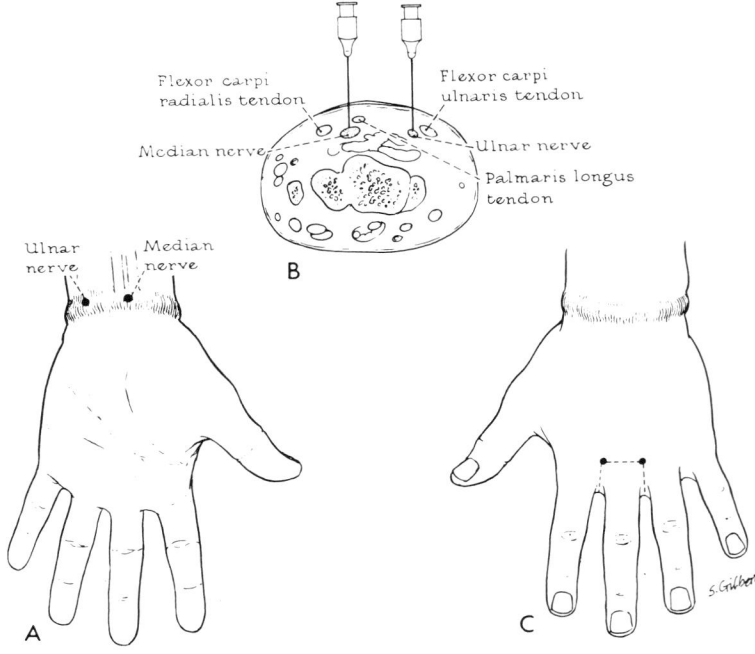

relaxation for surgery or manipulation of fractures and dislocations of the hip joint and parts of the body distal to this. Blocks in this area are not completely analogous to those for the upper extremity, however. The differences are that the lumbosacral plexus is not blessed with the same envelope of prevertebral fascia as the brachial plexus, which is a disadvantage, and that the lumbosacral plexus is situated at the termination of the cord so that blockade of the nerve fibers within the vertebral column does not have the same hazards as this procedure at a higher level, an advantage.

Subarachnoid Block

This is an excellent block, as it provides profound analgesia and muscle relaxation. It is reliable for all ages. It is technically quite straightforward, requiring the skills of lumbar puncture, which most physicians have practiced at one point in their training (Figs. 8–8 and 8–9). Block duration can be guaranteed for 30 minutes to two hours, depending on the agents used, so this technique as it is usually practiced is not suitable for prolonged surgery. The blockade itself leads to some cardiovascular instability, which makes its use more hazardous in poor-risk patients and in less experienced hands. The well publicized problem of postspinal headache is rare at present, with the use of small-gauge needles for dural puncture.

For those wanting more information on this technique, the paramedian and midline approach to the subarachnoid space, drugs used and their dosages, complications and treatment are all well explained in reference texts.[3, 4]

Epidural Block

Like the subarachnoid or "spinal" block just listed, this form of blockade is close to

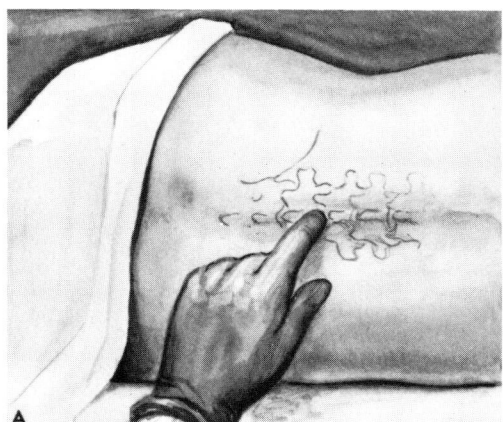
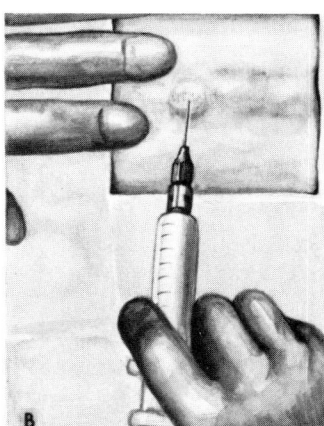
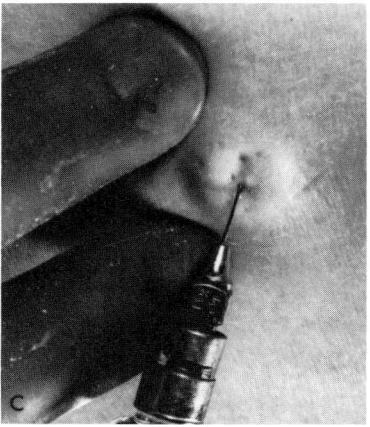

Figure 8–8 The technique for midline lumbar puncture. A. Palpation of the tips of the lumbar spines. Note that an imaginary line connecting the two iliac crests passes over the spinous process of the fourth lumbar vertebra. B and C. The formation of an intracutaneous wheal to anesthetize the skin. In C note that the second and third fingers straddle the midline to immobilize the skin. (Courtesy of J. J. Bonica and F. A. Davis, Philadelphia. *Principles and Practice of Obstetric Analgesia and Anesthesia*, 1957.)

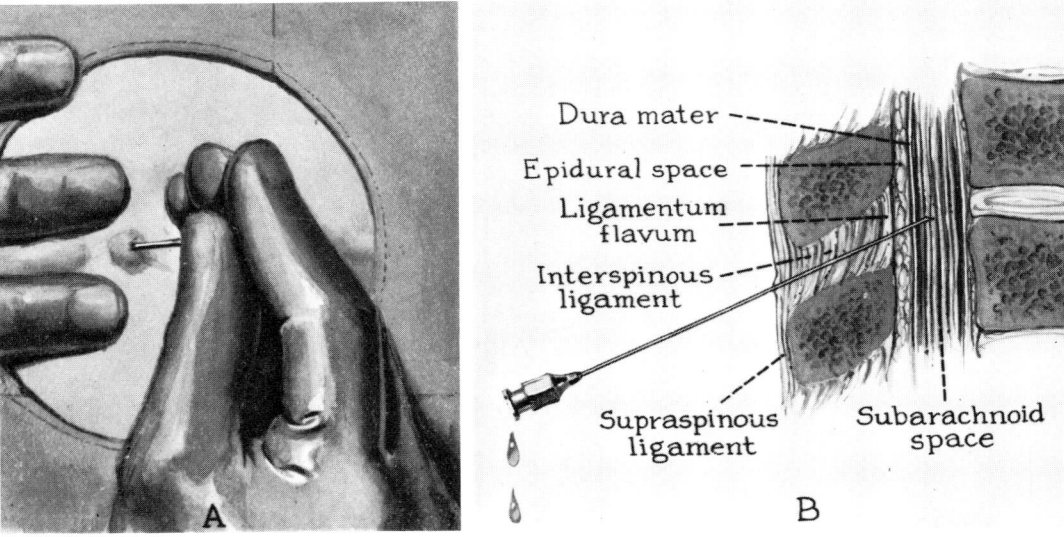

Figure 8–9.   A. The spinal needle is held like a dart in the right hand with the index finger over the top of the stylet to prevent displacement. The patient's skin is held taut as in Figure 8–8C to prevent movement of the dermal layers. The needle is then introduced through the same wound that was made for the skin wheal. The bevel of the subarachnoid needle should be positioned parallel to the longitudinal fibers of the dura so that as it pierces the dura it spreads the fibers like a wedge rather than cutting them. After piercing the skin, the needle is advanced perpendicular to the skin in a side-to-side plane at an angle of about 100 degrees to the skin cephalad to it and 80 degrees to the skin caudad to it. As soon as the needle has entered the interspinous ligament the position should be checked. If it is not correct, it should be changed before much of the needle is fixed in the firm ligament. Absolute resistance to advance indicates contact with bone and requires readjustment of the needle, best done by withdrawal to the subcutaneous tissues. When the point of the needle passes through the ligamentum flavum, marked resistance is often experienced, but when it enters the narrow peridural space, a sudden lack of resistance is felt. The needle is then advanced about 5 mm to the position shown in *B* and the stylet is removed to allow free flow of cerebrospinal fluid. Information on drugs, dosages, the alternate paramedian approach, and complications of this technique are given in standard textbooks. (Courtesy of J. J. Bonica and F. A. Davis, Philadelphia. *Principles and Practice of Obstetrical Analgesia and Anesthesia,* 1957.)

the neuraxis. It provides less profound but usually adequate analgesia with good muscle relaxation for orthopedic procedures involving the hip and lower limb. It is more difficult to perform and less reliable in older individuals. Technically more complicated than subarachnoid block, it requires careful placement of the needle tip in the potential space between the dura and the inner boundary of the neural arch. At this point, local anesthetic drug or a fine catheter or both are placed in the epidural space. With the use of an epidural catheter, a continuous blockade is possible for long orthopedic procedures and postoperative analgesia, this usually being limited to a 48 hour period.

For hip and pelvis, the catheter is usually placed in the lumbar region. For operative and manipulative procedures of the knee, lower leg, and foot, this approach may be used, or the catheter may be placed in the sacral epidural space via the sacral hiatus.

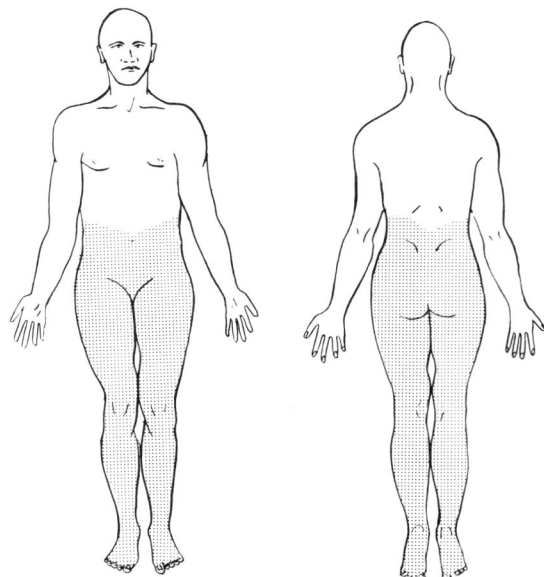

Figure 8–10.   The area of block produced by lumbar epidural blockade adequate for lower limb surgery.

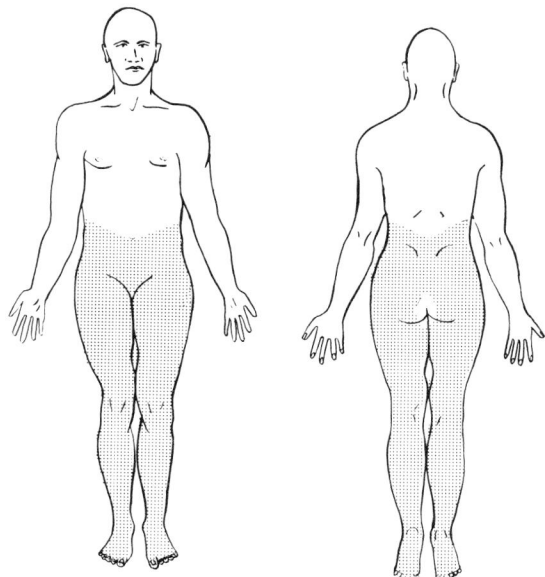

Figure 8–11. The area of block produced by caudal epidural blockade adequate for lower limb surgery.

This technique is often referred to as "caudal" anesthesia (Figs. 8–10 and 8–11).

Epidural anesthesia is fraught with the same problems of cardiovascular instability as spinal anesthesia. It is technically more difficult, and more experience is necessary for its successful mastery than for subarachnoid anesthesia. Referenced texts explain the different techniques, the complications and their treatment, and the drugs and dosages.[2, 3, 4] This skill, however, is best learned from an experienced practitioner and mastered by supervised practice, not undertaken on one's own.

Sciatic-Femoral Block

Blockade of these two nerves gives good analgesia and muscle relaxation for surgery or manipulation of the lower leg and foot when a thigh tourniquet is not needed. The addition of obturator and lateral femoral cutaneous nerve blocks allows the knee to be included in the surgical field and also allows a thigh tourniquet to be used.

A combination of these blocks that will allow the needed surgery or manipulation to take place is technically more difficult to perform than, say, spinal (subarachnoid) block, but it has advantages. It avoids much of the cardiovascular trespass involved in subarachnoid or epidural blockade but still obviates the need for central sedation. It leaves the patient with control of the hip and opposite leg so that postoperative supervision is less critical while the block is still in effect. Winnie is a proponent of the so-called "3-in-1" block, blocking the femoral, lateral femoral cutaneous, and obturator nerves with a single-needle lumbar plexus block.[6] This saves anesthesia time and is less unpleasant for the patient. It is also more frequently successful in blocking the obturator nerve than the standard approach.

Sciatic Nerve Block. The sciatic nerve may be blocked as it appears in the sciatic notch by a posterior approach with the patient in a prone position or a lateral position with the leg flexed. With the patient supine, the nerve may also be blocked from an anterior approach as it passes medial to the femur in traversing from posterior to the neck to posterior to the shaft (Fig. 8–12).

The classic approach to the sciatic nerve is the posterior one with the patient prone. With a skin marker a line is drawn between the posterior superior iliac spine and the superior border of the greater trochanter. A perpendicular is dropped from the midpoint 5 cm. The end of this perpendicular should overlie the sciatic notch. After local anesthetic is used to raise a skin wheal, a 3 to 4 inch needle is advanced perpendicular to the skin to elicit a sciatic paresthesia. Once this has been found, the deposition of 15 ml of local anesthetic solution will produce blockade of the sciatic nerve and numbness in its distribution.

Femoral Nerve Block. A very easy block to perform, this involves simply bathing the nerve with local anesthetic in the femoral triangle just below the inguinal ligament. The nerve is found approximately 1 cm lateral to the arterial pulse. Paresthesiae may be somewhat difficult to elicit. The deposition of 15 ml of local anesthetic solution about 1 cm below the skin in this area will provide anesthesia in the distribution of the femoral nerve. The Winnie modification of this procedure is very easy to perform and will produce obturator and

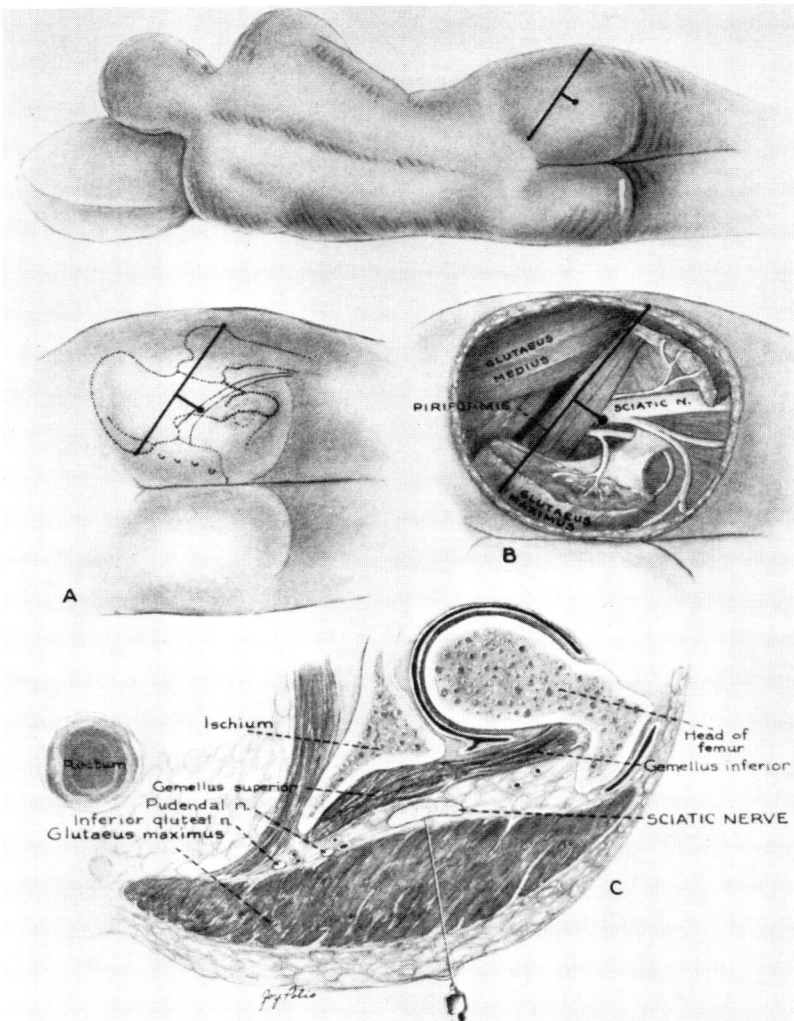

Figure 8-12   The technique of blocking the sciatic nerve with the patient in the lateral position. (This block may also be performed in the prone or supine positions.) *A* and *B.* A line is drawn from the middle of the greater trochanter to the posterior superior iliac spine and a perpendicular is dropped. A skin wheal is raised 3.5 to 5.0 cm along this line and a needle inserted perpendicular to the skin to contact the nerve as it passes through the greater sciatic notch and crosses posterior to the spine of the ischium. A paresthesia should be elicited before injection of solution. *C.* A cross section at the level of the block. (Courtesy of J. J. Bonica, and Lea and Febiger, Philadelphia. *The Management of Pain*, 1953.)

lateral femoral cutaneous nerve block along with femoral nerve block with one injection. To do this the needle should be advanced cephalad at a 45 degree angle beneath the inguinal ligament 1 cm lateral to the femoral pulse. A paresthesia should be elicited to verify correct needle placement. At this time, compression across the femoral triangle is produced distal to the needle, and 25 to 30 ml of local anesthetic solution is injected through the needle.

This will track back along the femoral nerve to the nerve roots to produce a lumbar plexus block (Fig. 8–13).

Obturator and Lateral Femoral Cutaneous Nerve Blocks.   Classically these nerves are blocked separately. The obturator nerve is blocked in its foramen as it passes through the pelvis. This is done through the perineum and is not an easy block to do nor is its success rate high except in very experienced hands. The lateral femoral

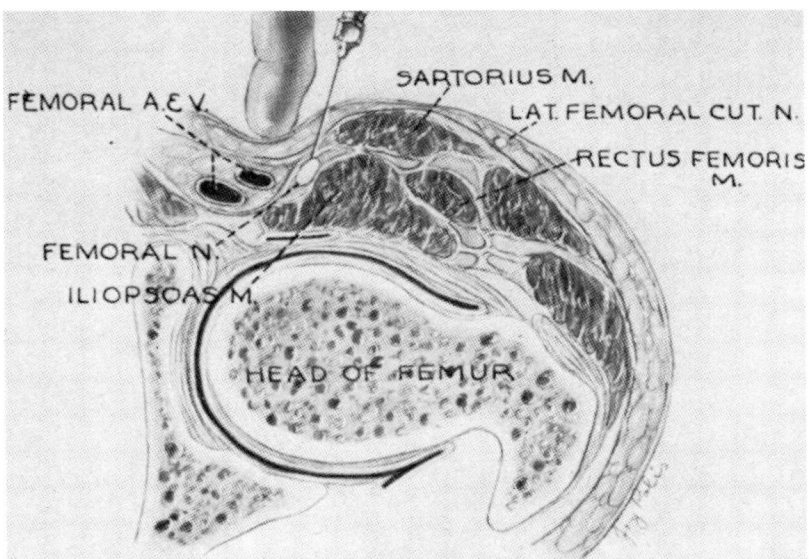

Figure 8–13 A cross section of the thigh just below the inguinal ligament. The needle for blockade of the femoral nerve is introduced 1 cm lateral to the femoral artery and perpendicular to the skin at the level of the top of the symphysis pubis. If a paresthesia is elicited, the solution is injected. If no paresthesias are elicited, injection while advancing the needle in a fanwise manner in a plane at right angles to the axis of the nerve will produce good blockade. (Courtesy of J. J. Bonica and Lea and Febiger, Philadelphia. *The Management of Pain*, 1953.)

cutaneous nerve of the thigh is blocked very simply by infiltrating the abdominal wall at a point 2 cm medial and 2 cm inferior to the anterior superior iliac spine. This produces a variable patch of numbness over the lateral border of the thigh. Both of these blocks are used with sciatic and femoral nerve blocks to supply anesthesia so that a thigh tourniquet may be used or to allow surgery to be performed in the region of the knee.

Again we urge use of the references for more explanation of these blocks and an awareness of the specific techniques and their complications. They may be found in references 3, 4, and 6.

Ankle Block

This is suitable for surgery on the forefoot when no tourniquet on the leg or lower leg is needed. It may be done easily as an outpatient procedure, as a long recovery period is not necessary. It involves superficial injection to block the tibial nerve, sural nerve, superficial and deep peroneal nerves, and saphenous nerve (Fig. 8–14).[1, 3, 4] The tibial nerve is blocked just posterior to the medial malleolus. It is located adjacent to the posterior tibial artery, and a blocking needle advanced just lateral to the posterior tibial artery will usually elicit a paresthesia and 5 ml of local anesthetic solution will effectively block this nerve. The sural nerve is found on the posterior aspect of the ankle as well, as it passes subcutaneously between the lateral malleolus and the Achilles tendon. Raising a wheal of local anesthetic subcutaneously between these two structures will effectively block impulses traveling with this nerve. The superficial peroneal nerve is also a subcutaneous structure and may be blocked by a subcutaneous wheal of local anesthetic extending from the anterior border of the tibia to the lateral malleolus. The deep peroneal nerve at the ankle is found between the anterior tibial muscle and tendon and extensor hallucis longus muscle and tendon. Inserting a needle between these structures and infiltrating while advancing and withdrawing will effectively block this nerve.

These procedures are relatively simple to do and suitable for outpatient surgery on the toes or forefoot.

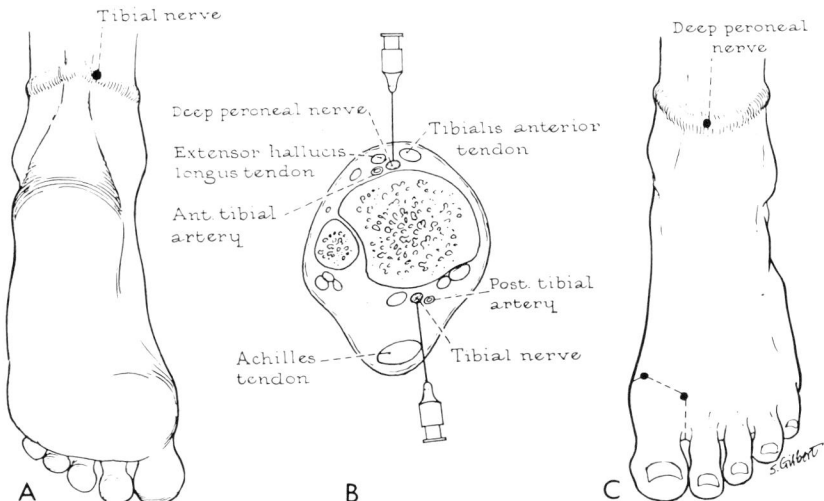

Figure 8–14 The technique of ankle and toe blocks. A. The site of injection for the tibial nerve and the posterior subcutaneous anklet for anesthetizing the cutaneous nerves. B. Note the needle for blocking the tibial nerve is inserted between the Achilles tendon and the posterior tibial artery, the needle for blocking the deep peroneal nerve is inserted between the extensor hallucis longus tendon and the tibialis anterior tendon. C. The sites of injection of the deep peroneal nerve and the anterior portion of the subcutaneous anklet and also those for anesthetizing the great toe. (Courtesy of J. J. Bonica and *Postgraduate medicine*. Regional anesthesia for surgery of the extremities, 28:324–332, 1960.)

Intravenous Block

The technique is the same as used to block the upper extremity. It may be used for surgery or manipulation of the ankle and foot with the tourniquet positioned around the calf. It may also be used for operative work on the knee in which a thigh tourniquet is used. One disadvantage of this second application is that because of the large volume of drug necessary for blockade of the complete leg, side effects from tourniquet failure or release of the tourniquet following a short operative procedure are more severe than with the arm block. Because of its technical simplicity, however, it is a very useful block for the surgeon without good anesthetic back-up.

REGIONAL ANESTHESIA FOR THE SPINE

Regional anesthesia is possible for use with operative intervention on spinal fractures but is seldom used. In some areas of North America, spinal or subarachnoid block was the preferred anesthetic for back surgery some years ago. The techniques of epidural or subdural block are not to be recommended, however, because of difficulties in positioning these patients for blockade and possible mechanical problems leading to inadequate or inappropriate spread of the anesthetic agents. Blocks in the cervical or thoracic region can lead to respiratory and cardiovascular problems difficult to manage with the patient in a prone position for spinal surgery.

REGIONAL ANESTHESIA FOR THE THORAX

Fractures of the bony thorax other than the vertebrae are likely to be ignored except in those patients with advanced acute or chronic pulmonary disease. This is because they tend to heal and stabilize fairly rapidly. Fractures of ribs especially are extremely uncomfortable, however, and an intercostal block with long-acting agents is easy to perform despite the ever-present danger of pneumothorax (Fig. 8–15).

The upper ribs are difficult to block in the standard way but are rarely fractured and, if they are, are not painful because there is little movement of the upper thorax with normal breathing and coughing. Ribs from the fifth on down are more easily blocked, and this is the area where discomfort is

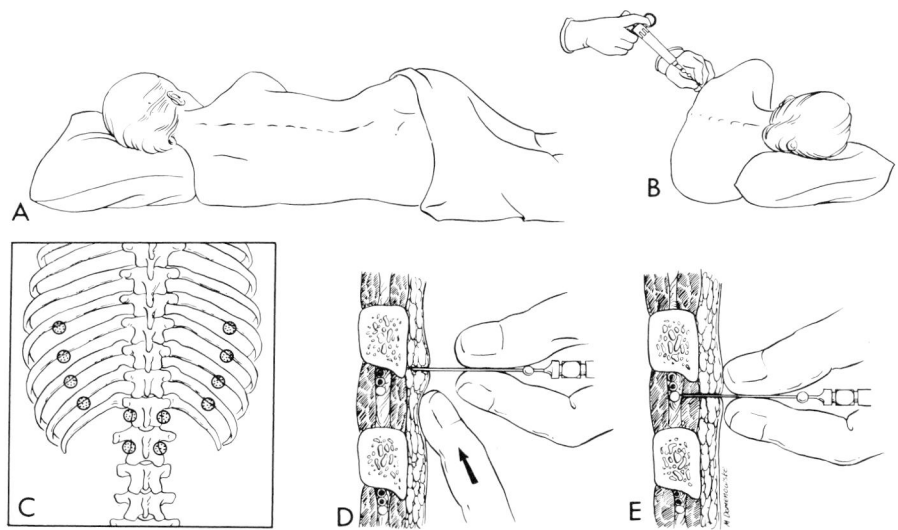

Figure 8–15 *A* and *B*. In this intercostal block, the patient is positioned at an angle of 45 degrees with the horizontal plane to make it possible to block both sides of the thorax without moving her. A true lateral position and a sitting position with the arms folded across a support in the lap are also used. *C*. Sites of injection for easily reached lower ribs. The intercostal block is carried out at the angle that is the most prominent point of the posterior part of each rib and can be easily palpated. *D* and *E*. Details of the block. Notice that the index finger of one hand pushes the skin cephalad and comes to overlie the intercostal space so that it can palpate the lower edge of the rib above and at the same time immobilize the skin over the rib. This finger also protects the interspace and thus decreases the risk of passing the needle too far and into the lung. As soon as the needle contacts the rib, the skin is moved caudad so that the needle just slips over the lower border of the rib and is then advanced 5 mm. With a long needle, this distance is measured by grasping the shaft between the thumb and index finger of the left hand about 5 mm from the skin so that it will not be advanced too deeply. (Courtesy of J. J. Bonica and F. A. Davis, Philadelphia. *Principles and Practice of Obstetric Analgesia and Anesthesia,* 1957.)

worse. The angle of the rib is its most prominent and accessible part. When this is palpated, a fine-gauge needle is passed through the skin to impinge upon the rib. The needle is then grasped between the thumb and index finger about .5 cm from the skin, and then moved over the lower edge of the rib and advanced until the fingers are flush with the skin. This prevents the needle from being advanced too deep and producing a pneumothorax. At this point 3 to 5 cc of local anesthetic solution is injected to block the intercostal nerve in that segment. Two or three sessions of blockade in a 24 hour period can keep most patients comfortable and very grateful, and can simplify their course for all involved.

SYMPATHETIC DYSTROPHY

Finally, we would like to provide information about a fairly frequent painful sequel to injury, accidental or surgical. The cycle of pain-immobility-vasospasm-pain is often ignored after accident or after surgery. This painful condition classically is associated with a cool sweaty extremity, smooth shiny skin, edema, hair loss, hyperesthesia, and dysesthesia. The cycle can be and often is broken with a course of physical therapy and analgesics (Fig. 8–16). Sympathetic blockade of the limb at frequent intervals such as every two days for two weeks will, however, accelerate recovery when used in conjunction with physical therapy. The blockade is best done prior to physical therapy, as it usually abolishes the pain and enables the patient to perform more effectively during the therapy session.

For the arm and shoulder, sympathetic blockade is usually accomplished by stellate ganglion block, but axillary block or paravertebral block can also temporarily abolish sympathetic hypertonus as well. For the leg and hip, lumbar sympathetic block with single- or multiple-needle technique paravertebrally is commonly used, but epi-

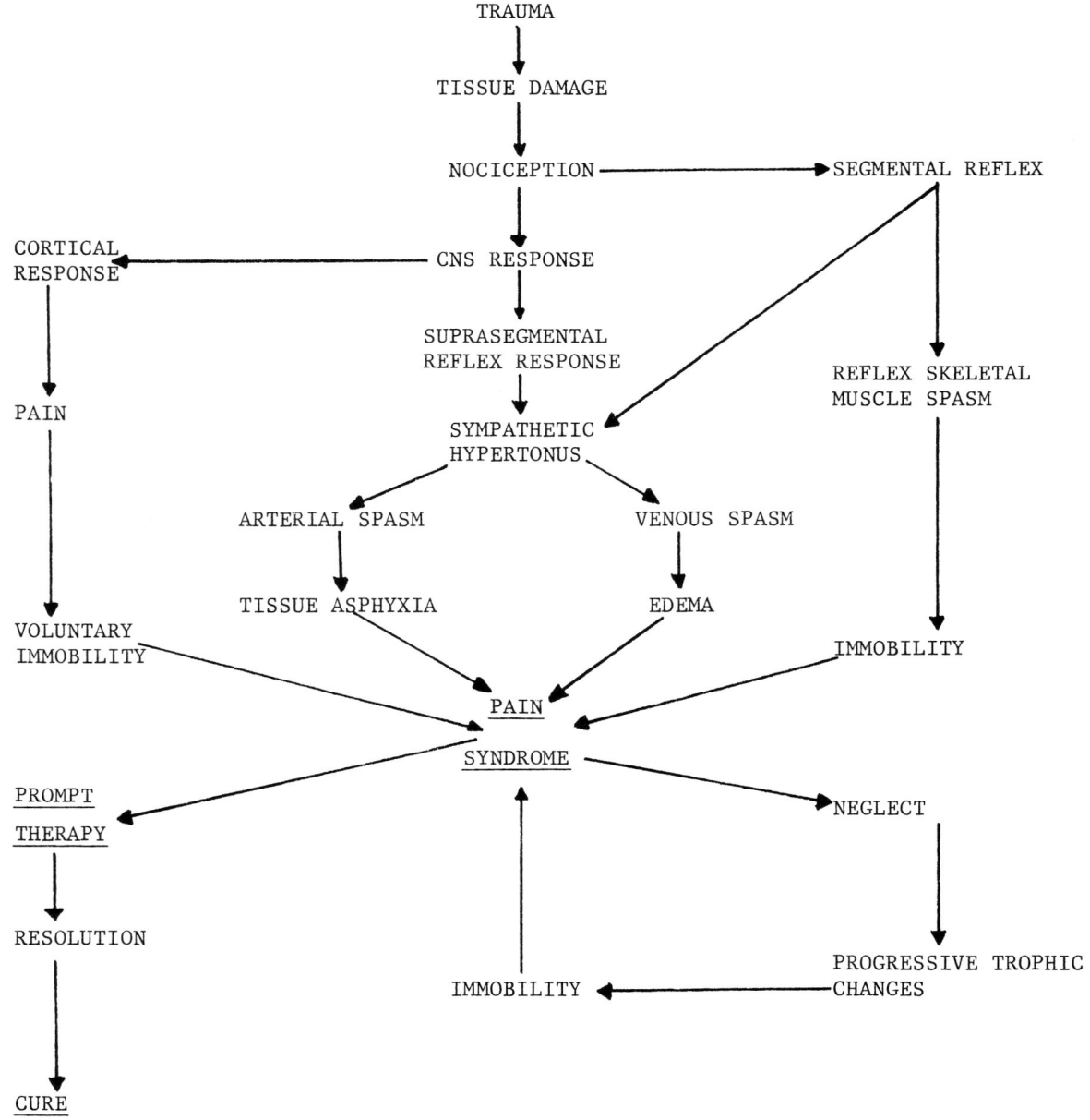

Figure 8–16   Mechanisms of Sympathetic Dystrophy.

dural or subarachnoid block may also be used effectively.[1, 3, 4]

This problem should always be kept in mind when painful immobility continues longer than should be expected after injury or surgery.

REFERENCES

1. Bonica, J. J.: Clinical Application of Diagnostic and Therapeutic Nerve Blocks. Springfield, Ill., Charles C Thomas, 1959.

2. Bonica, J. J.: Principles and Practice of Obstetric Analgesia and Anesthesia. Philadelphia, F. A. Davis, 1967.

3. Eriksson, E. (ed.): Illustrated Handbook of Local Anesthesia. Copenhagen, Munksgaard, 1969.

4. Moore, D. C.: Regional Block. 4th Ed. Springfield, Ill., Charles C Thomas, 1969.

5. Winnie, A. P.: Interscalene brachial plexus, Anesth. Analg. (Cleve.), 49:455–466, 1970.

6. Winnie, A. P., Ramamurthy, S., and Burrani, Z.: The inguinal paravascular technique of lumbar plexus anesthesia: The "3-in-1 block." Anesth. Analg. (Cleve.), 52:989–996, 1973.

ROBERT B. SALTER, M.D.

Birth and Pediatric Fractures[*]

9

Before considering specific injuries in children, it would be wise to consider some of the *special features* of fractures and dislocations in the growing years. Just as in all other clinical fields of medicine and surgery, so also in the field of fractures, children cannot be considered simply as "little adults." Fractures in children and the reaction of children's tissues to these fractures differ greatly from those in adults. Blount deserves special credit for emphasizing the fact that *fractures in children are different.*

SPECIAL FEATURES OF FRACTURES AND DISLOCATIONS IN CHILDREN

The special features of fractures and dislocations are first listed and then discussed individually. These differences are most striking in the infant and young child and become progressively less striking as the child approaches adulthood. Comparative terms, such as "more" and "less," refer to a comparison between fractures and dislocations in children and those in adults.
1. Fractures more common.

2. Stronger and more active periosteum.
3. More rapid fracture healing.
4. Special problems of diagnosis.
5. Spontaneous correction of certain residual deformities.
6. Differences in complications.
7. Different emphasis on methods of treatment.
8. Torn ligaments and dislocations less common.
9. Less tolerance of major blood loss.

Fractures More Common

The higher incidence of fractures in children is explained by the combination of their relatively slender bones and their carefree capers. Some of these injuries, such as crack or hairline fractures, buckle fractures, and greenstick fractures, are not serious, whereas others, such as intraarticular fractures and epiphyseal plate fractures, are very serious indeed.

Stronger and More Active Periosteum

The stronger periosteum in children is less readily torn across at the time of fracture, and consequently there is more often an intact periosteal hinge that can be utilized during closed reduction of the fracture. Furthermore, the periosteum is much more osteogenic in children than it is in adults (Fig. 9–1).

*Courtesy of the Williams & Wilkins Co., Baltimore, Md. *From:* Salter, R. B.: Textbook of Disorders and Injuries of the Musculoskeletal System, 1970.

189

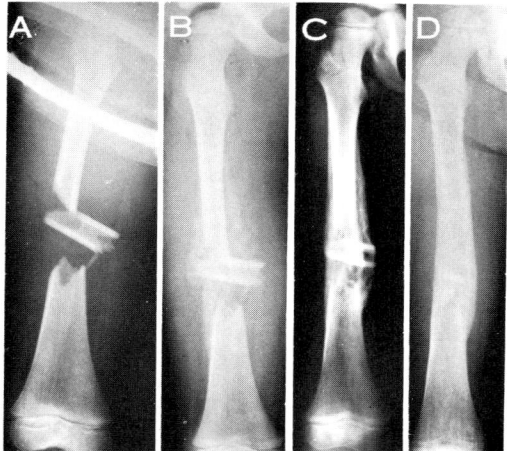

Figure 9–1 The importance of the strong and actively osteogenic periosteum in the healing process of children's fractures is demonstrated in this series of radiographs of a fractured femoral shaft in a 4-year-old child. *A.* The day of injury; a double fracture with the middle segment lying almost transversely. The strong periosteal sleeve, however, would not be completely torn across. Note the metal ring of the Thomas splint. *B.* Three weeks after injury abundant callus is forming from the actively osteogenic periosteum; at this stage traction was replaced by a hip spica cast. *C.* Ten weeks after injury the middle segment is well incorporated in the callus and is being resorbed; the fracture was clinically united at this stage and the child was allowed to walk. *D.* Six months after injury the contour of the femur is returning to normal through the process of remodeling.

More Rapid Fracture Healing

Age is a much more important factor in the rate of healing in bone than in any other tissue in the body, particularly during childhood. This is closely related to the osteogenic activity of the periosteum and endosteum, a process that is remarkably active at birth, becomes progessively less active with each year of childhood, and remains relatively constant from early adult life to old age.

Fractures of the shaft of the femur serve as an example of this phenomenon. A femoral shaft fracture occurring at birth will be united in 3 weeks; a comparable fracture at the age of 8 years will be united in 8 weeks; at the age of 12 years it will be united at 12 weeks; and from the age of 20 years to old age it will be united in approximately 20 weeks.

Nonunion of children's fractures is rare, unless an unnecessary open operation has damaged the blood supply to the fracture fragments or has introduced the complication of infection.

Special Problems of Diagnosis

The varying radiographic appearance of a given epiphysis, both before and after the development of a secondary center of ossification, can be quite confusing; although the various secondary centers of ossification appear at relatively constant ages, these are not easy to remember. Likewise, the radiographic appearance of the various epiphyseal plates may be puzzling to the inexperienced and may be mistaken for fracture lines. These radiographic problems of diagnosis, however, can be readily overcome in limb injuries. Just as an injured limb should be compared with its normal uninjured mate during the clinical examination, so too should they be compared during the radiographic examination (Fig. 9–2).

Spontaneous Correction of Certain Residual Deformities

In adults the deformity of a malunited fracture is permanent. In children, however, certain residual deformities tend to correct spontaneously, either by extensive remodeling or by epiphyseal plate growth,

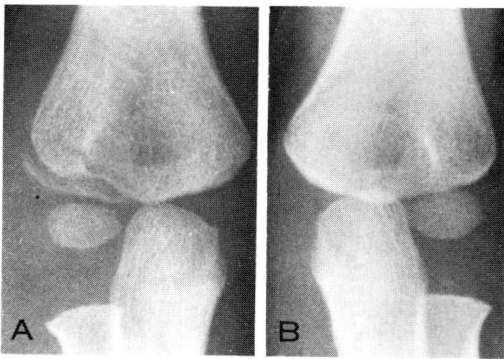

Figure 9–2 The value of a comparable radiographic examination of the opposite uninjured limb. *A.* Does the radiolucent line just proximal to the capitellum of this child's right humerus represent a fracture or just part of the epiphyseal plate? *B.* Comparison with the radiograph of the opposite elbow clarifies the situation; the child has a relatively undisplaced fracture of the lateral condyle of the right humerus, a potentially serious fracture.

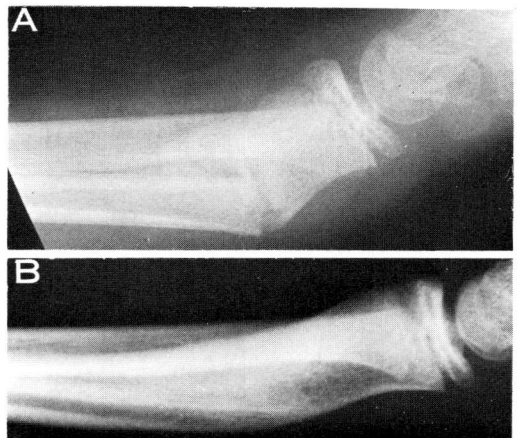

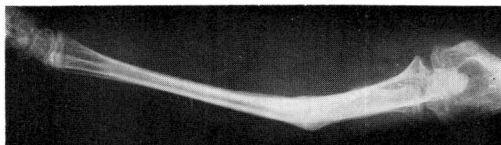

Figure 9–5 Failure of spontaneous correction of a residual fracture deformity. The fractures of the middle third of the radius and ulna of an eight-year-old girl had been allowed to unite in the unsatisfactory position of 35° of posterior angulation one year previously. This deformity of malunion is permanent.

Figure 9–3 Spontaneous improvement in a residual fracture deformity with subsequent growth. A. Lateral projection of the distal end of the radius of a 10-year-old boy six weeks after injury. Unfortunately the metaphyseal fracture had been allowed to unite with 35° of anterior angulation. B. Six months later there is only 15° of anterior angulation and the corners of the angulation deformity have remodeled. Note that the epiphysis has grown away from the fracture site during these six months.

or sometimes by a combination of both. Just how much spontaneous correction of the healed fracture deformity can be anticipated depends upon the age of the child (and the number of years of skeletal growth remaining) and the type of deformity (angulation, incomplete apposition, shortening, rotation). This phenomenon is therefore best considered in relation to specific deformities.

Angulation. Residual angulation near an epiphyseal plate will tend to correct spontaneously with subsequent growth *provided* that the plane of the deformity is the same as the plane of motion in the nearest joint. For example, residual anterior angulation at the site of a healed fracture in the distal end of the radius is in the same plane as the flexion and extension motion in the wrist joint; thus, in a young child it can be expected to correct to a large extent (Fig. 9–3). By contrast, residual angulation at right angles to the plane of motion of the nearest joint (for example, a lateral angulation or varus deformity in the supracondylar region of the humerus, which is at right angles to the flexion and extension motion of the elbow) cannot be expected to correct (Fig. 9–4). Furthermore, angulation in the middle third of a long bone, being well away from an epiphyseal plate, cannot be expected to correct spontaneously (Fig. 9–5).

Incomplete Apposition. With incomplete apposition of the fracture fragments or even side-to-side (bayonet) apposition in children, the contour of the healed fracture improves greatly through the active process of remodeling—an example of Wolff's law (Fig. 9–6).

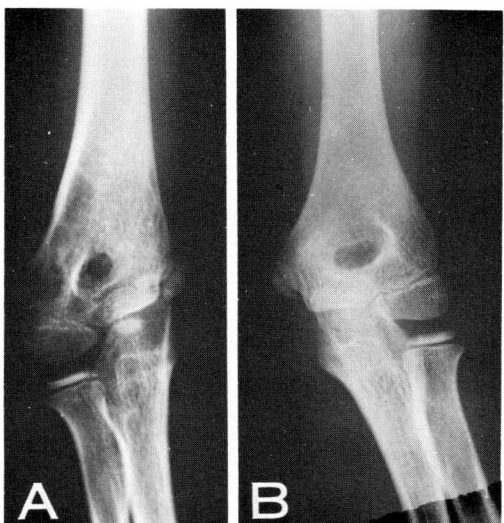

Figure 9–4 Failure of spontaneous correction of a residual fracture deformity. A. A supracondylar fracture of the humerus in a nine-year-old girl had been allowed to unite with 20° of lateral angulation two years previously. B. The opposite elbow has a normal carrying angle of 15°. Thus, on the injured side the normal carrying angle has not only been lost but also reversed so that there is 5° of varus deformity, which is permanent.

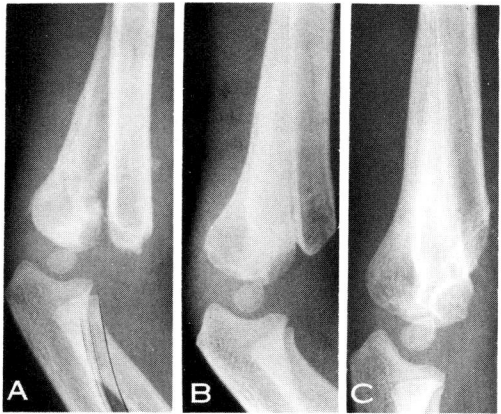
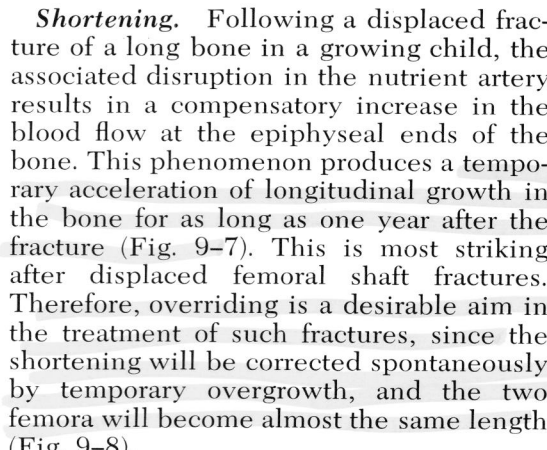

Figure 9-6 Spontaneous correction of incomplete apposition through remodeling. *A.* An unreduced supracondylar fracture of the humerus in a four-year-old child three weeks after injury; note the new bone formation in the periosteal tube through which the proximal fragment is protruding. *B.* Five months after injury the periosteal tube has formed a new shaft and the original shaft is becoming resorbed. *C.* One year after injury the contour of the fracture site has been markedly improved by the process of remodeling. Note that the epiphysis has grown away from the fracture site.

Shortening. Following a displaced fracture of a long bone in a growing child, the associated disruption in the nutrient artery results in a compensatory increase in the blood flow at the epiphyseal ends of the bone. This phenomenon produces a temporary acceleration of longitudinal growth in the bone for as long as one year after the fracture (Fig. 9–7). This is most striking after displaced femoral shaft fractures. Therefore, overriding is a desirable aim in the treatment of such fractures, since the shortening will be corrected spontaneously by temporary overgrowth, and the two femora will become almost the same length (Fig. 9–8).

Rotation. Residual rotational deformity at the site of a healed fracture in a long bone does not correct spontaneously regardless of the child's age or the site of the deformity.

Differences in Complications

Growth disturbances after epiphyseal plate injuries occur of course only in chil-

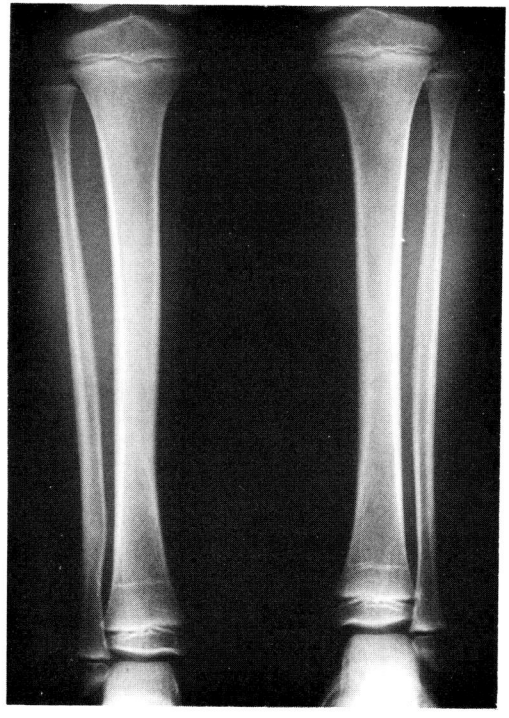

Figure 9-7 Overgrowth of a long bone after a displaced fracture. One year previously the right tibia of this eight-year-old boy had been fractured and during the ensuing year it had overgrown 1 cm. The transverse radiopaque lines in the distal tibial metaphyses represent the site of the epiphyseal plate at the time of injury; note that there has been more growth from the epiphyseal plate of the right tibia than from that of the left. The resultant leg length discrepancy will be permanent.

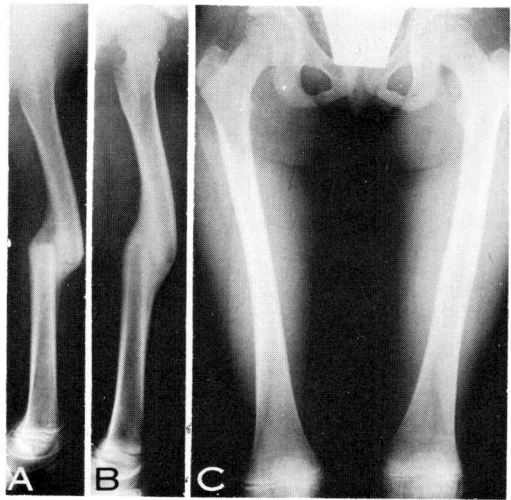

Figure 9–8 Overgrowth of the left femur after a displaced fracture of the shaft in a nine-year-old girl. *A.* Lateral projection eight weeks after injury; the fracture had been allowed to unite with 1 cm. of overriding intentionally. *B.* Six months after injury the united fracture is becoming remodeled. *C.* Eighteen months after injury the femora are virtually equal in length as a result of overgrowth of the left femur. If the fracture had been allowed to unite end-to-end, the femur would have been 1 cm. too long 18 months later and the leg length discrepancy would have been permanent.

dren. Osteomyelitis secondary to either an open fracture or an open reduction of a closed fracture tends to be more extensive in a child, and the infection may even destroy an epiphyseal plate, with resultant growth disturbance. Volkmann's ischemia of nerves and muscles is much more common in children as are posttraumatic myositis ossificans and refracture.

By contrast, persistent joint stiffness after fracture is relatively uncommon in children unless the fracture has involved the joint surface; consequently, physiotherapy and occupational therapy are seldom required in the aftercare of children with fractures. Likewise, fat embolism, pulmonary embolism, and accident neurosis are rare in childhood.

Different Emphasis on Methods of Treatment

Although the *principles* of fracture treatment are equally applicable to children and adults, there is a different emphasis on the *methods* of treatment in the two age groups. Virtually *all* fractures of the long bones in children can and indeed should be treated by means of closed reduction, either manipulation or continuous traction. Of course, the emotional exuberance and physical vigor of children recovering from fractures demand that their plaster of Paris casts be particularly strong.

Certain fractures in children do, however, necessitate open reduction and internal skeletal fixation; for example, displaced intraarticular fractures, femoral neck fractures, and certain types of epiphyseal plate injuries, which are described in a subsequent section. There is no indication for excision of a fracture fragment and replacement by a prosthesis in children.

Torn Ligaments and Dislocations Less Common

Children's ligaments are strong and resilient. Since they are stronger than the associated epiphyseal plates, sudden extension on a ligament at the time of injury results in a separation of the epiphyseal plate rather than a tear in the ligament (Fig. 9–9). This is also true to a lesser extent of fibrous joint capsules. For example, the type of injury that would produce a traumatic dislocation of the shoulder in an adult will produce a fracture–separation of the proximal humeral epiphysis in a child.

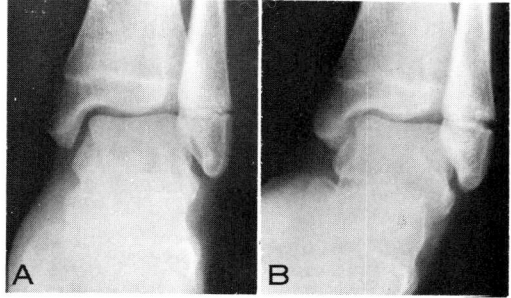

Figure 9–9 Traumatic separation of the distal fibular epiphysis in a 14-year-old boy. *A.* This radiograph appears normal because after the injury the fibular epiphysis had returned to its normal position. *B.* In this stress radiograph (taken while a varus stress is being applied to the ankle joint with the child under anesthetic) there is a tilt of the talus and the separation of the fibular epiphysis is apparent.

Less Tolerance of Major Blood Loss

The total blood volume is proportionately smaller in a child than in an adult. A formula for estimating the average blood volume in a child is 75 ml per kg of body weight. Thus, the average blood volume of a child who weighs 20 kilos (44 lb) is 1500 ml. Consequently, external hemorrhage of 500 ml in such a child represents 33 per cent of the total blood volume, whereas a similar hemorrhage in an average adult would represent only 10 per cent of the total blood volume of 5000 ml.

SPECIAL TYPES OF FRACTURES IN CHILDREN

In addition to *stress fractures* and *pathological fractures*, which occur in both children and adults, there are two special types of fractures that are limited to childhood, namely, *fractures that involve the epiphyseal plate and birth fractures.*

FRACTURES OF THE EPIPHYSEAL PLATE

Epiphyseal plate fractures present special problems in both diagnosis and treatment. Furthermore, they carry the risk of becoming complicated by a serious disturbance of local growth and the consequent development of progressive bony deformity during the remaining years of skeletal growth.

Anatomy, Histology, and Physiology

The types of epiphyses are shown in Figure 9–10. The weakest area of the epiphyseal plate is the zone of calcifying cartilage; when the epiphysis is separated by injury, the line of separation is through this zone (Fig. 9–11). Thus, the epiphyseal plate, which is radiolucent and therefore not radiographically visible, always remains attached to the epiphysis.

The blood supply of the epiphyseal plate enters from its epiphyseal surface. If the epiphysis loses its blood supply and becomes necrotic, the plate likewise becomes

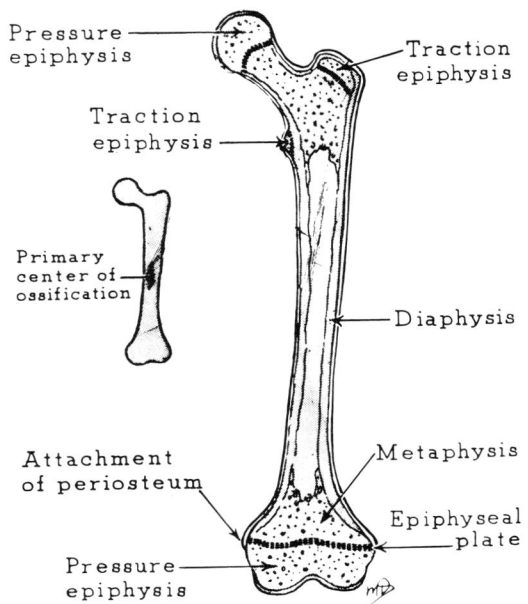

Figure 9–10 Types of epiphyses (secondary centers of ossification) in the femur. Note the attachment of the periosteum to the epiphysis.

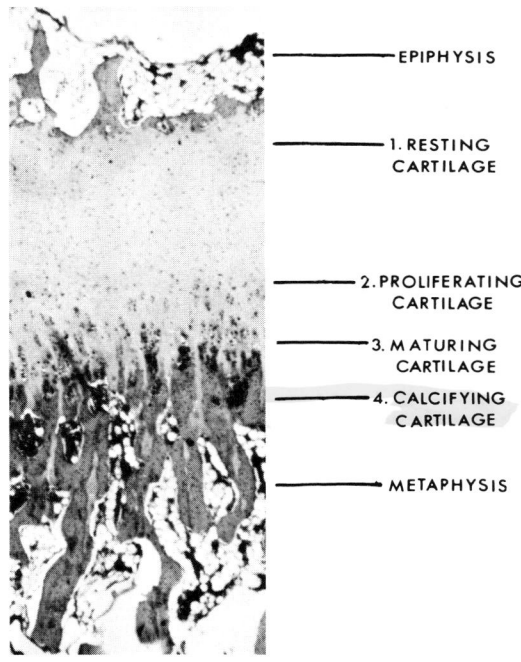

Figure 9–11 Low-power photomicrograph of an epiphyseal plate from the proximal end of the tibia of a child.

necrotic and growth ceases. In most sites the blood supply to the epiphysis is not damaged at the time of injury, but in the proximal femoral epiphysis and the proximal radial epiphysis the blood vessels course along the neck of the bone and cross the epiphyseal plate peripherally. Consequently, in these sites epiphyseal separation frequently damages the blood supply and leads to avascular necrosis of the epiphysis as well as of the epiphyseal plate.

The cartilaginous epiphyseal plate is weaker than bone, and yet epiphyseal injuries account for only 15 per cent of all fractures in childhood. The explanation for this apparent paradox is that the epiphysis is firmly attached to its metaphysis peripherally by the union of perichondrium and periosteum (Fig. 9–10). Nevertheless, as mentioned previously, epiphyseal plates are weaker than their associated ligaments and joint capsule. For this reason injuries that would result in a torn ligament or a dislocation in an adult usually produce a traumatic separation of the epiphysis in a child (Fig. 9–9).

In the lower limb more longitudinal growth takes place at the epiphyseal plates in the region of the knee than in the region of the hip or ankle. By contrast, in the upper limb more growth takes place in the region of the shoulder and wrist than in the region of the elbow.

Diagnosis of Epiphyseal Plate Injuries

An epiphyseal plate fracture should be suspected in any injured child who exhibits signs suggestive of a fracture near the end of a long bone, a dislocation, or a ligamentous injury (including a sprain). Precise diagnosis, however, depends upon radiographic examination; at least two projections at right angles to each other are essential and comparable projections of the same region of the opposite uninjured limb should also be obtained (Fig. 9–2).

Classification of Epiphyseal Plate Injuries

The following classification is based on the mechanism of injury as well as on the

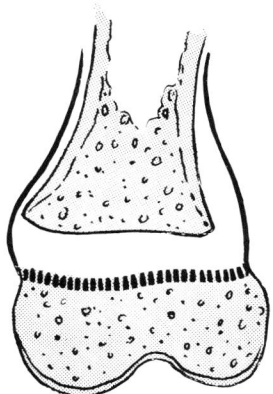

Figure 9–12   Type 1 epiphyseal plate injury. Separation of epiphysis.

relationship of the fracture line to the growing cells of the epiphyseal plate. It is also correlated with the method of treatment and the prognosis of the injury concerning growth disturbance.

Type 1 (Fig. 9–12). There is complete separation of the epiphysis without any fracture through bone; the growing cells of the epiphyseal plate remain with the epiphysis. This type of injury, the result of a shearing force, is more common in newborns (from birth injury) and in young children in whom the epiphyseal plate is relatively thick.

Closed reduction is not difficult because the periosteal attachment is intact around most of its circumference. The prognosis for future growth is excellent, provided the blood supply to the epiphysis is intact, which it usually is in sites other than the proximal femoral epiphysis and the proximal radial epiphysis.

Type 2 (Fig. 9–13). In this, the commonest type, the line of fracture–separation extends along the epiphyseal plate to a variable distance and then out through a portion of the metaphysis, producing a triangular-shaped metaphyseal fragment. The growing cells of the plate remain with the epiphysis. This type of injury, the result of shearing and bending forces, usually occurs in the older child in whom the epiphyseal plate is relatively thin. The periosteum is torn on the convex side of the angulation but is intact on the concave side. Thus, the intact periosteal hinge is always on the side of the metaphyseal fragment.

Closed reduction is relatively easy to

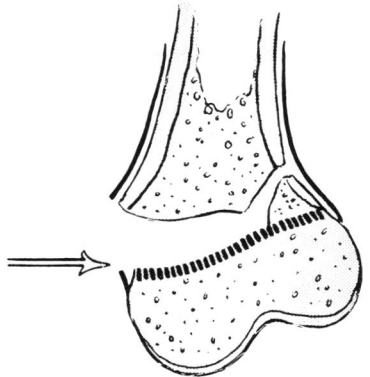

Figure 9–13 Type 2 epiphyseal plate injury. Fracture-separation of epiphysis.

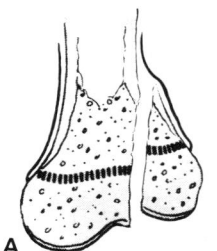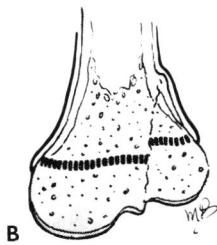

Figure 9–15 Type 4 epiphyseal plate injury. *A.* Fracture of epiphysis and epiphyseal plate. *B.* Bony union will cause premature closure of the plate.

obtain as well as to maintain; the intact periosteal hinge and the metaphyseal fragment both prevent overreduction. The prognosis for growth is excellent provided the blood supply to the epiphysis is intact, which it nearly always is at sites of type 2 injuries.

Type 3 (Fig. 9–14). The fracture is intraarticular and extends from the joint surface to the deep zone of the epiphyseal plate and then along the plate to its periphery. This uncommon type of injury is caused by an intraarticular shearing force and is usually limited to the distal tibial epiphysis.

Open reduction is usually necessary to restore a perfectly normal joint surface. The prognosis for growth is good provided the blood supply to the separated portion of the epiphysis has not been disrupted.

Type 4 (Fig. 9–15). The fracture, which is intraarticular, extends from the joint surface through the epiphysis, across the entire thickness of the epiphyseal plate, and through a portion of the metaphysis. The commonest example of a type 4 injury is the fracture of the lateral condyle of the humerus.

Open reduction and internal skeletal fixation are necessary not only to restore a normal joint surface but also to obtain perfect apposition of the epiphyseal plate. Indeed, unless the fractured surfaces of the epiphyseal plate are kept perfectly reduced, fracture healing occurs across the plate and renders further longitudinal growth impossible. Thus the prognosis for growth after a type 4 injury is bad unless perfect reduction is achieved and maintained.

Type 5 (Fig. 9–16). This relative uncommon injury results from a severe crushing force applied through the epiphysis to one area of the epiphyseal plate. It is most

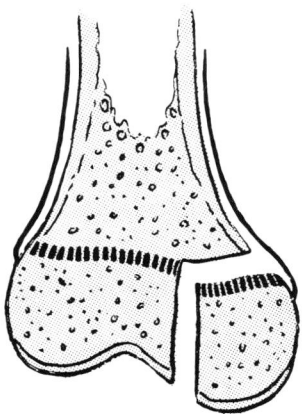

Figure 9–14 Type 3 epiphyseal plate injury. Fracture of part of epiphysis.

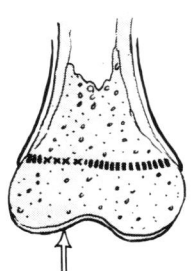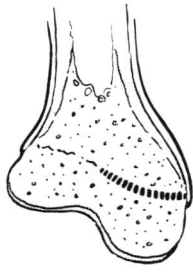

Figure 9–16 Type 5 epiphyseal plate injury. *(left)* Crushing of epiphyseal plate. *(right)* Premature closure of the plate on one side with a resultant angulatory deformity.

likely to occur in the region of the knee and ankle.

Because the epiphysis is not usually displaced, the diagnosis of a type 5 injury is difficult. Weight bearing must be avoided for at least three weeks in the hope of preventing further compression of the epiphyseal plate. The prognosis of type 5 injuries is decidedly poor since premature cessation of growth is almost inevitable.

Healing of Epiphyseal Plate Injuries

After reduction of a separated epiphysis, of type 1, 2, or 3, endochondral ossification on the metaphyseal side of the epiphyseal plate is only temporarily disturbed. Thus, within two or three weeks of replacement of the epiphysis, endochondral ossification has resumed and has united the epiphyseal plate to the metaphysis. This special type of fracture healing accounts for the clinical observation that these three types of epiphyseal separations heal in only half the time required for union of a fracture through the metaphysis of the same bone in a child of the same age. Type 4 and type 5 injuries, by contrast, must heal through cancellous bone, in the same manner as any other fracture.

Prognosis Concerning Growth Disturbance

The following factors will help in estimating the prognosis of a given epiphyseal plate injury in a child.

Type of Injury. The prognosis for each of the five classified types of epiphyseal plate injury has been discussed earlier.

Age of the Child. This is really an indication of the amount of growth normally expected in the particular epiphyseal plate; obviously, the younger the child at the time of injury, the more serious any growth disturbance will be.

Blood Supply to the Epiphysis. Disruption of the blood supply to the epiphysis is associated with a poor prognosis for reasons already discussed.

Method of Reduction. Unduly forceful manipulation of a displaced epiphysis may crush the epiphyseal plate and increase the likelihood of growth disturbance.

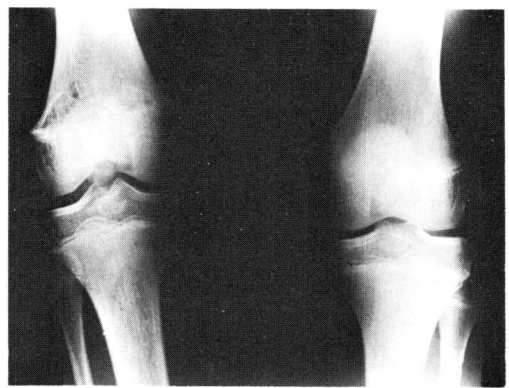

Figure 9–17 Progressive leg length discrepancy secondary to premature cessation of growth in the entire distal femoral epiphyseal plate. A type 4 epiphyseal plate injury had occurred two years previously in this 11-year-old boy; the discrepancy will continue to increase during the remaining years of growth.

Open or Closed Injury. Open injuries of the epiphyseal plate carry the risk of infection, which in turn is likely to destroy the plate and result in premature cessation of growth.

Possible Effects of Growth Disturbance

Fortunately, 85 per cent of epiphyseal plate injuries are uncomplicated by growth disturbance. In the remaining 15 per cent, however, the clinical problem associated with the dread complication of premature cessation of growth depends on several factors including the bone involved, the extent of the disturbance in the epiphyseal plate, and the amount of growth normally expected from that particular epiphyseal plate.

If the entire epiphyseal plate ceases to grow in a single bone, the result is a progressive limb length discrepancy (Fig. 9–17). If, however, the involved bone is one of a parallel pair (such as tibia and fibula, or radius and ulna), progressive length discrepancy between the two bones will produce a progressive angulatory deformity in the neighboring joint (Fig. 9–18). If growth ceases in only one part of the plate (for example, on the medial side) but continues in other parts, the result will be a progressive angulatory deformity (Fig. 9–19).

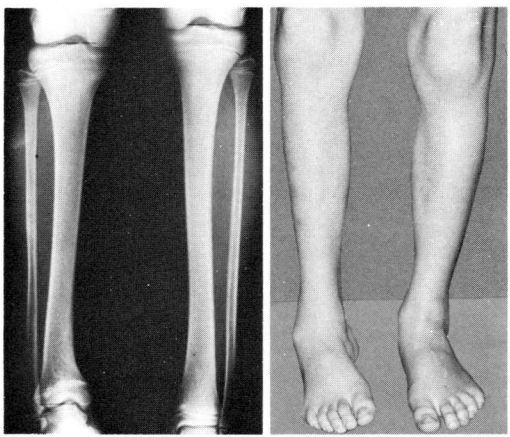

Figure 9–18 Progressive leg length discrepancy and progressive angulatory deformity in a nine-year-old girl 18 months after a type 4 epiphyseal plate injury of the right medial malleolus. Growth has ceased in the medial part of the tibial epiphyseal plate and has continued in the lateral part, as well as in the epiphyseal plate of the fibula. The result is a varus deformity of the ankle. Note also that the right tibia is shorter than the left.

Premature cessation of growth does not necessarily occur immediately after an injury to the epiphyseal plate; indeed, growth may be only retarded for a period of six

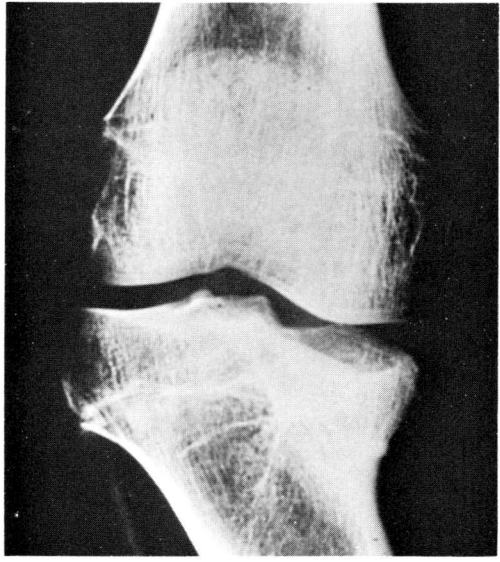

Figure 9–19 Progressive angulatory deformity of the knee in a 15-year-old boy three years after a type 5 injury involving the medial part of the upper tibial epiphyseal plate. Growth has ceased on the medial side but has continued on the lateral side with a resultant progressive varus deformity of the knee.

months or even longer before it ceases completely.

Special Considerations in the Treatment of Epiphyseal Plate Injuries

Injuries involving the epiphyseal plate must be treated gently and as soon after injury as possible. Type 1 and 2 injuries can nearly always be treated by closed reduction. Type 3 injuries frequently require open reduction, and type 4 injuries always require open reduction and internal fixation. The period of immobilization required for types 1, 2, and 3 injuries is only half that required for a metaphyseal fracture of the same bone in a child of the same age.

It is advisable to give the parents of a child who has sustained an epiphyseal plate injury some indication of the prognosis concerning future growth without causing them undue anxiety. The child should be carefully examined both clinically and radiographically at regular intervals for at least one year and often longer to detect any growth disturbance.

Specific epiphyseal plate injuries are discussed on a regional basis along with specific fractures and dislocations in a subsequent section of this chapter.

Avulsion of Traction Epiphyses

A sudden traction force applied through either a ligament or a tendon to a traction epiphysis (apophysis) may result in an avulsion of the epiphysis through its epiphyseal plate. Examples of such injuries are avulsion of the medial epicondyle of the humerus and the lesser trochanter of the femur. Since the epiphyseal plates of these traction epiphyses do not contribute to the longitudinal growth of the bone, such injuries are not complicated by a growth disturbance.

BIRTH FRACTURES

During the difficult delivery of a large baby (especially a breech presentation) when the threat of fetal anoxia may necessitate rapid extraction of the baby, one limb may be difficult to disengage from the birth canal, and a bone may be inadvertently fractured or an epiphysis separated. Only rarely is a previously normal joint dislocated by a birth injury. This usually unavoidable mishap is uncommon, but when it does occur it is usually the proximal bones of the limbs that are injured.

Multiple birth fractures are nearly always pathological and the commonest cause is osteogenesis imperfecta. Birth fracture of the tibia is rare, and when it does occur it is nearly always a pathological fracture—congenital pseudarthrosis of the tibia.

When either the humerus or the femur is fractured during delivery, the obstetrician feels and usually hears the bone break. When an epiphysis is separated, however, it tends to slide off the metaphysis, and the obstetrician may neither feel nor hear it. Thus, the diagnosis of epiphyseal separations necessitates careful and repeated physical examination of the newborn.

Parents are understandably distressed when their new baby has sustained a birth fracture—and so is the obstetrician. The physician or surgeon who treats the newborn infant's injury, however, should gently inform the parents not only that such an injury is unavoidable under the circumstances but also that it is much less serious than fetal anoxia, which the obstetrician had undoubtedly prevented by rapid extraction of the baby.

Specific birth injuries are discussed below in order of decreasing incidence.

Specific Birth Fractures

Clavicle. The slender newborn clavicle is the bone most susceptible to fracture during delivery, particularly in a broad-shouldered baby. The infant tends not to move the affected limb during the first week; this "pseudoparalysis" can be differentiated from the true paralysis of a brachial plexus injury by clinical examination (although, of course, the two may coexist). Radiographic examination confirms the presence of a fractured clavicle.

The fracture unites with remarkable rapidity, a strikingly large callus becoming apparent both clinically and radiographically within 10 days. Simple protection with a sling and bandage is the only treatment required.

Humerus. The humeral shaft is particu-

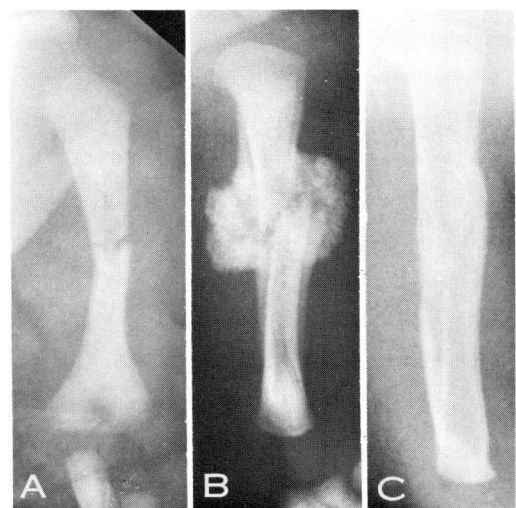

Figure 9–20 Birth fracture of the humerus. *A.* The day of birth. *B.* Ten days later there is profuse callus formation; the fracture at this stage was clinically united. *C.* Ten weeks later a remarkable amount of remodeling has occurred.

larly susceptible to a birth fracture during a difficult breech delivery. The complete fracture is in the shaft and is frequently associated with a radial nerve injury; the latter, being only a neuropraxia, recovers completely. The newborn infant's fractured arm is obviously floppy, and the diagnosis is readily confirmed radiographically (Fig. 9–20).

The infant's arm should be bandaged to the chest for a period of two weeks, by which time the fracture is always clinically united. Mild residual angulatory deformities improve with subsequent growth, but rotational deformities are permanent.

Rarely, the proximal humeral epiphysis is separated by a birth injury.

Femur. Birth fractures of the femur are most likely to occur during the delivery of a baby who has presented as a frank breech. The clinical deformity and floppiness of the lower limb are apparent, and radiographic examination confirms the diagnosis of a fracture, usually in the midshaft. Overhead (Bryant's) skin traction on both lower limbs provides adequate alignment of the fracture which is clinically united within three weeks.

Traumatic separation of the distal femoral epiphysis is more difficult to recognize clinically and may escape detection until the knee becomes enlarged by extensive

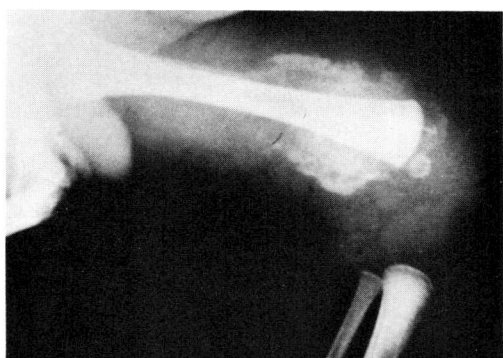

Figure 9-21 Birth injury of the distal femoral epiphysis. In this radiograph taken 10 days after birth, the center of ossification of the distal femoral epiphysis is seen to be displaced posteriorly (normally it is in line with the central axis of the femoral shaft). The marked new bone formation from the elevated periosteum would have taken approximately 10 days to develop and therefore, by deduction, this Type 1 epiphyseal plate injury probably occurred at birth. The injury had been unsuspected at the time of the difficult breech delivery but the radiograph was taken 10 days later because of the gross clinical swelling of the infant's knee.

new bone formation (Fig. 9-21). Overhead (Bryant's) skin traction is required for two weeks. Since it is a type 1 epiphyseal plate injury in an epiphysis that has a good blood

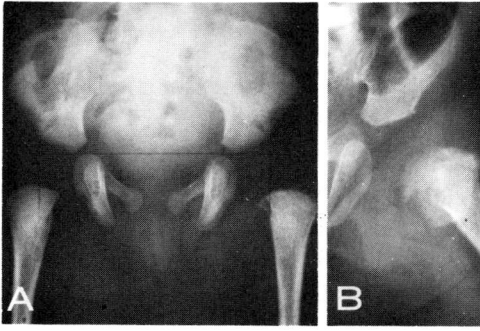

Figure 9-22 Birth injury of the proximal femoral epiphysis. *A.* Six days after birth there is obvious lateral displacement of the metaphysis of the left femur in relation to the acetabulum (the normal hip serves as a helpful comparison). Clinically, the infant was thought to have congenital dislocation of the left hip. The center of ossification does not appear until approximately six months of age. Note the slight new bone formation, however, around the metaphysis; this differentiates an epiphyseal plate injury from a dislocation of the hip. *B.* Eight weeks later there is further new bone formation and early remodeling.

supply, it has an excellent prognosis for subsequent growth.

Traumatic separation of the proximal femoral epiphysis is difficult to differentiate clinically from dislocation of the hip, but the latter is rare as a birth injury. The differentiation may also be difficult radiographically, since at birth the head, neck, and greater trochanter are completely unossified; indeed, at birth the radiographic differentiation from a congenitally dislocated hip may require an arthrogram. Within three weeks, however, radiographic examination reveals evidence of new bone formation in the metaphyseal region, indicating a traumatic epiphyseal separation (Fig. 9-22). Treatment consists of immobilization of the hip in abduction and flexion in a spica cast for two weeks. The prognosis for subsequent growth is good, since at birth the proximal femoral epiphysis consists of the head, neck, and greater trochanter, and therefore, at this stage, separation of the entire epiphysis does not jeopardize its blood supply.

Spine. Fortunately, birth injuries of the spine are rare, but they are extremely serious since they may be complicated by complete paraplegia.

SPECIFIC FRACTURES AND DISLOCATIONS

THE HAND

Apart from the crush injuries of the distal phalanges, fractures of the hand are much less common in children than in adults. In children, a hyperflexion injury of the distal interphalangeal joint may produce a fracture–separation through the epiphyseal plate, a *childhood type of mallet finger*, which can be differentiated from avulsion of the extensor tendon by a lateral radiograph. The finger should be immobilized with distal joint in extension for three weeks.

Phalangeal fractures must be accurately reduced to avoid a persistent angulatory deformity (Fig. 9-23A). Rotational deformity in a finger, which is most likely to occur through a *separation of the proximal phalangeal epiphyseal plate*, should also be corrected, since such deformity seriously impairs function of the hand (Fig. 9-23B).

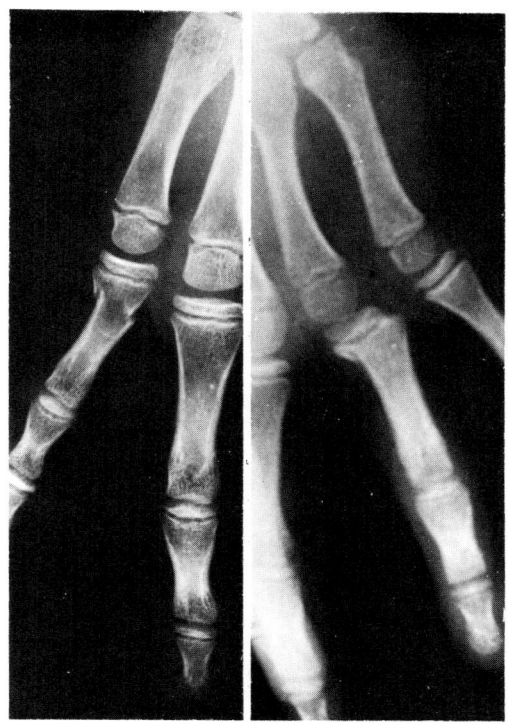

Figure 9–23 A. Fracture through the metaphysis of the proximal phalanx of the little finger with angulation. If this angulatory fracture deformity is not reduced, there would be a permanent deformity of the finger. *B.* Type 2 fracture-separation of the epiphysis of the proximal phalanx of the ring finger. Only slight displacement is apparent in this radiograph, which was taken three weeks after injury. Clinical examination at this time, however, revealed a 45° rotational deformity of the finger; as a result, this finger crossed over its neighbor during flexion. Since the epiphyseal plate injury had unfortunately been allowed to heal with this deformity, a corrective osteotomy of the phalanx was required to restore normal function in the child's hand.

Displaced *intraarticular fractures of finger* joints merit open reduction and internal fixation with fine Kirschner wires to restore a perfect joint surface.

Metacarpophalangeal dislocation of the thumb is not uncommon in children as a result of a hyperextension injury (Fig. 9–24). The first metacarpal head escapes through a small tear in joint capsule which then tends to grip the narrow neck of the metacarpal and act as a button hole. For this reason the dislocation may be frustratingly difficult to reduce by closed manipulation and frequently requires open reduction followed by immobilization of the joint in

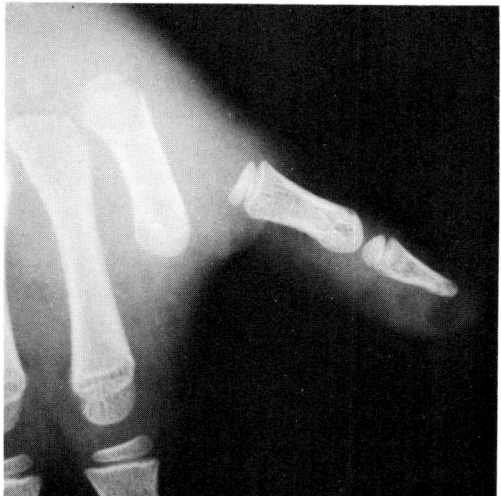

Figure 9–24 Traumatic dislocation of the metacarpophalangeal joint of the thumb of a child. In this particular child the dislocation could not be reduced by closed manipulation and consequently open reduction was required.

the stable position of moderate flexion for three weeks.

Older boys who fight with more force than finesse may sustain a *fracture of the neck of the mobile fifth metacarpal.* This fracture responds well to closed reduction; the depressed metacarpal head can be elevated by pressure along the axis of the proximal phalanx with the metacarpophalangeal joint flexed to a right angle. The fracture should be immobilized for four weeks with the finger in moderate flexion.

Fractures of the carpal bones are rare in childhood, possibly because of relatively large cartilaginous component in bone during the growing years. Nevertheless, *fractures of the carpal scaphoid* sometimes occur in older boys and may require the same prolonged immobilization as they do in adults.

Severe injuries of the hand, particularly tendon injuries and open fractures, should be treated by a surgeon who has a special interest and skill in surgery of the hand.

THE WRIST AND FOREARM

Fractures in the region of the wrist and forearm are extremely common in childhood because of frequent falls in which the

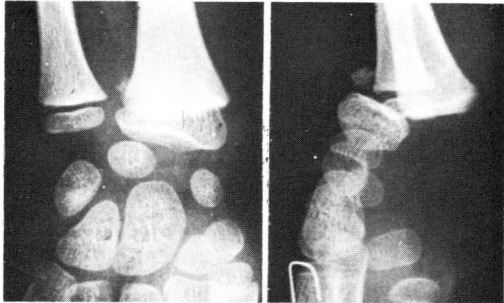

Figure 9-25 Type 2 fracture-separation of the distal radial epiphysis. In the anteroposterior projection the epiphyseal plate of the radius is not apparent because the epiphysis is displaced and angulated. In the lateral projection the backward displacement and angulation of the epiphysis are apparent. Note the small triangular metaphyseal fragment that is attached to the epiphysis and its epiphyseal plate.

forces are transmitted from the hand to the radius and ulna.

Distal Radial Epiphysis

Fracture–separation is by far the commonest epiphyseal plate injury in the body, ac-counting for approximately half of the total. This injury occurs frequently in older children and may be accompanied by a greenstick fracture of the ulna. It is a type 2 injury, as indicated by the separation of the entire epiphysis with a small triangular-shaped metaphyseal fragment (Fig. 9–25). Since this fracture–separation results from a forced hyperextension and supination injury, it can be reduced by a combination of flexion and pronation. The reduced fracture–separation should be immobilized in an above-elbow cast, with the forearm in pronation for a period of three weeks (epiphyseal separations heal twice as rapidly as fractures through the cancellous area of the same bone in the same child). Because it is a type 2 injury, the prognosis for subsequent growth is excellent.

Distal Third of Radius and Ulna

Incomplete Fractures. In young children the most frequent fracture in this region is the *buckle type* (Fig. 9–26), which requires protection alone for three weeks.

Greenstick fractures of the distal metaphyseal region of the radius and ulna require closed reduction by manipulation if the angulation is significant. The angulation is gradually corrected to the point at which the remaining intact part of the cortex is heard and felt to crack through (Fig. 9–27).

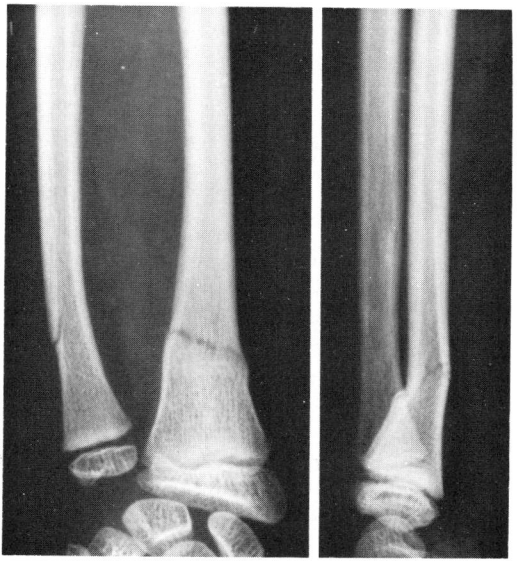

Figure 9-26 Buckle fracture of the distal metaphysis of the radius and a crack fracture of the ulna in a child. The angulation deformity with buckling, or crumpling of the thin dorsal cortex is apparent in the lateral projection. This is sometimes referred to as a "torus" fracture because of the ridge on the cortex (torus, L. means ridge or protuberance).

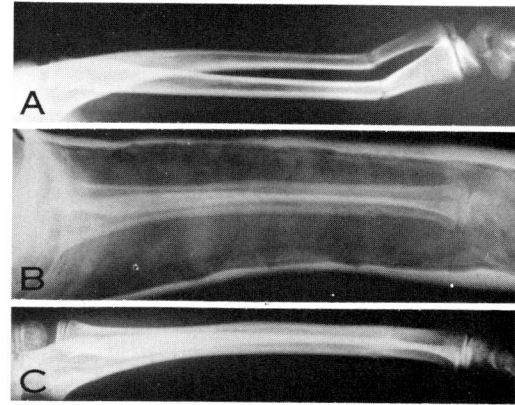

Figure 9-27 Greenstick fractures of the distal third of the radius and ulna with anterior angulation in a seven-year-old boy. *B.* Reduced position of the fractures in a plaster cast; the remaining intact portion of the cortex of each bone was deliberately cracked through at the time of reduction. *C.* Six weeks later both fractures have united in a satisfactory position.

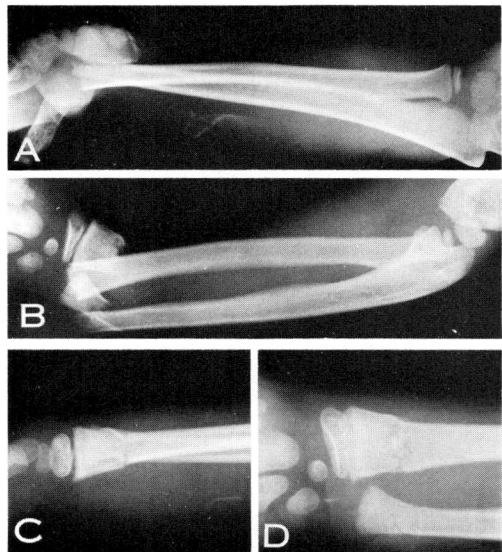

Figure 9-28 Displaced fractures of the distal metaphysis of the radius and ulna with marked overriding. *A* and *B*. Before reduction. *C* and *D*. Immediately after closed reduction utilizing the intact periosteal hinge.

Indeed, if this is not done, the angulatory deformity will not be completely corrected and may even recur during the period of immobilization.

Complete Fractures. *Displaced fractures of the distal metaphyseal region of the radius and ulna* are particularly common in childhood (Fig. 9-28). They may be difficult to reduce unless the significance of the intact periosteal hinge is appreciated. When the radius alone is fractured, the injury has been one of supination; consequently, the reduction is most stable in pronation. When both the radius and ulna are fractured, the reduction may be more stable with the forearm in the neutral position. In either case, a well-molded, above-elbow plaster cast is required for six weeks.

Moderate residual angulation, either anterior or posterior, though not desirable, is acceptable, since it tends to correct spontaneously with subsequent growth, mentioned earlier (Fig. 9-3).

Middle Third of Radius and Ulna

Greenstick fractures of the middle third of the radius and ulna can be completely reduced by a closed manipulation provided the practice of cracking through the remaining intact part of the cortex is utilized (Fig. 9-29). Indeed, unless the angulatory deformity is well corrected, the normal rotation of the radius around the ulna during supination and pronation will be permanently restricted.

Displaced fractures of the middle third of the radius and ulna are unstable and may be difficult to reduce and to keep reduced. Just how much of the fracture deformity is due to angulation and how much is due to rotation is often better assessed by looking at the child's two forearms than by looking at the radiographs.

Both angulation and rotation at the fracture site must be corrected, but side-to-side (bayonet) apposition of both fractures is acceptable. Nevertheless, it is usually possible to obtain end-to-end apposition first of one fracture and then of the other, after which the most stable position of the reductions can be assessed. It is usually, but not invariably, the midposition between supination and pronation. Immobilization in a well-molded, above-elbow cast, with

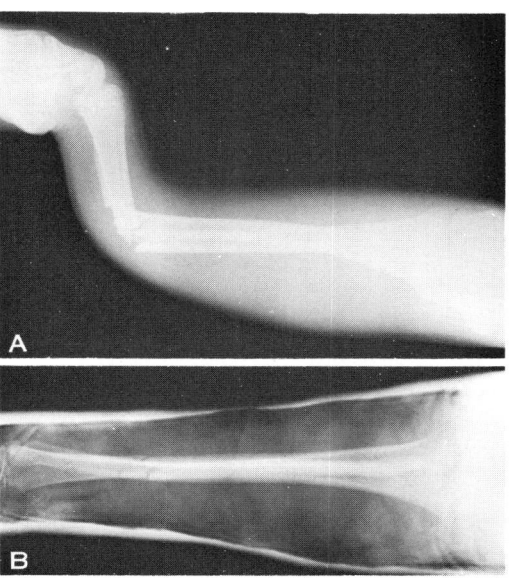

Figure 9-29 Greenstick fractures of the middle third of the radius and ulna of a 14-year-old boy. *A.* Note the gross angulation. *B.* Reduced position of the fractures in a plaster cast; the remaining intact portion of the cortex of each bone was deliberately cracked through at the time of reduction.

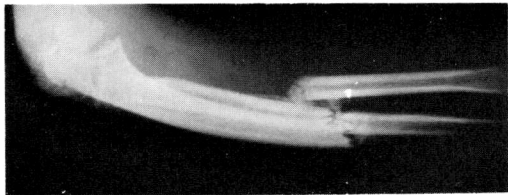

Figure 9–30 Displaced fractures of the middle third of the radius and ulna of a 15-year-old child. Six weeks after injury, the position of the fragments is obviously unsatisfactory; the ulna is out to length but there is marked overriding of the radial fracture and a rotational deformity at both fractures. At this time (after six weeks of healing) the fractures could not be reduced by closed manipulation and consequently open reduction and internal fixation were required. Closed reduction would have been possible at an earlier stage had the loss of position of the fragments been detected by repeated radiographic examinations during the first few weeks.

the forearm in the most stable position, should be maintained for eight weeks (healing through cortical bone is slower than through cancellous bone).

Unstable fractures of both bones of the forearm should be examined radiographically each week for at least four weeks in order to detect any deterioration in the position of the fragments (Fig. 9–30). If angulation recurs during the period of immobilization, remanipulation is best performed about two weeks after the injury, at which time the fracture sites have become

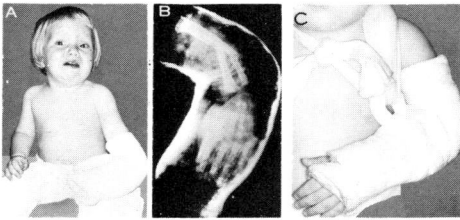

Figure 9–31 Avoidable pitfall in the treatment of fractures of both bones of the forearm in a child. *A.* This two-year-old child has reason to cry. The incorrectly applied above-elbow cast for her fractured forearm had been gradually slipping off during the preceding three days. Note that the fingers have disappeared into the cast and that the elbow of the cast is no longer at the level of the child's elbow. It is on the way to becoming a "shopping bag cast," one that the mother brings back in her shopping bag. *B.* The child's fractures have become angulated, since they are now at the level of the elbow of the cast. A second reduction was required. *C.* After the second reduction a well-molded cast was applied and was suspended from the child's neck; these precautions prevent the cast from slipping off.

"sticky" and the reduction is likely to be more stable. Loss of apposition with resultant overriding should be corrected by remanipulation as soon as it is recognized.

Fractures of both bones of the forearm in children may be difficult to treat and often are not treated well. There is virtually no indication for open reduction of these fractures in children. Some of the pitfalls of treatment are depicted as examples in order to show how to avoid them (Figs. 9–31 and 9–32).

Proximal Third of Radius and Ulna

Fracture of the shaft of the ulna combined with dislocation of the radiohumeral joint (Monteggia fracture–dislocation) is a serious injury not only because it is a fracture–dislocation but also because the dislocation component of the injury so often goes unrecognized and consequently remains untreated (Fig. 9–33). Because of the firm attachment of the radius of the ulna through the fibrous interosseous membrane, a fracture of the middle or proximal third of the ulna cannot become angulated unless its attached mate, the radius, either fractures or dislocates at its proximal end. Thus, the radiographic examination of a child with an angulated fracture of the ulna must include the full length of the forearm.

In children, closed reduction of a Monteggia fracture–dislocation can usually be obtained by correcting the angulation of the ulnar fracture and placing the radial head in proper relationship with the capitellum (Fig. 9–34). Immobilization of the limb in a cast, with the elbow in acute flexion, is necessary for six weeks to maintain the reduction. Active exercises may be required to help regain elbow motion after removal of the cast.

Neglected residual dislocation of the radiohumeral joint is difficult to treat even a few months after the injury and necessitates an extensive reconstructive operation (Fig. 9–33). If six months or more have elapsed since the time of injury, the dislocation is better left unreduced, since elbow stiffness after surgical correction may be more troublesome than the joint instability associated with the residual dislocation.

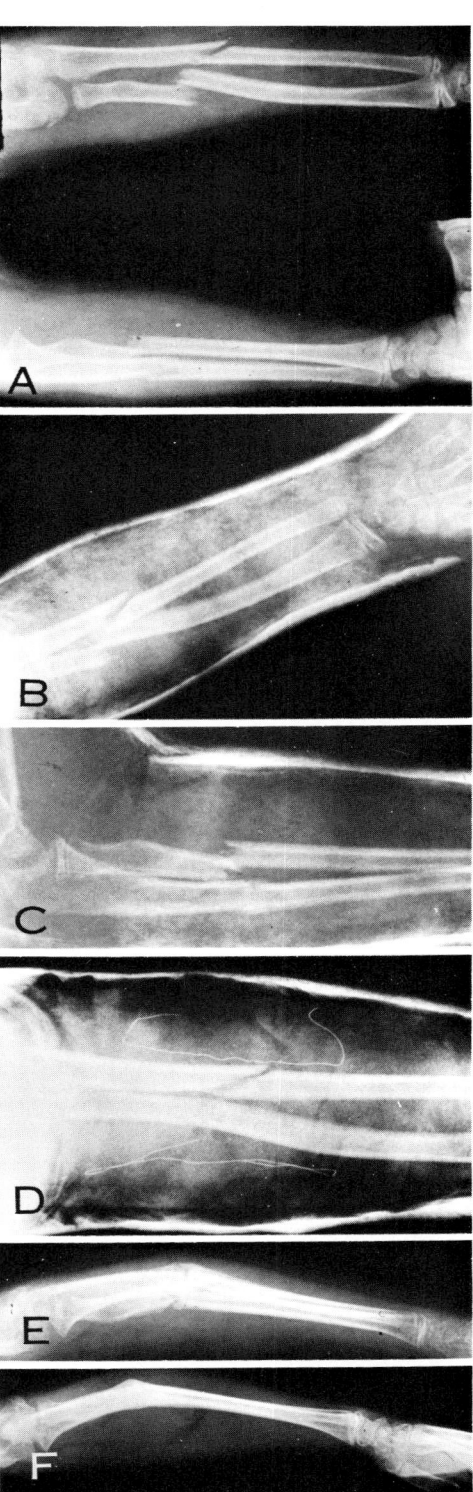

Figure 9–32 Avoidable pitfalls in the treatment of unstable fractures of both bones of the forearm in an eight-year-old girl. *A.* Initial radiographs. *B.* and *C.* The position obtained by closed reduction was unsatisfactory. The surgeon did not appreciate the rotational deformity at the fracture sites. *D.* The surgeon then performed an open reduction of both fractures but failed to secure the reduction by means of internal fixation. *E.* Six weeks after injury the fractures have united with an unacceptable amount of angulation (malunion). The surgeon apparently felt this would correct spontaneously with subsequent growth. *F.* One year later the angulation remains unchanged. In addition to an ugly clinical deformity, there was gross restriction of pronation and supination of the forearm.

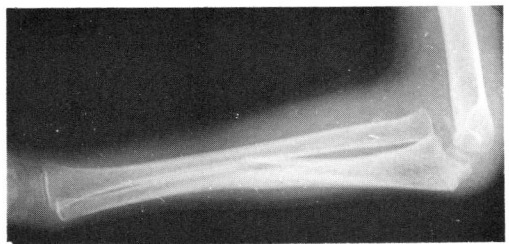

Figure 9–33   Healed fracture of the shaft of the ulna combined with dislocation of the radial head (Monteggia fracture-dislocation). The radial head should always be opposite the capitellum. The child had been treated for the fractured ulna three months previously, but the dislocated radial head had not been recognized. Unfortunately, at this stage reconstructive surgery on the ulna and radiohumeral joint is required.

THE ELBOW AND ARM

Fractures and dislocations of the elbow in children are common injuries. They are also serious, not only because of inherent difficulties in obtaining adequate reduction but also because of the high incidence of complications.

One very common but minor injury "pulled elbow," merits discussion here.

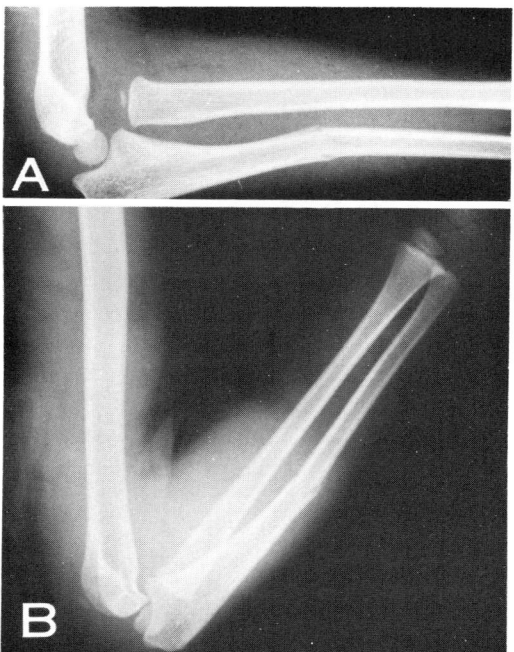

Figure 9–34   Fresh fracture of the shaft of the ulna combined with dislocation of the radial head. *A.* Before reduction. *B.* After closed reduction of the angulated ulna and the dislocated radial head.

Pulled Elbow

Children of preschool age are particularly vulnerable to a sudden pull or jerk on their arms and frequently sustain the common minor injury well known to family physicians and pediatricians as *pulled elbow.*

Clinical Features.   The history is characteristic; a parent, nursemaid, or older sibling, while lifting the small child up a step by the hand or pulling the child away from potential danger, exerts a strong pull on the extended elbow. The resulting injury of pulled elbow is sometimes referred to as nursemaid's elbow; although the nursemaid may cause the injury, it is the child who suffers it (Fig. 9–35).

The child begins to cry and refuses to use the arm, protecting it by holding it with the elbow flexed and the forearm pronated. Understandably, the parent fears that "something must be broken" and seeks medical attention.

Diagnosis.   Physical examination reveals a crying or fretful child, but the only significant local finding is painful limitation of forearm supination. Radiographic examination is consistently negative.

Pathological Anatomy.   Pulled elbow is essentially a *transient subluxation of the radial head.* For years it was assumed that

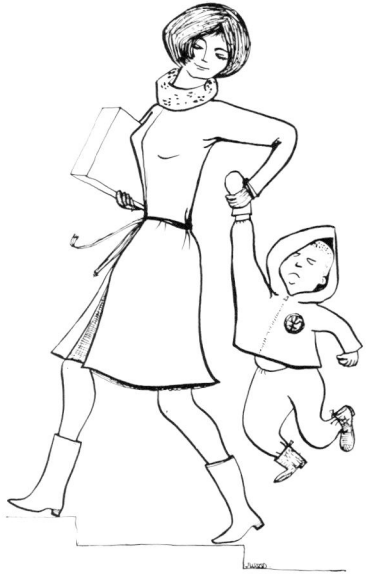

Figure 9–35   The mechanism of injury that produces a "pulled elbow" in a young child.

in children under the age of five years, the diameter of the cartilaginous radial head was no larger than that of the radial neck, and that consequently the radial head could easily be pulled through the annular ligament. This assumption, however, is incorrect. Anatomical studies post mortem reveal that in children of all ages the diameter of the radial head is always larger than that of the neck. In young children, however, the distal attachment of the annular ligament to the radial neck is thin and weak.

Post mortem studies conducted with the elbow joint exposed demonstrated that in young children a sudden pull on the extended elbow while the forearm is pronated produces a tear in the distal attachment of the annular ligament to the radial neck. The radial head penetrates part way through this tear as it is distracted from the capitellum. Then the proximal part of the annular ligament slips into the radiohumeral joint where it becomes trapped between the joint surfaces when the pull is released (Fig. 9–36). The subluxation, therefore, is transient, and this explains the normal radiographic appearance of the elbow. The source of pain is the pinched annular ligament. The post mortem studies also revealed that with the elbow flexed, sudden supination of the forearm frees the incarcerated part of the annular ligament which then resumes its normal position.

Treatment. On the basis of the pathological anatomy of pulled elbow, its treatment consists simply of a deft supination of the child's forearm while the elbow is flexed. A slight click can usually be felt over the anterolateral aspect of the radial head as the annular ligament is freed from the joint. Within moments the pain is relieved and the child begins to use the arm again.

If the child has been sent to the radiology department prior to treatment, the radiographic technician frequently and unwittingly "treats" the pulled elbow while the forearm is being passively supinated to obtain the anteroposterior projection.

Aftertreatment consists of a sling for two weeks to allow the tear in the attachment of the annular ligament to heal. In addition, parents are advised of the harmful effects of pulling or lifting their small child by the hand.

Proximal Radial Epiphysis

Fracture–separation of the proximal radial epiphysis is produced by a fall that exerts a compression and abduction force on the elbow joint. It is a type 2 epiphyseal

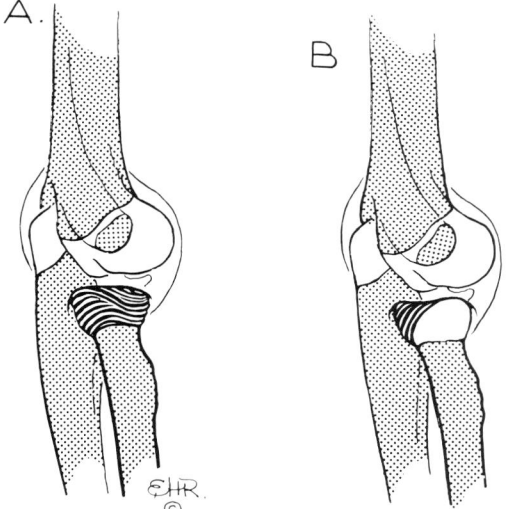

Figure 9–36 Schematic representation of the pathological anatomy of a "pulled elbow." *A.* Normal arrangement of the annular ligament. *B.* In the "pulled elbow" there is a tear in the distal attachment of the annular ligament through which the radial head has protruded slightly; the proximal portion of the annular ligament has slipped into the radiohumeral joint where it has become trapped.

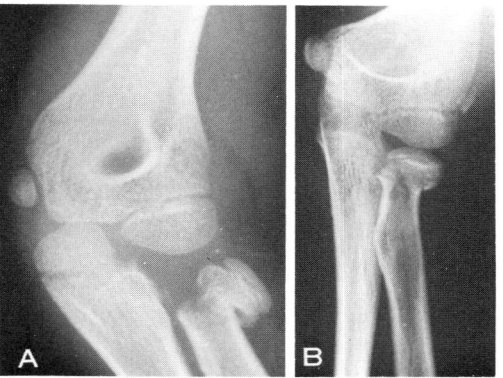

Figure 9–37 Type 2 fracture-separation of the proximal radial epiphysis in a child. *A.* Note the valgus deformity of the elbow, the angulation at the fracture site, and the loss of contact of the radiohumeral joint surfaces. *B.* The position of the fragments after closed reduction is satisfactory.

plate injury with a characteristic metaphyseal fragment, and the radial head becomes tilted on the neck (Fig. 9–37).

Treatment. Satisfactory closed reduction can usually be obtained by pressing upwards and medially on the tilted radial head while an assistant holds the arm with the elbow extended and adducted.

Residual angulation of less than 40 degrees is compatible with acceptable function. Occasionally, open reduction is necessary to restore congruity between the joint surfaces of the radial head and the capitellum. Internal fixation is not necessary. Even if it has lost all soft tissue attachments, the radial head should never be excised during childhood. Indeed, removal of the radial head also includes its epiphyseal plate from the proximal end of the radius. This produces a progressive discrepancy in length between the radius and ulna owing to relatively less growth in the radius. Consequently, the hand becomes progressively deviated toward the radial side. After reduction (either closed or open), the child's elbow should be immobilized for three weeks at a right angle with the forearm supinated, since this is the most stable position.

Complications. Since the blood supply to the intraarticular radial head is precarious, displaced fracture–separations through the epiphyseal plate may be complicated by avascular necrosis of the epiphysis. The small volume of the radial epiphysis, however, permits fairly rapid revascularization and regeneration. Little deformity of the replaced radial head ensues, but necrosis of the epiphyseal plate results in premature cessation of growth at this site and a discrepancy in length between the radius and ulna. Nevertheless, this is far superior to the results of removing the radial head in children.

Dislocation of the Elbow

Posterior dislocation of the elbow joint occurs relatively frequently in young children as a result of a fall on the hand with the elbow flexed. The distal end of the humerus is driven through the anterior capsule as the radius and ulna dislocate posteriorly (Fig. 9–38).

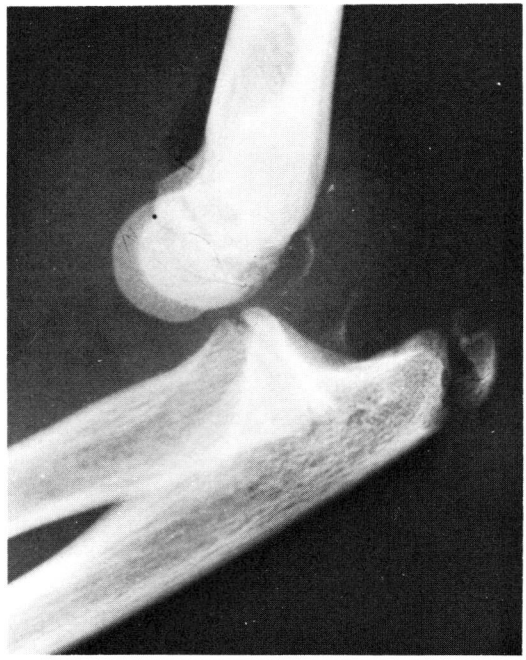

Figure 9–38 Posterior dislocation of the elbow joint in a child. The apparently separated fragment of bone at the proximal end of the ulna is a traction epiphysis rather than a fracture fragment.

Treatment. Closed reduction is readily accomplished by reversing the mechanism of injury; traction is applied to the flexed elbow through the forearm which is then brought forward. The reduced elbow should be maintained in the stable position of flexion above a right angle in a plaster cast for a period of three weeks, after which gentle active exercises are begun. *Post traumatic myositis ossificans* may develop after dislocation of the elbow.

Fracture–dislocations of the elbow are discussed in relation to the specific fractures of the medial epicondyle and lateral condyle of the humerus.

Medial Epicondyle

Avulsion of the medial epicondyle (a traction epiphysis) results from sudden traction through the attached medial ligament in association with two types of injuries. In one type the medial epicondyle is avulsed at the time of a posterior dislocation of the elbow and is therefore carried posteriorly; as the dislocation is reduced, so

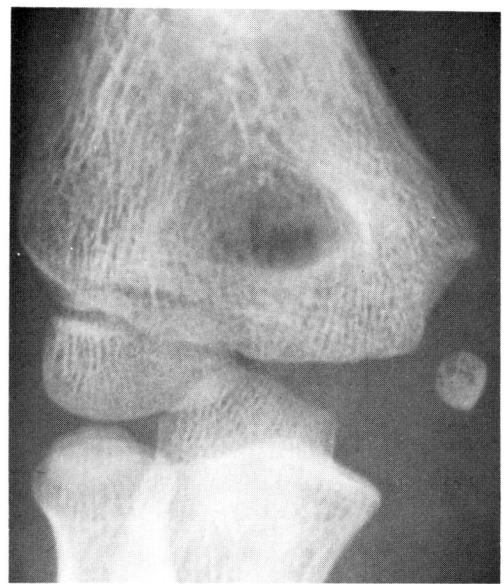

Figure 9–39 Avulsion of the medial epicondyle (a traction epiphysis) from the distal end of the humerus in a six-year-old child. The medial epicondyle has shifted distally approximately 1 cm to reach the level of the joint line of the elbow.

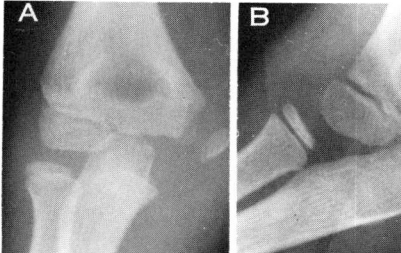

Figure 9–40 Instability of the right elbow joint of a seven-year-old boy in association with avulsion of the medial epicondyle. A. Anteroposterior projection of the elbow showing moderate separation of the medial epicondyle. B. This stress radiograph taken with the boy under anesthetic and with an abduction force being applied to the elbow reveals gross instability of the joint; the medial epicondyle has been pulled further distally.

also is the separation of the medial epicondyle.

More frequently, however, the injury that avulses the medial epicondyle is severe abduction of the extended elbow with or without a transient lateral dislocation of the joint; the medial epicondyle is carried distally. There is marked local swelling and tenderness. In the absence of a permanent lateral dislocation of the elbow, radiographic examination reveals only moderate separation of the medial epicondyle from the distal end of the humerus (Fig. 9–39). If there is doubt about the diagnosis, comparable radiographic projections of the opposite elbow are helpful.

Treatment. Stability of the elbow joint is the most important aspect of this second type of avulsion injury. It should always be assessed while the patient is under general anesthesia, in order to determine the optimum form of treatment. If the elbow is stable when subjected to an abduction force, the relatively slight separation of the medial epicondyle requires only immobilization with the elbow in flexion for three weeks. Under these circumstances, even if the epicondyle heals by fibrous union, there

is no growth disturbance, and the long-term result will be satisfactory. If, however, the elbow is grossly unstable when subjected to an abduction force, open reduction and internal fixation are indicated to restore stability of the joint (Fig. 9–40).

Complications. A *traction injury of the ulnar nerve* is a frequent complication of the abduction type of avulsion of the medial epicondyle. The prognosis for recovery of the nerve lesion is excellent, and the presence of such a lesion is in itself not an indication for open reduction.

Occasionally, at the moment of spontaneous reduction of a lateral dislocation, the avulsed medial epicondyle is trapped in the elbow joint. Under these circumstances, the medial epicondyle can be freed from the joint by closed manipulation. However, since open reduction and internal fixation are indicated to restore stability to the elbow, the trapped medial epicondyle is best freed at the time of operation.

Lateral Condyle

Fractures of the lateral condyle of the humerus in children are relatively common, frequently complicated, and regrettably often inadequately treated. The fracture line begins at the joint surface, passes through the cartilaginous portion of the epiphysis medial to the capitellum, crosses the epiphyseal plate, and extends into the metaphysis. Thus, a fracture of the lateral condyle represents a type 4 epiphyseal

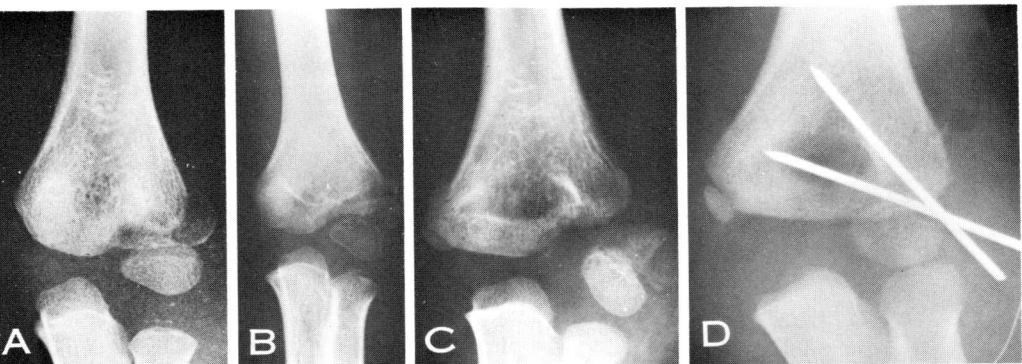

Figure 9–41 Fractures of the lateral condyle of the humerus in children, a Type 4 epiphyseal plate injury. *A.* Relatively undisplaced. *B.* Moderately angulated. *C.* Completely distracted and rotated. *D.* After open reduction and internal fixation of the fracture with Kirschner wires.

plate injury, the seriousness of which was discussed earlier (Fig. 9–15).

These fractures are inherently unstable since they are predominantly intraarticular. The only periosteal covering is on the metaphyseal fragment, and this is frequently completely disrupted. Consequently, even when the fracture appears undisplaced initially, it has a tendency to become displaced subsequently with serious sequelae.

Radiographically, an undisplaced fracture of the lateral condyle may escape detection unless comparable projections of the opposite elbow are obtained (Fig. 9–2). The lateral condyle (which includes the capitellum and the lateral portion of the metaphysis) may be relatively undisplaced, moderately angulated, or even completely distracted and rotated (Fig. 9–41). With severe injuries, there even may be an associated dislocation of the elbow and hence a fracture–dislocation.

Treatment. Even undisplaced fractures of the lateral condyle are potentially serious because of their instability. They may be treated initially by immobilization of the arm in a plaster cast with the elbow at a right angle. During the first two weeks, repeated radiographic examinations are essential, since even during immobilization the fracture may become displaced, in which case immediate open reduction and internal fixation are indicated.

Displaced fractures of the lateral condyle represent one of the relatively few absolute indications for open reduction and internal

fixation in children. Since these fractures are type 4 epiphyseal plate injuries, even relatively minor displacement must be perfectly reduced, and the reduction must be constantly maintained by internal fixation to avoid an otherwise inevitable growth disturbance (Fig. 9–41D). After operation, the arm should be immobilized in a plaster cast, with the elbow at a right angle, for three weeks. The metallic internal fixation (usually Kirschner wires) should then be removed, and gentle active exercises should be started.

Complications. If the union is delayed because of inadequate fixation, the associated hyperemia may cause an overgrowth

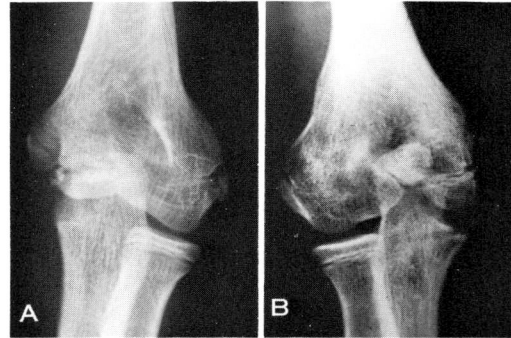

Figure 9–42 Growth disturbances complicating fractures of the lateral condyle of the humerus. *A.* Cubitus varus one year after a fracture of the lateral condyle due to overgrowth of the lateral part of the epiphyseal plate. *B.* Notch in the distal end of the humerus two years after a fracture of the lateral condyle (due to premature cessation of local epiphyseal plate growth).

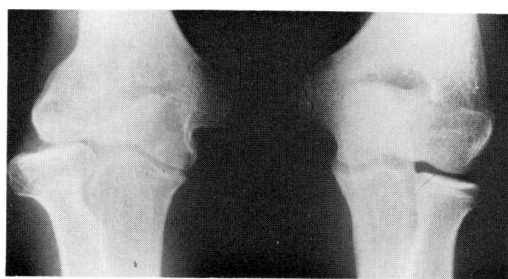

Figure 9–43 The late effects of avascular necrosis of the right capitellum that occurred five years previously as a complication of a fracture of the lateral condyle of the humerus. Note the growth disturbance of the distal end of the humerus, the deformity of the capitellum and the secondary enlargement of the radial head.

on the lateral side of the elbow with resultant cubitus varus (loss of carrying angle) (Fig. 9–42A). Failure to obtain and maintain perfect reduction of a fractured lateral condyle of the humerus leads to serious growth disturbance at the epiphyseal plate (Fig. 9–42B). If the fracture is complicated by avascular necrosis of the capitellum, there is not only a growth disturbance and deformity but also a marked

secondary enlargement of the radial head (Fig. 9–43). Inadequate treatment of a fractured lateral condyle may even result in a complete nonunion, one of the few examples of this complication in childhood (Fig. 9–44). The resultant cubitus valgus (increased carrying angle) is eventually further complicated by the gradual development of a tardy ulnar palsy.

Supracondylar Fracture of the Humerus

Of the significant injuries about the elbow, displaced supracondylar fractures of the humerus are the most common and certainly the most serious. Not only are they associated with a high incidence of malunion with residual deformity but also with the serious risk of Volkmann's ischemia of nerves and muscles of the forearm with resultant contracture.

The following discussion refers to the extension type of supracondylar fracture which comprises 99 per cent of the total.

Pathological Anatomy. The flared but flat distal metaphysis of the humerus is indented posteriorly (the olecranon fossa) and anteriorly (the coronoid fossa). Consequently, it is a relatively weak site in the upper limb. As a result of either a hyperextension injury or a fall on the hand with the elbow flexed, the forces of injury are transmitted through the elbow joint, which grips the distal end of the humerus like a right-angled wrench. Thus, the resultant fracture is consistently immediately proximal to the elbow joint. When the injury is severe, there is considerable follow-through of the fragments at the moment of fracture. The jagged end of the proximal fragment is

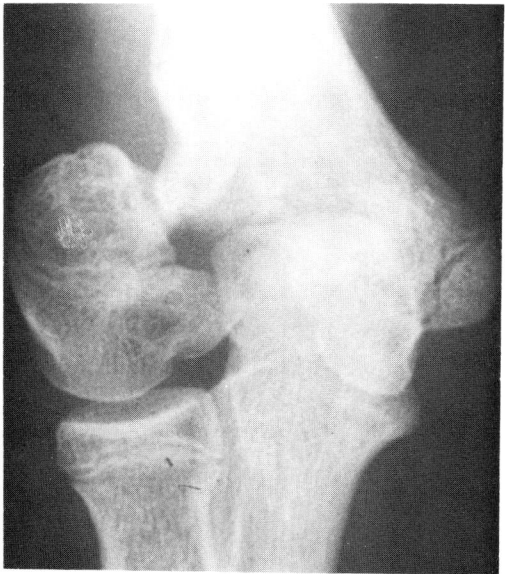

Figure 9–44 Nonunion of a fracture of the lateral condyle in a 12-year-old boy six years after an injury that had been thought to be a "sprained elbow." The boy's elbow was deformed and unstable but had a reasonable range of motion. Reconstructive surgery at this stage would be unlikely to improve the unfortunate situation.

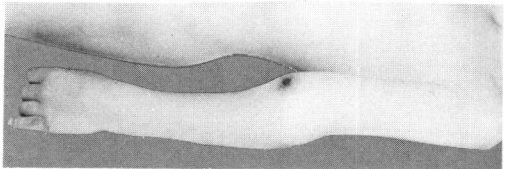

Figure 9–45 Clinical appearance of a child's arm with an open supracondylar fracture of the humerus. Note the wound in the antecubital fossa (the fracture was open from within), the gross swelling, and the striking extension deformity just proximal to the elbow joint.

driven through the anterior periosteum and the overlying brachialis muscle into the plane of the brachial artery and median nerve, coming to rest in the subcutaneous fat of the antecubital fossa. It may even penetrate the skin from within, thereby creating an open fracture (Fig. 9–45).

Diagnosis. Clinically, there is an obvious deformity in the elbow region which soon becomes grossly swollen and tense as a result of extensive internal hemorrhage. The state of the peripheral circulation and the function of the peripheral nerves should be assessed immediately; impairment of the circulation demands urgent reduction of the fracture. Radiographic examination provides striking evidence of the displacement of the fragments but little evidence of the severe soft tissue damage (Fig. 9–46). The distal fragment lies posteriorly, and hence there is an intact posterior hinge of periosteum. In addition, the distal fragment is displaced either medially or laterally, more often the former. When it is displaced medially there is an intact medial hinge of periosteum, whereas when it is displaced laterally there is an intact lateral hinge; these facts are important in relation to treatment.

Treatment. Undisplaced supracondylar fractures require only immobilization of the arm, with the elbow flexed, for three weeks. Most displaced supracondylar fractures of the humerus can be treated by closed reduction, which is made possible by utilizing the intact periosteal hinge. Thus, gentle traction on the forearm (with the elbow slightly flexed to avoid traction on the brachial artery) brings the fragments into general alignment, after which any rotational deformity and any medial or lateral displacement are corrected. At this stage – and not before – the elbow is flexed beyond a right angle. This maneuver tightens the posterior hinge of periosteum and helps to maintain the reduction. If the distal fragment was originally displaced medially, the forearm is pronated since this tightens the medial hinge and closes the fracture line on the lateral side, thereby preventing any varus deformity at the fracture site. If, however, the distal fragment was displaced laterally, the forearm is supinated, since this tightens the lateral hinge and closes the fracture on the medial side, thereby preventing any valgus deformity at the fracture site.

After reduction of the fracture, anteroposterior and lateral radiographs are obtained by rotating the tube of the x-ray machine (rather than by rotating the child's arm) so that the reduction is not lost (Fig. 9–47). The peripheral circulation is again as-

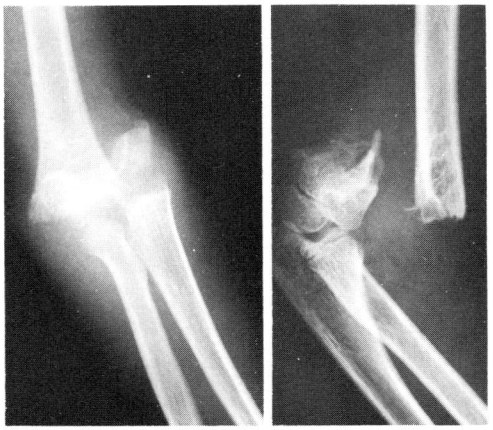

Figure 9–46 Displaced supracondylar fracture of the right humerus in a seven-year-old girl. *A.* In the anteroposterior projection the distal fragment of the humerus is displaced medially and proximally. *B.* In the lateral projection the distal fragment is displaced posteriorly and proximally. The jagged end of the proximal fragment is lying in the soft tissues of the antecubital fossa.

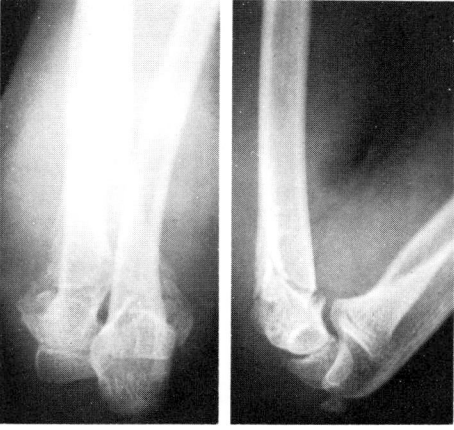

Figure 9–47 After closed reduction of the supracondylar fracture shown in Figure 9–46, the position of the fragments is satisfactory. *A.* The anteroposterior projection is taken with the elbow flexed. *B.* The position of the arm has not been altered for the lateral projection. Flexion of the elbow helps to maintain the reduction.

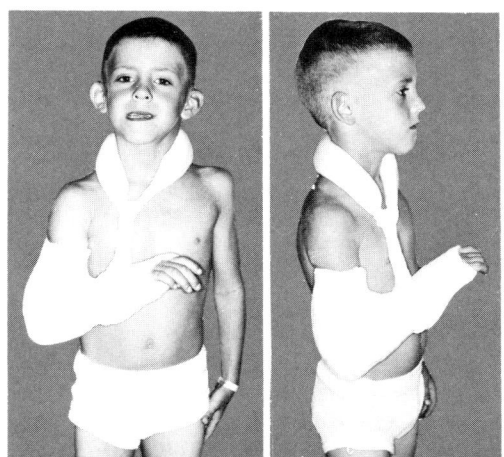

Figure 9–48 Above-elbow cast with neck sling attached for immobilization of a reduced supracondylar fracture of the humerus. The cast maintains the elbow in flexion and the forearm in pronation. Note that it does not extend into the antecubital fossa and therefore does not constrict the soft tissues in the region of the elbow.

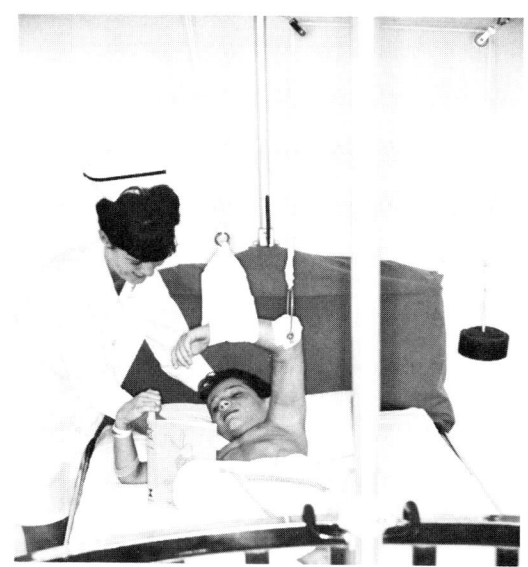

Figure 9–49 Continuous skeletal traction through a pin in the olecranon for a grossly unstable supracondylar fracture of the humerus. The position of the fragments must be monitored every few days by radiographic examination during the first two weeks so that the line and amount of traction may be adjusted as necessary to prevent malunion.

sessed, and if it is inadequate the elbow must be allowed to extend slightly. The child's arm is then immobilized in a special type of cast that does not constrict the area of maximal swelling (Fig. 9–48).

Children who require closed reduction of a supracondylar fracture of the humerus should be admitted to the hospital for at least a few days of observation, with particular reference to peripheral circulation in the limb. A well-reduced fracture is stable and hence comfortable; persistent pain may be a warning signal of ischemia and should not be masked by sedation. Repeated radiographic examinations are required during the first 10 days to assess the position of the fracture fragments within the cast.

Healing of supracondylar fractures is rapid, and consequently the cast should always be removed after three weeks. Immobilization for a more prolonged period is nearly always followed by prolonged elbow joint stiffness, even in children, because of the extensive soft tissue damage.

After removal of the cast, the child's elbow always lacks extension. Active exercises are the only safe way of regaining joint motion and may have to be carried out for several months or even longer before a full range of motion is regained. Passive

stretching of the joint is decidedly deleterious and should always be avoided.

Supracondylar fractures in which the reduction is grossly unstable as well as those with excessive soft tissue swelling or impairment of circulation are best treated by continuous skeletal traction through a pin in the olecranon (Fig. 9–49).

The rare flexion type of supracondylar fracture in which the distal fragment is displaced anteriorly is not serious. It requires closed reduction and immobilization of the elbow in extension.

COMPLICATIONS

Volkmann's Ischemia. The most serious complication of displaced supracondylar fractures of the humerus in children is Volkmann's ischemia of nerves and muscles of the forearm. The brachial artery may be caught and kinked in the fracture site, a complication that can be relieved only by reduction of the fracture. Moreover, the brachial artery, often contused at the moment of fracture is likely to develop severe arterial spasm, particularly if the subsequent manipulation of the fracture has been forceful or if there is rapidly progressive swelling within the unyielding fascial compartment of the arm. Excessive flexion of the elbow aggravates the tightness of the deep fascia in the antecubital fossa and may compress the brachial artery. A tight encircling cast may have the same effect.

The dread complication of Volkmann's ischemia, its recognition and urgent treatment as well as subsequent Volkmann's contracture, are fully discussed in Chapter 33 with other arterial complications. It is particularly pertinent to supracondylar fractures of the humerus in children.

PERIPHERAL NERVE INJURY. Although the median nerve and less commonly the radial and ulnar nerve may be injured at the moment of fracture, they are not divided, and consequently the prognosis for recovery is excellent.

MALUNION. A common complication of displaced supracondylar fractures of the humerus is malunion, particularly residual *cubitus varus* (Fig. 9–50). Once thought to be the result of an epiphyseal growth disturbance, this unsightly deformity is now known to be the result of fracture healing in an unsatisfactory position (malunion). It can and should be *prevented* by accurate reduction of the fracture.

Malunion, if sufficiently severe, necessitates a supracondylar osteotomy of the humerus after the child has regained a full range of elbow motion.

Shaft of the Humerus

Fractures of the humeral shaft are not common in childhood, and when they do occur they are the result of a fairly severe injury. The fracture is usually in the midshaft, less commonly in the proximal metaphysis, and tends to be unstable (Fig. 9–51).

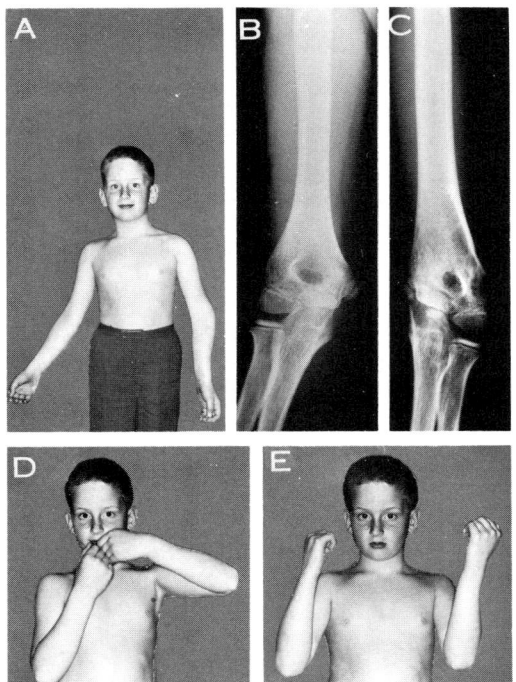

Figure 9–50 Cubitus varus (reversal of the carrying angle) of the left elbow of a nine-year-old boy due to malunion of a supracondylar fracture of the humerus one year previously. *A.* Note the unsightly deformity (sometimes referred to as a "gun stock" deformity). *B.* and *C.* Radiographs of this boy's upper limbs. Unfortunately the supracondylar fracture of the left humerus had been allowed to unite in a varus position. *D.* Because of the altered plane of the elbow joint the boy cannot put the left hand to his mouth without abducting his shoulder. *E.* For the same reason his hand and forearm are deviated laterally when he keeps his elbow to his side (this could create problems for a dinner partner seated on his left side). The appearance and function of this boy's arm can be improved by a supracondylar osteotomy of the humerus.

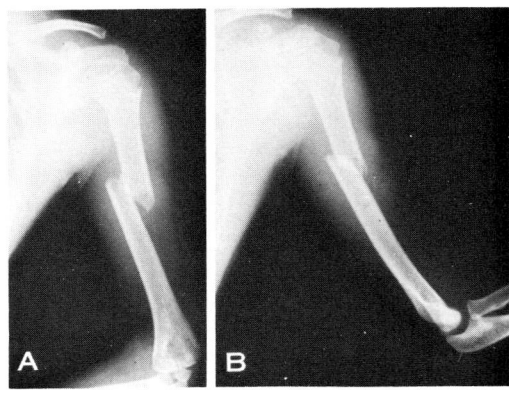

Figure 9–51 Unstable fracture of the midshaft of the left humerus in a seven-year-old boy. Prior to the radiographic examination, this boy's arm should have been splinted so that his arm could not be moved through the fracture site. *A.* An anteroposterior projection of both the proximal and the distal fragments. *B.* This is a lateral projection of the distal fragment but almost an anteroposterior projection of the proximal fragment. Obviously, between the two exposures the child's arm has been rotated approximately 90° through the unstable fracture site by the technician. The child would have experienced much pain at this time and might even have sustained further injury to the related soft tissues.

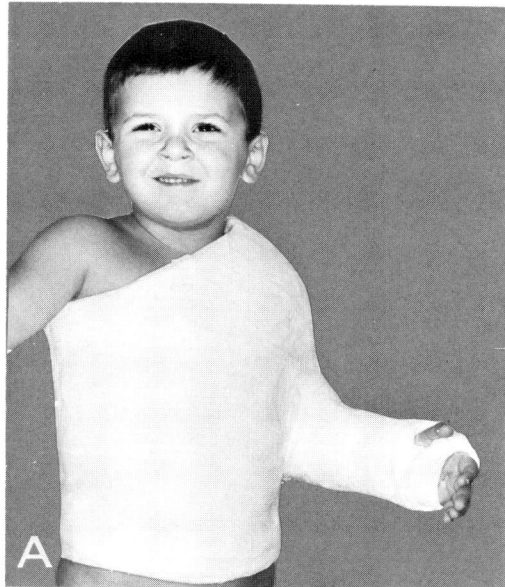

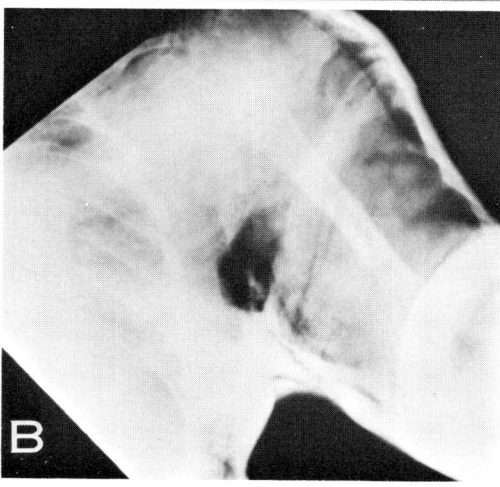

Figure 9–52 A. Shoulder spica cast for immobilization of an unstable fracture of the midshaft of the humerus in a five-year-old boy. *B.* Anteroposterior projection through the cast showing the satisfactory position of the fragments.

Relatively undisplaced stable fractures of the humeral shaft or proximal metaphysis can be adequately treated by a sling and a thoracobrachial bandage that binds the arm to the chest. Most displaced fractures can be managed by closed reduction followed by a shoulder spica cast for six weeks (Fig. 9–52). Markedly unstable fractures, particularly those in older children, may require continuous skeletal traction (Fig. 9–49) for a few weeks to maintain alignment and cor-

rect rotation, after which the fracture is sufficiently "sticky" for the traction to be replaced by a shoulder spica cast. An above-elbow cast suspended by a loop around the neck ("hanging cast") is an inefficient method of providing traction during the first few weeks, especially during sleep, and is uncomfortable for a child.

The commonest complication of a fracture of the midshaft of the humerus is an associated injury of the radial nerve, which winds around the humerus at this level; the prognosis for spontaneous recovery, however, is good.

THE SHOULDER

Proximal Humeral Epiphysis

The type of injury that in an adult would produce a dislocation of the shoulder produces a type 2 *fracture–separation of the proximal humeral epiphysis* in a child, since the joint capsule is stronger than the epiphyseal plate (Fig. 9–53).

If the displacement is slight, closed re-

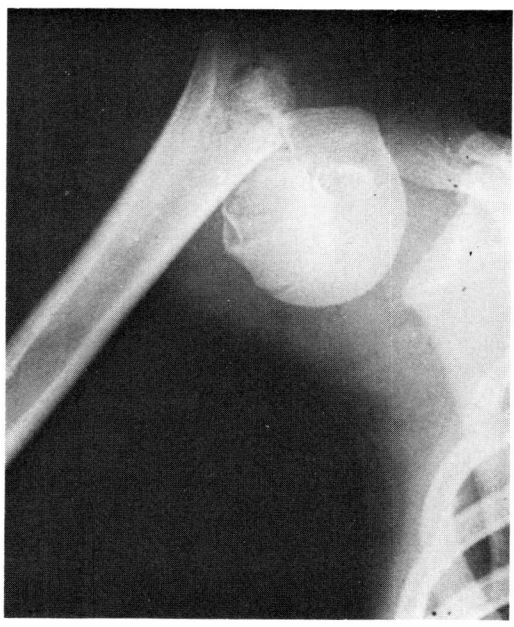

Figure 9–53 Type 2 fracture-separation of the right humeral epiphysis in a 14-year-old boy. Note the large metaphyseal fragment and the marked displacement of the fracture. The humeral head has retained its normal relationship with the glenoid cavity of the scapula.

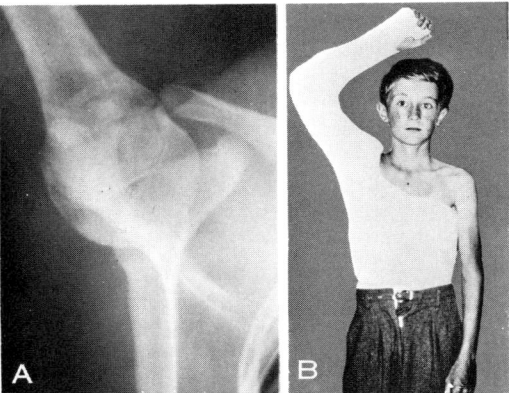

Figure 9–54 A. Reduced Type 2 fracture-separation of the right proximal humeral epiphysis in the boy whose initial radiograph is shown in Figure 9–53. Note that the arm is in the overhead position. B. Shoulder spica cast for immobilization of this boy's arm in the overhead position.

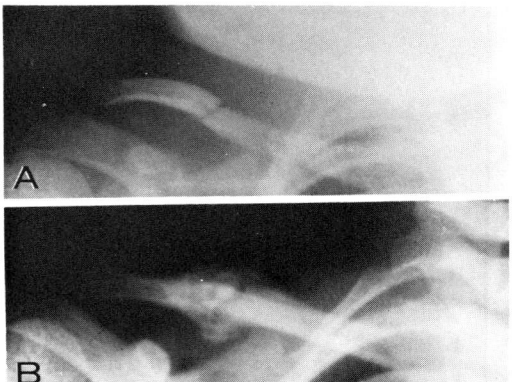

Figure 9–55 A. Undisplaced fracture of the right clavicle in a two-year-old boy. B. Three weeks after injury there is abundant callus formation; the fracture callus was both visible and palpable as a lump.

duction can usually be obtained, after which a sling and thoracobrachial bandage are used to immobilize the shoulder for three weeks.

If the displacement is marked, closed reduction can be difficult unless the intact periosteal hinge is utilized. This necessitates applying traction to the arm while it is held directly over the child's head in line with the trunk, a maneuver that pulls the distal fragment into line with the epiphysis. The reduction is frequently most stable in this position. In this case, the shoulder is immobilized in the overhead position in a shoulder spica cast for two weeks, after which the spica cast can be replaced by a sling for an additional week (Fig. 9–54).

Even with imperfect reduction of the separated epiphysis, union occurs through the intact portion of the periosteal tube. Spontaneous correction of deformity and remodeling of the proximal end of the humerus usually produce a satisfactory result. There is virtually no indication for open reduction of these type 2 epiphyseal injuries.

Clavicle

Fractures of the clavicle are the most common but the least serious of all childhood fractures. Preschool children in particular tumble almost daily, and when they land on their hands, elbows, or shoulders their slender clavicles are subjected to indirect forces that may produce a fracture. These common fractures are not serious, however, since virtually all of them unite rapidly, and there are almost never any permanent sequelae (Fig. 9–55).

Greenstick fractures of the clavicle require only a sling for three weeks, to provide protection from further injury. Displaced fractures of the clavicle in young children (under the age of 10 years) usually do not require reduction; they are best treated by a snug figure-of-eight bandage, not so much to hold the fragments in perfect position as to hold them relatively still and thereby to make the child comfortable (Fig. 9–56). The parents are instructed to tighten the bandange each day as it stretches. Within two weeks fracture callus is abundant in young children. The callus is

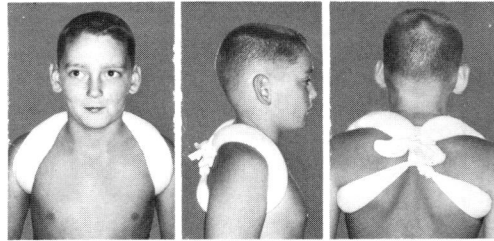

Figure 9–56 Figure-of-eight bandage for treatment of a fractured clavicle in a child; the bandage, which consists of stockinette filled with cotton wool, is adjustable so that the parent can tighten it each day.

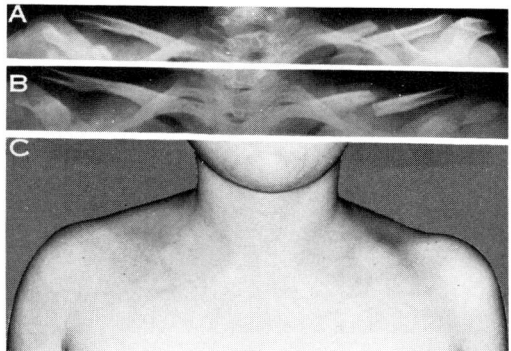

Figure 9–57 A. Displaced fracture of the left clavicle in a 15-year-old girl. Note the marked overriding of the fracture fragments. *B.* Three weeks after closed reduction and application of a snug figure-of-eight bandage, the clavicle is almost out to normal length; the side-to-side (bayonet) apposition of the fragments is satisfactory, callus formation is apparent and at this stage the fracture was clinically united. *C.* The same girl three weeks after injury showing a lump over the left clavicle. This became inconspicuous over the ensuing six months.

automobile accidents and falls from considerable heights, injuries to the spine during childhood tend to be less violent than those during adult life.

When a spinal injury is suspected clinically by local tenderness, muscle spasm, and deformity, radiographic examination must be thorough; at least four projections are required (anteroposterior, lateral, right and left oblique) and sometimes special projections, tomograms (laminograms), or even cineradiography are indicated.

Cervical Spine

Rotatory Subluxation of the Atlantoaxial Joint. Movement at the atlantoaxial joint (C1–C2) is principally rotation that allows the head to turn from side to side. If this joint is forced beyond its normal range of rotation by a sudden twisting type of injury,

even apparent clinically as a lump, but remodeling of the healed clavicle is remarkably complete within six months.

In children over the age of 10 years, fractures of the clavicle are more often displaced. With this age group an attempt should be made to align the fracture fragments by pulling the shoulders up and back before applying the figure-of-eight bandage (Fig. 9–57). For older boys, particularly those who are very active, the addition of plaster of Paris over the figure-of-eight bandage provides additional stability of the fracture. Even in older children the clinical results are consistently good, and any residual deformity corrects spontaneously by growth and remodeling during the ensuing year.

There is absolutely no justification for open reduction and internal fixation in closed uncomplicated fractures of the clavicle in children.

THE SPINE

The spinal column is much more flexible in children than it is in adults, and therefore it is less susceptible to fractures or dislocations. Furthermore, with the exception of

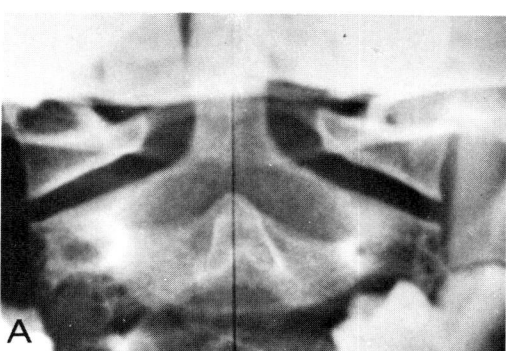

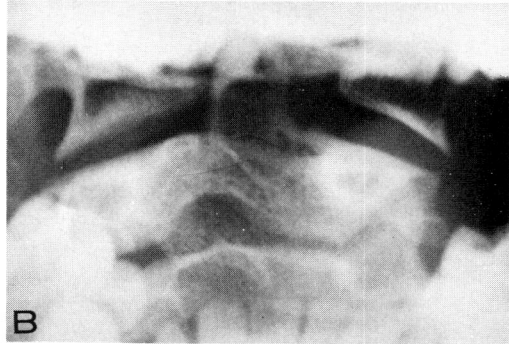

Figure 9–58 Anteroposterior projections of the atlantoaxial joint taken through the open mouth. A. Normal atlantoaxial joint. Note the symmetrical relationship of the lateral masses of the atlas (C1) to the odontoid process as well as to the lateral masses of the axis (C2). *B.* Rotatory subluxation of the atlantoaxial joint. Note the asymmetrical relationship of the lateral masses of the atlas to the odontoid process as well as to the lateral masses of the axis.

it may become locked in a position of *rotatory subluxation*, a phenomenon that is relatively common in childhood. Rotatory subluxation of the atlantoaxial joint is particularly likely to develop in a child who has had a recent throat infection. Secondary inflammation in the deep cervical glands may soften the ligaments of the upper cervical spine and render the antlantoaxial joint less stable than normal. Under these circumstances, a rotatory subluxation may occur even without injury.

DIAGNOSIS. The child develops an acute and painful wryneck deformity which persists because of muscle spasm. The uncomfortable child may prefer to support his head with his hands or to lie down. The radiographic examination may be difficult to interpret, but a projection taken through the open mouth usually reveals persistent asymmetry at the atlantoaxial joint (Fig. 9–58).

TREATMENT. Although it is possible to reduce the rotatory subluxation by manipulation of the neck, there is a slight risk of producing further displacement and even spinal cord injury, particularly when the ligaments have been previously softened by inflammation. The safest form of treatment, therefore, is mild continuous traction through a head halter. Spasm soon subsides as the subluxation is reduced, and in a few days the child's neck can be supported by a cervical "ruff" for a few weeks (Fig. 9–59).

Anterior Subluxation of the Atlantoaxial Joint. A severe fall on the top of the head may cause a forward subluxation of the atlas (C1) on the axis (C2). Such injuries may be incurred from dives into shallow water, from falls on the head from a considerable height, and from body contact sports.

Since the spinal cord is jeopardized by the injury, reduction of the subluxation and maintenance of the reduction are essential. Reduction is more effectively obtained by continuous traction through skull tongs than through a halter. After reduction, the C1–C2 joint should be stabilized by arthrodesis to prevent recurrence of the subluxation or even a dislocation from a subsequent injury.

Subluxations at Other Levels of the Cervical Spine. After any neck injury in children, cervical radiographs must be interpreted with caution. The increased mobility

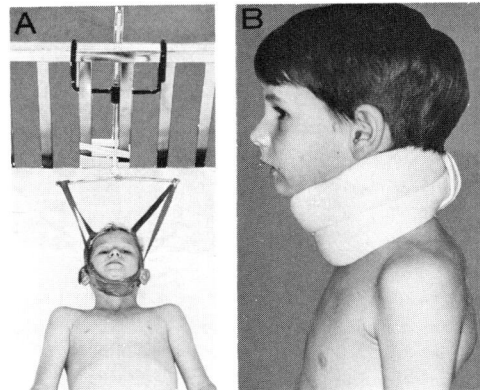

Figure 9–59 A. Continuous traction on the cervical spine through a leather head halter. B. A cervical "ruff" made of stockinette filled with cotton wool to provide temporary support for the cervical spine.

of the child's cervical spine may produce an appearance of subluxation, particularly between C2 and C3. Nevertheless, true subluxations or even dislocations may occur as the result of a severe injury (Fig. 9–60A).

Such injuries are best reduced by skull tong traction; the reduction is maintained by means of a body and head (Minerva) cast for eight weeks. If the injured segment is still unstable at the end of this time, local spinal arthrodesis is indicated (Fig. 9–60B).

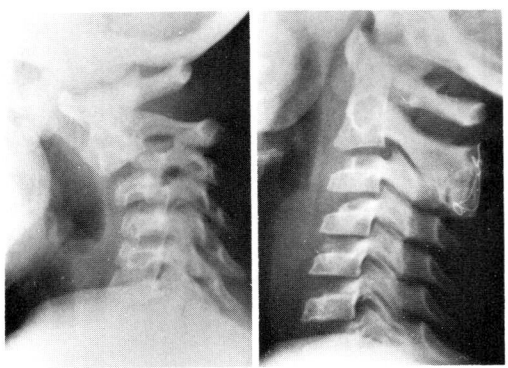

Figure 9–60 A. Traumatic anterior subluxation of C2 on C3 in a five-year-old boy who had fallen on his head during a fight. He had marked muscle spasm in his neck and a tingling sensation (paresthesia) in one arm. B. The anterior subluxation of C2 on C3 had been reduced by skull tong traction, but was still unstable despite eight weeks' immobilization in a Minerva cast. Consequently, a local posterior spinal arthrodesis was performed to provide permanent stability of the joint.

Thoracic Spine

Since fractures of the normal thoracic spine are relatively uncommon in childhood, the presence of such a fracture should always raise the possibility that it is of the pathological type.

A compression fracture of a thoracic vertebral body may result from a severe fall (Fig. 9–61). The posterior longitudinal ligaments of the spine remain intact, hence there is no injury to the spinal cord. The prognosis is excellent, and no attempt at reduction of the slight deformity is necessary. Although such an injury in a responsible adult can be treated by protection alone, in active, uninhibited children it is wiser to immobilize the spine in a body cast for eight weeks.

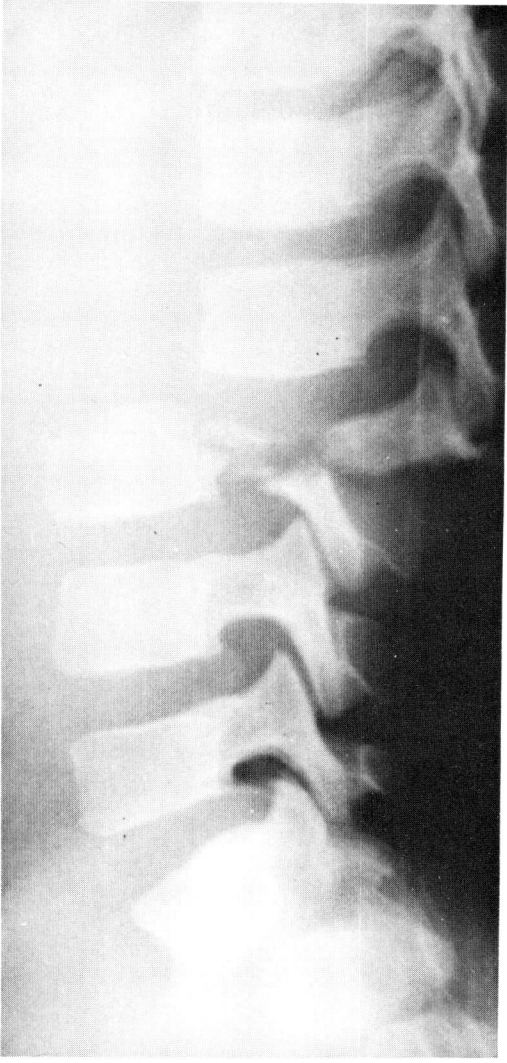

Figure 9–61 Compression fractures of two thoracic vertebrae in a 14-year-old boy who had sustained a severe fall while skiing. Note that the two vertebral bodies have been crushed anteriorly and are consequently somewhat wedge-shaped.

Figure 9–62 Severe fracture-dislocation of the lumbar spine in a child who had been struck by an automobile. The injury was complicated by damage to the cauda equina.

Lumbar Spine

In children, the lumbar segments of the spine are particularly mobile; thus, violent trauma is required to produce either a fracture or a dislocation in this region. Such violent trauma tends to produce a fracture–dislocation of the lumbar spine with resultant injury to the cauda equina (Fig. 9–62).

After closed reduction of the displacement, immobilization in a body cast for eight weeks may be sufficient to stabilize the spine, particularly if there has been an associated fracture. If there is any residual instability of the spine at the end of this time, spinal arthrodesis is indicated.

THE FOOT

Fractures of the Metatarsals

An isolated fracture of a single metatarsal is not common in childhood. More common are fractures of several metatarsals, usually the result of a crushing injury, such as a heavy object dropping on the child's foot; the local arteries and veins are usually injured also. Realignment of the metatarsals by manipulation is important, but even more important is elevation of the foot to minimize soft tissue swelling, which tends to be excessive. Tight encircling bandages and casts are contraindicated because of the associated vascular injury and the risk of ischemia. Furthermore, the child should avoid weight bearing for at least three weeks, after which a walking cast should be applied and retained for an additional three weeks.

Avulsion Fracture of the Base of the Fifth Metatarsal. Occasionally, in an older child a sudden inversion injury of the foot causes an avulsion of the bony insertion of the peroneus brevis tendon into the base of the fifth metatarsal, an insertion that may be into a separate center of ossification. Local tenderness and comparable radiographic projections of the opposite foot are helpful in assessing the injury. A walking cast applied with the foot in a position of eversion provides comfort for the child during the four weeks required for healing.

Fracture of the Os Calcis. In children the cancellous bone of the os calcis is relatively resistant to fracture. Nevertheless, a crush or compression type of fracture may occur when a child falls from a considerable height and lands on the heels. Under these circumstances, the child's spine should also be examined both clinically and radiographically because of the high incidence of a coexistent compression fracture of a vertebral body.

After a few days of bed rest with the foot elevated, the child may be allowed up on crutches without bearing weight on the injured foot for several weeks. Active exercises during this period help to regain a normal range of motion in the subtalar joint. In older children, as in adults, an intraarticular fracture of the os calcis may require open reduction.

THE ANKLE AND LEG

During childhood all significant fractures about the ankle involve an epiphyseal plate and therefore should be considered in relation to the particular type of epiphyseal plate injury as classified earlier.

Type 1 Injury of the Distal Fibular Epiphysis

Avulsion of the distal fibular epiphysis may be caused by a sudden inversion injury of the ankle. If the epiphysis returns immediately to its normal position, the child may seem to have merely sprained the ankle, since radiographic examination will be negative. Marked local tenderness at the site of the epiphyseal plate is an indication to obtain stress radiographs which may reveal evidence of occult joint instability due to separation of the epiphysis, as previously described (Fig. 9–9).

Treatment consists of a below-knee walking cast for three weeks. The prognosis for subsequent growth is excellent.

Type 2 Injury of the Distal Tibial Epiphysis

Even severely displaced type 2 epiphyseal plate injuries around the ankle can be readily reduced by closed means. Furthermore, the reduction can be well maintained provided there is appropriate molding of

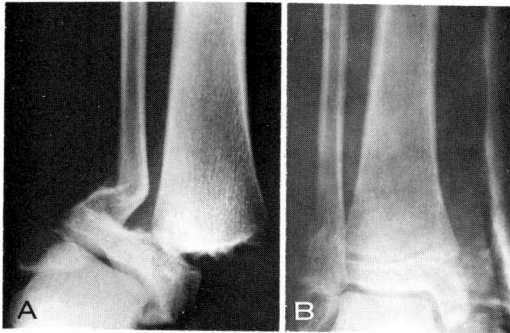

Figure 9–63 A. Severely displaced Type 2 fracture-separation of the distal tibial epiphysis combined with a greenstick fracture of the distal third of the fibula in a 13-year-old boy. The intact periosteal hinge is on the lateral aspect of the tibia. B. After closed reduction the fragments are in satisfactory position and the reduction is maintained by a well-molded plaster cast.

the plaster cast (Fig. 9–63). Healing is usually complete within three weeks, and the prognosis for subsequent growth is excellent.

Type 3 Injury of the Distal Tibial Epiphysis

In older children who are almost fully grown, a severe ankle injury may fracture the anterolateral corner of the distal tibial epiphysis—the last part of the epiphysis to become fused to the metaphysis.

This injury is more readily detected in the lateral radiographic projection than in the anteroposterior projection (Fig. 9–64). Since the fracture is intraarticular, open reduction is indicated to obtain perfect restoration of the joint surfaces.

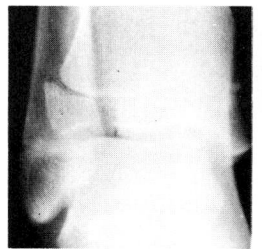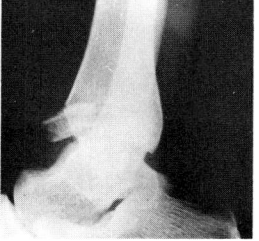

Figure 9–64 Type 3 injury of the distal tibial epiphysis in a 14-year-old boy. Note that the displacement of the anterolateral corner of the epiphysis is more obvious in the lateral projection than in the anteroposterior projection.

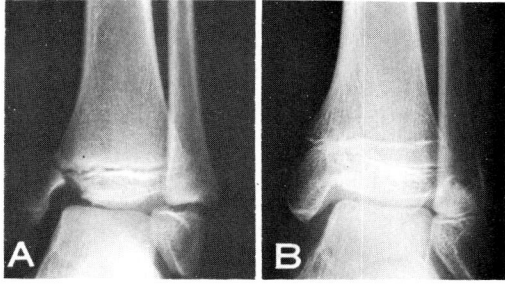

Figure 9–65 Type 4 injury of the distal tibial epiphysis. A. Note that the fracture line begins at the joint surface, crosses the epiphyseal plate, and extends into the metaphysis. The entire medial malleolus is shifted medially and proximally. This fracture should have been treated by open reduction and internal fixation. Also notice the Type 1 injury of the distal fibular epiphysis. B. One year after injury a growth disturbance is apparent; the medial part of the distal tibial epiphysis has ceased growing while the lateral part has continued to grow. The varus deformity of the ankle will be progressive.

Type 4 Injury of the Distal Tibial Epiphysis

A severe inversion injury of the ankle may produce a type 4 fracture through the medial portion of the distal tibial epiphyseal plate. The fracture line, which begins at the ankle joint surface, crosses the epiphyseal plate and extends into the metaphysis. Like type 4 injuries elsewhere, the fracture is unstable.

This is a treacherous injury, which requires open reduction and internal fixation to obtain and maintain perfect apposition of the fracture fragments. Indeed, even a slight residual disparity at the level of the fractured surfaces of the epiphyseal plate leads inevitably to a serious growth disturbance (Fig. 9–65).

Type 5 Injury of the Distal Tibial Epiphysis

When a child gets one foot caught, for example, between the pickets of a fence and then falls, the severe angulation of the ankle produces a tremendous compression force on the distal tibial epiphysis and epiphyseal plate. The result may be a type 5 epiphyseal plate injury.

Despite the paucity of clinical and radiographic evidence of the injury, the prognosis for subsequent growth is very poor

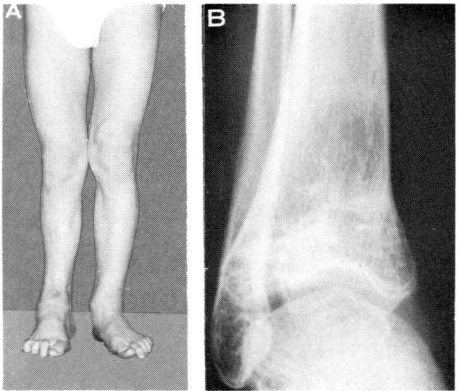

Figure 9–66 Type 5 injury of the distal tibial epiphysis. *A.* Clinical varus deformity of the ankle in a nine-year-old boy five years after a fall from a considerable height. He landed on his right foot and was thought to have sustained "only a sprained ankle." One year later he began to develop a progressive deformity of his ankle. Note also the shortening of the right leg. *B.* A radiograph of the ankle reveals a growth disturbance of the distal tibial epiphysis. Growth had ceased in the medial part of the epiphyseal plate because of a Type 5 crushing injury but had continued in the lateral part and also in the fibular epiphysis with a resultant varus deformity and shortening.

indeed (Fig. 9–66). When a type 5 injury is supected, the child should be kept from bearing weight on the ankle for at least three weeks in an attempt to prevent further compression of the epiphyseal plate. Regardless of treatment, however, subsequent growth disturbance is almost inevitable.

Fracture of the Tibia

The majority of tibial shaft fractures in children are relatively undisplaced, and this may be explained in part by the strong periosteal sleeve which is not readily torn across. Consequently, such fractures are relatively stable and can be adequately treated by closed reduction. Widely displaced open fractures of the tibia and fibula, however, can result from major trauma, such as an automobile accident (Fig. 9–67).

Closed reduction of a fractured tibial shaft must correct both angulatory and rotational deformities. The reduction is best maintained by the application of a long leg cast with the knee flexed to a right angle, not only to control rotation but also to prevent the child from bearing weight. After four weeks in such a cast the fracture is usually sufficiently healed that a long leg walking

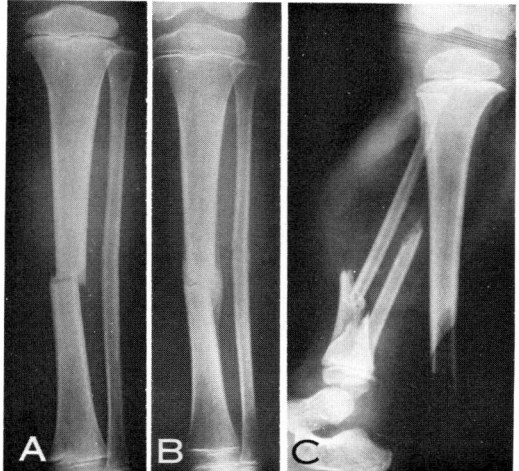

Figure 9–67 Fractures of the tibial shaft. *A.* Relatively undisplaced and stable fracture of the tibial shaft in a six-year-old girl. No reduction was required. *B.* Six weeks later the fracture is clinically united. *C.* Widely displaced open fracture of the tibia and fibula of a five-year-old boy who was run over by a truck. The skin was split open from the ankle to the knee and there was extensive soft-tissue damage. Note the marked overriding and external rotation at the fracture site. After thorough debridement the fractures were reduced and the soft tissues were repaired. Both bones and soft tissues healed without infection.

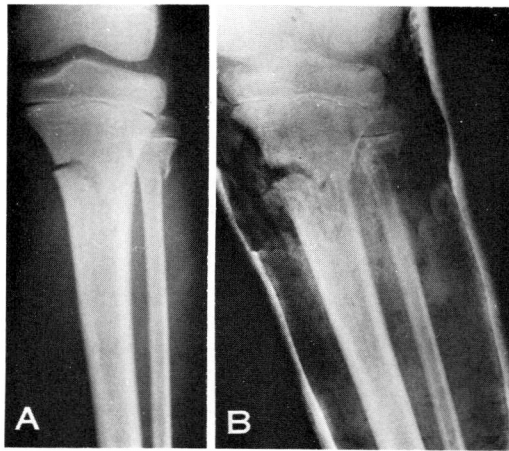

Figure 9–68 *A.* Slightly angulated fracture in the metaphyseal region of the upper end of the left tibia of a nine-year-old boy. Even this slight angulation should be corrected by manipulation, and no weight bearing should be allowed in the early stages of healing. Regrettably, the boy was treated with a long-leg walking cast. *B.* With weight bearing the angulation increased over the ensuing six weeks. This angulatory deformity cannot be expected to correct spontaneously.

cast can be applied and retained for an additional four weeks. There is virtually no indication for open reduction of an uncomplicated fracture of the tibial shaft in children.

Correction of alignment is particularly important when the fracture is in the proximal metaphysis of the tibia, since neither valgus nor varus deformities can be expected to correct spontaneously with subsequent growth (Fig. 9–68).

Fractures of the proximal third of the tibia and fibula are potentially serious because of the risk of injury to the anterior and posterior tibial arteries at the upper border of the interosseous membrane.

THE KNEE AND THIGH

The most significant injuries about the knee in children involve the epiphyseal plate of either the proximal tibial epiphysis or the distal femoral epiphysis.

Type 2 Injury of the Proximal Tibial Epiphysis

The attachment of the proximal tibial epiphysis to the metaphysis is particularly strong because of its irregular contour; consequently, a severe injury is required to separate it. A severe hyperextension injury of the knee may produce a type 2 fracture–separation of the proximal tibial epiphysis which, though not common, is serious because of the risk of injury to the popliteal artery (Fig. 9–69).

Type 2 Injury of the Distal Femoral Epiphysis

The distal femoral epiphysis is more often separated from its metaphysis than is the proximal tibial epiphysis. A hyperextension injury may produce a type 2 fracture–separation of the epiphysis. The metaphysis of the femur tears the posterior periosteum and is driven posteriorly into the soft tissues of the popliteal fossa where it may injure the popliteal artery as well as the medial or lateral popliteal nerves.

Clinical examination reveals a grossly swollen knee because of the associated hemarthrosis; radiographic examination re-

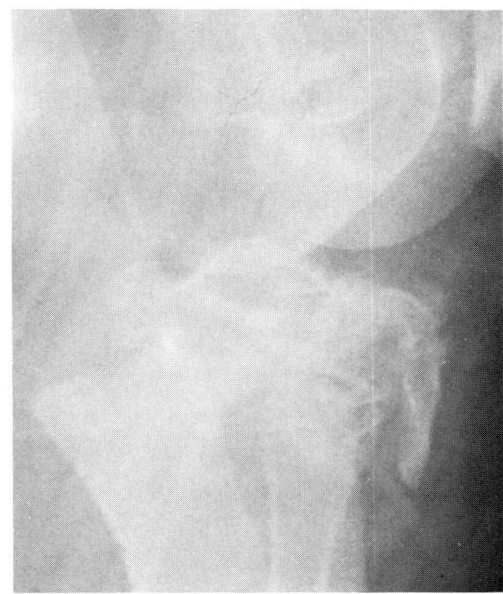

Figure 9–69 Type 2 injury of the proximal tibial epiphysis in a 14-year-old boy who was hit on the anterior aspect of the tibia by an automobile. This injury was complicated by severe damage to the popliteal artery, which necessitated local resection of the damaged portion of the artery and replacement by a vein graft.

veals a striking displacement of the epiphysis (Fig. 9–70).

This fracture–separation may be difficult to reduce unless the child is lying face down. Reduction then becomes comparable to that for a supracondylar fracture of the

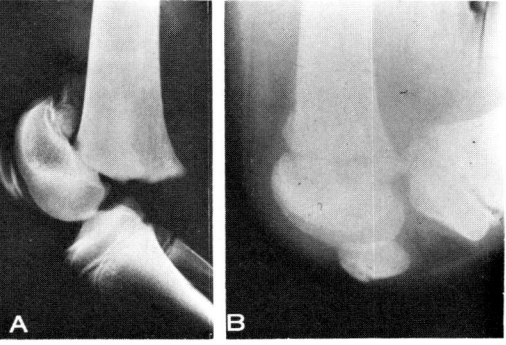

Figure 9–70 A. Type 2 injury of the distal femoral epiphysis in a 13-year-old boy as the result of a hyperextension injury of the knee. Note the large triangular fragment anteriorly, the side of the intact periosteal hinge. *B.* After reduction the epiphysis is in good position and the reduction is maintained by the flexed position of the knee.

humerus. Traction is applied to the leg with the knee slightly flexed, after which the epiphysis can be pushed into its normal position. The reduction is maintained by completely flexing the knee, since this tightens the intact anterior hinge of periosteum. The lower limb is immobilized in a cast in this position for only three weeks, after which active exercises are begun. Since this is a type 2 injury, the prognosis concerning subsequent growth is excellent.

Type 4 Injury of the Distal Femoral Epiphysis

Fortunately, this serious type of epiphyseal plate injury is uncommon at the knee. Because it is a type 4 fracture that traverses the joint surface as well as the epiphyseal plate, the prognosis for subsequent growth is very poor unless the reduction is perfect (Fig. 9–71).

This type of injury is extremely important to recognize, because with accurate open reduction and secure internal fixation the otherwise inevitable growth disturbance can be prevented.

Traumatic Dislocation of the Patella

Older children and adolescents, particularly girls who have some degree of genu valgum and generalized ligamentous laxity, may sustain a lateral dislocation of the patella owing to an abduction, external rotation injury to the knee. The patient experiences sharp pain, her knee gives way completely, and she falls.

Diagnosis. Physical examination reveals a grossly swollen knee as a result of a gross hemarthrosis. The patella can be felt lying on the lateral aspect of the knee. Sometimes, however, the patella has already slid back spontaneously into its normal position before the patient is seen.

Radiographic examination must include a tangential superoinferior (skyline) projection to detect the presence of an associated osteochondral fracture of either the medial edge of the patella or the lateral lip of the patellar groove, the site of impact as the patella dislocates laterally.

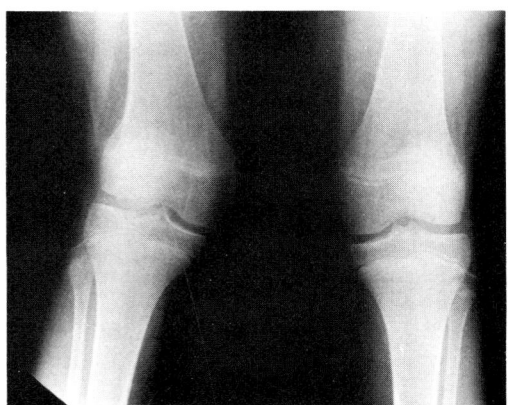

Figure 9–71 Type 4 injury of the right distal femoral epiphysis of a 12-year-old boy one year after injury. The fracture began at the joint surface of the lateral femoral condyle, crossed the epiphyseal plate, and extended into the metaphysis. The lateral condyle was displaced proximally and should have been treated by open reduction and internal fixation, but unfortunately it was not. One year after injury growth has ceased in the lateral part of the epiphyseal plate but has continued in the medial part with a resultant progressive valgus deformity.

Treatment. If there is no osteochondral fracture, the dislocated patella can be reduced by closed manipulation with the knee in the extended position. The knee is then immobilized in a cylinder cast (ankle to groin) in extension for six weeks. The presence of an osteochondral fracture is an indication for open operation, with removal of the fragment and repair of the torn soft tissues. During and after the period of immobilization, quadriceps exercises are important in attempting to prevent recurrence of the dislocation.

Complications. Recurring dislocation of the patella is a troublesome complication of this injury (Fig. 9–72). Moreover, with each dislocation the articular cartilage of the patella is injured, and this leads to the development of chrondromalacia of the patella and eventually to degenerative joint disease of the knee. Thus, recurring dislocation of the patella is an indication for a reconstructive operation that involves the release of tight structures on the lateral side of the joint, repair of the fibrous joint capsule on the medial side, and redirection of the line of pull of the patellar tendon by means of a tenodesis (using the semitendinosus tendon). In a growing child this type of operation is safer than that in which the

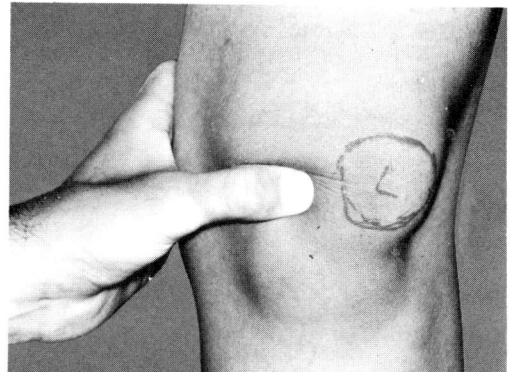

Figure 9-72   Recurring dislocation of the left patella in a 14-year-old girl who exhibited generalized ligamentous laxity. The patella could almost be dislocated by simply pushing it laterally with the thumb.

tibial tubercle is transplanted, since interference with the tibial tubercle (which includes part of the proximal tibial epiphyseal plate) may cause a serious growth disturbance.

Internal Derangements of the Knee

The semilunar cartilages (menisci) of the knee in children are resilient and relatively resistant to disruption. For this reason torn menisci are uncommon in young children. Nevertheless, they may occur in older children and adolescents as a result of injuries incurred in such sports as skiing, football, and hockey. Meniscal injuries and their treatment are discussed in Chapter 24.

Fractures of the Femoral Shaft

Displaced fractures of the femoral shaft are common in childhood and merit special consideration. Usually involving the middle third of the femur, the fracture may be transverse, oblique, spiral, or even comminuted, depending on the mechanism of injury. Even with marked displacement of the fragments, however, at least part of the strong periosteal sleeve remains intact, a point of considerable importance in relation to treatment and healing of the fracture.

Diagnosis. The diagnosis is obvious from clinical examination alone because of the typical deformity (Fig. 9-73). Since

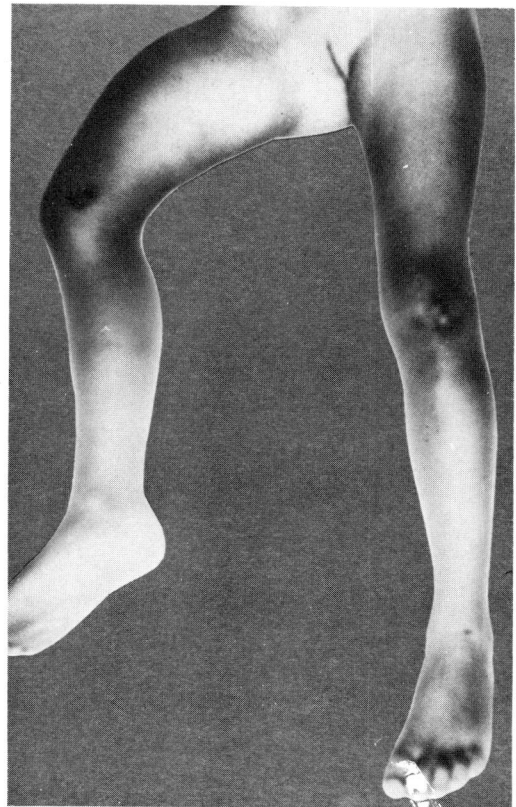

Figure 9-73   Clinical deformity in the thigh of a child with a displaced fracture of the right femoral shaft. Note the angulation, external rotation, and shortening.

these fractures are extremely unstable, it is essential to apply a temporary splint before radiographic examination is undertaken, not only to spare the child unnecessary pain but also to prevent further injury to the femoral artery.

Treatment. The basis of treatment for unstable fractures of the femoral shaft in children is continuous traction until the fracture is "sticky" (partially healed and hence relatively stable and painless), after which the healing femur is immobilized in a hip spica cast until it is clinically united. There is virtually no indication for open reduction of an uncomplicated femoral shaft fracture in a child. The type and duration of traction depends on the age of the child.

Children under the age of two years can be treated by overhead (Bryant's) skin traction which is applied to both lower limbs (Fig. 9-74). In children over the age

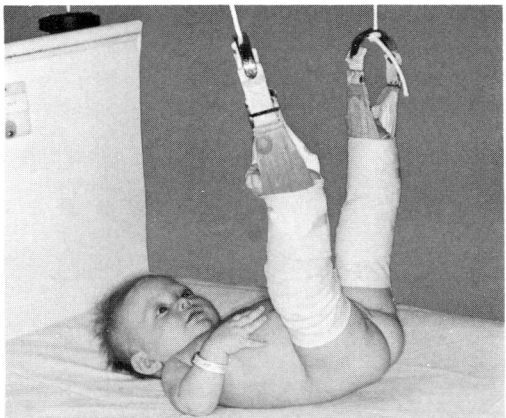

Figure 9–74 Continuous overhead (Bryant's) skin traction in the treatment of a fracture of the shaft of the left femur in a six-month-old baby girl. Note that both lower limbs are included in the traction and that the baby's buttocks are just clear of the bed.

of two years, however, overhead traction is potentially dangerous because of the risk of femoral arterial spasm and consequent Volkmann's ischemia of nerves and muscles (comparable to that seen in the upper limb as a complication of supracondylar fractures of the humerus).

Thus, in children over the age of two years, fractures of the femoral shaft are best treated by continuous traction of the fixed type in a Thomas splint which is slightly bent at the knee with the child lying on an inclined frame (Fig. 9–75).

Reduction of femoral shaft fractures in children is achieved gradually by the traction apparatus rather than by manipulation.

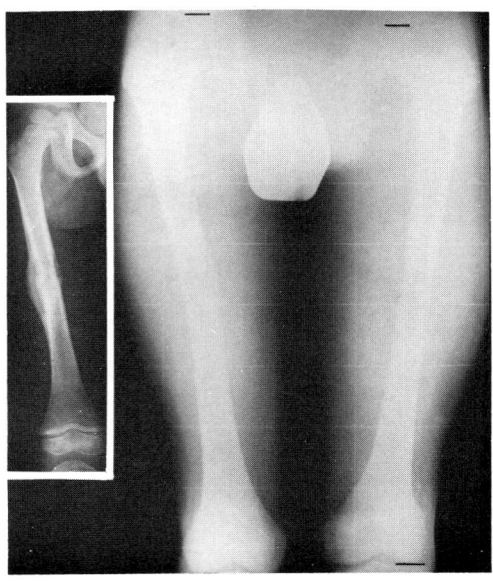

Figure 9–76 Overgrowth of the right femur after a perfectly reduced fracture of the midshaft at age five years (*inset*). Eight years later the right femur is 1.2 cm longer than the left.

Angulatory and rotational deformities must be completely corrected since these deformities do not correct spontaneously. For reasons discussed at the beginning of this chapter, temporary overgrowth always occurs after displaced fractures of the femoral shaft. The average amount of overgrowth is 1 cm, and any residual discrepancy in length one year after the fracture is

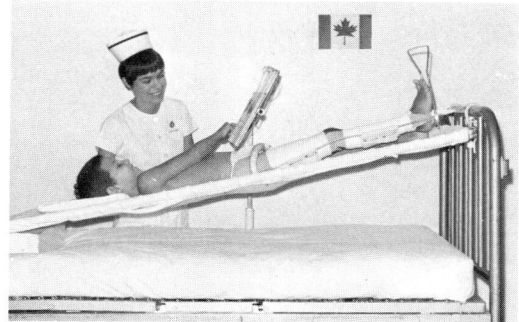

Figure 9–75 Continuous skin traction combined with a Thomas splint slightly bent at the knee for the treatment of an unstable fracture of the midshaft of the right femur in an eight-year-old boy.

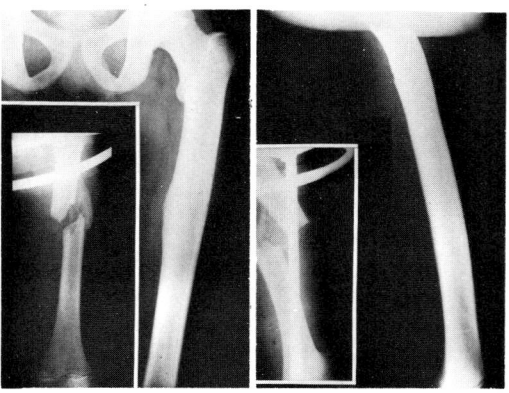

Figure 9–77 Remodeling after a displaced fracture of the femoral shaft at age six years (*insets*). Seven years later the fracture deformity has been beautifully remodeled.

permanent (Fig. 9–76). It is obvious that the ideal position in which to allow the fragments to unite is side-to-side (bayonet) apposition with approximately 1 cm of overriding. This intentional shortening is compensated within one year by the overgrowth, as discussed earlier (Fig. 9–8).

Remodeling of the healed femoral shaft fracture is remarkable during the growing years. Although residual angulation and rotation at the fracture site do not correct spontaneously, side-to-side apposition is beautifully remodeled over a period of years (Fig. 9–77).

Complications. The most serious complication of femoral shaft fractures in children is Volkmann's ischemia of nerves and muscles due to femoral arterial spasm. The spasm, which in turn may be secondary to a tear of the intima, is further aggravated by excessive traction on the fractured limb. The clinical manifestations of impending Volkmann's ischemia in the lower limb are the same as those in the upper limb—pain, pallor, puffiness, pulselessness, paresthesia, and paralysis. Thus, children being treated for a fracture of the femoral shaft should not be given analgesics. A well-controlled fracture should not be a source of pain, and therefore if the child has severe and constant pain—especially pain in the calf—the most likely cause is impending ischemia. Analgesics may mask this important warning signal and for this reason are contraindicated.

The moment impending Volkmann's ischemia is suspected, all encircling bandages should be removed immediately. The skin traction should be replaced by skeletal traction through the distal metaphysis of the femur, with the hip and knee flexed. If the

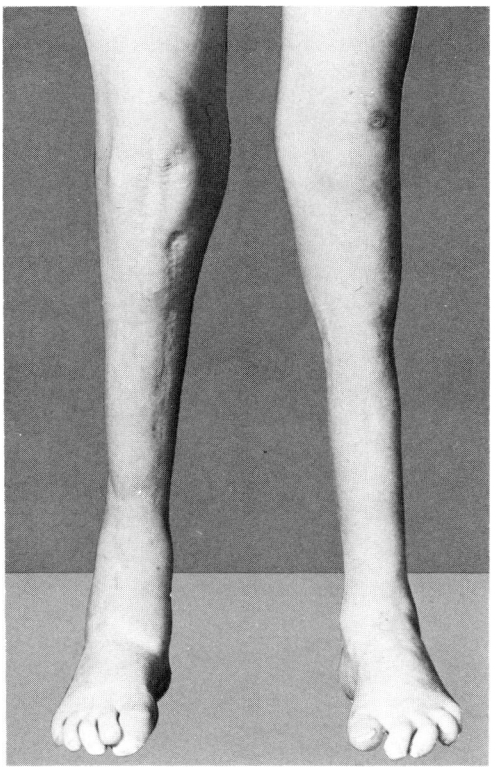

Figure 9–78 Residual Volkmann's ischemic contracture of both lower limbs in a seven-year-old boy who had been treated in overhead (Bryant's) traction for bilateral fractured femora at age five years, much beyond the age when overhead traction is safe. During the first two days of traction the boy had complained of severe pain in both legs. The ill-advised use of analgesics relieved the pain somewhat and this masked the relentless development of severe Volkmann's ischemia until the nerve and muscle damage was irreversible. This is a preventable tragedy.

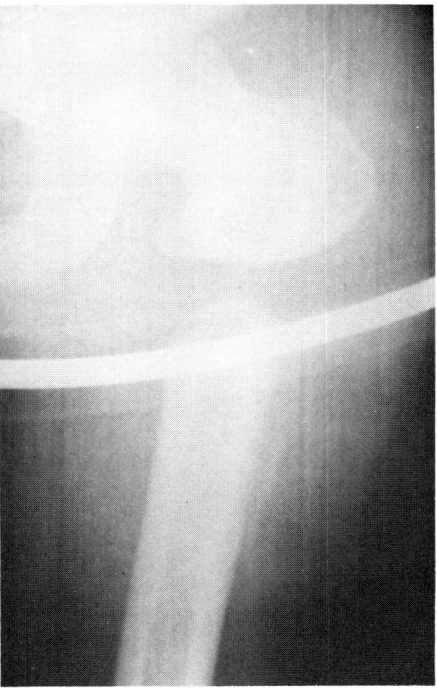

Figure 9–79 Subtrochanteric fracture of the left femur in a 14-year-old girl. Note the ring of the Thomas splint. In this anteroposterior projection the proximal fragment is flexed to 90 degrees; you are looking into its medullary cavity, which is represented by the round radiolucent area.

peripheral circulation has not been reestablished within half an hour, exploration of the artery is indicated, as described in Chapter 33 in relation to Volkmann's ischemia. The permanent effects of Volkmann's ischemia and subsequent Volkmann's ischemic contracture are tragic (Fig. 9–78).

Fractures of the Subtrochanteric Region of the Femur

When the femoral fracture is just distal to the trochanters, the muscles inserted into the proximal fragment, particularly the iliopsoas and the glutei, pull it into a position of acute flexion, external rotation, and abduction (Fig. 9–79). Therefore, in order to obtain correct alignment of the fracture fragments, continuous traction must be so arranged as to bring the distal fragment up to and in line with the proximal fragment. This is best accomplished by continuous skeletal traction through the distal metaphysis of the femur, with the thigh flexed, externally rotated, and abducted (Fig. 9–80). The remainder of the treatment is

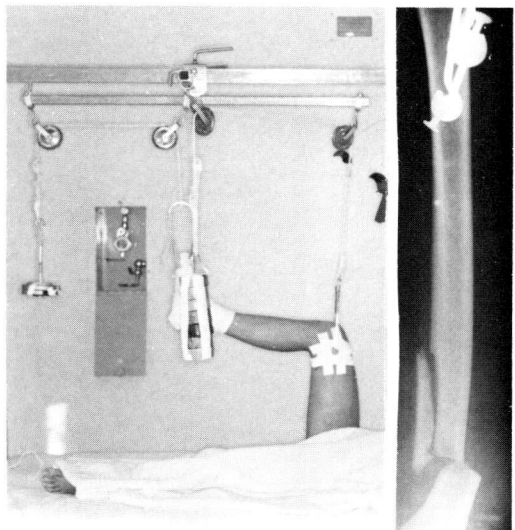

Figure 9–80 A. Continuous skeletal traction through a pin in the distal metaphysis for treatment of a subtrochanteric fracture of the femur. The distal fragment is thereby brought into line with the flexed proximal fragment. B. Lateral projection of the same fractured femur. Note the metal pin and stirrup in the region of the distal end of the femur. The distal fragment has been brought into line with the flexed proximal fragment. The comminution was not apparent in the anteroposterior projection.

comparable to that for a fracture of the midshaft of the femur in a child of the same age.

THE HIP AND PELVIS

Fractures of the Femoral Neck

The femoral neck in the child, unlike that in the elderly adult, is extremely strong, and consequently a severe injury is required to fracture it. Fractures of the femoral neck, therefore, are not common in childhood, but they are serious. The combination of the severe injury and the precarious blood supply to the femoral head lead to a high incidence of posttraumatic avascular necrosis. Moreover, as with femoral neck fractures in adults, they are extremely unstable and cannot be adequately treated either by closed reduction and external immobilization or by continuous traction.

Treatment. Displaced femoral neck fractures in children represent an absolute indication for internal skeletal fixation (Fig. 9–81). Since a child cannot be expected to refrain from weight-bearing during the healing phase of the fracture, it is necessary to supplement the internal fixation with a hip spica cast until the fracture is clinically united; this usually requires three months.

Complications. If internal skeletal fixation has not been used or if it has been

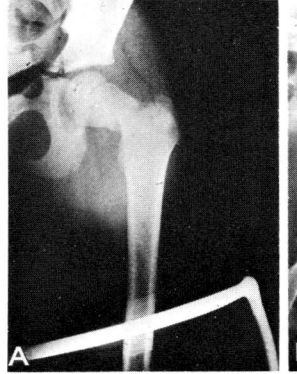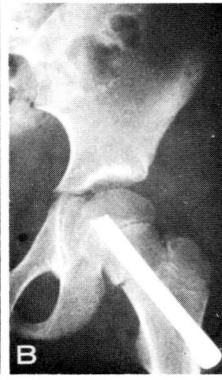

Figure 9–81 A. Fractured neck of femur in a 10-year-old boy. Note the ring of the Thomas splint. B. After closed reduction and percutaneous nailing, the fragments are in satisfactory position. Three threaded pins would have been equally satisfactory for internal fixation of this fracture.

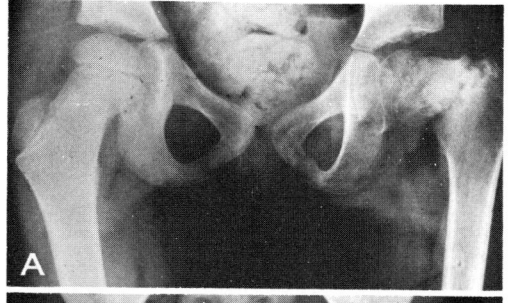

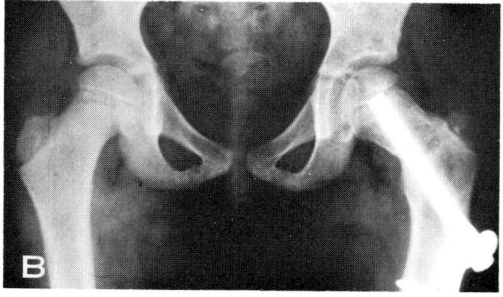

Figure 9–82 A. Nonunion of a fracture of the left femoral neck in a nine-year-old boy. Note the sclerosis at the fracture site and the coxa vara deformity with resultant shortening of the limb. This fracture should have been treated by internal skeletal fixation. *B.* Correction of the deformity and union of the fracture were obtained by means of an operation that included bone grafting and the use of a nail and plate.

inadequate, fractures of the femoral neck in children are likely to be complicated by *nonunion* and a progressive coxa vara deformity (Fig. 9–82).

When the femoral head has lost its blood supply by disruption of its vessels at the time of a fracture, the result is *posttraumatic avascular necrosis*, a complication that occurs in approximately 30 per cent of children with this injury. There is little radiographic evidence of this complication until several months have elapsed. The ossific nucleus stops growing for at least six months after injury and at first appears *relatively* radio-opaque (relative to the posttraumatic osteoporosis of the living bone in the acetabulum and femoral shaft). Later, when the ossific nucleus is being revascularized and reossified, it appears *absolutely* radio-opaque as new bone is laid down on dead trabeculae. Subsequently, the femoral head may become deformed. The treatment of the complication of posttraumatic avascular necrosis of the femoral

head in children is the same as that for Legg-Perthes' disease.

Type 1 Injury of the Proximal Femoral Epiphysis

This uncommon but serious injury carries the same risk of avascular necrosis of the femoral head as do fractures of the femoral neck and for the same reasons (Fig. 9–83). Like the femoral neck fracture, a type 1 injury of the proximal femoral epiphysis should be treated by internal skeletal fixation, usually with two or more threaded wires. After the injury has healed, the

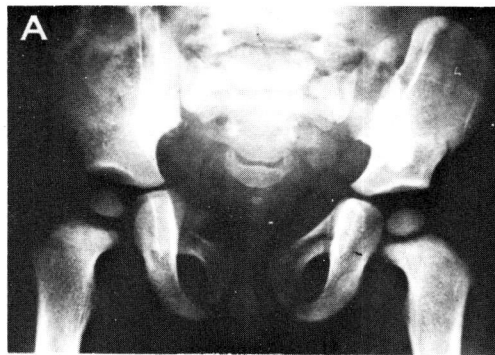

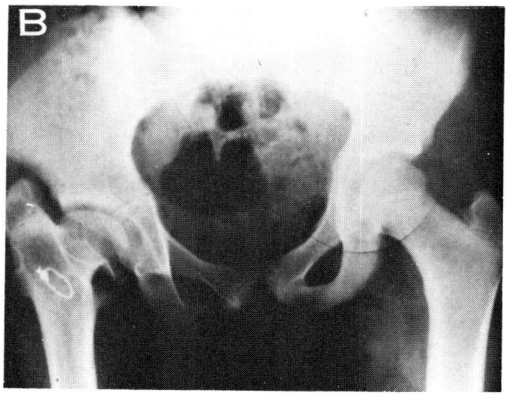

Figure 9–83 Type 1 injury of the proximal femoral epiphysis in a one-year-old child who had been struck by a truck. A. Note the obvious fractures of the pelvis. Less obvious is the increased distance between the proximal femoral epiphysis and metaphysis on the right side indicating a type 1 epiphyseal separation. *B.* Ten years later there is deformity of the femoral head (coxa plana), marked shortening of the femoral neck and coxa vara. (The wire loop is at the site of a previous osteotomy of the femur.)

threaded wires should be removed to avoid a growth disturbance.

Traumatic Dislocation of the Hip

The normal hip joint is most vulnerable to dislocation when it is in a position of flexion and adduction. In this position, a force transmitted along the shaft of the femur (as may occur from a dashboard injury or a fall on the flexed knee) may drive the femoral head posteriorly over the labrum, or lip, of the acetabulum to produce a posterior dislocation. Since the femoral head escapes through a rent in the capsule, it is an extracapsular type of dislocation.

Diagnosis. The clinical deformity of a posterior dislocation of the hip — flexion, adduction, and internal rotation — is characteristic (Fig. 9–84). Traumatic anterior dislocation of the hip is rare in childhood, but when it does occur the hip is held in the opposite position — extension, abduction, and external rotation. Posterior dislocation is obvious radiographically (Fig. 9–85).

Treatment. As long as the hip is dislo-

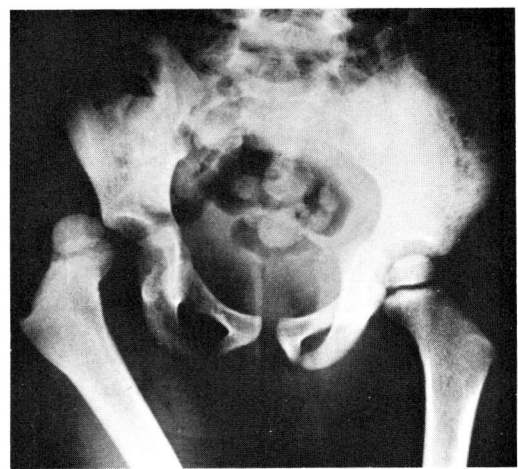

Figure 9–85 Traumatic posterior dislocation of the right hip suffered by the patient shown in Figure 9–84.

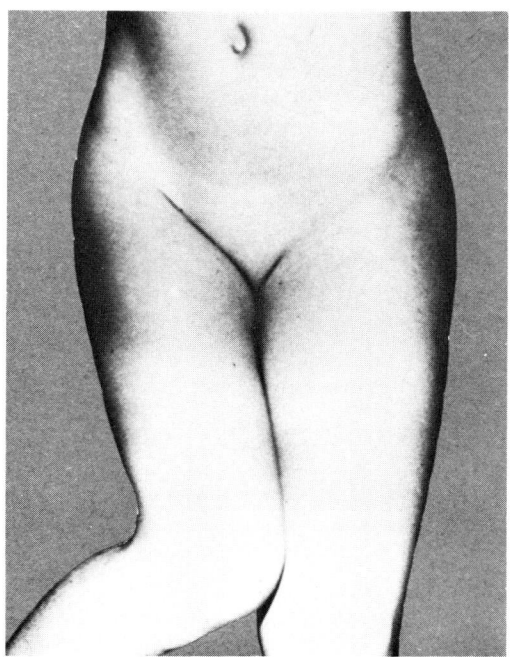

Figure 9–84 The typical clinical deformity of a child with traumatic posterior dislocation of the right hip — flexion, adduction, internal rotation, and apparent shortening.

cated, the torn capsule and surrounding structures constrict the femoral neck vessels, thereby jeopardizing the blood supply to the femoral head. For this reason traumatic dislocation of the hip represents an emergency. The dislocation should be reduced as soon as possible in an attempt to prevent the serious complication of avascular necrosis of the femoral head. Indeed, in children whose hips are reduced within eight hours of the time of injury, the incidence of avascular necrosis is low. However, in those whose hips have remained unreduced for longer than eight hours, the incidence of this complication is high (approximately 40 per cent).

Closed reduction is accomplished by applying upward traction on the flexed thigh and by forward pressure on the femoral head from behind. After reduction, which must be perfect both clinically and radiographically, a hip spica cast is applied with the hip in its most stable position — extension, abduction, and external rotation. Immobilization of the reduced hip is maintained for eight weeks to allow strong healing of the torn capsule.

Complications. The acetabular margin, being largely cartilaginous in children, is seldom fractured, and the sciatic nerve is seldom injured. The complication of post-traumatic avascular necrosis of the femoral head has been described earlier in relation to fractures of the femoral neck.

PELVIS

The pelvis of a child is more flexible and hence more yielding than that of an adult because of the cartilaginous components at the sacroiliac joints, triradiate cartilages, and symphysis pubis. Consequently, serious fractures of the pelvis are not common in childhood, although they do occur as the result of a severe injury, such as an automobile accident.

The most important aspects of fractures of the pelvis in children are not the fractures themselves but rather the associated complications—especially extensive internal hemorrhage from torn vessels, and extravasation of urine from rupture of the bladder or urethra.

Diagnosis. Physical examination reveals local swelling and tenderness. In unstable fractures there may also be deformity of the hips as well as instability of the pelvic ring. Special radiographic projections are required to assess the precise nature of a pelvic fracture, since the anteroposterior projection provides only a two-dimensional image of the injury. The lateral projection, which would normally provide the third dimension, is unsatisfactory because of overlap of the two innominate bones. Thus, in order to obtain a three-dimensional view of the disturbed anatomy of the injury, it is necessary to obtain: (1) an anteroposterior projection, (2) a tangential projection in the plane of the pelvic ring (with the tube directed upward 50 degrees and, (3) an inlet projection looking down into the pelvic ring with the tube directed downwards 60 degrees.

Treatment. The *emergency care* of a child with a fractured pelvis centers on the two major complications.

The pelvis is a particularly vascular area, and displaced fractures of the pelvis may tear vessels (such as the large superior gluteal artery) with resultant major hemorrhage. A child may lose as much as 60 per cent of circulating blood volume into the peripelvic and retroperitoneal tissues and develop severe hemorrhagic shock.

While the child is being treated for shock, a catheter should be inserted into the bladder to investigate the possibility of associated injury to the bladder or urethra. If there is blood in the urethra and a catheter cannot be passed, the urethra is almost certainly torn. Hence, a suprapubic cystotomy must be performed pending surgical repair of the urethra. If the catheter can be passed into the bladder and the urine contains blood, a cystogram should be carried out immediately to determine if the bladder has been ruptured, in which case it should be repaired as soon as possible.

Since the bone of the pelvis is principally cancellous and since its blood supply is abundant, fractures of the pelvis unite rapidly. Treatment of the various types of fractures is aimed at correcting significant fracture deformities in order to prevent malunion and resultant disturbance of function.

Stable Fractures of the Pelvis

Fractures that do not transgress the pelvic ring do not interfere with stability of the pelvis in relation to weight bearing and do not require reduction.

In children, particularly in athletic boys, a sudden violent pull on the hamstring muscles may avulse their origin, the ischial apophysis. This injury usually heals well but may result in a fibrous union.

Isolated fractures of the ilium are of little significance and require only protection from weight bearing until pain subsides, within a few weeks.

A "straddle" injury of the pelvis (which may occur as a child loses his footing while

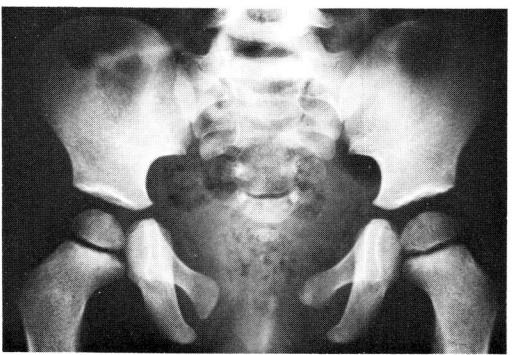

Figure 9–86 Traumatic separation of the symphysis pubis in a two-year-old child. Both sacroiliac joints have been spread open also. The separation was reduced by internal rotation of both hips, and the open internal rotation was maintained in a hip spica cast.

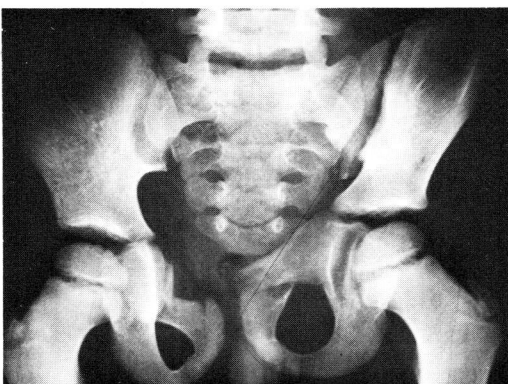

Figure 9–87 "Bucket-handle" type of unstable fracture of the pelvis of a nine-year-old boy who was run over by a truck. Note the vertical fracture just lateral to the left sacroiliac joint and the fractures of the superior pubic rami. The left half of this child's pelvis has been displaced forward and inward. The displacement was reduced by external rotation of the left hip, and the reduction was maintained in a hip spica cast.

Unstable Fractures of the Pelvis

Complete separation of the symphysis pubis and opening out of the pelvic ring is best reduced by internally rotating both hips; the reduction is maintained in a well-molded hip spica cast (Fig. 9–86).

Lateral compression of the pelvis may produce a "bucket handle" fracture, in which the fractured half of the pelvis rolls forward and inward (Fig. 9–87). In children this type of fracture can usually be managed by externally rotating the lower limb, and the reduction can be maintained by the application of a well-molded hip spica cast.

Unstable fractures in which one half of the pelvis is driven proximally by an upward thrust require continous skeletal traction through the femur to obtain and maintain reduction.

walking along the top of a fence) may cause one or more fractures of the inferior pubic rami but, more important, is likely to produce a tear of the urethra.

CHILD ABUSE

Distasteful and difficult to understand as it may be, the tragic truth remains that some

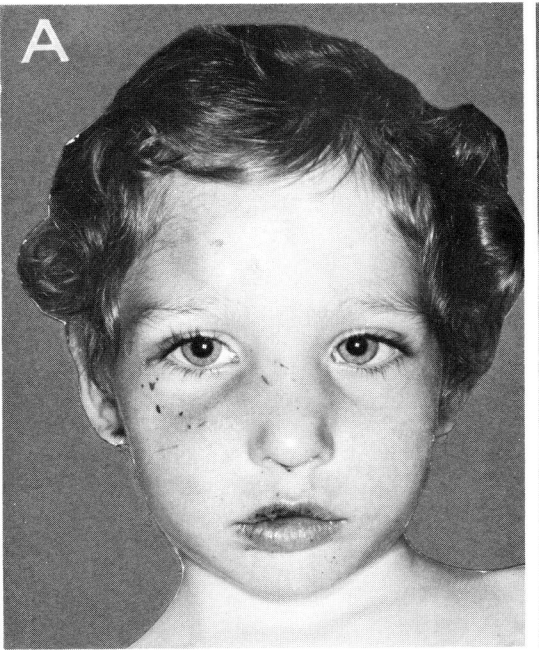
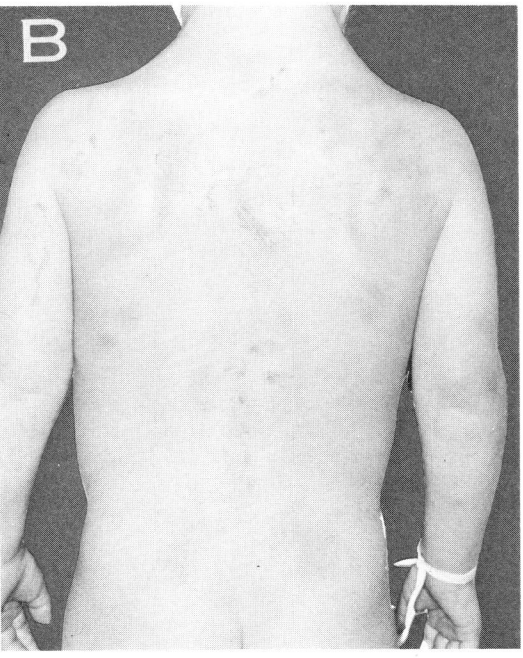

Figure 9–88 Child abuse. This sad looking five-year-old girl was brought to hospital with a history of having "fallen in the garden." Note the bruising and abrasions over the right side of her face. Further examination revealed multiple bruises in various stages of resolution over the girl's trunk and limbs. These physical findings suggest repeated assaults.

infants and small children are physically abused within their own homes by a disturbed parent or even an older brother or sister. Such *child abuse* tends to be repeated and often results in multiple musculoskeletal injuries, frequently referred to as "battered baby syndrome," a repulsive yet realistic term.

Diagnosis. The victim of such pathological behavior may not be brought for medical attention immediately. When the child is brought in, the history of injury given by the parents is often evasively vague and may even be deliberately misleading.

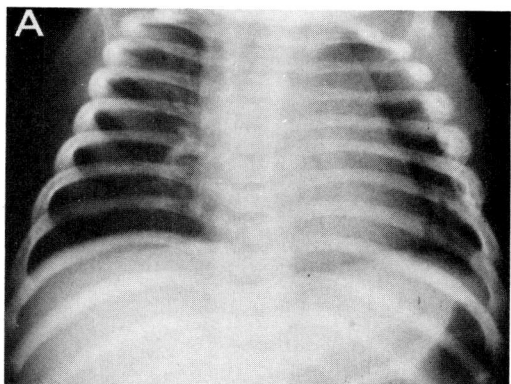

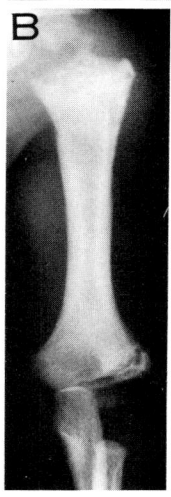
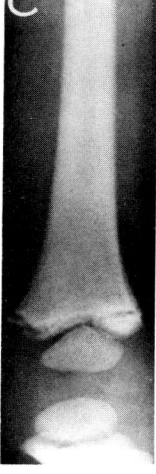

Figure 9–89 Child abuse. A one-year-old child suspected of being the victim of child abuse. A. Note the multiple rib fractures on the left side of the chest, some of which are fresh and others of which are partially healed. B. Note the callus formation in the region of the proximal metaphysis of the humerus as well as the partially healed fracture of the lateral condyle. C. A healing epiphyseal plate injury is apparent in the child's femur. These multiple radiographic findings are typical of child abuse.

There is usually something mysterious about the mishap which should arouse suspicion.

Physical examination may reveal multiple bruises, often in varying stages of resolution, which suggests multiple assaults over a period of time. The child usually has a sad countenance—and for good reason (Fig. 9–88).

Radiographic examination under such circumstances needs to be extensive and should include the skull, chest, and all four limbs. Skull fractures, multiple rib fractures, and epiphyseal separations in the limbs are the most characteristic skeletal injuries. These multiple injuries may also be in varying stages of healing, an observation that usually indicates repeated assaults (Fig. 9–89).

Treatment. Infants and children suspected of having been physically abused should be admitted to the hospital for complete investigation (as well as photographic documentation). The physician or surgeon who suspects child abuse has a moral, and indeed a legal, obligation to report the *suspicion* of such abuse to the local authorities who then proceed with the necessary investigation and action. Records of previous attendance at the hospital should be studied. If a central registry of physically abused children is kept in the community, this should also be consulted, since the parents may not consistently bring their child to the same hospital, particularly in a large community.

Regrettably, if these protective and preventive steps are not taken, a significant percentage of these helpless and hapless little victims will eventually succumb to multiple injuries—particularly cerebral injuries—that are wittingly and willfully inflicted upon them.

REFERENCES

1. Baker, R. H., Carroll, N., Dewar, F. P., and Hall, J. E.: The semitendinosus tenodesis for recurrent dislocation of the patella. J. Bone Joint Surg., *54B*:103, 1972.
2. Banerjee, S., and Bobechko, W. P.: Growth acceleration after femoral shaft fracture in children. Can. J. Surg., in press.
3. Blount, W. P.: Fractures In Children. Baltimore, Williams & Wilkins, 1955.

4. Boyd, H. B., and Boals, J. C.: The Monteggia lesion: a review of 159 cases. Clin. Orthop., 66:94, 1969.
5. Braunstein, P. W., Skudder, P. A., McCarroll, J. R., et al.: Concealed haemorrhage due to pelvic fracture. J. Trauma, 4:832, 1964.
6. Bright, R. W.: Surgical correction of partial epiphyseal plate closure in dogs by bone bridge resection and use of silicone rubber implants. J. Bone Joint Surg., 54A:1133, 1972.
7. Casey, B. H., Hamilton, H. W., and Bobechko, W. P.: Reduction of acutely slipped upper femoral epiphysis. J. Bone Joint Surg., 54B:607, 1972.
8. Charnley, J.: The Closed Treatment of Common Fractures. 3rd Ed. Edinburgh, E. & S. Livingstone, 1970.
9. Cooper, R.: Fractures in children: fundamentals of management. J. Iowa Med. Soc., 54:472, 1964.
10. Dale, G. C., and Harris, W. F.: Prognosis in epiphyseal separation. An experimental study. J. Bone Joint Surg., 40B:116, 1958.
11. Devas, M. B.: Stress fractures in children. J. Bone Joint Surg., 45B:528, 1963.
12. Engh, C. A., Robinson, R. A., and Milgram, J.: Stress fractures in children. J. Trauma, 10:532, 1970.
13. Evans, E. M.: Fractures of the radius and ulna. J. Bone Joint Surg., 33B:548, 1951.
14. Fielding, J. W.: Radio–ulnar union following displacement of the proximal radial epiphysis. J. Bone Joint Surg., 46A:1277, 1964.
15. Fraser, R. L., Haliburton, R. A., and Barber, J. R.: Displaced epiphyseal fractures of the proximal humerus. Can. J. Surg., 10:427, 1967.
16. Gaul, R. W.: Recurrent traumatic dislocation of the hip in children. Clin. Orthop., 90:107, 1973.
17. Griffin, P. P., Anderson, M., and Green, W. T.: Fractures of the shaft of the femur. Orthop. Clin. North Am., 3:213, 1972.
18. Griffiths, S. C.: Fracture of odontoid process in children. J. Pediatr. Surg., 7:680, 1972.
19. Haddad, R. J., Saer, J. K., and Riordan, D. C.: Percutaneous pinning of displaced supracondylar fractures of the elbow in children. Clin. Orthop., 71:112, 1970.
20. Hunter, G. A.: Non-traumatic displacement of the atlanto–axial joint. J. Bone Joint Surg., 50B:44, 1968.
21. Irani, R. N., Nicholson, J. T., and Chung, S. M. K.: Treatment of femoral fractures in children by immediate spica immobilization. J. Bone Joint Surg., 52A:1567, 1972.
22. Jackson, D. W., and Cozen, L.: Genu valgum as a complication of proximal tibial metaphyseal fractures in children. J. Bone Joint Surg., 53A:1571, 1971.
23. Kay, S. P., and Hall, J. E.: Fracture of the femoral neck in children and its complications. Clin. Orthop., 80:53, 1971.
24. Kempe, C. H., and Helfer, R. E.: Helping the Battered Child and his Family. Philadelphia, J. B. Lippincott, 1972.
25. Kleiger, B. and Mankin, H. J.: Fracture of the lateral portion of the distal epiphysis. J. Bone Joint Surg., 46A:25, 1964.
26. Melzak, J.: Paraplegia among children. Lancet, 2:45, 1969.
27. Murphy, A. F., and Stark, H. H.: Closed dislocation of the MPJ of the index finger. J. Bone Joint Surg., 49A:1579, 1967.
28. Mustard, W. T. and Simmons, E. H.: Experimental arterial spasm in the lower extremity produced by traction. J. Bone Joint Surg., 35B:437, 1953.
29. Neer, C. S., Francis, K. C., Marcove, R. C. et al.: Treatment of unicameral bone cyst. J. Bone Joint Surg., 48A:731, 1966.
30. Patrick, J.: A study of supination and pronation with especial reference to the treatment of forearm fractures. J. Bone Joint Surg., 28:737, 1946.
31. Pearson, D. E., and Mann, R. J.: Traumatic dislocation of the hip in children. Clin. Orthop., 92:189, 1973.
32. Pennsylvania Orthopaedic Society: Traumatic dislocation of the hip in children. J. Bone Joint Surg., 50A:79, 1968.
33. Rang, M.: Children's Fractures. Philadelphia, J.B. Lippincott, 1974.
34. Ratliff, A. H. C.: Traumatic separation of the upper femoral epiphysis in young children. J. Bone Joint Surg., 50B:757, 1968.
35. Ratliff, A. H. C.: Complications after fractures of the femoral neck in children and their treatment. J. Bone Joint Surg., 52B:175, 1970.
36. Rorabeck, C. H., Macnab I., and Waddell, J. P.: Anterior tibial compartment syndrome: a clinical and experimental review. Can. J. Surg., 15:249, 1972.
37. Salter, R. B.: Textbook of Disorders and Injuries of the Musculoskeletal System. Baltimore, Williams & Wilkins, 1970.
38. Salter, R. B., and Best, T.: The pathogenesis and prevention of valgus deformity following fractures of the proximal metaphyseal region of the tibia in children. J. Bone Joint Surg., 55A:1324, 1973.
39. Salter, R. B., and Harris, W. R.: Injuries involving the epiphyseal plate. J. Bone Joint Surg., 45A:587, 1963.
40. Salter, R. B., and Zaltz, C.: Anatomic investigations of the mechanism of injury and pathologic anatomy of "pulled elbow" in young children. Clin. Orthop., 77:141, 1971.
41. Sharrard, W. J. W.: Pediatric Orthopedics and Fractures. Oxford, Blackwell, Scientific Publications, 1971.
42. Siffert, R. S.: Displacement of the distal humeral epiphysis in the new born infant. J. Bone Joint Surg., 45A:165, 1963.
43. Tachdjian, M. O.: Pediatric Orthopedics. 2nd Ed. Philadelphia, W.B. Saunders, 1972.
44. Tator, C. H.: Acute spinal cord injury: a review of recent studies of treatment and pathophysiology. Can. Med. Assoc. J., 107:143, 1972.
45. Thompson, S. A., and Mahoney, L. J.: Volkmann's ischemic contracture and its relationship to fracture of the femur. J. Bone Joint Surg., 33B:336, 1951.
46. Wortzman, G., and Dewar, F. P.: Rotary fixation of the atlanto-axial joint. Radiology, 90:479, 1968.

E. STEPHEN GURDJIAN, M.D.

and

EDWIN S. GURDJIAN, M.D.

Head ——————————————— *10*
Injuries

Between the ages of 2 and 42, accidental injuries are the most important cause of death, and head injury is a major cause of lethality and morbidity. In vehicular accidents, 70 per cent of victims have head injuries, 50 per cent extremity injuries, 38 per cent chest injuries, and 10 per cent neck injuries. In 1974 there was a significant drop of 9 per cent in accidental deaths compared with 1973, with motor vehicle deaths down by 17 per cent. According to *Accident Facts*, accidental deaths reached a total of 105,000 in 1975. Motor vehicle deaths accounted for 46,200; 13,400 were job-related; 25,500 occurred in the home; and over 24,000 were public accidental deaths. In addition, disabling injuries totaled 11 million. It is hoped that with lowered speed limits, better education, and mitigating methods, deaths and disabilities will become less frequent.

In this chapter, the biomechanics and treatment of impact head injury, scalp lesions, concussion, skull fracture, and traumatic intracranial hemorrhage will be discussed.

IMPACT INJURIES

An impact injury may be produced when a moving object strikes the body (impact acceleration) or the moving body runs into a nonmoving or slowly moving object (impact deceleration). The result of an impact injury may be a tearing of the scalp from compression, tension, or shearing.

There may be deformation of the skull, resulting in linear fracture or depression. Relative movements (inertial stress propagation) of intracranial contents may take place. There may also be changes in intracranial pressure, with high pressure around the point of impact and low pressure at the antipole. All of these occur successively or simultaneously. Impact injuries may cause acceleration or deceleration of the impacted portion of the body and compression of the area of impact. Thus, impact injuries may have primarily a compressive effect if the injured part is relatively fixed or if it is caught been slowly moving objects. A compression of the head may occur when the head on the ground is caught under a heavy object that has fallen upon it. In compressive injuries, acceleration and deceleration are minimal, whereas when the head is free to move, impact injuries cause obvious acceleration or deceleration.

In blunt impacts, inertial stress propagation is an important mechanism of injury. The skull and brain are of different densities, the skull being more solid. The brain is surrounded by the subarachnoid space and cerebrospinal fluid and hence can move during impact. Relative movements or mass movements of the brain may result in contusions, intracerebral bruises, and contrecoup lesions. Impact acceleration may cause contrecoup tears of the cerebral surface with little or no bruising on the cerebral surface in the area of impact. With the head free to move, the brain may not receive the total effect of inbending of the skull sufficient to cause more extensive bruising in the impacted area (coup lesion). The movement of the brain against the internal irregular surface of the base of the skull is the usual cause of contrecoup contusions.[3]

EARLY MANAGEMENT AND ANATOMOPATHOPHYSIOLOGY OF IMPACT HEAD INJURY

Initial evaluation will reveal whether the patient sustained an isolated head injury or suffered damage to other systems as well. The responsive patient may cooperate sufficiently to rule out cervical spine, chest, and skeletal injuries. In an unconscious and disoriented patient, initial evaluation may be incomplete, and he should be transported to a hospital with care to avoid

further injury. An open chest wound should be packed and taped, and ventilation should be facilitated by positioning or intratracheal intubation. Obvious external bleeding should be controlled by bandaging, tourniquet, or compression, as indicated. At the scene of the accident the unconscious patient should be immobilized in the supine position to protect the neck and extremities during transport. Both at the scene of the accident and during transport, blood pressure, pulse, and respiration should be monitored. Obvious pupillary inequality and weakness or paralysis of any of the extremities should be noted.

Many patients arriving in the emergency room may have recovered consciousness. Others may remain unconscious and unresponsive. In the emergency room, the head injury status of a patient may be evaluated on the basis of the state of consciousness, changes in vital functions, and focal neurological abnormalities. These patients may be classified as follows: (1) minimal injury with no obvious neurological disorders, (2) minimal injury with complications (lacerations, depressed fracture, skeletal fracture,

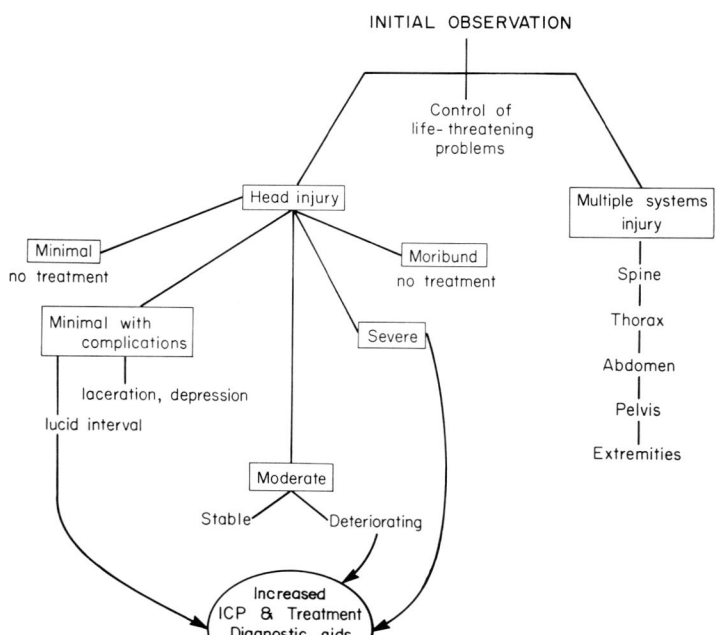

Figure 10-1 This figure summarizes initial observation and classification of injuries into life-threatening problems, multiple systems injuries, and head injuries. Head injuries are further subdivided into minimal, minimal with complications, moderate, severe, and too severe for recovery (moribund). The need for treatment of increased intracranial pressure (ICP) of whatever cause, diagnostic aids, and exploration is noted. Multiple system injuries include involvement of spine, thorax, abdomen, pelvis, and extremities.

lucid interval, deteriorating state), (3) moderate injury that stabilizes, (4) moderate injury with evidence of deteriorating, (5) severe injury with increasing deterioration, and (6) severe injury beyond hope (moribund). Of the six categories, (1) and (6) require little or no treatment; (2) and (4) may deserve diagnostic and surgical management; (3) may be treated symptomatically; and (5) will need special measures to control the increase in intracranial pressure. This grouping of cases may be simplified by their classification into minimal, moderate, and severe injuries. These classes will not be considered (Fig. 10–1).

Minimal Head Injury

A minimal head injury patient is responsive, and the vital functions are normal and stable. Such a patient may have complications, however. X-rays should be made of the skull and neck, lacerations should be repaired, and an extremity fracture should be evaluated and treated. If there is a history of unconsciousness, he should be hospitalized for 24 hours, if possible. Because such a patient occasionally deteriorates, it is important to observe him and to monitor vital functions and state of consciousness.

Moderate Head Injury

The patient with moderate head injury is unconscious or poorly responsive and may be disoriented. His vital functions are stable, and his condition may remain stable and improve, with recovery in a few days. He may have an open fracture or depression, and there may be lateralizing signs. A clear airway should be maintained.

This patient requires repair of lacerations and evaluation and management of skeletal injuries. He should also have x-rays of the skull and neck, stomach (nasogastric) intubation, gasometric studies of PaO_2 and $PaCO_2$, complete blood count (CBC), urinalysis, and blood electrolyte determination. Angiography, echoencephalography, scan, electroencephalography, and lumbar puncture, should be performed as indicated. A patient with moderate head injury will be hospitalized for several days. It is important

during that time to note any deterioration and institute management as needed.

Severe Head Injury

The patient with severe head injury is unconscious and may have pupillary abnormalities and evidence of a disconnection syndrome, such as decerebration or decortication. He may also have hemiparesis or paraparesis. The vital functions may show abnormalities, with initial slow pulse and respirations and elevated blood pressure. This patient requires a nasogastric tube, a Foley catheter, venopuncture and intubation for intravenous administration of fluids and drugs, and arterial puncture (radial or femoral) for gasometric studies. He is a candidate for management in the intensive care unit, and he may also be a candidate for angiography, lumbar puncture, and management by hypertonic diuretics and cerebrospinal fluid pressure monitoring. There may be some stabilization in patients with severe head injury. Others in this group may be moribund and die with tachypnea, slow pulse followed by an increased rate, hypertension, attacks of decerebration, pupillary inequality, dilatation and nonreactive pupils. Patients with minimal and moderate injury may deteriorate, showing signs and symptoms seen in the severely injured.

Many severely injured patients have increased intracranial pressure. This may be due to cerebral edema, resulting from diffuse brain injury. Increased intracranial pressure may also be due to a traumatic mass lesion, an epidural, subdural, or parenchymatous hemorrhage, or a combination of these. A mass lesion may be present in association with diffuse brain injury and cerebral edema. If there is a traumatic mass lesion, immediate surgical treatment is imperative. Corticosteroids and hyperosmolar diuretics given intravenously may be used while computerized tomography or cerebral angiography is performed to rule out a mass lesion.

In the next section, various types of head injury and their diagnosis and treatment will be described. They include scalp injuries and skull fractures, concussion and traumatic intracranial hemorrhages.

SCALP INJURIES

The scalp may be 3 to 5 mm. thick; it becomes thin and atrophic in old age. Although the scalp consists of six layers, it behaves as a one-layer structure from the cutis to the subgaleal space. It may be bruised by compression and torn by sharp-ended objects or by being pulled apart in tension. At times, large areas may be avulsed. Avulsion may be complete but usually involves only the frontoparietal scalp (Fig. 10–2).

Extensive lifting of the scalp may cause bleeding into the subaponeurotic space. Such a collection is usually absorbed, although occasionally needling or incisional drainage followed by a well-fitting scalp compression bandage is indicated.

Cephalhematoma is a subpoeriosteal collection of blood resulting from injury during parturition. It is usually unilateral and parietal in location, although, it may also be seen in the frontal and occipital areas. Cephalhematoma is absorbed in two to three weeks. Occasionally, it may calcify and some cases may require incisional drainage with aseptic precautions.

Caput succedaneum is an edema and a serous collection overlying the periosteum, which is caused by pressure on the scalp in the birth canal.

SKULL FRACTURE

In a large series of cases, about 30 per cent of patients with craniocerebral injuries

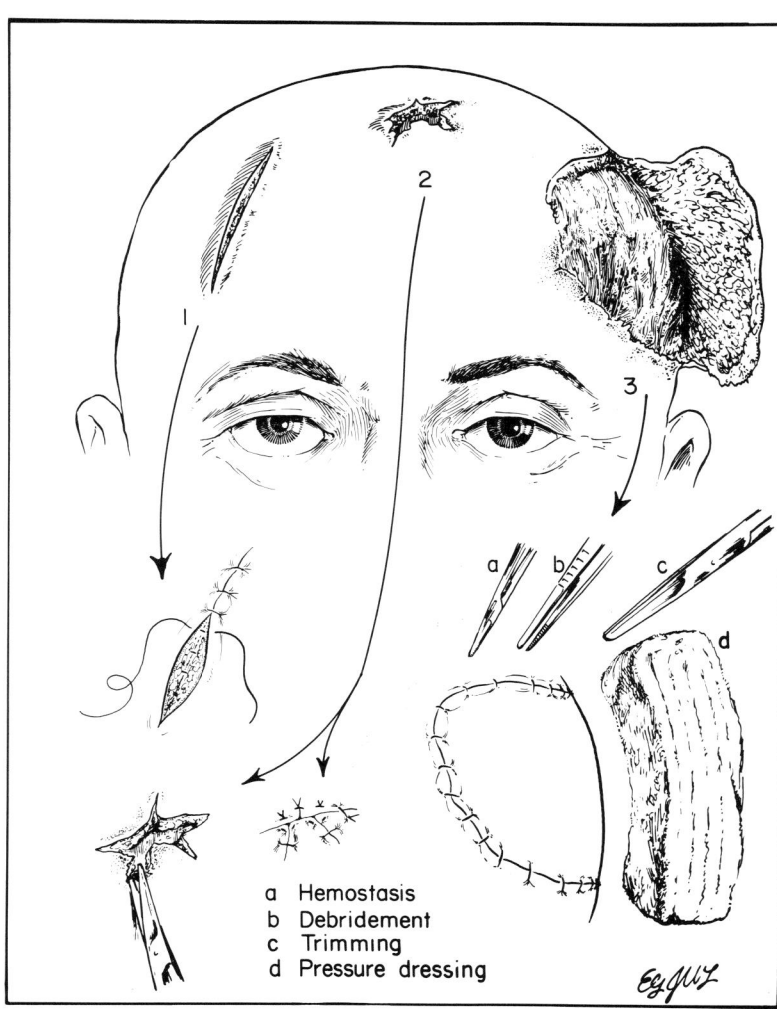

a Hemostasis
b Debridement
c Trimming
d Pressure dressing

Figure 10–2 Laceration of the scalp, 1, a punctate laceration, 2, and avulsion, 3, are shown as well as methods of debridement and repair. a, Hemostasis; b, debridement; c, trimming; d, pressure dressing.

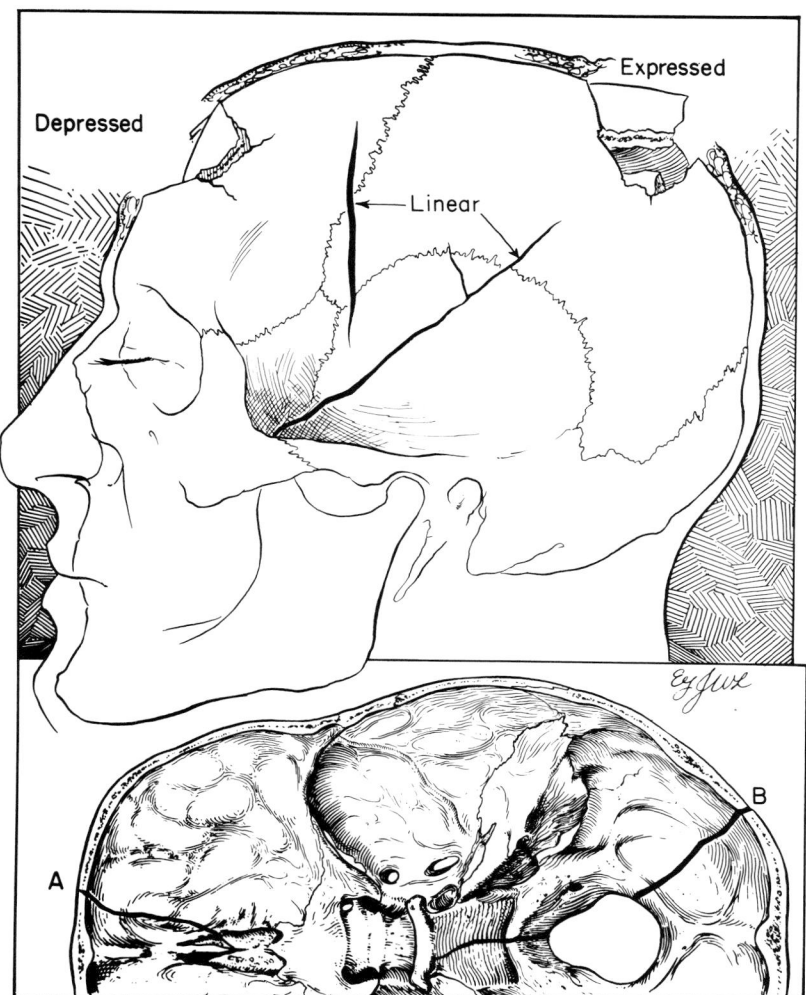

Figure 10-3 Depressed fractures are shown in the upper portion of the figure, fracture of the base of the skull in the lower portion. The posteriorly shown skull deformity is an expressed fracture in which fragments of bone have been pulled outward after comminution. The anteriorly shown skull deformity is a depressed fracture in which fragments of bone are pushed into the skull cavity. Typical linear fractures are shown in the coronal plane and in the parietotemporal area extending downward into the temporal fossa. A, A frontal fracture extending into the cribriform plate; B, a lateral occipital fracture extending into the foramen magnum and clivus all the way to the pituitary fossa.

have skull fractures. These fractures may be linear, depressed, expressed, comminuted, diastatic, or stellate. There may be multiple fractures and combinations of fractures. In some injuries, the calvarial fracture extends into the base; basilar fractures involve the base of the skull. Fractures may be open (compound) when the overlying scalp and mucous membranes are lacerated or torn but the dura is intact. In closed (or simple) fractures, the scalp, mucous membranes, and dura are intact. In closed brain injury,

the dural lining is intact, whereas in open brain injury, there is scalp laceration, skull fracture, and dural tear.

A linear fracture, which constitutes about 70 per cent of skull fractures, results from elastic deformation of the skull following impact. The area of impact is inbended, and farther out the skull outbends selectively. The outbended portion tears apart from tension, forming a fracture that extends toward the area of impact and toward the base of the skull. It extends toward the area of impact because following initial inbending this area becomes outbended and thus constitutes an area of stress concentration. Heavy impacts may cause depression, and depending upon the size of the injuring object, there may be stellate depression or more discrete areas of depression or perforation. The shape of the injuring object is extremely important (Fig. 10–3). With the same amount of energy, a flat object will cause a linear fracture, and a more pointed object will cause a depression.[5, 6]

Basilar fractures may result in cerebrospinal fluid (CSF) rhinorrhea when the anterior fossa and cribriform plate are involved. There may be CSF otorrhea with petrous bone injury. Occipital fractures and frontal fractures of the base may involve the clivus and pituitary fossa. In this case, injury of the pituitary gland and its blood supply may occur, and diabetes insipidus is sometimes seen.

Tissues may be entrapped in expressed fractures and in some linear fractures. At the time of fracture formation, the intracranial contents at the base may bulge into the fracture site during impact, with fracture edges snapping together and entrapping piarachnoid substance, brain tissue, and blood vessels. This may cause thromboses or the formation of aneurysms in arteriovenous communications. The same may occur in linear fractures of the calvarium when the dura is torn by the forming fracture.[2, 3]

A fine linear fracture may heal in 6 to 12 months. Comminuted and diastatic fractures may remain open for several years. A progressive skull fracture enlarges over a period of time. This may be the result of the pulsatile force of cerebrospinal fluid in spurious cranial meningocele, or of traumatic destruction of the periosteal lining in some cases of craniocerebral injury.

REPAIR OF LACERATION AND OPEN AND CLOSED DEPRESSION

Lacerations of the scalp should be carefully cleansed and debrided before closure. In some cases, adhesive dressing to approximate the skin edges may be used, particularly with superficial and short cuts. With an open linear fracture, the wound should be cleansed, and if the fracture site does not appear to be contaminated by hair or foreign matter the wound may be closed. Otherwise, linear craniectomy may be performed for bone debridement (Fig. 10–4).

Surgical treatment of open depression should be done within 24 hours. Closed

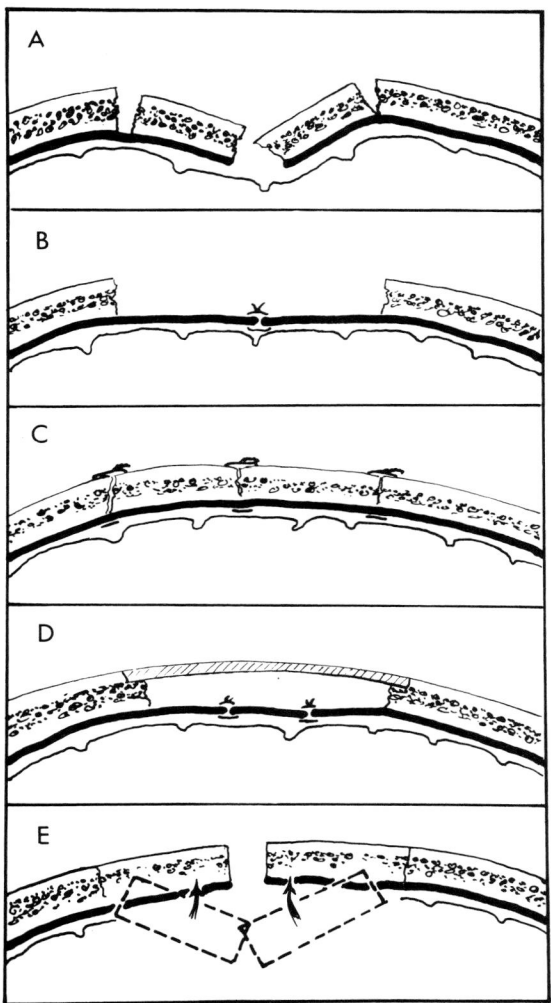

Figure 10–4 A. Open depressed fracture. B. Treatment by removal of bone fragments. C. Reconstructive work with the bone fragments. D. A clean depression. The skull defect has been repaired with methyl methacrylate. E. Depressed fracture is elevated. There may be need for removal of some bone tissue to elevate the depression more effectively with a bone elevator. It is important to note dural tears and inspect the surface of the brain, if this is indicated by the presence of the underlying discoloration due to a bruise or hematoma. In extensive open depression with laceration of the brain careful excision of destroyed brain tissue is performed under magnification.

depression may be elevated in two to three days. If the depressed pieces of bone can be used for reconstruction, they should be. If not, methyl methacrylate cranioplasty may be performed, either during the initial operation with closed depressions, or two to four months later with open, soiled depressions (Fig. 10–4).

Surgical treatment of CSF otorrhea is not normally indicated, unless the otorrhea persists. With CSF rhinorrhea, repair of the communicating channels between the cranial and nasal cavities is indicated. Conservative therapy of CSF rhinorrhea with bed rest and antibiotic medication may be used successfully in some cases. However, if the rhinorrhea recurs several days to weeks later, the patient should have operative repair.

If the patient survives a penetrating wound from a high-velocity missile, treatment by careful debridement of scalp, skull, and brain is indicated. Clots and organic matter in the path of the missile should be removed, and the missile itself should be removed if possible. In cases of perforating wounds, both the entrance and the exit tears should be debrided.

With low-velocity wounds, treatment is by careful debridement and removal of the foreign body. Antibiotic and chemotherapeutic measures are employed to prevent infection, osteomyelitis, and brain abscess.

CONCUSSION

Concussion is an immediate posttraumatic brain dysfunction characterized by unconsciousness, visual disturbance, disturbance of equilibrium, or other dysfunction of the brain due to mechanical forces. While concussion is usually reversible, it may result in neurological disability of long duration, and in some cases it may be fatal.

The patient with concussion may have anterograde and retrograde amnesia and possibly headaches, dizziness, and some personality disorders. The condition usually improves over a period of a few weeks to a few months. Occasionally, a concussive blow will cause no complaints. It is important to remember that a concussed individual may develop an intra-

cranial hematoma which manifests itself several days to several weeks after injury. Appropriate diagnostic evaluation is therefore important in those with complaints. Surgical treatment may be indicated when the presence of a mass lesion has been determined.

TRAUMATIC INTRACRANIAL HEMORRHAGES

Acute traumatic intracranial hemorrhages include subarachnoid hemorrhages, epidural, subdural, and parenchymatous hematomas, and subdural accumulation of cerebrospinal fluid, which may be bloody. In some cases, a combination of lesions is seen. The clinical manifestations of epidural and subdural hematomas will be discussed in some detail.

EPIDURAL HEMATOMAS

Clinical and Mechanistic Features

Epidural hematoma due to low-velocity impact has characteristic clinical manifestations. A short period of unconsciousness followed by a lucid interval and eventual deterioration of consciousness, with focal findings, is a classic picture. However, with higher velocity traffic injuries this picture is infrequently seen. In most series, 20 per cent or less have classic manifestations. In some patients there may be no initial unconsciousness; deterioration of the conscious state occurs several hours to days after injury. In a few, the state of consciousness remains intact, and the patient's focal abnormalities (pupillary dilatation, progressing hemiparesis, or hemiplegia of slow or sudden onset) point to the correct diagnosis. During the past few decades the typical patient whose condition is due to a vehicular accident (higher velocity impacts) has demonstrated a multiplicity of lesions. The typical syndrome of epidural hematoma resulting from a fall or a low-velocity impact may not be seen. The formation and development of an epidural hematoma has been described in previous publications.[8, 9]

The development of an epidural collection may be a result of (1) fracture with tear

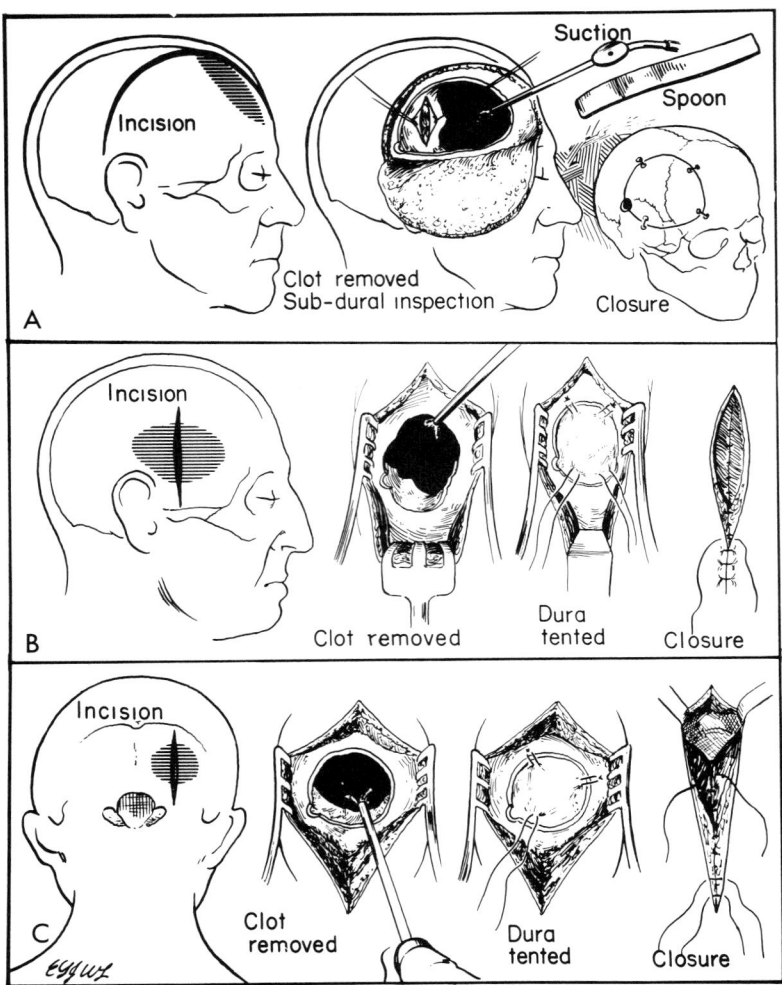

Figure 10–5 Diagrammatic representation of frontal, temporal, parietal, and posterior fossa epidural hematomas and their surgical management. *A.* A frontal epidural hematoma is excised through a bone flap in the right frontoparietal area. The bone flap may be bilateral if necessary. Usually the dura is opened to inspect a subdural collection or extensive brain contusion and softening. Such areas of brain softening may be excised by suction and electrocoagulation A drain my be used, epidurally and subdurally, after the dura has been closed. *B.* A temporal hematoma is excised through a subtemporal opening. The dura is tented after excision to control bleeding. A form of suction drainage may be used in such cases to control bleeding. *C.* A suboccipital epidural hematoma in the posterior fossa has been exposed through a straight paramedian incision with craniectomy of the occpital squama. It may be necessary to open the dura if indicated. The dura may be tented to control bleeding. A drain may be used or Hemovac drainage with suction may be utilized. Drains, if used, are removed in 12 hours.

of meningeal vessels and dural sinuses, (2) fracture with comminution and escape of blood from diploë and emissary veins into an epidural position and (3) separation of the dura from the skull convexity during skull deformation without fracture.

Lake and Pitts[10] have presented a number of cases without fracture of the skull. However, the usual patient has a parietal or temporal fracture tear of the middle meningeal vessels. The absence of a fracture in epidural collection may be due to inadequate inspection at the time of surgery or inadequate x-ray examination. In some unusual cases a separation of the dura from the skull may occur at the time of impact and during the elastic deformation of the skull, causing epidural collection but no fracture.

Many patients may have an associated tear of the dural membrane, so that bleeding may occur both intradurally as well as extradurally. Consequent formation of a large subdural hematoma and a small or insignificant epidural hematoma (or vice versa) may be seen in the operating room. Angiographic contrast material may escape and be seen on x-ray examination in a subdural position or over the convexity of the brain. Extravasation of contrast material from a torn middle meningeal artery or branches with subdural clots was described by Galligioni and his associates in 1968. It has also been reported that some subdural hematomas are due to arterial bleeding, and this is well substantiated when epidural and subdural hematomas coexist. A tear of the middle meningeal artery associated with a tear of the dura may result in a significant subdural accumulation and a small non-symptomatic epidural collection. At times, a communication between torn epidural artery and the diploë may be shown by angiography.

In some patients the condition may have a subacute course, with no history of unconsciousness but with manifest symptoms of changes in the conscious state and in focal signs. Operative intervention usually takes place from several days to about six weeks following the injury; in many cases, the lesion is localized with appropriate contrast studies. Subacute epidural hematomas may undergo a lysis of the clot by liquefaction, with no definite organization on the internal calvarial surface. Some organization by the dura may be surmised at the time of surgery by the obvious adhesions and connective tissue proliferation between the clot and the dural membrane.

The development of an epidural hematoma is aided by bleeding from veins and arterial channels. In the patient with a subacute course, the clot may slowly form from venous bleeding. With arterial bleeding, a symptomatic clot is formed within two or three hours or earlier. Epidural collection from venous sinuses and emissary veins is augmented by bleeding from dural venous channels. Rupture of occipital emissary veins may cause an epidural hematoma in the mastoparietal area. A sagittal sinus tear may be associated with a midline vertex hematoma, causing a deformation of the sinus which is seen during the venous phase in a lateral angiogram. If torn, the lateral sinus and the confluence may cause epidural hematomas in the posterior fossa, with some extending above the tentorial level. Venous bleeding may result from the tearing of channels between the dura and the bone as the dura is dissected off the skull by the enlarging clot. During changes

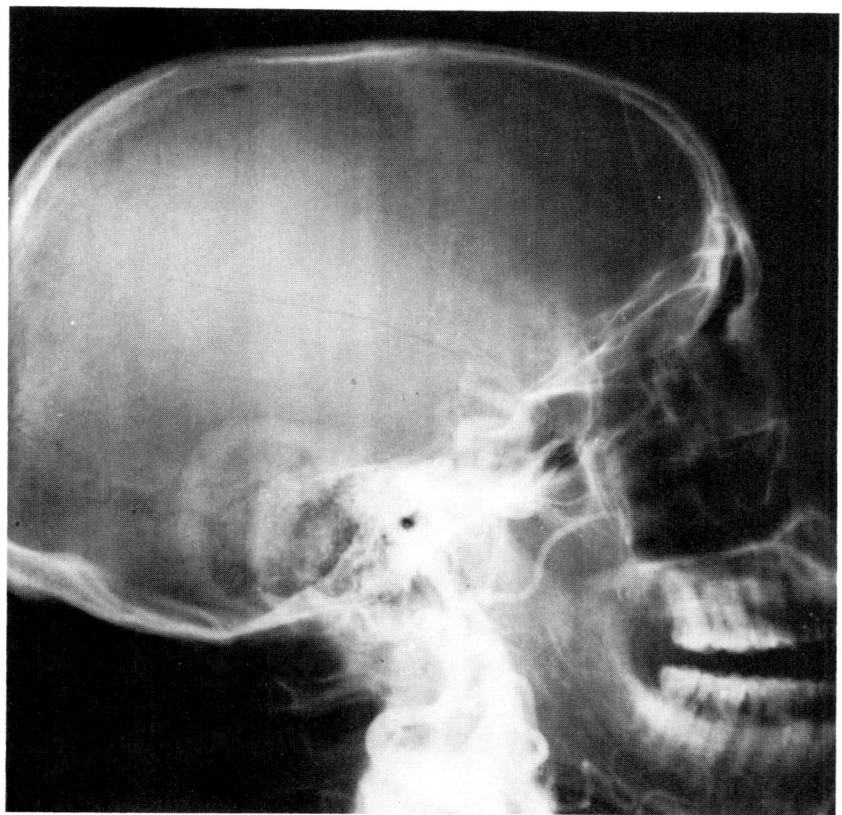

Figure 10–6   A right pareietotemporal linear fracture associated with a temporal parietal epidural hematoma.

in intracranial pressure associated with breathing or coughing, more venous bleeding may accumulate.

The prognosis in epidural collection is better if a lucid interval or a relatively normal state of consciousness post-injury lasts for 12 to 24 hours. Such may be operated on with impunity and with excellent results. The patient who deteriorates rapidly after injury is a surgical emergency of the first order. A normal state of consciousness on admission to the hospital followed by a deteriorating state due to epidural hematoma may spell a poor prognosis unless prompt and appropriate intervention is practiced (Figs. 10–4 to 10–6).

Diagnostic Evaluation

A dilated pupil and/or oculomotor involvement on the side of the epidural mass, and weakness, and pyramidal tract signs on the contralateral side are seen in the typical case. Many epidural hematomas can be diagnosed clinically with little labo-

ratory assistance. In the patient who is rapidly deteriorating surgical evacuation of the clot must be accomplished with dispatch. In general, radiographs of the skull, echoencephalogram, and angiogram are needed in emergency situations (Fig. 10–7). While these tests are being conducted, intravenous hyperosmolar solutions aid in control of the increased intracranial pressure.[9]

Pneumoencephalography, ventriculography, electroencephalography, radioisotope scan, and computerized axial tomography (CAT scan), if available, are additional aids. These may be useful in clarifying the status of patients who do not present a clear-cut picture or who need further evaluation for diagnostic accuracy.

Treatment

Epidural hematomas can be excised by subtemporal decompression or appropriate bone flap. More than one exploratory burr

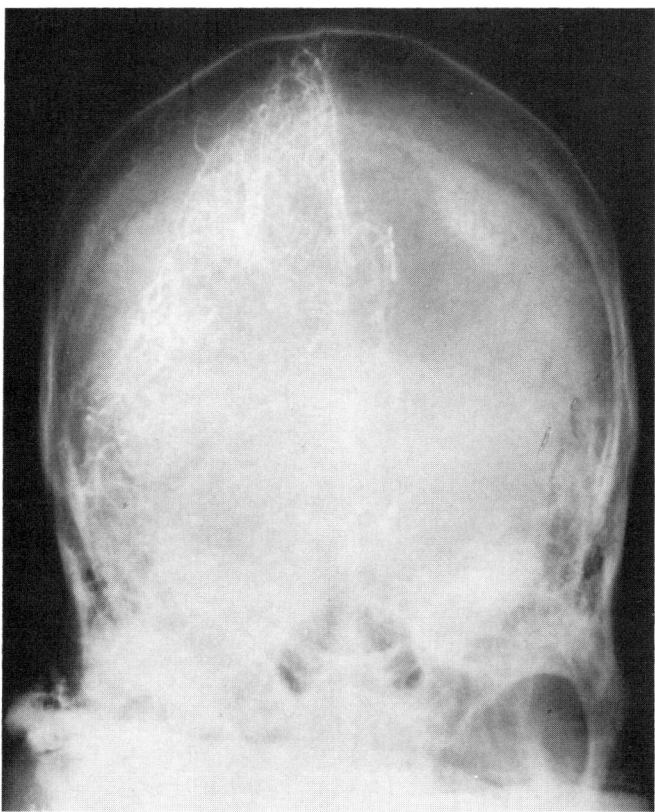

Figure 10–7 Angiogram in the case shown in Figure 10–6 demonstrating an epidural hematoma of the temporoparietal area. There is marked shift of the anterior cerebral artery below the midline dura separating the two hemispheres.

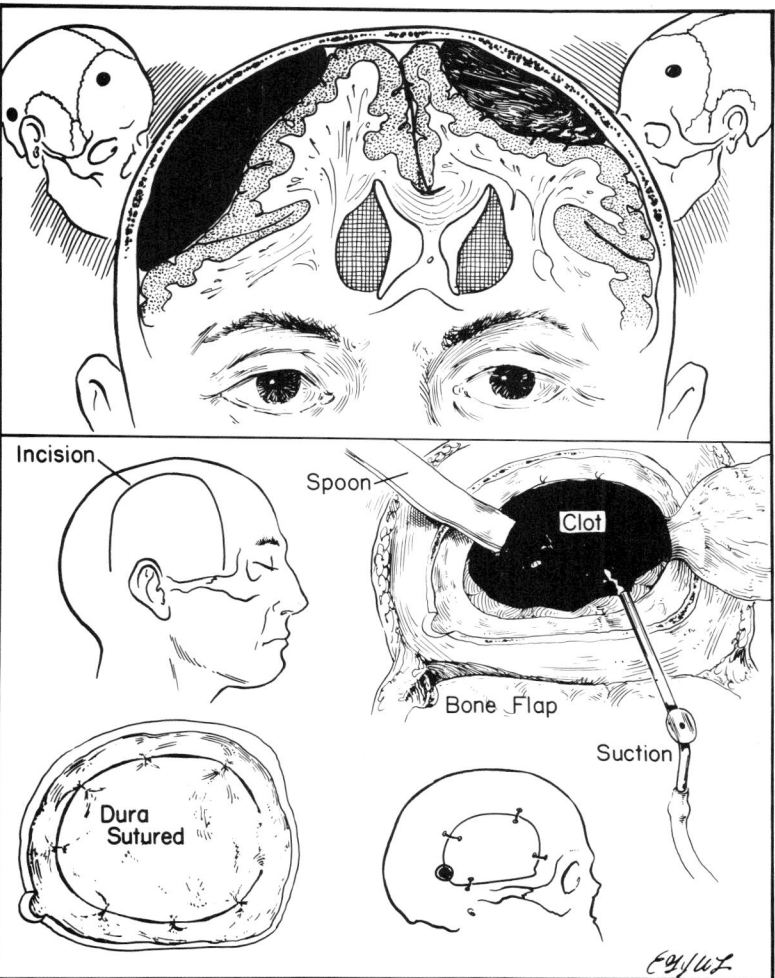

Figure 10–8 Management of subdural hematoma by two or more trephine openings or by bone flap. An acute subdural hematoma is best treated by appropriate bone flap. In all cases bilateral trephine openings should be used to ascertain whether bilateral hematomas are present. Subacute subdural hematoma may be treated with multiple trephine openings and drainage. In some cases a bone flap may have to be utilized later. Chronic subdural hematoma may be treated by multiple trephine openings or by bone flap initially or after exploration and drainage.

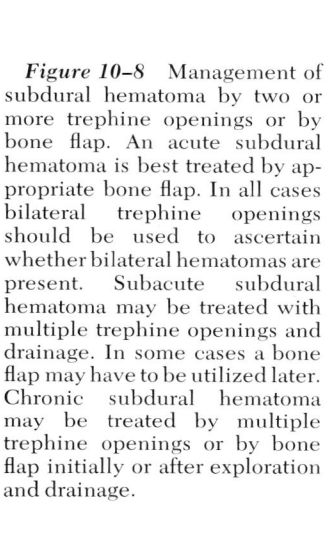

hole may be needed to locate the clot if preoperative angiography has not been performed. During surgical intervention there may be a need for intradural inspection for subdural hematoma, subdural accumulation of CSF, or parenchymatous hemorrhage. With a middle meningeal epidural hematoma, there may be a temporal lobe hematoma requiring excision in order to control bleeding and to prevent the formation of large areas of infarction. Occasionally, the epidural collection may be bilateral.

The use of some forms of drainage under pressure (Hemovac) may be desirable and is suggested by Lake and Pitts. This is particularly true of subfrontal and subtemporal collections. After removal of the clot, a large space is left which does not disappear rapidly owing to the deformation and pos-

terior and superior migration of the brain. The use of Hemovac and controlled breathing during the immediate postoperative period may be worthwhile in the attempt to obliterate the dead space. Dural stitching to extracranial tissues, in conjunction with drainage under negative pressure, may also be utilized.

SUBDURAL HEMATOMAS

Clinical and Mechanistic Features

Recent classification of subdural hematomas by a committee of the Congress of Neurological Surgeons is based on the prognosis and clinical course of the pathological process. Acute, subacute, and chronic forms are recognized.

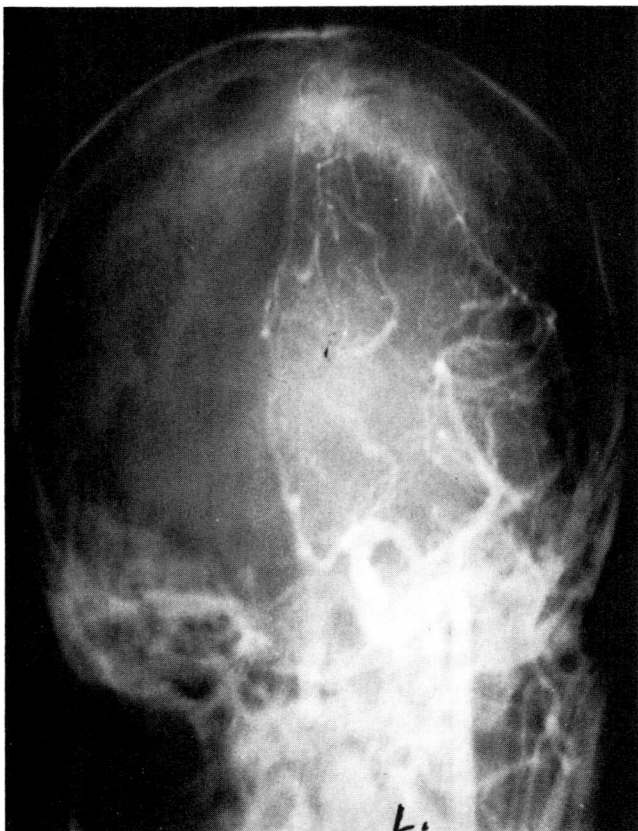

Figure 10-9 Angiogram in a 30-year-old black man with an acute subdural hematoma of the left parietal frontal temporal region following a car accident. The patient was operated on within one hour of injury. He was unconscious and had right-sided decerebrate rigidity attacks. The left pupil was large, and there was right-sided hemiparesis. Decadron and hypertonic mannitol were used as he was prepared for operation. Bilateral burr holes and left bone flap were performed. The patient made a satisfactory recovery.

Acute subdural hematomas cause signs and symptoms (deteriorating consciousness and focal manifestations) that necessitate intervention in 24 hours or less. The subacute variety causes signs and symptoms necessitating intervention in two to ten days. The chronic type includes cases that deserve intervention in 11 days or later. Acute subdural hematomas caused a mortality of 63 to 81 per cent whereas the chronic form may account for a mortality of 3 to 12 per cent, depending upon the author and the number of cases reported. The mortality rate for the subacute variety has been reported to be 12 to 25 per cent.

The cause of rapid development of signs of pressure may be the large size of the hemorrhagic mass or the combination of hemorrhage and brain edema. The age of the patient may also be an important factor in the development of subacute or chronic hematomas. Since in the older individual there may be a larger potential space available in the subdural region, a large subacute or chronic hematoma may not cause rapidly developing symptoms and signs. In the younger person, a small hematoma can cause both a large increase in intracranial pressure and intercompartmental herniations.

The neuropathological picture of acute, subacute, and chronic subdural hematoma is as follows: Organization and absorption of the clot begins a few hours after the bleed. If the clot is tolerated by the patient, it may cause no serious symptoms. As it enlarges by the addition of cerebrospinal fluid, tissue fluids, and blood from organizing vessels that rupture, it becomes symptomatic. An initially large bleed may cause a rapid onset of symptoms (acute subdural), or deterioration may occur over a few days (subacute subdural). In still other cases, the symptoms may appear from eleven days to one to three months later.

The older the clot, the greater the organization, with eventual formation of a cystic mass. A fairly thick membrane (½ to 2 mm) is formed on the dural side of the clot, and a thin membrane is formed on the arachnoid side. This clot is partially liquefied. In some chronic cases it may be almost entirely liquid. In unusual instances, absorption and organization cause the clot to be quite solid, and in very chronic cases it may calcify. In the acute variety the clot is mostly solid, and in the subacute variety it consists of solid and liquid portions.

The source of the bleeding may be venous or arterial or both. In the usual case, cerebral veins emptying into the saggital sinus may be torn. Ruptured sphenoparietal veins may cause a collection over the temporoparietal area and in the vicinity of the sphenoid sinus. Tears of the sagittal and lateral sinuses may cause subdural as well as epidural collections, supratentorially and infratentorially. Arterial bleeding has been proven in some cases by the contrast material spilling into the surface of the hemisphere. Many examples of subdural collection from hemorrhage of middle meningeal artery origin have been recently described.[11]

Subdural hematomas may be caused by linear and rotational accelerations. The amount of energy needed to cause a tear of a venous channel may be small. This depends upon the state of inflation of the specific vascular channel and relative movements (inertial stress propagation) necessary to tear this blood vessel. In many cases subdural hematomas are not associated with fracture of the skull. More often the fracture, if present, is on the side opposite the hematoma. In some situations, subdural hematomas form without trauma. A hydrocephalic patient with a ventriculoatrial or ventriculoperitoneal shunt may develop a migration of the brain downward when

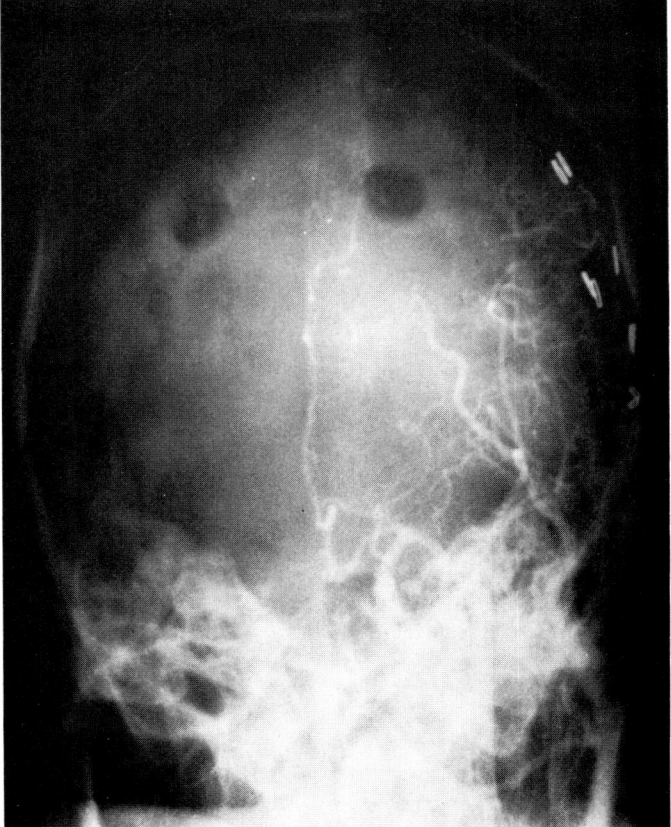

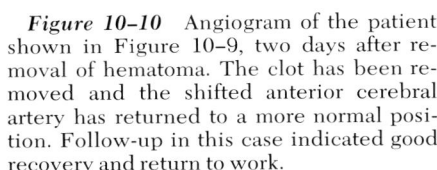

Figure 10–10 Angiogram of the patient shown in Figure 10–9, two days after removal of hematoma. The clot has been removed and the shifted anterior cerebral artery has returned to a more normal position. Follow-up in this case indicated good recovery and return to work.

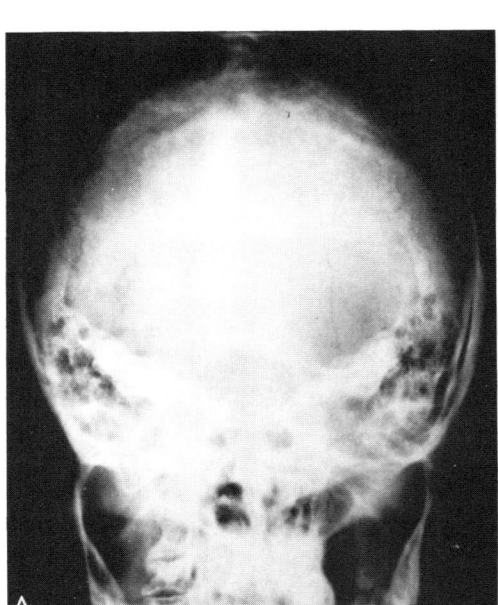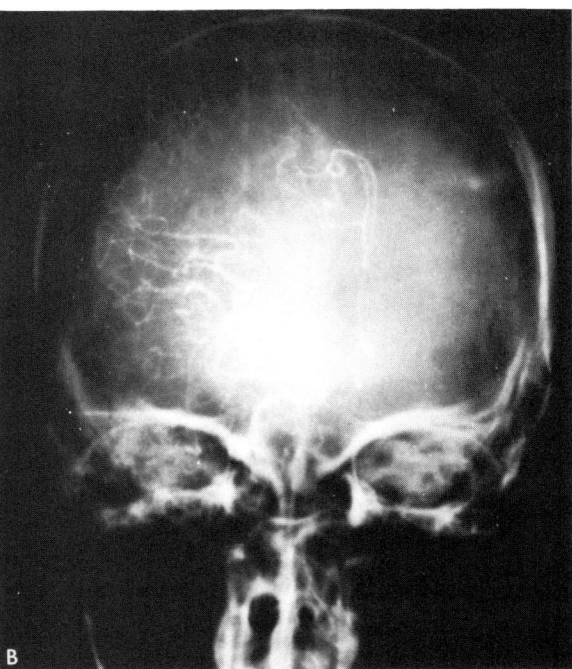

Figure 10–11   *A.* A patient, age 20, with a fracture of left lamboid suture. *B.* Biparietal and right temporal burr holes were performed. Left side was clear. On the right side a mostly liquid clot was found. It was evacuated by using irrigation through a rubber tube. Rubber catheter drains were inserted, brought out through scalp stab wounds, and removed 18 hours later. Patient made a satisfactory recovery. This was a subacute clot removed five days after injury.

sitting up or standing, with resultant tear of connecting veins and subdural bleeding. In some shunt series, 25 to 35 per cent of patients develop subdural hematomas from this mechanism.[12]

In football injuries, subdural hematomas represent an important cause of death. In 1972, there were 18 deaths from injuries in high school and college football. The use of a padded helmet prevents abrasions, lacerations of the scalp, and fractures of the skull during impact. However, relative movements (inertial stress propagation) of the brain, with tears of connecting veins, continue to cause the formation of subdural hematomas. Owing to freedom of neck motion and deceleration with bottoming out of the helmet cushioning material during impact, relative movements of the brain and its coverings result in the development of subdural hematomas.[5, 13]

Subdural hematoma also may be caused by laceration and contusions of the brain. At times, intracerebral hematomas may become partly subdural in position as a result of rupture of the hemorrhagic cyst into the subdural space.

Unusual locations of subdural hematomas include interhemispheric collections and posterior fossa hematomas. Acute, subacute, and chronic forms have been described in the posterior fossa. In a 12-year period, Wright[15] found 17 infratentorial hematomas in 361 patients harboring traumatic intracranial lesions. There were six epidural, five subdural, and six intracerebellar collections. Posterior fossa fracture was present in all six epidural and in four of five subdural collections. The site of trauma was in the occipital area in 16 of 17 cases.

Subdural hematoma in infancy and childhood is important and ranks second to hydrocephalus as an intracranial problem in the first year of life.[16] Subdural taps followed by craniotomy have been an effective form of management (Figs. 10–8 to 10–14).

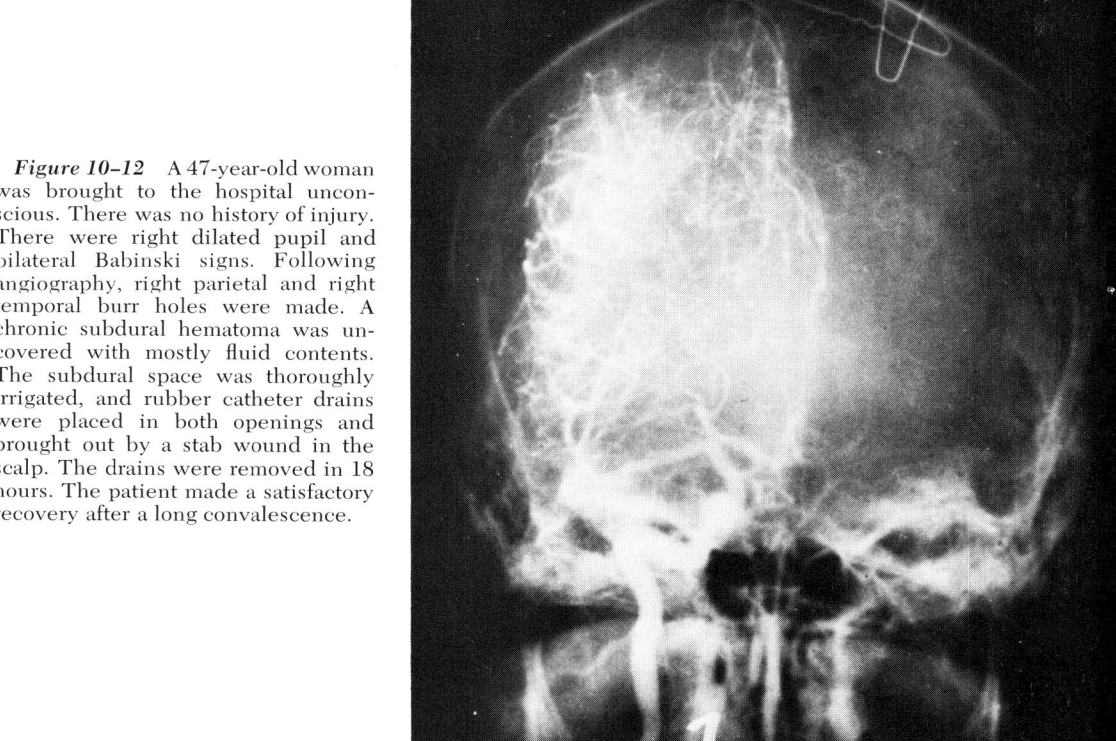

Figure 10–12 A 47-year-old woman was brought to the hospital unconscious. There was no history of injury. There were right dilated pupil and bilateral Babinski signs. Following angiography, right parietal and right temporal burr holes were made. A chronic subdural hematoma was uncovered with mostly fluid contents. The subdural space was thoroughly irrigated, and rubber catheter drains were placed in both openings and brought out by a stab wound in the scalp. The drains were removed in 18 hours. The patient made a satisfactory recovery after a long convalescence.

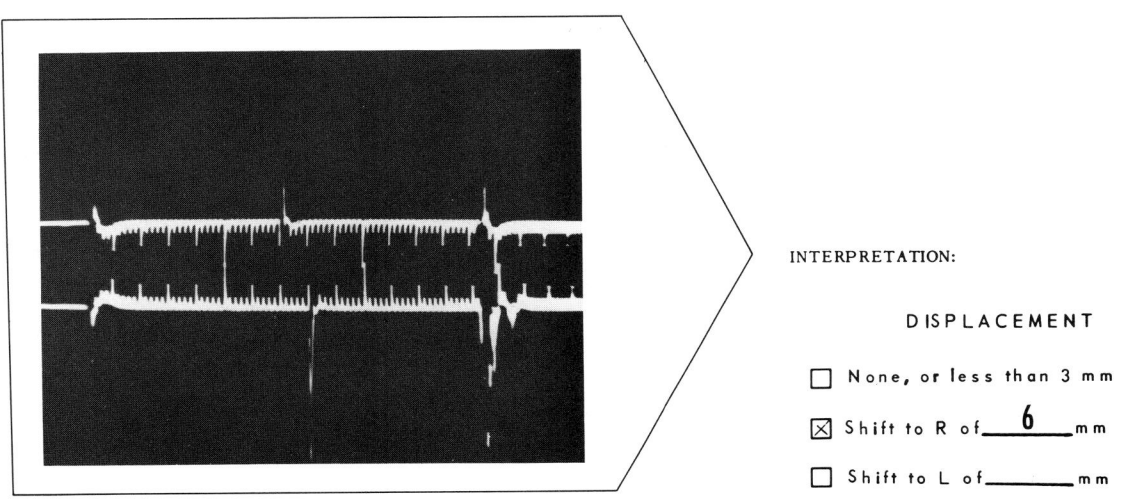

INTERPRETATION:

DISPLACEMENT

☐ None, or less than 3 mm

☒ Shift to R of __6__ mm

☐ Shift to L of _____ mm

Figure 10–13 Echoencephalogram showing a 6-mm shift to the right due to a left subdural hematoma.

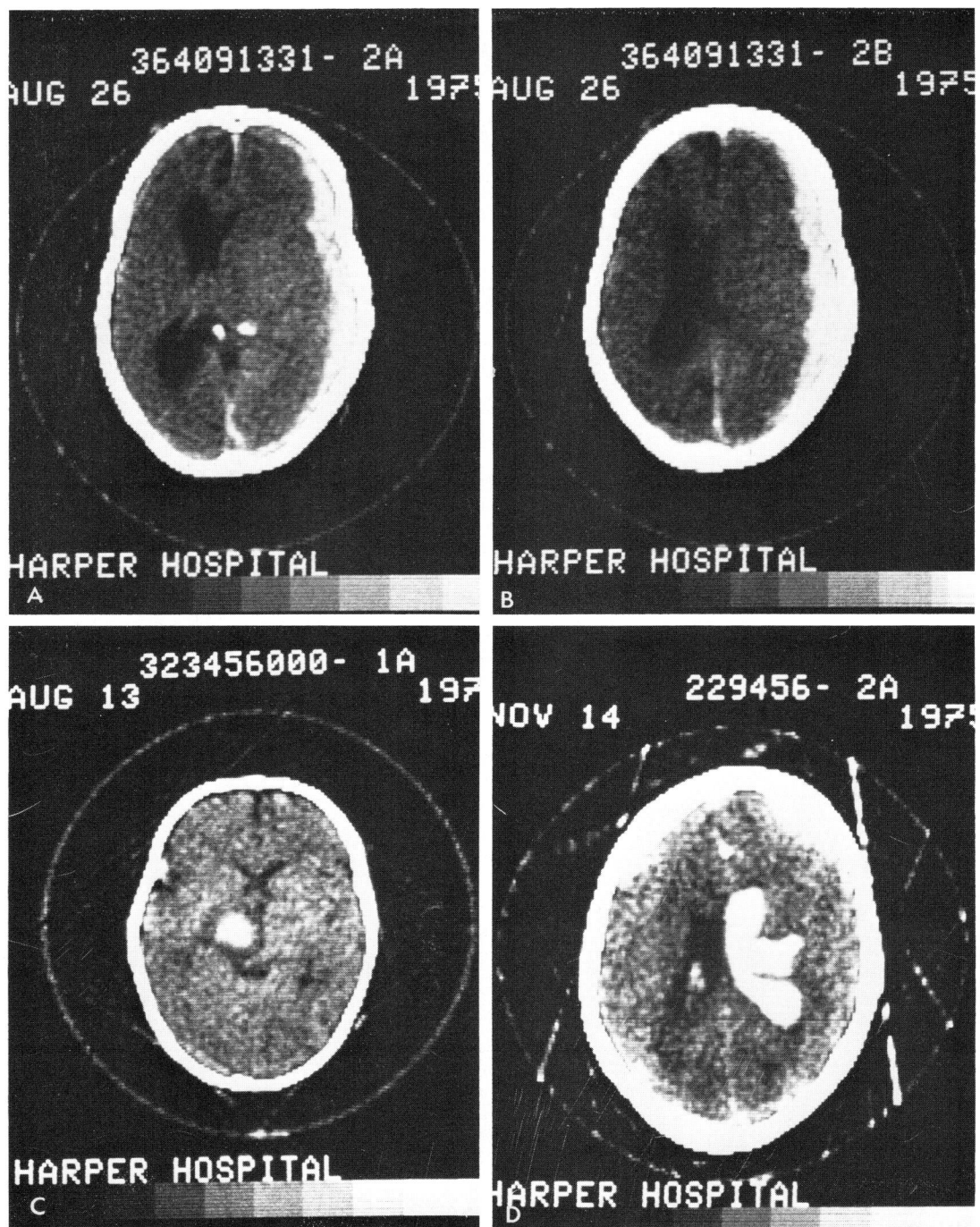

Figure 10–14 Computed tomographic scans of chronic subdural hematoma and intracerebral hemorrhages. *A* and *B*. Right chronic subdural hematoma. Note the displacement of the ventricular cavities. *C*. An area of hemorrhage in the left posterior thalamus. *D*. A right intracerebral hematoma extending into the lateral ventricle. The facility should be in the emergency care area of a hospital. Serial tomography may be invaluable in showing rebleeding in a postoperative case. A new bleed not previously seen may be shown in subsequent scans.

Diagnostic Evaluation

Pupillary abnormalities are important from a diagnostic and prognostic standpoint. A dilated pupil is almost always on the same side as the mass lesion. In both the epidural and subdural hematoma pupillary dilatation may become a complete oculomotor paralysis if it is untreated. A weakness of the opposite half of the body may be seen. Occasionally, the weakness or hemiparesis may be on the same side as the intracranial mass lesion. This is due to displacement of the brain stem and compression of its contralateral side against the incisural border, with pyramidal tract dysfunction on the same side as the hematoma. Such a paradoxical manifestation may be appreciated preoperatively by a pineal body displaced toward the paralyzed side or by contrast studies.

Pupillary abnormalities have prognostic significance. In the Jamieson and Yelland series, bilateral pupillary dilatation and fixation presented a mortality of 85 per cent. More than two out of three cases with bilaterally fixed pupils were associated with decerebrate rigidity. The mortality in this group (i.e., fixed pupils with decerebrate rigidity) was 95 per cent. The mortality of all cases of decerebrate rigidity was 87 per cent. When decerebration is due to an epidural or subdural hematoma, surgical excision may save life and function, if it is performed before irreversible changes take place.

Evaluation by skull x-ray, echoencephalography, and CAT scan may suffice in the acute subdural hematoma. In subacute and chronic forms, there may be the time and need for additional studies, such as angiography, repeat CAT scan, air studies, EEG, and radioisotope scan. (Fig. 10–14).

Treatment

Treatment of subdural hematoma may utilize multiple trephine openings, subtemporal decompression, and exposure of the intracranial space by appropriate bone flap. A fluid clot may be treated with burr holes. An acute subdural hematoma responds somewhat better with excision of bone flap. This permits a good exposure of the clot and bleeding area and enables more complete excision. Extensive contused areas with brain softening should be surgically treated by careful excision with magnification.

MEDICAL MANAGEMENT

Throughout this chapter, management of head injuries has been discussed in appropriate sections. As noted previously, the minimally injured patient does not need special management. Moderately and severely injured cases deserve careful observation. Their treatment may include administration of fluid and food via nasogastric tube. Decadron and antiacid medication may be helpful. Care of the respiratory system is extremely important, and intermittent positive pressure breathing (IPPB) may be useful. Increasing the positive end-expiratory pressure (PEEP) above 10 cm of water may be deleterious since it may cause a collapse of pulmonary capillary bed, resulting in more shunting and consequently increasing the hypoxia. Moderate increase of PEEP may overcome some of the right-to-left pulmonary shunting.[17]

Intravenous fluids, plasma, and blood transfusion are used if indicated. Usually, impending shock is seen when the head injury is associated with multiple injuries of the body.

CSF rhinorrhea should be treated with prophylactic doses of antibiotics. In the presence of infection (infected wound, osteomyelitis, meningitis, brain abscess, or pneumonitis), appropriate antibiotics should also be used. With open wounds of the brain, anticonvulsant medication is frequently required.

REFERENCES

1. Accident Facts, 1968–1975. Chicago, National Safety Council, 1976.
2. Gurdjian, E. S., and Gurdjian, E. S.: Reevaluation of the biomechanics of blunt impact head injury. Surg. Gynecol. Obstet., *140*:845–850, 1975.
3. Gurdjian, E. S., and Gurdjian, E. S.: Cerebral contusions. J. Trauma, *16*:35–51, 1976.
4. Gurdjian, E. S., Bartl, G. R., and Thomas, L. M.: Emergency care of patients with trauma of the nervous system. *In* Emergency Care. Philadelphia, Hahnemann Medical College, 1972.

5. Gurdjian, E. S.: Impact Head Injury—Mechanistic, Clinical and Preventive Correlations. Springfield, C C Thomas, 1975.

6. Hodgson, V. R., Brinn, J., Thomas, L. M.: and Greenberg, S. W.: Fracture behavior of the skull frontal bone against cylindrical surfaces. Proceedings of 14 Stapp Conference, pp. 341–355, 1970.

7. Ommaya, A. K., Corrao, P. B., and Latcher, F. S.: Head injury in the chimpanzee. Part I. Biomechanics of traumatic unconsciousness. J. Neurosurg., 39:152–166, 1973.

8. Gurdjian, E. S., and Webster, J. E.: Head Injuries. Mechanisms, Diagnosis and Management. Boston, Little, Brown, 1958.

9. Hooper, R. S.: Observations on extradural hemorrhage. Br. J. Surg., 47:71–87, 1959.

10. Lake, P. A., and Pitts, F. W.: Recent experience with epidural hematomas. J. Trauma, 11:397–411, 1971.

11. Galligioni, F., Bernardi, R., Pellone, M., and Iraci, G.: Angiographic signs of rupture of middle meningeal artery without epidural hematoma. Am. J. Roentgenol., 104:71–74, 1968.

12. Portnoy, J. D., Schulte, R. R., Fox, J. L., Croissant, P. C., and Tripp, L.: Anti-siphon and reversible occlusion valves for shunting of hydrocephalus and preventing post-shunt subdural hematomas. J. Neurosurg., 38:729–738, 1973.

13. Schneider, R. C.: Head and Neck Injuries in Football, p. 279. Baltimore, Williams & Wilkins, 1973.

14. Ciembroniewicz, J. E.: Subdural hematoma of the posterior fossa. J. Neurosurg., 22:465–473, 1965.

15. Wright, R. L.: Traumatic hematomas in the posterior cranial fossa. J. Neurosurg., 25:402–409, 1966.

16. Mealey, J., Jr.: Pediatric Head Injuries, p.243. Springfield, C C Thomas, 1963.

17. Laver, M. B., and Lowenstein, E.: Lung function following trauma in man. Clin. Neurosurg., 19:84–97, 1972.

JOHN MARQUIS CONVERSE, M.D.,
and
DANIEL C. BAKER, M.D.

Maxillofacial ————————————— 11
Fractures

In the twentieth century facial injuries, particularly fractures, have progressively increased in severity as the speed and number of automobiles have increased. The relatively simple fracture of bygone days has been replaced by the comminuted, often open, type of fracture that frequently involves the middle third of the facial skeleton, including orbital cavities, anterior cranial fossa, and brain (Table 11–1).

PHYSICAL BASIS OF FACIAL FRACTURES

Fractures of the facial bones are the result of direct or indirect injury. A fist blow to the face is an example of direct injury; the forward projection of the face onto the dashboard in an automobile crash is an example of indirect injury. The type of fracture depends upon the severity and direction of the impact. The striking force may result in fracture of a single bone without displacement, comminution of bone, or fractures involving a number of bones. The overlying soft tissues also influence the type of fracture as well as the displacement of fragments.

In automobile crash injuries, the direction of the blow is determined in part by the position of the victim at the time of impact. In striking the dashboard or windshield, the head is tilted forward, backward, or to one side, and the site of impact on the face varies (Fig. 11–1).

Timing of Treatment

The primary goal of the physician treating facial injuries is the restoration of normal

TABLE 11–1   Location of Facial Fractures by Cause of Injury*

Type	Auto	Athletic	Home	Other	Intended	Work	Total
Nasal bones	208	66	45	29	25	9	382
Zygoma and arch	105	13	7	12	14	8	159
Mandible	74	10	7	5	9	7	112
Orbital floor	76	12	6	6	10	2	112
Maxilla	67	3	4	5	2	3	84
Teeth	48	10	3	5	2	3	71
Sinuses	37	3	1	3	3	3	50
Supraorbital area	31	0	2	1	0	2	36
Alveolus	19	2	1	1	1	1	25
Total	665	119	76	67	66	38	1031
Per cent	65	12	7	6	6	4	100

*Courtesy of R. C. Schultz and Yearbook Medical Publishers, Chicago. *Facial Injuries*, 1970.

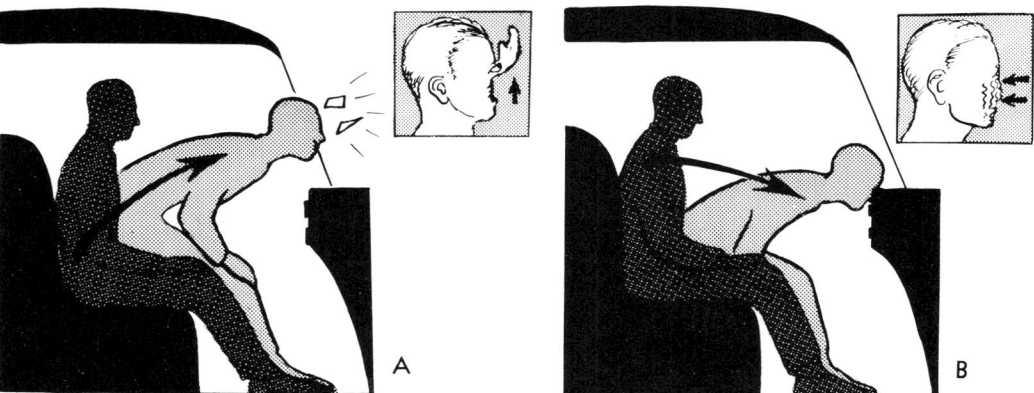

Figure 11–1 Two mechanisms of injury in automobile accident. *A.* Occupant is projected forward through windshield. Lower edge of broken windshield may cause avulsion of soft tissues of face (inset). *B.* Projection of occupant against dashboard produces a variety of fractures of the facial skeleton (inset). (Courtesy of J. M. Converse and *Medical Tribune.* An auto tragedy, Med. Trib., 1964.)

function and appearance. Although early treatment is especially important in minimizing cosmetic and functional disability, facial soft-tissue and bone injuries are rarely surgical emergencies. Except for control of hemorrhage and establishment of a satisfactory airway, treatment of intracranial, thoracic, and intraabdominal trauma takes precedence over the management of facial injuries. Furthermore, lacerations covered with sterile saline soaked dressings can still be closed primarily within 24 hours.

Early treatment of facial fractures is initiated either immediately or within 48 hours of the injury. Sometimes, when extensive edema and hematomas are present, it is better to delay treatment. Delayed treatment usually extends over the first few weeks of the injury, before consolidation of bone occurs. Purposeful delay in the reduction of facial fractures is decided upon when the condition of the patient is too critical. Late treatment is required if the fractured fragments have consolidated in faulty relationships and resulted in a malunited fracture; organized tissue must then be removed from the fracture site or osteotomy must be performed.

Healing of Maxillofacial Fractures

The healing of facial fractures is governed by the same biological factors involved in fractures of other bones. Most fractures of the facial bones, other than the mandible, heal rapidly because the fragments are not subjected to strong muscular activity. The rapidity with which fractures heal depends upon many factors: the age of the patient (fractures of the mandible in children usually heal within three weeks), the severity of the initial damage, and the bones involved (nasal bone fractures heal in seven days, maxillary fractures in four weeks, and mandibular fractures in four to six weeks). In older patients a fixation period of six to eight weeks may be required.

Reduction and Fixation

There is a wide choice in the methods of reduction and fixation of facial fractures. Each case must be considered individually; the treatment selected should be the one that will achieve good results in the simplest and most rapid manner. The most commonly used and preferred methods are described here.

It must be emphasized that fractured bone fragments will not heal and consolidate, nor will bone grafts be successful, unless they are covered with well-vascularized soft tissues, inasmuch as the bones depend upon the blood supply from the soft tissues for osteogenic potential. Realigned bony fragments assured of adequate fixation and covered with well-vascularized soft tissues should heal without complications.

The Importance of Dental Occlusion

Any fracture that involves the mandible or maxilla disrupts the alignment of the teeth. Anyone treating maxillofacial fractures must be aware of the normal occlusal relationships of dentition, as this serves as a guide in the reestablishment of displaced fragments and restoration of the masticatory efficiency of the teeth. Although several millimeters of displacement might be considered good reduction of a tibial fracture, this is not true of mandibular and maxillary fractures. When dental occlusion has been reestablished, the bone fragments have usually been placed in good functional alignment.

Immobilization and fixation of the fragments are facilitated when sound teeth are present on one or both sides of a fractured jaw, for the teeth provide an ideal means of anchorage. The edentulous patient requires special methods of fixation.

In what is usually considered normal occlusion, a vertical line drawn between the two central incisors and extended downward falls between the two lower incisors; the two midincisor points are on a vertical line (Fig. 11–2). The medial buccal cusps of the maxillary first molar fit into the buccal

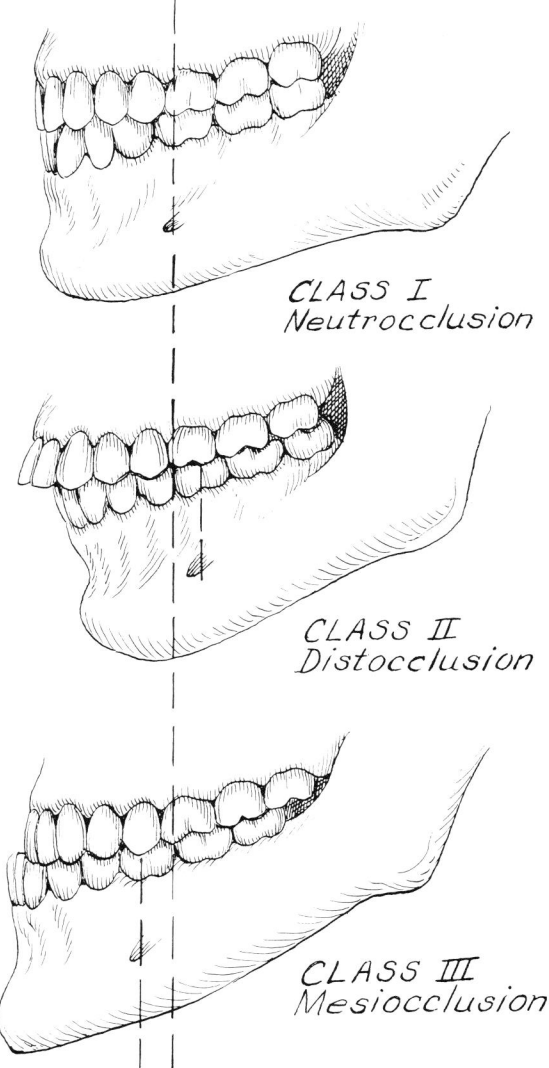

Figure 11–3 Angle classification of malocclusion. A. Simplified version of the Angle classification is useful in diagnosis of malocclusion in fractures. Class I (neutrocclusion) in which the mesiobuccal cusp of the first maxillary molar is occluded into the mesiobuccal groove of the first mandibular molar tooth. In Class II malocclusion, the mesiobuccal cusp of the first maxillary molar is in an anterior relationship with the first mandibular molar tooth. In Class III malocclusion, the mandibular dental arch is in an anterior relationship to the corresponding maxillary molar tooth. (After R. O. Dingman: The management of facial injuries in fractures of facial bones. In J. M. Converse (ed.): *Reconstructive Plastic Surgery*, Philadelphia, W. B. Saunders Co., 1964.)

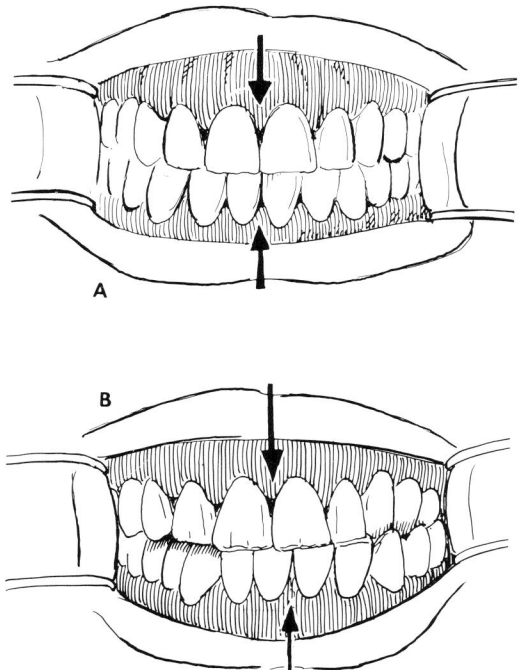

Figure 11–2 Midincisor points. A. Midincisor points lie within the midsagittal plane of the face. B. Deviation of the lower midincisor point from the midline, indicating deviation of the mandible resulting from the fracture or from developmental malformation. (Courtesy of V. H. Kazanjiian and J. M. Converse and The Williams & Wilkins Co., Baltimore. *Surgical Treatment of Facial Injuries.* 3rd Ed., 1974.)

groove of the mandibular first molar (Fig. 11–3). The disruption of these occlusal relationships is an important sign of fracture of the jaws; in a suspected fracture, a deviation of the midincisor points or a crossbite is indicative of a fracture with medial or lateral displacement; when the upper teeth are situated posteriorly or in lingual occlusal relationships with the mandibular teeth, a push-back maxillary fracture may be suspected.

FRACTURES OF THE MANDIBLE

The mandible, the largest bone of the face, consisting of a body and two rami, is a moveable bone articulated with the cranium by means of the temporomandibular joints and connected with other bones of the face and cranium by ligaments and muscles. Mandibular movements play a role in mastication, deglutition, respiration, and speech. Although the mandible is a strong bone with a thick cortex and contains but little spongiosa, it is frequently exposed to trauma because of its position and prominence.

CLASSIFICATION OF MANDIBULAR FRACTURES

Fractures of the mandible are variously classified by different authors. The following classification is based on the presence or absence of serviceable teeth in relation to the line of fracture, because the teeth and their supporting structures serve as anchorage for intermaxillary fixation appliances. Three groups or classes of mandibular fractures are distinguished, each requiring a different method of treatment (Fig. 11–4).[16] Class I fractures are those in which teeth are present on each side of the fracture; in Class II fractures teeth are present on one side only; in Class III fractures the mandible is edentulous.

SURGICAL PATHOLOGY

The mechanism of mandibular fractures is complex because of the arch shape of the mandible, which distributes the force of

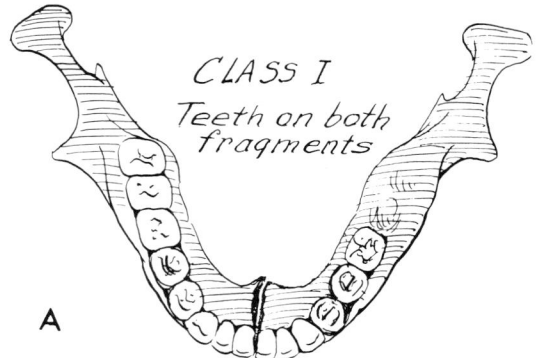

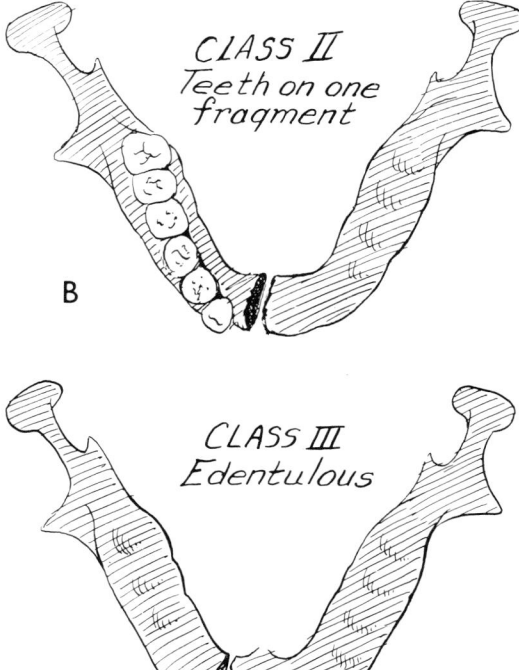

Figure 11–4   Classification of mandibular fractures. *A.* Class I fractures. *B.* Class II fractures. *C.* Class III fractures. (Courtesy of V. H. Kazanjian and J. M. Converse and The Williams & Wilkins Co., Baltimore. *Surgical Treatment of Facial Injuries,* 3rd Ed., 1974.)

impact throughout its length. The distributed force seeks out the weakest point in the arch and causes bending and tensile failure at that point.[14] Frequently there is a fracture at the impact point when the blow is to the mandibular body.

Displacement of the fragments is influenced by the direction of muscle pull, the direction and bevel of the fracture line, the presence or absence of teeth, the extent of soft-tissue wounds, and the direction and intensity of the traumatic force. The successful treatment of mandibular fractures requires an appreciation of all these factors.

CLINICAL EXAMINATION

The signs of mandibular fracture vary according to the severity of the injury. In most fractures, the dental occlusion is disrupted (Fig. 11–5). The patient complains that the teeth do not meet as before the accident and that attempts to masticate cause pain. Localized tenderness, ecchymosis, and abnormal mobility and crepitus between the teeth on each side of the fracture line may be noted on close examination (Fig. 11–6). Anesthesia of the lower lip on the affected side may result from damage or compression of the inferior alveolar nerve. Other signs include swelling, edema, trismus, and drooling because the patient has difficulty controlling saliva and swallowing.

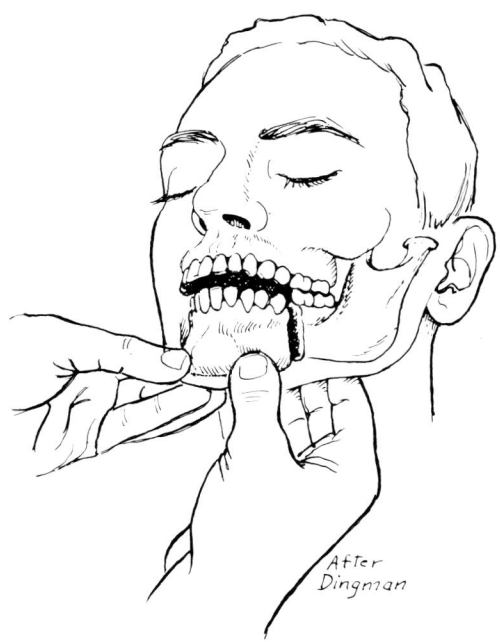

Figure 11–6 Palpation of the fractured mandible demonstrates mobility, pain, and crepitus. (Courtesy of V. H. Kazanjian and J. M. Converse and The Williams & Wilkins Co., Baltimore. *Surgical Treatment of Facial Injuries,* 3rd Ed., 1974.)

ROENTGENOGRAPHIC EXAMINATION

Careful roentgenographic examination is necessary to obtain a more accurate picture of the direction and extent of the fracture and to evaluate the teeth. Particular attention should be given to the condyles, and stereoscopic views may be helpful.

TREATMENT OF MANDIBULAR FRACTURES

The importance of early reduction and immobilization of bone fragments cannot be overemphasized; these procedures should be initiated as soon as the patient's condition permits. Local or inferior alveolar block anesthesia is usually adequate when treatment consists of closed reduction and immobilization by intermaxillary fixation alone. When multiple facial fractures are present and open reduction is required, general anesthesia with endotracheal intubation or tracheostomy is preferred.

The fragments usually prove to be in correct alignment when the teeth are immobilized in adequate occlusion. Any

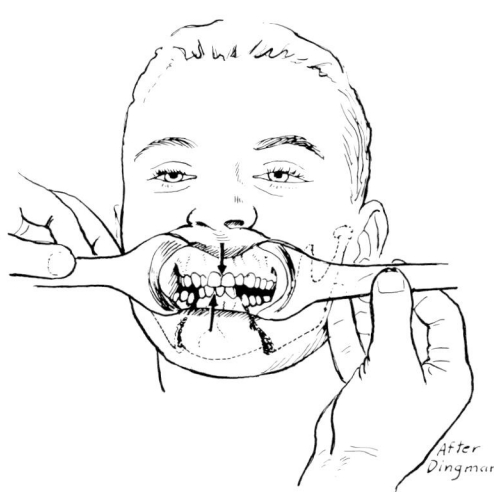

Figure 11–5 Examination of the teeth in a bilateral fracture of the body of the mandible shows an upward and backward displacement of the central fragment with deviation to the right, as demonstrated by the displacement to the right of the lower midincisor point. (Courtesy of V. H. Kazanjian and J. M. Converse and The Williams & Wilkins Co., Baltimore. *Surgical Treatment of Facial Injuries,* 3rd Ed., 1974.)

method of reduction should be based on this principle; otherwise the resulting deformities may not only affect the symmetry of the face but also result in functional impairment of mastication and speech.

Methods of Reduction and Fixation

Reduction of the displaced fragments can be performed either immediately or progressively. Immediate reduction is obtained by placing the fragments in alignment and splinting them in occlusion with the maxilla, using a variety of dental fixation appliances. Progressive reduction by means of steady traction with wires or elastic bands extending between the fractured fragments and the upper jaw may be achieved in a few hours or may require continuous elastic traction for one or two days.

In the treatment of the fractured mandible, the teeth serve as abutments for fixation appliances. Sound teeth may be compared to pegs fastened to bone, an ideal anchorage. If the long bones bore knobs or structures mechanically similar to teeth, the orthopedic surgeon would surely make use of them. If the teeth are neither sound nor numerous, the supporting alveolar process may be utilized for anchorage.

Intermaxillary (Bimaxillary) and Monomaxillary Fixation. Intermaxillary, or bi-maxillary, fixation consists of wiring the mandibular teeth to those of the maxilla in adequate dental occlusal relationships; the jaw is immobilized in a fixed mouth-closed position. Monomaxillary fixation appliances provide fixation of the jaw fragments without intermaxillary fixation; with this method movements of the mandible are possible during the healing period. The guiding principle—the assurance of correct occlusal relationshps—must always be observed, however, in monomaxillary fixation.

Although numerous methods and techniques to accomplish intermaxillary fixation have been described, the most popular methods when sufficient teeth are present are eyelet wiring, the arch bar technique, and splinting by means of bands around the teeth connected by a wire arch similar to the appliance used by the orthodontists (Figs. 11–7, 11–8, and 11–9).

Interosseous Fixation. Comminuted mandibular fractures, unstable and displaced fractures in the edentulous mandible, and some condylar fractures may require direct interosseous fixation to maintain adequate reduction. The most popular methods are direct interosseous wiring and bone plate fixation. Open reduction and direct interosseous wiring provide anatomical reduction and positive fixation at the site of fracture. In severely comminuted frac-

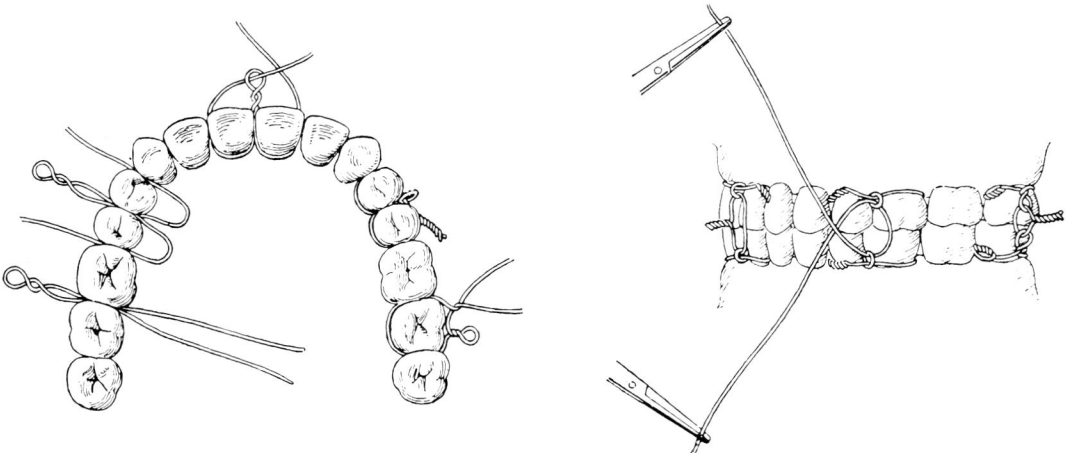

Figure 11–7 Eyelet method. The various steps in constructing eyelets and joining the upper and lower jaws together in intermaxillary fixation are shown. (After R. H. Ivy: Observations of fractures of the mandible J.A.M.A., 79:295, 1922. Courtesy of J. M. Converse and W. B. Saunders Co., Philadelphia. Reconstructive Plastic Surgery, 2nd Ed., 1977.)

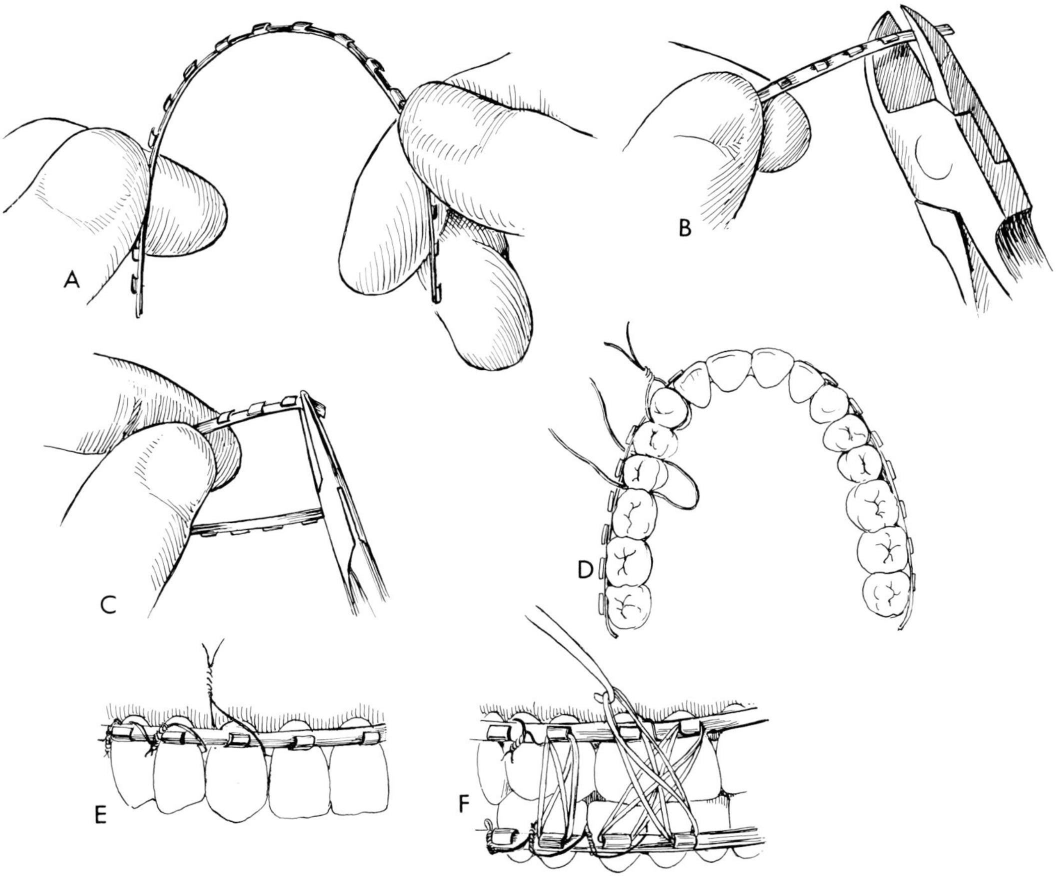

Figure 11–8 Arch bar technique. *A.* Malleable arch bar for intermaxillary fixation. *B.* Arch bar is cut to a suitable length. *C.* Arch bar is bent to adapt to the curvature of the teeth. *D.* Fixation of the arch bar to the dental arch by means of wires passed around the necks of selected teeth. *E.* Method of placing wire around neck of the tooth to prevent downward slippage of the arch bar. *F.* Intermaxillary fixation is provided by intermaxillary elastic bands. (Courtesy of J. M. Converse and W. B. Saunders Co., Philadelphia. *Reconstructive Plastic Surgery,* 2nd Ed., 1977.)

tures, there may be occasional indication for bone plate fixation of the fragments (Fig. 11–10).

Fractures of the Mandibular Condyle

Fractures of the condylar process are the most frequent of all mandibular fractures, since the neck of the condyle is the weakest part of the mandible.[23] Because of the protection from direct injury afforded by the zygomatic arch, condylar fractures generally result from a traumatic force applied to the body of the mandible, often the mental symphysis.

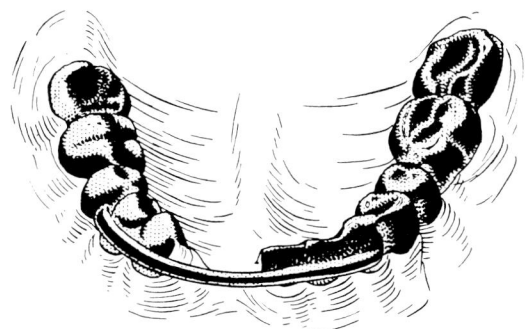

Figure 11–9 Swaged cap splint is cemented to the teeth on both sides of the fracture. The two halves of the splint are joined by the wire arch. (Courtesy of J. M. Converse and W. B. Saunders Co., Philadelphia. *Reconstructive Plastic Surgery,* 1st Ed., 1964.)

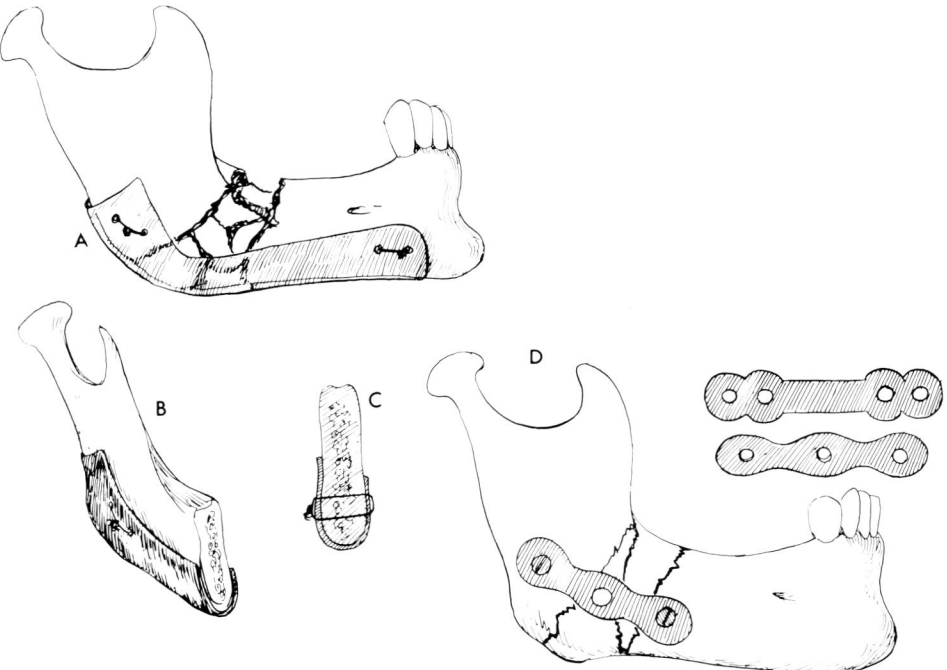

Figure 11–10   Bone plate fixation in comminuted Class II fractures. *A, B,* and *C.* Molded metal splint maintained by transosseous wiring. *D.* Another type of bone plate fixed to the mandible by means of bone screws. These appliances are rarely indicated in fractures of the mandible with the exception of badly comminuted fractures. (Courtesy of J. M. Converse and W. B. Saunders Co., Philadelphia. *Reconstructive Plastic Surgery,* 1st Ed., 1964.)

Because of the structural complexity of the temporomandibular joint, fractures in this area are often best treated by simple methods. Unless serious damage affects the joint surfaces of the condyle, the temporomandibular joint may be subjected to prolonged periods of immobilization without becoming ankylosed.

Mandibular displacement is usually lateral and backward in unilateral fracture, the most common of condylar fractures. The chin is deviated toward the injured side, normal occlusion is disturbed, and swelling and tenderness are present over the temporomandibular joint (Fig. 11–11). Roentgenographic examination may reveal an overriding of the fragments and forward or backward displacement of the neck of the condyle. Laminograms may be necessary to demonstrate fractures with minimal or no displacement.

Intermaxillary fixation alone achieves acceptable reduction in the majority of sub-

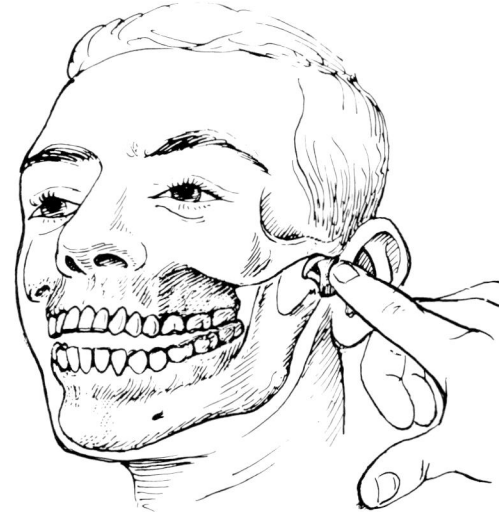

Figure 11–11   Pain elicited by digital palpation over the condylar area (and also within the external auditory canal) is one of the signs of fracture of the neck of the condyle. (Courtesy of J. M. Converse and W. B. Saunders Co., Philadelphia. *Reconstructive Plastic Surgery,* 2nd Ed., 1977.)

condylar fractures. Although this type of conservative treatment does not correct the position of the medially displaced condylar head, the maintenance of bony contact between the condylar fragment and the ramus results in consolidation. It is not essential to achieve perfect anatomical relationships in this type of fracture, for good function is restored by drawing the lower jaw forward until the teeth occlude. The occlusion must be maintained by intermaxillary fixation until union is established; four to five weeks of immobilization are usually sufficient.

Although some surgeons advocate open reduction in order to realign the fragment by means of interosseous wire fixation, a greater number feel that conservative treatment affords satisfactory results.[2, 9, 11, 19, 22] Open reduction is indicated, however, when the head of the condyle is luxated out of the glenoid fossa. Removal of the head of the condyle may be necessary in such cases, and also in comminuted fractures followed by wound sepsis, suppuration, fibrosis, or ankylosis.

Test for Consolidation of Jaw Fractures

Radiological evidence of healing is usually not present until several months after the injury. The only valid test for estimating consolidation of a jaw fracture is to release intermaxillary fixation and actually test the solidity of the union by digital manipulation. If the fracture appears to be consolidated, intermaxillary fixation is released for a few days. If a slight shift occurs in the occlusal relationships of the teeth, intermaxillary elastic bands are replaced for a week or two.

After the release of fixation, the patient should be advised to avoid attempting to eat hard foods, as he may develop temporomandibular pain. The muscles of mastication that have been long immobilized fatigue easily at this stage. It is interesting that the temporomandibular joint, if uninjured, appears to be the only joint in the body that can be immobilized for long periods of time without undue discomfort or resulting ankylosis.

COMPLICATIONS IN MANDIBULAR FRACTURES

Early complications following fracture of the mandible include primary hemorrhage, respiratory complications, infection, avascular necrosis of denuded bone, osteitis, osteomyelitis, and trismus.

Delayed union, nonunion, malunion, trismus and ankylosis of the temporomandibular joints, scar adhesions of the oral tissues, inferior alveolar nerve anesthesia, and concomitant deformities are late complications in mandibular fractures.

FRACTURES OF THE MAXILLA

The maxilla is the largest and the central bone of the midface skeleton, and along with the other bones of the midfacial area, it forms a protective shell for the brain. The midfacial area lodges the organs of vision and olfaction. The clinical importance of middle third fractures is explained not only by the deformity they cause and the danger of intracranial complications but also by the functional disturbances resulting from inadequate treatment.

SURGICAL PATHOLOGY

Partial, or alveolar, fractures are almost always caused by direct impact from a relatively narrow object, such as the rim of

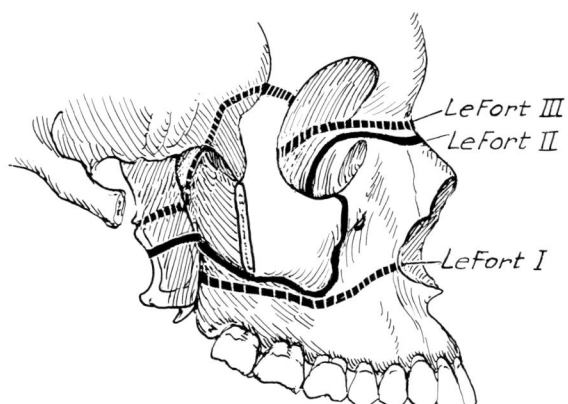

Figure 11–12 Le Fort's lines of fracture. (Courtesy of J. M. Converse and W. B. Saunders Co., Philadelphia. *Reconstructive Plastic Surgery*, 2nd Ed., 1977.)

an automobile steering wheel. Only a portion of the alveolar process or adjacent portion of the body of the maxilla is affected, the main segment of the maxilla remaining attached to the cranium.

Complete transverse fractures of the maxilla are transverse fractures that detach a portion of or the entire maxilla from the cranial base. The location and common sites of fracture were determined in experiments conducted by Le Fort.[20]

LeFort I, or Guérin's, Fracture

The alveolar process, the vault of the palate, and the pterygoid processes usually form a single detached block in lower maxillary fractures (Figs. 11–12 and 11–13).

LeFort II, or Pyramidal, Fractures

A transverse fracture line through the middle portion of the nasal bones may extend through the frontal process of the maxilla, cross the lacrimal bones, double back through the orbital plate of the maxilla and infraorbital margin, descend laterally through the anterior wall of the maxillary sinus near the zygomatic-maxillary junction, cross the posterior wall of the maxilla into the pterygomaxillary fissure, and extend through the pterygoid processes as shown in Figures 11–12 and 11–13. The zygomas are often not involved in the pyramidal fracture. The interorbital space, however, may be penetrated and splayed out in such fractures when they are associated with backward displacement and nasoorbital fractures.

Le Fort III Fracture, or Craniofacial Disjunction

The frontal process of the maxilla and the zygoma may remain attached to the maxilla, the bones of the middle portion of the face being completely detached from the cranium at the level of the floor of the orbits (Figs. 11–12 and 11–14).

Displacement in Maxillary Fractures

The maxilla, unlike the mandible, does not give origin to muscles sufficiently powerful to cause displacement, but offers only points of origin for the muscles of facial expression. Displacement, therefore, is the

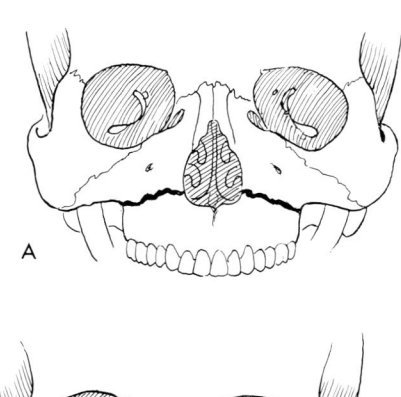
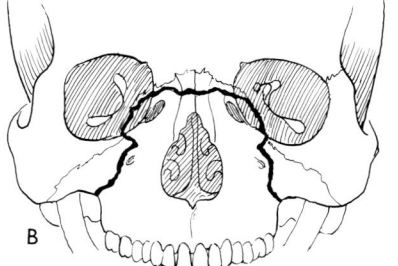

Figure 11–13 A. Low maxillary (Le Fort I or Guerin's fracture. B. Pyramidal (Le Fort II) fracture. (Courtesy of J. M. Converse and W. B. Saunders Co., Philadelphia. *Reconstructive Plastic Surgery*, 2nd Ed., 1977.)

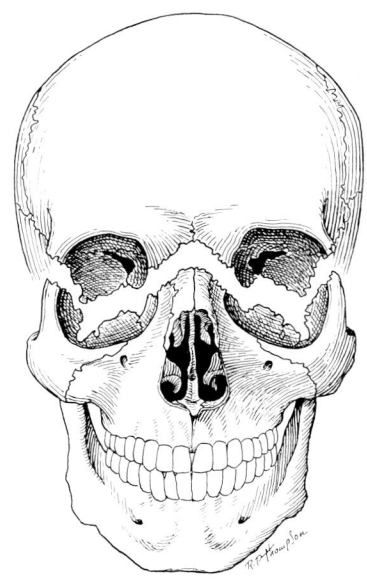

Figure 11–14 Craniofacial disjunction (Le Fort III). (Courtesy of J. M. Converse and W. B. Saunders Co., Philadelphia. *Reconstructive Plastic Surgery*, 2nd Ed., 1977.)

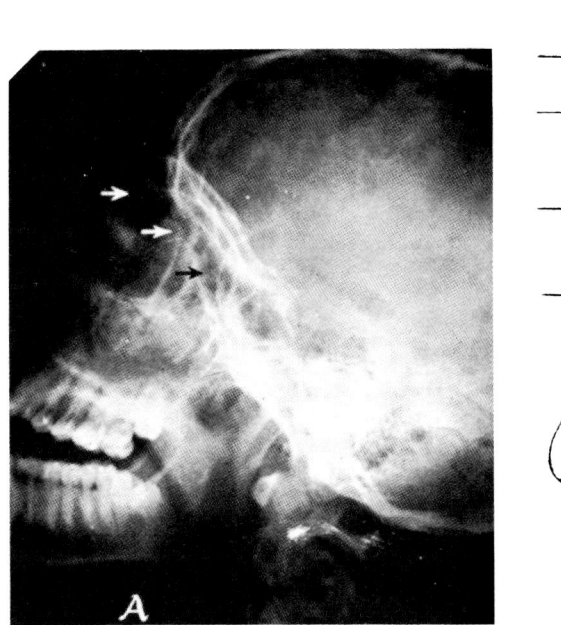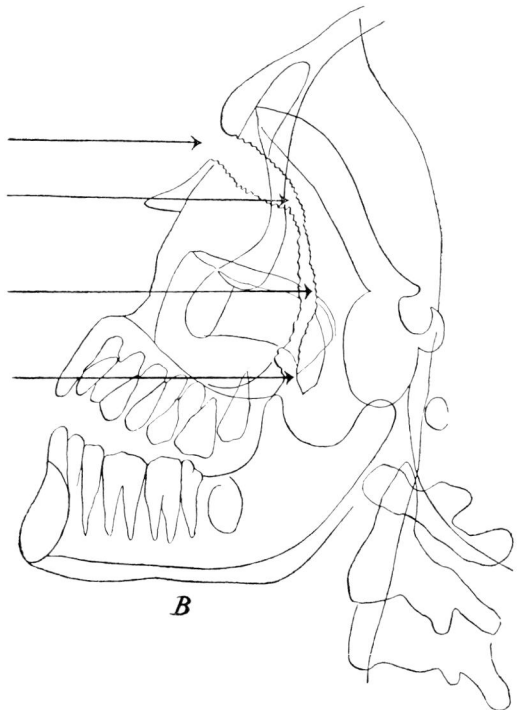

Figure 11–15   A. Craniofacial disjunction with backward and downward displacement of the maxilla. *B*. Tracing of roentgenogram showing the lines of the fracture. (Courtesy of J. M. Converse and W. B. Saunders Co., Philadelphia. *Reconstructive Plastic Surgery*, 2nd Ed., 1977.)

result of the direction and point of impact plus the severity of the traumatic force that has caused the fracture. Displacement occurs downward and laterally, or downward, laterally, and backward (Fig. 11–15).

CLINICAL EXAMINATION

The patient often presents a typical appearance with symmetrical swelling of the face, bilateral orbital ecchymosis, subconjunctival hemmorhage, and swollen eyelids. When there is severe retroposition of the maxilla, the face appears flat and longer or shorter than normal despite the swelling (Fig. 11–16). In high maxillary fractures involving the cribriform plate and anterior cranial fossa, cerebrospinal fluid may discharge from the nostrils and backward into the pharynx.

Inspection of the teeth usually shows disturbance in the occlusal relationships. When the displacement is vertical and downward only, the teeth may meet in normal occlusion even though the entire maxilla is freely moveable. Complete disarrangement of occlusion occurs, however, when the displacement is backward and downward, or backward and upward, or when the maxilla is twisted laterally.

Palpation demonstrates mobility and crepitation at the site of the fracture lines. Bimanual palpation elicits additional information. By grasping the teeth and alveolar process between the thumb and forefinger of one hand, one may feel movement by palpating the face with the fingers of the other hand (Fig. 11–17). The position of the lines of fracture can be elicited in Le Fort II fractures; in Le Fort III fractures, the area of craniofacial separation at the central frontonasal area and at the lateral frontozygomatic areas can also be identified by bimanual palpation.

It is important, in high maxillary fractures, to determine whether the fracture extends to the cranium. A telescoping of the nose backward into the ethmoid, associated with widening of the intercanthal distance, may

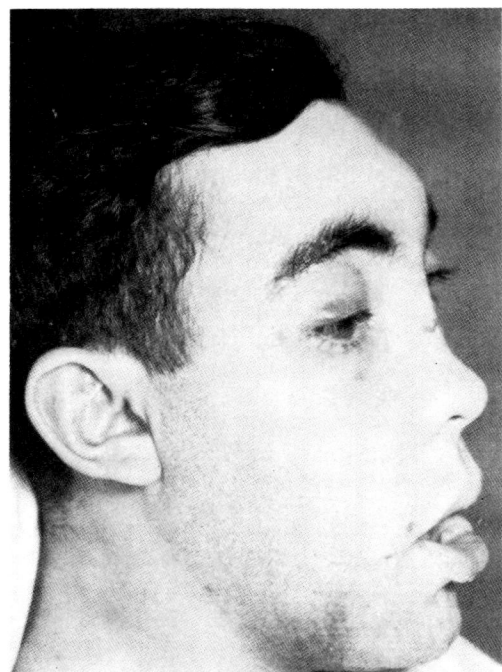

Figure 11–16 Elongation of the face caused by the downward displacement of the maxilla in craniofacial disjunction (Le Fort III fracture). (Courtesy of J. M. Converse and W. B. Saunders Co., Philadelphia. *Reconstructive Plastic Surgery,* 2nd Ed., 1977.)

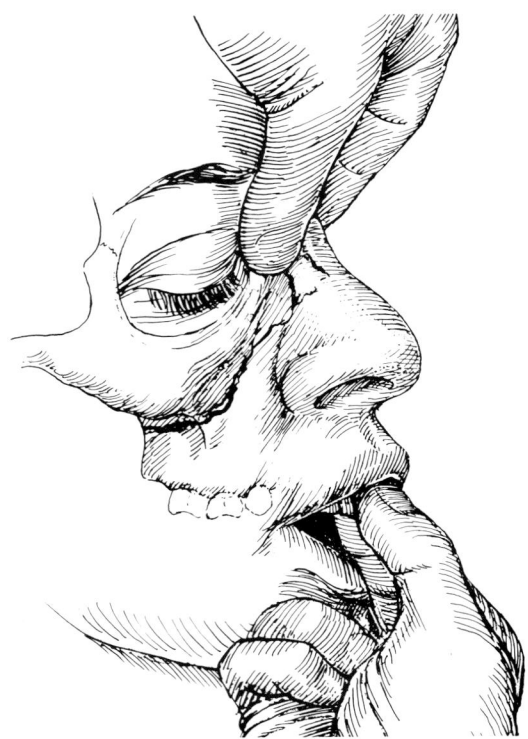

Figure 11–17 Bimanual palpation provides valuable information, for movement at the fracture lines indicates their location. (Courtesy of J. M. Converse and W. B. Saunders Co., Philadelphia. *Reconstructive Plastic Surgery,* 2nd Ed., 1977.)

occur in severe crash injuries with nasoorbital fracture. Positive diagnosis of cerebrospinal fluid rhinorrhea is evidence of cribriform plate involvement.

ROENTGENOGRAPHIC EXAMINATION

The clinical diagnosis of maxillary fracture is verified by roentgenographic examination, which may disclose unsuspected fractures of other bones of the middle portion of the face. The Waters view is excellent for demonstrating fractures of the maxilla and adjacent bones.

TREATMENT OF MAXILLARY FRACTURES

As fractures of the maxilla heal quite readily, reduction and fixation should not be delayed. The entire facial substructure may be grossly distorted in severe fractures, and permanent deformity will be the price to pay for inadequate treatment.

Although each type of fracture requires a specific technique based upon available points of anchorage for fixation appliances, treatment of the fractured maxilla essentially consists of two procedures: (1) reduction of displaced fragments and their replacement, using normal occlusal relationships as a guide; and (2) fixation of the reduced fragments against the base of the cranium until consolidation occurs.

Complete Transverse Fractures of the Maxilla

A feature of the transverse fracture is the complete separation of the lower maxillary fragment from its attachments to the remainder of the maxilla or the separation of the entire maxilla from the cranium. The fragmented segments may be separated and loose, the "floating" maxilla, or firmly

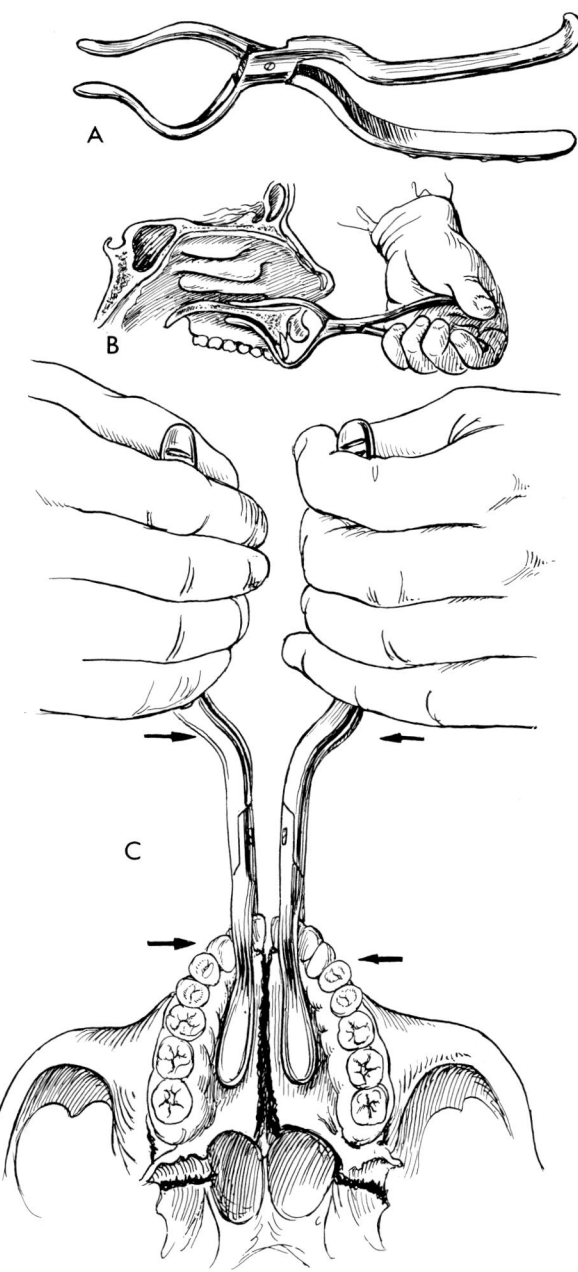

Figure 11–18   A. Rowe's forceps for disimpaction of the maxilla. *B*. Position of the forceps in maxillary fracture disimpaction. *C*. Two forceps can be employed to approximate maxillary fragments in a sagittal fracture. (Courtesy of J. M. Converse and W. B. Saunders Co., Philadelphia. *Reconstructive Plastic Surgery*, 2nd Ed., 1977.)

impacted at the line of fracture. Another feature, which is particular to complete transverse fractures of the maxilla, is that intermaxillary fixation does not suffice to ensure consolidation of the fracture, as movements of the mandible will displace the bone. It is necessary, therefore, either to immobilize the mandible or to provide cranial fixation of the maxilla independent of the mandible.

Treatment follows the pattern outlined for all fractures: first, reduction of the displaced maxilla must be accomplished in order to reestablish the occlusal relationships of the maxillary and mandibular teeth; second, fixation must be provided to permit consolidation at the fracture line. Reduction can be either immediate or progressive.

Immediate Reduction. In severe maxillary fractures, particularly in those cases with associated fractures of other bones of the face, general anesthesia is usually required and immediate reduction is often the most efficient method of treatment. Gentle manipulation is sufficient in loose fractures; in impacted fractures and in partially consolidated fractures, more energetic disimpaction may be required. Various forceps can be employed for this purpose, such as the Rowe forceps (Fig. 11–18). One branch of the forceps is applied through the anterior naris to the floor of the nose, and the other branch of the forceps is applied to the hard palate. Lateral movements combined with a forward and downward displacement will provide satisfactory reduction.

Progressive Reduction. Most fractures of the maxilla, when seen early, can be treated by progressive reduction with elastic traction, which is the simplest form of treatment. Reduction can be assisted by manipulation.

Cranial Fixation by Internal Wiring. Methods of fixation are varied and have undergone considerable evolution as the result of the increase in severity of maxillary and middle third facial bone fractures. Internal wiring is the technique most commonly employed for cranial fixation of maxillary fractures, and it is also the method of choice for the fixation of dentures, bite-blocks, or other prosthetic appliances required in edentulous or comminuted cases. Through an incision of the lateral portion of the eyebrow on each side, a wire is threaded down through the temporal fossa beneath the zygomatic arch, along the lateral wall of the maxilla, and into the mouth. The wires are grasped with a hemostat and looped around the arch bar at the level of the first or second molar (Figs. 11–19 and 11–20). The internal wires may also be looped around the zygomatic arch.

In a Le Fort III craniofacial disjunction, direct interosseous fixation is also established at the frontozygomatic fracture line in the lateral wall of the orbit.

Internal wire fixation is remarkably well

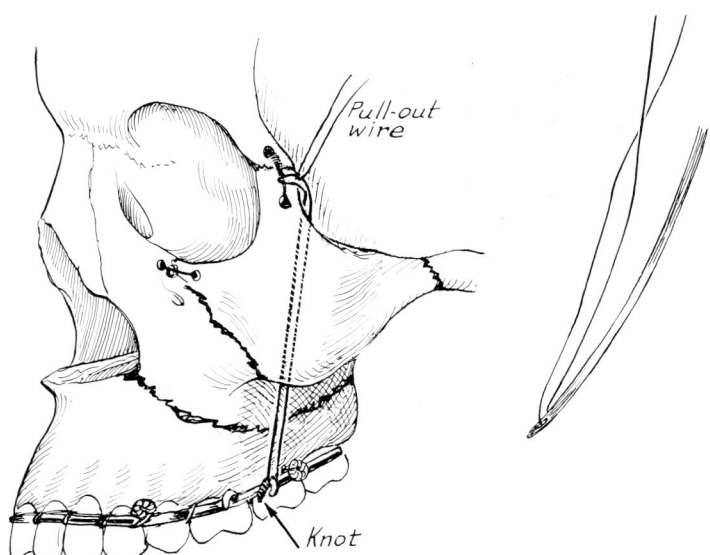

Figure 11–19   Internal wiring combined with interosseous fixation in fracture of the zygoma and maxilla. Note internal wire looped through the frontozygomatic interosseous wire. Note also the vertical position of the internal frontomaxillary wire. The vertical position of the internal wires allows for early release of intermaxillary fixation without the danger of maxillary recession. (Courtesy of J. M. Converse and W. B. Saunders Co., Philadelphia. *Reconstructive Plastic Surgery,* 2nd Ed., 1977.)

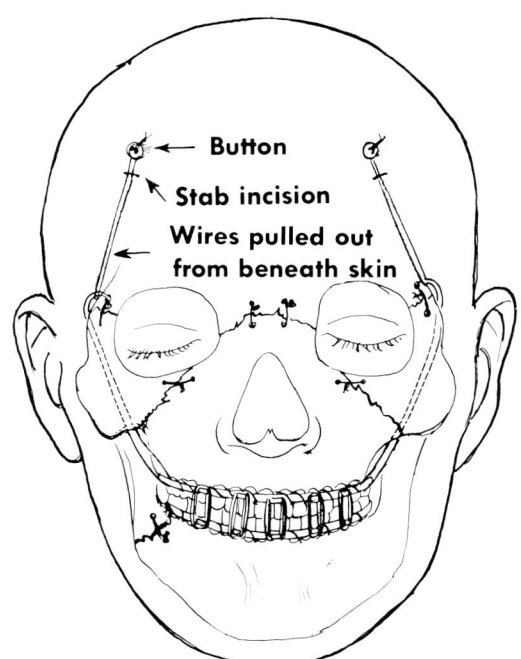

Figure 11–20 Use of interosseous wiring and internal wiring with pull-out wires in maxillary fracture with associated mandibular fracture. (Courtesy of J. M. Converse and W. B. Saunders Co., Philadelphia. *Reconstructive Plastic Surgery*, 2nd Ed., 1977.)

tozygomatic junction and the nasofrontal junction is a useful procedure in Le Fort III craniofacial disjunction and in comminuted fractures. Subperiosteal exposure of the line of fracture permits drilling of holes in the bone above and below the fractured area. Stainless steel wire is passed through the holes, and the fractured surfaces are brought together by twisting the wires; the cut wire ends may remain buried indefinitely. One should not depend upon this procedure alone, however, for although the upper end of the fractured bone is held securely on each side, the occlusal relation of the teeth is not controlled; intermaxillary wiring of the teeth of the upper and lower jaws in correct dental occlusion is a prime requisite.

tolerated and can be maintained over periods extending up to 8 to 12 weeks. To remove the fixation wires, a pull-out wire can be brought out through the scalp. This serves as a means of traction upon the internal wires after they have been cut free from their attachments in the oral cavity. Usually a short, light anesthesia is given for removal of these wires. Circumzygomatic wires can be pulled out through the oral cavity.

Open Reduction and Interosseous Fixation. The present trend is toward more frequent employment of open reduction and direct interosseous wiring in the treatment of comminuted fractures of the facial skeleton. This procedure is especially suitable for severe injuries in which the external wound permits inspection of the fracture sites and verification of the reduction and fixation under direct vision. Otherwise, selective sites for cutaneous incisions afford good exposure with minimal resultant scarring (Fig. 11–21).

Direct interosseous wiring at the fron-

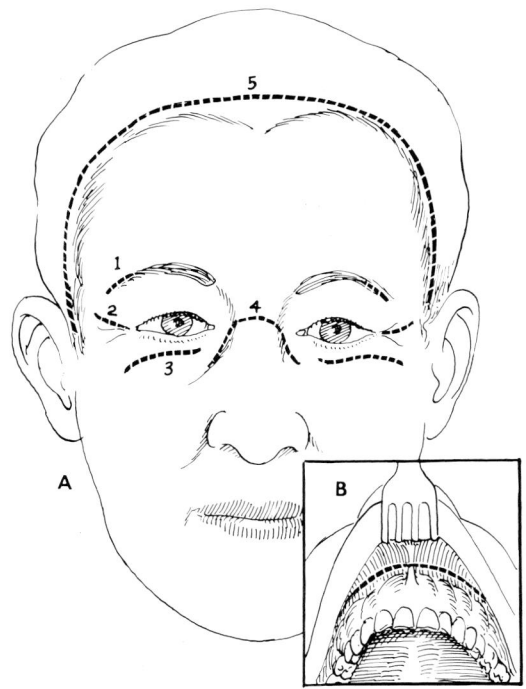

Figure 11–21 Various incisions for exposure of the midfacial skeleton. *A.* 1, Supraorbital eyebrow incision; 2, lateral canthal incision; 3, lower eyelid incision; 4, transverse incision across the nasal frontal junction (this incision is extended laterally by vertical incisions over the lateral nasal wall; lateral nasal wall incisions may be adequate to provide exposure of the fracture); 5, incision for scalp flap. *B.* Incision on the buccal aspect of the oral vestibule for intraoral exposure of the midfacial framework. (Courtesy of J. M. Converse and W. B. Saunders Co., Philadelphia. *Reconstructive Plastic Surgery*, 1st Ed., 1964.)

COMPLICATIONS IN MAXILLARY FRACTURES

Early complications after fractures of the maxilla include primary hemorrhage, respiratory complications, and those due to infection, such as secondary hemorrhage, osteitis, and osteomyelitis.

Late complications of maxillary fractures include delayed union, nonunion, malunion, infraorbital anesthesia, and interference with lacrimal function.

FRACTURES OF THE ZYGOMA

The zygoma or malar bone, referred to in the vernacular as the "cheek bone," is a strong buttress in the lateral portion of the middle third of the facial skeletal framework (Fig. 11–22). Because of this position, it is a bone that is frequently fractured, either singly or in conjunction with fractures involving the maxilla and other bones of the midfacial area.

SURGICAL PATHOLOGY

Zygomatic bone fractures are usually caused by direct impact to the bone or to one of its processes. A direct blow often causes a dislocation of the solid body of the bone from its weaker attachments to the maxilla and the frontal and temporal bones. Indirect impact fractures are unusual and occur when a force of unusual violence is applied to the opposite side of the facial skeleton, resulting in a lateral shift of the midfacial skeletal framework.

Although the zygoma is a sturdy bone, its processes are subject to separation from the frontal, temporal, sphenoid, and maxillary bones, with the zygoma usually being displaced downward, inward, and backward. Because the zygoma participates in the formation of the lateral orbital wall and floor, orbital complications are not infrequent.

Because the zygoma forms the bony wall of the superolateral portion of the maxillary sinus, its fracture causes tearing of the mucosal lining of the sinus, hemorrhage, and hematoma; bleeding from the nose may be an indication of blood escaping through the ostium in the middle meatus.

Crash injuries cause comminuted fractures in which the rim and floor of the orbit are reduced to splinters, the anterior wall of the maxillary sinus is shattered, bone fragments are lodged in the sinus, and the main fragment of the body of the zygoma is rotated into the sinus.

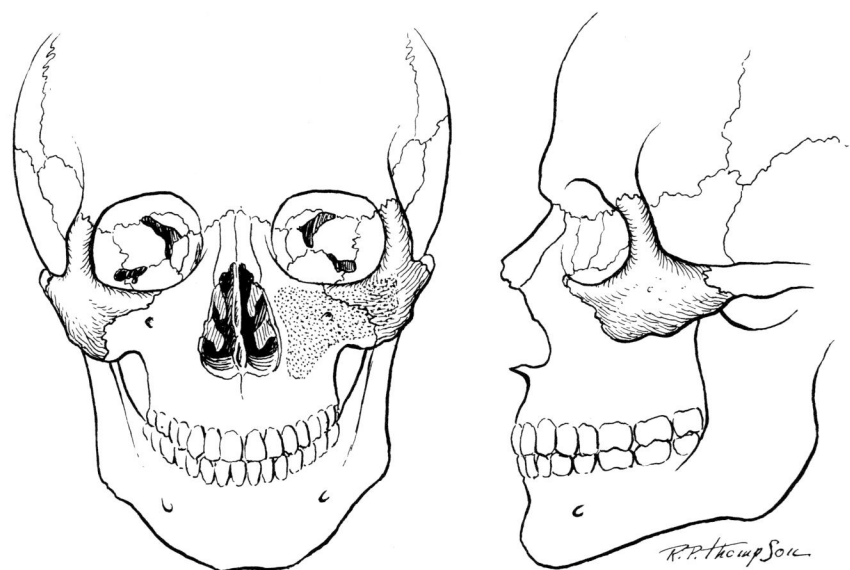

Figure 11–22   The zygoma articulates with frontal, sphenoid and temporal bones and the maxilla. (Courtesy of J. M. Converse and W. B. Saunders Co., Philadelphia. *Reconstructive Plastic Surgery,* 2nd Ed., 1977.)

TABLE 11–2   Classification of 120 Cases of Fracture of the Zygoma*

Group	Description	Per Cent
I	No significant displacement; fractures visible on roentgenogram but fragments remain in line	6
II	Zygomatic arch fractures; inward buckling of the arch; no orbital or maxillary sinus involvement	10
III	Unrotated body fractures; downward and inward displacement but no rotation	33
IV	Medially rotated body fractures; downward, inward and backward displacement with medial rotation	11
V	Laterally rotated body fractures; displacement is downward, backward and medialward with lateral rotation	22
VI	Includes all cases in which additional fracture lines cross the main fragment	18

*After J. S. Knight and J. F. North, The classification of malar fractures: an analysis of displacement as a guide to treatment. Br. J. Plast. Surg., *13*:325, 1961. (Courtesy of V. H. Kazanjiian and J. M. Converse and The Williams & Wilkins Co., Baltimore. *Surgical Treatment of Facial Injuries*, 3rd Ed., 1974.)

CLASSIFICATION OF ZYGOMATIC FRACTURES

Knight and North devised a classification of fractures of the zygoma based on the anatomy of the fracture (Table 11–2).[18] This is helpful in predicting the clinical features and planning treatment.

CLINICAL EXAMINATION

The striking feature noted in the first few hours after the accident in a patient who has suffered a fracture of the zygoma with displacement is the loss of normal prominence of the cheek bone (Fig. 11–23). The one-sided flatness of the face, however, is often concealed by soft-tissue swelling. The eyelids are swollen and ecchymotic, and there is subconjunctival hemorrhage. The patient may complain of pain, particularly when attempting to open the mouth.

Some patients have double vision, often of a transitory type, and enophthalmos may be present if not masked by edema. The patient may complain of numbness of the upper lip on the fractured side, and examination will disclose loss of sensibility in the area of distribution of the infraorbital nerve.

The face should be examined and palpated with the patient seated. Points of tenderness are elicited at the lines of fracture (Fig. 11-24). The fracture is defined by palpating the unaffected and the injured orbital margins simultaneously. It is often possible to detect a separation at the junction of the zygoma and the frontal bones on the injured side.

A slight depression noted in the area of junction of the temporal process of the zygoma with the zygomatic process of the temporal bone may be an indication of a depressed fracture in the zygomatic arch. If the patient has difficulty in opening the mouth, a diagnosis of zygomatic arch fracture is probable.

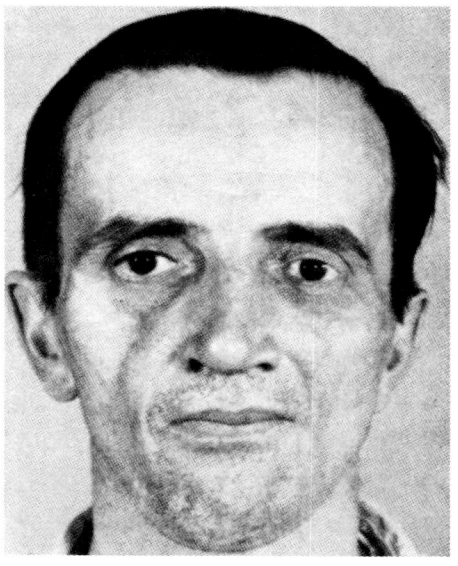

Figure 11-23 Depression at the zygomaticomaxillary junction resulting from depression of the zygoma into the maxillary sinus as a result of a fist blow. Rotation that occurred in fracture-dislocation has caused a prominence of the lateral portion of the zygoma. (Courtesy of J. M. Converse and W. B. Saunders Co., Philadelphia. *Reconstructive Plastic Surgery*, 2nd Ed., 1977.)

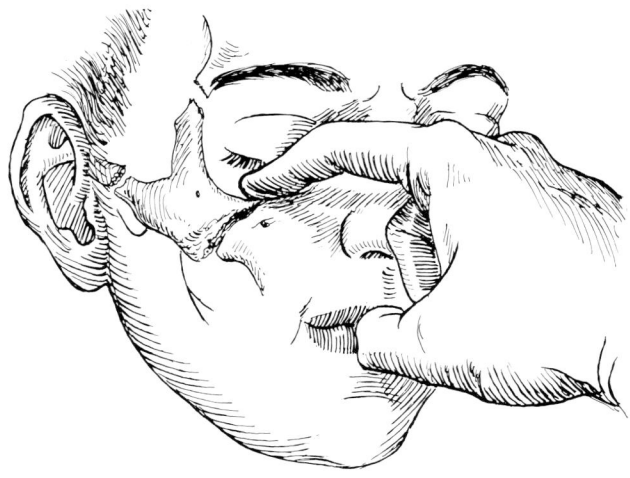

Figure 11–24 Palpation of a fractured zygoma elicits points of tenderness at the fracture site. Separation between the bones and bone irregularities may also be felt by the palpating finger. (Courtesy of J. M. Converse and W. B. Saunders Co., Philadelphia. *Reconstructive Plastic Surgery*, 2nd Ed., 1977.)

Abnormal mobility is rarely elicited in most of the fracture-dislocations of the zygoma that are impacted, but mobility and crepitation are observed in comminuted fractures. A technique for evaluating the displacement of the zygoma is to introduce the index finger into the upper oral vestibule on the fractured side, and palpate the area of junction of the zygoma and maxilla (Fig. 11–25). A groove felt between the zygoma and maxilla on the unaffected side is absent in a depressed fracture.

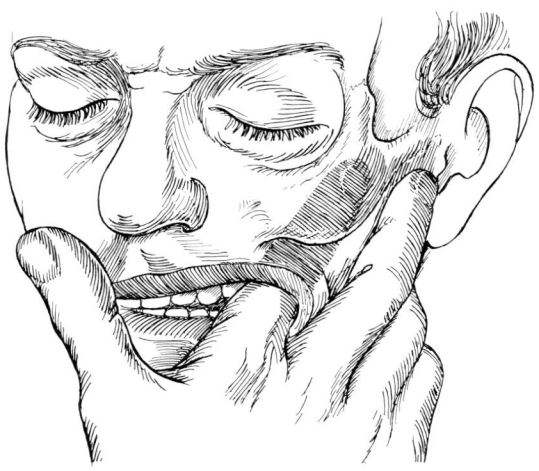

Figure 11–25 Finger palpation in the upper buccal sulcus will indicate the degree of depression of the fractured zygoma, for the groove between zygoma and maxilla, which is present on the unaffected side, is absent in a depressed zygomatic fracture. (Courtesy of J. M. Converse and W. B. Saunders Co., Philadelphia. *Reconstructive Plastic Surgery*, 2nd Ed., 1977.)

ROENTGENOGRAPHIC EXAMINATION

Two roentgenographic positions are of particular value, the Waters view and the Caldwell posteroanterior view. The Waters position is of assistance in detecting multiple fracture lines, separation at the frontozygomatic junction, and depression of the orbital floor. Tomograms are indispensable with a blow-out fracture of the orbital floor or a concomitant nasoorbital fracture, or when other complicating fractures are suspected.

TREATMENT OF FRACTURES OF THE ZYGOMA

Most simple fractures usually respond to reduction without fixation. Others require fixation after open reduction. Comminuted fractures of the floor of the orbit require the surgical reestablishment of the continuity of the orbital floor.

Fracture-Dislocation

Oral Approach. Under general anesthesia a short elevator is passed upward behind the fractured zygoma through an incision made in the buccal mucosa above the tuberosity of the maxilla on the affected side (Fig. 11–26). Reduction of the fracture is accomplished by elevating the bone upward and outward; a snapping sound may be heard when the bone is replaced. The

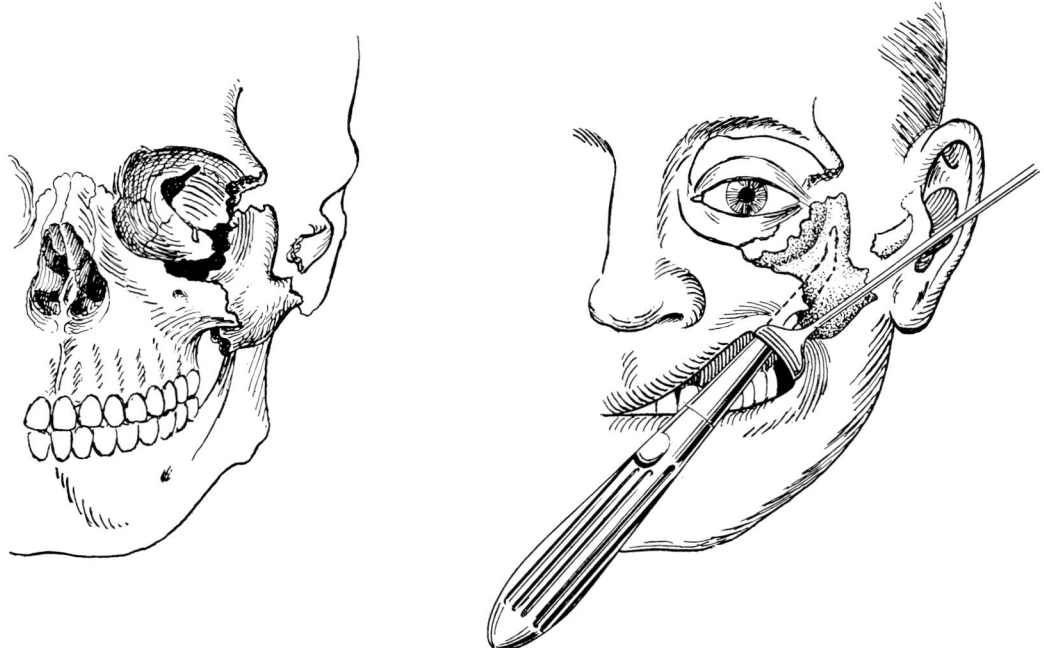

Figure 11–26 Oral approach for reduction of the fractured zygoma. (Courtesy of J. M. Converse and W. B. Saunders Co., Philadelphia. *Reconstructive Plastic Surgery*, 2nd Ed., 1977.)

procedure is simple, direct, and rapid. Infection has not been observed to result from passage through the oral cavity.[17]

Temporal Approach. This technique is indicated when the entire zygomatic arch is depressed and interferes with the free movement of the mandible because of pressure by the coronoid process. Through a temporal incision, an elevator is placed between the temporalis fascia and muscle (an instrument placed superficial to the fascia will not penetrate the zygomatic fossa). A cleavage plane, established between the muscle fibers and the temporalis fascia, leads directly under the zygomatic arch to the medial surface of the bone (Fig. 11–27). The zygoma is raised by using leverage with a long, flat elevator, following the movement of the bone and controlling it with the fingers. The operation is simple and rapid and is particularly effective when strong leverage is required to reduce a partially consolidated fracture.[13]

Supraorbital Approach. This approach is employed when interosseous wiring is required. An incision at the lateral aspect of the eyebrow provides exposure of the area

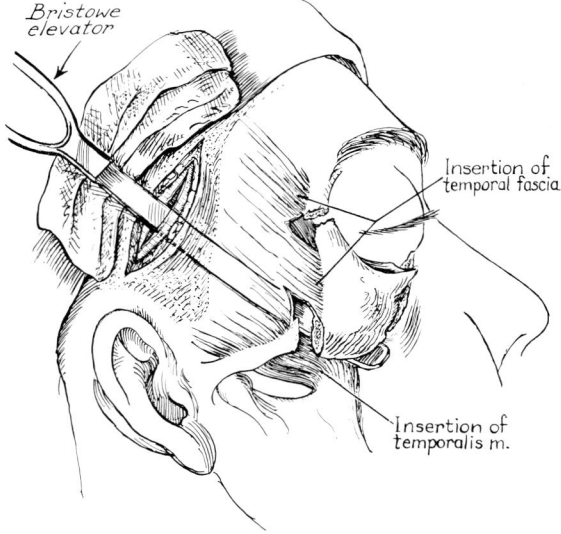

Figure 11–27 Attachment of the temporalis fascia along the upper margin of the zygomatic arch. To penetrate into the zygomatic fossa, the instrument must be placed on the deep surface of the temporalis fascia. (Courtesy of J. M. Converse and W. B. Saunders Co., Philadelphia. *Reconstructive Plastic Surgery*, 2nd Ed., 1977.)

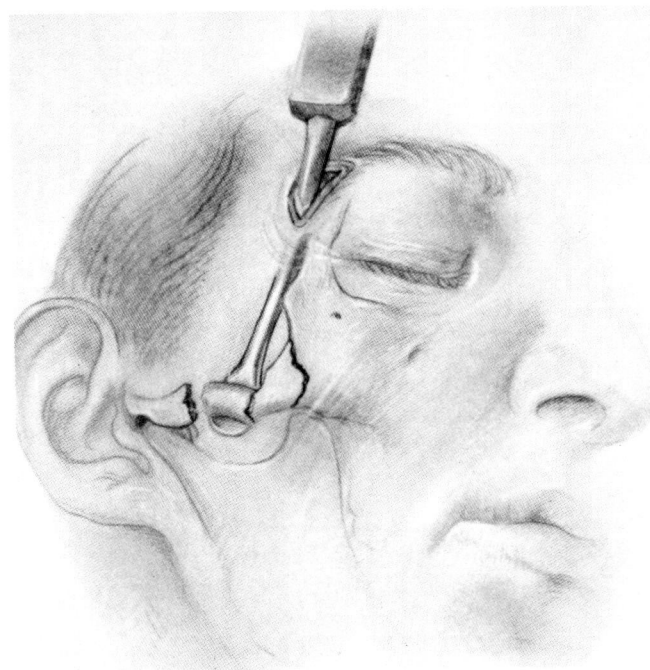

Figure 11-28 The supraorbital approach is useful when interosseous wiring is required at the frontozygomatic junction. Elevator is introduced, and the zygoma is elevated. This approach is particularly helpful in elevating zygomatic arch fractures (as shown in drawing). (Courtesy of J. M. Converse and W. B. Saunders Co., Philadelphia. *Reconstructive Plastic Surgery*, 2nd Ed., 1977.)

of the frontozygomatic suture. An elevator passed through this incision into the temporal fossa elevates the zygoma into a position of reduction. This is also an excellent approach for fractures of the zygomatic arch (Fig. 11–28).[10]

Open Reduction and Wire Fixation. Although open reduction and wire fixation are usually employed in comminuted fractures, the technique is also indicated in fracture-dislocation of the zygoma when the bone

fails to maintain its position of reduction, particularly in cases in which treatment has been delayed.

Various incisions similar to those employed for maxillary fractures are available for the approach to the zygoma and leave inconspicuous scars. After exposure of the fracture sites, stainless steel wire is passed through drill holes in the bones and tightened to maintain the fragments (Fig. 11–29).

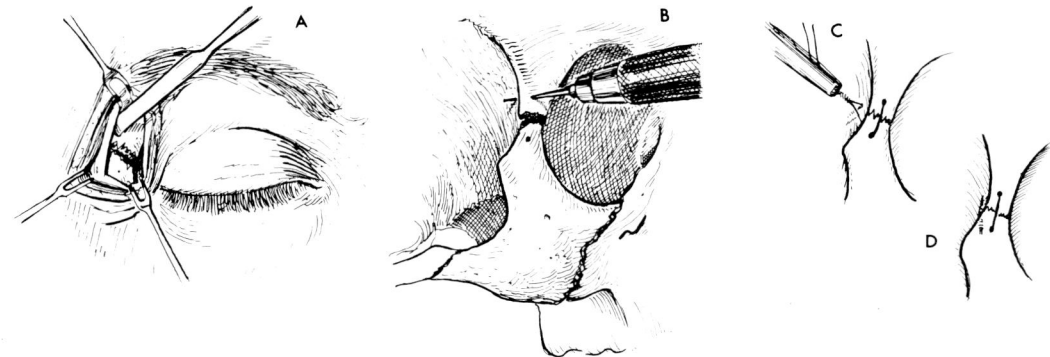

Figure 11-29 Interosseous wiring of the frontozygomatic junction. A. Subperiosteal exposure of the fracture. B. Drill holes are placed on each side of the fracture line. C. Wire has been passed and is being twisted and tightened. D. Interosseous wiring in position. (Courtesy of J. M. Converse and W. B. Saunders Co., Philadelphia. *Reconstructive Plastic Surgery*, 2nd Ed., 1977.)

COMPLICATIONS IN FRACTURES OF THE ZYGOMA

Diplopia is usually transitory in most zygomatic fractures, disappearing after hematoma has been absorbed and edema and reaction from injury of the extraocular musculature have subsided. Infraorbital nerve anesthesia is usually temporary, and infection is rare in simple fractures.

Late complications such as enophthalmos and diplopia are encountered more frequently in comminuted fractures that involve the zygoma, maxilla, and floor of the orbit.

Most complications are the result of malunited fractures. The resulting deformity may be slight or quite noticeable. Correction of the deformity from malunited fractures may require osteotomy and realignment of the zygoma or contour restoration by bone grafts.

FRACTURES OF THE FLOOR OF THE ORBIT

Fractures of the floor of the orbit are the most frequent of orbital fractures. Fractures of the medial orbital wall can occur in conjunction with fractures of the orbital floor. In fractures of the zygoma, in high maxillary fractures, and in nasoorbital fractures, the line of fracture traverses the orbital floor. A frequent special type of orbital floor fracture is the "blow-out" fracture.

The orbital contents are protected by strong bony abutments: the supraorbital arch of the frontal bone above, and the relatively thick rim of the orbital floor formed by the zygoma and maxilla medially and inferiorly (Fig. 11–30). Although the orbital rims are strong, the orbital walls consist of relatively thin bone throughout with the weakest area situated anterior to the inferior orbital fissure. This "weak area" is continued medially by the lamina papyracea of the ethmoid, a portion of the medial orbital wall and, as its name implies, a plate of bone of paperlike thinness. The medial half of the orbital floor is further weakened by the infraorbital canal or groove. The area of junction between the floor of the orbit and its medial wall forms a wide angle, an inclined plane that seems to constitute an

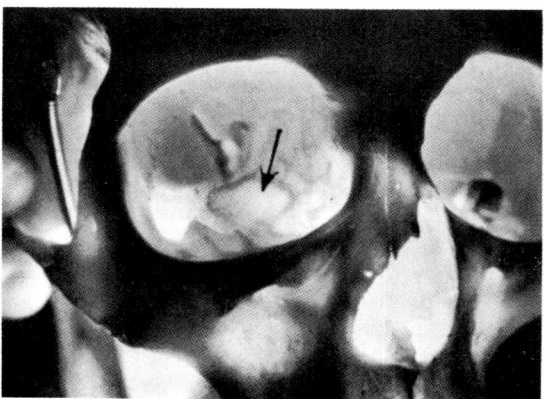

Figure 11–30 Transilluminated dried skull. Area of thin bone (arrow) is flanked by the inferior orbital fissure posterolaterally and the lacrimal groove anteromedially. (Courtesy of J. M. Converse and W. B. Saunders Co., Philadelphia. *Reconstructive Plastic Surgery*, 2nd Ed., 1977.)

inferomedial wall of the orbit. This anatomical characteristic explains the frequency of medial blow-outs through the lamina papyracea. A blow-out fracture of the medial orbital wall should be suspected when there is concomitant nasoorbital fracture.

SURGICAL PATHOLOGY

Orbital fractures occur in association with zygomatic and nasoorbital fractures, and in high maxillary fractures in which the line of fracture traverses the orbital floor. The backward displacement of the fractured thick inferior orbital rim produces a comminuted fracture of the thinner portion of the orbital floor; downward displacement of the zygoma results in a separation of the frontozygomatic junction; and in nasoorbital fractures, backward displacement of the nasal bones and frontal processes of the maxilla into the interorbital space comminutes the medial orbital wall.

Fracture of the orbital bones may have minimal functional consequences when there is little displacement of the fragments, with the notable exception of the blow-out type of fracture, in which a simple linear fracture of the orbital floor suffices to arrest rotary movements of the eyeball. In another, fortunately rare, occurrence, a linear fracture may extend into the optic canal, causing consequent blindness.

Orbital Blow-Out Fractures

A blow-out fracture is caused by a sudden increase in intraorbital pressure resulting from the application of a traumatic force to the soft tissue of the orbit area. It may be associated with diplopia due to a vertical muscle imbalance caused by the entrapment of the inferior rectus and inferior oblique muscles in a dehiscence in the orbital floor. The escape of orbital fat through the blow-out dehiscence is a major cause of enophthalmos.

After application of a traumatizing force over the orbital contents by a nonpenetrating object, such as a large ball or a human fist, the orbital contents are pushed backward into the smaller portion of the orbital cone (Fig. 11–31). The increased intraorbital pressure thus exerted causes a blow-out at the weakest area of the orbit without fracturing the orbital rim. This type of fracture may be referred to as a "pure" blow-out fracture. The traumatic object, a tennis ball or human fist, for example, is sufficiently large to produce increased orbital hydraulic pressure, but usually does not cause destructive damage to the ocular globe as can occur with smaller objects

Pure and Impure Blow-out Fractures. In the typical automotive injury in which the passenger's face is projected against the dashboard, the thick orbital rim is fractured and displaced backward, resulting in an "eggshell" comminution of the orbital floor. The continuing momentum and the pressure against the dashboard raises the pressure of the intraorbital contents producing a superimposed blow-out fracture. It is to this type of orbital fracture that the term "impure blow-out" may be applied (Fig. 11–32). Impure blow-out fractures often occur as one of many associated midfacial fractures. Pyramidal maxillary fractures (Le Fort II) and craniofacial disjunction (Le Fort III) are characterized by fracture lines extending through the orbital floor, which further contribute to the comminution of the bone produced by the fracture of the orbital rim. Orbital fractures with massive ptosis of the floor into the maxillary sinus can be explained on the basis of this type of injury.

One should not be induced into the

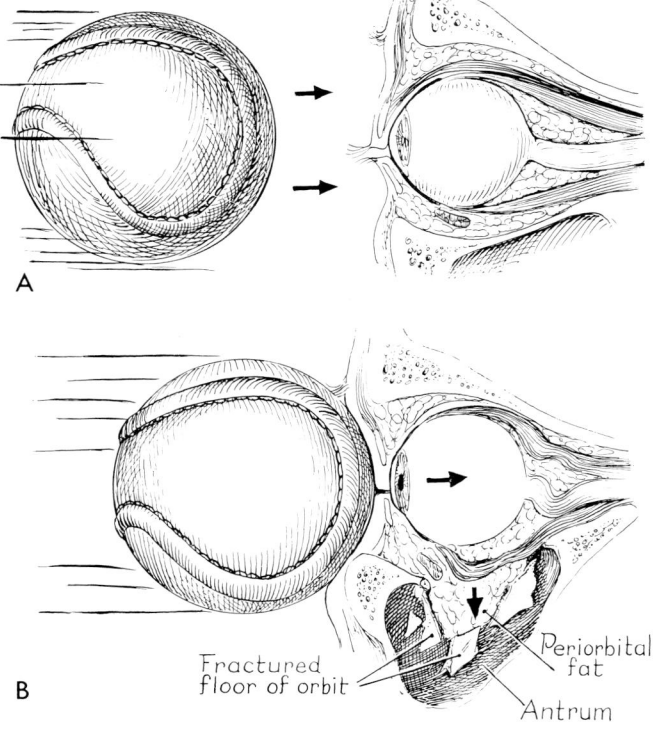

A

B

Fractured floor of orbit

Periorbital fat

Antrum

Figure 11–31 External pressure forcing blow-out fracture of the orbital floor with incarceration of the inferior oblique and the inferior rectus muscles and facial expansion. Our first patient in whom a diagnosis of a blow-out fracture was made was hit by a hurtling ball, here represented. (Courtesy of J. M. Converse and W. B. Saunders Co., Philadelphia. *Reconstructive Plastic Surgery*, 2nd Ed., 1977.)

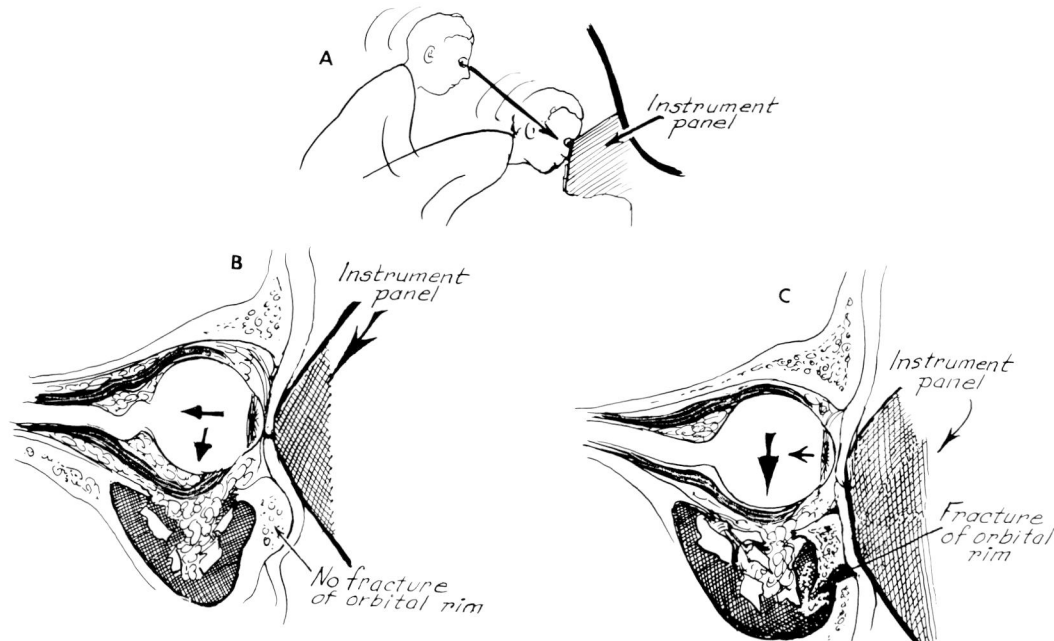

Figure 11–32 Pure and impure blow-out fractures. *A.* Impact of the orbit against the padded dashboard of the automobile. *B.* Protuberance of the dashboard may compress the orbital contents without injury to the rim; a pure blow-out fracture. *C.* When the impact is over the orbital rim, the rim is fractured and subjected to a posterior displacement that comminutes the thin portion of the orbital floor. Continued momentum of impact then reaches the orbital contents, which are compressed and entrapped in the area of the fracture: an impure blow-out fracture. (Courtesy of J. M. Converse and W. B. Saunders Co., Philadelphia. *Reconstructive Plastic Surgery,* 2nd Ed., 1977.)

fallacy of referring to all orbital fractures as blow-out fractures. The term "blow-out fracture" defines one mechanism of fracture and does not apply to all orbital fractures. As stated earlier, orbital floor fractures occur in fractures of the zygoma and in upper maxillary fractures.

CLINICAL EXAMINATION

In the typical blow-out fracture, the patient complains of diplopia, particularly on upward gaze. The patient may not recognize diplopia early if the eye is temporarily closed by edema of the lids, by dressings, or because of intraocular injury. Examination shows varying degrees of ecchymosis and edema, and the ocular globe gives the appearance of being displaced backward and downward. Oculorotary movement is restricted by the entrapment of the orbital contents in the floor of the orbit, and the superior oblique and rectus muscles cannot rotate the globe because of the resistance offered by the short rein of the incarcerated muscles.

Sensory nerve loss, anesthesia or hypoesthesia in the area of distribution of the infraorbital nerve, is evidence suggestive of blow-out fracture involving the infraorbital canal or groove. This sign is useful in making a diagnosis when the orbital rim is not fractured and also assists in locating the site of the blow-out; normal infraorbital nerve conduction implies that the fractured area is either lateral or medial to the infraorbital groove or canal.

An ophthalmological examination should investigate the possibility of *intraocular injuries* such as vitreous hemorrhage, dislocated lens, or rupture of the sclera, which may require immediate attention. Jabaley and associates found a 20 per cent incidence of ocular injuries in orbital fractures.[15]

ROENTGENOGRAPHIC EXAMINATION

Early diagnosis of blow-out fracture of the orbital floor established by roentgenography and its interpretation is important before surgical treatment. The Waters view and supine anteroposterior tomograms are essential diagnostic aids. Radiological diagnosis of blow-out fracture of the orbit is frequently missed if the examination is not comprehensive. Fracture lines may be mistaken for superimposed bony septa or suture lines, or they may be hidden by disease processes in the underlying maxillary sinus. The thin orbital floor, partially transparent on radiographs, may be obscured against the background of other bones of the skull. Tomograms may demonstrate fractures of the orbital floor with greater clarity or verify a clinically suspicious orbital blow-out fracture not seen on the routine Waters views.

The common roentgen findings are: (1) fragmentation of the bones of the orbital floor; (2) depression of bony fragments; and (3) prolapse into the subjacent maxillary sinus of the orbital soft tissue.[24, 25] The x-ray is also an important medicolegal document in case of litigation.

TREATMENT OF THE BLOW-OUT FRACTURE

There is controversy concerning the indications for surgical exploration in blow-out fractures of the floor of the orbit.

The principal indications for surgical treatment of a blow-out fracture are: (1) the patient's inability to rotate the ocular globe in upward gaze because of the structures entrapped in the fracture site (diplopia is present in the upward gaze and often in the forward gaze); (2) the forced duction test (the inferior rectus muscle is seized by forceps 6 mm from the limbus; an unsuccessful attempt to rotate the globe upward confirms the diagnosis of entrapment); (3) the presence of enophthalmos with deepening of the orbitopalpebral fold, which is noticeable in the early hours following the fracture (in massive comminuted fractures with collapse of the orbital floor, enophthalmos may be severe if the orbital floor is not restored); enophthalmos of more than 5 mm relative to the opposite globe is dis-

figuring;[8] and (4) further confirmation by radiography (polytomography defines the location and extent of the fracture).

The objectives of treatment are the prevention of permanent diplopia and disfiguring enophthalmos.

There are three basic methods of open reduction: the direct eyelid approach to the floor of the orbit and restoration of continuity, the Caldwell-Luc approach to the maxillary sinus and packing of the sinus, and a combined approach.

Eyelid Approach. The eyelid approach is preferred because it permits disengagement of the entrapped orbital tissues and reconstruction of the defect under direct vision. An incision is made along the lower border of the tarsus of the lower lid, the fibers of the orbicularis oculi muscle are split at a slightly lower level than the skin incision; the septum orbitale is now exposed, and the dissection extends to the orbital rim where the periosteum is incised and the periorbita is raised from the orbital floor until the area of the blow-out fracture is reached and identified (Fig. 11–33). The entrapped orbital contents are disengaged, and the continuity of the orbital floor is restored by placing an inorganic implant such as Teflon, Supramid, or Silastic over the area of the blow-out fracture (Fig. 11–34). Bone grafts, the anterior wall of the maxillary sinus in the canine fossa, septal cartilage, and ethmoid plate are available organic transplants. The purpose of the orbital floor insert, whether inorganic or organic, is to reestablish the continuity of the floor, which seals off the orbit from the maxillary sinus and restores the volume of the orbital cavity to what it was before injury.

Caldwell-Luc Approach. This approach to the orbital floor through the canine fossa and the maxillary sinus is indicated for the removal of bone fragments in the maxillary sinus and has merit in cases of severely comminuted fracture of the maxilla and other bones of the midfacial area.

Combined Approach. When the orbital structures are entrapped, their disentrapment is difficult through the maxillary sinus approach alone. For this reason, a dual approach is required, the eyelid incision providing the surgeon with a direct view of the fractured orbital floor.

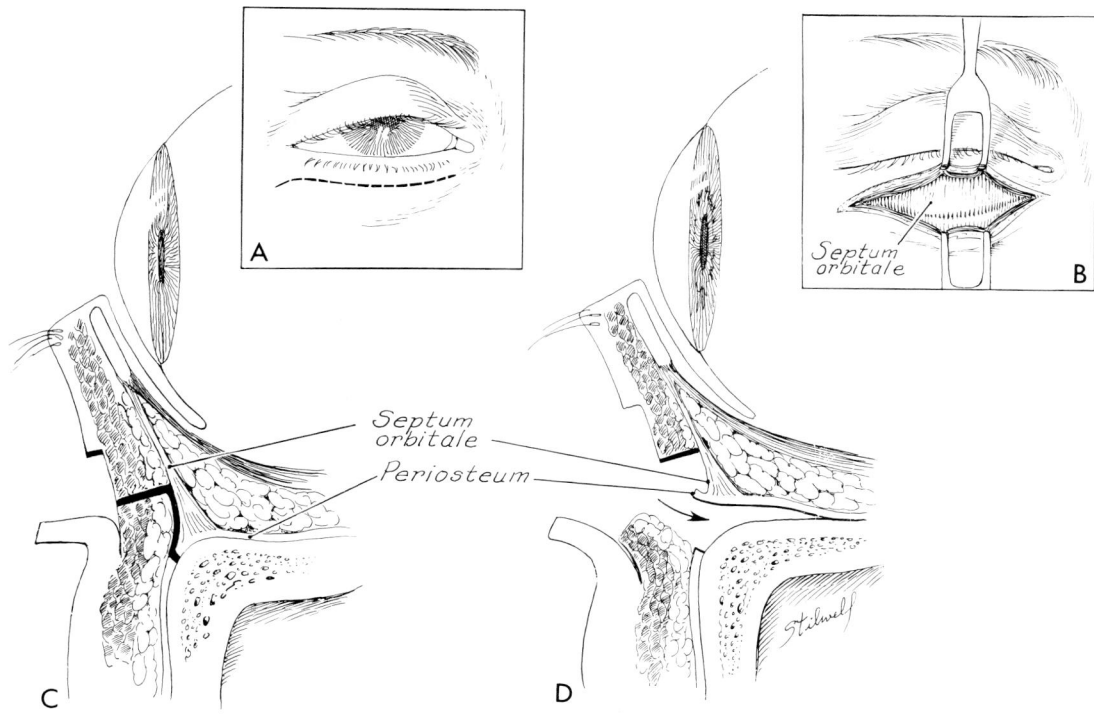

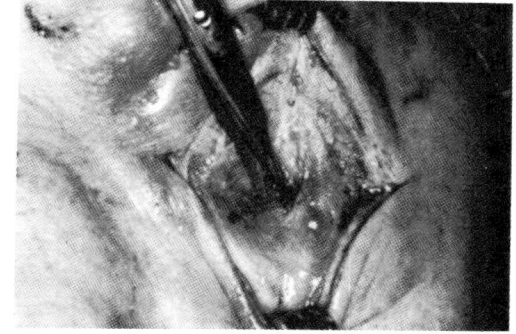

Figure 11–33 Technique for exposing the orbital floor. *A.* Outline of the eyelid incision. *B.* Septum orbitale is exposed. *C.* Sagittal section showing the skin incision through the orbicularis oculi muscle, path of dissection over the septum orbitale to the orbital rim. *D.* Periosteum of the orbit (periorbital) is now raised from the orbital floor. *E.* Scissors dissecting tissues anterior to the septum orbitale as far downward as the orbital rim. (Courtesy of J. M. Converse, J. G. Cole, and B. Smith and *Plastic and Reconstructive Surgery.* Late treatment of blowout fracture of the floor of the orbit, Plast. Reconstr. Surg., 28:183, 1961.)

COMPLICATIONS OF ORBITAL FRACTURES

The complications of orbital blow-out fractures are summarized in Table 11–3. Deformities and functional impairment are late complications that can be reduced by early diagnosis and treatment, but often the diagnosis is obscured by more severe cranial and facial injuries that demand primary treatment. The unconscious patient cannot experience diplopia, and orbital edema, hemorrhage, and ptosis can mask the enophthalmos. After several weeks fibrosis cicatrization has set in, and reconstruction of the architecture of the orbital cavity and restoration of symmetrical ocular function,

in a malunited fracture, must be done under more difficult conditions.

FRACTURES OF THE BONES AND CARTILAGES OF THE NOSE

The nose occupies the most prominent position on the face, and consequently the nasal bones are the most frequently fractured of the facial bones (see Table 11–1). Although usually referred to as "fractures of the nasal bones," in reality the fracture involves not only the nasal bones themselves but also the frontal process of the maxilla and the cartilages and bones form-

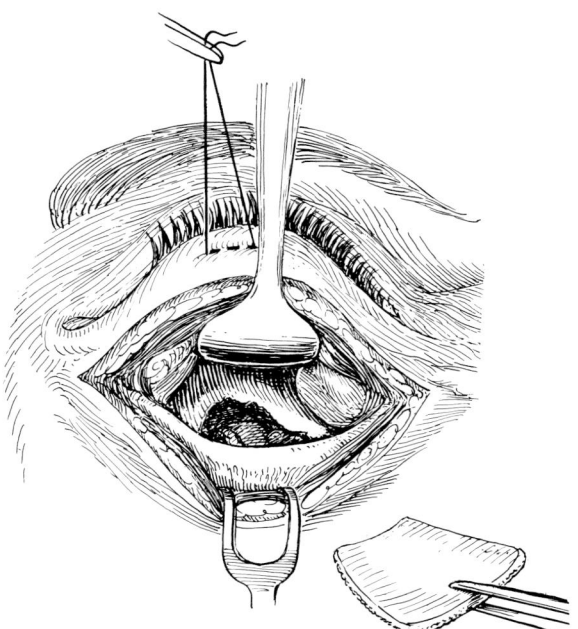

Figure 11-34   Orbital contents are raised, and continuity of the orbital floor is restored by placing of an insert over the area of blow-out fracture. (Courtesy of J. M. Converse and W. B. Saunders Co., Philadelphia. *Reconstructive Plastic Surgery*, 2nd Ed., 1977.)

ing the septum. In severe fractures the structures in the interorbital space may be penetrated by the backwardly displaced nasal skeletal framework.

SURGICAL PATHOLOGY

Most nasal fractures are due to blows that strike the nose from the side. In such cases

both nasal bones are fractured at a horizontal level and dislocated to one side as shown in Figure 11-35; the septum is also fractured, and the upper fragment of the septum is displaced laterally with the nasal bones. The level at which most of these fractures occur is accounted for by the structure of the nasal bones, the thick upper part of the bones being more resistant than the lower, thinner portion.

Head-on injuries are the cause of depressed nasal fractures, and a violent blow may cause comminution of the nasal bones and flattening of the entire dorsum.

The most severe fractures are due to a direct anterior blow on the nasal bridge resulting in nasoorbital fractures with comminution and projection of fragments into the interorbital space. These nasoorbital fractures, if neglected, result in severe deformities.

CLINICAL EXAMINATION

Nasal hemorrhage is usually of short duration and ceases spontaneously. A deviation or a flattening of the nose may be seen, but as swelling progressively increases, the deformity may be obscured. Periorbital ecchymosis appears with subconjunctival hemorrhage. Besides causing pain, breathing through the nose may be difficult because of blood clots, edema of the mucous membrane, and displacement of intranasal structures. Subcutaneous emphysema may be noted in patients who have attempted to clear the nasal airway by blowing through the torn mucoperiosteum

TABLE 11-3   Complications of Orbital Fractures Persistent after Floor Repair (50 Cases)*

Complications	Preoperative	Postoperative	
		3 Months	1 Year
Extraocular muscle imbalance	43	30	20
Enophthalmos	27	15	11
Ptosis	12	3	2
Medial canthal deformity	12	12	9
Lacrimal obstruction	3	3	0
Vertical shortening of the lower lid	4	4	2†
Visual impairment	5	5	5
Trichiasis-symblepharon	2	1	0

*Courtesy of J. M. Converse, B. Smith, M. F. Obear, and D. Wood-Smith, and *Plastic and Reconstructive Surgery*. Orbital blow-out fractures: A ten-year study. Plast. Reconstr. Surg., 39:20, 1967.
  †Repaired later.

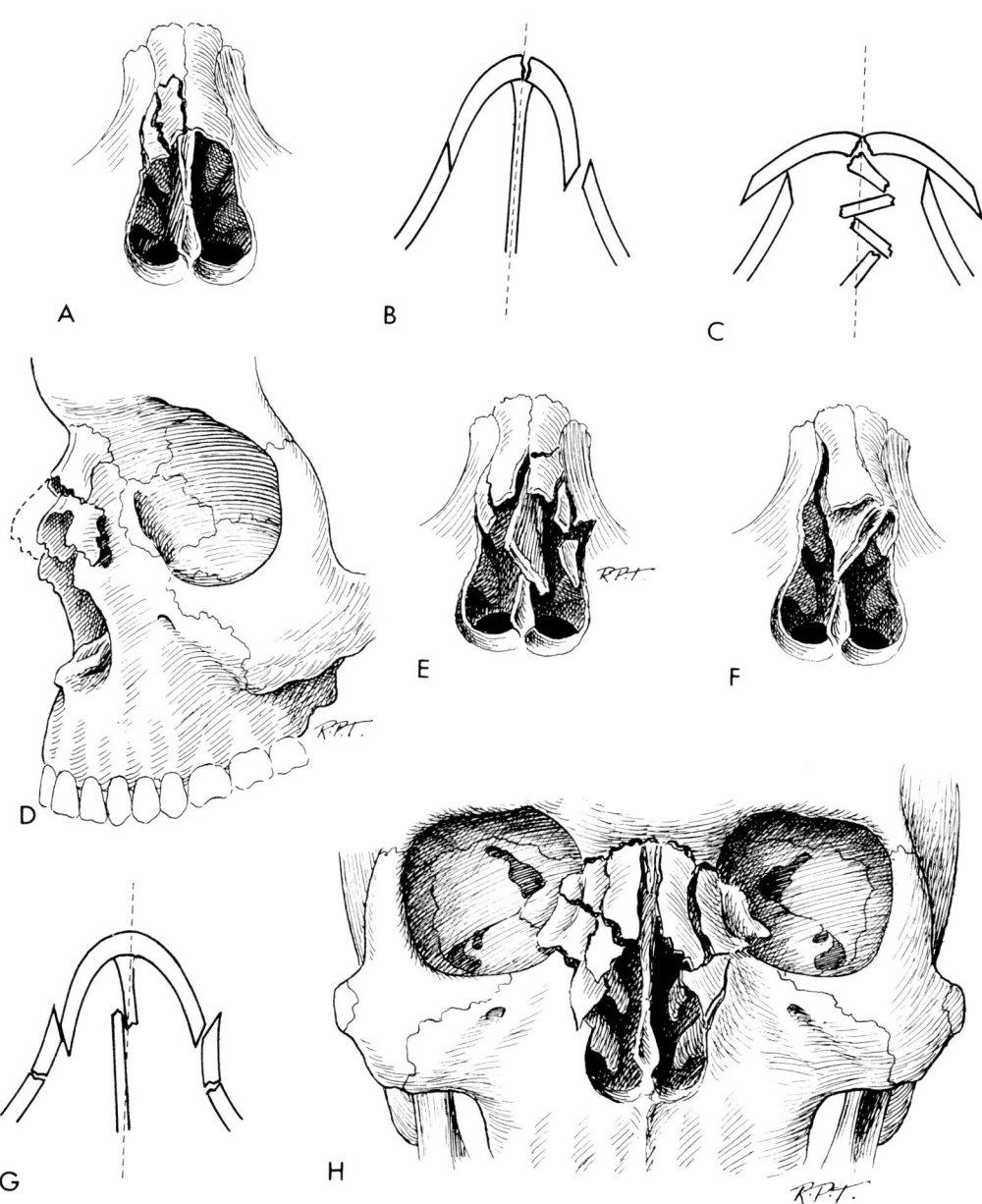

Figure 11–35   Various types of fractures of the nasal bones. *A* and *B*. Depressed fracture of one nasal bone. *C*. Open-book type of fracture seen in children. *D*. Fracture of the nasal bones at the junction of the thick upper and thin lower portions. *E*. Comminuted fracture. *F* and *G*. Fracture-dislocation. *H*. Comminuted fracture of the nasal bones involving the frontal processes of the maxilla. (Courtesy of J. M. Converse and W. B. Saunders Co., Philadelphia. *Reconstructive Plastic Surgery*, 2nd Ed., 1977.)

of the fractured nasal bones into the subcutaneous space overlying the bone adjacent to the nose.

Palpation of the nasal bones reveals mobility and tenderness, and crepitus caused by the loose fragments may be present. After examination of the external nose, a complete intranasal examination is essential to rule out a septal hematoma.

ROENTGENOGRAPHIC EXAMINATION

Roentgenograms of the nasal bones are important diagnostic and medicolegal measures, for they may show a linear fracture without displacement or with only slight displacement that is unaccompanied by distinctive clinical manifestations. The roentgenogram helps to furnish information concerning the degree of displacement in comminuted nasal fractures.

TREATMENT OF NASAL FRACTURES

The goal in the treatment of nasal fractures is to restore an adequate nasal airway and realign the nasal bones for an acceptable esthetic appearance. Reduction of fractured nasal bones is usually a simple

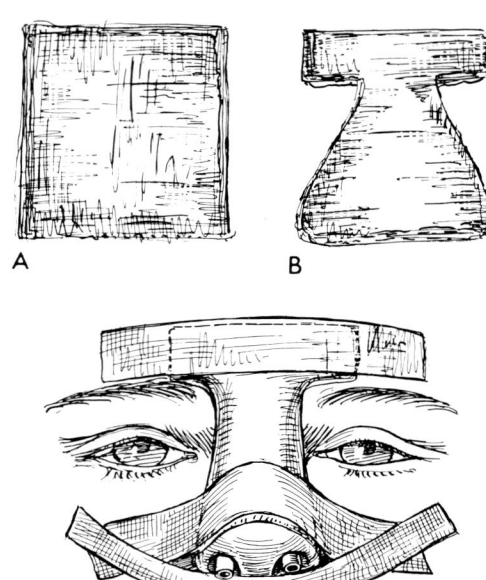

Figure 11–37   Plaster splint. A. A sufficient number of layers of plaster of Paris bandage to insure adequate strength is prepared. B. Plaster is cut to an hourglass shape. C. After being soaked in water, plaster is molded to the nose. After it has hardened, it is maintained in position with adhesive tape. (Courtesy of J. M. Converse and W. B. Saunders Co., Philadelphia. *Reconstructive Plastic Surgery*, 2nd Ed., 1977.)

procedure if undertaken soon after injury and before the onset of swelling. Local anesthesia using a 5 per cent cocaine solution on soaked cotton is usually sufficient for adult patients, whereas in children short general anesthesia is preferred (Figs. 11–36 and 11–37).

Purposeful delay in fracture reduction is justified when the entire nasal area and a large portion of the adjacent facial region is edematous and all landmarks are lost, as they are when the patient with a fractured nose is seen later than 24 hours after the fracture. The swelling is caused by edema and hematoma under the soft tissues of the nose. The method of treatment in such cases consists of administering antibiotic therapy, draining the hematoma, and treating the patient expectantly until the swelling is reduced. This may entail a delay of three or four days, but the nasal reduction can then be done under more favorable circumstances.

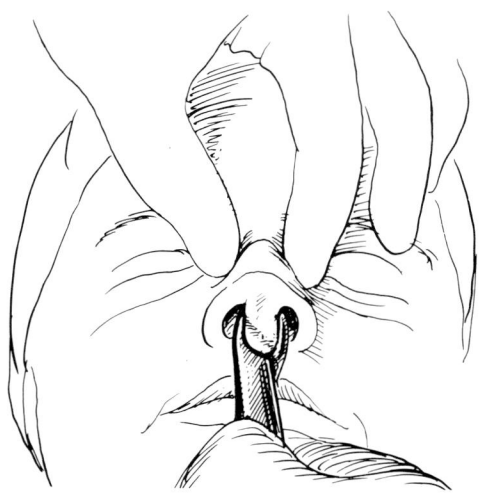

Figure 11–36   Use of Asche forceps to straighten the septum, correcting overriding fragments. External manipulation during this procedure assists in realigning the bony fragments. (Courtesy of J. M. Converse and W. B. Saunders Co., Philadelphia. *Reconstructive Plastic Surgery*, 2nd Ed., 1977.)

COMPLICATIONS OF NASAL FRACTURES

Simple fractures do not usually result in serious complications. Epistaxis at the time of injury usually ceases spontaneously, but if it persists or recurs, the usual measures of packing and cautery are employed. Septal hematoma must be treated early to avoid abscess and necrosis of the septal cartilage with eventual depression of the dorsum of the nose. Osteitis and osteomyelitis are unusual after nasal bone fractures.

Delayed union is unusual, for most nasal bone fractures consolidate within a week. Malunion of nasal fractures resulting in deviations or depressions requires corrective plastic surgery.

FRACTURES OF THE NASOORBITAL FRONTOETHMOIDAL REGIONS

Severe injuries of the midfacial area with fractures of the maxilla, nasal bones, zygoma, or orbits may be associated with fractures of the bones of the frontoethmoidal area of the facial skeleton. The bones of the middle third of the face are related to one another through the frontal sinuses and the cribriform plate, the floor of the anterior cranial fossa, and the frontal lobes of the brain, which may also be injured (Figs. 11–38 and 11–39).

SURGICAL PATHOLOGY

The bones forming the skeletal framework of the nose may be projected backward between the orbits when subjected to a strong traumatic force. The term "nasoorbital" designates this type of fracture.[5-7] The usual cause of nasoorbital fracture is an impact force applied over the upper portion of the bridge of the nose that projects the face against the dashboard or steering column of an automobile when it comes to a crash stop. A crushing injury with comminuted fractures is thus produced.

In addition to disorganization of the skeletal framework produced by the backward displacement of the bony structures between the orbits (interorbital space), fractures involving the cribriform plate and the anterior cranial fossa may result in cerebrospinal rhinorrhea and brain damage. Lacerations of the soft tissues may sever the levator palpebrae superioris muscle or penetrate through the medial canthal area, severing the medial canthal tendon and the lacrimal canaliculi or sac.

In severely injured patients, an associated

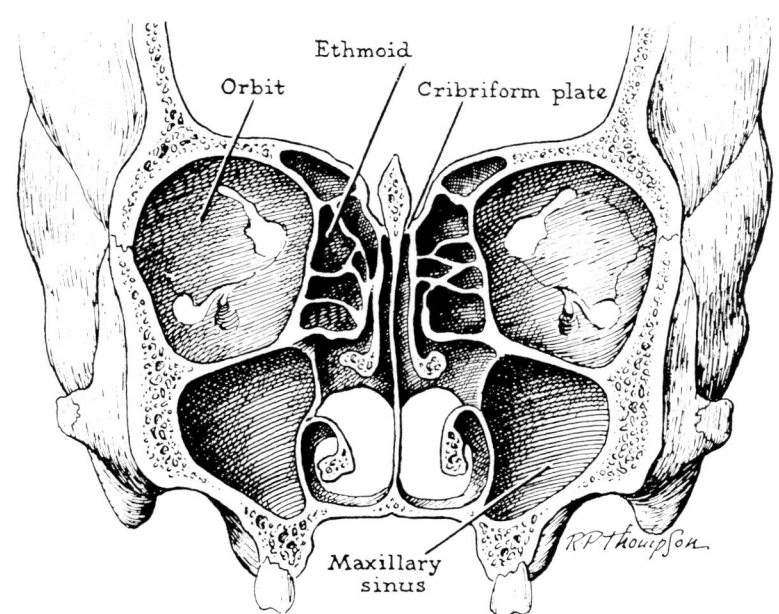

Figure 11–38 Interorbital space. (Courtesy of J. M. Converse and W. B. Saunders Co., Philadelphia. *Reconstructive Plastic Surgery*, 1st Ed., 1964.)

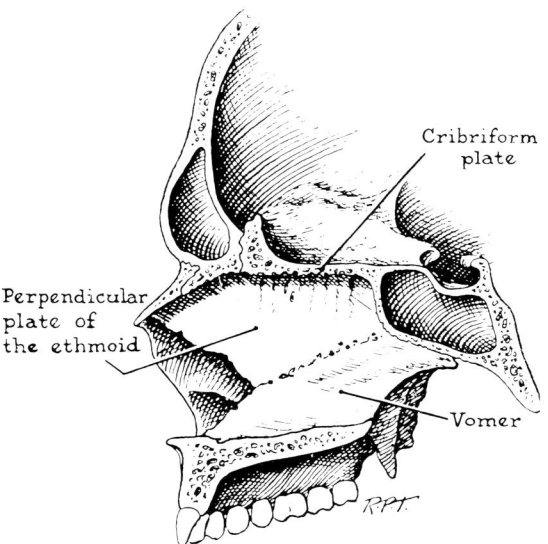

Figure 11–39 Sagittal section of a fragment of skull lateral to the nasal septum. Relationship of perpendicular plate of the ethmoid to the cribriform plate is shown. (Courtesy of J. M. Converse and W. B. Saunders Co., Philadelphia. *Reconstructive Plastic Surgery*, 1st Ed., 1964.)

fracture of the orbital floor, often a blow-out fracture, is also observed; fractures of other facial bones, particularly of the middle third of the face, are frequently seen. In some patients the frontal bone may be involved.

CLINICAL EXAMINATION

The appearance of the patient who has a nasoorbital fracture is typical; the nose is flattened, appearing to have been pushed between the eyes; the medial canthal areas are swollen and distorted, and ecchymosis and subconjunctival hemorrhage are usual findings (Fig. 11–40).

There may be little evidence of deformity because of hematoma or swelling. In some cases, however, when the frontal bone has been crushed in or the nasal structures have been conspicuously pushed backward, the deformity is evident. The bones may be loose, and crepitation may be felt when they are mobilized. If there is an associated fracture of the maxilla, the entire upper jaw may be movable, and the motion may be felt in the bones of the interorbital space. A portion of the forehead skin may be avulsed in compound fractures, exposing bone and revealing the site of fractures.

Clear fluid escaping from the nose is strongly suggestive of cerebrospinal fluid rhinorrhea, and appropriate diagnostic tests should be performed to verify this.

ROENTGENOGRAPHIC EXAMINATION

Stereoscopic roentgenograms and tomograms are required to estimate the amount

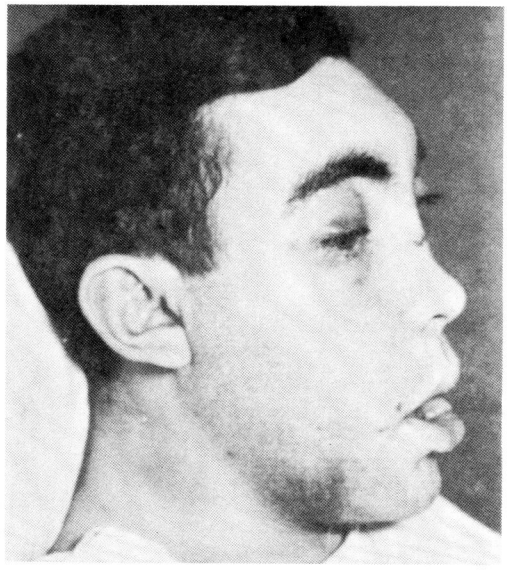
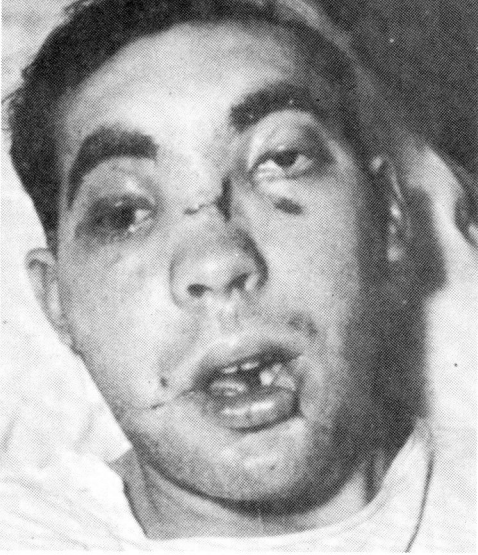

Figure 11–40   Five days after the nasoorbital fracture and high maxillary (Le Fort III) fracture. Note the flattening of the nasal dorsum, traumatic telecanthus, elongation of the middle third of the face, and openbite. (Courtesy of J. M. Converse and W. B. Saunders Co., Philadelphia. *Reconstructive Plastic Surgery*, 2nd Ed., 1977.)

of damage, for fractures of the cribriform plate may be impossible to detect by ordinary radiographic examination. The presence of air in the subdural space, the subarachnoid space, or the ventricle is a sign of communication with the nasal cavity or sinuses, establishing a direct pathway for infection, and is an absolute indication for operation. Fragmentation and a "buckled" appearance of the cribriform plate are suggestive of penetration of fragments of ethmoidal cells into the brain; this is a further indication for operation.

TREATMENT OF NASOORBITAL FRACTURES

Prior to treatment of nasoorbital fractures, careful neurological and radiological examination is required. Cerebrospinal fluid

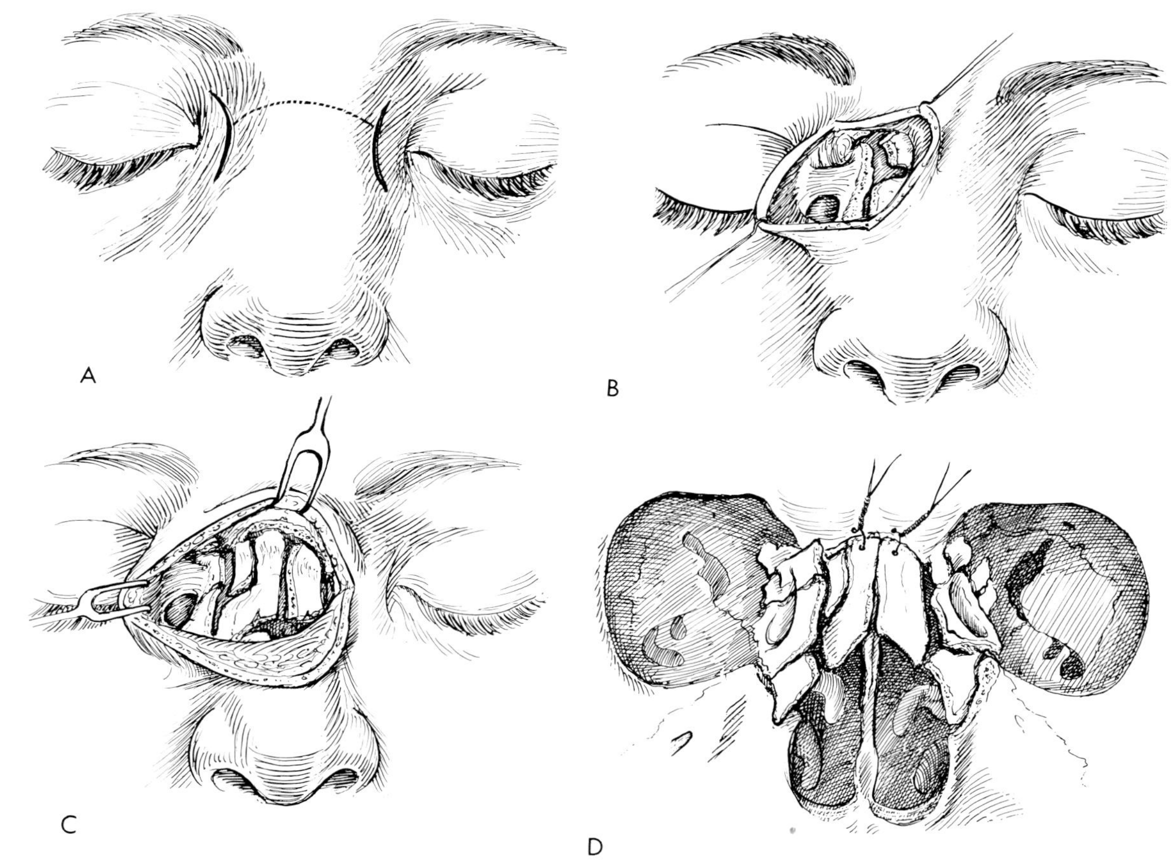

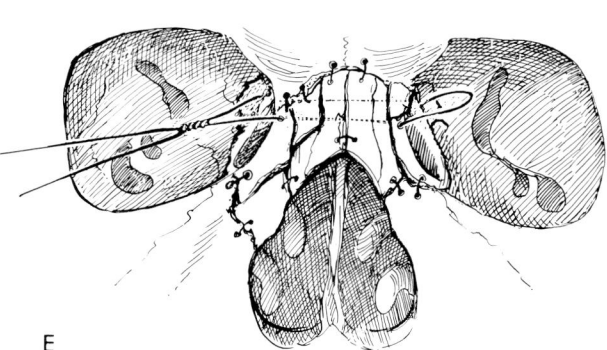

Figure 11–41   Open-sky technique in treatment of nasoorbital fractures. A. Lateral nasal incisions, which can be joined if necessary by a transverse incision. B. Exposure obtained through external incision. C. Comminuted fragments are visualized, as well as the lacrimal sac and the medial canthal tendon. D. Interosseous wiring of the main fragments of the nasal bones is established, providing initial stability. E. Other fragments have been drawn together by interosseous wiring, and a through-and-through wire maintains the anatomical position of the medial orbital walls. (Courtesy of J. M. Converse and V. M. Hogan and *Plastic and Reconstructive Surgery.* Open-sky approach for reduction of naso-orbital fractures. Case report. Plast. Reconstr. Surg., *46*:396, 1970.)

rhinorrhea should not, as a rule, be a contraindication to treatment of the fractures. A delay of a number of days may be required to allow for subsidence of swelling and hematoma and clarification of the neurological status of the patient; such a delay does not jeopardize the ultimate success of early treatment.

The modern approach to the treatment of severe nasoorbital fractures consists of exposing the fractured area through cutaneous incisions placed in judicious positions. Vertical incisions placed through the cutaneous tissues overlying the frontal process of the maxilla on each side may be adequate for exposure of the fractured skeletal structures. The vertical incisions can be joined by a horizontal incision at the nasofrontal angle. A trap-door flap can thus be reflected downward, exposing the bones and the medial canthal structures, the lacrimal sacs, and the medial canthal tendons. Realignment of the bones after disimpaction, wiring of the

fragments, reinsertion of a severed medial canthal tendon, verification of the patency of the lacrimal system, repair of a lacerated lacrimal sac, primary iliac bone grafting of the bony dorsum, or reconstruction of a medial orbital wall by bone grafting, all of these procedures done under direct vision restore the architecture and the function of the nasoorbital area (Fig. 11–41).

Concomitant fractures of the glabella, the anterior wall of the frontal sinus, and the frontal bone require raising a coronal scalp flap for adequate exposure and treatment. Craniotomy may be indicated.

COMPLICATIONS IN FRACTURES OF THE FRONTOETHMOIDAL AREA

Complications that occur as a result of frontal bone fractures and fractures of the bones of the interorbital space are numerous and varied. Some of these include

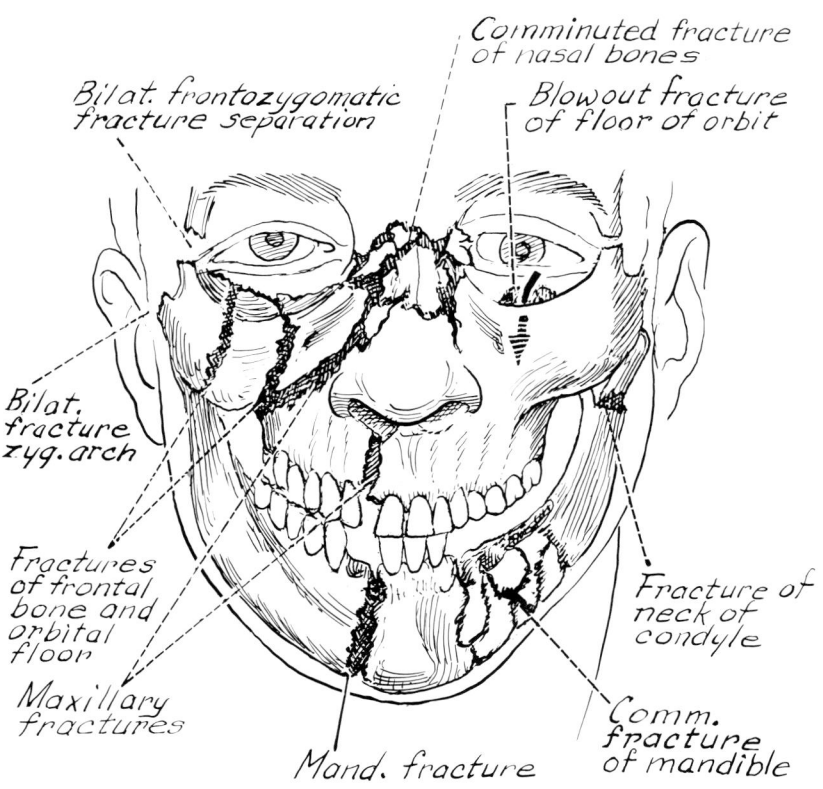

Figure 11–42   Typical complex fracture: multiple comminuted maxillary, mandibular, and nasoorbital fractures. (Courtesy of J. M. Converse and W. B. Saunders Co., Philadelphia. *Reconstructive Plastic Surgery*, 2nd Ed., 1977.)

diplopia, which is usually temporary, interference with lacrimal function because of damage to the lacrimal sac, and traumatic telecanthus. Sinusitis and osteomyelitis occur infrequently, but all patients with fractures in the frontoethmoidal area should receive broad-spectrum antibiotics.

COMPLEX FRACTURES OF THE FACIAL BONES

In high-speed accidents, "complex" or multiple fractures of the facial bones are often encountered. According to Georgiade, 20 per cent of individuals who have sustained injuries to the facial skeleton have multiple facial bone fractures.[12] McCoy and associates reported that 41 per cent of their cases of midfacial fractures were associated with fractures of the mandible.[21]

The methods previously described for treatment of individual facial bone fractures must be combined effectively and efficiently for proper management of the patient with multiple facial fractures (Fig. 11–42).

Associated orthopedic, thoracoabdominal, and craniocerebral injuries may take priority over facial injuries and fractures. Although early treatment before massive edema occurs is preferred, purposeful delay may be decided upon when the patient's condition is too critical or edema obscures normal anatomical landmarks.

REFERENCES

1. Angle, E. H.: Classification of Malocclusion. Dent. Cosmos, *41*:248, 1899.
2. Chalmers J. Lyons Club (Members): Fractures involving mandibular condyle; post-treatment survey of 120 cases. J. Oral Surg., *5*:45, 1947.
3. Converse, J. M.: Facial disfigurement: A national tragedy. Med. Tribune, 1964.
4. Converse, J. M., and Hogan, V. M.: Open-sky approach for reduction of naso-orbital fractures. Case report. Plast. Reconstr Surg., *46*:396, 1970.
5. Converse, J. M., and Smith, B.: Naso-orbital fractures (Symposium: Midfacial Fractures). Trans. Am. Acad. Ophthalmol. Otolaryngol., *67*:622, 1963.
6. Converse, J. M., and Smith, B.: Deformities of the eyelids and orbital region. *In* Converse, J. M. (ed.): Reconstructive Plastic Surgery, Chapter 20, pp. 645–661. Philadelphia, W. B. Saunders Co., 1964.
7. Converse, J. M., and Smith, B.: Naso-orbital fractures and traumatic deformities of the medial canthus. Plast. Reconstr. Surg., *38*:147, 1966.
8. Converse, J. M., Cole, J. G., and Smith, B.: Late treatment of blowout fracture of the floor of the orbit. A case report. Plast. Reconstr. Surg., *28*:183, 1961.
9. Cook, R. M., and MacFarlane, W. I.: Subcondylar fracture of the mandible—a clinical and radiographic review. Oral Surg., *27*:297, 1969.
10. Dingman, R. O.: The management of facial injuries and fractures of the facial bones. *In* Converse, J. M. (ed.): Reconstructive Plastic Surgery, Vol. 11, Chapter 17. Philadelphia, W. B. Saunders Co., 1964.
11. Dingman, R. O., and Natvig, P.: Surgery of Facial Fractures. Philadelphia, W. B. Saunders Co., 1964.
12. Georgiade, N. G.: Complex and External Fixation of Multiple Facial Fractures. *In* Plastic and Maxillofacial Trauma Symposium of the Educational Foundation of the American Society of Plastic and Reconstructive Surgery. St. Louis, C. V. Mosby Co., 1969.
13. Gillies, H. D., Kilner, T. P., and Stone, D.: Fractures of the malarzygomatic compound; with description of a new x-ray position. Br. J. Surg., *14*:651, 1927.
14. Huelke, D. F., and Burdi, A. R.: Location of mandibular fractures related to teeth and edentulous regions. J. Oral Surg., *22*:396, 1964.
15. Jabaley, M. E., Lerman, M., and Sanders, H. J.: Ocular injuries in orbital fractures, review of 119 cases. Plast. Reconstr. Surg., *56*:410, 1975.
16. Kazanjian, V. H., and Converse, J. M.: The Surgical Treatment of Facial Injuries. Baltimore, The Williams & Wilkins Co., 1949.
17. Keen, W. E.: Surgery, Its Principles and Practice. Philadelphia, W. B. Saunders Co., 1909.
18. Knight, J. S., and North, J. F.: The classification of malar fractures: An analysis of displacement as a guide to treatment. Br. J. Plast. Surg., *13*:325, 1961.
19. Kristen, K.: Zur Prognose der Luxations Fracturen des Processus articularis im Wachstumsalter. Fortschr. Kiefer. Gesichtschir., *11*:47, 1966.
20. LeFort, P.: Étude expérimentale sur les fractures de la machoire supérieure. Rev. Chir., *23*: 208,360,470, 1901.
21. McCoy, F. J., Chandler, R. A., Magnan, C. G., Jr., Moore, J.R., and Siemsen, G.: An analysis of facial fractures and their complications. Plast. Reconstr. Surg., *29*:381, 1962.
22. Rowe, N. L., and Killey, H. C.: Fractures of the Facial Skeleton. 2nd Ed. Baltimore, Williams & Wilkins Co., 1968.
23. Swearingen, J. J.: Tolerances of the Human Face to Crash Impact. Oklahoma City, Federal Aviation Agency, 1965.
24. Zizmor, J., Smith, B., Fasano, C., and Converse, J. M.: Roentgen diagnosis of blowout fractures of the orbit. Am. J. Roentgenol. Radium Ther. Nucl. Med., *88*:1009, 1962.
25. Zizmor, J., Smith, B., Fasano, C., and Converse, J. M.: Roentgen diagnosis of blowout fracture of the orbit. Trans. Am. Acad. Ophthalmol., Otolaryngol., *66*:802, 1962.

R. BRUCE HEPPENSTALL, M.D.

12 _____ _Injuries_
of the Chest

Isolated injuries of the chest wall resulting in fractures of one or several rib segments are commonly caused by direct trauma. The more severe type of crushing injury has been associated with high-speed automobile accidents; the frequency of such injuries has been on the increase over the past several decades. The most significant advance in treatment is appreciation of the pulmonary hypoxia that may result from these injuries. There has been a definite trend toward aggressive "pulmonary toilet." This is extremely important in the elderly patient if significant pulmonary complications are to be avoided. The old method of taping the chest wall to provide an adequate splint for the management of fractures has been replaced by aggressive pulmonary therapy.

SURGICAL ANATOMY

The chest cavity is surrounded by the osseous thorax, which functions to protect the lung and heart from injury. The sternum is located anteriorly, the ribs on the lateral aspect, and the spine posteriorly.

The sternum is composed of three distinct portions. The uppermost is the manubrium sterni. The middle portion is known as the body or gladiolus, and the inferior portion is referred to as the xiphoid process. The manubrium is the largest part of the sternum in terms of width and thickness. Facets along the proximal portion of the manubrium function for articulation with the clavicle. The costocartilage of the first rib attaches along the peripheral portion.

The body of the sternum accounts for its length. The manubrium is united to the body of the sternum through a synchondrosis which may ossify in adult life. The second through the eighth ribs articulate with the body of the sternum through the costocartilage. The xiphoid process is a wedge-shaped cartilagenous plate projecting in a distal direction. The first seven ribs have been referred to as the true ribs, and the eighth through the twelfth ribs as false ribs.

FRACTURES OF THE STERNUM

In the past, fractures of the sternum were considered a rare injury. However, they are seen with increasing frequency in association with automobile accidents. Their importance lies in the fact that significant trauma is required to produce a fracture of the sternum, and therefore a careful evaluation for associated injuries is essential.

MECHANISM OF INJURY

The most common mechanism of injury is direct trauma along the anterior aspect of the chest, such as that produced by the impact of a steering wheel or a forceful direct blow. A second, less frequent, mechanism is crushing or hyperflexion. As stated, a fracture of the sternum is an injury of significant magnitude. It is interesting that the sternum is rarely fractured in children, owing to the elasticity of the anterior costocartilage and the ribs.

286

PHYSICAL EXAMINATION

Visible swelling and definite tenderness over the fracture site are evident with isolated fractures of the sternum. The examiner can usually elicit pinpoint tenderness directly over the fracture, and if there is significant displacement an actual step-off deformity may be palpable. The customary deformity in a fractured sternum is the displacement of the distal portion to a more anterior position than the proximal portion.

If the sternal fracture is associated with rib fractures a true flail segment of the anterior portion of the chest wall may be present. Under these conditions a paradoxical motion of the anterior portion of the chest wall will be noted on respiration. It is mandatory for all patients with fractures of the sternum to be thoroughly evaluated for associated cardiac, pulmonary, or great vessel injuries.

ROENTGENOGRAPHIC EVALUATION

It is important to obtain anteroposterior, lateral, and oblique chest roentgenograms in all patients sustaining major chest trauma. The majority of sternal fractures are located in the body of the sternum in close proximity to its junction with the manubrium (Fig. 12–1). The lateral roentgenogram is frequently helpful in delineating these fractures. The typical deformity present in displaced fractures is anterior displacement with overriding of the distal fragment owing to the normal fixation of the manubrium sterni. Interestingly, in spite of overriding the periosteum of the posterior aspect of the sternum usually remains intact. Fractures of the xiphoid process are uncommon because of its position between the flare of the costal margins which provides some protection.

TREATMENT

Treatment of associated intrathoracic injuries takes precedence over management of the sternal fracture. If a significant injury has occurred a thoracotomy may be indicated, and the sternal disruption may be

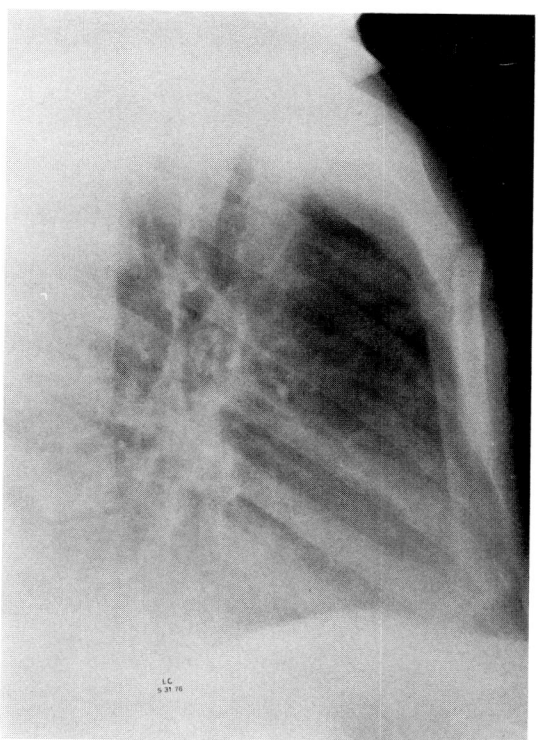

Figure 12–1   A lateral view of the chest wall demonstrating a fracture of the sternum on the right-hand side of the roentgenogram, with typical anterior displacement of the distal portion.

repaired at the end of the procedure. If an undisplaced fracture of the sternum occurs without significant associated injury the mainstay of treatment is to administer analgesics for comfort. Occasionally it is necessary to inject a local anesthetic into the fracture site for relief of pain. Operative management of these fractures should be undertaken in all patients with severely displaced fractures. The fracture site is exposed through a vertical incision over the body of the sternum. Towel clips are placed on the proximal and distal fragments, and the fracture is openly reduced by extending the patient and manipulating the fracture ends with the towel clips. Internal fixation is accomplished with the use of two or three simple through-and-through sutures of number 20 stainless steel wire.

Nonunion of sternal fractures is rare. If a patient presents with a definite nonunion, that is painful and unresponsive to local injection, some consideration may be given to operative fixation with the use of a sliding slot bone graft.

FRACTURES OF THE RIB

Rib fractures occur in approximately 40 to 50 per cent of patients who sustain significant nonpenetrating thoracic trauma. As with fractures of the sternum, fractures of the rib are seen more frequently in adults, owing to the resilient nature of the cartilage in children. Fractures of the rib may be isolated, or they may be seen in association with multiple fractures.

Mechanism of Injury

Fractures of the rib may occur secondary to a direct or indirect injury. Those resulting from direct injury frequently have associated pulmonary damage, since the rib fragment may be driven directly inward against the lung. In indirect trauma the force may be applied to a wider area, possibly causing the ribs to buckle outward. This can produce a fracture in the midportion of the rib without associated injury to

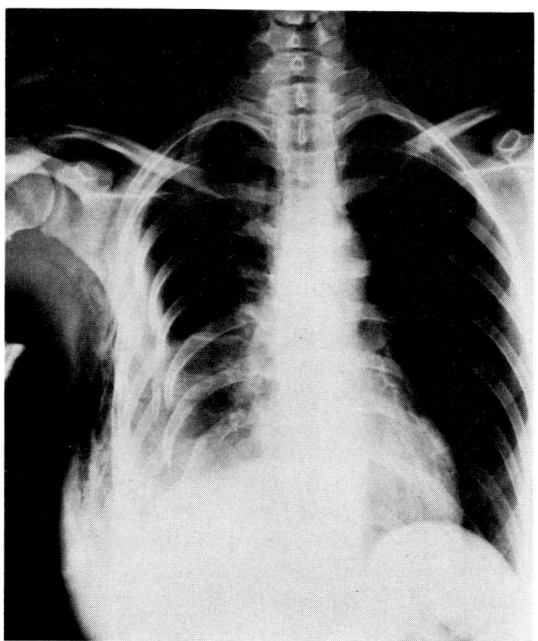

Figure 12–2 An anteroposterior view of the chest demonstrating multiple rib fractures on the right side, with evidence of subcutaneous emphysema.

the pulmonary structures. Structurally, the rib is weakest at the posterior angle. Rib fractures are usually located from the fifth to the ninth rib. Fractures of the first two ribs are rare, owing to the protective shield of the shoulder girdle and surrounding musculature. The opposite is true of the lower two ribs which are very mobile. Therefore, fractures of the 11th and 12th ribs are not seen as frequently.

Fractures of the rib may be associated with a subcutaneous emphysema (Fig. 12–2). This is produced by the rib fragment piercing the lung, causing an air leak. The air may then pass directly into the subcutaneous tissues where it may be palpable and noted on routine roentgenograms of the chest.

Physical Examination

Physical examination in isolated rib fractures will frequently elicit pinpoint tenderness directly over the fracture site. Patients will splint this portion of the chest in an attempt to limit the excursion of the fracture fragments, thus diminishing the pain. Swelling of the soft tissue structures may be evident over the fracture area. If multiple ribs are fractured, patients will markedly splint that portion of the rib margin, as they have lost the protective function of an intact rib above and below the level of the fracture. Respirations are usually very shallow under these conditions. Crepitus may be palpable in the subcutaneous tissues and may be an indication of gas within the tissues secondary to subcutaneous emphysema. It is important to obtain routine blood gas values and appropriate roentgenograms during the initial examination of these patients.

Roentgenographic Evaluation

Standard anteroposterior and lateral roentgenograms may not reveal the extent of the rib fractures. For this reason right and left anterior oblique views must be obtained if the rib margins are to be properly evaluated. It is also important to obtain an anteroposterior roentgenogram in the sitting or standing position to rule out an associated pneumothorax or hemothorax.

The most common location of single and multiple rib fractures is along the lateral rib margin. Mild displacement at the fracture site is not uncommon. Air may be visible in the soft tissue structures, indicative of subcutaneous emphysema.

TREATMENT

An associated pneumothorax or hemothorax demands aggressive early treatment. A large pneumothorax with significant embarrassment of respiration may be managed by the immediate insertion of a large-bore needle through the chest wall into the pleural cavity. This will convert a tension pneumothorax to an open pneumothorax, which will improve respiration until a chest tube can be inserted. In a similar fashion a hemothorax may be drained through a thoracentesis.

Isolated rib fractures are usually managed with analgesic medication sufficient to control the pain but still allow the patient to continue normal respiration. These fractures are usually tolerated, because the presence of an intact rib above and below the fracture site tends to splint the area. However, multiple rib fractures have lost this splinting capacity and are frequently extremely painful. It is important to provide for adequate analgesia under these conditions, or the patient will definitely splint the rib margin which may lead to pneumonia or atelectasis of the underlying lung.

Occasionally an intercostal nerve block may be advisable in order to provide adequate analgesia. This is performed by locally preparing the area and injecting 0.5 per cent lidocaine in the form of a cutaneous wheal at the posterior rib margin. It is important to include two ribs above and two ribs below the fracture site. A number 23- or 25-gauge needle may be introduced through the local subcutaneous skin wheal until the tip of the needle strikes the rib. The needle is then withdrawn slightly and slid under the rib where approximately 5 ml of a 2 per cent lidocaine solution is injected if an attempt at aspiration is negative. It is customary to observe at least a four to six hour interval for the patient to obtain significant relief of pain. It is vitally important to provide for vigorous pulmonary toilet during this time. The blocks may have to be repeated at various intervals to insure the maintenance of proper pulmonary toilet.

The application of adhesive chest strapping has decreased over the past decade because this type of splinting significantly reduces expansion of the chest wall, thereby subjecting the patient to the possibility of pneumonia or atelectasis. Therefore, an aggressive course of pulmonary toilet is preferred, even if intermittent injections of a local anesthetic are required to prevent these complications. The pain is usually significantly decreased three to four days postfracture, and the fractured rib is usually healed by six weeks.

CARTILAGINOUS INJURIES

Fractures at the costochondral or chondrosternal junction are commonly associated with fractures of the sternum. However, they can occur as isolated entities. The most common mechanism of injury is direct trauma, such as that caused by a steering wheel injury. Physical examination will usually reveal an area of pinpoint tenderness over the injured segment. These injuries may be more painful than rib fractures, with pain persisting over an extended period of time. A clicking sensation may be noted with respiration. Treatment is similar to the management of rib fractures.

FLAIL CHEST

This injury is not uncommon following automobile accidents in which the steering wheel is pushed directly into the anterior chest wall. It is a difficult injury to treat, and if not managed properly may result in a high incidence of morbidity and mortality.

MECHANISM OF INJURY

The most common mechanism of injury of a flail chest is direct trauma from a high-speed automobile accident, when the individual is suddenly thrust forward against the steering wheel. This frequently results in multiple fractures of the ribs, such that a segment of the chest wall loses continuity with the intact portion. This injury results in definite paradoxical respiration. The flail portion of the chest wall may be located in the anterior, lateral, or posterior part of the chest. However, the lateral portion is the area most frequently involved. If the injury occurs in the posterior aspect of the chest wall, paradoxical motion is decreased owing to the support provided by the scapula and surrounding musculature.

PHYSICAL EXAMINATION

On physical examination a definite paradoxical respiratory pattern is evident. The intact portion of the rib cage expands during normal inspiration, causing air to be drawn into the lungs. The flail portion of the chest wall does not expand, since it is no longer in continuity with the intact portion. This results in atmospheric pressure forcing the unstable segment in an inward direction. This inward migration is increased by the gradient produced by the negative intrapleural pressure. On expiration the normal intact chest wall decreases as air is forced out of the lungs. However, the unstable flail portion of the chest wall is pushed outward because intrathoracic pressure exceeds atmospheric pressure. Alveolar ventilation and perfusion of the lung are severely hampered by this mechanism. The ultimate result is hypoxia as a result of decreased alveolar ventilation. The patient is also unable to cough up secretions, and this will ultimately lead to further pulmonary problems.

A specific pattern of breathing, known as a seesaw pattern, is noted with flail chest along the anterior chest wall. In other words, as the patient attempts to inspire, the anterior chest wall moves in an inward direction and the abdominal wall moves in an outward direction. Arterial blood gas measurements are essential in evaluating these patients. Routine blood studies should also be obtained at this time.

ROENTGENOGRAPHIC EVALUATION

As a rule, a standard roentgenographic examination will reveal the severity of the rib fractures. The flail portion of the chest is usually obvious. Again, it is important to evaluate for the presence of air within the subcutaneous tissues and also for hemothorax.

TREATMENT

The emergency treatment of a patient with paradoxical respiration is to provide pressure over the flail segment during transportation to an appropriate care facility. This may be performed by direct pressure of the examiner's hand over the flail segment, by application of a light sandbag against the flail segment, or by turning the patient onto the injured side, so that the flail segment is splinted by the patient's chest being placed against a firm surface. This will limit the paradoxical motion of the chest wall and may help to improve ventilation. Definitive management involves the insertion of an endotracheal tube as soon as possible to provide for adequate suction of retained secretions in the bronchi and also to implement positive-pressure respiration. This has been referred to as providing a pneumatic splint for the flail segment of the chest wall. One of the common ventilators selected for the management of these injuries is a volume-cycled respirator. If it is important to stabilize the chest wall in an outward direction, this may be accomplished with the use of surgical towel clips. These are inserted subcutaneously around the involved rib segments and then connected to an overhead pulley which provides constant traction with the aid of a light weight. This was a common mechanism in the past to provide for adequate stabilization of the flail segment. However, more modern methods using improved artificial ventilators have largely replaced external fixation devices.

If a thoracotomy is required to manage the associated pulmonary or cardiac injury, it may be advantageous to provide for internal fixation of the fractured rib segments with the use of through-and-through wire or small compression plates.

REFERENCES

1. Ashbaugh, D. G., Peters, G. N., and Halgrimson, C. G.: Chest trauma. Analysis of 685 patients. Arch. Surg., 95:546–555, 1967.

2. Conn, J. H., Hardy, J. D., and Fain, W. R.: Thoracic trauma. Analysis of 1022 cases. J. Trauma, *3*:22–40, 1963.
3. D'Abreu, A. L.: Thoracic injuries, critical review. J. Bone Joint Surg., *46B*:581–597, 1964.
4. Fowler, A. W.: Flexion-compression injury of the sternum. J. Bone Joint Surg., *39B*:487–497, 1957.
5. Helal, B.: Fracture of the manubrium sterni. J. Bone Joint Surg., *46B*:602–607, 1964.
6. Kirsh, M. M., and Sloan, H.: Blunt Chest Trauma. General Principles of Management. Boston, Little, Brown, 1977, pp. 1–229.
7. LeRoux, B. T.: Maintenance of chest wall stability. Thorax, *19*:397–405, 1964.
8. Ransdell, H. T., Jr.: Treatment of flail chest injuries with a piston respirator. J. Trauma, *5*:412–420, 1965.
9. Williams, G.: The management of stove-in chest J. Bone Joint Surg., *46B*:598–601, 1964.

13 _____ *Fractures and Dislocations of the Cervical Spine*

In the past, the diagnosis of a "broken neck" carried a very grave prognosis. This bleak attitude was justified by the poor results obtained in treating these injuries. Only in the past few decades has a more rational and scientific approach been taken to patients with injuries of the cervical spine, a new approach that has greatly improved the outlook for the patients. A definite step forward was the realization that "routine laminectomy" is an aggressive approach whose benefits are unproved in this type of problem except in the case of a complete spinal cord syndrome and progressive neurological deterioration. This change of attitude was one of the most significant contributions to the management of patients with fractures and dislocations of the cervical spine. In the past, many patients were treated with wide decompressive laminectomy, which not only resulted in an increased neurological loss but also produced instability of the spine with progressive gibbus formation. A decompressive laminectomy is still applicable in the face of a progressing neurological deficit. If a complete neurological deficit is present at the time of the injury, however, the benefit derived from such a procedure is minimal

and the procedure itself compounds the problem by producing an increased instability of the spine that may be difficult to manage.

Present-day treatment includes early reduction of the fractured spine and stabilization by operative methods or by an external fixation device. An improved understanding of the mechanisms of injury and the biomechanical forces involved has aided the modern physician in determining which patients require continued conservative treatment and which patients require operative management. The halo external fixation device developed at Rancho Los Amigos in California has greatly facilitated the conservative approach.[50, 80] It allows for early reduction and immobilization of the injury while allowing the patient to be out of bed, preventing secondary complications. This device has received enthusiastic acceptance for treatment of these injuries.

Many new operative techniques have allowed early fixation of the fracture in patients with and without associated spinal cord injuries. Progressive gibbus formation, seen in patients with neurological involvement in the past, has been seen less frequently in recent times owing to these

292

improved surgical techniques. Many of the metabolic complications also have been eliminated.

Significant new research has enhanced our understanding of the physiological aspects of the neurological deficit associated with these injuries. Intravenously administered steroids in large doses along with local hypothermia of the spinal cord have demonstrably reduced the spinal cord edema and improved return of function in experimental animals. In many centers large doses of steroids continue to be administered intravenously in the hope that the spinal cord edema will be reduced. In clinical practice, however, it is impractical to provide early cooling of the spinal cord following these injuries. It has been adequately demonstrated that the cooling must be performed within the first four to six hours if any benefit is to be derived. In most cases, transportation to a hospital and preparation for a surgical procedure cannot be performed within this time interval. It is for this reason that this form of treatment has not gained widespread acceptance in clinical practice at the present time. It is to be hoped that, with continued research in this area, significant advances will make it possible to reduce the amount of permanent neurological deficit produced. At present we must realize that it is impossible to reverse an established neurological deficit associated with complete spinal cord lesions entirely.

The bright side of this picture is that many patients presenting with fractures of the cervical spine do not have neurological deficits. Following appropriate treatment, these patients may be returned to an active role in society without physical impairment.

SURGICAL ANATOMY

A thorough understanding of the pertinent anatomy is essential to understand the mechanism of injury and to formulate a rational approach to treatment of lesions of the cervical spine. The osseous elements comprise seven vertebrae, of which the first two, the atlas (C1) and the axis (C2), have unique anatomical features that allow flexion, extension, and rotatory motion. The atlas consists of a ring of bone without a central body but with large lateral masses that provide weight-bearing articulation between the skull and the vertebral column (Fig. 13–1). The superior facets articulate with the occiput, and the inferior facets with the axis. Spanning the lateral masses anteriorly is the slender arch of the atlas, lying in front of the odontoid process. The odontoid is held against the arch by the strong transverse ligament posteriorly as well as by the alar and apical ligaments. This anatomical configuration provides a check rein to limit the amount of rotation and anteroposterior excursion of C1 on C2. The posterior arch is longer than the anterior and bears a small posterior tubercle in place of a spinous process. Sulci are found along the upper surface for the vertebral arteries.

The axis, or second cervical vertebra, has a characteristic projection known as the odontoid process, or dens, which was developmentally the body of the first vertebra (Fig. 13–2). This anatomical configuration allows rotation at the superior articulation

Figure 13–1   Anatomy of the atlas. A ringlike structure. The odontoid is situated behind the anterior position of the ring. (Courtesy of J. Langman and M. W. Woerdeman and W. B. Saunders Co., Philadelphia, Pa. Atlas of Medical Anatomy, 1978.)

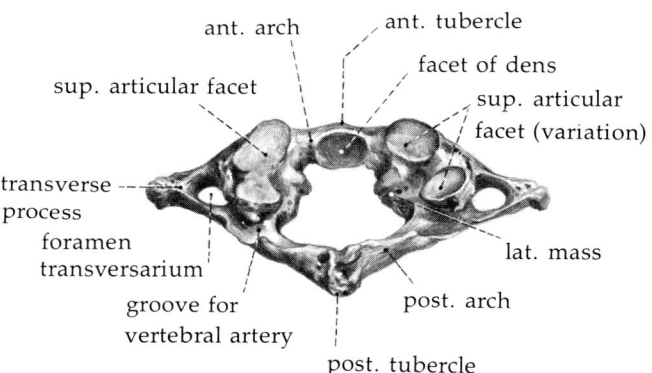

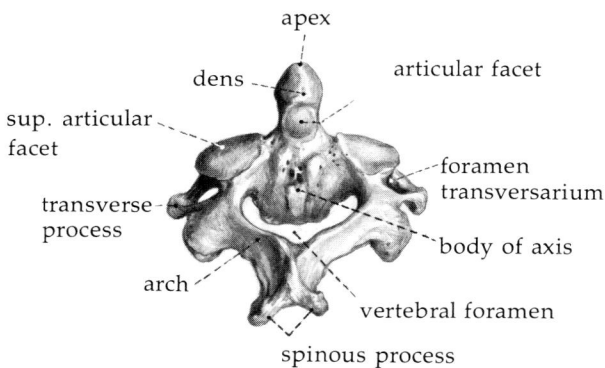

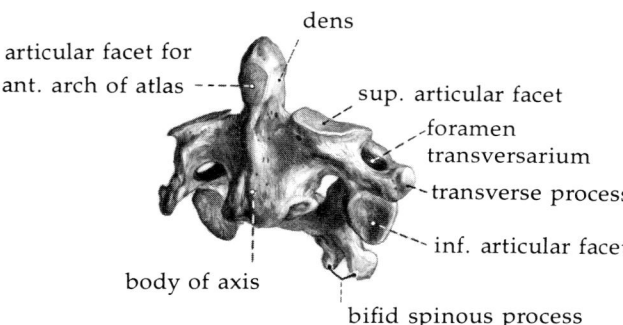

Figure 13-2 Anatomy of the axis. The odontoid originates from the body of the axis. (Courtesy of J. Langman and M. W. Woerdeman and W. B. Saunders Co., Philadelphia, Pa. Atlas of Medical Anatomy, 1978.)

with the atlas and limited flexion, tilt, and rotation at the inferior articulation with C3. Superior articular surfaces are large and face upward, posteriorly, and laterally. These in turn, originate on heavy masses arising from the body and pedicles. The powerful transverse ligament along with the alar and apical ligaments stabilizes the superior projection of the odontoid to the ring of the atlas (Fig. 13-3). Apertures are

present along the lateral masses of the axis for the vertebral artery. The spinous process of the axis is elongated and bifid. The blood supply of the odontoid process has recently been demonstrated by Schiff and Parke, who showed that three main groups of arteries supply the odontoid and its ligaments. They named the arteries the anterior ascending artery of the axis, the posterior ascending artery of the axis, and the cleft perforators. The anterior and posterior ascending arteries originate from the vertebral arteries, while the cleft perforators originate from the internal carotid artery.[60]

The remainder of the cervical vertebrae, C3 to C7, have a similar anatomical appearance (Fig. 13-4). Their function is to provide limited flexion, extension, tilt, and rotation. They also provide anatomical stability to support the cranium. Their vertebral bodies articulate with one another via superior and inferior articular facets. The intervertebral discs, contained by the anterior and posterior longitudinal ligaments, are located between the vertebral bodies.

The vertebral artery passes upward

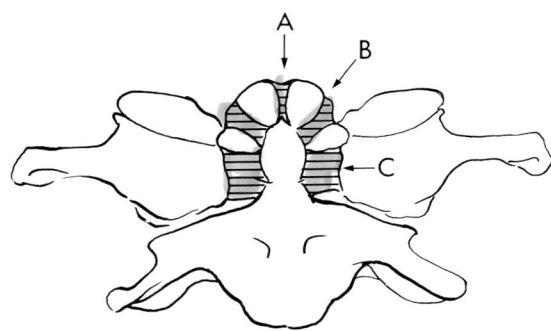

Figure 13-3 Coronal section through the first and second cervical vertebrae demonstrating the apical ligament (A), the alar ligament (B) and the transverse ligament (C).

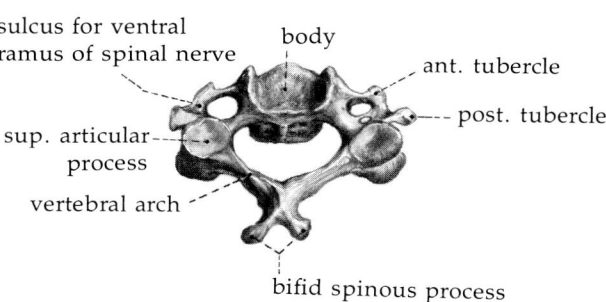

Figure 13-4 Typical cervical vertebra demonstrating that the articular surfaces of the superior facets face upward and posteriorly while those of the inferior facets face downward and anteriorly. (Courtesy of J. Langman and M. W. Woerdeman and W. B. Saunders Co., Philadelphia, Pa. Atlas of Medical Anatomy, 1978.)

through the vertebral foramen in the lateral masses from C6 to C1. The seventh cervical vertebra does have a small transverse foramen, but this does not usually transmit the vertebral artery. The nerve roots traverse behind the vertebral artery in a groove along the superior aspect of the lateral mass. The facet joints are found directly posterior to the nerve root canal. The articular surfaces of the superior facets face upward and posteriorly, while those of the inferior facet face downward and anteriorly. The posterior root of the transverse process arises from about the junction of the pedicle with the lamina, while the anterior root, developmentally a rib, arises from the side of the body. The transverse foramen is formed between the two roots of the transverse process. The lamina of C2 is heavy, while the laminae of C3, C4, and C5 are thin; heavy laminae reappear at C6 and C7. The spinous process of the cervical vertebrae except the sixth and seventh are typically short; those of the third through the sixth are typically bifid.

A few surface landmarks are useful in identifying structures in the cervical spine. The spinous processes of C2 and C7 are palpable posteriorly. The most prominent spinous process, however, is that of the first thoracic vertebra.

Neuroanatomy. In adults the spinal cord extends from the foramen magnum to the second lumbar vertebra. It is suspended by the dentate ligaments, nerve roots, and blood vessels, all within a shock-absorbing cerebrospinal fluid sac. The arachnoid and tough fibrous dura protect the spinal cord. According to Steel's rule of thirds, the spinal cord and contents occupy approximately one third of the area enclosed by the arch of the atlas. In the remainder of the cervical area, the spinal cord and contents occupy approximately 50 per cent of the spinal canal. A typical nerve root is formed from ventral and dorsal rootlets. Although there are seven cervical vertebrae, there are eight cervical nerves. The root of the first cervical nerve exits in the canal between the occiput and first cervical ring. Each succeeding nerve root exits above its corresponding vertebra. For example, the second cervical nerve root exits between C1 and C2; the eighth cervical nerve root exits between C7 and T1.

The spinal cord is protected by the surrounding vertebral structures as well as by the hydraulic system within the subarachnoid space, which has excellent shock-absorbing capacity. The blood supply of the spinal cord is provided by a single anterior spinal artery and two posterior spinal arteries, running longitudinally. The anterior spinal artery originates by fusion of paired branches rising from two vertebral arteries. Posterior spinal arteries originate from the posterior inferior cerebellar arteries or the vertebral arteries. They are reinforced by branches that reach the spinal cord by way of the nerve roots.

In cross section the gray matter of the spinal cord resembles the shape of a butterfly or an H. The gray matter contains anterior horn cells that innervate the muscles of the neck and upper extremities. The peripheral white matter relays sensation and motor impulses to and from the trunk and lower extremities. It is important to bear in mind that the lower motor neuron fibers to the upper extremities exit from the cervical portion of the cord, while the upper motor neuron fibers to the lower extremities traverse the cervical portion of the spinal cord.

NORMAL MOTION OF THE CERVICAL SPINE

Motion in the cervical spine occurs through three distinct mechanisms. These include sliding, tilting, and rotation. The sliding mechanism comes into play when one vertebra slides over the vertebra below—seen primarily in the sagittal plane and involving a forward and backward displacement during motion. The tilting mechanism on the other hand occurs in both frontal and sagittal planes. In lateral bending the vertebral body tends to tilt in the direction of the lateral displacement. Rotation occurs through a vertical axis between two vertebrae.

The principal motions in the cervical spine include flexion, extension, lateral bending, and rotation.

Flexion. Most flexion occurs in the mid and lower segments of the cervical spine—approximately 15 degrees at both the atlantooccipital and atlantoaxial joints, and the remainder, which allows the chin to approximate the chest, through the mid and lower cervical segments. There is normally some lordosis in the cervical spine. With flexion this normal lordotic pattern is gradually abolished. The segments that allow the greatest mobility in the lower cervical spine are C4–C5, C5–C6, and C6–C7. In this area the intervertebral discs are taller and are wedge-shaped. The anterior disc height is greater than the posterior. Thus, as flexion is initiated, sliding occurs between the vertebral bodies, the disc is displaced posteriorly, and an additional tilting occurs between the vertebrae. The greatest amount of tilt occurs at the C6–C7 segment.

Extension. Extension produces the reverse of the foregoing pattern. With this motion the normal cervical lordosis is accentuated. Fifteen degrees of extension occurs at the atlantooccipital and atlantoaxial joints. The intervertebral discs are displaced anteriorly, and there is tilting of each vertebral body.

Lateral Bending. In the cervical spine, lateral bending is produced by tilting of the vertebrae toward the side of the bend combined with compression of the corresponding discs. The atlas displaces laterally on the axis when the head is tilted to the side. At the atlantoaxial joint, true lateral displacement cannot occur because of the anatomical restrictions. In this area extension is usually combined with rotation. If the head is bent more than 30 degrees to the side, the spinous process of the axis will deviate in the opposite direction, which indicates that a greater degree of rotation is occurring.

Rotation. Fifty per cent of rotation, a complex and vital movement, occurs in the upper cervical spine, where the atlantoaxial complex is responsible for the motion. The atlas tends to pivot around the odontoid, permitting rotation of 45 degrees in the axial plane to both right and left. A mild telescoping type of motion also occurs with rotation at this level. Owing to the configuration of the surface of the facets, the atlas tends to slide downward on the convex slope of the axis, and a mild upward and downward pistoning action occurs with alternating directions of rotation. From a biomechanical standpoint, instant centers of rotation may be calculated for the cervical spine. This allows an analysis of the amount of rotation in the sagittal plane. The instant center of rotation for each cervical vertebra is located in the body of the vertebra below. For example, the center of rotation about which the second vertebra rotates is located in the posterior and inferior portion of the body of the third cervical vertebra. Continuing in a distal direction, each center tends to assume a location anterior and superior to the one in the vertebra below. For example the instant center for the sixth cervical vertebra is at the level of the upper endplate of the seventh body and anterior to it. The importance of this finding is that if the instant center of rotation is found near the vertebra, then the motion associated with this vertebra is primarily that of tilt. On the other hand, if the center is removed from the vertebral body, as occurs in the second cervical vertebra, the motion of that particular body contains a large element of sliding. This helps to explain why the second cervical vertebra tends to slide while the sixth cervical vertebra tends to tilt.

HISTORY

As a general rule, all patients with serious injuries to the cervical spine will complain of significant pain in the cervical area. This symptom should not be taken lightly, given the history that the patient was involved in an accident. Occasionally, unfortunately, patients who come to an emergency room complaining of neck pain following an injury are released after a very superficial examination. A thorough history is vital in evaluating patients with neck pain following an accident. The examining physician should ask several specific questions in regard to the injury:

Were you stationary at the time of injury to the neck?

If involved in an automobile accident, were you the passenger in the front or rear seat or were you the driver of the automobile?

Were you wearing a hat or glasses at the time of the accident and if so were they knocked off during the accident?

Were there any neurological alterations immediately following the accident?

Did you experience radiating pain or numbness?

Were you knocked unconscious at the time of the accident?

Were there associated injuries to the extremities or the trunk?

Do you remember whether the neck injury was of an extension, flexion, or lateral rotation type?

Did you have trouble swallowing following the accident?

Were there alterations in vision?

Did you experience ringing in the ears or dizziness?

It is also important to document whether the patient was thoroughly evaluated in a nearby hospital emergency room following the accident or waited a few hours prior to being seen.

Recently, a number of these patients have presented with a history of diving into water and injuring the cervical spine, with or without neurological impairment. It is important to obtain appropriate information from the patient as to the height of the dive and the approximate depth of the water.

PHYSICAL EXAMINATION

A careful well-documented physical examination is of paramount importance in the evaluation of these injuries. Patients fre-

quently have to be transferred from temporary stretchers when they are brought in by emergency rescue squads. It is important to maintain mild gradual traction on the neck while the person is being transferred from a rescue cot to a stretcher or bed.

Associated injuries should be noted and recorded. Lacerations or abrasions over the forehead, along the temporal region, or in the occipital region will frequently furnish a clue to the mechanism of injury. The postural attitude of the head on the trunk is noteworthy. Frequently patients with spasms of the sternocleidomastoid muscle will present with the head tilted to the side. Associated spasm of the trapezius muscle complex will cause the shoulders to be elevated in a protective fashion. Careful observation of whether the patient is able to move the upper and lower extremities during the initial evaluation is essential. The blood pressure is carefully recorded, and the presence or absence of hypotension is noted. It is important to differentiate between hypotension on the basis of spinal shock and that associated with hypovolemia secondary to hemorrhagic loss. A key factor in this determination is whether the pulse rate is increased: in spinal shock it is not, but in hypovolemia the rate is definitely elevated.

Careful palpation of the anterior structures in the neck will reveal whether there is abnormal tenderness along the belly of the sternocleidomastoid muscle and whether the trachea is displaced and tender. Retropharyngeal hematoma will frequently produce this localized tenderness. Careful rotation of the neck is performed under mild traction to determine whether the patient experiences pain with rotation. This maneuver must be very gentle and must be discontinued if it causes pain or abnormal sensation. The spinous processes are carefully palpated along the posterior neck region. Localized tenderness along the spinous processes and a step-off deformity should immediately alert the examiner to a definite injury of the cervical spine.

Neurological Evaluation

A careful sensory and motor examination is essential in evaluating these patients.

The sensory modalities, including pinprick, position, touch, vibration, and deep pain, must be thoroughly tested. Sensory levels for each cervical spinal cord segment must be recorded. It may be difficult to differentiate between spinal cord and nerve root signs at the level of injury, as there is a little disparity between the sensory level and the corresponding spinal cord segment. Figure 13–5 shows a useful diagram for documenting sensation in cervical nerves with which the neurological deficit may be "mapped out." The sensory pattern corresponding to the apparent level of injury should be carefully tested to determine whether there is any discrimination between a sharp and a dull sensation, as this may well indicate an incomplete lesion, which obviously carries a better prognosis. Sensory examination of the anal, perianal, and scrotal areas is important in the differentiation of complete and incomplete lesions. Intact perianal sensation usually indicates an incomplete lesion, while discrimination between sharp and dull indicates preservation of the lateral spinal cord columns, which usually indicates an eventual recovery. Anterior column function is usually evaluated by the presence or absence of light touch, and posterior column function is indicated by the presence or absence of deep pressure, vibration, and position sense.

Motor function proximal and distal to the level of involvement should be recorded. Spinal lesions proximal to the C4 level usually result in immediate death due to paralysis of all respiratory muscles. The cell bodies for the phrenic nerves are located at about the C4 spinal level, and cord injury at this level or above will interfere with phrenic nerve function. If the lesion is below C5, both intercostal and abdominal musculature will be flaccid, which will leave only the phrenic-innervated diaphragmatic muscles functioning. Remember the old mnemonic "C3, 4 and 5 keep the diaphragm alive." The following guide has been useful in determining the exact level involved: C5 function is indicated by activity in the deltoid, biceps, and brachialis muscles. C6 function is indicated by activity in the abductor pollicis longus, the extensores pollicis brevis and longus, the extensores carpi radialis longus and brevis. C7 function is indicated by activity in the

triceps, the finger extensors, and the flexor carpi radialis. C8 function is indicated by activity of the flexores digitorum sublimus or profundis. T1 function is indicated by activity in the lumbricals or interossei. The remainder of the neurological examination related to the lower extremities and abdominal musculature is carried out in a routine fashion to determine motor function in these areas.

Rectal Examination

The rectal examination is extremely important in the evaluation of spinal injuries. It is frequently not carried out properly, with the result that the examiner is unable to determine whether the lesion is complete or incomplete. The old medical saying "if you do not put your finger in it, you will put your foot in it," certainly applies to this examination in spinal injuries. If sensation is absent around the anal area or immediately within the rectum, a complete sensory lesion is present. If there is no voluntary contraction of the anal sphincter during a rectal examination and no voluntary motor control below the upper extremities, complete motor paralysis is present. The bulbocavernosus reflex deserves special attention. This is produced by a pull on the urethral catheter, which stimulates the trigone of the bladder, producing a reflex contraction of the anal sphincter around the gloved finger. If the patient is in spinal shock the reflex may be absent and the sphincter flaccid. This is important because if the reflex is present and the patient is out of spinal shock (usually less than 24 hours postinjury) with no sensory or motor sparing, then a complete cord lesion is present. This is, therefore, an extremely important prognostic sign that should be recorded for all patients with neurological deficit following spinal injury.

ROENTGENOGRAPHIC EXAMINATION

If the examiner feels that a patient does have a cervical spinal injury, he must then make arrangements for the patient to have a thorough roentgenographic examination.

Patients with this type of injury frequently are brought to the emergency room

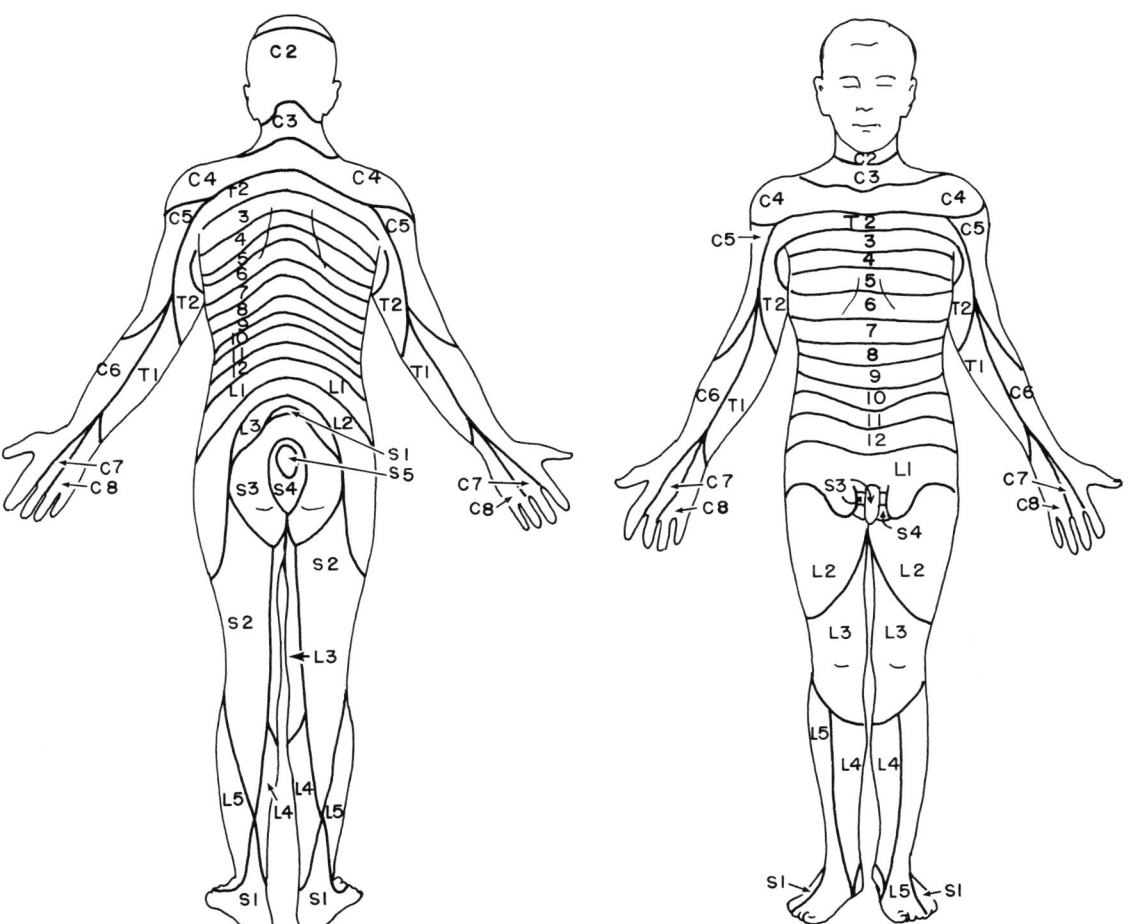

Figure 13-5. Cervical nerve evaluation. The sensory dermatomes can be used as the function of the various cervical nerve roots.

C2 – posterior aspect of the scalp
C3 – anterior aspect of the neck
C4 – clavicles to second rib interspace
C5 – lateral aspect of proximal arm
C6 – radial border of forearm, thumb, index and long fingers
C7 – long finger
C8 – ring and little fingers, ulnar border of forearm and hand
T1 – medial aspect of proximal arm

during the early hours of the morning. It is imperative that a physician accompany the patient to the radiology department in order to supervise the movement of the patient during roentgenographic examination. It is best to leave the patient on the examining stretcher and obtain a straight lateral view of the cervical spine. Once the lateral view has been obtained, if it does not reveal a definite fracture of the cervical spine, the patient may be moved — with gentle traction maintained on the cervical area — to a proper roentgenographic table for further evaluation of his associated injuries.

A common error is to accept roentgenograms that do not reveal all seven cervical vertebrae (Fig. 13–6). *Never accept roentgenographic examination of the cervical vertebrae without viewing all seven cervical vertebrae.* Patients will frequently elevate the shoulders in a reflex protective muscle spasm, which will interfere with visualization of C5–6 and C6–7. Gentle downward traction on the upper extremities can usually overcome this. If the shoulder shadow is still present after this maneuver, the patient may be placed in gentle head-halter traction, and downward traction may be applied to the upper extremities. It is not advisable to administer muscle relaxants or any other medication, as these patients may well have associated head injuries and the medication will only cloud the clinical picture. If the C7–T1 interval is still not well visualized with the foregoing measures, a "swimmer's view" may be obtained. This particular view is helpful in visualizing the C7–T1 articulation, as it abducts the arm 180 degrees with the opposite arm along the side; the beam is then directed at a 60 degree oblique angle. A complete roentgenographic examination should include regular anteroposterior, open-mouth, and oblique projections. If there is any question about the presence or absence of a fracture, further roentgenographic evaluation is indicated, including pillar views and laminograms if necessary.

It must be reemphasized that a physician should be present during the initial roentgenographic evaluation to determine whether the patient can tolerate the various procedures. If a lateral view demonstrating all seven cervical vertebrae does not reveal any gross fracture or dislocation in a multiply injured patient, then further roentgenographic evaluation can be postponed, as emergency measures for his immediate care may have to be instituted. It must also be kept in mind that many patients suffering multiple trauma including head injury may also have a fracture-dislocation of the cervical spine. All such patients should have a routine lateral roentgenogram of the cervical spine. The sequence of roentgenograms obtained, however, and the judgment whether additional roentgenograms are necessary to evaluate a particular patient can only be determined by an attending physician. It is for this reason that a patient should never be sent to the radiology department for routine roentgenographic evaluation of a suspected cervical fracture accompanied only by an orderly or radiology technician.

Roentgenographic Signs of Cervical Injury

Several roentgenographic signs are indicative of prior cervical injury. It is important not only to evaluate the osseous evidence of injury but also to evaluate the soft-tissue structures that may be indicative of an osseous injury. This is also important in other areas, as for example, a positive fat-pad sign indicates a probable osseous injury around the elbow.

Lateral View. A lateral roentgenogram of the cervical spine may reveal a prevertebral soft-tissue abnormality that is indicative of a cervical spine injury. At the level of the anterior inferior border of the third cervical vertebral body, the prevertebral soft-tissue thickness should be less than 4 to 5 mm. If the soft-tissue density between the pharynx and the vertebral body measures 5 mm or more, this is indirect evidence of a cervical spine injury — a rough rule, but very useful in assessment of patients with cervical injuries. If this finding is present, the attending physician should perform additional studies to rule out a fracture. Fractures of the odontoid process and of the pedicle of C2 notoriously cause little or no alteration in alignment and may well be overlooked if the soft-tissue shadow is not observed. In children the soft-tissue space is normally about two thirds of the thickness of the second cervical vertebra. It also must

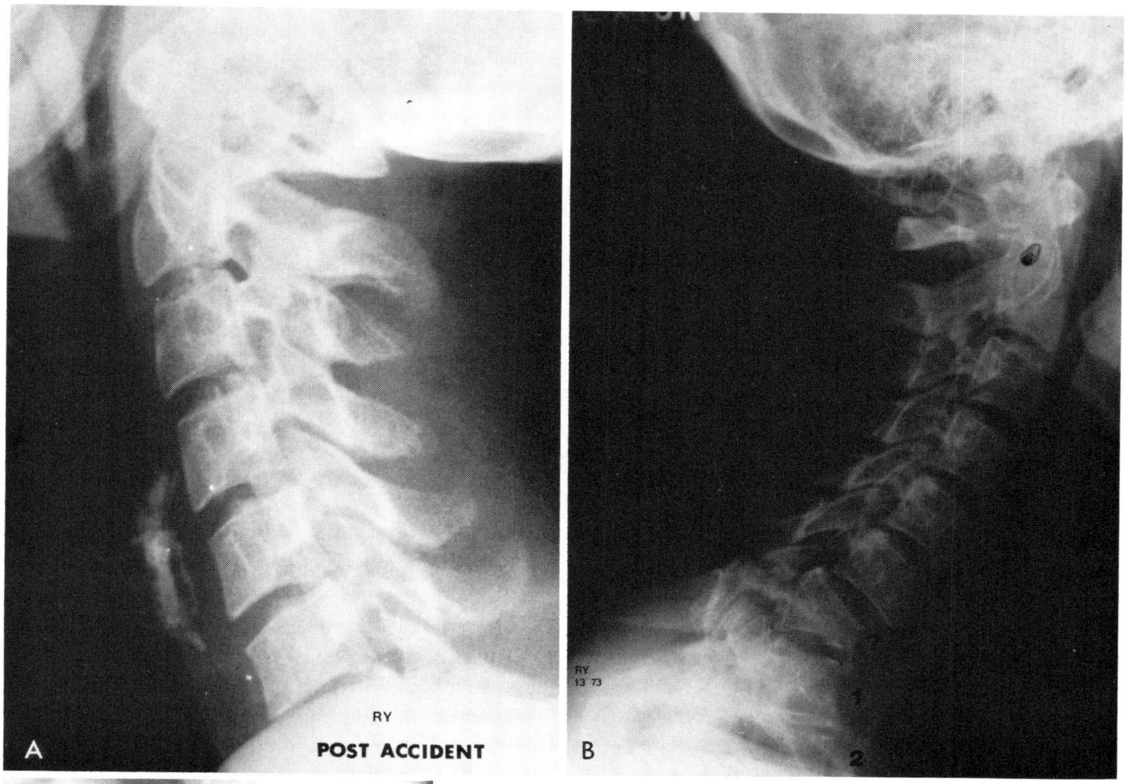

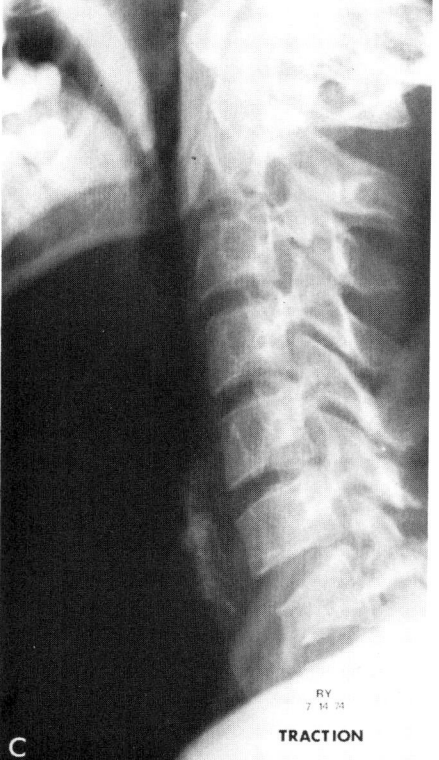

RY

POST ACCIDENT

RY
13 73

1

2

RY
7 14 74

TRACTION

Figure 13–6   *A.* Lateral roentgenogram of the cervical spine of
a nurse involved in an automobile accident. Only six cervical
vertebrae are visualized because of the elevation of the shoulders.
B. One month postaccident, after essentially no treatment, there is
definite evidence of instability of C6 on C7. *C.* Skeletal traction
produced improvement in vertebral alignment.

be kept in mind that in children this density varies with inspiration and expiration. With inspiration the pharyngeal wall is close to the vertebra, while forced expiration produces a marked physiological increase in the size of the shadow. A child who is crying may displace the hyoid bone and larynx forward, which will increase the width of the shadow. Therefore, it is important in evaluating pediatric injuries to make sure that the child is not crying at the time the roentgenogram is made. This is often difficult, because children who are in pain secondary to the injury are frequently crying at the time of the examination.

A loss of the normal cervical lordotic curve is common with cervical spine injuries. It is felt that this posture is due to secondary reflex muscle spasm around the shoulder. It must be borne in mind, however, that a normal patient can obliterate the lordotic curve in the lateral view simply by depressing the chin. Therefore, the "poker" spine may be due not to reflex muscle spasm but to positioning of the chin during the roentgenographic examination.

A unilateral anterior interfacet dislocation of one vertebral body upon another will produce a 25 per cent anterior displacement of the one vertebral body upon the other, while a bilateral interfacet dislocation will produce a 50 per cent forward displacement of the one upon the other.

White and co-workers have demonstrated that a greater than 3.5 mm horizontal displacement of one vertebra upon another or a greater than 11 degree angulation of two adjacent vertebrae is direct evidence of instability.[84]

An avulsion-type injury with a small fleck of bone removed from the anterior superior aspect of a vertebral body may be indicative of a previous extension injury. A fragment off the anterior inferior portion of a vertebral body may indicate a teardrop type of injury with disruption of the posterior complex.

Finally, as I have stated previously, it is absolutely essential that all seven cervical vertebrae be visualized in the lateral projection.

Anteroposterior View. In this view the mid and lower cervical vertebrae are visualized for evidence of fracture within the vertebral body or in the lateral processes. Horizontal displacement in a lateral direc-tion is indicative of an unstable fracture-dislocation. The upper cervical vertebrae are usually not visualized in this view and a special open-mouth view is necessary.

Open-Mouth View. The open-mouth view, in which the atlas and the axis (including the odontoid process) can be visualized, is essential in evaluating all cervical spine injuries. A Jefferson fracture of the ring of the atlas may be evidenced by an overhang of the lateral masses of the atlas. There may also be unequal distances between one lateral mass of the axis and the odontoid and the opposite lateral mass and the odontoid. This disparity in the distances between the lateral masses and the odontoid may also be seen with rotary subluxation.

Odontoid fractures are evident in this view. There may or may not be associated displacement of the odontoid secondary to the fracture. The odontoid joins the neural arches and the body of the axis between the third and sixth years of age. Therefore, a radiolucency in the open-mouth view of a patient more than six years old probably represents an odontoid fracture.

Flexion-Extension Views. The range of vertebral body excursion in flexion and extension depends upon the age of the patient and the level considered. Vertebral body displacement is greater in children under the age of 10 years. In adults the range of forward motion of one vertebral body on the other usually progressively increases in degree from the level of the second cervical vertebra down to the C6 level, with the C6 and C7 levels demonstrating the least excursion. Offset of one vertebral body upon the other of 2 to 3 mm is within the normal range, particularly in degenerative disc disease. Excursion greater than 3.5 mm is indicative of instability. In children, however, excursion of the vertebral bodies up to 4 or 5 mm at the C2–C3 level is considered normal.

Oblique View. This view is obtained by having the patient in the supine position with the head held straight. The x-ray tube is placed in the horizontal plane with a 45 degree tilt toward the midline and centered over the midcervical area with a 5 degree cephalic angulation of the primary beam. The roentgenographic film is placed behind the neck and inclined 45 degrees so that the

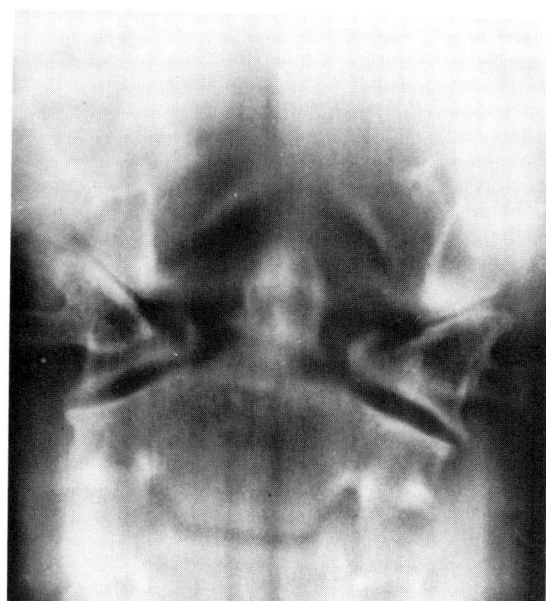

Figure 13–7 Tomogram of the upper cervical vertebra reveals a fracture at the base of the odontoid.

primary roentgenographic beam forms a 90 degree angle with it. The projection is repeated for the opposite side. The left posterior oblique projection visualizes the right pedicle. The right posterior oblique projection outlines the left pedicle.

Pillar View. The pillars are anatomical structures between the inferior and superior facets that may be fractured by hyperextension and rotation or other forces. Since the articular facets are angled about 35 degrees from the horizontal, the roentgenographic beam must be directed 35 degrees from the horizontal for proper visualization. This view is obtained with the patient supine. The central ray is centered over the mid-cervical area with a 35 degree cephalocaudal tilt. The head is rotated about 45 degrees to the right to visualize the left articular pillars. A similar view is taken of the right pillars with the head rotated to the left. If the patient cannot rotate his head, the exposure may be obtained with a 35 degree cephalocaudal angulation of the roentgenographic beam. This will demonstrate both pillars simultaneously in the midcervical area.

Tomograms. If there is a suggestion of a fracture of the odontoid, articular facets, pedicles, or lamina, tomograms may be helpful in making a definitive diagnosis (Fig. 13–7). These views should be obtained for all patients who are suspected of having a fracture that is not definitely demonstrable with routine views. The tomogram provides the physician with varying depth of cut of the roentgenographic beam, and with it, incomplete fractures may be visualized.

ADDITIONAL DIAGNOSTIC STUDIES

Queckenstedt Test

This controversial procedure has definite proponents and opponents. It is not to be considered routine in the evaluation of all cervical injuries. Some surgeons employ the Queckenstedt test to determine whether surgical exploration is indicated for a patient who has an acute spinal injury with the presence of a spinal manometric block. Patients with complete spinal cord injury do not always have complete blocks, however, and patients with incomplete syndromes may not have normal cerebrospinal fluid dynamics. The Queckenstedt test is used to determine the flow of spinal fluid in the subarachnoid space at the area of the cord injury. The patient is placed on his side, a spinal puncture is performed with an 18 gauge spinal needle in the lumbar area, and cerebrospinal fluid pressure is determined. A Valsalva maneuver will cause a pressure rise secondary to an increase in abdominal venous pressure. The pressure recorded in the manometer should rise and fall with the heartbeat. Pressure is then applied to both jugular veins, obstructing venous outflow from the brain. The normal response is a rapid rise in cerebrospinal fluid pressure in the lumbar manometer; failure of the pressure to rise indicates a block in the cerebrospinal fluid channels between the ventricles and the puncture site. As mentioned previously, the Queckenstedt test has limited usefulness in the routine evaluation of cervical spine injuries.

Myelography

Myelography is not a routine part of the evaluation of a patient with cervical injury. The only possible indication for a myelogram is the failure of a patient with an incomplete lesion to demonstrate progressive improvement and in whom there may be signs of external pressure on the spinal cord from an osseous fragment.

MECHANISMS OF INJURY

Controversy does exist about the exact mechanisms of injury that produce fractures of the spine, and many excellent reviews have attempted to classify these injuries on the basis of their mechanisms. It is important to have a thorough understanding of the forces involved if a rational approach is to be found for a classification and mode of treatment.

Pure Flexion

In this type of injury the flexion force is dissipated through compression of the cancellous portion of the vertebral body. In general we know that bone fails in tension. This is the sort of situation that exists with this type of injury. With extreme flexion, were the force not dissipated by the compression mechanism, it is conceivable that the posterior ligament complex would fail through a tension mechanism. In the usual flexion-type injury in the cervical spine, however, the energy is dissipated with the production of a flexion compression deformity of the anterior portion of the vertebral body. In general, the posterior ligament complex remains intact. This injury is not associated with a neurological deficit, as the spinal cord is not injured. The spine remains stable.

Flexion-Rotation

This type of injury results when a rotatory component is combined with flexion (Fig. 13–8). The combination of the two forces results in a more serious injury than does a pure flexion force. The rotation component disrupts the posterior ligament complex, producing an unstable spine. The capsule of the facet joint may be disrupted, producing a unilateral dislocation of the facet joint, or both facet joints may be dislocated, producing anterior displacement of the vertebrae of 50 per cent or more on the corresponding

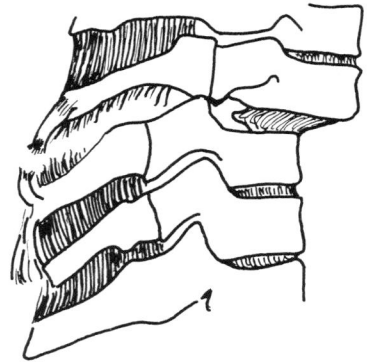

Figure 13–8 Flexion-rotation injury with disruption of the posterior ligamentous complex. (Courtesy of F. W. Holdsworth and Journal of Bone and Joint Surgery. Fractures, dislocations, and fracture-dislocations of the spine J. B. J. S., 45B:6–20, 1963.)

lower vertebrae. Fractures may occur through the facet joints, pedicle, lamina, or vertebral body. Schneider coined the term "teardrop" fracture to describe this type of injury (Fig. 13–9).[63] He chose this term because of the characteristic roentgenographic picture of a fracture of the anterior inferior portion of the vertebral body. There may or may not be posterior displacement of the remainder of the body into the spinal canal, and there is frequently neurological deficit produced, with a sad result.

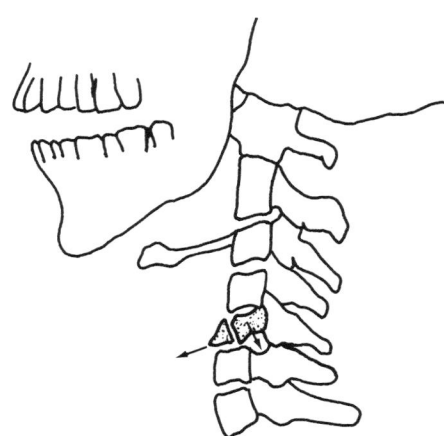

Figure 13–9 "Tear-drop" fracture–dislocation. (Courtesy of R. C. Schneider and E. A. Kahn and Journal of Bone and Joint Surgery. Chronic neurological sequelae of acute trauma to the spine and spinal cord. Part I. The significance of the acute flexion or "tear-drop" fracture-dislocation of the cervical spine. J. B. J. S., 38A:985–997, 1956.)

Flexion–Axial Load

A combination of flexion and axial load forces may produce incomplete disruption of the posterior ligamentous complex. The importance of this injury is that it may also be unstable.

Axial Load

Axial loading of the spine is not an uncommon source of injury. It occurs in any type of accident in which the top of the head strikes a firm object, producing an axial load without a flexion component. Typically, this injury occurs in diving accidents or automobile accidents. The axial load is transmitted to and produces a fracture through the central portion of the vertebral body with an anterior displacement of the anterior portion of the vertebral body and a posterior displacement of the posterior portion of the body. The posterior ligamentous complex remains intact. There may be a neurological deficit secondary to the posterior displacement of the vertebral body into the spinal canal. The typical roentgenographic picture is that of a "burst" fracture of the vertebral body.

Extension

In a pure extension injury the posterior ligamentous complex remains intact. The force may produce disruption of the anterior longitudinal ligament that may or may not be associated with an avulsion fracture from the anterior superior portion of the vertebral body. Usually there is no neurological deficit. In an arthritic spine, however, occasionally a fracture will not be produced by this injury but a neurological deficit will be present. Here the injury is due to osteophyte formation with infolding of the ligamentum flavum and narrowing of the spinal canal. The sudden hyperextension may then injure the spinal cord through a "pinching" mechanism. The posterior elements are usually not fractured, as they tend to abut with this type of injury, which tends to dissipate the force involved (Fig. 13–10).

Extension–Axial Load

An axial load added to hyperextension force may well produce disruption of the posterior elements along with an avulsion fracture of the anterior superior portion of the vertebral body. This injury is unstable and requires appropriate treatment. The axial force loads the posterior elements beyond their capacity and they fail.

Lateral Bending

This injury is produced by forced lateral bending of the cervical spinal column. The abnormal loading of the lateral masses may produce a fracture through the pedicles or facet joints. It is unusual for this type of injury to affect the spinal cord, but it may produce a peripheral nerve entrapment syndrome. These are considered stable injuries.

CLASSIFICATION OF CERVICAL INJURY – SPINAL STABILITY

If we keep in mind the foregoing mechanisms, it is possible to evolve a working

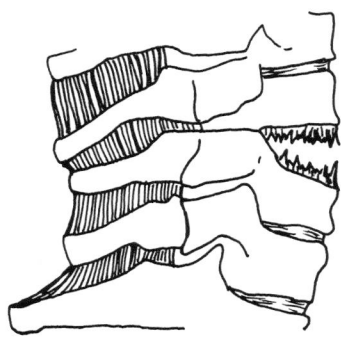

Figure 13–10 Diagramatic representation of an extension injury of the cervical spine revealing that the posterior element complex is intact. (Courtesy of F. W. Holdsworth, and Journal of Bone and Joint Surgery. Fractures, dislocations, and fracture-dislocations of the spine. J.B.J.S., 45B:6–20, 1963.)

TABLE 13–1 Cervical Spine Stability

Stable Injuries
  Flexion
  Extension
  Axial loading
  Lateral bending

Unstable Injuries
  Flexion–axial loading
  Flexion–rotation
  Extension–axial loading

classification of these injuries into those that are stable and those that are unstable. This becomes extremely important, as the methods of treatment are obviously different. The stable injury requires conservative treatment, while the unstable injury requires a more aggressive approach. The injuries that may be considered stable are flexion, extension, axial loading, and lateral bending; the unstable injuries include flexion–axial loading, flexion-rotation, and extension–axial loading (Table 13–1).

White and co-workers have recently performed biomechanical tests on cadaver spines to evaluate spinal stability. They found that the spine should be considered unstable if (1) either all the anterior elements or all the posterior elements are destroyed or unable to function; (2) there is more than 3.5 mm horizontal displacement of one vertebra in relation to an adjacent vertebra, anteriorly or posteriorly, measured on resting lateral or flexion-extension roentgenograms of the spine; or (3) there is more than 11 degrees of rotational difference from either adjacent vertebra, measured on a resting lateral or flexion-extension roentgenogram. If instability as determined by the foregoing criteria is present, surgical fusion or another method to achieve stability should be seriously considered.

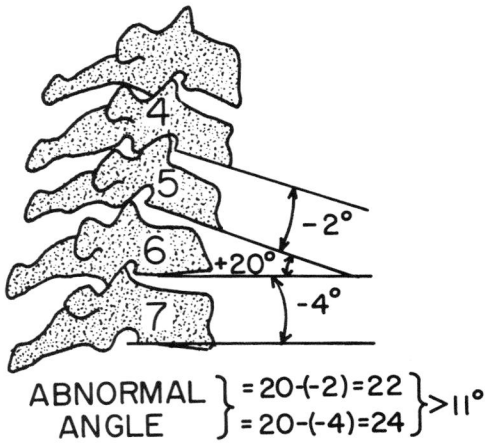

Figure 13–12 If there is more than 11 degrees of rotational difference from either adjacent vertebra, an unstable spine exists. (Courtesy of A. A. White, R. M. Johnson, M. D. Panjabi, and W. O. Southwick and *Clinical Orthopaedics and Related Research.* Biomechanical analysis of clinical stability of the cervical spine. Clin. Orthop., *109*:85–96, 1975.)

TREATMENT OF CERVICAL INJURIES

Skeletal Traction

All physicians dealing with the treatment of cervical injuries should have a thorough knowledge of the various devices for skeletal traction. In general there are four types available at the present time: three general types of tongs—the Vinke, the Crutchfield, and the Barton—and the recently developed halo skeletal traction device. This last has largely supplanted the various tongs. The author prefers the halo traction device because of its simplicity and ease of application. It was originally designed at Rancho Los Amigos, and extensive clinical application in that institution has demonstrated its particular value. It may be applied in the emergency room with local anesthesia. The device consists of a circular metal structure in the form of a halo that surrounds the skull and is attached to it by four heavy threaded pins extending from the halo into the outer table of the skull (Fig. 13–13). It is customary to insert two pins through the anterior portion of the halo and two pins through the posterior portion. The ring of the halo is commercially available in several sizes, and a universal halo that can be adjusted to the size of the patient is also available.

Only the surgeon and an assistant are

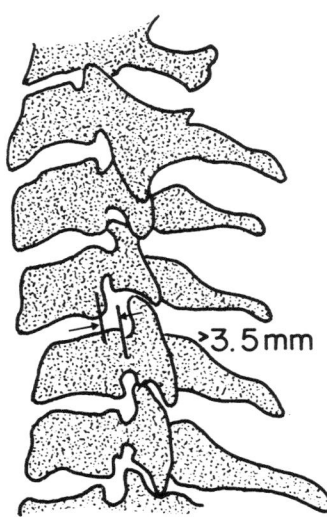

Figure 13–11 If more than 3.5 mm horizontal displacement is present, an unstable spine exists. (Courtesy of A. A. White, R. M. Johnson, M. D. Panjabi, and W. O. Southwick and *Clinical Orthopaedics and Related Research.* Biomechanical analysis of clinical stability of the cervical spine, Clin. Orthop., *109*:85–96, 1975.)

Figure 13–13 A. Anteroposterior view of a patient in a halo–body jacket device. Note that the halo is attached to an overhead outrigger that is then attached to a body jacket. *B.* Lateral view of the halo demonstrating the outrigger device and the body jacket.

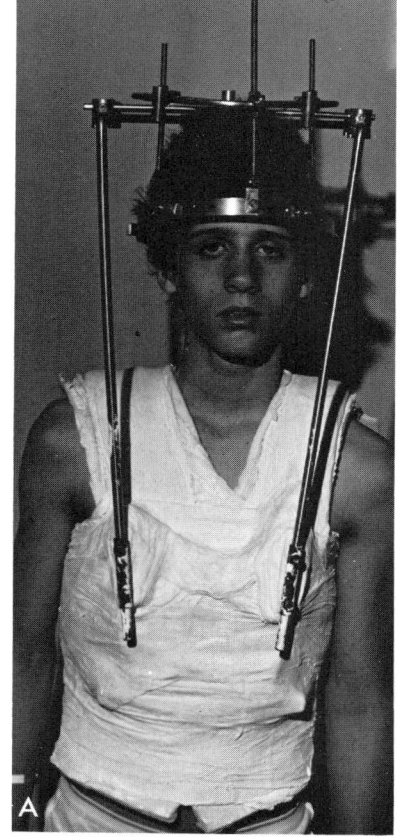
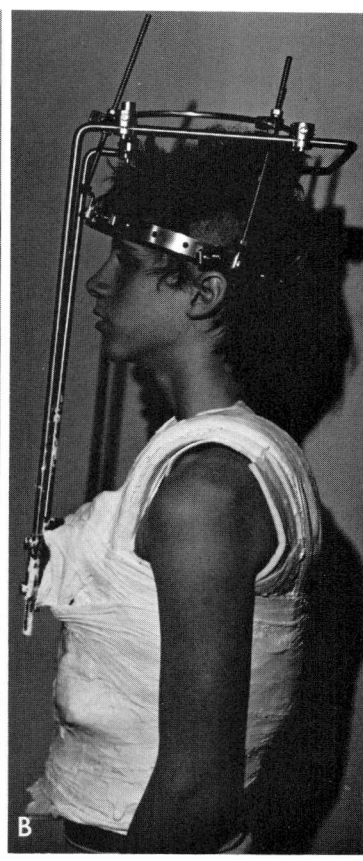

required for the application of the halo. The patient is maintained in the supine position on the stretcher, the head supported at the end of the stretcher by the assistant. The ring of the halo is approximated over the skull to determine the position of the skull pins. The placement of the ring portion of the device is extremely important; it must be just above the level of the eyebrows and pass posteriorly just above the level of the tips of the earlobes. If the halo is not applied in this low position, the skull pins do not gain purchase in the greatest diameter of the skull and there is danger that the device will pull out. There is some controversy over whether the hair should be shaved in the vicinity of the skull pins. The author feels that the hair should be removed locally around the site of insertion of the pins. The skin is properly cleansed with a Betadine solution, and is then infiltrated with 1 per cent lidocaine (Xylocaine) solution at all four sites of insertion of the pins. It is important to infiltrate the local anes-

thetic down to the outer table of the skull. The two anterior and two posterior skull pins are then advanced through the appropriate holes in the ring of the halo, through the skin, and into the outer table of the skull. It is not necessary to provide an opening in the skin for insertion of the pins, as they are tapered at the ends and can easily be inserted without a skin incision. The opposite pins are then tightened simultaneously to insure proper tension between anterior and posterior. A specifically designed torque screwdriver is available commercially for insertion of the skull pins. This is a very important aspect of the procedure. The pins are tightened to a maximum torque of 5 lb of resistance. It has been adequately demonstrated that with this degree of torque the sharp portion of the pin perforates the outer table of the skull, but the broad shoulder of the tip prevents migration of the pin through the outer table. These four pins provide adequate fixation through their tips anchored in the outer table. Locknuts are then applied over the skull pins to fasten them securely to the ring of the halo device.[50]

Thereafter, the pins are tightened with the torque screwdriver to a maximum of 5 lb resistance daily for one week. This may be performed regularly during ward rounds. The screwdriver and the wrench for tightening the locknuts are kept on the ward with the patient. The halo device allows for application of heavy skeletal traction if necessary to reduce fractures and dislocations. The author has applied 60 lb of skeletal traction for a short time without experiencing any difficulty in regard to fixation of the device, and the patients also tolerated the heavy skeletal traction very well. The pin sites are treated with Betadine solution daily.

It is extremely important to observe eye movement daily following insertion of the halo device. If excessive distraction forces are applied, an abducens nerve palsy may result. This will produce nystagmus, and extraocular motion will not be symmetrical. If this physical abnormality is evident, the traction force on the halo device should be diminished.

In general there is very little skin reaction around the skull pins over the extended time interval required for treatment of these injuries, but the pins can be repositioned around the ring of the halo if necessary. If a local skin infection develops at the site of one pin, that pin should be removed and placed in another position along the ring of the halo. In general, this problem may be alleviated by the local application of Betadine solution around the pins.

If it is determined that the treatment program requires the patient to remain supine in bed, a special device is available to place under the halo in order to insure that the posterior part of the ring remains

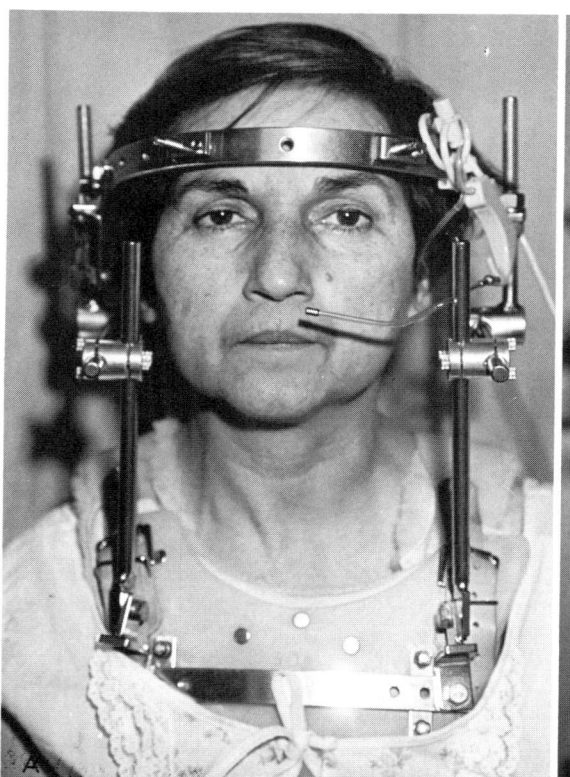
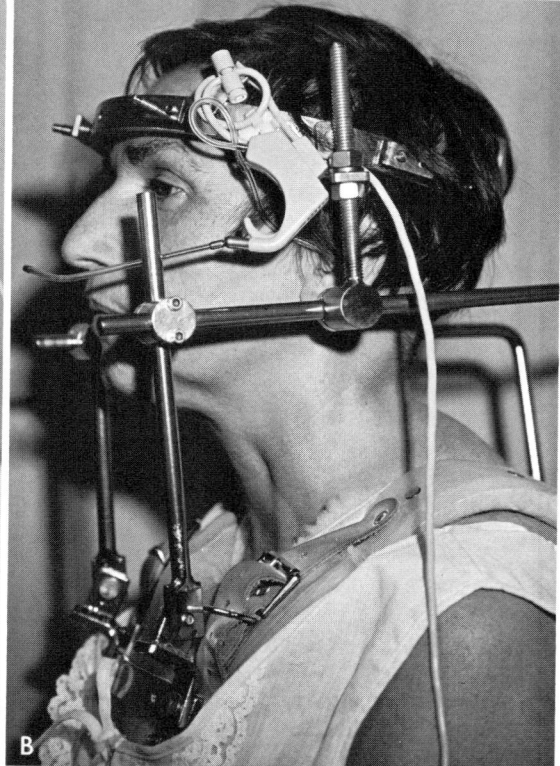

Figure 13–14 A. Anteroposterior view of patient in a "low-profile" halo with a plastic body jacket. The ring of the halo is situated just above the eyebrows for maximum purchase on the skull. Note also the telephone transmitter receiver that this patient had placed on the ring of the halo, as she was a telephone operator. B. Lateral view of the "low-profile" halo revealing the level of the halo ring just above the eyebrows and just above the tip of the ear. The metal uprights connect the halo to the plastic body jacket.

free of the bed, allowing uninterrupted longitudinal traction. This has been referred to as the cranial halo. The patients are usually maintained on a Stryker frame, and the traction rope is passed through the small hole at the head of the frame.

If it is determined that the fracture or dislocation can be treated while the patient is ambulatory, the halo device can be attached to a body jacket. This will allow for uninterrupted skeletal traction while allowing the patient to be freely mobile and out of bed. In general, two types of body jackets are available. The first is a standard plaster body jacket carefully molded over the iliac crest to allow secure fixation. The plaster is extended to the pubic area and halfway to the greater trochanter along the lateral aspects. The halo is then secured to the plaster jacket through an outrigger overhead attachment. Roentgenograms are obtained immediately following application of this device. It is important to obtain adequate reduction of the fracture or dislocation following attachment of the outrigger, which occasionally requires minor adjustments to maintain proper alignment.

The second type of body jacket is of molded plastic and consists of two form-fitted portions—an anterior and a posterior—that are joined by means of Velcro straps and buckles (Fig. 13–14). The advantage of this type of body jacket is that the plastic can be heavily lined with a thick sheepskin type of material that will prevent bedsores in paralytic patients. It also has the advantage of being very light compared with a regular plaster body jacket. The plastic body jacket is attached to the halo device through an external outrigger apparatus. A new low-profile halo has been designed for use with this type of body jacket and virtually eliminates the large overhead outrigger. The danger in utilizing this type of device is that it can be removed at will. Therefore, the plastic body jacket should only be applied to a very trustworthy patient who will tolerate this type of external fixation and will not remove it.

As stated previously, the halo external fixation device has largely replaced the various types of skull tongs for treatment of cervical fractures and dislocations. The ease of application, minimal complications, and significant advantage of mobilization of the patient have been a real step forward in the treatment of these injuries.

Spinal Fusion for Atlantoaxial Instability

The three commonest clinical indications for cervical spinal fusion are a deficient odontoid process, a deficient transverse and alar ligament complex, and a rotatory fixation of the atlas on the axis. Fielding and co-workers have recently outlined the technique of spinal fusion for atlantoaxial instability. A Gallie-type fusion of the first and second cervical segments is preferred. The patient is positioned on the operating table prone with his head resting in a cerebellar headrest. If he is already in a halo-cast device, he is maintained in this device intraoperatively and postoperatively. A midline incision is utilized. The dissection proceeds down to the posterior bifid spine of the axis. Blunt finger palpation will identify the posterior tubercle of the atlas. The spinous process and the laminae of the axis are then decorticated. The arch of the atlas is exposed through a longitudinal incision over the posterior tubercle of the first cervical segment with transverse incisions to each side of the midline. Extreme caution must be exercised not to carry exposure further than 1.5 cm laterally from the midline in adults and 1 cm in children so that damage to the vertebral artery may be avoided. Attention is then focused on the posterior arch of the atlas. The anterior portion of this segment is dissected free of periosteum so that a loop of 22 gauge wire may be passed through this area. The wire is passed from below upward under the arch, usually with the aid of a silk suture. A large cortical graft is then removed from the iliac crest and is notched in its inferior portion to conform to the contour of the spine of the second cervical segment, straddle this segment, and extend across the posterior arch of the first cervical vertebra. The 22 gauge wire is then brought over the graft and through the spinous process of the second cervical vertebra. Strips of cancellous bone graft are placed around the exposed area. Several arrangements of the wire holding the graft in place have been advocated. In the commonest and most popular method, the wire extends under the

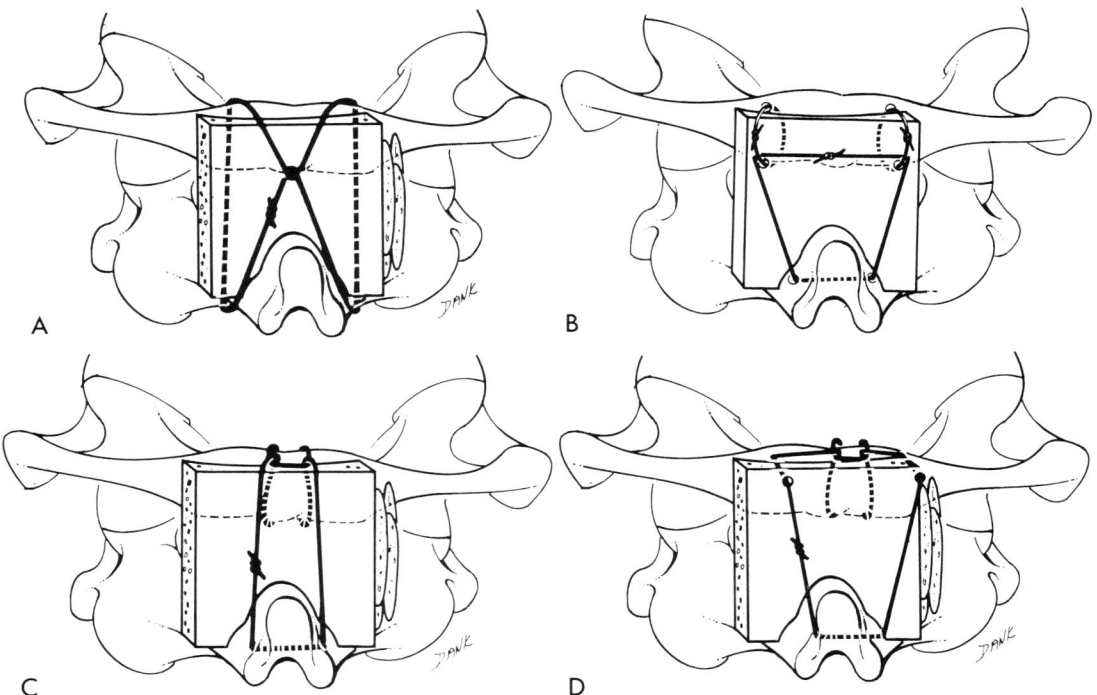

Figure 13–15 *A.* The wire passes under the lamina of the atlas and axis and is tied over the graft. *B.* The wire passes through drill holes in the lamina of the atlas and through the spine of the axis; holes are drilled through the graft. *C.* Wire passes under the lamina of the atlas and through the spine of the axis, and is tied over the graft. *D.* Wire passes under the lamina of the atlas and through the spine of the axis; holes are drilled through the graft. (Courtesy of J. W. Fielding, R. J. Hawkins, and S. A. Ratzan and *Journal of Bone and Joint Surgery.* Spine fusion for atlanto-axial instability, J. B. J. S., 58A:400–407, 1976.)

arch of the first cervical vertebra, passing over the graft itself, and then extends through the spine of the second cervical vertebra (Fig. 13–15). The various wire arrangements are depicted in Fielding's illustrations.[30]

The patient is kept in the halo-cast immobilization apparatus postoperatively or, alternatively, is placed in a Minerva jacket within one to two weeks postoperatively. During the interim, sandbags may be used to provide immobilization. If skeletal traction is not employed, however, a semi-rigid type of collar similar to the Philadelphia collar should be used prior to application of the Minerva jacket. If a halo device has been utilized the patient is maintained in the halo for 12 weeks postoperatively before progressing to a Philadelphia-type collar. If a Minerva jacket has been the initial form of postoperative treatment, the jacket is removed at three months and the patient wears a collar or brace for an additional six to eight weeks.

The fusion should be extended up to the posterior aspect of the occiput if there is a deficiency in a portion of the posterior arch of the atlas. In this situation, there will be insufficient fixation for the wire loop holding the bone graft; hence the fusion must be extended to the occiput. If it is felt that immediate relative stability is required, a wire loop may be positioned between the spinous process of the second cervical vertebra extending up through two drill holes at the base of the occiput and back down to the spinous process of C2 (Fig. 13–16). Bone graft is then placed along the lateral gutters. This type of fixation occasionally must be employed in a patient with Morquio's syndrome in whom the odontoid is deficient or absent and the posterior arch of the atlas is deficient (Fig. 13–17).

Anterior versus Posterior Cervical Fusion

Posterior cervical fusion is the treatment of choice for cervical spine injuries when fusion is felt to be necessary, usually

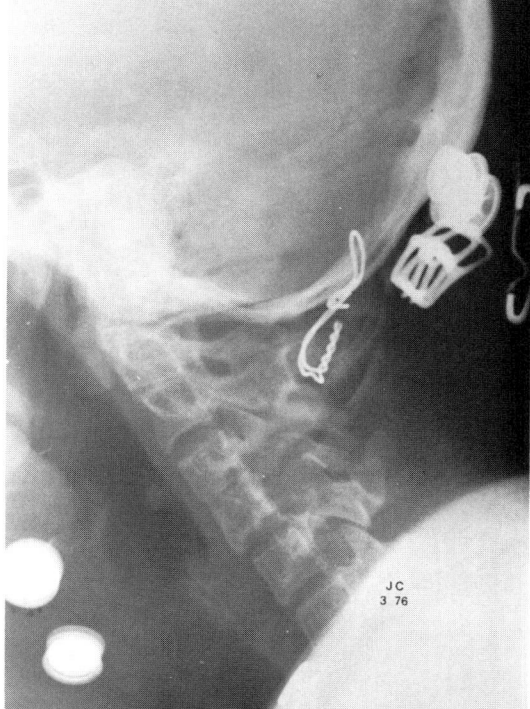

Figure 13–16 Lateral roentgenogram of a patient requiring fusion of the occiput to C2. It shows the proper position of the wire passing through the base of the skull and the spinous process of C2.

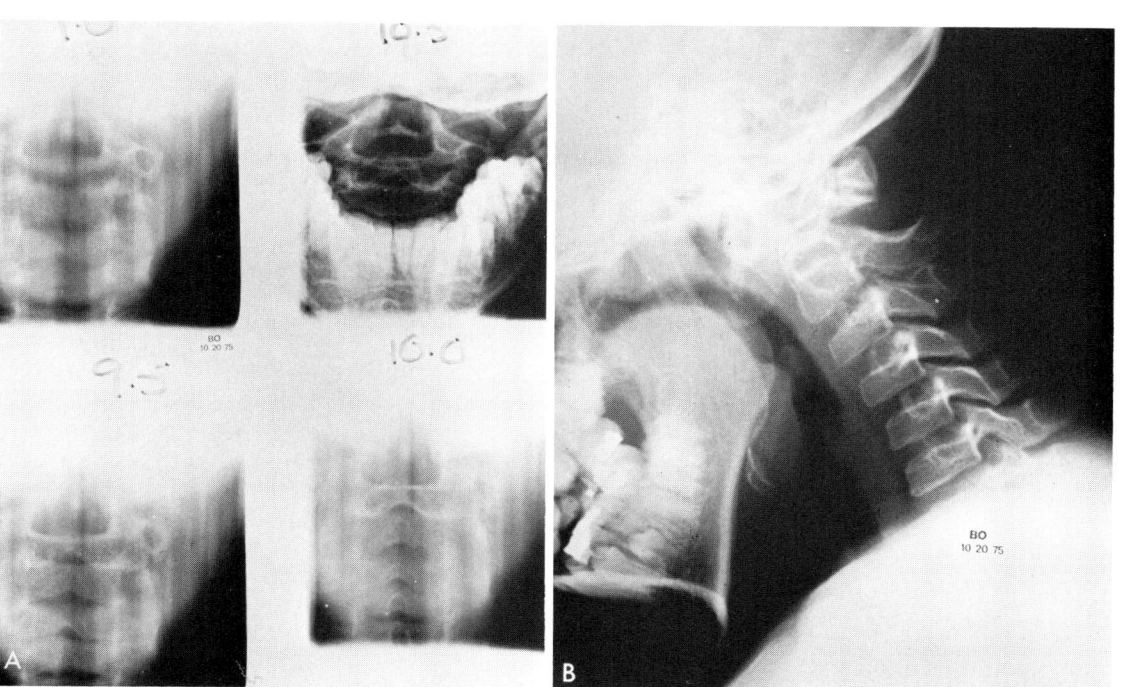

Figure 13–17 *A.* Tomograms of a patient with Morquio's disease with absence of the odontoid process. *B.* Lateral roentgenogram of the same patient. This patient required a posterior cervical fusion of C1 to C2.

because of injury to the posterior element complex. The only remaining stability in these injuries is derived from the anterior longitudinal ligament. It does not make sense to the author to attempt an anterior fusion that will destroy these last remaining elements. Several recent studies on the effect of early anterior cervical fusions have not produced completely satisfactory results. Clawson and co-workers found that anterior cervical fusions for cervical spine wedge and burst deformities did not prevent angulation.[18] Stauffer and Kelly reviewed 16 patients with fracture-dislocations of the cervical spine treated by the anterior dowel interbody fusion method. All had postoperative instability with recurrence of angular deformity, and all 16 were shown to have disruption of the posterior ligaments.[73] These investigators concluded that anterior fusion should not be performed as primary surgical treatment for fractures of the cervical spine when there is either evidence of disruption of the posterior ligaments or a strong presumption that such disruption exists.

One of the few primary indications for an anterior approach to cervical spine injuries involves trauma caused by an axial bursting mechanism. If a neurological deficit is present owing to posterior migration of the posterior portion of the vertebral body through a bursting mechanism and the patient presents with a progressing neurological deficit, then an anterior approach may be indicated. This would involve resection of the entire vertebral body to relieve the anterior compression on the spinal cord. Osseous strut grafts could then be inserted into the vertebral space and set into both the vertebra above and the one below to provide some stability. Fibular strut grafts appear to be ideal for this purpose. This is one of the very few primary indications for an anterior cervical fusion associated with a fracture of the cervical spine.

Role of Laminectomy

The only role for laminectomy in the treatment of spinal fractures and dislocations is in the presence of a progressing neurological deficit. Recognition of this has been one of the major advances made in the treatment of these injuries. In the past, laminectomies were performed with the idea that everything possible should be done to relieve pressure on the spinal cord and permit neurological recovery. This did not happen, however. Instead of helping the patients recover from the neurological deficit, the laminectomy not only did not provide for recovery of the neurological deficit but it further increased the instability of the spine. Many patients had to have further operative procedures in an attempt to obtain some stability of the spine at a later date. The author feels that, if a complete neurological deficit is present immediately following the accident, that is a definite contraindication for laminectomy. Osterholm and Mathews have provided us with a beautiful demonstration of the sequential changes within the spinal cord due to trauma. If there is a complete neurological deficit at the time of injury, then further hemorrhagic necrosis occurs within the cord and relief of external pressure on the cord does not improve the neurological picture.[53] Breig also has questioned the role of dentate ligament section to provide decompression of the spinal cord.[15]

FRACTURES AND DISLOCATIONS OF THE UPPER CERVICAL SPINE (Odontoid–C1–C2)

Occiput–C1 Dislocation

This is a relatively rare injury that is usually fatal. The mechanism of injury involves a severe rotational component, which produces gross ligamentous disruption between the occiput and C1. If the patients do survive, rigid immobilization is required because of the serious nature of the injury and the susceptibility of the spinal cord in this location. Since this is a grossly unstable injury with severe ligamentous disruption, skeletal traction is contraindicated. The halo device is probably the best type of fixation for this particular injury and, with accompanying body jacket, will allow secure fixation. Surgical stabilization through a posterior approach is definitely necessary and may be performed while the patient is in the halo device. The procedure involves early posterior bone grafting from the occiput down to C2.

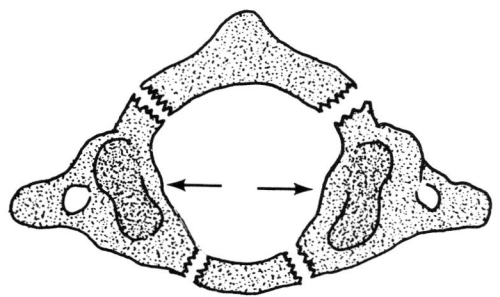

Figure 13–18 Diagramatic representation of a Jefferson fracture of the ring of the atlas.

Additional stabilization may be obtained through wires extending from the posterior aspect of C2 up through drill holes in the skull and back down to C2.

C1 Fracture (Jefferson's Fracture)

In 1920 Jefferson published a review of fractures of the atlas and discussed four personal cases that he had observed. This fracture occurs through the ring of the atlas (Fig. 13–18). The mechanism of injury is an axial load that is transmitted through the

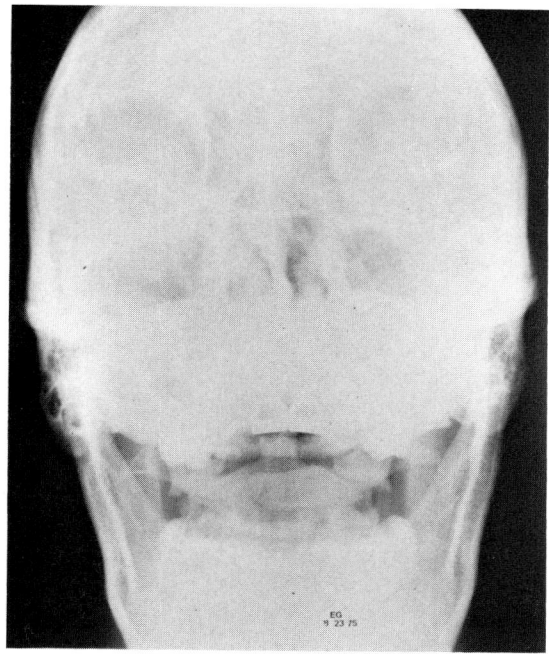

Figure 13–19 An anteroposterior open-mouth roentgenogram revealing the break in the ring of the atlas.

skull to the atlas, producing disruption of the atlantal ring. The fracture tends to occur in the thinnest and weakest point of the ring where the posterior arch joins the lateral masses (Fig. 13–19). It produces an explosion-type injury of the ring, and for this reason there is usually no neurological deficit, as the osseous fragments tend to migrate outward rather than impinging on the spinal cord. In the rare instance of neurological deficit, the injury is almost universally fatal owing to the level of the cord involved. The typical Jefferson fracture may be treated with the use of the halo device with accompanying body jacket. The halo device is maintained in position for a total of eight weeks. It is then removed and the patient is placed in a cervical brace (the author prefers the Philadelphia brace) for six to eight weeks. The brace is then removed and gentle flexion-extension roentgenograms are obtained; if no displacement is evident, bracing may be discontinued. The advantage of using the halo device for this fracture is that the patient can be mobile and can be discharged from hospital early in the treatment program and followed in the office at periodic intervals. An important point to remember in regard to these fractures is that approximately one third are associated with fractures of the axis. It is interesting that rupture of the vertebral artery rarely occurs with this type of fracture despite the close proximity of the structures.

Odontoid Fractures

Fractures of the odontoid continue to be a perplexing clinical problem. The exact mechanism of injury is still controversial. It is felt that this fracture does not result from simple shear or avulsion, but probably from a combination of several forces, with displacement of the odontoid occurring through a shearing force. The blood supply of the odontoid, which has been carefully defined by Schiff and Parke, is felt to be an important factor, as the incidence of nonunion of odontoid fractures continues to be relatively high.[60] It must also be borne in mind that fusion of the base and apex of the odontoid occurs by 12 years of age but osseous union is not complete until adult life. If the apex does not fuse to the body of

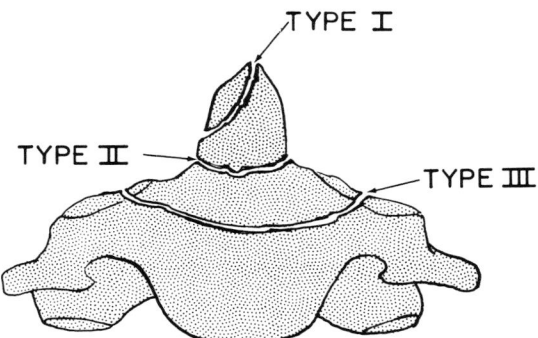

Figure 13-20 Anderson classification of odontoid fractures. Type 1, through the upper process proper; type 2, through the base of the odontoid, and type 3, extending downward into cancellous bone. (Courtesy of L. D. Anderson, and R. T. Alonzo and *Journal of Bone and Joint Surgery.* Fractures of the odontoid process of the axis. J.B.J.S., 56A:1663–1674, 1974).

the odontoid, an os odontoideum results. This is not to be confused with an acute fracture.

Following an excellent review at their institution, Anderson and Alonzo recently classified fractures of the odontoid (Fig. 13-20). A *type 1* odontoid fracture is an oblique fracture through the upper portion of the odontoid process itself and in all likelihood represents an avulsion fracture where the alar ligament attaches to the tip of the odontoid process. A *type 2* fracture occurs at the junction of the odontoid process with the body of the second cervical vertebra. A *type 3* fracture extends downward into the cancellous portion of the body and is really a fracture through the body of the axis.[4] This is an excellent classification and is useful in regard to management.

Neurological deficits occur in only approximately 5 per cent of odontoid fractures. The reason for the low percentage of neurological complications is probably related to Steel's rule of thirds, which correlates the amount of space available for spinal cord and odontoid process at this level: one third of the space is occupied by the odontoid process, one third is occupied by the spinal cord, and one third allows for displacement.[75] It is because of this anatomical configuration that neurological deficits are not frequently seen with this type of injury. The injury is, however, definitely unstable and if not properly treated may result in a severe neurological deficit.

The treatment of type 1 fractures of the odontoid follows a conservative route. A collar or brace may be used until the acute reaction from the fracture subsides. This particular fracture is located too high on the odontoid process to lead to instability of the first cervical vertebra on the second. Even if it progresses to nonunion, no particular problem should exist.

Treatment of type 2 fractures is much more controversial (Fig. 13-21). Schatzker and co-workers found that the incidence of nonunion was definitely linked to the displacement and the presence of a significant gap between the fracture surfaces. In experimental investigation on dogs as well as clinical evaluation in humans, they found that the incidence of nonunion with conservative treatment approached 64 per cent. They also noted that 60 per cent of the fractures treated by open operative fusion failed to unite, and that in 54 per cent of those treated by solid atlantoaxial fusion, the dens failed to unite.[58,59] This is not particularly significant, as once atlantoaxial fusion has been secured, a shearing motion of C1 on C2 cannot occur. Finding such a high incidence of nonunion of the odontoid fracture despite a solid C1 to C2 fusion does, however, bring out the high rate of nonunion of type 2 fractures. Anderson and Alonzo also found a high rate of nonunion with type 2 fractures — 36 per cent. They felt that primary fusion of C1 to C2 should be considered in these patients because of the frequency of nonunion when they are treated conservatively.[4] If primary fusion of C1 to C2 is elected, patients must be informed that they will lose 10 to 15 per cent of rotation. If the occiput is included in the fusion, an additional loss of 30 per cent of flexion-extension will result. The author has continued to treat this type of injury conservatively with a halo incorporated in a body jacket, allowing for early mobilization of the patient. If at the end of five months there is no evidence of spontaneous healing of the odontoid fracture, then a C1 to C2 fusion is elected and the patients are maintained in the halo device. If an initial conservative treatment program is followed, however, the percentages of healing must be thoroughly explained to the patient as well as the ultimate necessity for surgical intervention if conservative treatment fails.

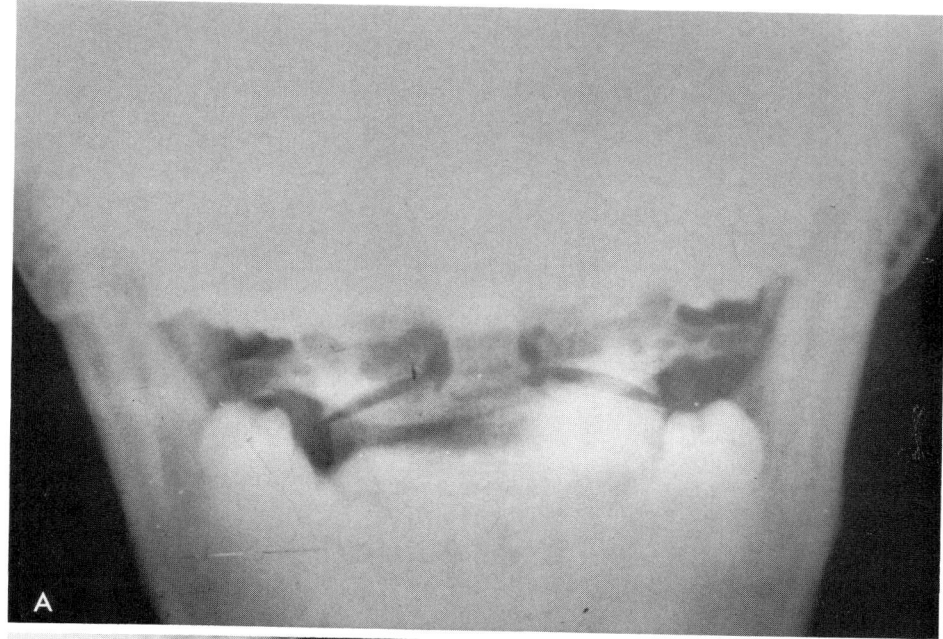

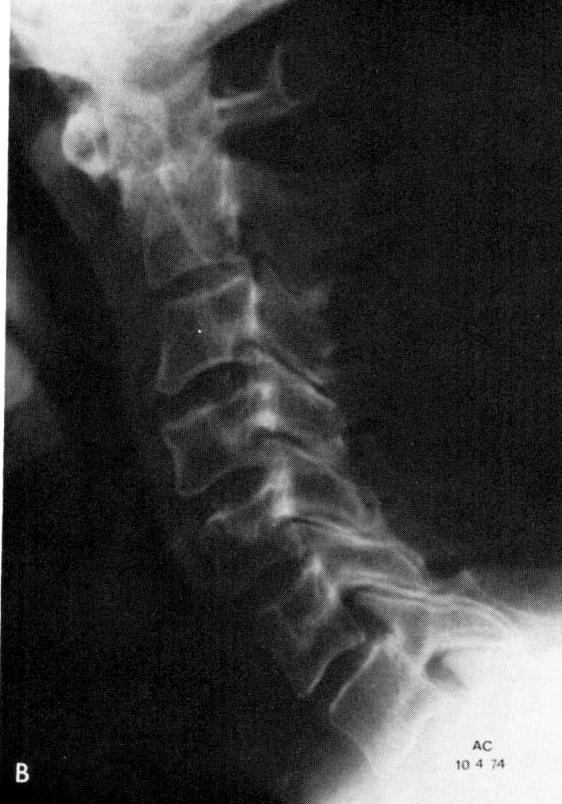

Figure 13–21 A. Open-mouth odontoid view revealing a Type 2 fracture. *B.* Lateral roentgenogram revealing forward displacement of C1 on C2 due to the odontoid fracture.

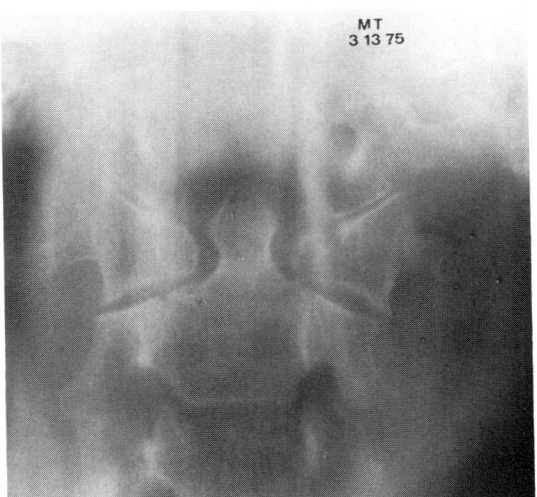

Figure 13–22. Tomogram of the upper cervical vertebra revealing a type 3 odontoid fracture through the cancellous portion of the body of C2.

The particular types of posterior cervical fusion are discussed elsewhere in this chapter.

Type 3 odontoid fractures are treated conservatively. These fractures extend down into the cancellous portion of the body of C2 and provide an excellent surface for fracture healing (Fig. 13–22). They can therefore be treated in the halo–body cast type of fixation device until they are healed, which takes from three to five months. Primary posterior cervical fusion is not justified in this group because spontaneous union can be expected with conservative treatment.

Tears of the Transverse Ligament of the Atlas

Fielding and associates have provided us with excellent studies on this particular subject. The transverse ligaments are largely responsible for maintaining anterior stability of the first cervical vertebra in relation to the second. They are supported in this function by the alar and apical ligaments. The normal joint space between the odontoid process and the anterior arch of the atlas should not exceed 3 mm in adults in the presence of intact atlantoaxial ligaments. Flexion and extension do not significantly increase this distance if the ligamentous structures are intact. No corre-

lation has been found between ligament strength and age. The transverse ligament tends to rupture if displacement of 3 to 5 mm occurs between the odontoid process and the anterior arch of the atlas. If the transverse ligament ruptures, the alar ligament is usually inadequate to prevent further significant displacement of the first on the second cervical vertebra. It must be kept in mind that there is a serious risk of damage to the spinal cord if there is an anterior shift of the atlas with an intact normal odontoid process. This danger is decreased if the odontoid process is fractured and carried forward with the atlas. Surgical stabilization by posterior C1 to C2 fusion should be considered if there is evidence of a forward displacement of 5 mm of the atlas on the axis, particularly if the odontoid process is intact.[31]

Atlantoaxial Rotatory Fixation

With this type of problem there is frequently a delay in diagnosis. Patients present with torticollis and a diminished range of motion. They may or may not have facial flattening. The typical head position is 20 degrees of tilt to one side, 20 degrees of rotation to the opposite side, and slight flexion. This particular position has been compared to that of a robin listening for a worm and has been dubbed the "cock-robin position." Cervical extension is frequently diminished by 50 per cent. In an open-mouth anteroposterior roentgenographic projection the lateral mass of the axis that is rotated forward appears wider and closer to the midline while the opposite mass appears narrower and farther away from the midline (Fig. 13–23). If the spinous process of the axis (which is the best indicator of axial rotation) is tilting in one direction and rotated in the opposite direction, rotatory fixation or torticollis is present and usually the chin and spinous process are on the same side of the midline. The most useful procedure to demonstrate atlantoaxial rotatory fixation, however, is cineroentgenography in the lateral projection. This particular procedure demonstrates that the posterior arches of the atlas and axis move as a unit during attempted neck rotation. Normally the atlas clearly rotates independently on the relatively immobile axis. The

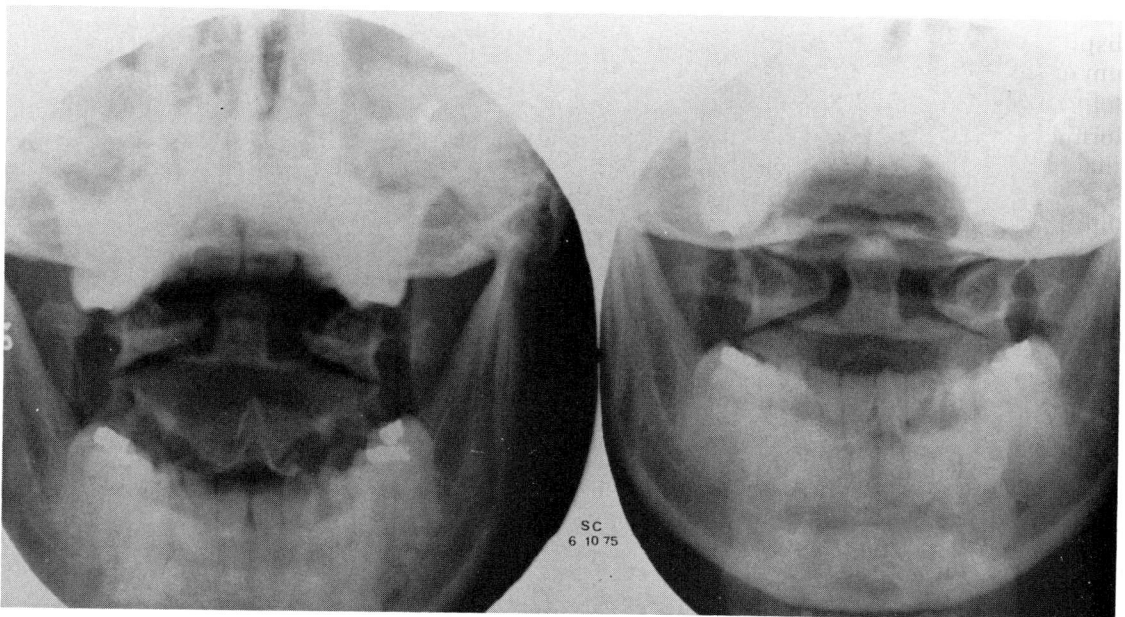

Figure 13–23   An open-mouth view revealing evidence of rotatory fixation with definite increase in distance between the odontoid process and the ring of the atlas on one side.

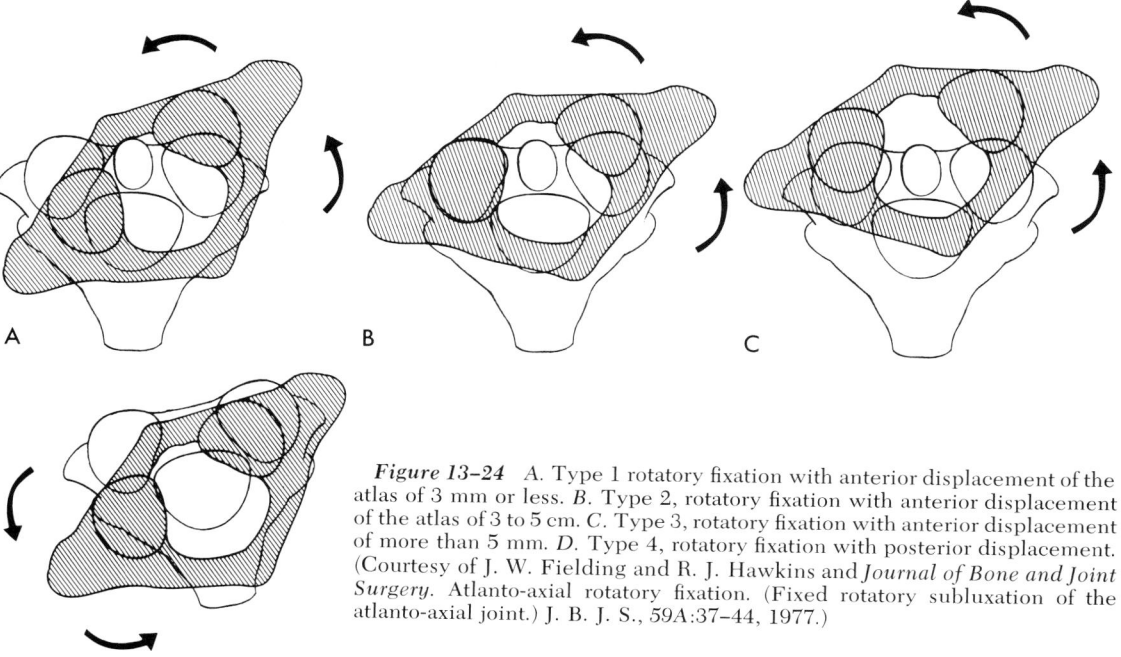

Figure 13–24   A. Type 1 rotatory fixation with anterior displacement of the atlas of 3 mm or less. *B.* Type 2, rotatory fixation with anterior displacement of the atlas of 3 to 5 cm. *C.* Type 3, rotatory fixation with anterior displacement of more than 5 mm. *D.* Type 4, rotatory fixation with posterior displacement. (Courtesy of J. W. Fielding and R. J. Hawkins and *Journal of Bone and Joint Surgery.* Atlanto-axial rotatory fixation. (Fixed rotatory subluxation of the atlanto-axial joint.) J. B. J. S., 59A:37–44, 1977.)

importance of recognizing this entity is that it may indicate a compromised atlantoaxial complex with the potential to cause neural damage or death.

Fielding and Hawkins classified four distinct types of this entity (Fig. 13–24). *Type 1* is rotatory fixation without anterior displacement of the atlas (displacement of 3 mm or less). This is the commonest type of deformity. The fixed rotation is within the normal range of atlantoaxial rotation with an intact transverse ligament, so the dens acts as a pivot. *Type 2* is rotatory fixation with anterior displacment of the atlas of 3 to 5 mm. This is the second most common lesion. It is associated with a deficiency of the transverse ligament and unilateral anterior displacement of one lateral mass of the atlas while the opposite, intact, joint acts as the pivot. These patients present with an abnormal anterior displacement of the atlas on the axis and an amount of fixed rotation in excess of normal maximum rotation. *Type 3* is rotatory fixation with anterior displacement of more than 5 mm. In this type a deficiency exists in both the transverse and secondary ligaments. Both lateral masses of the atlas are displaced anteriorly, one more than the other, producing the rotated position. *Type 4* is rotatory fixation with posterior displacement. This is the rarest lesion. Fielding and Hawkins found one patient with a deficient dens that allowed posterior shift of one or both lateral masses of the atlas, one of them shifting more than the other so that the atlas was rotated on the axis.[29]

Prognostically, type I is the most benign because the transverse ligament is intact and patients with this lesion can be treated more or less expectantly.

Type 2, with a deficient transverse ligament, is potentially dangerous. Types 3 and 4 are extremely rare fortunately, as they have a catastrophic potential.

The exact etiology of this condition remains obscure. It was Fielding and Hawkins' belief that reduction was probably obstructed in the early stages by swollen capsular and synovial tissues and by associated muscle spasm.

The characteristic clinical picture is that of a persistent torticollis that began spontaneously following trivial trauma or occurred after an upper respiratory tract infection. An important differentiating finding in spasmodic torticollis is that the shortened sternocleidomastoid muscle is the deforming force and is characteristically in spasm. In rotatory fixation the elongated sternocleidomastoid may be in spasm as if attempting to correct the deformity.

Treatment should be aggressive, particularly if anterior displacement is present along with rotatory fixation, since the atlantoaxial stability may be compromised and a catastrophic result may follow a minor neck injury. Skeletal skull traction has been advocated. The author prefers the halo traction device. Once the deformity has been corrected, the reduction must be maintained by immobilization in a device such as the halo or a Minerva jacket for approximately three months. Patients with long-standing fixation (longer than three months) are probably best treated by a C1 to C2 fusion. Manipulation of the fixed deformity is not recommended.

Hangman's Fracture (Neural Arch of the Axis)

This fracture occurs through the neural arch of the second cervical vertebra and has occasionally been referred to as traumatic spondylolisthesis of the axis. This lesion is similar to the one noted in judicial hanging, which lead Schneider and associates to coin the term, "hangman's fracture."[64] The results of use of the subaural knot for judicial hanging in Medieval times were unsatisfactory in terms of the purpose it was meant to serve. Instead of producing an acute fracture of the cervical spine with resulting neurological deficit not compatible with life, it was reported to cause death by asphyxiation. The submental knot, however, produced a characteristic fracture through the neural elements of the atlas through a mechanism of acute extension and distraction of the cervical spine. There was also acute displacement of the second on the third vertebral body with the characteristic resultant immediate cord deficit.

The usual mechanism of injury in the fractures seen in civilian practice today is extension and axial compression of the cervical spine. It characteristically occurs in automobile accidents in which the automobile turns over or the patient is thrown from

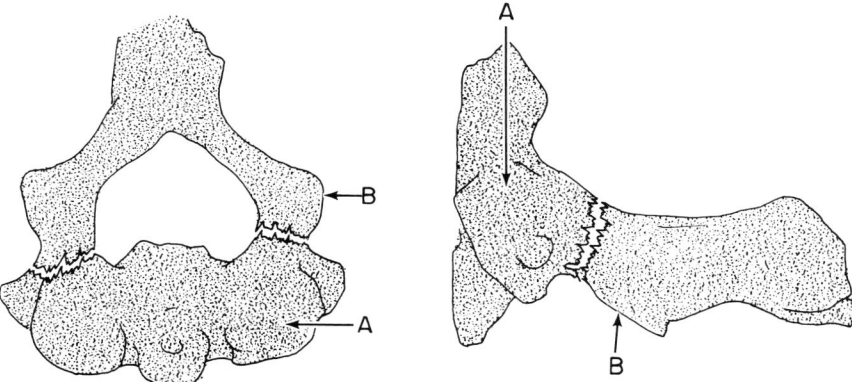

Figure 13-25 Hangman's fracture through the neural arch of the axis. Note in this diagram that the superior articular process (A) is situated anterior to the inferior articular process (B) on the right, a lateral diagramatic view revealing that the fracture separates the superior (A) from the inferior (B) articular process.

the vehicle. Anatomically the superior articular facets are well anterior to the inferior facets and a longitudinal axial compressive force may produce a shearing stress on the neural arch of the axis (Fig. 13-25). If the disc and anterior ligaments between C2 and C3 have been grossly disrupted by the force, the body of the axis will then displace in a position of flexion and forward subluxation on the body of the third cervical vertebra. A final but less common mechanism of injury is a flexion force associated with an axial compression fracture of the body of the third vertebra. The force will cause a collapse of the body of C3, which will effectively unload the anterior structures, shifting the force posteriorly to the facet area and creating a shear stress across the isthmus similar to that in hyperextension-compression injuries. This, however, is seen very infrequently and is added for completeness' sake. The commonest mechanism is the hyperextension-axial compressive force.

There is a surprising paucity of neurological findings in association with this injury. Significant spinal cord injury is usually not evident. Examination of these patients may reveal an abrasion or laceration across the forehead or chin, which is in keeping with the usual mechanisms of injury. Examination of the posterior structures reveals definite point tenderness along the spinous processes of C2 and C3. The injury is very difficult to visualize with an anteroposterior roentgenographic view but is easily visual-

ized in the lateral projection (Fig. 13-26). The atlantoaxial joint and the dens remain intact. Bilateral fractures of the neural arch of the axis are seen anterior to the inferior facets. The fracture pattern is an oblique line extending from superoposterior to in-

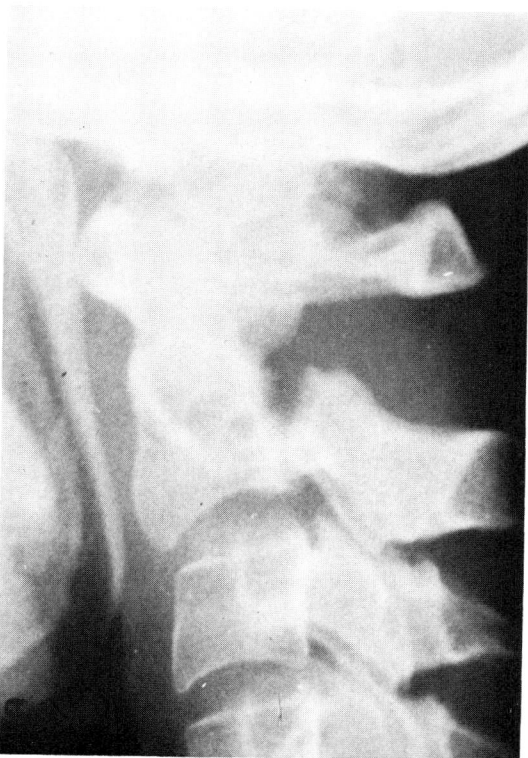

Figure 13-26 Lateral roentgenogram of a hangman's fracture.

feroanterior. There is usually evidence of forward displacement of C2 on C3. Occasionally an avulsion fracture of the anterior inferior margin of the axis or anterior superior margin of C3 will identify the site of rupture of the anterior longitudinal ligament. As with all significant cervical injuries, a retropharyngeal soft-tissue swelling is present roentgenographically. The fractures can also be well demonstrated through oblique roentgenographic views.

The treatment for this type of injury is a halo device and body jacket for six to eight weeks followed by a rigid cervical collar similar to the Philadelphia collar or a four-poster brace. Skeletal traction must be employed very carefully. Minimal traction is necessary to reduce the majority of these fractures but excessive skeletal traction is to be avoided, especially if there is evidence of anterior longitudinal rupture. Traction under these circumstances could conceivably distract the second from the third cervical vertebra and produce a lesion similar to the type seen in judicial hanging. Careful adjustment of the halo device may be necessary to reduce this fracture satisfactorily. Therefore, daily roentgenograms are indicated until satisfactory reduction has been obtained. It is difficult to justify posterior or anterior cervical fusion as an initial form of treatment for these injuries, as the majority will go on to spontaneous fusion of the neural arch fracture or C2 will spontaneously fuse to C3. It is for this reason that surgical fusion is not recommended unless nonunion develops across the fracture site. As stated, however, this is indeed rare.

FRACTURES OF THE LOWER CERVICAL VERTEBRAE (C3–C7)

Both motion and excursion are greater in the lower cervical spine than in the upper cervical spine. Approximately 80 degrees of flexion occurs in the mid and lower cervical spine, allowing the chin to approximate the chest. The greatest amount of mobility occurs from C4 through C7. While approximately 50 per cent of rotation occurs in the upper cervical segments, only 15 degrees of extension is present in that area, the remainder occurring in the lower cervical spine.

Although the increased mobility of the lower segments may compensate for increased loads on the cervical spine, fractures and dislocations with displacement of one cervical vertebra forward on the other occur when significant mechanical forces are applied.

Flexion Injuries

A flexion force in the lower cervical spine may result in a compression fracture of the vertebral body. The load is absorbed by the compression of the vertebral body, preventing formation of significant tension shearing force, and therefore the posterior elements remain intact. This type of fracture may be treated expectantly with a soft cervical collar or a more rigid collar similar to the Philadelphia collar. Patients frequently are more comfortable in the collar for four to six weeks. The collar can then be gradually removed for extended periods during the daytime.

Another type of injury that may result from acute muscle contraction force is avulsion of the spinous process of C7, commonly referred to as "clay shoveler's" fracture. This injury is due to an avulsion mechanism secondary to contracture of the paraspinal musculature. It was commonly encountered in patients who were employed as clay diggers. The clay would stick to the shovel, as the digger, with neck in extension, hoisted it above his shoulder, sudden contracture of the trapezius complex and the paraspinal ligaments would avulse the spinous process of C7. This injury may also result from a direct blow over the spinous process. In either event the treatment is conservative with a soft cervical collar for four to six weeks for comfort. If a fibrous union results and the patient has pain directly over the area, the small avulsed portion of the spinous process may be surgically excised for pain relief. Prior to surgical excision, however, it is customary to attempt to relieve the pain with local injections.

Facet Dislocations

If rotation is added to the flexion force, a more serious injury results. The capsule of the facet joint may be disrupted, producing a unilateral dislocation of the facet joint (jumped facet), or both facets may dislocate, producing anterior displacement of the vertebra of 50 per cent or more on the corresponding lower vertebra. Calcification of the anterior longitudinal ligament may occur at the point of rupture. A rough rule of thumb in regard to displacements and fractures or subluxations of the facets is that if 25 per cent forward displacement of the vertebra occurs, one can assume that a fracture or subluxation of one facet is present. If a 50 per cent forward displacement of one vertebral body on the vertebra below occurs, then one can assume that a bilateral facet dislocation is present.

It is important to remember the biomechanical studies performed by White and co-workers. They were able to demonstrate that any horizontal displacement greater than 3.5 mm of one vertebra in relationship to an adjacent vertebra anteriorly or posteriorly, measured on resting lateral or flexion-extension roentgenograms of the spine, indicated spinal instability. They further pointed out that more than 11 degrees of rotational difference from either adjacent vertebra, measured on a resting lateral or flexion-extension roentgenogram, was indicative of spinal instability.[84]

The unilateral facet dislocation is treated by application of a cranial halo and an attempt at closed reduction with increasing skeletal traction weight. It is best to begin with at least 15 to 20 lb of weight. This amount is increased sequentially if roentgenograms do not reveal satisfactory reduction of the dislocation. Occasionally, weights of up to 50 lb will be necessary to reduce the facet dislocation. The author feels that weights over 50 lb should not be used for this type of injury. If reduction is not obtained with weights up to 50 lb, consideration should be given to open reduction and internal fixation. It is dangerous and not a common practice in the United States to perform a closed reduction of the facet dislocation under general anesthesia. It is possible that a major neurological deficit could result from this type of manipulation. If the surgeon feels that closed reduction should be attempted prior to open reduction, then this is performed in the operating room with the patient under light anesthesia but awake. The maneuver consists of longitudinal traction with gentle flexion and extension manipulation. Even so, this is a risky procedure, and it is probably best to perform an open reduction under direct vision under these circumstances. If the unilateral facet dislocation can be reduced with longitudinal traction through the cranial halo, the patient is then kept in the halo for a total of 12 weeks with the neck in slight extension, allowing for healing of the posterior ligament complex. At the end of this time, if spontaneous ankylosis has not occurred and there is still evidence of instability, a posterior spinal fusion with internal wiring should be performed. In the event that an open reduction and internal fixation are required to treat this problem, a rigid collar may be worn postoperatively or the patient may continue in the halo and jacket device for two to three months.

Bilateral facet dislocations are more difficult to treat, as the ability to reduce them decreases with bilateral involvement. The initial treatment is the same as for a unilateral dislocation in that a cranial halo is immediately applied. Skeletal traction of 15 to 20 lb is initiated and increased in increments up to 50 lb in an attempt to reduce the bilateral facet dislocation. The author has found it best to treat these problems with early open reduction and internal wiring if there is no definite evidence of early reduction following this amount of skeletal traction. The rationale for this approach is that far less damage is done by definitive reduction under direct vision than by several manipulative attempts at reduction. These difficult problems are best managed through a posterior approach. Once the dislocation has been openly reduced, the spinous process of the involved vertebra and the vertebra below are wired together to provide some stability. Bone graft is utilized to stimulate early fusion of these segments.

Braakman and Vinken have adequately demonstrated that if the dislocation is less than six weeks old, open reduction and internal fixation with application of a bone graft is the treatment of choice. If an interval greater than six weeks has passed from the date of the accident, however, it is probably best to treat these injuries with fusion in situ.[13]

Teardrop Fracture. In 1956 Schneider and Kahn described a characteristic type of

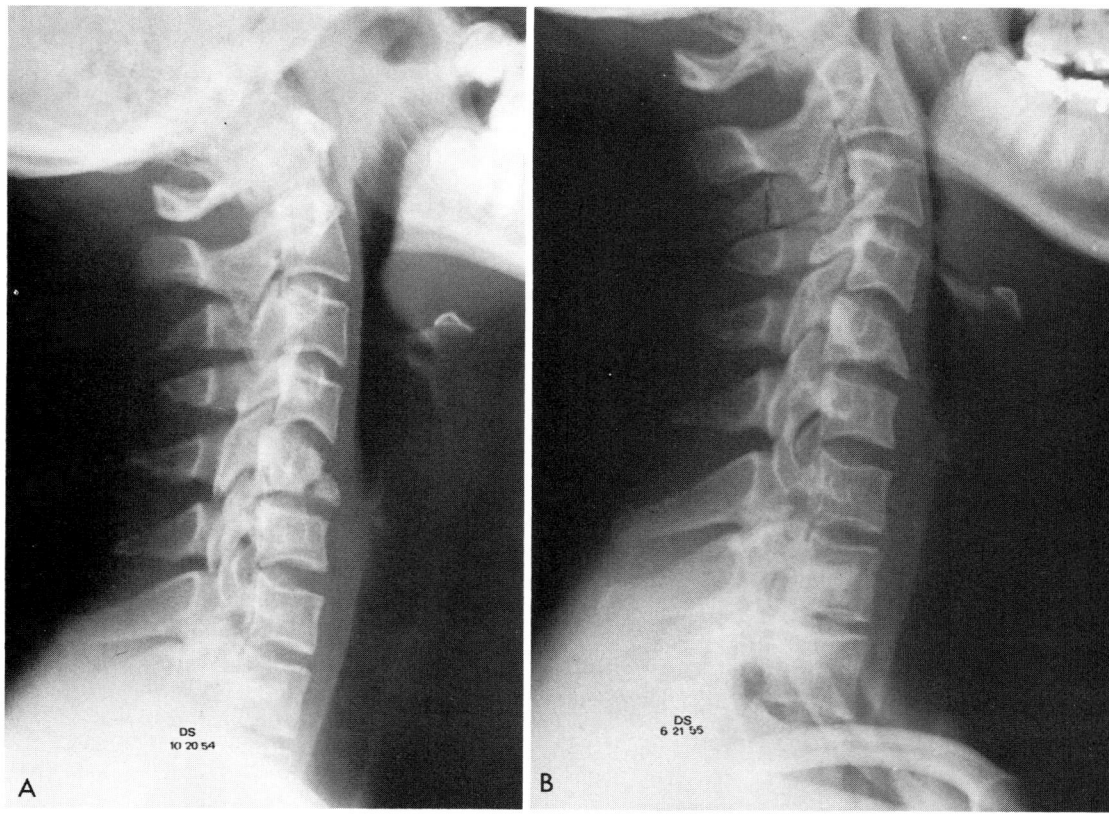

Figure 13–27 Lateral roentgenogram demonstrating a "teardrop" fracture of C5. *B.* Healed teardrop fracture following treatment by skeletal traction.

fracture-dislocation of the lower cervical spine due to excess flexion and rotation forces. They termed this the "teardrop fracture" (Fig. 13–27). This lesion is characterized by the crushing of one vertebral body by the vertebral body superior to it in such a manner that the anterior portion of the involved vertebra is not only compressed but is frequently broken away from the major portion. Because this fragment resembles a drop of water dripping from the vertebral body and has been associated with dire circumstances so frequently, the term "teardrop" was coined to describe the lesion and also to suggest the mechanism of injury. The most important feature of this injury is the displacement of the inferior margin of the fractured vertebral body backward into the spinal canal, which often causes compression or destruction of the anterior portion of the cervical spinal cord. This may produce an anterior spinal cord syndrome due to retropulsion of either the portion of the vertebral body or the intervertebral disc. This is an extremely unstable injury and usually presents with forward translation of one vertebra upon the other. It is important to attempt to reduce this fracture-dislocation as soon as possible to avoid further neurological sequelae. Partial or complete neurological deficit is not an uncommon initial manifestation. In patients who present without a neurological deficit or with a nonprogressing deficit the treatment of choice is a cranial halo until the acute reaction around the spinal cord subsides. This usually requires an interval of one to two weeks. Following this, a posterior spinal fusion is performed to provide stability at this particular level. It must be emphasized that it is best to wait long enough to allow the edema around the cord to subside. Early active intervention may increase this edema, and further damage to the cord may result. The patients are then maintained in the halo and body jacket postoperatively for three to four months until evidence of spinal stability is present. In the meantime they may be up and about in the halo and jacket. Spinal fusion has also been advocated for patients with a complete neurological deficit below this level in order to stabilize the lower cervical spine. This active form of treatment permits earlier rehabilitation in these serious injuries.

Extension Injuries

Extension injuries are seen more frequently than flexion injuries in civilian practice. Selecki and Williams concluded that extension injuries occurred three times as frequently as flexion injuries in the cervical spine. They also emphasized that the degree of ligamentous and intervertebral disc injury was greater than initially anticipated from the roentgenographic examination.[66] A characteristic feature of extension injuries is a small triangular chip of bone from the anterior inferior angle or the superior end-plate of the vertebral body seen on a lateral roentgenogram. This chip is secondary to a tear in the anterior longitudinal ligament that causes avulsion of the anterior osseous fragment. In follow-up, calcification of the ligament at the point of rupture may frequently be visualized. Several mechanisms have been proposed for the type of central cervical spinal cord injury that infrequently accompanies this injury. Taylor felt that the infolding and forward bulging of the ligamentum flavum, as produced by a hyperextension injury, may be the cause of damage to the cervical spinal cord.[79] Others, however, have felt that the most likely explanation is a minor mechanical insult within the cord followed by progressive central hemorrhagic destruction, as outlined by Osterholm and Mathews.[52, 53] This is not a frequent lesion, and most hyperextension injuries present without a neurological deficit. These may be treated by a soft cervical collar or a Philadelphia collar worn for six to eight weeks for comfort and then gradually discontinued.

Injuries produced by an extension–axial load force disrupt the posterior elements and make the spine unstable. They usually present with an avulsion fracture along the anterior superior portion of the vertebral body and evidence of disruption of the posterior elements. This is an unstable injury and requires active treatment, initially in a cranial halo that is then converted into a halo–body jacket arrangement. If at the end of three months there is no evidence of spinal stability, a posterior cervical fusion should be performed. Initial operative fusion shortly after the injury is not indicated, as the majority of these patients will obtain spinal stability with three to four months of conservative treatment in a halo and body jacket.

Lateral Bending Injuries

Lateral bending injuries are for the most part confined to the pediatric age group. The mechanism of injury is a direct force on the lateral aspect of the cervical spine and skull. A wedging type of injury occurs along the lateral aspect of the vertebral body and its associated lateral mass. This injury is considered stable and may be treated with a soft cervical collar for four to six weeks providing comfort.

SPINAL CORD INJURY AND CERVICAL FRACTURES AND DISLOCATIONS

PROGNOSIS FOLLOWING CERVICAL SPINAL CORD INJURY

The early mortality rate following operative intervention in these patients varies from 10 to 15 per cent. In Guttmann's large series of nonoperatively managed patients, the death rate was 7.6 per cent.[38] In a series that included operatively and nonoperatively managed patients with severe neurological deficit, Harris reported an 18 per cent mortality rate.[41]

If a complete traumatic lesion is present at 24 hours following injury, it is irreversible. Particularly poor prognostic signs include a tonic flexor plantar response with a short interval between the stimulus and the response, or priapism. In 1972 Osterholm and Mathews explained the pathophysiology of progressive autodestruction of the traumatized spinal cord. Large increases in the norepinephrine levels in the injured tissues were universally associated with massive central hemorrhages. The increased levels of norepinephrine were noted immediately following the spinal cord injury, and they reached a maximum level when central hemorrhages appeared. Osterholm and Mathews then hypothesized that the norepinephrine liberated earliest at the injury site depressed or halted electrical transmission, but higher levels of norepinephrine produced basal spasm, which arrested spinal cord perfusion and thus resulted in autodestruction. They were able to control accumulation of norepinephrine at the injury site by utilizing alpha-methyltyrosine, which significantly reduced norepinephrine synthesis. This had a potent protective effect against the development of the progressive hemorrhagic necrosis that he had demonstrated previously.[53] Alphamethyltyrosine cannot be employed in humans, however, as it is extremely toxic.

Albin and co-workers demonstrated the beneficial effect of local cord cooling employed within specific time intervals in reversing experimental traumatic parapalegia. They felt that the beneficial effect was due to prevention of edema by the hypothermia.[2, 3] In some institutions this procedure is still advocated for acute spinal cord injury. Because it is often impossible to expose the spinal cord within the first four hours following injury and then to perfuse it with the hypothermic solution, this is generally impractical in the routine management of patients with spinal injury.

Several investigators have advocated the administration of large doses of dexamethasone in the treatment of the patient with spinal cord injury. The feeling is that the large doses of steroids will suppress the inflammatory response. This procedure is advocated in most spinal centers.

Spinal Cord Syndromes

The anterior spinal cord syndrome is due to direct pressure or damage to the anterior portion of the spinal cord. This syndrome may be seen in association with "teardrop" and axial burst fracture with posterior displacement of the vertebral body. It presents with total motor paralysis associated with sensory anesthesia except for deep pressure

and proprioception, which is present because of sparing of the dorsal columns. The prognosis for recovery from an anterior cord syndrome is extremely poor.

The central cord syndrome is commonly seen with hyperextension injuries in patients with osteoarthritis of the spine. It is felt that this syndrome is produced by infolding of the ligamentum flavum posteriorly and a pinching effect of the osteophytes anteriorly. This is the most common incomplete cord syndrome. Patients present with a flaccid type of lower motor neuron paralysis of the upper extremities. A different picture is seen in the trunk and lower extremities. The corticospinal and spinal thalamic long tracts in the white matter are damaged, and this produces an upper motor neuron spastic paralysis of the trunk and lower extremities. Since the sacral trunks are anatomically located on the periphery of the spinal cord, they are usually not damaged in this type of injury. Therefore, even though patients present with gross quadriplegia, they demonstrate sacral sparing due to preservation of the sacral tract. The prognosis in this syndrome is considered fair.

The posterior cord syndrome is rare. Since the posterior portion of the spinal cord has been damaged, the patients present with loss of deep pressure, deep pain, and proprioceptive sensation. They have full motor power. Pain and temperature sensations are unaffected. A good prognosis for complete recovery exists.

The Brown-Séquard syndrome results from a discrete injury that is limited to one lateral half of the spinal cord. Owing to its anatomical location, it produces ipsilateral paralysis with contralateral hypesthesia to pain and temperature sensations. Approximately 90 per cent of patients with the Brown-Séquard syndrome recover all function.

GENERAL CARE OF THE PATIENT WITH SPINAL INJURY

Aggressive pulmonary toilet and care have largely accounted for the improved statistics achieved in treating patients with spinal cord injuries. Some of these patients will present with problems of pulmonary insufficiency but will also have problems related to direct injuries to the chest wall. Abdominal distention secondary to paralytic ileus will further compound the problem and limit diaphragmatic excursion. The danger is that patients presenting with this clinical picture will regurgitate and will develop aspiration pneumonia. Some of these victims are also unable to cough and therefore cannot clear the normal secretions. It is important to evaluate the spinal fracture prior to instituting corrective pulmonary measures such as endotracheal intubation. If this has to be performed, the nasal route is often the safest. Volume pressure respirators are extremely important in the care of these patients, and almost all patients with severe cervical spinal cord injury require this type of treatment. The patient's ventilatory status is guided by the serial quantification of the blood gases. In the event of infection, it is best to withhold antibiotic coverage until a specific organism has been cultured from the pulmonary tract. Once the organism is identified, however, the infection is treated very aggressively in conjunction with the ventilation provided by the respirator.

Respiratory Care

A specific syndrome that has occurred with the acute cervical spinal cord injury is known as sleep apnea. This syndrome presents with vague subjective sensations of lethargy associated with a sighing respiratory pattern. The patients may be confused and may complain about their breathing. This progresses until they begin to hypoventilate and then become apneic while asleep. This complication must be recognized immediately. If the patient is awakened his normal breathing will resume. The hypoventilation remains, however, and the sleep apnea recurs. It is due to a faulty respiratory control mechanism that is manifested by a decreased response to carbon dioxide. Therefore, the administration of oxygen may well be injurious to these patients. It is for this reason that their breathing patterns must be closely monitored. If there is any tendency towards hypoventilation or irregular breathing, an endotracheal tube should be introduced and the patient maintained on a controlled mechanical respirator. The periods for which the respirator is required vary from 3 to 10 days.

Urinary Management

Urinary care plays a very significant role in the treatment of patients with acute spinal cord injury. The drainage is best provided by Guttmann's intermittent no-touch technique, which requires a scrubbed and gowned physician.[39] The problem with administering this type of care is that it usually requires specialized paramedical personnel. The worst treatment for a patient with a spinal cord syndrome is to insert a permanent indwelling urethral catheter. All this produces is a constant series of significant urinary tract infections, and it is therefore to be condemned. Intermittent catheterization is to be advocated. Comarr has recently analysed the urinary status of a significant number of patients with spinal cord lesions. Intermittent catheterization was initiated at four-hour intervals and the time was extended, depending upon the progress of the bladder. He also noted that several patients who had established urinary tract infections and were then started on the intermittent catheterization technique developed sterile urine. Of the group that had intermittent catheterization started at the time of the injury, 78 per cent became catheter-free.[20]

Decubitus Ulcers

This particular problem should not occur if patients are treated adequately and properly. This requires specific attention to detail on the part of the nursing staff. Since these patients lack sensation, they must be turned at least every two hours around the clock. If this is not performed, the patients will develop decubitus ulcers. The author therefore considers this a specific nursing problem; if the patients develop this problem, it is due to inadequate nursing care. This may seem to be a straightforward problem that should be treated routinely, but a review by Wilcox and co-workers revealed that one third of patients being transferred to Rancho Los Amigos Hospital from other referring hospitals presented with decubitus ulcers.[87] This is definitely an unacceptable figure. Patients with spinal cord injury may be treated in a regular bed and turned from side to side, or they may be treated on a Stryker frame, which allows them to be turned from back to front periodically. The circle electric bed is contraindicated for patients with this type of problem. This is related to the mechanics of turning patients with this type of frame; the traction alters sequentially as the patient is being turned. Patients have also fallen out of this type of apparatus.

Gastrointestinal Care

The majority of the patients with injury of the cervical spine will also have paralytic reflex ileus and will present with abdominal distention. The first order of business in managing the gastrointestinal tract is to pass a nasogastric tube into the stomach. Stress ulcers may occur in these patients, and this complication must be closely monitored. The exact etiology of the acute multiple stress ulcers has never been adequately evaluated. The drainage from the gastrointestinal tract must be provided early or patients may regurgitate, producing aspiration pneumonia. It is best to withhold oral fluids until the patients' bowel sounds are adequate. Antacids should be administered in an attempt to decrease gastric irritation.

Nutritional Care

Nutrition is extremely important for patients suffering transection of the spinal cord, as they are subject to a profound systemic catabolism. The serum protein and hematocrit may decrease significantly. These patients also frequently develop profound hyponatremia, which will, however, usually respond to intravenous sodium replacement. A specific problem to be aware of in their management is hyperkalemia, which may result in ventricular fibrillation following the administration of succinylcholine. This is a very dangerous and specific syndrome and should always be kept in mind when treating these patients. The hyperkalemia has been felt to be due to an alteration in the denervated muscle cell membrane that results in an atypical response to depolarization produced by succinylcholine. Another type of

specific syndrome is that of inappropriate antidiuretic hormone secretion. This syndrome presents with hyponatremia, renal excretion of sodium, evidence of hyperosmolar serum, and normal renal and adrenal function. This problem may be treated by withholding fluids until the hyponatremia has reversed itself.

ACCELERATION-EXTENSION INJURIES ("Whiplash")

This syndrome is presented for completeness' sake. The injury is a major source of litigation in modern times. The classic history is that the patient was seated in a stationary automobile that was struck from the rear by another automobile. Since the present legal system demands that a driver have complete control of his automobile, the person in the rear car is automatically at fault. Regrettably, the inaccurate but easily remembered term "whiplash" was coined by Crowe in 1928. It is often extremely difficult to sort out the patients who are litigation-conscious from the one who suffers a true injury via this particular mechanism. It is important to understand the mechanism of injury and the pathophysiological changes that occur in the cervical region. Primarily owing to the excellent experimental work performed by MacNab, we can now understand the basic changes that occur.[49]

MECHANISM OF INJURY

When an automobile is struck from the rear, a sudden forward acceleration is produced and the passenger's trunk is thrust forward by the acceleration force. The forward acceleration force is, however, also applied to the cervical spine. If a headrest is not present, the cervical spine must extend because of the forces applied. The backward rotation of the head is checked by the anterior cervical muscles, the anterior longitudinal ligament, and the anterior fibers of the annulus. The amount of injury produced will depend on the rate of stretch of the anterior cervical muscles and the anterior longitudinal ligament. If the elastic limit is exceeded, a muscle rupture may well occur.

Therefore, the degree of injury is dependent on the rate of acceleration. The head will rebound forward when the car stops accelerating. According to basic physical principles, the acceleration is dependent on the force supplied and the inertia of the stationary vehicle. The force applied to the cervical spine will be significantly altered if the seat tilts backward. This will allow partial resolution of the force and decrease the fulcrum.

PATHOLOGY

MacNab's animal experiments with monkeys have led to an understanding of the pathological processes involved. He demonstrated that various lesions could be produced by placing an animal on a platform and then dropping the platform over varying distances. The animal's head would suddenly extend when the platform struck the bottom of the runway. Minor tears of the sternocleidomastoid muscle were frequently seen. With a more severe acceleration injury, tears of the longissimus colli muscles were seen. Tears of the longissimus colli produced a retropharyngeal hematoma. Hemorrhages were also seen in the esophagus. If the acceleration injury was of greater severity, a tear of the anterior longitudinal ligament with separation of the disc from the associated vertebra was seen. It was of interest that the disc injury in the animals could not be detected on roentgenograms even with passage of time.[49]

It is difficult to correlate the significance of the animal studies as applied to the clinical situation. MacNab's studies do, however, illustrate the severity of lesions produced with an acceleration injury to the cervical spine.

CLINICAL PRESENTATION

Frequently patients will experience immediate pain in the area of the cervical spine. There are some patients, however, who have no pain in the cervical area immediately following the accident but have gradual onset of pain developing over the next 24 hours. The pain may be localized to the neck or may radiate down one or both shoulders into the arms. Occipital headaches are common. Persistent suboccipital pain may be referred pain from the damaged cervical segment.

True disc herniation with nerve root irritation rarely results from a whiplash injury of the neck. Vague paresthesias produced may well be based on associated muscle spasm.

Dysphagia produced immediately following the accident is of prognostic significance. It is usually caused by pharyngeal edema or retropharyngeal hematoma. This symptom complex tends to point to a more severe injury.

Many patients complain of temporary tinnitus. The exact etiology of this complex has never been completely understood. It is usually temporary and is of no prognostic significance.

Patients frequently complain of intermittent blurring of vision. This is felt to be due to an alteration of the cervical sympathetic chain or to temporary damage to the vertebral arteries.

Vertigo is usually caused by vertebral artery spasm or by an inner ear disturbance. This symptom complex is frequently seen in older patients with atherosclerotic changes in the vertebral arteries.

The head is usually held rigidly, the normal cervical lordosis frequently abolished. There is spasm of the sternocleidomastoid and the trapezius muscle complex. Occasionally a hematoma is present within the sternocleidomastoid muscles. The patient is very apprehensive and fearful of gentle motion of the cervical spine, particularly rotation. Occasionally tenderness is present over the temporamandibular joints. Reflexes and sensation are usually intact in the upper extremities. Fine muscle control in the hands is normal.

As stated previously, it is extremely important to attempt to determine whether the patient is suffering from a psychological overlay or is experiencing a true injury. If the patient presents with a positive history and demonstrable physical findings, then appropriate treatment is indicated. The patient should be placed in a soft cervical collar (the rigid collars that hold the neck in extension are contraindicated). Bed rest is advised for the first 24 to 48 hours. Traction is not indicated at this stage. The attending physician should not be lured into overtreatment with sedatives. A short course of antiinflammatory medication may be prescribed early in the course. Most patients will achieve symptomatic relief with the application of moist heat. This is usually accomplished by standing in a hot shower or by applying hot moist packs to the cervical area. One of the most important aspects of the treatment of this injury is gentle, kind reassurance. It is also important to explain to the patient the expected duration of symptoms.

If the patient does not appear to be responding to conservative measures and no physical defect is demonstrated, then appropriate psychological evaluation should be instituted.

REFERENCES

1. Abbott, K. H., and Hale, N.: Cervical trapeze. An apparatus for ambulatory treatment of fractures of the cervical spine. J. Neurosurg., 10:436–437, 1953.
2. Albin, M. S., White, R. J., Acosta-Rua, G., and Yashon, D.: Study of functional recovery produced by delayed localized cooling after spinal cord injury in primates. J. Neurosurg., 29:113–120, 1968.
3. Albin, M. S., White, R. J., Yashon, D., and Harris, L. S.: Effects of localized cooling on spinal cord trauma. J. Trauma, 9:1000–1008, 1969.
4. Anderson, L. D., and Alonzo, R. T.: Fractures of the odontoid process of the axis. J. Bone Joint Surg., 56A:1663–1674, 1974.
5. Anderson, S., and Bradford, D. S.: Lo-profile Halo. Clin. Orthop., 103:72–74, 1974.
6. Babcock, J. L.: Cervical spine injuries. Diagnosis and classification. Arch. Surg., 111:646–651, 1976.
7. Bailey, R. W., and Kingsley, T. C.: Dislocation of cervical spine following laminectomy. J. Bone Joint Surg., 51A:1029, 1969.
8. Barton, L. G.: The reduction of fracture/dislocation of the cervical vertebra by skeletal traction. Surg. Gynecol. Obstet., 67:94–96, 1938.
9. Bellamy, R., Pitts, F. W., and Stauffer, E. S.: Respiratory complications in traumatic quadriplegia. J. Neurosurg., 39:596–600, 1973.
10. Bohlman, H.: The pathology and current treatment concepts of cervical spine injuries; a critical review of 300 cases. J. Bone Joint Surg., 54A:1353–1354, 1972.
11. Bosch, A., Stauffer, E. S., and Nickel, V. L.: Incomplete traumatic quadriplegia; a ten year review. J.A.M.A., 216:473–478, 1971.
12. Braakman, R., and Vinken, P. J.: Unilateral facet interlocking in the lower cervical spine. J. Bone Joint Surg., 49B:249–257, 1967.
13. Braakman, R., and Vinken, P. J.: Old luxations of the lower cervical spine. J. Bone Joint Surg., 50B:52–60, 1968.
14. Brashear, H. R., Venters, G. C., and Preston, E. T.: Fractures of the neural arch of the axis. J. Bone Joint Surg., 57A:879–887, 1975.
15. Brieg, A.: Biomechanics of the Central Nervous System. Stockholm, Almquist and Wiksell, 1960.
16. Burke, D. C., and Berryman, D.: The place of closed manipulation in the management of flexion-rotation dislocations of the cervical spine. J. Bone Joint Surg., 53B:165–180, 1971.
17. Chesire, D. J. E.: The stability of the cervical spine following the conservative treatment of fractures and fracture-dislocations. Paraplegia, 7:193–203, 1969.
18. Clawson, D. K., Gunn, D. R., and Friz, L.: Early anterior fusion of cervical spine injury. J.A.M.A., 215:2113–2115, 1971.
19. Comarr, A. E.: Neurogenic bladder. Paraplegia, 2:125–131, 1964.
20. Comarr, A. E.: Intermittent catheterization for the traumatic cord bladder patient. J. Urol., 108:79–81, 1972.
21. Comarr, A. E., and Kaufman, A. A.: A survey of the neurological results of 858 spinal cord injuries; a comparison of patients treated with and without laminectomy. J. Neurosurg., 13:95–106, 1956.
21a. Crowe, H. E.: Injuries to the cervical spine. Paper presented at 1928 Western Orthopaedic Association, San Francisco.
22. Crutchfield, W. G.: Skeletal traction for dislocation of the cervical spine. Report of a case. South. Surg., 2:156–159, 1933.
23. Crutchfield, W. G.: Treatment of injuries of the cervical spine. J. Bone Joint Surg., 20:696–704, 1938.
24. Ducker, T. B., Kindt, G. W., and Kempe, L. G.: Pathological findings in acute experimental spinal cord trauma. J. Neurosurg., 35:700–708, 1971.
25. Durbin, F. C.: Fracture/dislocations of the cervical spine. J. Bone Joint Surg., 39B:23–38, 1957.
26. Evarts, C. M.: Traumatic occipito-atlantal dislocation. J. Bone Joint Surg., 52A:1653–1660, 1970.
27. Feuer, H.: Management of acute spine and spinal cord injuries. Arch. Surg., 111:638–645, 1976.
28. Fielding, J. W.: Cineroentgenography of the normal cervical spine. J. Bone Joint Surg., 39A:1280–1288, 1957.
29. Fielding, J. W., Hawkins, R. J.: Atlanto-axial rotatory fixation. (Fixed rotatory subluxation of the atlanto-axial joint.) J. Bone Joint Surg., 59A:37–44, 1977.
30. Fielding, J. W., Hawkins, R. J., and Ratzan, S. A.: Spine fusion for atlanto-axial instability. J. Bone Joint Surg., 58A:400–407, 1976.
31. Fielding, J. W., Cochran, G. V., Lawsing, J. F., and Hohl, M.: Tears of the transverse ligament of the atlas. J. Bone Joint Surg., 56A:1683–1691, 1974.
32. Forsyth, H. F.: Extension injuries of the cervical spine. J. Bone Joint Surg., 46A:1792–1797, 1964.
33. Forsyth, H. F., Alexander, E., Jr., and Underdal, R.: The advantages of early spine fusion in the treatment of fracture-dislocation of the cervical spine. J. Bone Joint Surg., 41A:17–36, 1959.

34. Fried, L. C.: Atlanto-axial fracture/dislocations: Failure of posterior C1 to C2 fusion. J. Bone Joint Surg., 55B:490–496, 1973.
35. Gallie, W. E.: Fractures and dislocations of the cervical spine. Am. J. Surg., 46:495–499, 1939.
36. Grogono, B. J. S.: Injuries of the atlas and axis. J. Bone Joint Surg., 36B:397, 1954.
37. Guttman, L.: Early management of the paraplegic. Symposium on spinal injuries. J. Roy. Coll. Surg., 1963.
38. Guttmann, L.: Spinal Cord Injuries; Comprehensive Management and Research. London, Blackwell, 1973.
39. Guttmann, L., and Frankel, H.: The value of intermittent catheterization in the early management of traumatic paraplegia and tetraplegia. Paraplegia, 4:63–84, 1966.
40. Hall, R. D. M.: Clay-shoveler's fracture. J. Bone Joint Surg., 22:63–75, 1940.
41. Harris, P.: Some neurosurgical aspects of traumatic paraplegia. *In* P. Harris, ed.: Spinal Injuries. Edinburgh, Morrison & Gibb, Ltd., 1965, pp. 101–112.
42. Holdsworth, F.: Fractures, dislocations and fracture-dislocations of the spine. J. Bone Joint Surg., 52A:1534–1551, 1970.
43. Howorth, B., and Petrie, J. G.: Injuries of the Spine. Baltimore, Williams & Wilkins, 1964.
44. Hunter, G. A.: Non-traumatic displacement of the atlanto-axial joint. J. Bone Joint Surg., 50B:44–51, 1968.
45. Jacobs, B.: Cervical fractures and dislocations (C3–7). Clin. Orthop., 109:18–32, 1975.
46. Jefferson, G.: Fracture of atlas vertebra: Report of four cases and a review of those previously recorded. Br. J. Surg., 7:407–422, 1920.
47. Kahn, E. A.: On spinal cord injuries. J. Bone Joint Surg., 41A:6–11, 1959.
48. Lipscomb, P. R.: Cervico-occipital fusion for congenital and posttraumatic anomalies of the atlas and axis. J. Bone Joint Surg., 39A:1289–1301, 1957.
49. MacNab, I.: Acceleration injuries of the cervical spine. J. Bone Joint Surg., 46A:1797–1799, 1964.
50. Nickel, V. L., Perry, J., Garrett, A., and Heppenstall, M.: The halo: a spinal skeletal traction fixation device. J. Bone Joint Surg., 50A:1400–1409, 1968.
51. Norton, W. L.: Fractures and dislocations of the cervical spine. J. Bone Joint Surg., 44A:115–139, 1962.
52. Osterholm, J. L., and Mathews, G. J.: Treatment of severe spinal cord injuries by biochemical norepinephrine manipulation. Surg. Forum, 22:415–417, 1971.
53. Osterholm, J. L., and Mathews, G. J.: Altered norepinephrine metabolism following experimental spinal cord injury. Part 1. Relationship to hemorrhagic necrosis and post-wounding neurological deficits. J. Neurosurg., 36:386–394, 1972.
54. Perry, J., and Nickel, V. L.: Total cervical-spine fusion for neck paralysis. J. Bone Joint Surg., 41A:37–60, 1959.
55. Petrie, J. G.: Flexion injuries of the cervical spine. J. Bone Joint Surg., 46A:1800–1806, 1964.
56. Queckenstedt, M. E.: Zur diagnose der rukenmarks Kompression. Dtsch. Z. Nervenheilkd., 55:316, 1916.
57. Rogers, W. A.: Fractures and dislocations of cervical spine; an end-result study. J. Bone Joint Surg., 39A:341–376, 1957.
58. Schatzker, J., Rorabeck, C. H., and Waddell, J. P.: Fractures of the dens (odontoid process). An analysis of thirty-seven cases. J. Bone Joint Surg., 53B:390–405, 1971.
59. Schatzker, J., Rorabeck, C. H., and Waddell, J. P.: Non-union of the odontoid process; an experimental investigation. Clin. Orthop., 108:127–137, 1975.
60. Schiff, D. C. M., and Parke, W. W.: The arterial supply of the odontoid process. J. Bone Joint Surg., 55A:1450–1456, 1973.
61. Schneider, R. C.: The syndrome of acute anterior cervical spinal cord injury. J. Neurosurg., 12:95–122, 1955.
62. Schneider, R. C.: Trauma to the spine and spinal cord. *In* Kahn, E. A., et al.: Correlative Neurosurgery. Springfield, Ill., Charles C Thomas, 1969, p. 597.
63. Schneider, R. C., and Kahn, E. A.: Chronic neurological sequelae of acute trauma to the spine and spinal cord. Part I. The significance of the acute flexion or "tear-drop" fracture-dislocation of the cervical spine. J. Bone Joint Surg., 38A:985–997, 1956.
64. Schneider, R. C., Livingston, K. E., Cave, A. J. E., and Hamilton, G.: "Hangman's fracture" of the cervical spine. J. Neurosurg., 22:141–154, 1965.
65. Schneider, R. C., Cherry, G., and Pantek, H.: The syndrome of acute central cervical spinal cord injury with special reference to the mechanisms involved in hyperextension injuries of the cervical spine. J. Neurosurg., 11:546–577, 1954.
66. Selecki, B. R., and Williams, H. B. L.: Injuries of the Cervical Spine and Cord in Man. Glebe, N. S. W., Australian Medical Publishing Co., Ltd., 1970.
67. Shea, J. D.: Pressure sores. Clin. Orthop., 112:89–100, 1975.
68. Sherk, H. H., and Nicholson, J. T.: Fractures of the atlas. J. Bone Joint Surg., 52A:1017, 1970.
69. Southwick, W. O., and Keggi, K.: The normal cervical spine. J. Bone Joint Surg., 46A:1767–1777, 1964.
70. Southwick, W. O., and Robinson, R. A.: Surgical approaches to the vertebral bodies in the cervical and lumbar regions. J. Bone Joint Surg., 39A:631–644, 1957.
71. Stauffer, E. S.: Orthopedic care of fracture-dislocations of the cervical spine. Proceedings of the 17th V.A. Clinical Spinal Cord Injury Conference, September and October, 1969. Washington, Veterans Administration, 1970.
72. Stauffer, E. S.: Diagnosis and prognosis of acute cervical spinal cord injury. Clin. Orthop., 112:9–15, 1975.
73. Stauffer, E. S., and Kelly, E. G.: Fracture-dislocations of the cervical spine. Instability and recurrent deformity following treatment by anterior interbody fusion. J. Bone Joint Surg., 59A:45–48, 1977.
74. Stauffer, E. S., and Rhoads, M. E.: Surgical

stabilization of the cervical spine after trauma. Arch. Surg., *111*:652–657, 1976.

75. Steel, H. H.: Anatomical and mechanical considerations of the atlanto-axial articulations. *In* Proceedings of the American Orthopaedic Association. J. Bone Joint Surg., *50A*:1481–1482, 1968.

76. Stone, W. A., Beach, T. P., and Hamelberg, W.: Succinylcholine-danger in the spinal-cord-injured patient. Anesthesiology, *32*:168–169, 1970.

77. Stryker, H.: A device for turning the frame patient. J.A.M.A., *113*:1731–1732, 1939.

78. Suwanwela, C., Alexander, E., Jr., and Davis, C. H., Jr.: Prognosis in spinal cord injury, with special reference to patients with motor paralysis and sensory preservation. J. Neurosurg., *19*:220, 1962.

79. Taylor, A. R.: The mechanism of injury to the spinal cord in the neck without damage to the vertebral column. J. Bone Joint Surg., *33B*:543–547, 1951.

80. Thompson, H.: The "halo" traction apparatus. A method of external splinting of the cervical spine after injury. J. Bone Joint Surg., *44B*:655–661, 1962.

81. Verbiest, H.: Anterior operative approach in cases of spinal-cord compression by old irreducible displacement or fresh fracture of cervical spine. J. Neurosurg., *19*:389, 1962.

82. Vinke, T. H.: A skull fracture apparatus. J. Bone Joint Surg., *30A*:522–524, 1948.

83. Weir, D. C.: Roentgenographic signs of cervical injury. Clin. Orthop., *109*:9–17, 1975.

84. White, A. A., Johnson, R. M., Panjabi, M. D., and Southwick, W. O.: Biomechanical analysis of clinical stability of the cervical spine. Clin. Orthop., *109*:85–96, 1975.

85. White, R. J.: Pathology of spinal cord injury in experimental lesions. Clin. Orthop., *112*:16–26, 1975.

86. Whitley, J. E., and Forsyth, H. F.: A classification of cervical spine injuries. Am. J. Roentgenol., *83*:633–644, 1960.

87. Wilcox, N. E., Stauffer, E. S., and Nickel, V. L.: A statistical analysis of 423 consecutive patients admitted to the Spinal Cord Injury Center, Rancho Los Amigos Hospital, 1 January 1964 thru 31 December 1967. Paraplegia, 8:27–35, 1970.

88. Williams, T. G.: Hangman's fracture. J. Bone Joint Surg., *57B*:82–88, 1975.

89. Wortzman, G., and Dewar, F. P.: Rotary fixation of the atlanto-axial joint: rotational atlanto-axial subluxation. Radiology, *90*:479, 1968.

R. BRUCE HEPPENSTALL, M.D.

Fractures and ——————————————— 14
Dislocations
of the
Thoracolumbar
Spine

In the past, a diagnosis of a "broken back" carried a very grave prognosis similar to that of a "broken neck." As has been outlined in the preceding chapter, this attitude is not justified at the present time since it has been adequately demonstrated that 5 per cent or less of spinal fractures are associated with a neurological deficit. It is only in the past few decades that this changing attitude has become prevalent. A more thorough understanding of the mechanisms of injury as well as new therapeutic approaches to the problem have vastly improved the outlook. One of the more positive advances in the treatment of these patients is the concept that a "routine laminectomy" is a very aggressive approach to this type of problem and that its results are unproved, just as they are in cervical spine injuries, unless there is an incomplete spinal cord syndrome and progressive neurological deterioration. A second positive advance is the decline in the use of the hyperextension body jacket for treatment of these injuries—a treatment that is at present the exception rather than the rule. This is a major advance for both the patient and the surgeon, as the application of a hyperextension jacket under these conditions is at best difficult, and many patients immobilized in an unphysiological position end up with persistent back pain later.

The majority of thoracolumbar fractures are the direct result of hyperflexion injuries. The spine from T12 to L2 is definitely predisposed to vertebral fractures, more than 50 per cent of which occur in this area. This is because this is a transitional area where the relatively fixed thoracic spine adjoins the more mobile lumbar spine. This situation produces an area of stress concentration between T12 and L2. The most common type of hyperflexion injury seen in clinical practice is a compression fracture of the twelfth thoracic vertebra secondary to significant axial osteoporosis.

Fortunately, with modern treatment, victims of thoracolumbar spinal injuries can receive appropriate therapy and return to an active role in society. This is particularly true of patients presenting with spinal fractures unassociated with a neurological deficit. It must be borne in mind, however, that patients presenting with neurological deficits should not be viewed as "hopeless" cases, as these patients may be appropriately treated and still return to active roles in today's society.

Controversy still exists in regard to conservative versus surgical management of many of these injuries. Guttmann has championed the conservative approach to the treatment of patients with thoracolumbar injuries. Several spinal centers in the

331

United States, however, have been taking a more aggressive approach and advocating operative stabilization of the fractures and early mobilization of the patients in an attempt to prevent secondary complications. This approach is similar to the early-weight-bearing concept in the treatment of fractures that has emerged during the past two decades. There is no doubt that the theory of early mobilization in association with operative stabilization has significantly changed the outlook of many patients with spinal fractures. Recently, there has been enthusiastic support for the use of Harrington distraction rods or compression rods or both in selected cases. In the past, the Meuhrig-Williams plates were advocated for open reduction and internal fixation, but several follow-up studies have revealed that a significant amount of angulation occurs with the use of these plates. Therefore, their popularity has decreased in the past two decades.

Modern supportive treatment has helped to decrease the morbidity and mortality rates associated with the treatment of patients with this type of injury. Proper pulmonary toilet along with adequate nutritional support has been definitely beneficial. As with cervical spine injuries, careful attention must be paid to skin care in patients with neurological deficits. Intermittent catheterization rather than continuous indwelling catheterization has been another major advance in the management of these patients.

The majority of patients with spinal injuries are acutely anxious because they fear becoming completely incapacitated by their injuries. These patients require constant reassurance and must be placed in active rehabilitation programs.

ANATOMY OF THE THORACOLUMBAR SPINE

The thoracolumbar spine consists of 12 thoracic vertebrae and 5 lumbar vertebrae. The distal portion of the lumbar spine may be altered owing to sacralization of the fifth lumbar vertebra or the appearance of a transitional vertebra between it and the sacrum. The characteristic curvatures consist of a mild kyphosis in the thoracic region

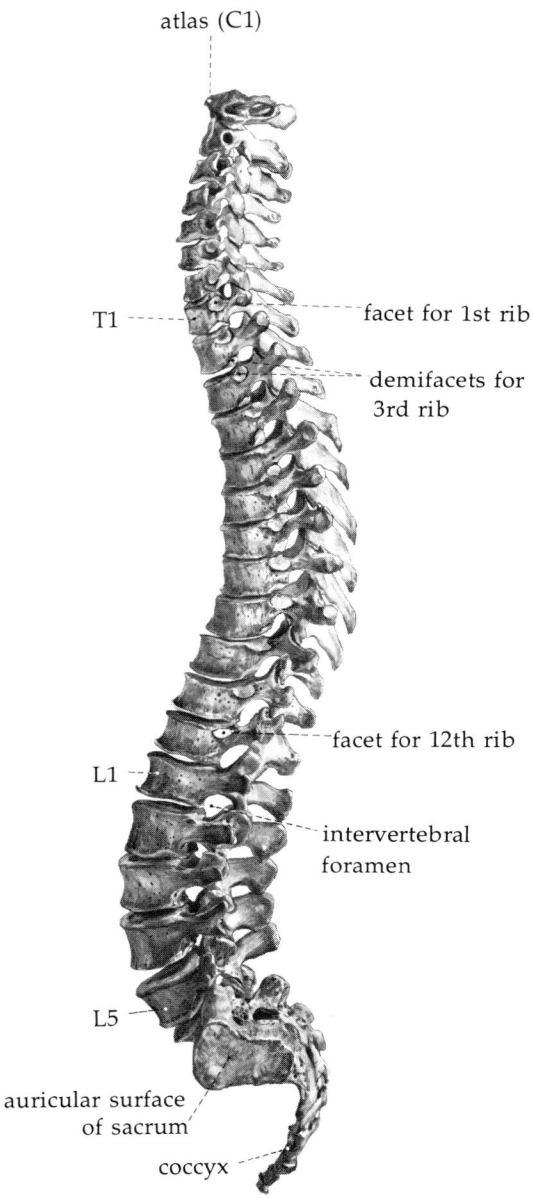

Figure 14–1 A lateral view of the spinal column demonstrating the normal thoracic kyphosis and lumbar lordosis. Note the increasing size of the vertebral bodies in a more distal direction. (Courtesy of J. Langman and M. W. Woerdeman and W. B. Saunders Co., Philadelphia. Atlas of Medical Anatomy, 1978.)

and a mild lordosis in the lumbar region. In comparison with those in the cervical spine, the vertebrae in the midthoracic and lumbar areas are significantly larger. The size of the vertebra increases in assocation with a more

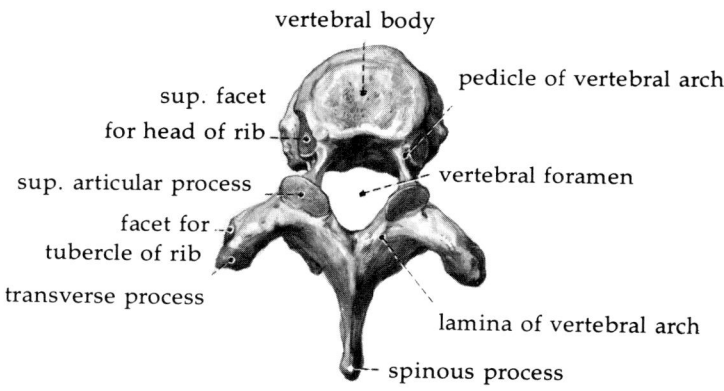

Figure 14–2 A typical thoracic vertebra. Note that facets are present for the articulation with the rib cage. The spinous processes are long and triangular. (Courtesy of J. Langman and M. W. Woerdeman and W. B. Saunders Co., Philadelphia. Atlas of Medical Anatomy, 1978.)

distal location in the spine. The typical body of a midthoracic vertebra is heart-shaped, and its dimensions in length and width are approximately halfway between those of a cervical and a lumbar vertebra. The thoracic spine also functions as an attachment for the rib cage. Facets are present for the diarthrodial articulations with this structure. The superior articular facets form a thick projection from the junction of the lamina and the pedicles. The articular surfaces of the facets face in a posterior direction in this area. The inferior articular facets are borne by the inferior edges of the lamina, and the articular surface faces anteriorly. The transverse processes arise between the superior and inferior facets at the junction of the pedicle and lamina, and project laterally and posteriorly. The spinous processes are long and triangular in section. The middle four are longer and directed downward so that the spines overlap the next lower segment.

The anterior and posterior longitudinal ligaments are thickest in the thoracic region. Therefore, in addition to stabilizing the spinal column, these thick ligaments restrict flexion and extension.

The lumbar vertebrae are larger than the thoracic vertebrae, having a width greater than the anterior-posterior diameter, and are slightly thicker anteriorly. Stout pedicles are situated on the dorsolateral aspects of the body, and together with the lamina they enclose a triangular vertebral foramen. The superior articular facets are concave and they face posteriorly and medially in such a fashion that they almost face each other. The articular surfaces of the inferior facets face anteriorly and laterally. This anatomical configuration of the superior and inferior articular facets restricts both flexion and rotation in the lumbar region. The transverse processes in this region are flat and stout.

The joints formed by the articular processes are true synovial joints with a joint capsule, which allows limited gliding articulation. The ligamentum flavum bridges the space between the lamina of adjacent vertebra. The fibers of the ligamentum flavum are almost vertical and are attached to the ventral surface of the upper lamina and to the superior lip of the lamina below. This very elastic structure derived its name from its characteristic yellow color. The intertransverse ligaments are fibrous connections between the transverse processes and are most developed in the lumbar region. The interspinal ligaments connect adjoining spinous processes. Their fibers are arranged obliquely and connect the base and superior spine with the superior ridge and apex of the next inferior spinous process. The supraspinal ligament runs along the apices of the spinous processes. Through the intervertebral foramen, the space between the pedicles of adjacent vertebrae, passes the spinal nerve with its dural sleeve, accompanying arteries, and veins. The anterior border is formed by the vertebral body and disc while the posterior border is formed by the articular facets.

The intervertebral disc is a fibrocartilagenous complex consisting of an internal semifluid mass, the nucleus pulposis, and a fibrous container, the anulus fibrosis. The summation of movements involved by each disc inparts to the spinal column its characteristic universal motion. The discs contrib-

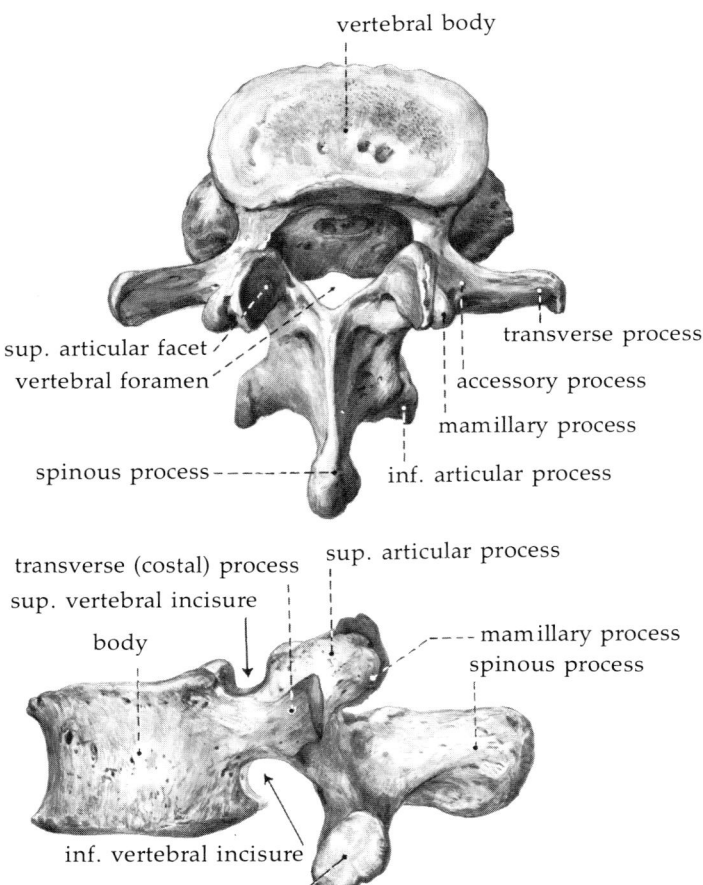

vertebral body

sup. articular facet
vertebral foramen

transverse process

accessory process

mamillary process

spinous process

inf. articular process

transverse (costal) process
sup. vertebral incisure
body

sup. articular process

mamillary process
spinous process

inf. vertebral incisure
inf. articular facet

Figure 14–3 A typical lumbar vertebra. Note the increased width of the
vertebra. The superior facets face posteriorly and medially while the inferior
facets face anteriorly and laterally.
(Courtesy of J. Langman and M. W.
Woerdeman and W. B. Saunders Co.,
Philadelphia. Atlas of Medical Anatomy,
1978.)

ute to lengthen the spinal column; they
provide approximately one fifth of the
length in the thoracic column and approximately one third of the length in the lumbar
column. The thickness and the horizontal
dimensions of the thoracic disc increase
caudally with corresponding increase in
size of the vertebral bodies. The characteristic lumbar lordosis is due to an equivalent increase in the differential between the
anterior and posterior thickness of the disc.
In other words, as one progresses distally in
the lumbar spine the anterior portion of the
disc is thicker than the posterior portion.
The nucleus pulposis receives vertical
forces from the vertebral bodies and then
redistributes them radially in a horizontal
plane. The distortion of the annulus by the
internal pressure of the nucleus supplies
the disc with its compressive quality. The
resilience is what allows the disc to recover

from applied pressure. The nucleus demonstrates a functional ability to absorb and
retain relatively large amounts of water. It is
the gradual loss of this ability to retain water
within the nucleus that accounts for some of
the structural changes with age. The disc
functions as a shock absorber between the
vertebrae. With advancing age it tends to
lose some of its water content and actually
shrinks in size, which accounts for the
decrease in stature with advancing old age.
The end-plates deform under compressive
loads, forcing blood out of the cancellous
bone and exerting a load dampening effect;
if the compressive loads are increased,
however, end-plate deformation also increases and failure occurs, resulting in a
fracture with invasion of the vertebral body.
This is commonly referred to as a traumatic
Schmorl's node. It has previously been
demonstrated that the end-plate fails prior

to rupture of the annulus in a "normal" spine.

Neuroanatomy. The spinal cord extends from the foramen magnum to the second lumbar vertebra and is suspended by the dentate ligaments, nerve roots, and blood vessels and surrounded by a shock-absorbing cerebrospinal fluid sac. The cauda equina begins at the L1–L2 interspace and extends to the sacrum. The dura mater consists of dense fibrous tissue extending from the foramen magnum to the middle of the second sacral vertebra. The dura is anchored firmly at the intervertebral foramina, where the dural sleeve surrounding each set of spinal nerve roots and dorsal root ganglia blends with the surrounding connective tissue. The surrounding dural sleeve protects the nerve roots; strain on the nerve at the foramen is transmitted through the dural sheath to the dural sac itself. The filum of the dura mater begins at the tapered lower end of the dural sac, with the dural sac itself ending at approximately the level of the second sacral vertebra. The second layer of tissue surrounding the spinal cord is the arachnoid, between the cellular surface of which and the pia mater lies the subarachnoid space. The arachnoid and the third lining membrane, the pia mater, are related to each other in a way similar to that of the visceral and the parietal peritoneum. The pia mater is a thin layer closely applied to the spinal cord and to the nerve roots as they cross the subarachnoid space. The arachnoid sac ends below at essentially the same level as the dural sac. The subarachnoid cavity is smaller in the thoracic region, where the spinal cord is also small. In the lumbar region, however, both the dura and arachnoid are large tubes, accounting for the large size of the subarachnoid cavity in the lumbar region. A segment of the subarachnoid space, the lumbar cistern, is occupied by the nerve roots of the cauda equina and by the filum terminale.

The tapered lower end of the spinal cord is known as the conus medullaris. It begins at the level of origin of the fourth sacral nerve, which is below the level of the nerves supplied to the limbs, and it ends below the origin of the coccygeal nerve. From its tapered point the conus medullaris continues as the filum terminale.

The L4–L5 level of the spinal cord is

situated at the T11–T12 interspace, the S2 level of the cord at the T12–L1 interspace, and the S4 cord level at the L1 vertebral body.

The average dimensions of the thoracic vertebral canal are 17.2 mm in width and 16.8 mm from anterior to posterior. The thickest portion of the thoracic spinal cord is located between T10 and T12 and measures

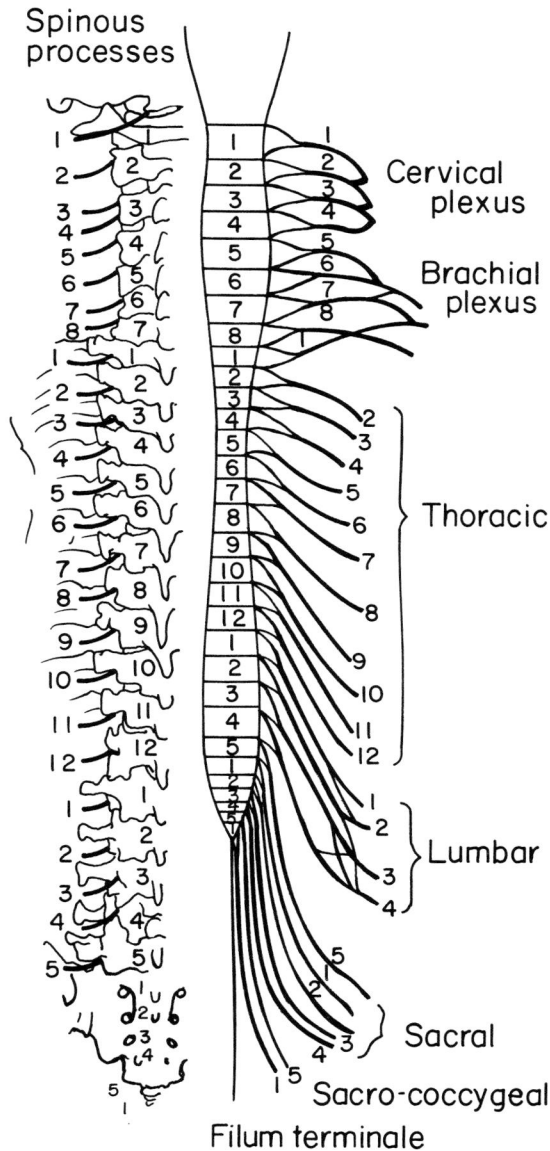

Figure 14–4 The spinal cord, including the conus medullaris and the distal portion known as the filum terminale. Note the different levels of spinal cord at various vertebral levels.

9.6 mm in width and 8.0 mm from anterior to posterior. As can be seen by these figures, the spinal cord occupies approximately half of the available space in the thoracic region.

In the lumbar region the average measurements of the canal are 23.4 mm in width and 17.4 mm from anterior to posterior. Since the spinal cord ends at the L1–L2 level and the roots of the cauda equina are the only neural contents of the spinal canal, a large amount of free space is available within the lumbar spinal canal in comparison with other regions. This accounts for the fact that significant displacement of the vertebral bodies in the lumbar spinal area is required to produce neurological impairment.

The sensory and motor roots of the spinal nerves remain separate in the spinal canal. The sensory root (dorsal) ganglion is located near the intervertebral foramen through which that root passes. The sensory root is not a peripheral nerve until it exits from the dorsal root ganglion. Since motor roots are the axons of the anterior horn cells, they are considered peripheral nerves all the way from the spinal cord origin to the terminus at the motor end-plate. Damage to motor roots carries a favorable prognosis.

Owing to the anatomical configuration in the thoracolumbar region, skeletal disruption above T10 is usually associated with cord damage; between T10 and L1, deficits may be due to both cord and root damage; and below L1, entirely to root damage.

As outlined previously for the cervical region, immediate and complete loss of neurological function following injury is usually due to an irreparable lesion of the spinal cord. This rule does not apply, however, if the deficit is due to cauda equina damage. The cauda equina does contain motor fibers, and the potential for recovery is present as long as the fibrous perineurium of the fasciculi remains intact. This does not apply to the sensory components of the cauda equina.

Blood Supply. The spinal cord is entirely dependent upon three longitudinal arterial trunks or channels for its blood supply. These consist of one anterior and two posterior spinal arteries. The anterior spinal artery originates from a fusion of branches from the vertebral artery and runs

the length of the spinal cord, lying in the anterior longitudinal fissure. This supplies the anterior and central portions of the cord. The two posterior spinal arteries originate from branches of the posterior inferior cerebellar arteries and run the length of the cord. They lie on the posterior aspect of the cord and supply its posterior and peripheral lateral portions. Additional blood supply to the cord in the thoracic and lumbar regions is derived from the spinal branches of the intercostal and lumbar segmental arteries, which pass through their respective intervertebral foramina, dividing into posterior and anterior radicular branches that contribute to the posterior and anterior spinal arteries respectively. There is a definite sparsity of these vessels in the midthoracic region. As demonstrated by Dommisse, it is this region of the cord that is particularly vulnerable to vascular insult.[10] At the thoracolumbar junction additional blood supply is received from anastomosing vessels entering most often at the T11 level on the left side. The segmental anterior radicular branch at this level is frequently called the artery of Adamkiewicz or the great radiculomedullary artery. Recently, significant importance has been attached to this artery.

NORMAL MOTION OF THE THORACOLUMBAR SPINE

Flexion of the spine is a highly significant motion throughout our regular daily activities. For flexion to take place, two events must take place simultaneously, anterior compression of the intervertebral disc and motion at the articular facets. The inferior set of facets tends to move upward and forward over the opposing superior set of an adjacent inferior vertebra. This motion is checked by the posterior ligaments and the dorsal musculature. Extension tends to be a more subtle motion, with posterior compression of the discs and motion of the articular facets. In this particular movement the inferior articular process glides posteriorly and downward over the superior set of the inferior vertebra. This motion is opposed by the anterior longitudinal ligament and all of the ventral musculature. For lateral flexion to take place, there has to be a degree of rotation. This involves a rocking motion of each vertebra upon the corresponding disc, a sliding separation of the diarthrosis of the convex side, and an overriding of that on the concave side. This motion moves the anterior surface of the body toward the convexity of the flexor and the spinous processes toward the concavity. Lateral flexion is opposed by the intertransverse ligaments and the extensions of the ribs.

Mobility of the thoracic region is not uniform throughout its entire length. The ribs and their corresponding attachments impair the range of motion of the thoracic spine. Rotation is the movement least restricted by the articular facets. Flexion and extension tend to increase in the lower thoracic region where the discs and vertebral bodies progressively increase in size. Axial rotation has been extensively investigated in human subjects by Gregersen and Lucas.[14] Considerable axial rotation can take place in the thoracic spine, depending on the orientation of the planes of the articular surfaces in the thoracic vertebrae. If the center of rotation falls within or anterior to the intervertebral disc, a considerable amount of axial rotation can occur. The opposite situation applies to a typical lumbar vertebra with the articular processes aligned in a more sagittal plane, as its center of rotation lies posterior to the disc. This limits the amount of axial rotation that can occur. In a standing position with the pelvis fixed an average of 74 degrees of rotation may occur between the first and twelfth thoracic vertebrae. The amount of axial rotation in the thoracic spine is somewhat less during sitting than during standing. During walking the lower thoracic spine rotation diminishes gradually up to the seventh thoracic vertebra. The amount of rotation in the upper thoracic spine increases gradually from the seventh to the first thoracic vertebrae. It appears that the seventh thoracic vertebral area represents the area of transition from vertebral rotation in the direction of the pelvis to rotation in the opposite direction, that of the shoulder girdle. Axial rotation in the lumbar spine is restricted compared with that in the thoracic spine. The articulations of the lumbar region allow flexion, lateral flexion, and

extension; but the facets of the synovial joints lie in a ventral medial to dorsal lateral plane that virtually locks them against rotation. Axial rotation at the lumbosacral junction is accomplished by lateral shearing of the fifth lumbar vertebral body on the first sacral segment. Lumsden and Morris have demonstrated that approximately 6 degrees of rotation occurs at the lumbosacral joint during maximum rotation with the patient standing or seated with the pelvis fixed. With normal walking approximately 1.5 degrees of rotation takes place at this level.[29]

It must be stressed that the location of the vertebrae in relation to the center of gravity of the spine directly influences the amount of motion and stability of the spine. The normal thoracic kyphosis places the thoracic vertebrae posterior to the center of gravity. In the lumbar spine the normal lumbar lordosis brings the middle lumbar vertebrae anterior to the center of gravity. Therefore, it is the transitional vertebrae between the two regions that intersect the center of gravity, and this is the most unstable region of the spine. For this reason the T10 to L2 area is where fractures and dislocations of the thoracolumbar spine most frequently occur. This also applies to the lumbosacral articulation. The sacral vertebral angle produces an abrupt change of direction of the spinal column, and the center of gravity passes through the fifth lumbar vertebra, falling anterior to the sacrum. The result is a marked tendency for the fifth lumbar disc to give way to the shearing vector that the lumbosacral angularity has produced. It is this type of stress that produces the condition known as spondylolisthesis, which may in fact be further aggravated by a chronic stress fracture at the pars interarticularis area. It is not difficult to understand why the forward displacement of the fifth lumbar vertebra occurs when such a defect is present in the pars interarticularis and the aforementioned stress patterns are present.

HISTORY

As with cervical spine injuries, the history is frequently very helpful in determining the extent and location of the injury. In general, patients with these injuries complain of thoracic or lumbar spinal pain. This complaint should not be taken lightly, as frequently it may be a specific aid to the diagnosis. It is true that many patients will complain of vague back pain following injury, trivial or major. It is important, however, to extract this information from the patient, as the exact location of the back pain may help to make the diagnosis. Occasionally, a patient will present with a history of back pain following an accident in which he is not able to remember the exact mechanism of injury. If the patient has been in an automobile accident, it is important to include the following questions: Were you stationary at the time of the injury to your back? Where were you located in the automobile at the time of the accident? Did you notice any loss of sensation or pins and needles feeling following the accident? Were you unconscious? Do you remember the mechanism of injury at the time of the accident? Have you had problems with your bowel or bladder habits since the accident?

It is important to re-emphasize that a good history is important because it may help to locate and differentiate between regular low back pain and a true serious spinal injury.

PHYSICAL EXAMINATION

A careful, thorough examination of the patient is extremely important in evaluating the extent of spinal injury. Patients are frequently brought to the emergency room on a stretcher by the police or firemen. It is extremely important to apply mild longitudinal traction and support the buttock and lumbar area when they are to be moved onto a permanent stretcher or bed. Associated injuries of the extremities or skull should be noted and recorded. All clothing should be removed so that the entire trunk can be adequately inspected. A careful inspection of the anterior aspect of the chest wall and abdomen will reveal abnormal swelling or ecchymosis. The chest wall should be inspected for evidence of a flail chest; the abdominal wall, for evidence of guarding or rigidity. If deemed necessary, a four-quadrant tap can be performed to rule out a serious abdominal visceral injury.

The entire thoracolumbar spinal area is then inspected by log-rolling the patient into the lateral decubitus position. Palpation of the spinous processes of the entire thoracolumbar spine may reveal evidence of injury reflected by acute tenderness, swelling, a gap between the spinous processes or a step-off deformity. The normal thoracic kyphotic and lumbar lordotic postural pattern may be altered because of significant spinal injury. Characteristically, there will be paravertebral muscle guarding following this type of injury.

If a step-off deformity or a palpable gap is present between the spinous processes then the patient's injury must be considered unstable until proven otherwise.

Neurological Examination

The initial neurological examination begins with the upper extremities, as outlined in Chapter 13. It is extremely important to record the findings for future reference. All too frequently a superficial neurological examination is performed, the true nature of the injury is not recorded, and it is exceedingly difficult in follow-up to document spontaneous recovery or progression of the neurological deficit. This has been emphasized in the past by Rogers, who reported a 10 per cent incidence of spinal cord compression or increasing neurological deficit following an original injury during emergency care, during the time taken for the initial diagnosis, during definitive treatment for the injury, and finally following spinal reduction.[42] It is important to bear in mind that injuries to this portion of the spine may frequently involve both the conus medullaris (the terminal spinal cord) and the roots of the cauda equina. It is not only academic but of paramount importance to recognize the difference between a conus lesion and a cauda equina lesion, as the prognosis for recovery is different with each injury. Repeated neurological evaluation is necessary to determine whether there is any residual motor or sensory function of the sacral segments of the spinal cord, since their presence is a very good prognostic sign.

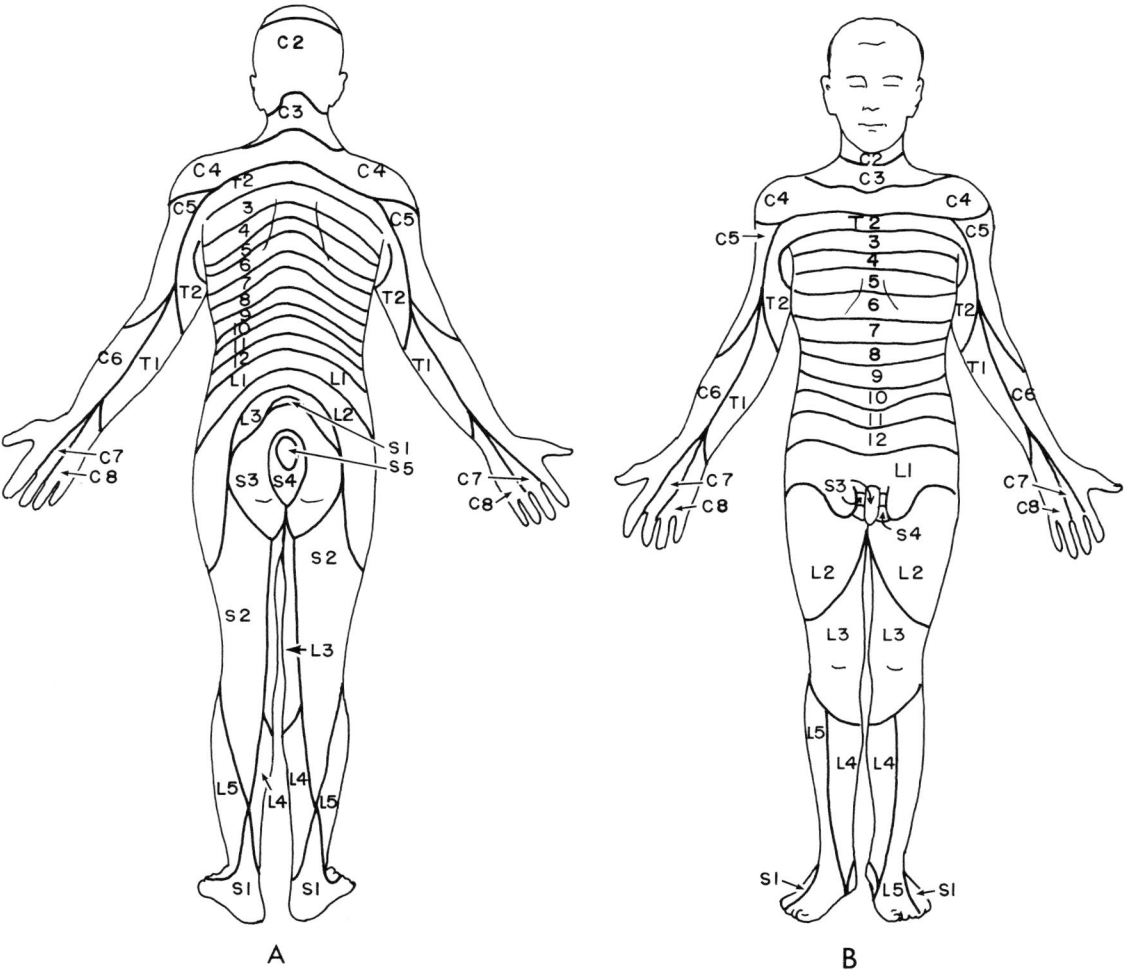

Figure 14–5 An outline of the sensory dermatomes. Note the cord levels present in the perianal area.

All voluntary motor control in the lower extremities is carefully recorded. In a similar manner the deep tendon reflexes are serially recorded. The abdomen is carefully inspected for the presence of abdominal cutaneous reflexes. The cremasteric reflex is carefully evaluated. Testing of the various dermatomes of the trunk and lower extremity is serially performed. The sensory dermatomes are outlined in Figure 14–5. Finally, a thorough evaluation of the motor and sensory function around the anal area is performed. As can be readily noted in Figure 14–5, several cord levels are represented in the small perianal area. A rectal examination will allow the examiner to determine the amount of anal sphincter tone present. The bulbocavernosus reflex is

examined, as outlined in Chapter 13. A favorable prognosis is reflected by muscle paralysis and concurrent absence of the deep tendon reflex, as this usually indicates a lower motor neuron lesion. Paralyzed muscles in the presence of intact deep tendon reflexes, however, usually indicate a spinal cord or upper motor neuron lesion and therefore are associated with a poor prognosis. The presence or absence of spinal shock must be determined, as outlined in the preceding chapter.

ROENTGENOGRAPHIC EXAMINATION

Patients with thoracolumbar spinal injuries, like those with cervical injuries,

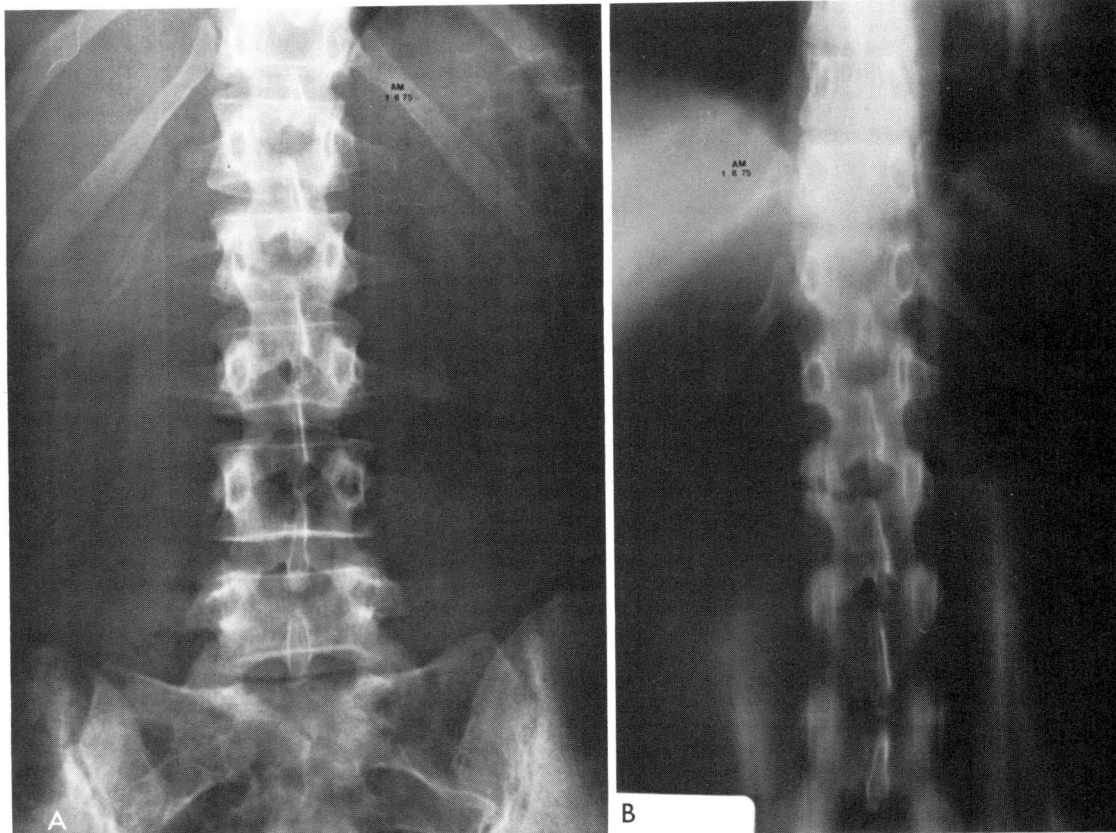

Figure 14–6 A. Anteroposterior roentgenogram of the lumbar spine with evidence suggestive of a defect through the pedicle at L2 on the right. B. Tomogram demonstrating definite disruption through the pedicle at L2 on the right.

frequently are brought to the emergency room during the early hours of the morning, and it is imperative that the physician accompany the patient to the radiology department in order to supervise the roentgenographic evaluation. It is best to leave the patient on the stretcher rather than to transfer him to the regular roentgenographic table. The first view that should be obtained is a straight lateral roentgenographic view of the thoracolumbar spine. This will provide insight into the presence of an unstable spinal fracture. If no evidence of a spinal fracture or dislocation is revealed, the technician can then proceed to a thorough evaluation of the entire thoracolumbar spine. The anteroposterior view must be obtained with the patient in supine position. If a physician does not supervise the roentgenographic evaluation, a patient

may inadvertently be placed in the seated position to obtain various roentgenographic views, which is contraindicated with this type of fracture. Both the lateral and anteroposterior views are then carefully scrutinized for evidence of disruption of the posterior complex. If there is evidence of such disruption, an unstable spine is present. The laminae, pedicles, and facet joints must be examined meticulously to rule out a fracture in this vital area. Occasionally tomograms are necessary to rule out a defect in the posterior complex as outlined in Figure 14–6.

The patient must not leave the radiology department until a thorough roentgenographic evaluation has excluded the possibility of an unstable spinal fracture. This is an additional reason why it is extremely important for the examining physician to be present during the performance of the roentgenographic examination. *Never send an unaccompanied patient to the radiology department for roentgenographic evaluation if an unstable spinal fracture is suspected.*

MECHANISMS OF INJURY

Injury to the thoracolumbar spine may be caused by local direct trauma or by peripheral indirect trauma. In military practice, many of the injuries to the spine were the result of direct trauma caused by missile wounds. A neurological deficit under these conditions is relatively common, as the force of the missile causes spreading and disruption of the spinal contents. These injuries are also complicated by being open injuries with direct communication between the exterior and the spinal cord and nerve roots.

In civilian practice, the majority of injuries are due to indirect trauma. The damage produced by indirect trauma is usually the result of excessive loading of the axial spine, sudden muscular contracture in a protective pattern, and excessive motion of the spine beyond the physiological limit. Several mechanisms of injury have been identified, among them hyperflexion, hyperextension, excessive lateral flexion, excessive rotation, axial load, distraction, and shear.

Flexion

As in the cervical spine, flexion injuries are the most common type. The deforming force characteristically injures that portion of the spine that is transitional between a fixed and mobile segment—in this area, the thoracolumbar junction and the lumbosacral junction. The flexion force tends to cause a compression-type injury to the anterior vertebral body, which dissipates a great portion of the energy, decreasing the amount of stress on the posterior ligaments. An explanation for the excessive anterior compressive force is found when we examine the fulcrums present with a flexion motion. In the thoracic region the distance between the tip of the spinous process and the flexion axis, compared with the distance

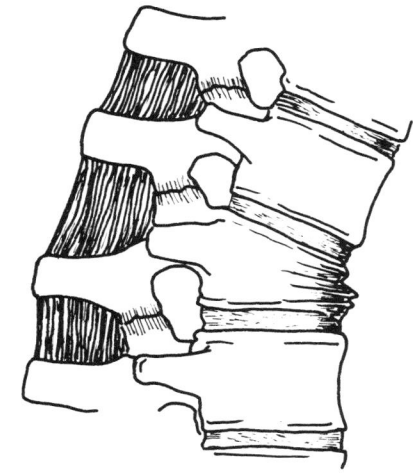

Figure 14–7 Diagrammatic representation of a flexion injury with compression of the anterior portion of the vertebral body. (Courtesy of F. W. Holdsworth and Journal of Bone and Joint Surgery. Fractures, dislocations and fracture-dislocations of the spine. J.B.J.S., *45B*:6–20, 1963.)

between the flexor axis and the anterior margin of the vertebral body, is 3 to 1. In the lumbar region this area is increased to a ratio of 4 to 1. In view of these ratios, it is not difficult to understand why the anterior margin of the vertebra experiences the greater portion of the load. If the anterior margin of the vertebra is not fractured and the energy was not partially dissipated, then there would tend to be a disruption of the posterior elements. In the usual sequence of events, however, with flexion injuries to the thoracolumbar spine the greater portion of the energy is dissipated in the production of an anterior marginal fracture, and the posterior ligamentous structures remain intact. These injuries are considered stable, as the posterior element complex is not affected. In general they are not associated with a neurological deficit.

Extension

Hyperextension injuries are infrequent in the thoracolumbar spine. When they do occur they may cause an avulsion fracture of the anterior portion of the vertebral body or a fracture through the pars interarticularis. The latter represents a true traumatic spondylolysis. Extension injuries are considered stable and are not associated with a neurological deficit. They are extremely rare in the thoracic region and occur very infrequently in the midlumbar region.

Lateral Flexion

Excessive lateral flexion will produce a compression fracture of the vertebral body similar to the anterior flexion lesion. The compressive load is placed on the lateral aspect of the vertebral body, and a typical compressive fracture is produced. These injuries, like the extension injuries, are very infrequent and when they do occur they occur similarly in the midlumbar region. They are considered stable and are not associated with a neurological deficit.

Rotation

A fracture produced by rotation alone is quite rare. A combination of rotation and flexion, however, is the most common cause of dislocation and fracture-dislocation in the thoracolumbar spine (Fig. 14–8). The rotation component of this injury increases the tensor component on the posterior element of the spine, causing failure. This type of injury occurs in the transitional area of the spine between T10 and L1. If the rotational

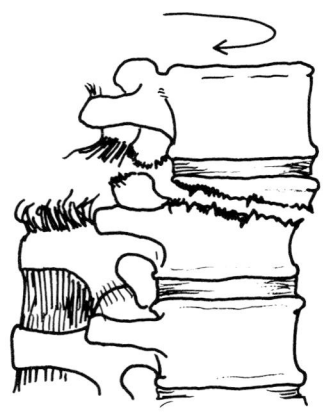

Figure 14–9 Diagrammatic representation of the more usual flexion-rotation injury with fracture of the facets. The upper vertebra swings upon the lower, carrying with it a typical slice fragment from the upper portion of the body of the lower vertebra. (Courtesy of F. W. Holdsworth and Journal of Bone and Joint Surgery. Fractures, dislocations and fracture-dislocations of the spine. J.B.J.S., *45B*:6–20, 1963.)

components involved with a rotation-flexion type injury are excessive, the lesion described by Holdsworth as "slice fracture-dislocation" may well be produced (Fig. 14–9). Fractures and dislocations caused by this mechanism of injury are unstable, and frequently a neurological deficit is present. A portion of this neurological deficit may be due to herniation of disc material compressing the neural elements. A roentgenogram will frequently reveal an oblique fracture of the vertebra with disruption of the posterior elements. Occasionally, the roentgenogram will be deceiving owing to spontaneous reduction of the fracture-dislocation, and unless the true extent of the injury is realized, an unstable spine will be unrecognized.

Shear

This type of injury is very deceiving when first seen roentgenographically; it is produced by a transverse shear force and it does not produce a wedge fracture of the vertebral body or angular displacement. It has the appearance of one vertebral body "jumped" forward over the inferior vertebral body without significant deformity of the inferior body. Because of the usual severe displacement produced, it is not

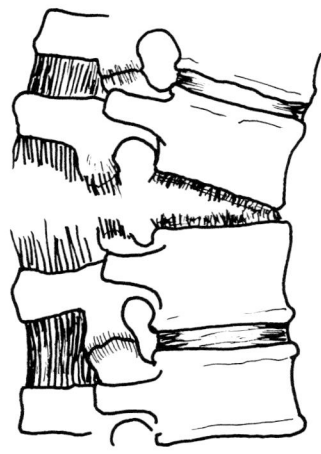

Figure 14–8 Diagrammatic representation of a flexion rotation injury in the lumbar spine demonstrating that a significant amount of flexion is required to disengage the large vertical articular processes in the lumbar spine. (Courtesy of F. W. Holdsworth and Journal of Bone and Joint Surgery. Fractures, dislocations and fracture-dislocations of the spine. J.B.J.S., *45B*:6–20, 1963.)

uncommon for this type of injury to present with a neurological deficit. In order to prevent further neurological deficit, the fracture must be reduced and stabilized.

Axial Load

Axial load fractures are produced by excessive vertical loading of the spinal segment. A variant of this type of injury may be seen in patients who are severely osteoporotic and in whom a compression fracture occurs secondary to spontaneous muscle contraction. The "cod fish" spine is also an expression of compressive stress on an osteoporotic spine. Occasionally a compressive force will produce a traumatic Schmorl's node due to protrusion of nuclear material through the vertebral end-plate. Holdsworth described the familiar "burst fracture" produced by an axial load force. The central portion of the vertebral body was severely compressed on both the superior and inferior aspects, and the result was a severely biconcave spine with a fracture line through the central portion. Occasionally displacement of the posterior portion of the vertebral body may cause a neurological deficit (Fig. 14–10).

Axial load fractures are considered stable but may be associated with a neurological deficit, although the majority are not.

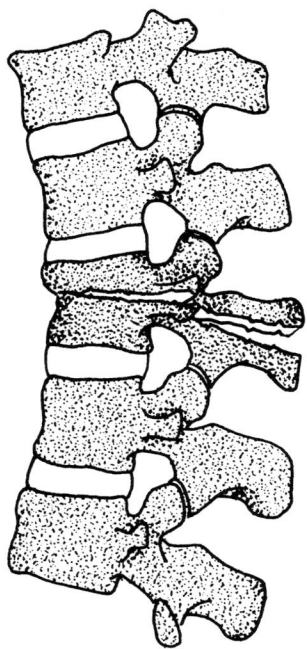

Figure 14–11 Diagrammatic representation of a Chance fracture of the vertebra. Note that it is essentially a horizontal fracture through the vertebral body and the posterior element.

Distraction

This type of injury is frequently seen in patients wearing lap seat-belts. It occurs between L1 and L4. In injury of this type the flexion axis is markedly altered. The point of contact between the seat-belt and the abdominal wall becomes the axis around which flexion occurs. This places all of the spinal column posterior to the flexion axis, and the vertebral body as well as the neural arch is exposed to a tensile stress. Roentgenographically, the spine appears as if it has been pulled apart. This entity was originally described by Dr. C. Q. Chance and has subsequently been referred to as the "Chance fracture." Although the vertebral body and the posterior elements are fractured, there is minimal damage to the major ligaments. Because of the remaining ligamentous structure and the coarse interdigitations across the fracture site, the spine is relatively stable. This is in marked contrast to the same type of injury with severe disruption of the ligamentous structures and a fracture-dislocation with displacement, which is definitely unstable and requires aggressive treatment.

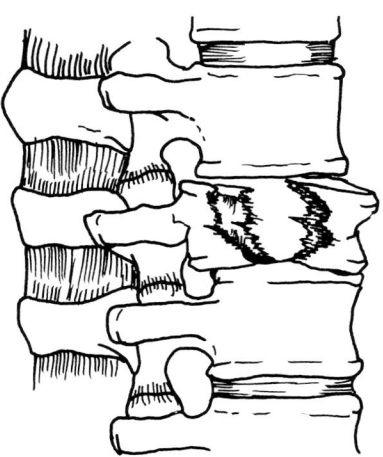

Figure 14–10 Diagrammatic representation of a "burst" fracture. (Courtesy of F. W. Holdsworth and Journal of Bone and Joint Surgery. Fractures, dislocations and fracture-dislocations of the spine. J.B.J.S., 45B:6–20, 1963.)

Muscle Contraction

For completeness' sake, violent muscle contraction must be included as a mechanism of injury in fractures of the lumbar process. These fractures are frequently multiple.

Fractures similar to the "clay shoveler's fracture" in the cervical spine are uncommon in the thoracolumbar spine.

CLASSIFICATION OF INJURIES — SPINAL STABILITY

It is extremely important during the assessment of a patient with a spinal fracture or fracture-dislocation to determine whether the spine is stable. The evaluation of spinal stability has received previous attention, particularly by Holdsworth.[16, 17] Stability of the spine is present if the fracture or dislocation will not become displaced during the repair. Instability of the spine is present if there is a possibility that during the course of treatment the fragments will shift position prior to the repair.

A useful method reported by Kelly and Whitesides for evaluating whether a spinal fracture or dislocation is stable is to consider the spine as composed of two structural columns. The anterior structural column consists of the vertebral bodies and disc. The posterior structural column comprises the neural arch, articular processes, and ligament. In concert, both of these structural columns maintain spinal stability. If both the structural columns have been disrupted, the spine is acutely unstable and is capable of significant displacement and neurological damage.[25]

TABLE 14–1   Thoracolumbar Spinal Stability

Stable
   Flexion (wedge fracture)
   Extension
   Axial load (burst)
   Lateral bending
   Pure distraction (Chance)
   Avulsion

Unstable
   Flexion-rotation
   Shear
   Distraction-dislocation

Table 14–1 gives a useful working classification for determining whether a spinal injury is stable or unstable.

TREATMENT OF THORACOLUMBAR INJURIES

Stable injuries of the thoracolumbar spine are fairly straightforward and do not present a therapeutic dilemma. This is not true, however, of unstable spinal fractures in the thoracolumbar area. At the present time there is a great deal of controversy about the exact management of patients with unstable injuries. Nicoll and Guttmann have been the major proponents of a conservative approach. Nicoll not only made a plea for conservative treatment but was also able to demonstrate that whether the spine was completely realigned did not appear to have any bearing on the incidence of significant low-back discomfort in follow-up. He was, in fact, able to demonstrate a negative correlation. Many patients, several years after their injury, complained of significant back pain in spite of roentgenographic evidence of good to excellent reduction of the spinal fracture. On the other hand, several patients without roentgenographic evidence of good alignment of their spinal fractures had very little back pain.[36]

Guttmann has also been a proponent of nonoperative conservative treatment of these injuries. He has also noted in follow-up that patients treated with bed rest and positional realignment of the fracture fragments obtained the best results. He compared long-term results in two groups of patients — the first group treated by his method of positional realignment in bed, and the second group operatively managed with open reduction and internal fixation with long spinal plates. The patients treated with spinal plates demonstrated evidence of progressive angulation at the fracture site with time in spite of adequate reduction immediately postoperatively. It was Guttmann's contention that patients should not be treated operatively for these injuries.[15]

On the other hand, at several centers in the United States, there have been experiments with early open reduction and internal fixation with various devices to allow early ambulation with the aid of plaster body jackets. A recent review by Flesch and co-workers of 40 patients treated with open reduction and internal fixation with Harrington rods along with a posterior fusion demonstrated excellent results.[13]

Weiss, in Poland, has developed a spring-loaded corrective device for the treatment of these injuries. She refers to the procedure as "dynamic spine alloplasty with the use of a spring-loaded device." Her results with the use of this device and early ambulation have been good.[49]

Stable Injuries

Flexion (Wedge-Fracture). The flexion fracture is a common injury seen in clinical practice (Fig. 14–12). The majority of the

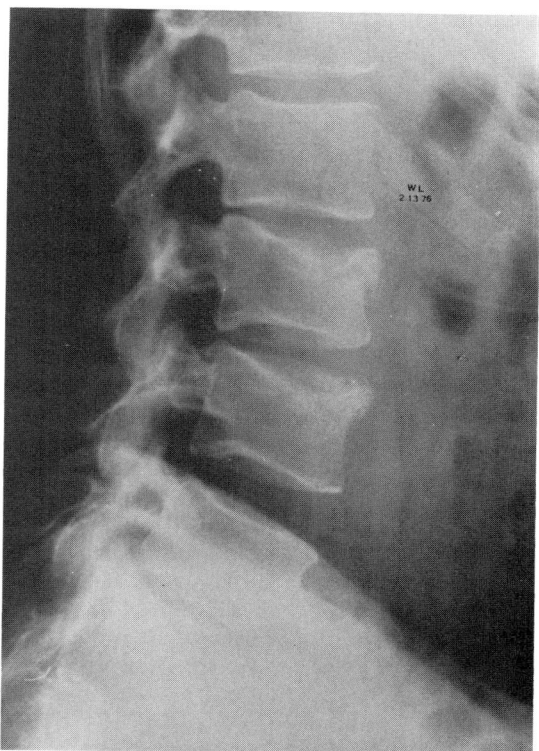

Figure 14–13 The flexion injury may occur at multiple levels, as indicated in this 20-year-old man.

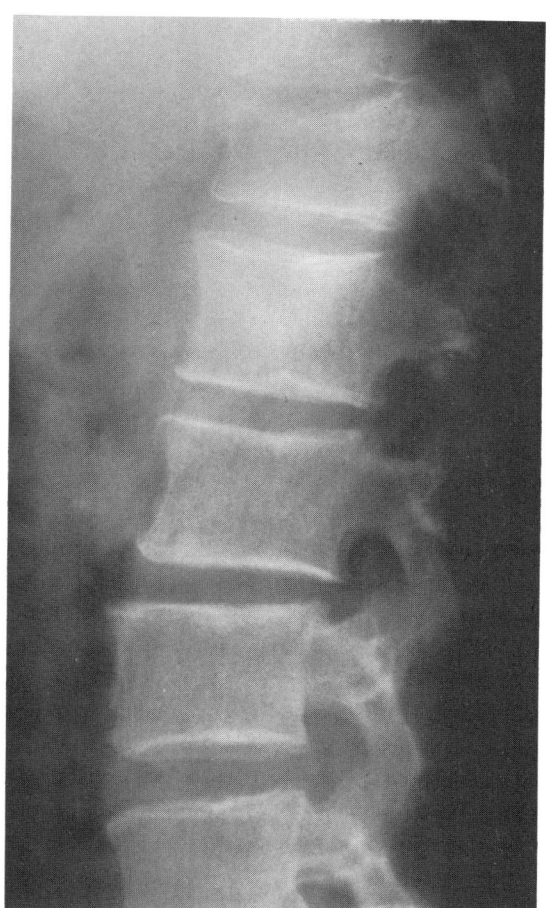

Figure 14–12 A flexion fracture of the T12 thoracic vertebra with compression of the anterior portion of the vertebral body.

patients present with evidence of axial osteoporosis. There is a very minimal history of flexion injury with the sudden onset of back pain that is usually localized to a single portion of the thoracolumbar spine. Occasionally these patients prove to have multiple flexion fractures, and under these conditions the pain is described as more diffuse (Fig. 14–13). Physical examination usually demonstrates localized tenderness to direct palpation directly over the involved spinous process. There is definite paraspinal reflex muscle spasm associated with the injury. Patients tend to assume an immobile posture in an attempt to splint the spine. Neurological deficits are not encountered with this type of injury. Patients are usually treated with bed rest in mild extension until they are comfortable, which usually requires two to three weeks. They are then gradually mobilized with the use of a spinal brace—the Knight-Taylor spinal brace is frequently employed. Every attempt should be made, however, to wean the patient from the spinal brace over a period of two to three months. Patients may become very dependent on the brace, which is the exact opposite of what the attending physician is trying to accomplish. The brace should be gradually discarded and the patient started on a course of Williams exercises for the spine. Since most of these patients suffer from axial osteoporosis, the only measure that can prevent these injuries is an aggressive course of spinal exercises to increase the spinal muscle tone as well as to decrease the amount of axial osteoporosis. Occasionally, patients will demonstrate an increased thoracic kyphosis secondary to flexion-compression fractures. This is because the anterior portion of the vertebral body absorbs the load from the flexion injury and is compressed, decreasing its anterior height. In this manner the posterior elements are unloaded and do not experience a severe tensile stress. It is this decrease in anterior vertebral body height that produces the increase in a thoracic gibbus. For this reason patients with this type of injury are initially treated with mild extension in an attempt to reduce the anterior vertebral body deformity that is present.

Extension. This injury is not as common in the thoracolumbar spine as it is in the cervical spine. Patients present with a similar history of sustaining a sudden extension injury to the thoracolumbar spine followed by back pain. Physical examination usually demonstrates a local area of pinpoint tenderness. There is paraspinal reflex muscle spasm present in the area. The commonest location in the thoracolumbar spine is in the midlumbar region. Lateral roentgenograms will occasionally reveal an avulsion fracture of the anterior portion of a vertebral body, produced by the anterior longitudinal ligament avulsing a portion of the vertebral body through its attachment.

Very occasionally patients will present with a history of a sudden extension injury to the thoracolumbar spine with low-back pain. Roentgenographic examination may reveal a stress fracture through the pars interarticularis, commonly known as true traumatic spondylolysis. Wiltse has written extensively on this type of injury. It is his feeling that the typical pars interarticularis defect that occurs at L5 may well be due to a stress fracture secondary to extension injuries of the lower lumbar spine. He feels that patients presenting with this history and injury should be treated with a body cast in order to place the spine at relative rest until the fracture has a chance to heal.[53, 54] Although the exact etiology of the typical pars interarticularis defect is still controversial, Wiltse's theory certainly appears attractive, particularly as applied to the patient with an extension injury.

In summary, extension injuries can be treated in a conservative fashion with bed rest for two to three weeks until the pain subsides followed by gradual mobilization with the aid of a spinal brace.

Axial Load (Burst Fractures). These fractures are produced by a sudden axial

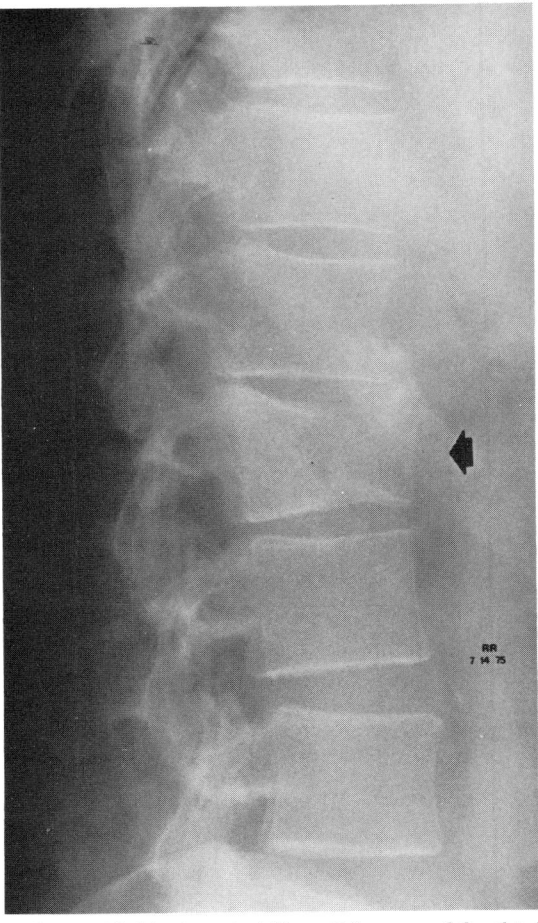

Figure 14-14 A typical "burst" fracture of the third lumbar vertebra.

load on the thoracolumbar spine. Holds-worth has described this type of fracture as a typical "burst" fracture.[16] The force is transmitted through the central portion of the vertebra, resulting in disruption of the end-plate and a fracture through the central portion of the vertebra. Comminution is frequently present. The anterior and posterior segments of the vertebral body may be separated. Occasionally the posterior portion of the vertebra may migrate into the spinal canal and result in a neurological deficit. The average case, however, does not present with a neurological deficit, and the injury is stable. Frequently, spontaneous fusion will occur owing to the gross comminution of the vertebral body with disruption of the end-plate. The treatment for this injury is immobilization of the lumbar spine until spontaneous fusion occurs. It is not uncommon to immobilize these patients for

10 to 12 weeks. They usually do not have back pain at follow-up.

Patients with posterior migration of the vertebral fragment and a resultant neurological deficit require a different form of treatment. The neurological deficit may be minimal initially, only to progress with time. In these patients it is extremely important to decompress the spine in order to relieve the pressure on the spinal cord. This involves an anterior approach to the lumbar fracture. The appropriate form of treatment is an anterior abdominal approach to the injured segment and removal of the vertebral fragments from the front. This will provide direct visualization of the spinal cord. Once the decompression has been completed, tibial or fibular strut bone grafts can be inserted between the vertebrae above and below to provide stability. It does not make sense to the author to attack

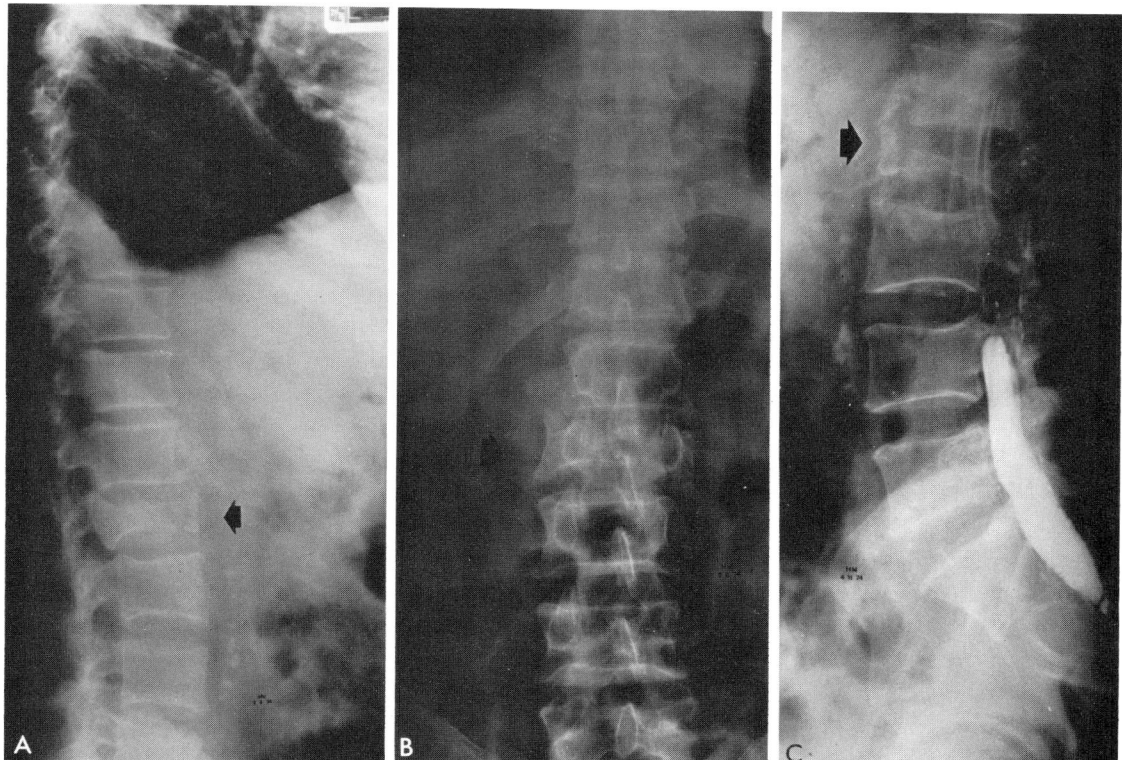

Figure 14–15   *A*. Lateral roentgenogram of a "burst" fracture with posterior migration of the vertebra into the spinal canal. *B*. Anteroposterior roentgenogram of the "burst" fracture revealing the significant disruption of the second lumbar vertebra. *C*. Follow-up lateral roentgenogram of the same patient, who was treated initially with open reduction, removal of the protruding posterior vertebral fragment from an anterior approach, and insertion of fibular strut grafts between the vertebrae to provide stability.

this problem from a posterior approach, as the posterior aspect would render the spine unstable. Also, the fragments cannot be removed as adequately from a posterior approach as they can from an anterior approach. The patients are then placed in a body jacket postoperatively and gradually mobilized by six weeks.

Lateral Bending. This injury is similar to a flexion wedge fracture but occurs in the lateral aspect of the vertebral body. It may be managed conservatively with bed rest until the acute pain subsides, followed by gradual mobilization with or without a spinal brace. These injuries as a rule do not cause problems in follow-up care.

Pure Distraction (Chance Fracture). This injury was originally described by C. Q. Chance in 1948.[7] He felt that it was a flexion-type fracture of the spine. In the present day this type of fracture is usually incurred by a person wearing a lap seat belt in an automobile accident. Smith and Kaufer have recently defined this fracture. It usually occurs between L1 and L4. The lap-type seat belt alters the flexion axis. A sudden deceleration causes the body to flex over the restraining belt, and the point of contact between the lap seat belt and the abdominal wall becomes the axis around which flexion occurs. Since the entire spinal column is posterior to the flexion axis, the entire vertebral complex including the neural arch is exposed to a tensile stress.[46] These injuries are felt to be stable, as there is minimal damage to the major ligaments. The interdigitation of the osseous irregularities on the opposing surfaces accounts for the fact that the Chance fracture is resistant to displacement. It usually heals rapidly through cancellous bone. Patients usually present without a neurological deficit, as there has not been any translational displacement of vertebral column. It is important to bear in mind that this type of fracture is completely different from the distraction-dislocation type of fracture that results in translational displacement of the vertebral column. This is discussed later under unstable injuries.

Avulsion. This type of fracture occurs in the lumbar transverse processes. It is due to sudden contraction of the surrounding musculature with avulsion of the transverse process proper. These injuries are painful

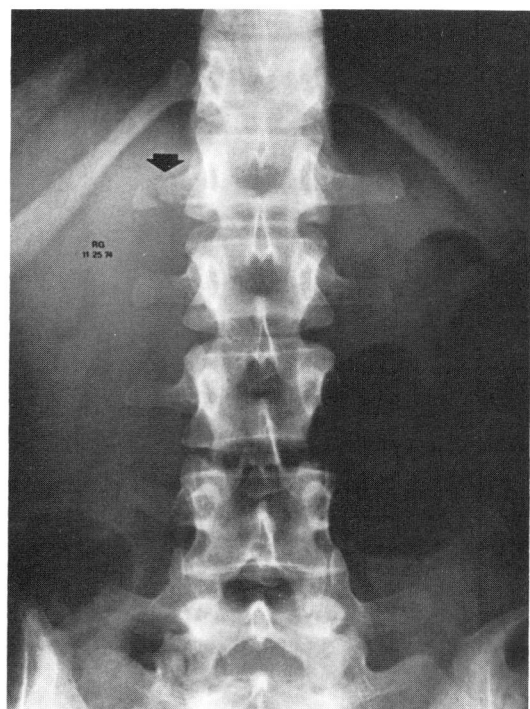

Figure 14–16 Avulsion fracture of the first lumbar transverse process on the right.

for three to four weeks, but they are stable and do not present any problem in follow-up. They may occur at multiple levels. Nonunion is frequent but does not appear to present any specific problem.

Avulsion fractures may be treated by initial bed rest for one to two weeks until the patient's acute pain subsides and then by gradual mobilization.

Unstable Injuries

Flexion-Rotation. This type of injury is the most common cause of dislocation and fracture-dislocation in the thoracolumbar spine. The majority of these injuries occur at the transitional area between T10 and L1, which is predisposed to them by the relative fixity of the thoracic area from T1 to T10 and the relative mobility of the lumbar area from L1 to L4 secondary to the orientation of the facet joints.

At least 70 to 80 per cent of patients with this injury present with a significant neurological deficit. This is due to the translational displacement of the vertebral body

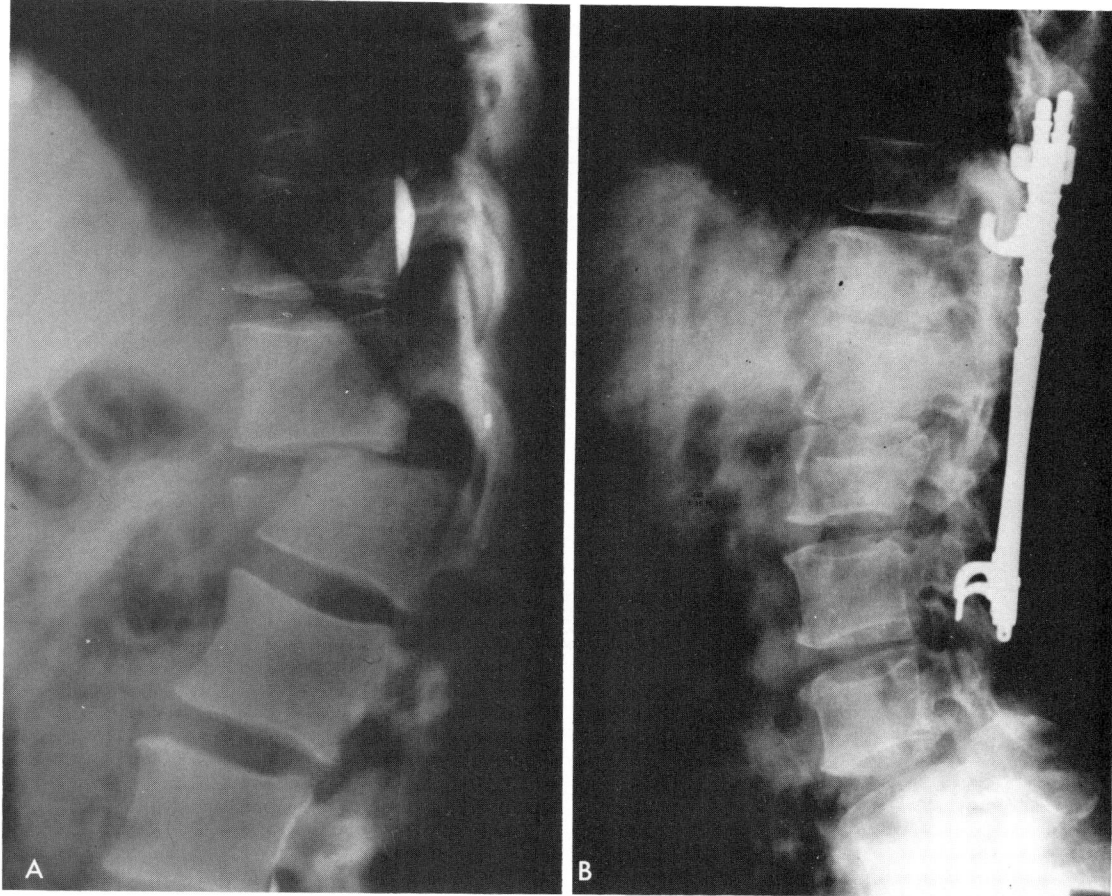

Figure 14-17 A. A typical "slice fracture-dislocation" as described by Holdsworth. *B.* The fracture was treated with open reduction and internal fixation with two Harrington distraction rods and a posterior fusion. Note that the distraction hooks have been placed two vertebrae above and two vertebrae below the fracture site. Anatomical alignment has been restored.

secondary to the fracture. Holdsworth originally coined the term "slice fracture-dislocation" for this type of injury.[16]

As stated in the beginning of this chapter, the management of these patients remains controversial. The author has been impressed with the results obtained by open reduction and internal fixation with two Harrington distraction rods and a posterior fusion. Initially, it is appropriate to treat the patient conservatively on a Stryker-type frame until the edema around the spinal cord has a chance to subside. This also means that a gentle attempt at reduction by mild extension of the area should be made on the Stryker frame. It is unwise to operate on these patients immediately, as they do

have a significant amount of edema and the surgery adds insult to the injury. Therefore, the surgery is generally usually performed five to seven days postinjury. In the meantime the patients have received large doses of dexamethasone. The author has administered 10 mg of dexamethasone initially followed by 4 to 6 mg every four hours. These are large doses, but the experimental evidence is very convincing that this is the dose required to reduce swelling. It is important to have good nursing care for these patients. They must be turned every two hours on the Stryker frame. As discussed in Chapter 13, the author condemns the circle electric bed for this type of injury.

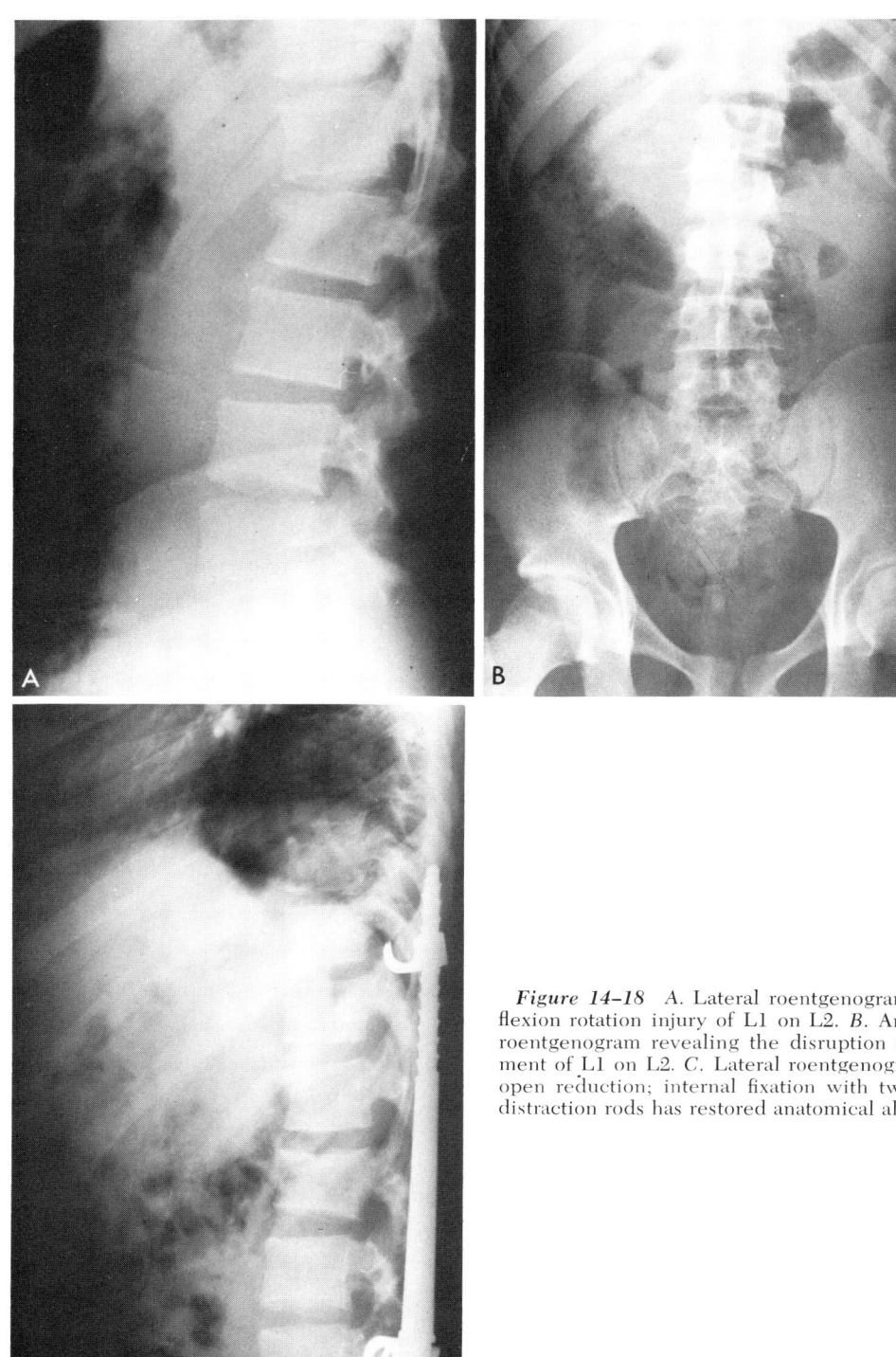

Figure 14–18 A. Lateral roentgenogram revealing a flexion rotation injury of L1 on L2. *B.* Anteroposterior roentgenogram revealing the disruption and malalignment of L1 on L2. *C.* Lateral roentgenogram following open reduction; internal fixation with two Harrington distraction rods has restored anatomical alignment.

At the end of five to seven days the patient is taken to the operating room on the Stryker frame, and a general anesthetic is administered. The patient is then gently rolled over on the operating table in a prone position. Positioning on the operating table is important, as some provision must be made to hyperextend the thoracolumbar spine if necessary. Following appropriate preparation and draping, a standard midline incision is utilized to expose the spinous processes of the vertebrae above and below the fracture site. If Harrington rods are to be employed in the treatment of these patients the rods must be secured at least two vertebrae above and two vertebrae below the fracture site to provide adequate three-point fixation. Generally, the spinous process is disrupted at the level of the fracture site and minimal dissection is required to expose the spinal cord at this level. A no. 1251 purchase hook is inserted in the standard fashion two vertebrae above the fracture site. A no. 1253 inferior purchase hook is inserted two vertebrae below the fracture site. The correct length of rod is then selected. The outrigger is applied to the purchase hooks and the spine is gradually distracted. A lateral roentgenogram is obtained in the operating room in order to evaluate the amount of distraction. The posterior spinous processes and laminae of the two vertebra above and below are then decorticated, and the Harrington rods are inserted in the standard fashion. A check roentgenogram is obtained following final distraction of the rods. The one contraindication to use of the Harrington distraction rods is the presence of definite destruction of the anterior longitudinal ligament. The rationale for utilizing Harrington distraction rods is that they normally restore the spine to reasonable alignment, allow reduction of the translational displacement, and maintain the reduction by three-point fixation by the purchase above and below the fracture site. The anterior longitudinal ligament acts as a checkrein to prevent overdistraction of the vertebral bodies. If the ligament is completely disrupted, it is possible to overdistract the vertebral bodies and injure the spinal cord directly.

It is for this reason that investigators at some centers in the United States have elected to use the Harrington compression

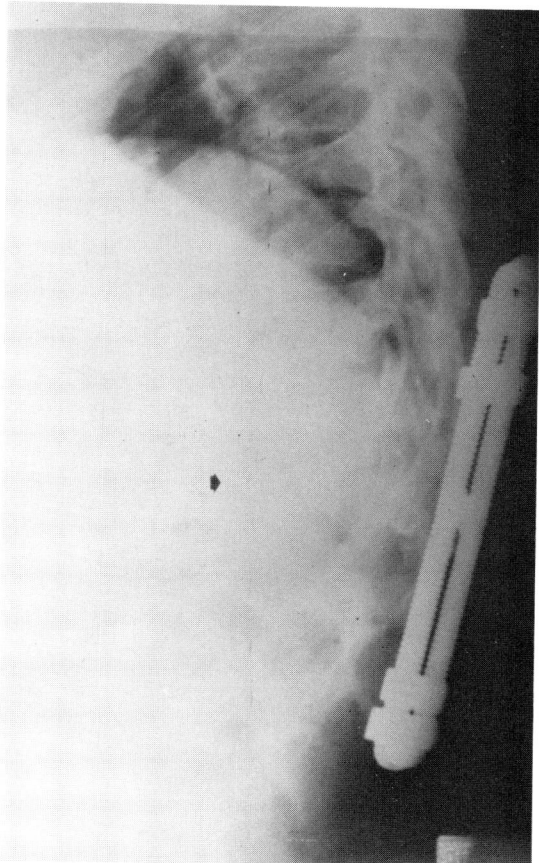

Figure 14–19 A patient was initially treated with open reduction and internal fixation with the Meuhrig-Williams spinal plate. Alignment was excellent immediately postoperatively. In follow-up, however, there is severe angulation at the fracture site.

rods rather than the distraction rods. These investigators feel that the compression rods provide better stability and the possible damage due to overdistraction is therefore avoided.

The Meuhrig-William spinal plate is to be condemned for treatment of these injuries. Several excellent studies have revealed that this device does not provide adequate fixation for the fractured spine. The majority of patients demonstrate increasing angulation at the fracture site despite the spinal plate. The author has seen several examples of this forward progressive translational deformity of the vertebral bodies following insertion of these spinal plates.

If the Harrington distraction rods have

been utilized to provide stability of the injured vertebra, the patient is placed in a posterior plaster shell postoperatively until the acute edema from the operative procedure subsides. The high-dosage dexamethasone maintenance program is continued. One of the problems with this high-dosage steroid therapy is that there is a definitely greater incidence of wound complications postoperatively. Therefore, the author feels that intraoperative and postoperative antibiotic coverage is essential for these patients. One week postoperatively the patients are taken to the cast room, where the sutures are removed and Steri-strips are applied to the wound. A body jacket is then applied by placing the patient on a Risser frame. Within one week after application of the plaster body jacket the patients are gradually mobilized with the use of ancillary devices.

Patients presenting with a complete neurological deficit in association with this injury are treated in a very similar manner. The only additional precaution is adequate padding of the plaster jacket that is applied. For these patients, the author has employed a molded plastic body jacket similar to that described for use in association with the low-profile halo in cervical spine fracture. In this manner pressure sores can be avoided.

Flesch and associates have recently reported their results in management of patients with unstable thoracolumbar spine fractures. Their group included 40 patients, 35 of whom had neurological deficit. Five were neurologically normal, twelve had complete cord lesions, and twenty-three had incomplete cord or cauda equina lesions. Twenty-one of these last appeared to improve with this treatment. They found that the average length of time for the body jacket to be worn was five months. Patients treated with the Harrington distraction rods tended to fare better than those treated with compression rods.[13] This is a very encouraging report.

The alternate form of therapy is postural reduction, first advocated by Hippocrates and then by Malgaigne, which has more recently been championed by Guttmann. This is a more conservative approach, and Guttmann felt that some degree of forward collapse was inevitable with unstable fractures and dislocations of the thoracolumbar spine; therefore he stated that a posterior spinal plate was futile.[15] Nicoll also felt that postural reduction and conservative treatment was the procedure of choice. It was his feeling that the majority of these patients went on to spontaneous anterior fusions following conservative treatment.[36] Kaufer and Hayes, however, in a recent review felt that only 14 per cent of patients progressed to a spontaneous anterior fusion. They recommended that these injuries should be treated with open reduction and internal fixation with wiring of the spinous processes.[23]

If the conservative nonoperative approach is selected, gradual postural reduction must be accomplished with the use of pillows or sandbags under the appropriate spinal level. The patients must then be kept in bed for at least 12 weeks prior to gradual mobilization with an external support. We must bear in mind, however, that Nicoll felt that a perfect anatomical reduction was not absolutely necessary. In fact, at follow-up, many of his patients with perfect alignment continued to have some back pain while patients without perfect alignment did not have severe back pain. This may have been because the patients with perfect anatomical alignment were placed in unphysiological positions to maintain the alignment. It is possible that this contributed to the persistent back pain. The problem with the conservative approach is that it requires meticulous nursing care. The patients must be turned at least every two hours to prevent bed sores. Many patients without a neurological deficit still find it difficult to void in the supine position following a vertebral injury. This requires repeated intermittent straight catheterization to avoid urinary tract infections. Pneumonia may develop in these patients owing to splinting of the spine and reduction in active pulmonary toilet due to the pain. The results obtained by both Nicoll and Guttmann with their conservative nonoperative approach to this problem were, however, certainly excellent.

Paraplegia may be present in association with a fracture-rotation-type injury. Investigators at several centers in the United States have recently advised an aggressive operative approach for these patients to prevent unstable spines in the long term. The overall feeling is that if the spine is stabilized with an internal fixation device, then the patients may be gradually mobilized, preventing the secondary complications and in particular preventing progressive angulation deformities secondary to these injuries. It is the author's feeling that the rehabilitation program may be improved by stabilization of the spine and future spinal deformities may be prevented. If the injury involves the lumbar spine, the neurological deficit may be due to nerve root damage and recovery of partial function may occur.

Shear Fractures. Shear fractures may occur without any evidence of a wedge deformity of the inferior vertebra. The initial roentgenograms may be deceiving, as the only evidence of this type of injury is translational displacement of one vertebra forward on the vertebra below without significant alteration of the inferior vertebral body. At the time of injury, however, there was probably more translational displacement than is present when the patient is initially evaluated in the hospital. Once the patient is placed on a stretcher in a supine position the displacement may gradually diminish. The great danger in management of this type of injury is that it may not be recognized initially. The majority of patients present with a neurological deficit secondary to the initial translational displacement. This is an extremely unstable injury, and it is the author's feeling that these patients should have open reduction and internal fixation to prevent further displacement. This is an ideal circumstance for the insertion of Harrington compression rods rather than distraction rods for internal fixation. Weiss compression springs have also been advocated in some centers for this type of injury. Paraplegia or a severe neurological deficit is not a contraindication for open reduction and internal fixation for the reasons mentioned in the preceding section.

Distraction-Dislocation. This type of injury is essentially a Chance fracture but with significant displacement of the upper portion of the vertebra over the lower portion. This is an extremely unstable fracture in contradistinction to the regular Chance hemivertebra fracture without displace-

ment. In this particular injury there is ligamentous disruption as well as the hemivertebral fracture. As in the shear fracture, the amount of displacement when initially seen is probably less than the amount of displacement at the time of the accident. It requires an aggressive approach to prevent further neurological injury from translational displacement. The Harrington compression rod is an excellent device for fixation of this particular fracture-dislocation. A neurological deficit due to the amount of initial displacement may well be present. The concept of stabilizing the spine and then mobilizing these patients with the use of external support appeals to the author.

Role of Laminectomy

As with cervical spine injuries, the role of laminectomy in the treatment of injuries of the thoracolumbar spine is very limited indeed; the only "absolute" indication for it is the presence of a progressing neurological deficit. This concept has been a major advance in the treatment of spinal fractures. In the past, many patients in whom the onset of complete paraplegia immediately followed their injury received laminectomies. It was felt by the attending surgeon that "all that was possible should be done." This attitude is no longer acceptable. Not only did the laminectomy not produce significant improvement in the neurological status but it also increased the instability of the spine. The attending surgeon was then faced with a grossly unstable spine along with a permanent neurological deficit, and frequently a secondary procedure was required to provide some spinal stability. Osterholm and White in separate studies have recorded the sequential changes in the spinal cord following injury. Osterholm[38a] was able to demonstrate that small areas of hemorrhage occurred within the spinal cord associated with release of norepinephrine. The hemorrhagic areas then coalesced, with almost complete destruction of the central portion of the spinal cord. White was able to document sequential histological changes in the spinal cord following a standard injury. The same sequence of events, beginning with small punctate areas of hemorrhage followed by hemorrhagic necrosis of the spinal cord, was demonstrated.[52] With these two studies in mind, it is very difficult for the author to visualize just how a laminectomy could improve the neurological picture. The damage to the spinal cord has already occurred at the time of the injury. The hemorrhagic necrosis that occurs in the cord is completely unrelated to any type of decompressive laminectomy. It would seem futile indeed to expect a laminectomy to provide decompression and relief of the neurological picture when there already is hemorrhagic necrosis occurring within the spinal cord itself. This is not the case when a patient presents initially without a neurological deficit or with a minimal neurological deficit that appears to progress over a period of time. Under these conditions, a decompressive laminectomy is certainly warranted and should be performed as soon as possible.

The foregoing rationale appears fairly straightforward, but many years passed before it was completely accepted. This has been a major advance in the management of patients with spinal injury.

REFERENCES

1. Albin, M. S., White, R. J., Acosta-Rua, G., and Yashon, D.: Study of functional recovery produced by delayed localized cooling after spinal cord injury in primates. J. Neurosurg., 29:113–120, 1968.
2. Aufdermaur, M.: Spinal injuries in juveniles. J. Bone Joint Surg., 56B:513–519, 1974.
3. Bedbrook, G. M.: Treatment of thoracolumbar dislocation and fracture with paraplegia. Clin. Orthop., 112:27–43, 1975.
4. Benassy, J., Blanchard, J., and Lecog, P.: Neurologic recovery rate in para- and tetraplegia. Paraplegia, 4:239–263, 1967.
5. Böhler, J.: Operative treatment of fractures of the dorsal and lumbar spine. J. Trauma, 10:1119–1122, 1970.
6. Carey, P. D.: Neurosurgery and paraplegia. Rehabilitation, 31:27–29, 1965.
7. Chance, C. Q.: Note on a type of flexion fracture of the spine. Br. J. Radiol., 21:452–453, 1948.
8. Davis, L.: Treatment of spinal cord injuries. Arch. Surg., 69:488–495, 1954.
9. Dewey, P., and Browne, P. S. H.: Fracture-dislocation of the lumbosacral spine with cauda equina lesion. J. Bone Joint Surg., 50B:635–638, 1968.
9a. Dickson, J. H., Harrington, P. R., and Erwin, W.: Results of reduction and stabilization of the severely fractured thoracic and lumbar spine. J. Bone Joint Surg., 60A:799–805, 1978.
10. Dommisse, G. F.: The blood supply of the spinal cord. A critical vascular zone in spinal surgery. J. Bone Joint Surg., 56B:225–235, 1974.
11. Ducker, T. B., and Hamit, H. F.: Experimental treatment of acute spinal cord injury. J. Neurosurg., 30:693–697, 1969.
12. Elliot, H. C.: Cross sectional diameters and areas of the human spinal cord. Anat. Rec., 93:287–293, 1945.
13. Flesch, J. R., Leider, L. L., Erickson, D. L., Chou, S. N., and Bradford, D. S.: Harrington instrumentation and spine fusion for unstable fractures and fracture-dislocations of the thoracic and lumbar spine. J. Bone Joint Surg., 59A:143–153, 1977.
14. Gregersen, G. G., and Lucas, D. B.: An in vivo study of the axial rotation of the human thoracolumbar spine. J. Bone Joint Surg., 49A:247–262, 1967.
15. Guttman, L.: Surgical aspects of the treatment of traumatic paraplegia. J. Bone Joint Surg., 31B:399–403, 1949.
16. Holdsworth, F. W.: Fractures, dislocations and fracture-dislocations of the spine. J. Bone Joint Surg., 45B:6–20, 1963.
17. Holdsworth, F. W.: Fractures, dislocations and fracture-dislocations of the spine. J. Bone Joint Surg., 52A:1534–1551, 1970.
18. Holdsworth, F. W., and Hardy, A.: Early treatment of paraplegia from fractures of the thoracolumbar spine. J. Bone Joint Surg., 35B:540–550, 1953.
19. Howland, W. J., Curry, J. L., and Buffington, C. G.: Fulcrum fractures of the lumbar spine. J.A.M.A., 193:240–241, 1965.
20. Huelke, D. F., and Kaufer, H.: Vertebral column injuries and seat belts. J. Trauma, 15:304–318, 1975.
21. Kahn, E. A.: Editorial on spinal cord injuries. J. Bone Joint Surg., 41A:6–11, 1969.
22. Kallio, E.: Injuries of the thoracolumbar spine with paraplegia. Acta Orthop. Scand., (Suppl. 60): 1963.
23. Kaufer, H., and Hayes, J. T.: Lumbar fracture-dislocation. A study of 21 cases. J. Bone Joint Surg., 48A:712–730, 1966.
24. Kelly, D. L., Jr., Lassiter, K. R., Calogero, J. A., and Alexander, E., Jr.: Effects of local hypothermia and tissue. Oxygen studies in experimental paraplegia. J. Neurosurg., 33:554–563, 1970.
25. Kelly, R. P., and Whitesides, T. E., Jr.: Treatment of lumbodorsal fracture-dislocations. Ann. Surg., 167:705–717, 1968.
26. Kilfoyle, R. M., Foley, J. J., and Norton, P. L.: Spine and pelvic deformity in childhood and adolescent paraplegia. A study of 104 cases. J. Bone Joint Surg., 47A:659–682, 1965.
27. Lafferty, J. F., Winter, W. G., and Gambaro, S. A.: Fatigue characteristics of posterior elements of vertebrae. J. Bone Joint Surg., 59A:154–158, 1977.
28. Lewis, J., and McKibbin, B.: The treatment of unstable fracture-dislocations of the thoracolumbar spine accompanied by paraplegia. J. Bone Joint Surg., 56B:603–612, 1974.
29. Lumsden, R. M., and Morris, J. M.: An in vivo study of axial rotation and immobilization at the lumbosacral joint. J. Bone Joint Surg., 50A:1591–1602, 1968.
30. Markolf, K. L.: Deformation of the thoracolumbar intervertebral joints in response to external

loads. A biomechanical study using autopsy material. J. Bone Joint Surg., *54A*:511–533, 1972.

31. Morgan, T. H., Wharton, G. W., and Austin, G. N.: The results of laminectomy in patients with incomplete spinal cord injuries. Paraplegia, 9: 14–23, 1971.

32. Morris, J. M.: Biomechanics of the spine. Arch. Surg., *107*:418–423, 1973.

33. Morris, J. M., Lucas, D. B., and Bresler, B.: Role of the trunk in stability of the spine. J. Bone Joint Surg., *43A*:327–351, 1961.

34. Munro, D.: The role of fusion or wiring in the treatment of acute traumatic instability of the spine. Paraplegia, 3:97–111, 1966.

35. Naffziger, H. C.: The neurological aspects of injuries to the spine. J. Bone Joint Surg., *20*:444–448, 1938.

36. Nicoll, E. A.: Fractures of the dorsolumbar spine. J. Bone Joint Surg., *31B*:376–394, 1949.

37. Norton, P. L., and Brown, T.: The immobilizing efficiency of back braces. J. Bone Joint Surg., *39A*:111–139, 1957.

38. Olsson, O.: Fractures of the upper thoracic and cervical vertebral bodies. Acta Chir. Scand., *102*:87–92, 1951.

38a. Osterholm, J. L., and Mathews, G. J.: Altered norepinephrine metabolism following experimental spinal cord injury. J. Neurosurg., *36*: 386–394, 1972.

39. Rennie, W., and Mitchell, N.: Flexion distraction fracture of the thoracolumbar spine. J. Bone Joint Surg., *55A*:386–390, 1973.

40. Roaf, R.: A study of the mechanics of spinal injuries. J. Bone Joint Surg., *42B*:810–823, 1960.

41. Roberts, J. B., and Curtiss, P. H., Jr.: Stability of the thoracic and lumbar spine in traumatic paraplegia following fracture or fracture-dislocation. J. Bone Joint Surg., *52A*:1115–1130, 1970.

42. Rogers, W. A.: Cord injury during reduction of thoracic and lumbar vertebral-body fracture and dislocation. J. Bone Joint Surg., *20*:689–695, 1938.

43. Schmorl, G., and Junghanns, H.: The Human Spine in Health and Disease. New York, Grune & Stratton, 1971.

44. Schneider, R. C.: Surgical indications and contraindications in spine and spinal cord trauma. Clin. Neurosurg., 8:157–184, 1962.

45. Schneider, R. C., Crosby, E. C., Russo, R. H., and Gosch, H. H.: Traumatic spinal cord syndromes and their management. Clin. Neurosurg., *20*: 424–492, 1973.

46. Smith, W. S., and Kaufer, H.: Patterns and mechanisms of lumbar injuries associated with lap seat belts. J. Bone Joint Surg., *51A*:239–254, 1969.

47. Stanger, J. K.: Fracture-dislocation of the thoracolumbar spine. With special reference to reduction by open and closed operations. J. Bone Joint Surg., *29*:107–118, 1947.

48. Stauffer, E. S., and Neil, J. L.: Biomechanical analysis of structural stability of internal fixation in fractures of the thoracolumbar spine. Clin. Orthop., *112*:159–164, 1975.

49. Weiss, M.: Dynamic spine alloplasty (spring-loading corrective devices) after fracture and spinal cord injury. Clin. Orthop., *112*:150–158, 1975.

50. Westerborn, A., and Olsson, O.: Mechanics, treatment and prognosis of fractures of the dorsolumbar spine. Acta Chir. Scand., *102*:59–83, 1951.

51. White, A. A., III, and Hirsch, C.: The significance of the vertebral posterior elements in the mechanics of the thoracic spine. Clin. Orthop., *81*:2–14, 1971.

51a. White, A. A., and Panjabi, M. M.: Clinical Biomechanics of the Spine. Pp. 1–534. Philadelphia, J. B. Lippincott Co., 1978.

52. White, R. J.: Pathology of spinal cord injury in experimental lesions. Clin. Orthop., *112*:16–26, 1975.

53. Wiltse, L. L.: The etiology of spondylolisthesis. J. Bone Joint Surg., *44A*:539–560, 1962.

54. Wiltse, L. L., Widell, E. H., and Jackson, D. W.: Fatigue fracture: The basic lesion in isthmic spondylolisthesis. J. Bone Joint Surg., *57A*:17–22, 1975.

55. Yocum, T. D., Leatherman, K. D., and Brower, T. D.: The early rod fixation in treatment of fracture-dislocations of the spine. (Abstr.) J. Bone Joint Surg., *52A*:1257, 1970.

56. Yosipovitch, Z., Robin, G. C., and Makin, M: Open reduction of unstable thoracolumbar spinal injuries and fixation with Harrington rods. J. Bone Joint Surg., *59A*:1003–1015, 1977.

57. Young, M. H.: Long term consequences of stable fractures of the thoracic and lumbar vertebral bodies. J. Bone Joint Surg., *55B*:295–300, 1973.

R. BRUCE HEPPENSTALL, M.D.

15 _____ Injuries of the Shoulder Girdle

Injuries to the shoulder girdle involve both the osseous structures and the surrounding soft tissue. They account for a significant number of the patients seen in an average orthopedic practice. A more thorough understanding of the biomechanics of shoulder function has aided in the recognition and management of these complex injuries.

Hippocrates recognized the problems in diagnosis of shoulder injuries and became interested in the management of shoulder dislocations.[2] He described the different types of shoulder dislocations as well as the anatomical variations involved. His method of reducing shoulder dislocations is still practiced today. Hippocrates also described a burning procedure for the treatment of shoulder dislocations in which the burning iron was inserted through the axilla to produce a scar in the distal portion of the shoulder joint. It is interesting that today we still attempt to produce some type of scar along the anterior aspect of the shoulder joint for the operative management of shoulder dislocations.

Fractures involving the shoulder girdle were also recognized during the time of Hippocrates, and it was common practice to immobilize the shoulder for an extended period until healing was complete. The problem with this type of management is that it frequently produces a very stiff and painful shoulder. This old concept has given way to the more modern approach of

attempting to return the injured part to functional activity as early as possible, as outlined in other sections of this book. That is not to state that aggressive physical therapy is the sole answer. Therapy has a place in the management of shoulder injuries, but forceful manipulation of the shoulder may hinder rather than aid progress. It is extremely important to have a thorough working knowledge of soft tissue and osseous wound healing if appropriate treatment programs are to be properly implemented. The shoulder is similar to the knee in that both these joints rely very heavily on surrounding soft tissue structures for function and stability.

The first portion of this chapter will deal with the recognition and management of fractures of the shoulder girdle; this will be followed by a discussion of the various dislocations of the shoulder girdle.

SURGICAL ANATOMY

The shoulder girdle involves the following structures: (1) the scapula, including the glenoid fossa, spine, and acromion process; (2) the acromioclavicular joint; (3) the clavicle; (4) the sternoclavicular joint; and (5) the associated ligamentous and muscular structures in the osseous configuration.

The scapula presents a dorsal and a costal surface for muscular attachments. The coracoid process extends in a proximal, forward and lateral position from the superior aspect of the scapula. This important osseous structure is the site of origin of the short head of the biceps and the coracobrachialis. It also is the site of insertion of the pectoralis minor. Two important ligaments are attached to the coracoid process. The coracoclavicular ligament, composed of the trapezoid and conoid ligaments, extends from the coracoid process to the clavicle. It anchors the clavicle in proper alignment at the acromioclavicular joint. The coraco-acromial ligament is a broad thick structure that extends from the coracoid process to the acromion. Its exact function has never been adequately defined. It forms a tight arch known as the coracoacromial arch which separates the deltoid muscle above from the supraspinatus muscle in the capsule of the shoulder joint below. Some investigators feel that this tight arch predisposes the rotator cuff to degenerative changes.

The acromion extends laterally from the spine of the scapula to form the roof of the shoulder joint proper (Figs. 15–1 and 15–2). The deltoid originates partly from the acromion, and the trapezius inserts on a portion of the acromion. Abnormal osseous forma-tion on the undersurface of the acromion may play a role in degeneration of the rotator cuff. The glenohumeral joint consists of the articulation of the humeral head with the glenoid fossa of the scapula. This is a non–weight-bearing joint, and its stability depends on the surrounding ligamentous, tendinous, and muscular structures. In an extensive study Saha found variation from individual to individual in the depth and tilt of the glenoid fossa.[166] The humeral head is normally in a slightly retroverted position, and this provides some stability at the glenohumeral joint. Since the shoulder joint has a wide range of motion, the articular surface of the humeral head must of neces-sity be very large. In fact, it is approximately three times the size of the articular portion of the glenoid fossa.

The capsule of the shoulder joint is a relatively thin structure, considering the fact that there is no inherent osseous stability of the shoulder joint proper. It extends from the scapula in a roughened area around the lip of the glenoid cavity over the humeral head, and is attached to the humerus at the level of the anatomical neck. It is a large and lax structure, which accounts for the free mobility at the glen-ohumeral joint. Three specific ligaments are

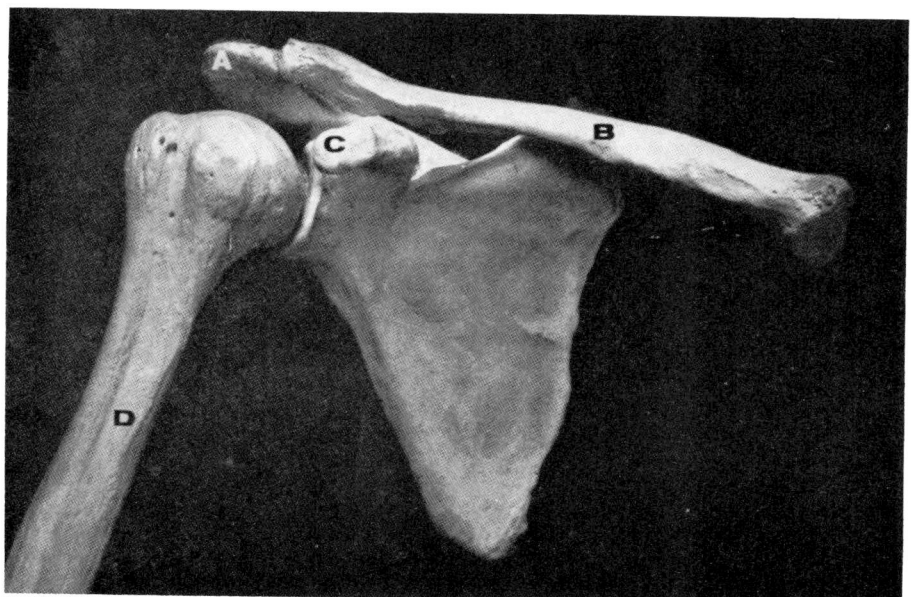

Figure 15–1   Anterior view of the skeletal components of the shoulder. *A.*   Acromion. *B.*   Clavicle. *C.*   Cora-coid process. *D.*   Humeral shaft.

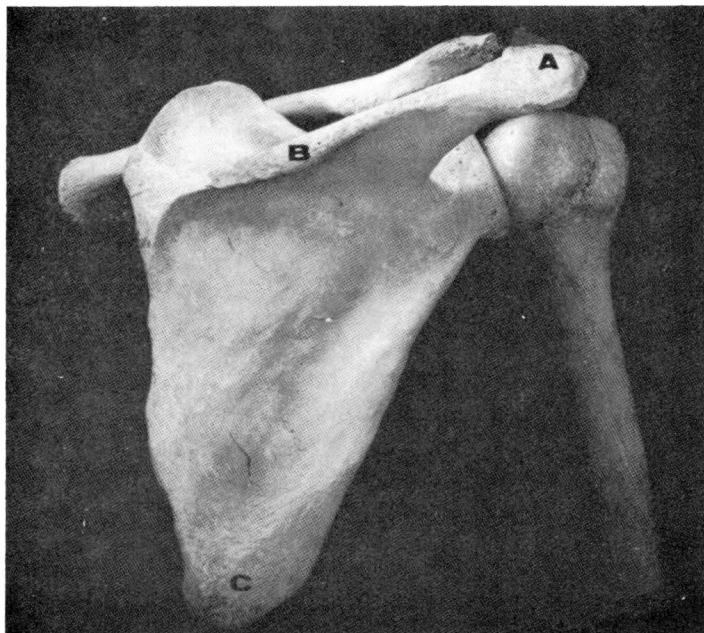

Figure 15-2 Posterior view of the skeletal components of the shoulder. *A.* Acromion. *B.* Scapular spine. *C.* Inferior scapular angle.

associated with the anterior capsule: These are the superior, middle, and inferior glenohumeral ligaments. The size of these ligaments is extremely variable, but they are usually visible as a slight thickening along the interior surface of the anterior capsule. These ligaments probably help strengthen the lax anterior capsule.

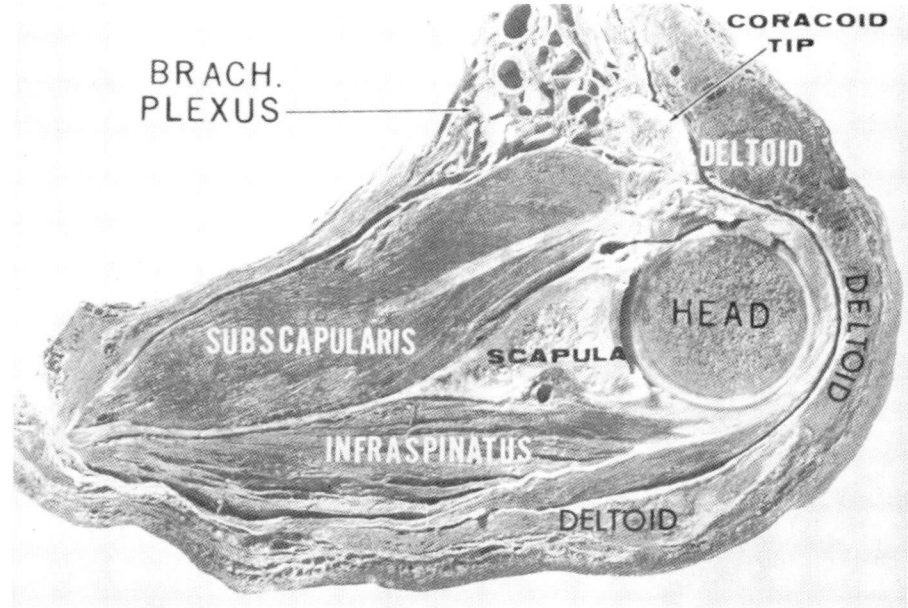

Figure 15-3 Transverse section of the right shoulder region viewed from above. The subscapular bursa communicates with the joint cavity. Note the intramuscular tendon in the subscapularis muscle. Also note that the subscapularis is the main structure along the anterior aspect of the shoulder. (Courtesy of J. J. Joyce, M. Harty, and the *Journal of Bone and Joint Surgery.* J. Bone Joint Surg., *49A:*547–554, 1967.)

Two other important ligaments are associated with the glenohumeral joint (Fig. 15–3). These are the coracohumeral ligament and the coracoacromial ligament, which was described earlier. The coracohumeral ligament is a rather thick structure that originates from the lateral aspect of the coracoid process and extends over the superior aspect of the shoulder joint to attach to the greater tuberosity. It functions as a suspensory ligament of the humeral head and also plays a role in limiting external rotation.

The subacromial or subdeltoid bursa is a large sac that extends over the glenohumeral joint. It extends from the rotator cuff and greater tuberosity to the undersurface of the acromion and the deltoid muscle. This important structure can account for significant pain and disability of the shoulder.

BIOMECHANICS OF THE SHOULDER

Our present knowledge of shoulder motion and function has been enhanced by a more thorough understanding of the biomechanics involved. In 1944 Inman, Saunders, and Abbott published a classic article on motion and function of the shoulder joint.[82] More recently, Freedman and Monroe contributed to this knowledge.[55]

Motion at the shoulder joint occurs through a series of very complex muscle interactions and coupled motion of several joints. Normal motion is recorded with the patient standing erect. At the zero reference point the arm is hanging by the side of the trunk. Abduction is the normal upward and outward motion of the arm away from the trunk in the coronal plane. It measures from 0 degrees in the neutral position to 180 degrees. Adduction is the opposite motion of the shoulder, in which the arm is directed toward the midline of the body or extends beyond it in an upward plane. This measures from the neutral 0 position to 75 degrees. Forward flexion as measured in a vertical plane occurs from the neutral position to 180 degrees and backward extension to 60 degrees.

Rotational motions of the shoulder may be gauged with the arm at the side of the body

and the elbow flexed to 90 degrees. Internal rotation is measured from this neutral position to approximately 80 degrees, when the arm strikes the trunk. External rotation occurs from the neutral position in an outward direction to 60 degrees. The elbow is held stationary at the side of the body, and the measured motion of the forearm and hand is recorded. A simple clinical test to measure rotation is to have the patient attempt to place his hand behind his back toward the tip of the scapula. Normally, the fingertips should be able to approximate the inferior border of the opposite scapula. For reference, this is a method of measuring internal rotation in a posterior direction. This type of motion is particularly important in females to attach or detach a brassiere strap. Frequently, asking the patient whether she is able to perform this function satisfactorily is a quick method of determining rotatory movement.

Elevation of the extremity during flexion or abduction occurs primarily through a combined glenohumeral and scapulothoracic motion. Therefore, it is important to record these two separate aspects of motion during examination of the shoulder. In the fully flexed or abducted position the scapula will be seen to rotate from a neutral position in an outward direction of 60 degrees. This outward rotation is initiated after 30 degrees of abduction or 60 degrees of flexion at the glenohumeral joint. Once outward rotation is initiated there is approximately a two to one ratio of glenohumeral motion to scapulothoracic motion.

We must also remember that motion of the shoulder joint involves motion of the entire shoulder girdle, including the sternoclavicular and acromioclavicular joints. With full flexion or abduction, approximately 40 degrees of elevation of the clavicle occurs at the sternoclavicular joint, most of it during the initial 90 degrees of glenohumeral motion. Twenty degrees of motion occurs at the acromioclavicular joint. Approximately 40 to 50 degrees of upward rotation of the clavicle takes place with full flexion or abduction of the shoulder. If we bear in mind the motion that occurs at the acromioclavicular joint and the rotation of the clavicle with motion, it is not difficult to understand why the shoulder must be immobilized if an internal fixation device has been placed across the acromioclavicular joint during the treatment of an acromioclavicular separation. If the shoulder is not immobilized with an internal fixation device across this joint, it will break under shoulder motion.

The short rotator muscles of the shoulder function to maintain the humeral head in the glenoid fossa during abduction. The deltoid muscle and the rotator cuff muscles act as a coupled force to elevate the upper extremity. The deltoid is the primary abductor of the shoulder. The electrical activity in the deltoid increases progressively during abduction to reach a maximum at between 90 and 100 degrees of elevation. The supraspinatus muscle reaches its peak activity during abduction at 100 degrees and acts together with the deltoid muscle throughout the range of motion. Therefore, the earlier concept of the supraspinatus muscle as the sole initiator of abduction is incorrect. The subscapularis, the infraspinatus, and the teres minor, (the depressors of the humerus) constitute a functional group that is necessary for abduction motion. Their activity rises in a linear fashion to reach a summit at 180 degrees for the infraspinatus, 90 degrees for the subscapularis, and 120 degrees for the teres minor. If

these three depressor muscles are summated it is found that there are two peaks of activity, one at 70 degrees and a second at 115 degrees of abduction. The first peak is due to the depressor action, and the second to the rotational activity of these muscles during the extreme of abduction.

During flexion of the shoulder the clavicular portion of the pectoralis major, the anterior fibers of the deltoid, and both heads of the biceps brachii are active. The pectoralis major, the latissimus dorsi, and the posterior fibers of the deltoid are active during adduction.

Basmajian has cast considerable light on the mechanism by which the shoulder is able to resist downward dislocation of the humeral head.[16] Interestingly, it is not those muscles that have a vertical orientation, such as the biceps, but rather the supraspinatus that is most active in this function. It is Basmajian's contention that during downward loading of the arm, stabilization of the humeral head is obtained by combining a slight upward inclination of the glenoid fossa with marked activity in the supraspinatus muscle, which supplements the passive force of the superior portion of the joint capsule.

Part I ———— **FRACTURES OF THE SHOULDER GIRDLE** ————

FRACTURE OF THE CLAVICLE

Fractures of the clavicle are commonly encountered in an orthopedic practice, particularly in the pediatric age group. Adolescents frequently present with clavicle fractures secondary to athletic activities. The incidence tapers off in adults, but this is still a common injury. Anatomically, the clavicle is not a straight structure. It has a typical S shape. The type of deformity produced with a fracture of the clavicle is determined by the shape and by the extent of disruption of the associated ligaments.

MECHANISM OF INJURY

The usual mechanism of injury is a fall on the extended arm or a direct blow to the

shoulder. The fracture most commonly occurs at the junction of the middle and distal thirds of the clavicle. This is the area in which the clavicle is changing direction from one curve to the other. This change in configuration creates an area that is more susceptible to fracture. There is also a change in cross-sectional thickness. The distal third presents a flattened thin horizontal surface, while the middle and inner portions of the clavicle are more rounded and thickened (Fig. 15–4). The typical deformity is a downward and inward displacement of the shoulder associated with elevation of the proximal portion of the clavicle. This is because the shoulder has lost part of its support owing to the fracture of the clavicle and tends to sag in a downward direction. The strong pull of the sternocleidomastoid muscle in a proximal

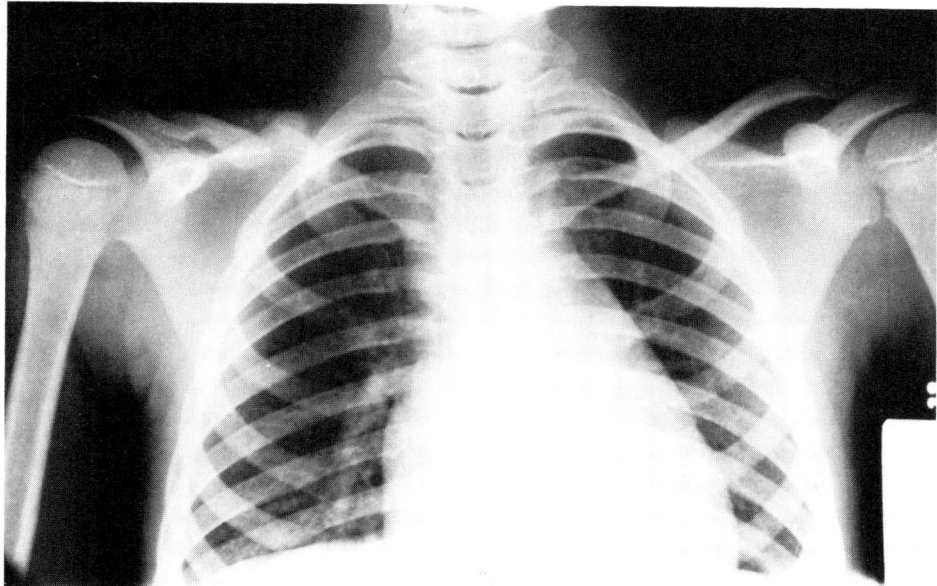

Figure 15–4 Anteroposterior view of the chest revealing a fracture of the midportion of the right clavicle.

direction produces the typical upward displacement of the proximal portion of the clavicle.

CLASSIFICATION

Anatomically, these fractures may be classified by three specific areas: (1) the inner third of the clavicle, (2) the middle third, and (3) the distal third. The most common fracture by far occurs in the middle third, accounting for at least 80 per cent of all clavicle fractures.

Neer has subdivided fractures of the distal third of the clavicle into a useful working classification (Fig. 15–5).[128] It was his feeling that fractures in this area behaved in a different manner from fractures in the proximal or middle third of the

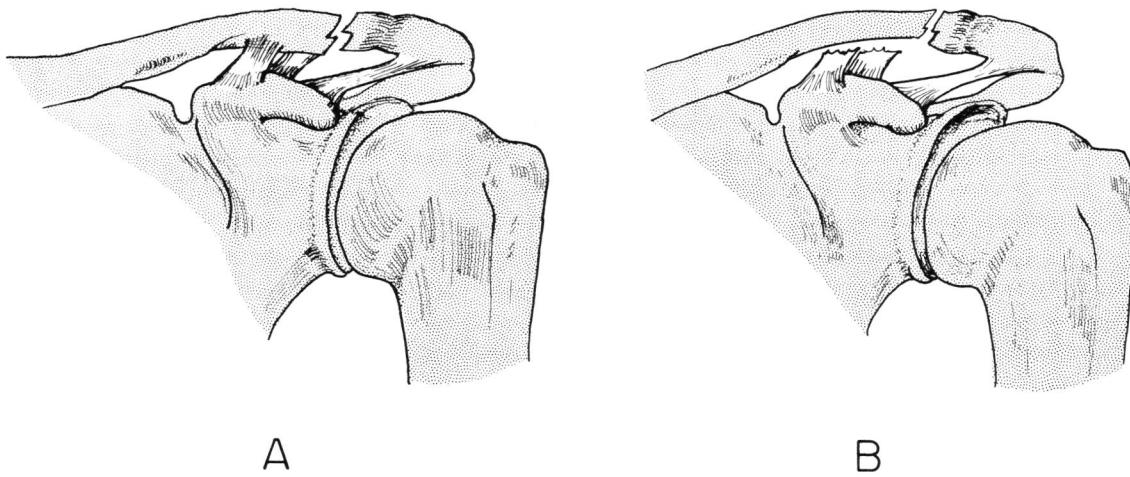

A   B

Figure 15–5 Classification of fractures of the distal third of the clavicle. (Courtesy of C. S. Neer, II, and *Clinical Orthopaedics*. Clin. Orthop., 58:43–50, 1968.)

clavicle, and therefore warranted a separate subclassification. Type 1 is a fracture with minimal displacement and intact coracoclavicular ligaments. Type 2 is a displaced fracture caused by detachment of the ligaments from the proximal fragment. Type I fractures will usually heal without significant difficulty. Type 2 fractures are much more difficult to treat owing to the displacement of the proximal portion of the clavicle.

PHYSICAL EXAMINATION

Patients presenting with a fracture of the clavicle have a typical deformity. In the typical middle third fracture the shoulder is in a slightly downward and inward position. The proximal portion of the clavicle may be elevated, producing an obvious deformity in the middle third. The patient tends to hold the injured extremity at the elbow and close to the trunk, since any motion of the upper extremity elicits pain caused by motion at the fracture site. Palpation will reveal a deformity at the fracture site if there is displacement of the fracture fragments. There is tenderness to direct palpation in this region. Crepitation is also usually present over the fracture site. A careful neurovascular examination of the upper extremity is important to rule out any damage to the major vessels or the brachial plexus, as the clavicle normally functions to protect these structures. Severe displacement of the fracture fragments may injure the neurovascular bundle. This is a relatively rare occurrence, but documentation during the initial examination is essential to rule out this possibility.

ROENTGENOGRAPHIC EVALUATION

The majority of fractures of the clavicle will be evident on a routine anteroposterior view. Very occasionally, the fracture will not be demonstrated with this view, and a 45 degree oblique view of the clavicle is necessary to visualize it. The majority of fractures in the middle portion of the clavicle will present with an oblique fracture line, but the fracture may take almost any direction. Fractures of the distal third with an intact ligamentous structure (type 1)

will frequently demonstrate a relatively vertical fracture line through the distal third of the clavicle. If the ligamentous structures are detached (type 2) the fracture line will often be oblique, extending from the undersurface of the clavicle in a lateral direction toward the superior aspect. Displacement at the fracture site is common owing to elevation of the proximal portion of the clavicle secondary to detachment of the ligamentous structures (Fig. 15–6).

In regard to treatment it is important to determine whether or not the coracoclavicular ligaments have been detached from the clavicle. The integrity of the ligamentous structures may be assessed by having the patient hold 10 lb of weight in each hand and then taking a routine anteroposterior view of the chest, including both shoulders. If there is detachment of the ligamentous structures the clavicle will be noted to be elevated in the proximal portion. The roentgenogram with the patient holding 10 lb will show increased width between the coracoid and clavicle compared with the regular roentgenogram without weights.

TREATMENT

The vast majority of clavicle fractures can be treated conservatively. The end result is usually a well-healed fracture with minimal deformity. Surgery does have a role in the management of these fractures, but it is a very minor one. It is almost never indicated for relatively nondisplaced fractures of the middle portion. In fact, it has been the author's experience that the majority of patients who present with nonunion of the clavicle have had a prior operative procedure. This does not pertain to fractures of the distal third of the clavicle which are very difficult to manage nonoperatively as outlined by Neer.[128]

Open fractures of the clavicle also necessitate operative intervention. Thorough irrigation and debridement are required in order to avoid severe infection and gas gangrene. A decision should be made at the time of operation as to whether or not internal fixation is required. In the author's experience, it is seldom needed. However, if it is the procedure of choice, both the

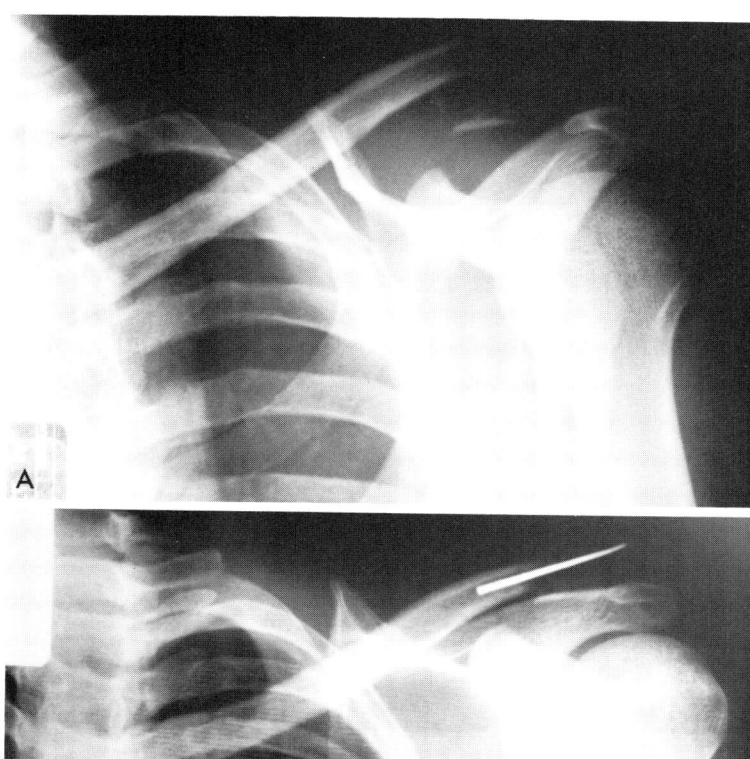

Figure 15–6 A. Anteroposterior view of the type 2 fracture of the distal third of the clavicle. Note the displacement at the fracture site. B. Following an open reduction and internal fixation with a threaded wire.

surgeon and the patient must realize that the risk of infection is increased.

Neurovascular compromise secondary to a fracture of the clavicle is also an indication for an operative approach. If an osseous fragment has been responsible for a laceration of the neurovascular structures, this will have to be removed and the damaged structures repaired. Although this is a rare event, it does occur, and the surgeon must be aware of the possibility and prepared to deal with it appropriately.

Nonunion of the clavicle is a definite indication for operative intervention. This may be managed by open reduction and internal fixation, as outlined by Rowe.[162] A 2-to 3-inch linear incision is made at the fracture site. A 3/32-inch Kirschner wire is then inserted into the distal clavicular fragment. The wire extends through the medullary canal to emerge behind the acromion without piercing the acromioclavicular joint. It is then drilled in a lateral direction until the blunt base of the pin is at the level of the fracture site. The drill is removed, and the fracture site is reduced. The drill is reattached to the Kirschner wire, and the wire is driven across the fracture site into the proximal clavicle. After a distance of 2 to 3 cm the tip of the wire will abut the cortex of the middle third of the clavicle. The blunt end of the pin must not be allowed to penetrate the cortex. The projecting portion of the pin along the lateral aspect of the shoulder is cut off, and the tip is bent over to prevent medial migration. The bone in the area of the fracture site is then decorticated. Cancellous bone graft is obtained from the iliac crest and placed in longitudinal strips along the fracture surface. The wound is closed in layers, and the Kirschner wire is left in place for 10 to 12 weeks, when it is removed.

Two alternative operative approaches are available. The first is open reduction and internal fixation with the use of dual onlay bone grafts held in position with fixation screws. The second procedure which may be considered in the future is the application of electrical current to stimulate fracture healing, as outlined in Chapter 3.

Fracture of the Inner Clavicle

These fractures are normally treated in a conservative manner with the use of a sling for three to six weeks (Fig. 15–7). Once the pain and tenderness to palpation have diminished, the sling may be discarded and gentle exercises initiated. However, heavy activity is not allowed for three months postinjury.

Fracture of the Middle Third

Almost all of these uncomplicated fractures may be handled conservatively. If significant overriding is present a closed reduction may be attempted. This can usually be accomplished by positioning the shoulders upward and backward, in the so-called soldier position. A fracture maintained in this way will usually reduce spontaneously. The problem is in holding this position until the fracture fragments are healed enough to discontinue support, which is usually at six weeks in the adult.

Several appliances and techniques are available to obtain and maintain this position. In children the simple figure-of-eight webbing, which can be made of Webril and Ace bandages, will provide support and comfort. Frequent adjustments are necessary to maintain the position. Careful attention must be given to the padding of this device in the axilla, because there is a danger of neurovascular compromise if it is pulled too tightly. Several commercial devices in the form of a figure-of-eight support are available. They also require frequent adjustments to maintain the position. A small pillow may be placed between the scapulae during sleep, so that the shoulders will fall naturally in a backward and upward position.

The Billington posterior figure-of-eight plaster bandage with a plaster yoke is another very efficient method of maintaining reduction.[19] Occasionally, local anesthetic must be injected into the fracture site. Following this, the shoulder is held in an upward, backward, and outward position to obtain reduction. Felt padding is placed in both axillae and over the tip of the acromion. Webril is applied over the skin areas, and a figure-of-eight plaster jacket is then constructed. This will maintain the shoulders in appropriate position. The plaster device is removed at four weeks in

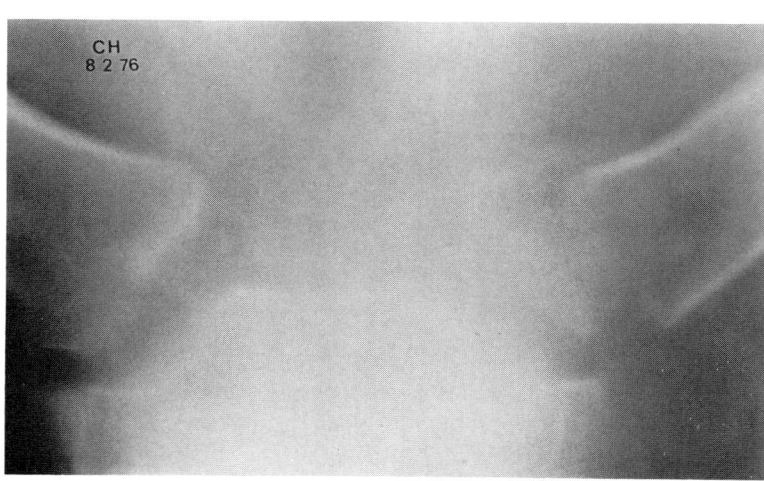

Figure 15–7 Tomogram of a fracture of the inner portion of the left clavicle.

adolescents and six weeks in adults. It must be reemphasized that it is rare indeed for an uncomplicated fracture of the middle third of the clavicle to require operative treatment. In fact, the majority of nounions of the clavicle probably result from operative intervention.

Fracture of the Distal Clavicle

As mentioned earlier, Neer's subclassification of fractures of the distal clavicle is very useful in regard to management.[128] Type 1 fractures have intact ligaments with minimal displacement, and these may be managed conservatively. All that is required is a sling to support the upper extremity and the curtailment of physical activities.

Type 2 fractures present with displacement secondary to disruption of the coracoclavicular ligaments and usually demand more aggressive treatment. The proximal portion of the clavicle is displaced in an upward and backward direction secondary to the pull of the sternocleidomastoid muscle. The distal fragment is noted to be in a downward and forward position. The remainder of the shoulder and the clavicle may be rotated by any motion of the scapula. Basically, three methods of treatment are available.

1. *Closed reduction with external support.* This method requires the intravenous administration of Valium and appropriate analgesics. The proximal fragment must be pulled in a forward and downward direction. The author has not been satisfied with the various forms of splints and strapping to maintain this reduction. Invariably, the proximal fragment resumes its posterior position, causing a high incidence of nonunion. For this reason this conservative form of treatment has been essentially abandoned.

2. *Excision of the outer fragment.* This method creates more problems than it solves. If the distal segment is excised without reconstruction of the coracoclavicular ligaments, the shaft is displaced upward and may become symptomatic. This situation differs from acromioclavicular dislocation (to be discussed), because bone-to-bone repair takes place if the other fragment is preserved.

3. *Open reduction and internal fixation.* This is essentially the same procedure as that described for nonunion, but without the application of a bone graft. A Kirschner wire, 3/32 inches in diameter, is selected for fixation. It is important to bend the distal portion of the wire to prevent medial migration. Patients are usually discharged on the third or fourth postoperative day with a sling. Movement of the shoulder must be prevented, because scapular motion will cause rotation and tilting at the fracture site, increasing the chance of a pin or wire complication. The wire is removed at six weeks, followed by a graded course of shoulder motion. This usually results in a high percentage of healed fractures.

FRACTURES OF THE SCAPULA

The scapula is a large, flat, broad-surfaced structure on the posterior aspect of the upper trunk. Because of its location it is exposed to injuries caused by direct trauma, such as a backward fall. Indirect trauma may also result in fractures of the scapula. In spite of its location and its large surface, fractures of the scapula are relatively uncommon. Injuries to this structure occur mainly in middle-aged individuals. Imatani has recently reviewed 53 fractures of the scapula. The majority were due to automobile or motorcycle accidents.[80]

FRACTURE OF THE BODY AND SPINE

Mechanism of Injury

Fractures in this area may occur by means of both direct and indirect trauma, the former being more frequent. The body and spine of the scapula are usually fractured by a fall from a height, with a direct landing on the posterior aspect of the trunk. This may result in a stellate fracture of the body of the scapula or in a fracture of the spine of the scapula associated with a comminuted fracture of the body. Since a force of great magnitude is required to produce these injuries, it is important to examine the patient for associated serious injuries.

Indirect trauma may also cause these fractures. This occurs from a fall on the

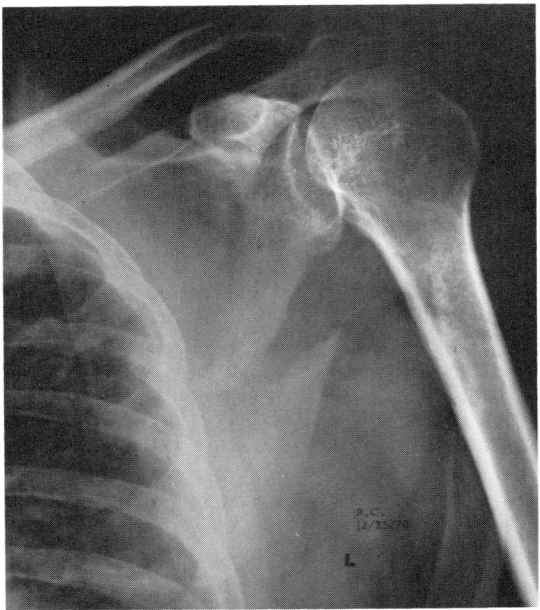

Figure 15–8 A fracture of the lower pole of the scapula.

outstretched upper extremity or shoulder, with the force transmitted in a retrograde direction through the humerus to the scapula. Isolated fractures of the body of the scapula occur, but isolated fractures of the spine of the scapula are not common. They are usually associated with a comminuted fracture of the body of the scapula.

Physical Examination

If the injury has been caused by direct trauma, it is imperative that a careful search be made of other systems for serious injury. Gross ecchymosis and swelling are usually present over the body and spine of the scapula. Crepitus may occasionally be palpable. The patients refuse to move the upper extremity, frequently immobilizing the arm against the trunk to prevent pain. The pain that occurs is due to the fact that the scapula must be fixed before any attempt is made to raise the upper extremity. This obviously pulls on the fracture fragments and elicits pain. In an injury seen shortly after the accident there may be a palpable gap between the fracture surfaces.

Roentgenographic Evaluation

A routine chest roentgenogram may demonstrate a fracture of the body of the scapula (Fig. 15–8). Anteroposterior and oblique views of the scapula are necessary to further evaluate these injuries. Occasionally, a single transverse or oblique fracture line may be evident, but the more common manifestation is a series of comminuted fracture lines. The most common location in the body is the lower angle; this may be seen in association with a fracture of the spine of the scapula. In general, there is usually not

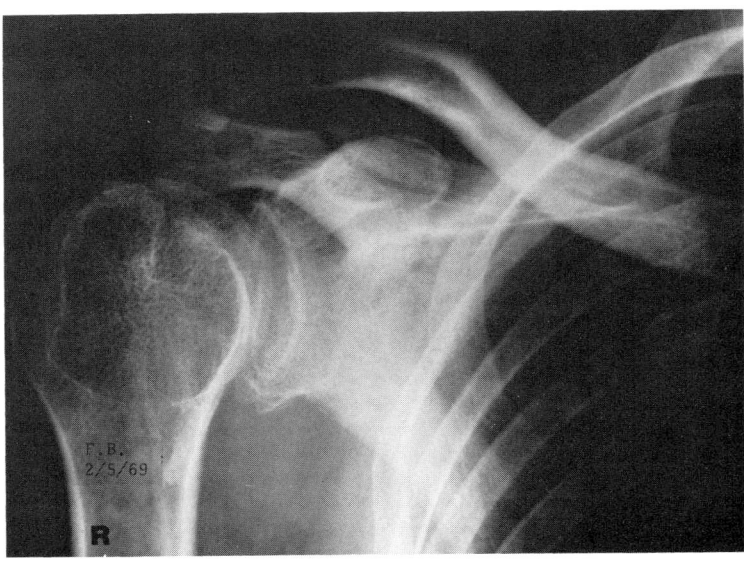

Figure 15–9 A fracture of the spine of the scapula.

wide separation of the fracture fragments owing to the muscular influence which tends to prevent it (Fig. 15–9).

Treatment

Almost all these fractures can be treated conservatively. A simple sling and swathe for two weeks is usually all that is necessary. If there is significant displacement of the fracture fragments, closed reduction should be performed. Traction of the involved arm along with adduction or abduction maneuvers will frequently decrease the displacement that may be present. If the displacement recurs on an attempt to bring the arm back into anatomical position, it may be necessary to immobilize the arm in the position that produces the most satisfactory reduction of the fracture fragments. This may require an abduction splint or a shoulder spica. Operative reduction is almost never indicated with these fractures, because slight displacement at the fracture site is compatible with good function in follow-up examination.

FRACTURE OF THE ACROMION

Mechanism of Injury

Since the acromion forms the roof of the shoulder joint, it is very susceptible to direct trauma from above or to an upward thrust of the head of the humerus. The majority of these injuries are the result of direct trauma from above which places significant force on the acromion. The superior dislocation of the humeral head is a relatively rare lesion, but it is possible to fracture the acromion through a superior migration of the humeral head. In any event, the acromion is a very strong structure, and considerable force is required to fracture its substance.

Physical Examination

Visible ecchymosis and swelling are usually present over the acromion. The patient will hold the arm immobile at the side, as any motion at the shoulder joint is painful. Palpable crepitus is usually present. If the injury is seen early, the examiner

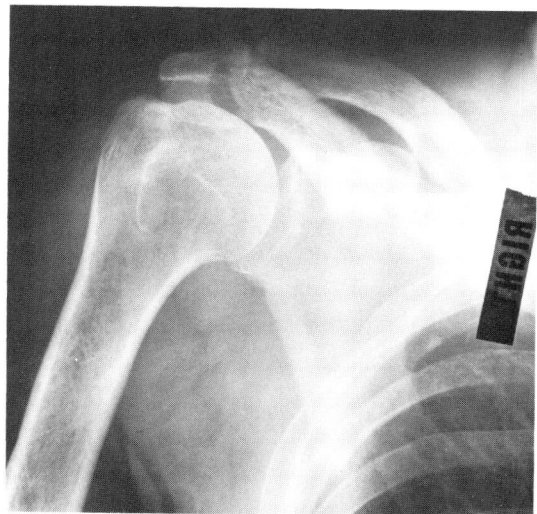

Figure 15–10 A fracture of the acromion.

may be able to move the fragment with gentle direct palpation.

Roentgenographic Evaluation

The acromion process may be fractured at the base or just lateral to the acromioclavicular joint (Fig. 15–10). The majority of the fractures occur in the latter position. Anteroposterior and axillary lateral views of the shoulder will usually demonstrate the fracture line. A point to remember is that the os acromiale (unfused acromial epiphyses) may be misdiagnosed as a fracture of the acromion. It is important to obtain roentgenograms of both shoulders, as this anomaly is bilateral in approximately 60 per cent of cases.

Treatment

The majority of these fractures are nondisplaced and may be managed with a sling and swathe for three to four weeks. Range-of-motion exercises are then initiated. The only exception is when there is significant displacement that might result in a compromise of the subacromial space. Under these conditions the fragment may have to be elevated and held in position with a transfixing wire. Acromionectomy should definitely be avoided, as this has been demonstrated to weaken the action of the deltoid muscle.

FRACTURE OF THE CORACOID PROCESS

Mechanism of Injury

Direct trauma may result in a fracture of the coracoid process. This may be produced by falling on a projecting object that strikes the body just under the clavicle, transmitting the force directly to the coracoid process. Indirect trauma may also result in fractures of the coracoid. Acute muscle contraction of the pectoralis minor, short head of the biceps, or coracobrachialis may cause an avulsion of the coracoid. Occasionally, with a complete acromioclavicular separation the coracoclavicular ligaments may remain intact and avulse a small portion of the coracoid.

Physical Examination

Flexion of the elbow will elicit pain caused by the pull of the short head of the biceps and the coracobrachialis on the avulsed fragment. A careful neurovascular examination must be performed, because if this injury is due to direct trauma there may also be associated injury to the neurovascular bundle. It is important to document this at the time of the initial evaluation. There may also be evidence of a complete acromioclavicular separation with a large palpable mass over the acromioclavicular joint.

Roentgenographic Evaluation

Anteroposterior and lateral axillary views will usually demonstrate the fracture (Fig. 15–11). The tip of the process may be avulsed, or the coracoid may be fractured through its base. There may also be evidence of a complete acromioclavicular separation if the injury was due to an avulsion with intact coracoclavicular ligaments.

Treatment

The majority of these injuries may be managed in a conservative fashion. A simple sling for comfort for the initial seven to ten days is probably indicated. Vigorous athletic activity is restricted for at least two months.

Good results may be obtained by primary open reduction and internal fixation if there is marked displacement of the fragment on initial evaluation. If the patient is young and athletic and has evidence of a complete acromioclavicular separation, it is not unreasonable to consider internal fixation of the coracoid fracture at the time of internal fixation of the acromioclavicular injury. If the patient is not a young athletic individ-

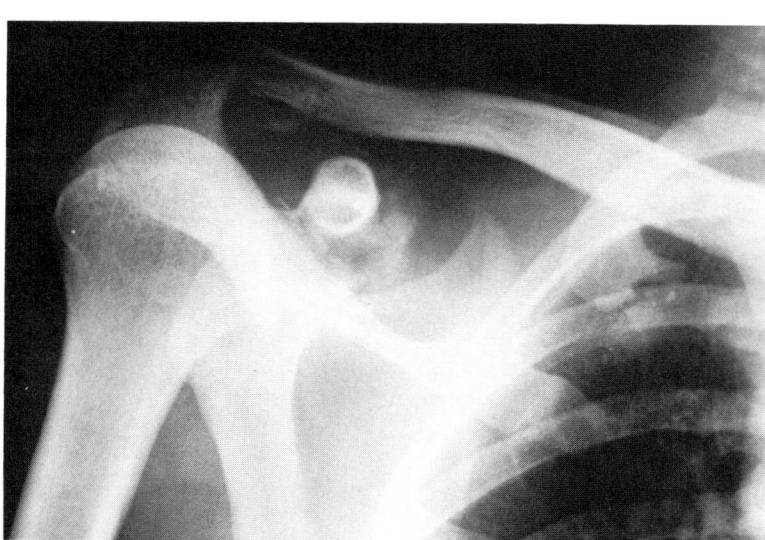

Figure 15–11 Comminuted fracture at the base of the coracoid.

ual, then both injuries may be treated conservatively and surgery performed at a later date if necessary.

FRACTURE OF THE SURGICAL NECK AND GLENOID FOSSA

These injuries are classified together, as it is common to encounter fractures of the surgical neck of the scapula associated with fractures of the glenoid fossa. However, a fracture of the glenoid fossa may occur as an isolated lesion.

Mechanism of Injury

The usual mechanism of injury is direct trauma to the anterior or posterior aspect of the shoulder. These fractures may also result from indirect trauma as a result of the force being transmitted down the humeral shaft through the humeral head into the glenoid fossa.

Physical Examination

If the fracture is associated with a disruption of the coracoclavicular and coraco-acromial ligaments, there is definite displacement of the fragment in a downward and inward direction. Under these circum-stances it may be very difficult to distin-guish this injury from a dislocation of the shoulder. There may be a loss of the normal shoulder contour owing to a downward and inward displacement of the humeral head. Although the patient is unable to move the shoulder, it can be passively moved by the examiner. Crepitus may be palpable, par-ticularly in association with an upward thrust of the humerus, which may reduce the fracture. However, the deformity recurs once the force is released.

Roentgenographic Evaluation

An anteroposterior and lateral axillary view will usually delineate these fractures (Fig. 15–12). The usual fracture line extends from the suprascapular notch in a down-ward and outward direction to a point on the axillary border beneath the glenoid. For this reason, the coracoid process and glenoid cavity appear detached from the rest of the body of the scapula. Therefore, there is a downward and inward displacement of the fracture fragments. The amount of displace-ment is directly related to the associated injury of the coracoclavicular and coraco-acromial ligaments. If these ligaments are intact, there is very little displacement. However, if they are disrupted, there is usually significant displacement. Fractures

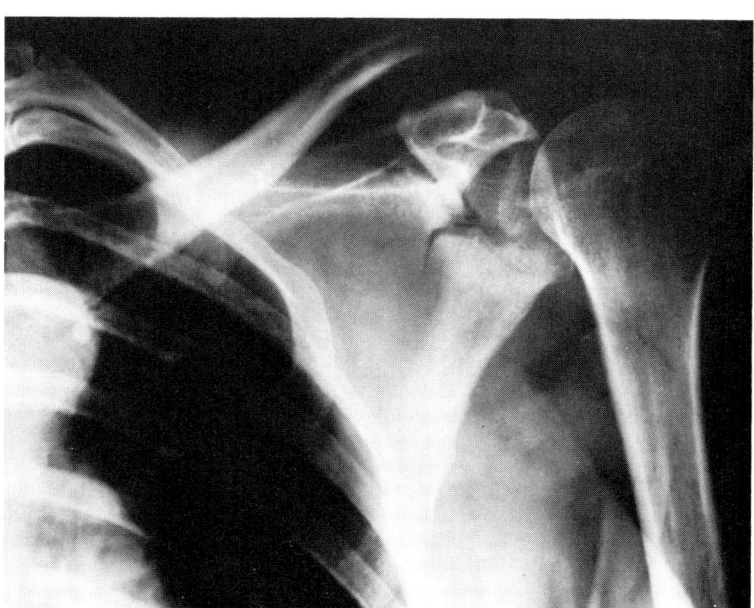

Figure 15–12 A fracture of the glenoid with the fracture line ex-tending into the surgical neck.

of the lip of the glenoid may also be seen in association with dislocations of the shoulder joint.

Treatment

The majority of patients may be managed conservatively. A sling and swathe is supplied for two to three weeks, followed by initiation of gradual motion of the shoulder. If there is significant downward and inward displacement of the glenoid cavity and coracoid process, this may be treated with a shoulder spica to immobilize the shoulder in abduction. This will realign the position of the glenoid cavity. The shoulder spica is maintained for six to eight weeks and then is discontinued, with gradual range-of-motion exercises instituted. If there is gross comminution of the glenoid cavity, it may be beneficial to treat the patient with lateral traction in bed through an olecranon pin. This treatment is maintained for two to three weeks, and the arm is then placed in a sling for an additional two to three weeks.

Isolated fractures of the glenoid rim may require operative removal if they become interarticular loose bodies. In the presence of subluxation or dislocation of the humeral head, traumatic fractures of the glenoid rim may require open reduction and internal fixation.

DISLOCATION OF THE SCAPULA

Mechanism of Injury

This very rare injury may result from a direct force applied to the posterior surface of the scapula or from forceful outward traction on the arm. The entire scapula may be dislocated in an outward direction, or the lower angle of the scapula may become entrapped between the ribs and remain in this position.

Physical Examination

Physical examination is not difficult under these conditions. The axillary border of the scapula is noted to be displaced in an outward direction. The scapula appears to be relatively fixed in this position, and pain is produced by any attempt at reduction.

Roentgenographic Evaluation

Anteroposterior and axillary views of the shoulder will reveal the abnormal position of the scapula.

Treatment

The trick is to unlock the scapula from its fixed position between the ribs. Key and Conwell advocate traction on the hyperadducted arm while the surgeon manually rotates the axillary border of the scapula forward and then pushes directly backward.[91] Once released, the scapula tends to resume its normal position. A piece of strapping is utilized to maintain the scapula against the chest wall. For comfort, the arm is also placed in a sling for two weeks.

FRACTURES OF THE PROXIMAL HUMERUS

Fractures of the proximal humerus are relatively uncommon in young adults, but occur with increasing frequency in the older age group, with a definite female predominance. Codman originally observed that fractures of the humeral neck separate one or more fragments from the rest.[37] These include segments of the head, lesser tuberosity, greater tuberosity, and shaft. Management of these frequently complex fractures is aided by a useful working classification, and requires a thorough knowledge of the anatomical relationships, underlying predisposing factors, and mechanisms of injury. There has been a definite trend toward early mobilization of these fractures in order to prevent the dread complication of frozen shoulder. However, as will be discussed, certain of these fractures require operative intervention owing to displacement of the fracture fragments or interference with the local blood supply.

The majority of fractures of the proximal humerus occur through the surgical neck rather than the anatomical neck. These injuries may or may not be associated with fractures of the greater or lesser tuberosities. The arterial blood supply to the adult humerus has been described previously by Laing.[96] A constant anterolateral artery formed by the ascending branch of the anterior humeral circumflex artery enters the humeral head either at the upper end of the bicipital groove or by its branches entering the greater and lesser tuberosities. This vessel has been described as the arcuate artery. The distribution of these vessels closely resembles that of the lateral epiphyseal arteries of the femoral head. Contributions to the blood supply of the humeral head have also been demonstrated from the posterior humeral circumflex artery as posteromedial arteries. An inconstant arterial supply enters the humeral head posteriorly and anteriorly via the region of the attachment of the rotator cuff. The importance of the vasculature lies in the fact that the blood supply of the humeral head enters anterolaterally above the common site of fractures of the surgical neck. Thus, both bone ends have a good blood supply, accounting for the rapidity of union of these fractures.

The major factor predisposing to fractures in this area is underlying osteoporosis. The trabecular pattern and osteoporotic changes in senescence have been documented by Hall and Rosser.[62] Sections of the proximal humerus have revealed the scar of the epiphyseal plate remaining in the medullary cavity, and the cavity stopping short of the plate in younger bone. However, with advancing age and osteoporosis the cavity has extended up to the plate, causing diminished mechanical support in this area. The cancellous bone in the greater tuberosity decreases in quantity, producing cavitation with a thin shell of external bone. The cortex of the head becomes a thin shell, and in its lower third, where the head merges into the surgical neck, a cancellous appearance is seen in the bone shell. In the upper end of the humerus two major rays of trabeculi are demonstrated. The medial ray passes into the inferomedial aspect of the head and aids in resisting deformation by static loading. The lateral humeral ray passes vertically to the tuberosities, with a second ray passing to the superolateral aspect of the head. These are also involved in static loading, as force is transmitted through the lateral ray between the supraspinatus muscle and the humeral shaft. The commonest site of fracture is through the surgical neck, which has been demonstrated to contain a decreased quantity of supporting osseous structure.

NEER CLASSIFICATION

The working classification originally outlined by Charles S. Neer in 1970 and modified in 1975 is preferred by the author (Fig. 15–13).[129, 131] Other classifications based solely on the anatomical location of the fracture line are not useful, as they do not take into account displacement of the fragments. The amount of displacement of the fragments is vitally important, since this has a direct bearing on both the type of treatment and the prognosis. The classification based on abduction and adduction type fractures also is misleading, because the apex of angulation is rarely in the coronal or scapular plane. Therefore, angulation of the fragments may appear as either an abduction or an adduction fracture, depending on the degree of rotation of the humerus.

Neer's classification was developed according to a four-segment concept. The four major segments of the proximal humerus include the articular segments, or "anatomical neck" level, the greater tuberosity, the

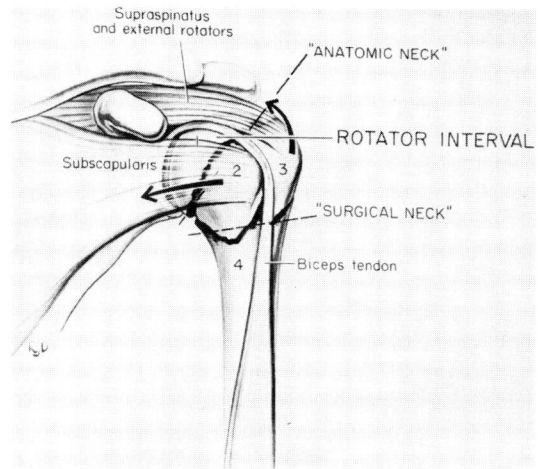

Figure 15–13 The rotator interval, a ligamentous area between the tendons of the supraspinatus and subscapularis, and the four major fragments of proximal humeral fractures: (1) head, (2) lesser tuberosity, (3) greater tuberosity, and (4) shaft. (Courtesy of C. S. Neer, II and the *Journal of Bone and Joint Surgery.* J. Bone Joint Surg., 52A:1077–1089, 1970.)

lesser tuberosity, and the shaft, or "surgical neck" level. If any of these is displaced greater than 1 cm or angulated greater than 45 degrees, the fracture must be considered displaced.

In summary, the following nomenclature is employed. A one-part fracture is one with minimal displacement. A two-part fracture occurs when one segment is displaced in relation to the three remaining segments. In a three-part fracture, two segments are displaced in relation to the two remaining undisplaced segments. A four-part fracture involves displacement of all four segments.

Two final concepts are involved in this classification. The first has to do with fracture-dislocation of the proximal humerus (Fig. 15–14). This occurs when the articular surface of the proximal humerus is located in a position that does not have direct contact with the articular surface of the glenoid fossa. These dislocations may be anterior or posterior, and they may be associated with two-, three-, and four-part lesions. Second, fractures of the articular surface per se of the humeral head are considered separately.

This classification is extremely useful because it offers the surgeon a more comprehensive understanding of the significance of the fracture; in this manner appropriate treatment may be determined. It is also useful in follow-up studies to determine the effect of various treatment programs. Since this classification is based upon roentgenographic evaluation of these serious injuries, Neer has outlined a trauma series of roentgenographic views obtained in the scapular planes.

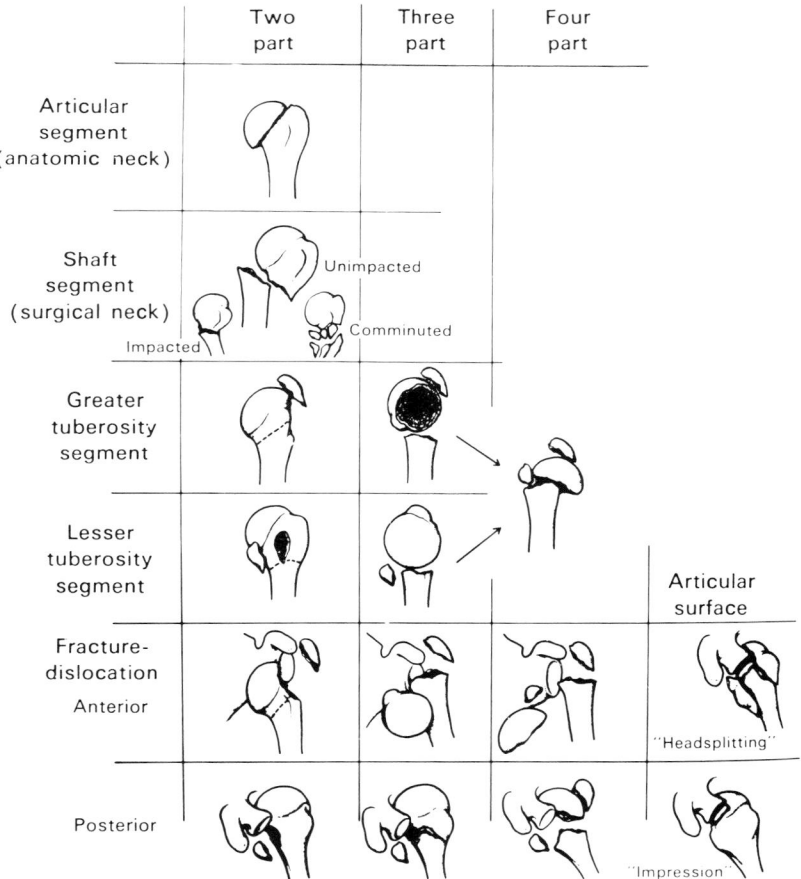

Figure 15–14 The Neer four-segment classification of displaced fractures. This classification describes only displaced segments. Courtesy of C. S. Neer, II and the *Journal of Bone and Joint Surgery.* J. Bone Joint Surg., 52A:1077–1089, 1970.

Mechanisms of Injury

The commonest mechanism of injury is indirect trauma as the result of a fall on the outstretched and pronated upper extremity. Since lateral rotation is required during full abduction of the shoulder, a fall on the pronated outstretched upper extremity may result in a fracture through the osteoporotic proximal humerus in the elderly female. The sudden excessive force exerted on structurally weak bone will result in both simple and comminuted fractures. An additional mechanism secondary to direct trauma is a blow to the anterior or posterolateral aspect of the shoulder. This may produce a traumatic avulsion of the greater tuberosity or a direct injury to the surgical neck. The greater tuberosity is also subject to an avulsion injury in association with a dislocation of the shoulder.

Physical Examination

The physical examination will depend in large part on the amount of displacement of the fracture fragments. The patient will have less discomfort with an impacted fracture than with one in which there is significant displacement of the fracture fragments. Most patients will present with evidence of gross swelling in the area of the shoulder joint, with the appearance of ecchymosis within 24 to 48 hours in a large percentage of cases. There is tenderness to direct palpation over the proximal humeral area. The posture of the patient is usually indicative. He will tend to rigidly immobilize the injured extremity next to the body and support the arm with the use of the uninvolved extremity.

In the presence of a fracture-dislocation of the proximal humerus the normal contour of the shoulder may be obliterated. This is because the humeral head is no longer in contact with the glenoid cavity. However, if there is gross hemorrhage in the soft tissues and displacement of the fracture fragments this gross defect may not be present. Any attempt at motion of the shoulder is usually painful and may produce crepitation.

It is vitally important to perform a careful neurovascular examination of the upper extremity with these injuries. Displacement of the fracture fragments may cause significant injury to the neurovascular bundle. This is not a common occurrence, but if a careful search is not made for this complication at the time of the initial evaluation the true seriousness of the injury may be overlooked.

Roentgenographic Evaluation

A careful and thorough roentgenographic evaluation is essential if the Neer classification is to be applied to these injuries. Neer has outlined the appropriate roentgenographic evaluation needed to assess these injuries. The basic views are known as the trauma series and are obtained in the scapular plane (Fig. 15–15). The rationale for these views is that the glenohumeral joint does not lie in a coronal or sagittal plane. Therefore, Neer advocates two-plane views obtained in the scapular plane rather than the coronal or sagittal plane. The patient may be supine, sitting, or standing.

For the anteroposterior view the patient is positioned against the cassette such that the scapula is parallel to the cassette. This is accomplished by tilting the patient 35 to 40 degrees as illustrated. The roentgenographic tube is then directed at a right angle to this plane. The lateral view is obtained by placing the cassette at a right angle to the plane of the scapula and then directing the roentgenographic tube in a plane parallel to the scapula. For this view the cassette is usually placed against the shoulder, and the roentgenographic tube is placed behind the patient directly along the scapular plane. These two views are excellent for the initial evaluation of patients with fractures of the proximal humerus.

The true axillary view of the glenohumeral joint is valuable in evaluating fracture-dislocations of the proximal humerus (Fig. 15–16). Since the humeral articular surface is no longer in contact with the glenoid cavity, it is extremely important to establish its exact position. The axillary view is helpful in making this determination and is particularly valuable in evaluating posterior fracture-dislocations. This simple view is obtained by abducting the patient's injured arm slightly and positioning the roentgenographic tube in close proximity to the ipsilateral hip with the beam directed into

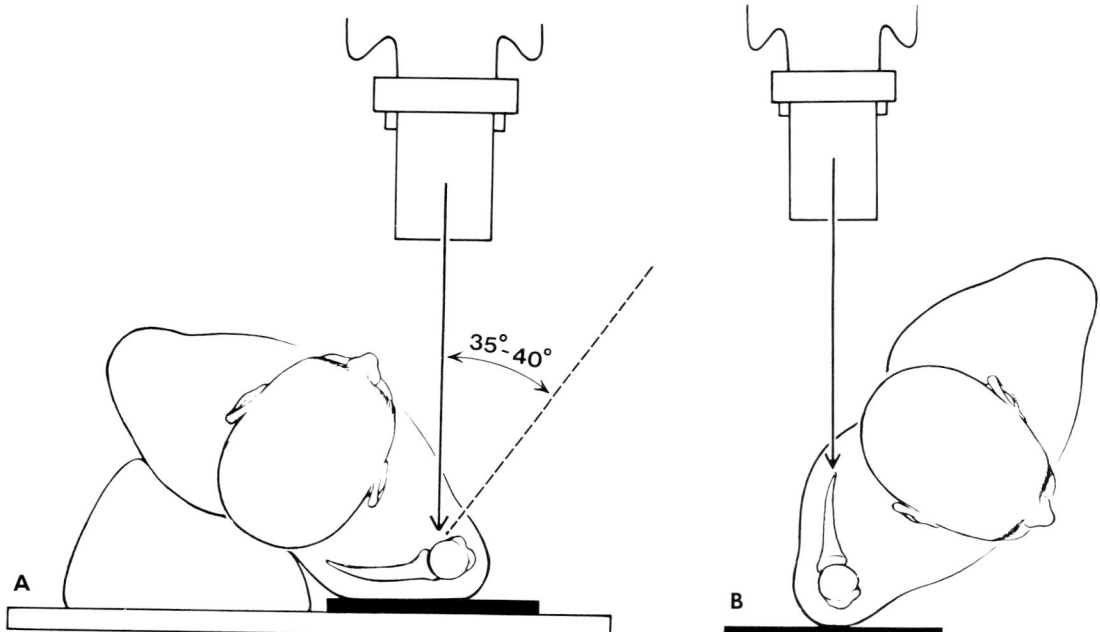

Figure 15–15   A and B. Trauma series includes two views of the shoulder made perpendicular and parallel to the scapular plane. The advantage is that roentgenograms may be obtained without moving the patient or removing the arm from the sling. (Modified from and courtesy of C. S. Neer, II and the *Journal of Bone and Joint Surgery.* J. Bone Joint Surg., 52A:1077–1089, 1970.)

the axilla. The cassette is then placed above the superior aspect of the shoulder at a right angle to the beam of the tube.

Additional roentgenographic views may

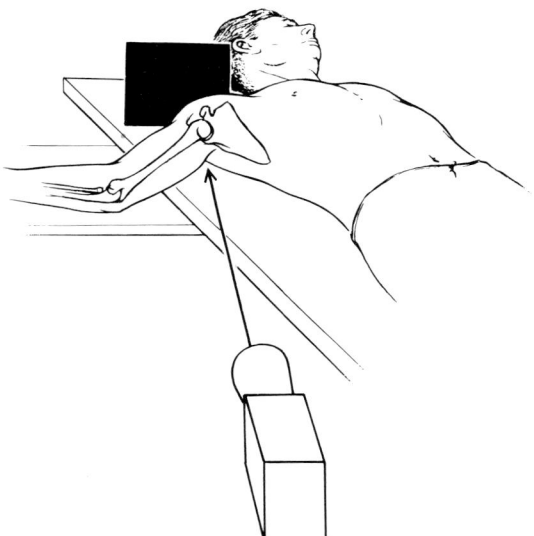

Figure 15–16   The method of obtaining a true axillary view of the glenohumeral joint. (Courtesy of C. S. Neer, II, AAOS Exhibit, 1978.)

be taken at the discretion of the attending physician. The transthoracic view is helpful in determining whether a dislocation is present. Tomograms of the shoulder may be useful in verifying a dislocation or assessing the degree of depression of the articular surface of the humeral head. Finally, anteroposterior views of the humeral head in various degrees of rotation may be beneficial in assessing the degree of displacement of the fracture fragments.

Treatment

It is generally agreed that fractures with minimal displacement, regardless of the level or number of fracture lines, can be satisfactorily treated with early functional exercises. This was the original conclusion by Roberts in 1930 and has not changed significantly over the years.[154] Early motion of the shoulder is essential in order to prevent scarring of the surrounding soft tissue structures and interarticular adhesions. This concept has been vital in obtaining satisfactory functional motion of the shoulder following these injuries. The hanging-arm cast has been advocated in the past for the management of these injuries. The author is opposed to this form of treatment, as the hanging-arm cast may cause distraction of the fracture fragments. The weight of the arm alone is probably enough to aid in the reduction of these fractures by gravity. If significant distraction is produced at the fracture site the incidence of nonunion will be increased.

Open reduction and internal fixation have a definite place in the management of these injuries. If there is significant displacement of the fracture fragments and associated tears of the rotator cuff, this type of treatment is certainly indicated. Prosthetic replacement of the humeral head when the head has lost its blood supply is also an established procedure.[125, 126]

In order to discuss the specific treatment of these injuries the author will follow Neer's classification.

Minimal Displacement

The fracture is minimally displaced (Fig. 15–17). There may be evidence of impaction at the fracture site, such that the entire

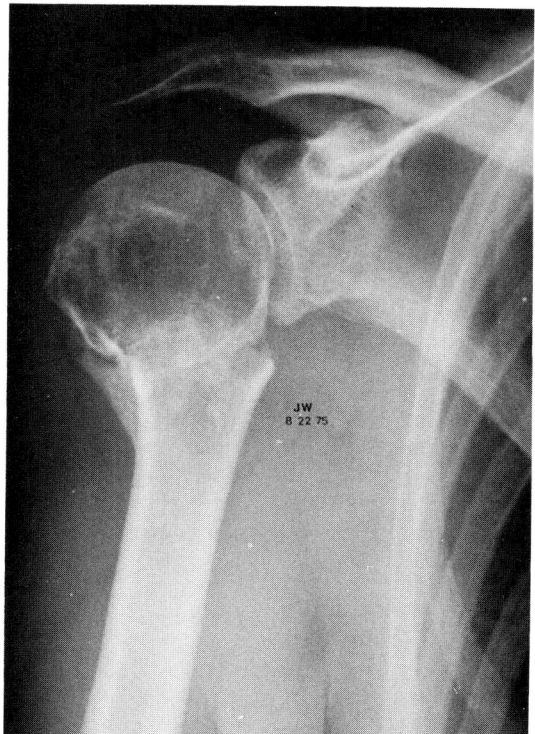

Figure 15–17 A minimally displaced humeral neck fracture.

humerus tends to move as one unit. On the other hand, there are fractures that present with evidence of impaction; if motion is initiated very early in these patients, movement at the fracture site will be noted. The author has found it useful to place patients with this injury in a simple sling or a sling-and-swathe type of immobilization for the first week following injury. This interval allows the acute hemorrhagic and inflammatory reaction to subside. At the end of one week the patient is removed from the immobilization apparatus, and gentle circumduction exercises are initiated. The object is to start off in a gradual small circle and then expand the circle each day as pain decreases in the shoulder. This is the first step in producing motion of the glenohumeral joint. It is true that this circumduction motion has a high component of scapulothoracic movement, but the patient is able to observe the progress he is making, and glenohumeral motion gradually increases. It is important not to aggressively force these exercises on the patient, as this may increase motion at the fracture site and increase the pain. It is uncommon for significant displacement to occur during the gradual initiation of these exercises.

At the end of one week, the patient is thoroughly comfortable performing the exercises and is advanced to forward wall-climbing. To perform this exercise the patient faces the wall and gradually "walks" the fingers up the wall. These exercises are performed eight to ten times a day in association with the circumduction exercises. At the end of each day the patient records the highest point on the wall that was achieved. The object of this therapy is to make a concentrated effort each day to surpass the height attained the previous day. Again, this creates an excellent mental attitude toward progress, in that the patient is able to observe his progress on a daily basis.

At the end of a further seven to ten days the patient has usually progressed to 90 degrees of flexion. At this time abduction exercises of the shoulder are initiated. These are performed by having the patient stand at a right angle to the wall. The hand is then walked up the wall as in the previous exercise. However, in this position the patient is performing active abduction, whereas when facing the wall he is performing active flexion. This motion is a little more difficult to achieve than forward flexion. Once the patient is comfortable performing this exercise, active and passive elevation, external rotation, and internal rotation of the arm are initiated.

The object of these exercises is to obtain an adequate functional range of motion of the shoulder. Once this is achieved, aggressive resistance exercises may be attempted to increase the strength of the involved extremity. Throughout the course of these exercise periods the patient must be monitored very closely. This can be done by regular attendance at physical therapy sessions. In this way the therapist is able to estimate the progress on a daily or every other day basis. The therapist should also be instructed in the type of program the physician prefers and encouraged to communicate with the physician regarding the progress of the patient.

For all intents and purposes, these simple fractures are usually healed by six to eight weeks. Vigorous activity, such as tennis, is restricted for an additional four weeks.

Two-Part Displacement

The majority of these patients may be managed by nonoperative methods. Isolated fractures through the anatomical neck with some displacement of the articular head fragment are uncommon. There are usually two alternatives to treatment in this situation. The first is a closed reduction to improve the position of the head fragment. It is probably worthwhile to try to improve the position of the fragment by closed manipulation. However, we have all seen terrible-appearing roentgenograms in follow-up studies of various shoulder fractures with excellent function maintained. Therefore, if gentle closed manipulation is unsuccessful the most appropriate course of action is to accept the position and initiate early range-of-motion exercises. The danger in this approach is that because the blood supply to the humeral head is probably affected, the patient may develop significant avascular necrosis with resorption in the future. Since this is not a weight-bearing joint, patients who do have mild avascular necrosis without large resorptive cavities are capable of excellent functional activity (Fig. 15–18).

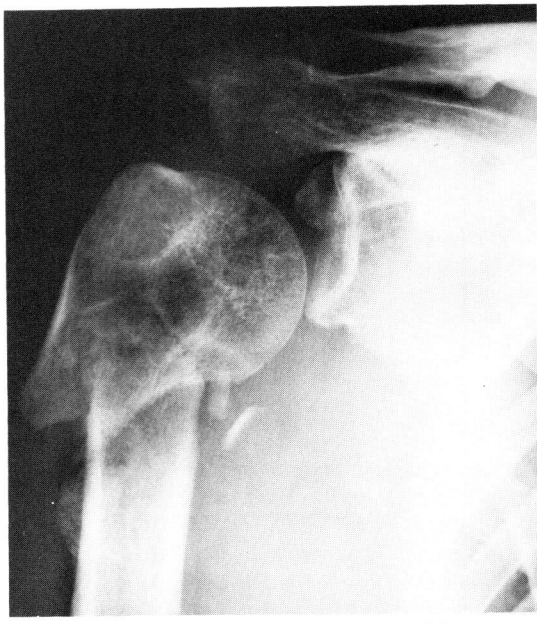

Figure 15–18   A two-part comminuted fracture.

The second alternative is to attempt open reduction and internal fixation with the use of a small blade plate or a compression screw device with a side plate. The author feels this method is probably too aggressive for the elderly patient. If patients develop significant avascular necrosis of the humeral head and are symptomatic at a later date following conservative treatment, this can always be managed with prosthetic replacement of the humeral head. For this reason the author prefers to treat these fractures in a more conservative manner when they are first evaluated.

Displaced surgical neck fractures may present a problem in management. If the fracture is impacted with significant angulation at the fracture site, the position may be accepted and early motion may be initiated or a closed reduction may be performed in an attempt to improve the angulation. The problem with accepting the angulation is that this may limit range of motion in the future. In a very elderly patient it is best to accept the angulation and initiate early range-of-motion exercises. However, in a middle-aged patient an attempt at closed reduction should be performed in the expectation of increasing future range of motion.

If this form of treatment is selected the impacted fracture must be disimpacted. Once this is accomplished by firm distal traction, the proximal portion of the shaft can be levered anteriorly under the humeral head. This maneuver is usually performed under general anesthesia. In this manner muscle contraction may be avoided, and the deforming forces may be temporarily obliterated. Once the reduction has been obtained the patient is placed in a sling-and-swathe immobilization apparatus. He is maintained in this device for at least three weeks, when gentle circumduction exercises are initiated.

Unstable surgical neck fractures are most often managed by closed reduction. Since the rotator cuff is usually uninjured in this fracture, the humeral head is held in a relatively normal position. It is the muscular pull of the pectoralis that displaces the shaft in a medial direction. The object of the reduction is to engage the proximal portion of the shaft of the humerus with the cancellous surface of the head fragment. A sling and swathe is used postreduction to immobilize the shoulder for at least three weeks. If closed reduction is unsatisfactory, open reduction should be performed and the head fragment held to the shaft with the use of two or three wire sutures through the tuberosities and into the humeral shaft. If an open reduction and internal fixation have been performed in this manner, motion may be initiated one to two weeks postoperatively. An alternative form of surgical treatment is the use of a rush rod to "lollipop" the head on the shaft.

Comminuted fractures of the humeral neck may be very difficult to treat, as they are extremely unstable. These fractures must be managed by lateral skin traction or by overhead skeletal traction with the use of an olecranon pin. Specific attention to detail is required, as overdistraction of these fractures may lead to nonunion.

GREATER TUBEROSITY DISPLACEMENT. In young individuals, displacement of the greater tuberosity may involve a large fragment (Fig. 15–19). If the fragment is in satisfactory position and is relatively undisplaced, this fracture may be treated in a conservative fashion. However, significant displacement of the greater tuberosity in a proximal direction indicates a tear in the

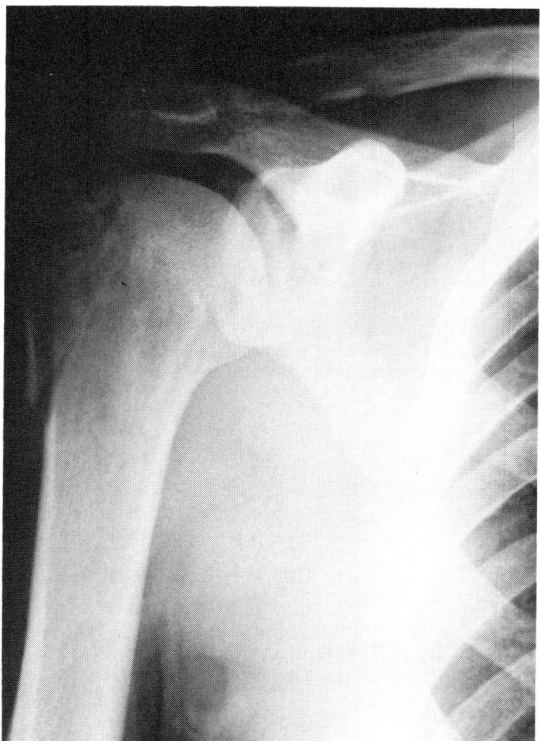

Figure 15–19 A relatively nondisplaced greater tuberosity fragment. This may be managed conservatively.

rotator cuff. In the presence of this displacement, operative intervention is necessary. This requires open reduction and internal fixation of the greater tuberosity fragment with the use of wire loops or a lag compression screw (Fig. 15–20). At the same time the tear in the rotator cuff should be surgically repaired. If this is not performed, abduction of the shoulder will be blocked by the large tuberosity fragment as it impinges on the acromion. The patient may also develop symptoms of rotator insufficiency.

LESSER TUBEROSITY DISPLACEMENT. This is not a very common lesion. It is managed in a conservative fashion with early range-of-motion exercises. The displacement of the lesser tuberosity does not appear to be a problem in follow-up examination.

Three-Part Displacement

These fractures have been referred to in the past as rotatory fracture-subluxations or rotatory fracture-dislocations.[129, 130] They in-

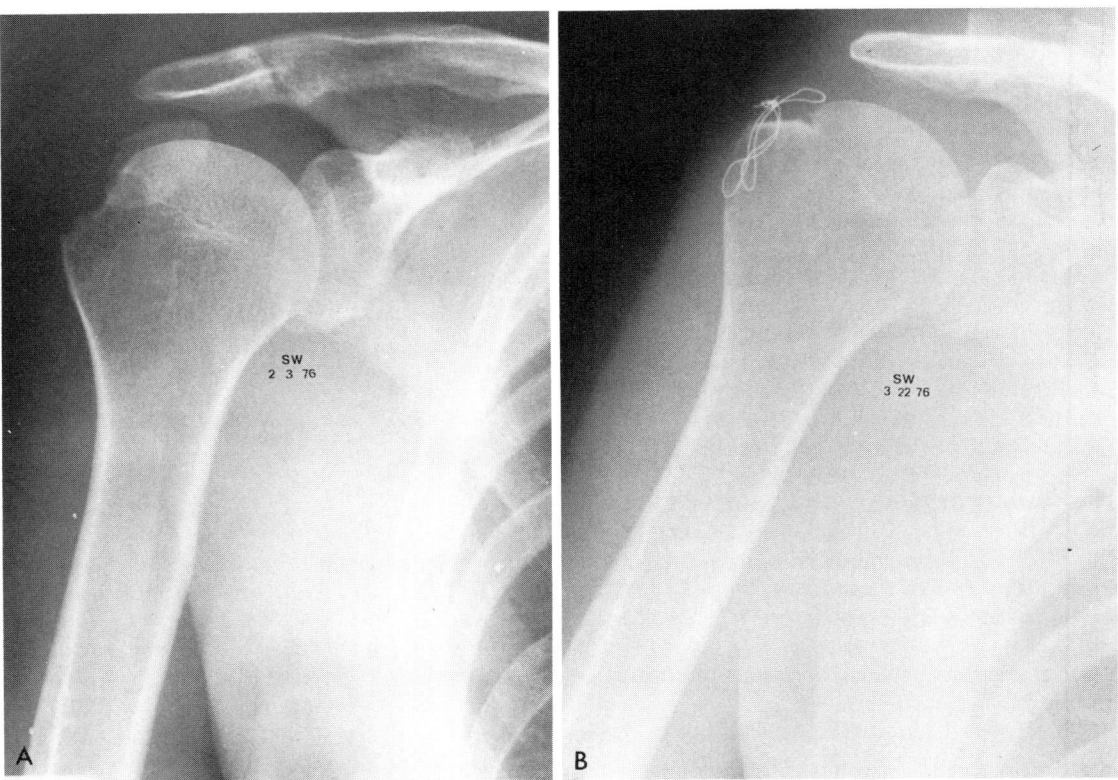

Figure 15–20 *A.* Displaced greater tuberosity fragment. This must be treated surgically since abduction motion will be blocked otherwise. *B.* Following open reduction and internal fixation with the use of a wire. There is evidence of complete healing at seven weeks.

volve a fracture through the surgical neck with displacement of one of the tuberosities. If the greater tuberosity is displaced, the head is rotated in a posterior direction by the pull of the subscapularis. As a result, the articular surface of the humeral head faces posteriorly. If the lesser tuberosity is displaced, the head is rotated anteriorly by the pull of the supraspinatus and external rotators. The articular surface of the humeral head is now facing in an anterior direction. These fractures must be treated by open methods for the following reasons: (1) The rotator cuff is torn owing to displacement of the involved tuberosity; (2) the articular surface of the humeral head has been rotated and is not in its normal articulating position with the glenoid fossa; and (3) these are unstable fractures. Operative treatment consists of a deltopectoral incision, with identification of the tuberosity involved, followed by suturing of the tuberosity back to the humeral head with wire loops. The head fragment is then attached to the shaft with additional wire

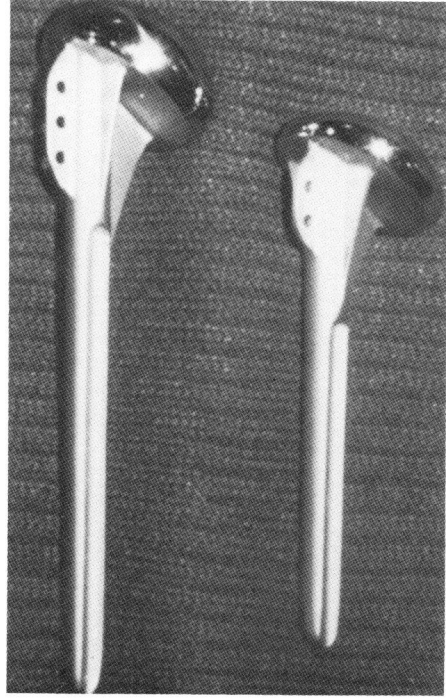

Figure 15–21 The new revised Neer prosthesis. (Courtesy of C. S. Neer, II and C. V. Mosby Co. Four-segment classification of displaced proximal humeral fractures. AAOS Instructional Course Lectures. Vol. XXIV, pp. 163–168. St. Louis, C. V. Mosby Co., 1975.)

loops. Postoperatively these patients are maintained in a sling-and-swathe device for at least three weeks, when motion is gradually initiated.

Four-Part Displacement

Since there is no source of blood supply to the humeral head in this type of fracture, the incidence of avascular necrosis is extremely high. This is the classic case for the use of a prosthetic replacement for the humeral head. Several devices are now available; the author prefers the Neer device which has recently been revised, as illustrated (Fig. 15–21).[131] If this treatment is undertaken it is important to place the device in appropriate retroversion. The reader is referred to Dr. Neer's articles for an explanation of the technique and the postoperative care that is vital in these cases.[125, 126, 130, 131]

Prior to the development of prosthetic replacement of the humeral head the Jones procedure was very popular.[87, 88] This involved resection of the humeral head and reattachment of the greater and lesser tuberosities to the humeral shaft. Pain was not a particular problem in follow-up examination but the function of the shoulder was significantly diminished. The development of improved prosthetic devices has largely replaced this procedure.

FRACTURE-DISLOCATION

It is important to recognize these serious injuries and treat them appropriately if severe disability is to be avoided. These involve anterior and posterior dislocations and may be associated with a two-, three-, or four-part fracture.

ANTERIOR FRACTURE-DISLOCATIONS

Two-Part

This is the most common type of fracture-dislocation encountered. It is interesting that in anterior dislocations the greater tuberosity may be fractured and displaced, while in posterior dislocations it is the lesser tuberosity that may be fractured and displaced. A two-part anterior fracture-dislocation may be managed by careful closed reduction of the dislocation. The usual sequence is that the greater tuberosity fragment is in satisfactory position following repositioning of the dislocation. The hippocratic method or the Stimson method may be utilized for the reduction. If the greater tuberosity fragment is not in satisfactory position, this is managed by open reduction and internal fixation of the fragment with the use of wire loops or a lag compression screw along with repair of the rotator cuff defect.

Three-Part

In this injury the blood supply to the head of the humerus is still intact, as the lesser tuberosity has not been fractured from the articular segment. This is a serious injury. If avascular necrosis of the humeral head is to be avoided, gentle open reduction is probably the method of choice. The head is located and placed back in appropriate position in the glenoid fossa. The greater tuberosity is then wired back to the head fragment, and the head fragment is wired to the shaft of the humerus. The shoulder is immobilized in a sling and swathe for three weeks, and then motion is initiated.

Four-Part

This is a relatively uncommon lesion (Fig. 15–22). However, in its presence the head is devoid of all blood supply. For this reason this lesion is probably best managed with the use of a prosthetic replacement.

POSTERIOR FRACTURE-DISLOCATIONS

Two-Part

A fracture of the lesser tuberosity may occur in association with posterior fracture-dislocations. This injury is managed in the standard fashion for treating an acute posterior dislocation. Longitudinal traction is applied to the arm in the adducted position with slight internal rotation of the humerus. Internal rotation may disengage the head from the posterior glenoid. Direct posterior pressure may be applied to the humeral head, and with a slight external rotation maneuver the humeral head will usually relocate in the glenoid fossa. Postreduction care involves immobilization in slight external rotation for four weeks.

Three-Part

In this injury the shoulder is dislocated in a posterior direction, and there is a fracture of the surgical neck associated with a fracture of the lesser tuberosity. The axillary view roentgenogram is very useful in establishing the correct diagnosis. Closed reduction, performed by longitudinal traction of the humerus while the arm is positioned in adduction, may be attempted. Direct pressure is applied to the humeral head, which is located posteriorly. If the reduction is satisfactory and the position of the fragment is acceptable, a sling and swathe is applied for four weeks. However, if a gentle closed reduction is not successful in reducing the dislocation or the position of the fragments is not acceptable, open reduction is indicated.

Four-Part

This involves posterior dislocation of the humeral head with wide separation of both tuberosities. In other words, the blood supply to the humeral head is completely disrupted. This is a prime indication for a prosthetic replacement. Fortunately, this is a rare injury.

Articular Surface Fractures

Impression fractures may result from acute dislocations of the humeral head, particularly posterior dislocations. The fracture results from pressure of the humeral head against the rim of the glenoid fossa, similar to the mechanism that produces a Hill-Sachs defect. The subchondral bone is acutely crushed. If the fracture involves less than a quarter of the articular surface it is reduced in the usual manner for a posterior dislocation. If there is 50 per cent involvement of the humeral head, this must be treated by primary prosthetic replacement. The cases that fall between these two extremes may be treated by reduction, but the head may be then unstable in the glenoid fossa. In the presence

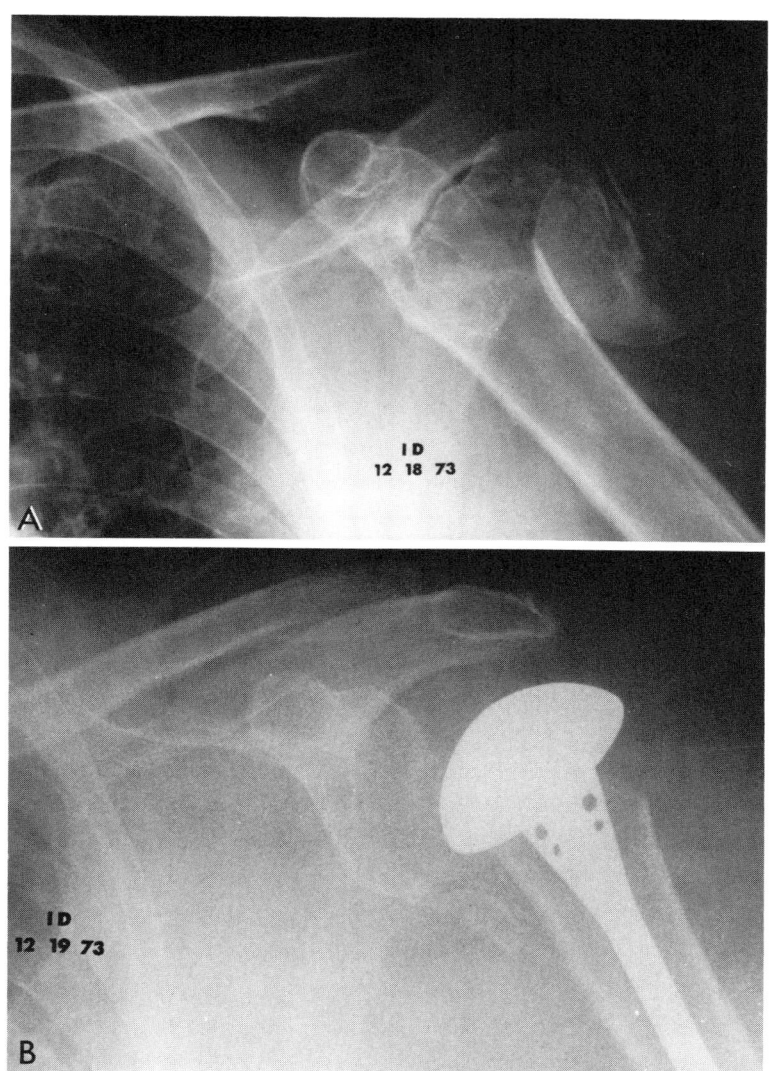

Figure 15-22   *A.*   A four-part displacement. The articular surface is completely detached from its circulation with separation of the tuberosities. *B.*   Treated with a primary Neer prosthetic replacement. The result is good.

of instability in a large defect, the subscapularis tendon may be transferred into the defect, as originally outlined by McLaughlin.

An uncommon head-splitting type of fracture may result from a violent thrust of the humeral head into the glenoid fossa. In this condition the humeral head is fragmented into several separate pieces. The management of this type of injury involves prosthetic replacement.

DISLOCATIONS OF THE SHOULDER GIRDLE

Part II

Dislocations about the shoulder girdle are frequently encountered in everyday orthopedic practice. They affect all age groups, with a definite male preponderance. Since this is a common injury, it is important to have a clear understanding of the mechanisms of injury and the appropriate treatment program for each patient. This is a large subject, and any discussion must involve subluxations and dislocations of the shoulder proper, the acromioclavicular joint, and the sternoclavicular joint. In the following sections each of these areas will be dealt with separately.

CLASSIFICATION OF SHOULDER DISLOCATIONS

The author has found it very useful to classify shoulder dislocations on an anatomical basis, designating four subtypes (Table 15–1). First, there is the anterior

TABLE 15–1   Shoulder Dislocations

Anterior
  Subcoracoid
  Subglenoid
  Subclavicular
  Intrathoracic

Posterior
  Subacromial
  Subglenoid
  Subspinous

Inferior
  Infraglenoid (*Luxatio erecta*)

Superior
  Supraglenoid

shoulder dislocation, which may be subdivided into subcoracoid, subglenoid, subclavicular, and intrathoracic. Second, posterior dislocations may be subdivided into subacromial, subglenoid, and subspinous. Third, inferior dislocations are also known as luxatio erecta and are located infraglenoid. Finally, superior dislocations occur in the supraglenoid area.

Other classifications based on the mechanism of injury are available, but the anatomical grouping outlined here is the simplest and most useful.

ANTERIOR SHOULDER DISLOCATIONS

Dislocations of the shoulder have traditionally been divided into traumatic and atraumatic types. The traumatic type occurs in approximately 85 per cent and the atraumatic type in 15 per cent. A traumatic dislocation is characteristically produced by a significant force being directly applied to the shoulder joint proper. This may occur as the result of a backward fall against a solid object, driving the humeral head anteriorly. Football injuries may account for this type of dislocation, which occurs when the individual falls directly onto the lateral or posterolateral aspect of the shoulder.

Atraumatic dislocations result from a minor injury to the shoulder joint proper. A subclassification of this type is the voluntary dislocation of the shoulder, which is a specific entity. In general, atraumatic dislocations are more unpredictable and difficult to treat. Rowe followed up 500 dislocations of the shoulder and noted a 96 per cent incidence of the traumatic type and a 4 per cent incidence of the atraumatic type.[159]

TRAUMATIC ACUTE ANTERIOR SHOULDER DISLOCATIONS

Mechanism of Injury

The mechanism of injury is slightly different for each type of anterior dislocation. The resultant deformity and dislocation of the humeral head is directly related to the force exerted to produce the injury.

The subcoracoid dislocation is the most common anatomical type and is caused by a combination of abduction and external rotation forces. The combination of these forces produces a typical subcoracoid dislocation, with the head of the humerus located in an anterior position in relationship to the glenoid fossa and slightly inferior to the coracoid process. A second mechanism of injury is most commonly encountered when an individual falls in a backward direction, striking the posterior aspect of the humerus directly against a solid object with force sufficient to produce an anterior dislocation. As previously stated, football injuries may be responsible for this type of dislocation.

The subglenoid dislocation occurs much less frequently than the subcoracoid type, but it is still the second most common acute anterior dislocation. The mechanism of injury is again abduction and external rotation, but with a greater amount of abduction force applied. This results in the humeral head being located in an anterior and inferior position in relationship to the glenoid fossa.

The subclavicular dislocation is uncommon and is produced by a combination of abduction and external rotation, with the addition of a direct lateral force. This results in the humeral head being located in a position just inferior to the midclavicle and medial to the coracoid process.

Finally, an intrathoracic dislocation is also a very uncommon injury. This results from a mechanism similar to that of the subclavicular dislocation, but with a more severe laterally applied force which tends to drive the humeral head into a more medial position. The result is that the humeral head may be driven into the thoracic cavity between the ribs. Fortunately, this is a rare injury, as it may produce significant morbidity.

Physical Examination

An acute traumatic anterior dislocation of the shoulder is very painful. In general, the patient will tend to immobilize the involved extremity in an effort to decrease the pain. He is very apprehensive about any attempt at motion of the shoulder joint during examination. The normal deltoid contour of the shoulder is altered with this type of dislocation. Instead of the normal round appearance of the deltoid region, there may be an abrupt alteration with flattening of the involved area. This is because the humeral head is displaced in an anterior direction, which anatomically alters the characteristic fullness of the shoulder. Palpation of the involved area will reveal a depression just under the acromion, where the humeral head is normally located. A palpable mass may be present in a more medial direction.

The specific attitude of the extremity is dependent on the exact type of dislocation. In general, with the most common type of subcoracoid dislocation the involved extremity is held in slight abduction, with the forearm located in close proximity to the trunk and supported by the uninvolved extremity. This is the typical attitude of the dislocated shoulder. However, the amount of abduction of the shoulder is increased with subglenoid dislocation. Finally, with the rare intrathoracic type there may be a significant amount of abduction owing to the location of the humeral head within the chest cavity.

It is extremely important to document the neurovascular status of the involved extremity. Depending on the location of the humeral head secondary to the applied force, there may be direct trauma to the neurovascular bundle with accompanying deficits. Therefore, the presence or absence of a neurovascular deficit must be ascertained prior to any type of treatment if significant repercussions are to be avoided. The axillary nerve function is tested by pinprick sensation along the lateral aspect of the humeral shaft area. The musculocutaneous nerve is tested by pinprick sensation along the dorsal aspect of the forearm. This is not always 100 per cent reliable, as has been outlined by Blom,[20] but a definite attempt to estimate the gross neurological status of the extremity should be made.

The vascular status of the extremity may be assessed by the presence of a brachial pulse in the antecubital area and the presence or absence of radial and ulnar pulses at the wrist. It is extremely important to assess the capillary flow of the nailbeds to determine if an adequate blood supply is present. Again, it is impossible to overemphasize the importance of performing these simple physical examinations prior to reduction if significant problems are to be avoided later.

Roentgenographic Evaluation

The "trauma series," as advocated by Neer and described in the beginning of this chapter, is an excellent set of roentgenograms for evaluating shoulder injuries.[129] A characteristic deformity of the posterolateral aspect of the humeral head is fre-

quently present following anterior dislocations of the shoulder. This lesion was outlined in the English literature by Hill and Sachs in 1940.[72] They attributed the characteristic deformity to a compression fracture of the humeral head produced by the dense cortical bone of the anterior glenoid rim against the posterolateral aspect of the humeral head (Fig. 15–23). In the English literature this defect has come to be known as the Hill-Sachs lesion. Interestingly, the mechanism producing this lesion as well as the general description of the lesion itself was documented by Hermodsson in the German literature in 1934.[70, 71]

This particular defect is found along the posterolateral aspect of the humeral head and is of variable size, although it is almost always found during surgical exploration. It is generally accepted that the longer the head remains dislocated, the larger the Hill-Sachs lesion will be. Special roentgenographic techniques will adequately demonstrate this defect. The key to demonstrating the lesion is in obtaining an anteroposterior view with internal rotation of the involved extremity. In regular an-

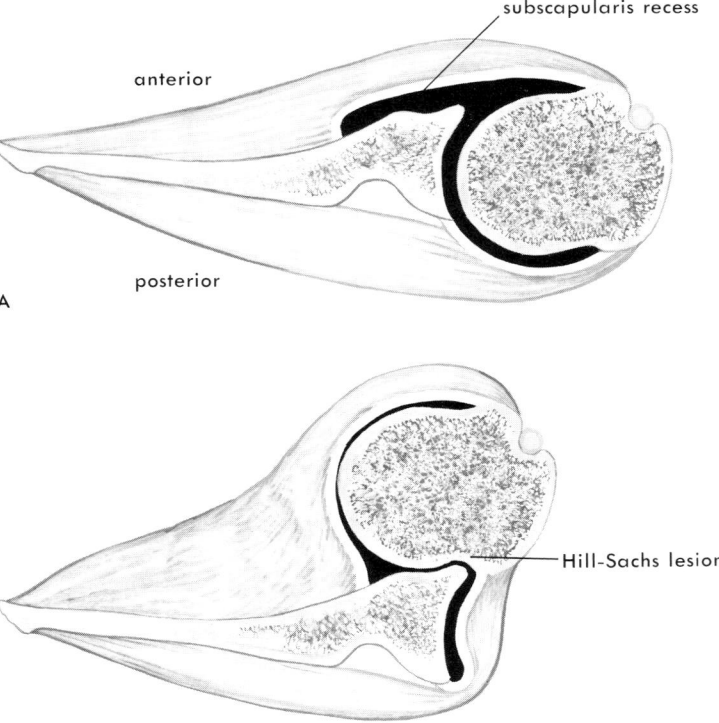

Figure 15–23 A. A large subscapularis recess with insertion of the anterior capsule far medially along the neck of the glenoid. This permits easy anterior dislocation of the shoulder. *B.* This drawing illustrates the creation of a compression fracture in the posterolateral aspect of the humeral head by the rim of the glenoid during anterior dislocation and the position of the humeral head in the subscapularis bursa. (Courtesy of R. H. Rothman, J. P. Marvel, R. B. Heppenstall and *Orthopaedic Clinics of North America.* Orthop. Clin. North Am., 6:415–422, 1975.)

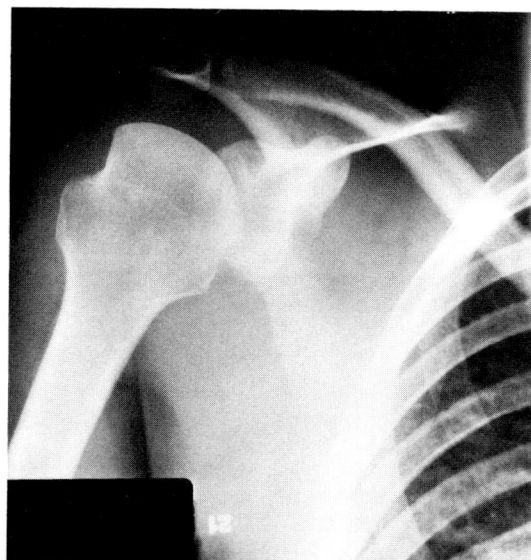

Figure 15–24 A Hill-Sachs lesion demonstrated in the anterolateral aspect of the humeral head.

teroposterior views the defect is present in only 50 per cent of cases. However, if special views are obtained, the defect may be present in from 69 to 87 per cent of cases. The Hill-Sachs view is an anteroposterior roentgenogram of the shoulder with the involved extremity held in a position of excessive internal rotation.

Hermodsson also recommended an anteroposterior view with internal rotation.[69, 70] In this technique the involved extremity is in a position of adduction with the humerus internally rotated at least 45 degrees. The roentgenographic beam is then positioned at a 15 degree angle toward the feet, and the beam is centered over the humeral head.

Stryker advocated a different technique to demonstrate the defect.[62] The patient is placed supine on the x-ray table with a cassette under the involved shoulder. The involved extremity is then gradually elevated such that the palm is placed on the crown of the posterior aspect of the head. The elbow is positioned so that it is pointing in an upward direction. The x-ray beam is then centered and tilted 10 degrees toward the head. This technique has obvious limitations for the initial evaluation of a dislocated shoulder owing to the associated muscle spasm, but is very useful for delin-

eating the posterolateral defect in the head in follow-up examination.

Treatment

A dislocated shoulder should be reduced as soon as possible. However, with a dislocation the blood supply to the humeral head is not as precarious as the blood supply to the femoral head. Therefore, it is not quite as urgent to reduce the humeral head as it is to reduce the femoral head in order to prevent avascular necrosis. Nevertheless, early reduction will prevent the marked muscle changes associated with the dislocation and may decrease the size of the posterolateral humeral head defect. Early reduction may also prevent secondary neurovascular changes from occurring as a result of the dislocation. The majority of these injuries may be reduced in the emergency room under appropriate parenteral medication. A 5 to 10 mg dose of intravenous Valium is an excellent muscle relaxant prior to reduction. If this is coupled with intramuscular administration of appropriate analgesics the patient will be more relaxed, and the associated muscle spasm will be less, allowing an easier reduction. However, if this medication is not successful in relaxing the patient adequately, general anesthesia should be considered. It is probably better to switch to a general anesthetic than to make several attempts at reduction under parenteral analgesics. If too vigorous methods are applied to the reduction, there is always the danger of producing an associated fracture of the humeral shaft, humeral head, or glenoid rim.

At the present time four general methods are frequently employed to accomplish a closed reduction of a dislocated shoulder.

Hippocratic Method. This is the oldest technique that is still in use today.[2] It involves positioning the patient supine on the edge of the examining table. The involved extremity is grasped by the physician at the forearm and wrist, and the physician's foot is placed in the axilla. The reduction is accomplished by the physician's applying longitudinal traction to the involved extremity, while at the same time applying countertraction through the foot in the patient's axilla (Fig. 15–25). It is ex-

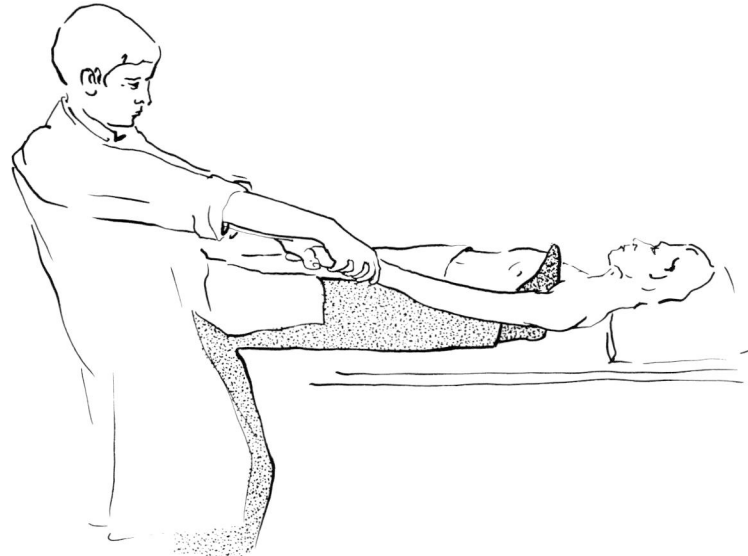

Figure 15-25 A pictorial representation of the classic hippocratic method for reduction of anterior dislocations.

tremely important not to drive the heel of the foot into the axilla, as this may cause neurovascular damage. Rather, the entire foot must span the axilla such that the midportion of the foot lies across the axilla. The secret of this method is in applying gradual and gentle traction along with countertraction. The added advantage is that the method may be accomplished by one person. It is also safe in that associated fractures about the shoulder joint are almost unheard of with this method. There is no question that this is an excellent way to reduce the dislocation. However, it is esthetically unacceptable to some patients to have the surgeon's foot placed in the axilla for countertraction.

Modified Kocher Method. This excellent technique has been used frequently by the author. The original Kocher method called for four specific steps for the reduction.[93] The elbow was flexed to 90 degrees, and traction was applied in a longitudinal direction through the humeral shaft. While the traction was maintained the involved extremity was slowly placed in full external rotation (Fig. 15-26). The humerus was then adducted across the anterior aspect of the chest to approximately the midline, and the arm was internally rotated until the hand was placed on the opposite shoulder. The mechanism involved was direct leverage of the humeral head against the anterior

glenoid rim. It was felt that the external rotation brought the humeral head over to the glenoid rim, and the associated adduction and internal rotation of the humerus accomplished the reduction. However, the author has found that the modified Kocher technique is associated with fewer complications than the original method. The criticism leveled against the original technique is that if the maneuver is performed rapidly, a fracture of the humeral shaft, humeral head, or glenoid rim may occur.

In the author's experience fractures are never encountered with the modified technique. It is accomplished by having the patient lie supine on a stretcher or bed. The physician then holds the involved extremity at the elbow with one hand and at the wrist with the other hand. If the right shoulder is to be reduced, the physician's right hand is placed on the patient's right elbow, and the physician's left hand is placed around the patient's right wrist. The reverse is true for reduction of the left shoulder. Longitudinal traction is applied through the humeral shaft, and the humerus is held in a position of adduction against the patient's trunk. The second and most important phase of the reduction involves *gradual* external rotation of the patient's forearm with the humerus held in a position of adduction.

Emphasis is placed on the slow, gradual position of external rotation of the involved

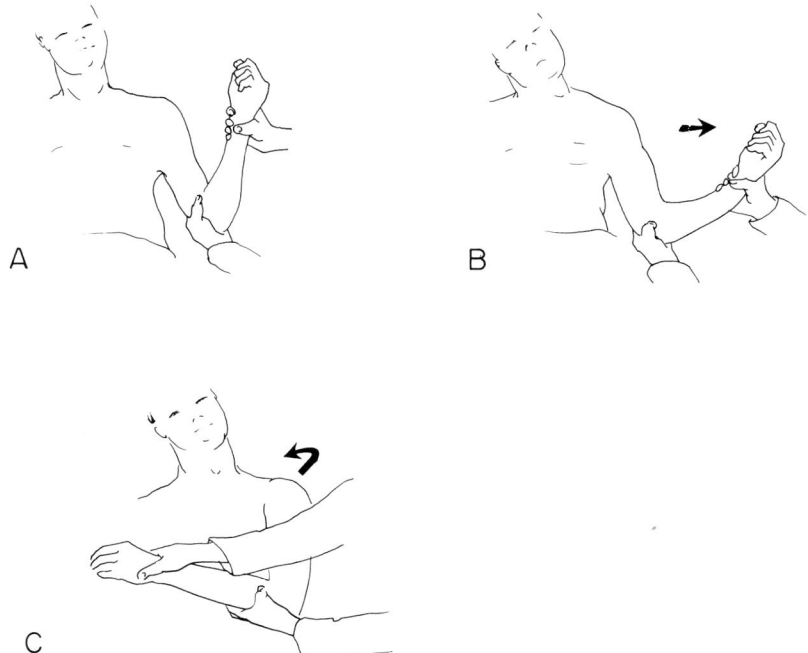

Figure 15–26 The Kocher method for reduction of an anterior dislocation.

extremity. The goal is to produce full external rotation, such that the patient's extremity touches the bed or stretcher. If this portion of the maneuver is performed too quickly, associated muscle spasm about the shoulder may limit the external rotation, and an attempt at forced external rotation may produce an associated fracture. Once full external rotation of the involved extremity is accomplished, the physician will frequently feel the shoulder gradually reduce spontaneously. In other words, the forced adduction of the extremity to the midline of the patient along with sudden internal rotation of the involved extremity, as advocated in the original method, is not necessary to accomplish the reduction.

Unfortunately, in the past, descriptions of the Kocher maneuver did not emphasize the fact that slow, gradual external rotation was the key to success. In fact, many readers have the erroneous impression that adduction and internal rotation of the patient's extremity may be the most important point. In the author's hands, the modified Kocher technique will produce greater than 95 per cent success in reducing shoulder dislocations without associated fractures.

Stimson Method. This is also an excellent technique for reducing a shoulder dislocation. It is based on the fact that gradual traction applied through a weight attached to the patient's upper extremity will provide the necessary force for reduction. The procedure is carried out by placing the patient in a prone position on the edge of an examining table or bed. The involved extremity is then allowed to hang free in a downward direction. The bed or stretcher must be high enough to allow the extremity to hang by gravity without touching the floor. A 10- to 15-lb weight is then attached to the patient's upper extremity and allowed to hang free, providing longitudinal downward traction of the extremity (Fig. 15–27). At least 20 to 25 minutes are allowed for the reduction to occur. This is a slow method, and the associated muscle spasm is gradually decreased with the longitudinal traction. This method has the advantage of not requiring actual manipulation by the physician. It is based on a very sound principle of gradual traction and is successful in a high percentage of cases. The author has been extremely satisfied with the results obtained by this method.

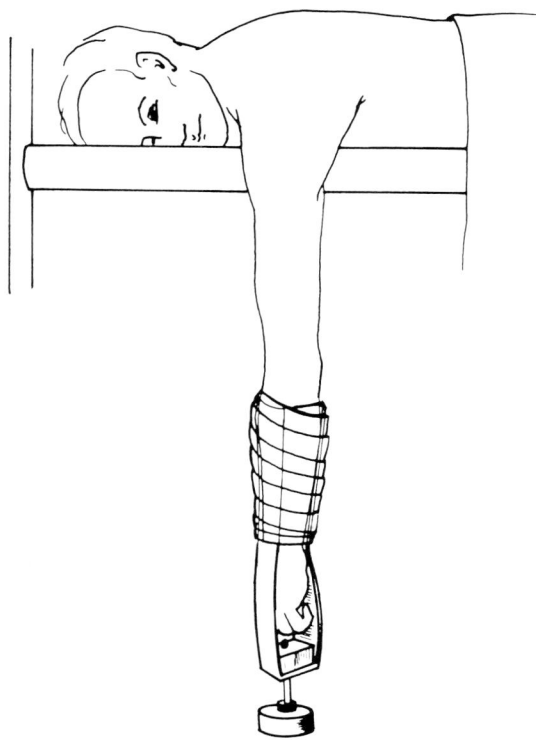

Figure 15–27 The Stimson method for reduction of an anterior dislocation.

Elevation Method. This maneuver is accomplished with the patient in a supine position. The involved extremity is then gradually elevated in forward flexion to a direct overhead position. This method does require the patient's cooperation. If the patient experiences paresthesia in the involved extremity the maneuver is abandoned. However, this has not been encountered to any extent. The physician first applies gentle outward and upward traction in approximately 25 to 30 degrees of abduction. He then positions his hand under the patient's humeral head, gently lifting it over the glenoid rim into the glenoid fossa. This is another excellent method that may be performed without assistance.

Other techniques are available for reduction, but the four methods described are popular in general orthopedic practice today.

Specific treatment is required for intrathoracic dislocations. This type of injury is usually associated with significant trauma. The humeral head is displaced within the chest cavity between the ribs. A general anesthetic is usually required to accomplish reduction with lateral traction.

Open Reduction. Rarely, a dislocation of the shoulder is resistant to the standard methods of closed reduction even under general anesthesia. Under these circumstances an open reduction of the dislocation is indicated. Soft tissue interposition usually accounts for failed attempts at closed reduction. The humeral head is exposed through a standard deltopectoral incision, and any interposed soft tissue is surgically released. It is rare that an open reduction is necessary, but any patient who is taken to the operating room for an attempted closed reduction should have an operative permit signed for possible open reduction if the closed reduction fails.

POSTREDUCTION. Rowe has demonstrated that recurrent dislocation drops off rapidly at 50 years of age.[159, 165] However, he also showed that a short time is all that is required for immobilization in the 50-year and older group. This may be a one-week period, followed by active range-of-motion exercises. The teenager and young adult have a significant incidence of recurrent dislocation. In this group Rowe found that three weeks of immobilization in a position of adduction together with internal reduction decreased the incidence of recurrent dislocation by 15 per cent. However, if more than three weeks of immobilization was instituted, the incidence of recurrent dislocation actually increased. It has become standard policy in most centers to restrict movement of the shoulder for three weeks in the young patient and for approximately one week in the older patient.

Several devices are available to accomplish the immobilization after reduction. A sling and swathe is a simple method of providing satisfactory immobilization. The Nicola shoulder harness is excellent for restricting motion; the author has used this device for postoperative management. However, for routine management of the simple closed reduction any of the commercial shoulder immobilizers is satisfactory. Once the immobilization has been discontinued, a graded course of exercises is important to regain motion of the shoulder. The Codman pendulum exercises are an excellent means of initiating motion. These are followed by active flexion and extension and finally by active abduction. Overhead pulley exercises are useful in strengthening the musculature about the shoulder. The most important point to remember is that any motion of the shoulder following an injury must be initiated gradually and if pain intervenes, forced manipulation of the shoulder must be avoided. Therapists are to be taught that gradual graded range of motion is a much more physiological goal than aggressive manual forced range of motion, which will actually hinder recovery in the long run.

ATRAUMATIC OR VOLUNTARY DISLOCATIONS

This type of injury is infrequent compared with traumatic dislocation. It usually occurs in young adolescents. The condition is twice as frequent in males as in females.

Mechanism of Injury

Many patients have no history of injury prior to the ability to voluntarily dislocate the shoulder; in some, spontaneous dislocation is preceded by a mild injury.

Physical Examination

The majority of patients do not demonstrate any other significant soft tissue laxity. However, a small percentage do demonstrate increased laxity of the soft tissue structures. In other words, in a minority of patients a defect in collagen metabolism or in the structure of the ground substance may account for the ability to voluntarily dislocate the shoulder. In any event, a connective tissue disorder should be ruled out as the cause of the dislocation. An example of this problem is seen in some patients with the Ehlers-Danlos syndrome.

The patient is able to dislocate the shoulder at will. It may be seen as a unilateral or bilateral dislocation. Frequently, the patient will derive some pleasure from demonstrating the voluntary nature of the dislocation. This is in some ways attention-seeking behavior. In fact, in many cases it reflects a definite emotional disturbance.

Roentgenographic Evaluation

Routine roentgenographic studies reveal that the shoulder may be voluntarily dislocated anteriorly, posteriorly, or inferiorly. There is usually no evidence of a Hill-Sachs lesion in these patients. Traumatic arthritis of the glenohumeral joint is usually absent in patients who have not received surgical treatment. On the other hand, traumatic arthritis of this joint is common in patients who have had repeated unsuccessful operative procedures.

Treatment

Rowe and co-workers demonstrated that in general, patients with an underlying psychological disorder have a poorer result with any type of surgical procedure.[164] They also felt that patients without psychological disorders have a much better result with a rehabilitation program designed to strengthen the surrounding shoulder musculature. This was particularly important in regard to the shoulder abductors as well as to the external and internal rotators. If the patient does not respond to the conservative rehabilitation program, surgical treatment is indicated, provided that any psychiatric problems have been resolved. It appears that a combination of surgical procedures, rather than a standard single operative approach, is necessary for the management of these injuries. Surgical exploration of the shoulder usually demonstrates some laxity of the anterior capsule, but there is a consistent absence of both the true Bankart lesion and the Hill-Sachs lesion. The surgery should probably include a procedure to tighten the subscapularis muscle as well as the capsule in the anterior aspect of the shoulder. A combination of a Magnuson-Stack procedure along with scarification of the anterior capsule is probably indicated. An alternative may be a combination of a Putti-Platt and a Bankart repair.

RECURRENT ANTERIOR DISLOCATIONS OF THE SHOULDER

Recurrent dislocation of the shoulder is seen regularly in an average orthopedic practice. Of all the joints in the human body, the shoulder is the one that is most subject to recurrent dislocation. This is a particularly troublesome affliction, since most affected individuals are young and athletically active. In fact, all studies reveal that the younger the patient, the more likely the incidence of recurrent dislocations. The true occurrence in the adolescent and young adult group is probably close to 80 per cent. On the other end of the scale, it has been noted that the incidence of dislocation decreases significantly after the age of 40. The accepted figure past 40 is probably close to 15 per cent. This condition is more commonly encountered in males compared with females, by at least a four to one ratio.

The length of time that a shoulder should be immobilized following reduction of the initial dislocation has long been a matter of debate. McLaughlin and Cavallaro felt that the immobilization time after the initial dislocation was not important in terms of the development of future dislocations.[112] On the other hand, Rowe has demonstrated that a three-week interval of immobilization is adequate in the young individual, and that further immobilization will not produce a lower incidence of recurrence; in fact, in his series there was a higher incidence of recurrence if immobilization was prolonged.[159, 165] Prolonged immobilization in the older age group is not only unnecessary but detrimental to restoration of function. Early mobilization following reduction of a primary dislocation in an individual over 40 years of age may be carried out without fear of recurrence.

Anatomical Lesions Associated with Recurrent Dislocation

The Glenoid Labrum. Perthes and later Bankart felt that anterior instability of the shoulder was due to detachment of the fibrocartilaginous labrum or detachment of the capsule from the glenoid rim.[13, 149] It was Bankart's contention that these structures were disrupted by the dislocating humeral head. Although it is true that these lesions are frequently seen upon inspection of the interior of the shoulder joint after repeated dislocations, it is also true that autopsy studies have clearly demonstrated that linear tears and detachment of the labrum are found in many individuals who have never had a history of dislocation.

It has also been shown by Townley that the anterior glenoid labrum can be removed by the posterior approach, and that if the anterior capsule is intact it is impossible to cause anterior dislocation of the joint.[181, 182] Fractures of the bony anterior rim have also been noted. It would seem that, although these lesions are associated with anterior dislocation and undoubtedly contribute to instability, they are neither essential nor exclusive to this disorder.

The Anterior Capsule and Glenohumeral Ligaments. The capsule of the shoulder joint is inherently lax to allow for its great mobility, and has a volume approximately double that of the humeral head. This volume may be further enlarged in recurrent dislocation. Anteriorly, the capsule may be thickened in three areas forming the superior, middle, and inferior glenohumeral ligaments. In the presence of three well-formed glenohumeral ligaments, there will undoubtedly be an excellent checkrein and buttress against anterior dislocation.

However, several excellent cadaveric and surgical studies have demonstrated that there is considerable variation in the arrangement of the glenohumeral ligaments and the synovial recesses found between them. The superior glenohumeral ligament arises from the supraglenoid tubercle and courses laterally to its insertion on the humerus near the tip of the lesser tuberosity. The middle and inferior glenohumeral ligaments evidence considerable variability. The middle glenohumeral ligament is absent or poorly defined in one third of the cases. In many individuals a prominent subscapular bursa is present that may extend for a variable distance anterior and medial to the glenoid rim, forming a pouch that would easily accept the humeral head.

It is thus evident that considerable variation exists in the configuration of the so-called anterior capsular mechanism. Although a strong anterior capsular mechanism buttresses and helps prevent anterior dislocation, individuals with absence of the middle and inferior glenohumeral ligaments and a large subscapular recess may never dislocate the shoulder. Again, skepticism must be cast on the theory that disruption of the anterior capsular support is the "essential lesion" of this disorder.

The Posterolateral Notch in the Humeral Head. It is now generally accepted that the posterolateral indentation in the humeral head found with recurrent dislocation is a compression fracture caused by impingement of the anterior glenoid rim on the posterior and lateral aspect of the humeral head during the process of dislocation. This notch, although of variable size, is almost always found during surgical exploration. It is a secondary rather than primary pathological lesion. Certainly a significant defect of this type would predispose to recurrences.

Excessive Anterior Tilt of the Glenoid and Excessive Retroversion of the Humeral Head. Saha has implicated excessive anterior tilt of the glenoid and excessive retroversion of the humeral head (excessive anteversion with the arm in full abduction) as possible causative factors in recurrent anterior dislocation of the shoulder.[168] Although his anatomical and radiographic studies appear to be well founded, his surgical procedures have not gained wide acceptance or confirmation. Correction of these defects could be obtained by osteotomy of the glenoid or rotational osteotomy of the humerus.

Laxity of the Subscapularis. Both Moseley and DePalma have demonstrated laxity of the subscapularis muscle and tendon in recurrent anterior dislocation of the glenohumeral joint.[45, 120, 121] It is obvious that in the shoulder joint the osseous configuration itself and the lax synovial capsule produce no inherent stability. If the inferior and middle glenohumeral ligaments are congenitally absent or elongated through trauma, only the subscapularis muscle remains as a buttress to prevent dislocation. Most recurrences of dislocation, in fact, occur not with extreme trauma, but rather when the shoulder is in an unguarded position with the subscapularis muscle relaxed. In summary, there is no one basic anatomical lesion that is solely responsible for the disorder known as recurrent anterior dislocation. Hence a search for the "essential lesion" is neither fruitful nor logical. It should also be stated that the subscapularis appears to be an important

dynamic anterior buttress, the loss of which permits recurrent anterior dislocations.

Mechanism of Injury

The mechanism of injury for recurrent anterior dislocations is similar to that for primary anterior dislocations. In other words, abduction and external rotation are the most common maneuvers producing recurrent anterior dislocations. The force required to produce a recurrent dislocation is much less than that required to produce the initial dislocation.

Physical Examination

Patients will usually describe some form of abduction and external rotation component in the production of the dislocation. The pain associated with a recurrent dislocation is not quite as severe as that of the initial dislocation. However, the patient will cautiously hold the involved extremity alongside the trunk in a protective manner. The deltoid fullness of the shoulder will be lost, as in an initial dislocation. The injured extremity will be supported by the uninvolved extremity.

Roentgenographic Evaluation

The location of the humeral head in routine roentgenographic examination is similar to that described previously for the initial dislocation. If there have been several episodes of dislocation, there may be definite evidence of degenerative changes within the glenohumeral joint (Figs. 15–28 to 15–31). A common finding with multiple recurrent dislocations is loose bodies along the inferior glenoid rim. A defect in the glenoid rim may also be evident. Roentgenograms will demonstrate evidence of a Hill-Sachs lesion in the humeral head in the majority of cases.

Treatment

A general rule of thumb is that at least two documented episodes of dislocation must occur prior to any surgical intervention. It is also important to have roentgenographic

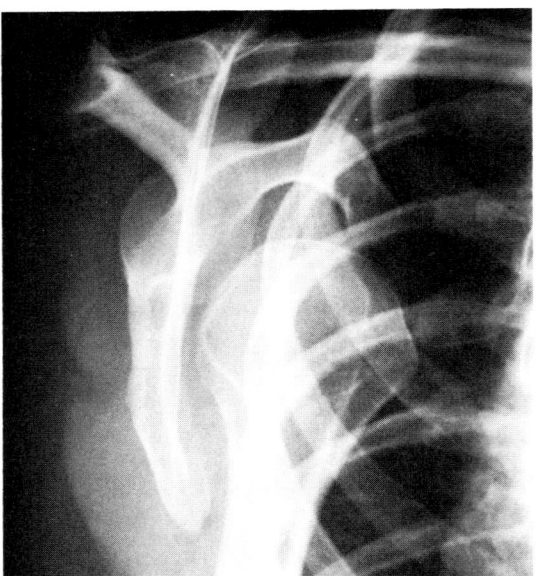

Figure 15-28   A lateral roentgenogram of the trauma series demonstrating a definite anterior dislocation.

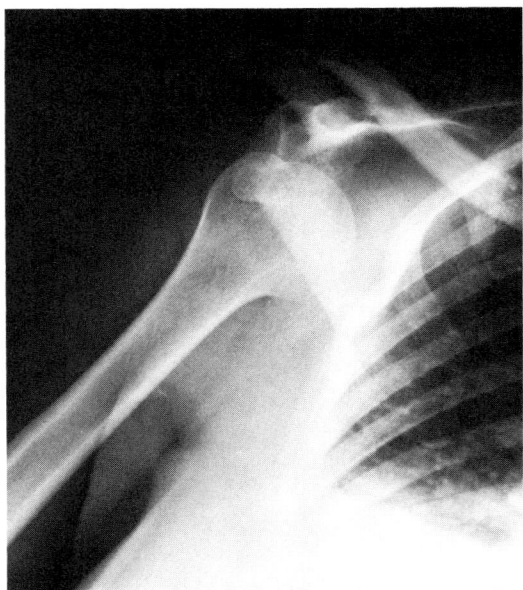

Figure 15-29   A subcoracoid anterior dislocation.

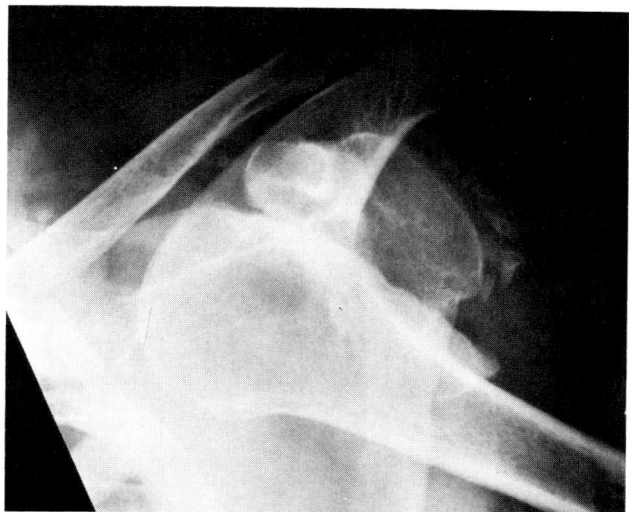

Figure 15–30   A subcoracoid anterior dislocation with defects from the glenoid rim.

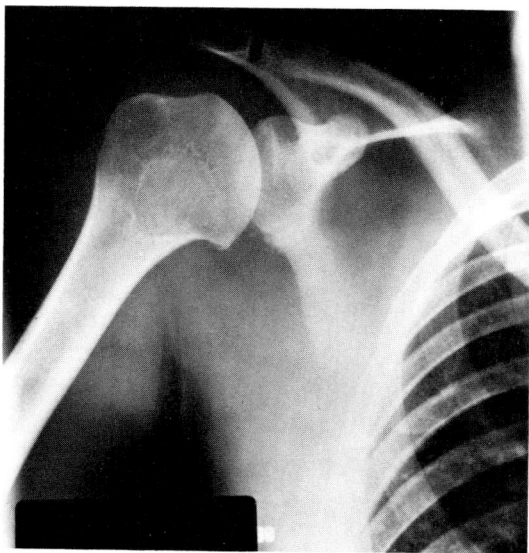

Figure 15–31   A recurrent dislocation of the shoulder with a Hill-Sachs lesion and a defect on the inferior rim of the glenoid.

evidence to prove that it is an anterior dislocation.

A wide variety of surgical approaches have been successful in the management of this disorder. In fact, more than 113 procedures have been described for operative repair of a recurrent dislocation. At the outset it must be recognized that no single operative procedure is universally applicable to all recurrent anterior dislocations of the shoulder. It is important to tailor the operative procedure to each patient. It is true that the majority of surgeons will favor the operative approach with which they have obtained the best results. However, it is rigid and inappropriate thinking to feel that one, and only one, procedure is indicated for all shoulder repairs. At the present time, there are five basic operations that are widely used. Each of these procedures will be described separately along with its advantages.

Modified Magnuson-Stack (Subscapular Transfer). The modified Magnuson repair is a simple, safe, and effective reconstructive surgical solution for operative repair of a dislocated shoulder.[107] The basic principle of this procedure is a distal and lateral transfer of the insertion of the subscapularis tendon in order to tighten and increase the effectiveness of this anterior buttress to the humeral head. Clearly, in transferring the insertion of the subscapularis tendon one is also tightening the glenohumeral ligaments, since the lateral portion of the anterior capsule and ligaments blend with the subscapularis tendon, and indeed in most individuals are inseparable. Properly performed, this maneuver will also obliterate the subscapularis bursa and pouch. The recurrence rate subsequent to this procedure has varied from 3 to 14 per cent. This method appears to have a lower recurrence rate than the Bankart operation, and 87 per cent of patients showed no evidence of restriction of external rotation.

The operation is performed under general anesthesia with endotracheal intubation. The patient is in a semisitting position with a folded sheet beneath the scapula. The shoulder projects well beyond the edge of the operating table, and the head is turned toward the opposite side. A curved anterior incision is utilized, beginning anterior to the acromioclavicular joint, curving slightly

medially, and then proceeding distally to a point just lateral to the anterior axillary fold. The cephalic vein is identified and retracted medially with a 1/4-inch strip of deltoid muscle. The dissection is then carried downward just lateral to the deltopectoral interval. Complete hemostasis is obtained until the subscapularis tendon and its overlying bursa are identified. The humerus can then be externally rotated and the upper and lower limits of the subscapularis tendon clearly identified. The bursa should be dissected from the anterior portion of this tendon, and the veins coursing over the tendon should be cauterized. The insertion of the subscapularis tendon together with the anterior joint capsule is then transferred.

A Kelly hemostat is placed beneath the subscapularis tendon at its insertion, and the insertion is freed by sharp dissection. Placement of the hemostat can be facilitated by nicking the tendon in line with its fibers 2 mm from its upper and lower margins with a scalpel. The full thickness of the tendon and joint capsule is then grasped with two Allis clamps and, with a heavy scissors, dissected medially well beyond the margin of the glenoid rim. The upper and lower incisions along the border of the subscapularis must be sufficiently extensive to allow easy distal transplantation of the insertion. If the origin of the middle glenohumeral ligament and joint capsule is in a medial location, or if it has been stripped medially by trauma, the capsule and anterior aspect of the bone should be roughened in order to cause adhesions and eliminate the subscapularis pouch.

The arm is then rotated internally, and the site of reimplantation of the subscapularis tendon is selected (Fig. 15–32). The site of insertion should be lateral to the biceps tendon and 1 to 2 cm distal to its original insertion. The periosteum is elevated as a laterally based flap. The cortical surface is freshened with a narrow gouge, but a full-thickness defect is not created, since adequate bone stock to hold the staple must be maintained. If the full thickness of the cortex is inadvertently violated, the tendon will be sewn rather than stapled in place. With the arm in full internal rotation, the first assistant pulls the tendon distally and laterally with the Allis clamp while the

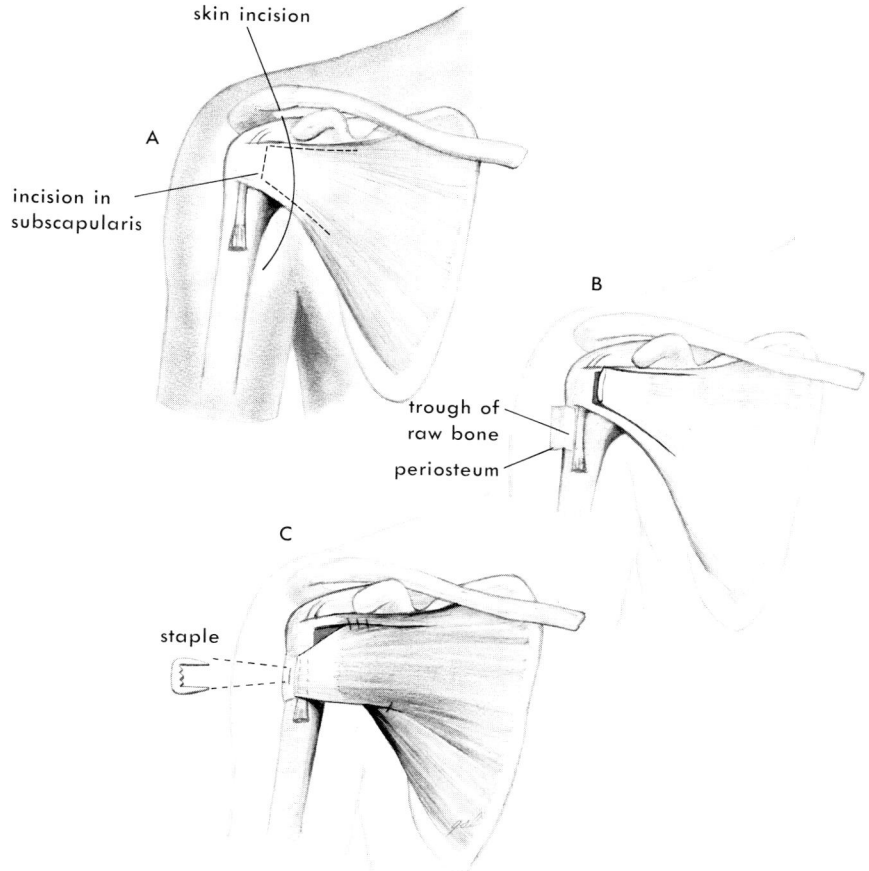

Figure 15–32 The modified Magnuson-Stack subscapularis transfer with a serrated staple. (Courtesy of R. H. Rothman, J. P. Marvel, R. B. Heppenstall and *Orthopaedic Clinics of North America.* Orthop. Clin. North Am., 6:415–422, 1975.)

surgeon inserts a serrated staple to hold the tendon in appropriate position. The upper and lower borders of the subscapularis muscle and the capsule may be repaired with number 1 chromic sutures. The wound is copiously irrigated and the skin closed, using fine subcuticular wire.

An alternative to the staple method is to place a small trough in the cortex with two or three drill holes through the cortex. The subscapularis tendon may be inserted into this defect and held in this position with heavy silk sutures through the tendon and the drill holes and tied on itself. However, the author has found the staple method to be both simple and quick, and associated with very low morbidity.

This is an excellent procedure for repair of a recurrent anterior dislocation. It is particularly applicable to shoulders that do not have a large defect in the inferior glenoid rim. Under these circumstances, a different type of procedure, such as a bone block operation, should be considered.

Bankart (Anterior Capsular Repair). This operative procedure was essentially designed to repair the Bankart lesion, which is a soft tissue defect along the glenoid rim.[13, 15] The term has come to be associated with any avulsion of the capsule or detachment of the glenoid labrum. The principle of the repair is to expose the capsular attachment to the glenoid from an anterior approach and to repair the detached capsule by drill holes through the glenoid rim. Rowe has devised several modifications for attachment of the capsule to the glenoid rim through the drill holes.

An anterior incision is utilized for exposure. The deltoid fibers are split and re-

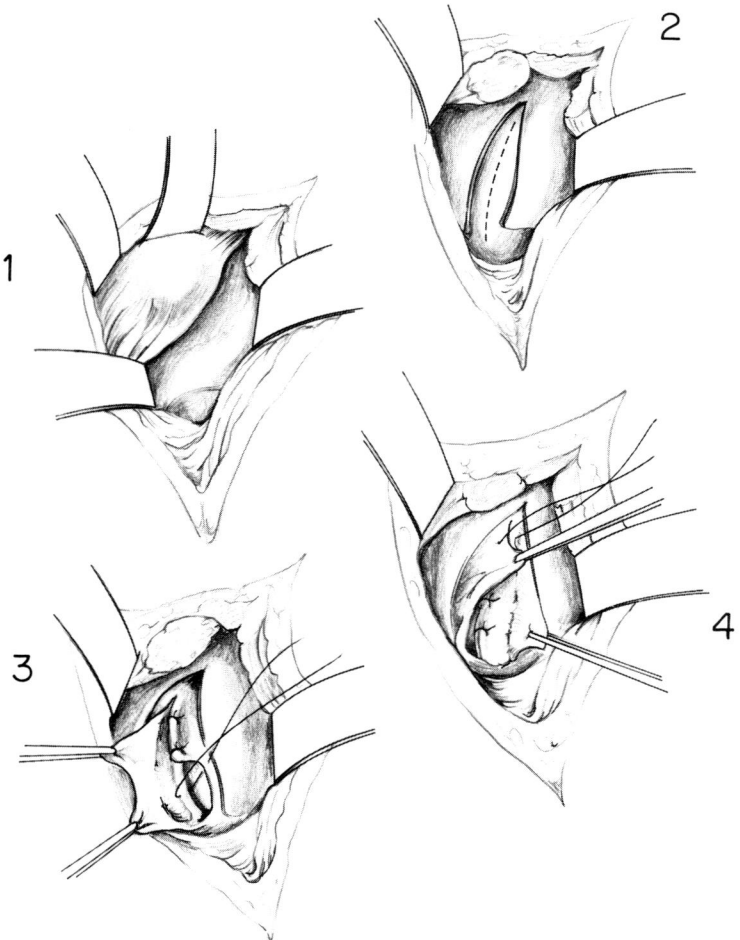

Figure 15–33 The Bankart anterior capsular repair.

tracted. The subscapularis will then come into view (Fig. 15–33). The subscapularis muscle is detached at the central portion of the tendon and retracted in a medial direction. The anterior and inferior aspect of the capsule is then adequately visualized. The detached capsule or labrum is reattached to the glenoid rim through drill holes that are placed in the margin of the glenoid. A humeral head retractor is very useful in gaining exposure to the rim of the glenoid for placement of the holes within the rim. It is probably best to decorticate the rim of the glenoid as well, to encourage scar formation around the anterior aspect of the capsule. It has been customary to fashion three separate holes in the glenoid rim for suturing the advanced lateral capsular flap into this

location. The capsular flap is sutured with heavy silk to encourage mild scar formation. The medial portion of the capsule is imbricated over the sutured lateral portion. The subscapularis is then reattached to the stump. This essentially completes the repair.

It is interesting that Rowe and co-workers in a recent review of 161 Bankart repairs found that there was a separation of the capsule from the anterior glenoid rim at the time of surgery in 85 per cent of their cases. A Hill-Sachs lesion was demonstrated in the humeral head in 77 per cent. There was damage to the anterior glenoid rim in 73 per cent. There was a 3.5 per cent recurrence rate following their repair. This was a long-term follow-up study that demonstrated the good results that may be obtained with the Bankart procedure properly applied.

The Bankart repair is a tried and proven repair for recurrent shoulder dislocations. However, it is technically difficult to place the drill holes in the glenoid rim for reattachment of the capsule. It definitely does tighten the anterior aspect of the shoulder and is very useful in this respect. However, if a large defect is present in the inferior glenoid rim, it is probably best to perform a bone block type of procedure.

Putti-Platt (Subscapularis Shortening). It is interesting that Sir Harry Platt of England and Vittorio Putti of Italy never really published their technique. The operative procedure was described by Osmond-Clarke, who credited both Putti and Platt with developing the procedure.[141, 142] The principle of this operation is to overlap and shorten both the capsule and the subscapularis. An anterior incision is utilized to expose the shoulder, as in the other procedures (Fig. 15–34).

The subscapularis muscle is identified and cut vertically approximately ½ inch from the musculotendinous junction through the muscle fibers. The stump of the muscle is retracted in a lateral direction, exposing the anterior capsule. The lateral aspect of the anterior capsule and the lateral

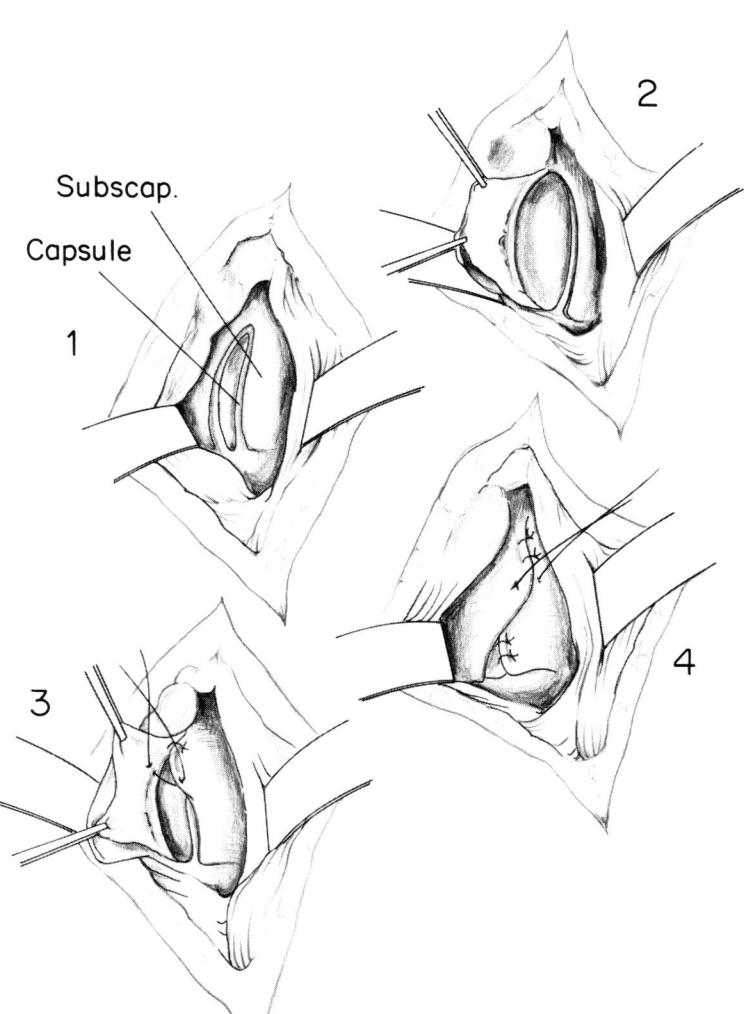

Subscap.

Capsule

Figure 15–34 The Putti-Platt subscapularis shortening procedure.

portion of the subscapularis are then sutured into the base of the medial capsular flap along the glenoid rim while the arm is held in marked internal rotation. The medial portion of the capsule is sutured over the lateral portion of the subscapularis tendon. The medial portion of the subscapularis is then imbricated in a pants-over-vest type of arrangement over the lateral subscapularis stump. This completes the repair.

This is a useful procedure, but again, if there is a defect in the anterior glenoid rim this should probably be treated with a different method, such as a bone block.

Recently, Morrey and Janes reported a long-term follow-up study of the Putti-Platt and Bankart procedures.[118] The average follow-up of 10.2 years revealed a recurrence rate of 11 per cent. It was their impression that in the presence of a Bankart lesion or erosion of the rim of the glenoid, the Putti-Platt procedure may not always be an adequate operation.

Bristow (Coracoid Process Transfer). Bristow never described the procedure that bears his name. It was first described in 1958 by Helfet, who named it after Rowley Bristow of South Africa.[65] The procedure involves the transplantation of the coracoid process with the attached conjoined tendon to the anterior surface of the glenoid (Fig. 15–35). The coracoid process is detached from the scapula just distal to the insertion of the pectoralis minor muscle, leaving the conjoined tendons attached. The subscapularis muscle is then isolated, and a vertical incision is placed within the substance of the subscapularis tendon. The joint is visualized, and the anterior portion of the neck of the scapula is decorticated. The coracoid process with the attached conjoined tendons is then transferred through the vertical incision in the subscapularis and is positioned in direct contact with the decorticated surface of the scapula. It is maintained in position by suturing the conjoined tendon to the incised edges of the subscapularis tendon. Helfet believed this procedure functioned in a dual capacity. First of all, it aided in supporting the anterior capsular portion of the joint; second, it functioned as a small bone block. Helfet reported good results

with the use of this technique and only one recurrence out of thirty cases.

In 1970, May reviewed the results of a modified Bristow procedure in 16 patients.[108] The operation was altered to the extent that the coracoid process was attached to the anterior edge of the glenoid rim and overlapped the superior half of the subscapularis tendon and muscle. All 16 of the patients were found to have a good functional range of motion, and none had limitation of external rotation greater than 15 degrees. It is felt that the transplanted coracoid process with the attached short head of the biceps and coracobrachialis functions as an anterior sling when the shoulder is abducted and externally rotated. It also serves as a modified bone block.

A deltopectoral type of incision is utilized to expose the shoulder. The coracoid process is identified and osteotomized with the use of a curved osteotome. The osteotomy site is selected to leave the pectoralis minor attached to the remaining portion of the coracoid process. In other words, a small portion of the coracoid process with the attached conjoined tendons is reflected off the main coracoid process. The short head of the biceps and the coracobrachialis, which are attached to the osteotomized coracoid process, are then mobilized. Special care is taken to protect the musculocutaneous nerve as it enters the posteromedial aspect of the coracobrachialis muscles approximately 6 cm distal to the tip of the coracoid process. A vertical incision is placed in the substance of the subscapularis muscle between its midportion and the lower third. The muscle is reflected in an inferior direction, providing adequate visualization of the glenoid rim for the placement of the coracoid process against the anterior glenoid. The surface is decorticated with the use of a gouge. A small drill hole, approximately 3.2 mm in size, is placed in the coracoid process and into the glenoid rim and directed posteriorly. A lag screw is utilized to transfix the coracoid process to the anterior portion of the glenoid.

This is an excellent procedure for the management of recurrent dislocations of the shoulder. It appears that this will continue to be a popular shoulder repair, particularly for the athletic individual who does not

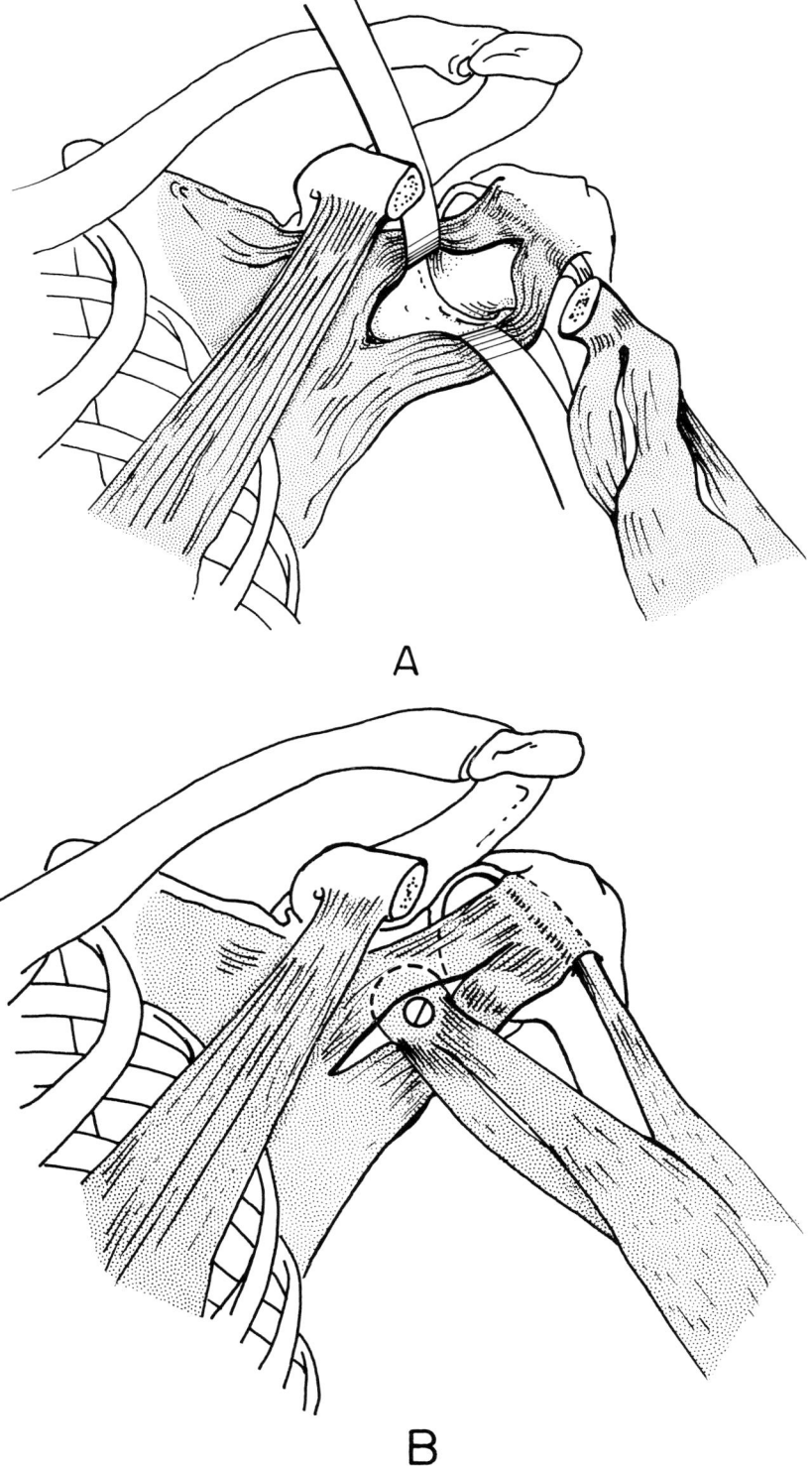

A

B

Figure 15–35   The May modification of the Bristow coracoid process transfer.

want to have a severe restriction of external rotation. Lombardo and co-workers recently reviewed 51 cases of the modified Bristow procedure.[102] Their redislocation rate was 2 per cent, with few complications. Their average limitation of motion was 11 degrees of external rotation. This procedure appears to have a definite place in the management of recurrent dislocations in individuals who require overhead motion for athletic endeavors. There is very little morbidity associated with the transplantation of the coracoid process and fixation with a lag compression screw.

Eden-Hybbinette (Anterior Bone Block). This procedure involves establishing an anterior bone block to prevent redislocation. It was developed independently by Eden and Hybbinette,[49, 79] and is extremely valuable in the presence of a large defect in the glenoid rim or a large Hill-Sachs lesion. The shoulder is exposed through a standard deltopectoral groove. The coracobrachialis is retracted in a medial direction. The subscapularis muscle is identified, and the subscapularis tendon is divided approximately 1/4 inch medial to the insertion of the tendon. The underlying capsule is also incised. The glenoid rim is then inspected along the inferior aspect. A subperiosteal pocket is created along the inferior portion of the anterior lip of the glenoid cavity. A bone graft is obtained from the iliac crest, 1 inch in length by 1/2 inch in width. The bone graft is positioned into the subperiosteal pocket so that the projecting portion of the graft is against the glenoid rim, thus forming an anterior wall or buttress of bone. No additional fixation was recommended. However, the author has found that the graft may be stabilized in position with a small lag compression screw. This adds little morbidity and provides for adequate fixation. The subscapularis tendon is then reapproximated.

Palmer and Widen felt that this is also an excellent procedure for the management of recurrent dislocation of the shoulder in association with a large posterolateral defect in the humeral head.[144]

POSTOPERATIVE IMMOBILIZATION. The author has found the Nicola sling to be very useful for immobilizing the shoulder postoperatively.[138] It provides for fairly rigid immobilization of the shoulder, yet allows for some access to the upper arm for hygienic purposes. Other commercial devices are available for immobilization, and the individual physician will usually select the device that works best for him. The duration of immobilization depends upon the physical activity of the individual. In a very athletic individual it may be preferable to maintain the immobilization for four to six weeks. If the patient is not very athletic or is in an older age group, three to four weeks are all that is required. Graded range-of-motion exercises are initiated following the immobilization period. This includes Codman pendulum exercises followed by forward flexion and then eventually by abduction range-of-motion exercises. Strengthening exercises are reserved until an adequate range of motion is obtained.

OLD ANTERIOR DISLOCATIONS

This type of injury is seen in two specific patient populations. The first and most frequent is the elderly patient. Many of these patients are debilitated and have an organic mental syndrome. Therefore, the dislocation is not apparent following the initial injury. The second population comprises young patients who have suffered multiple trauma with associated head injury. The obvious head injury and other vital organ injuries are recognized early and treated on an emergency basis. Unfortunately, the dislocated shoulder may not be recognized initially under these circumstances.

Physical Examination

In the elderly patient the loss of normal contour of the deltoid muscle may be evident. However, the active range of motion at the shoulder joint is usually adequate. This is because the associated scapulothoracic motion allows for apparent active flexion and abduction. It is important to record the neurovascular status of the involved extremity since 20 to 30 per cent of these patients may have a neurological deficit secondary to the dislocation. There may also be evidence of decreased blood flow in the axillary artery, as evidenced by decreased capillary filling time under the nailbeds.

In the young patient who has recovered from other major organ injuries, similar physical findings may be evident. However, in this age group there is usually significant limitation of motion of the shoulder owing to continued associated muscle contraction. The muscle mass is usually larger in these patients compared with the elderly, and this contributes to the restriction of motion in the young.

Roentgenographic Evaluation

The anteroposterior and axillary or transthoracic views will usually demonstrate the anterior dislocation (Fig. 15–36). The vast majority of patients will demonstrate subcoracoid location of the humeral head. They may also demonstrate an associated fracture. The true incidence is probably greater than one third of patients, and the fractures may involve the humeral neck, tuberosities, glenoid rim, or coracoid process. Schulz and co-workers found a greater than 50 per cent incidence of associated fractures in their series.

Treatment

A good rule of thumb is to consider an open reduction of the dislocation if three weeks have elapsed since the initial dislocation. Up until three weeks, a gentle closed reduction is indicated. However, this must be performed under general anesthesia to insure complete muscle relaxation. After a three week interval the risks of a closed reduction are increased, owing to the fact that considerable scarring has occurred in the vicinity of the dislocated humeral head. This condition may then bind the neurovascular bundle, and a forced closed reduction may lead to avulsion of the neurovascular bundle.

This is particularly true in the elderly in regard to the axillary artery, as there may already be evidence of arteriosclerosis in the vessel, and associated traction during reduction may have disastrous consequences. For this reason some consideration should be given to obtaining a preoperative arteriogram to visualize the status of the axillary vasculature. At the time of the

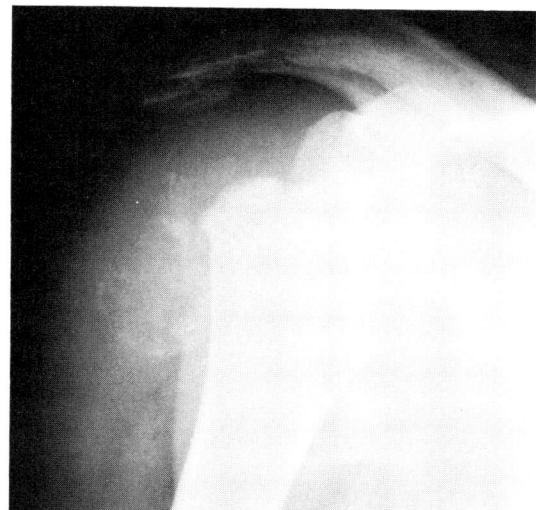

Figure 15–36 An old unrecognized anterior dislocation of the shoulder. Note the calcific reaction in the surrounding tissues.

operative procedure it is extremely important to isolate the proximal vessels in order to obtain control. If this is not performed and the soft tissue is released in an attempt to reposition the humeral head, some damage may occur to the axillary artery. Control of bleeding may be extremely difficult if the vessel has not been isolated proximally prior to release of the soft tissue structures.

If the humeral head has been dislocated for a five- to six-month period, it is probably appropriate to consider a rehabilitation program rather than an open reduction. Many patients at this stage will have a limited functional range of motion of the extremity with minimal pain. This is particularly true in the elderly and in injury of a nondominant extremity.

SUBLUXATION OF THE SHOULDER

Anterior subluxation of the shoulder is a relatively new entity. At the present time there are few articles in the literature regarding this subject. However, there is no question that this is a definite recognizable entity. It usually presents in the young athletic individual who has sustained an injury to the shoulder with a "popping" sensation at the time of injury. The main complaint in follow-up examination is a feeling of instability of the shoulder.

Physical Examination

The contour of the shoulder is normal. There is usually some limitation of the extremes of external rotation on examination. The patient will become very apprehensive as the shoulder is brought into a position of external rotation. The examiner may have the impression that the humeral head is riding up on the glenoid rim when the arm is in external rotation, and then that the humeral head is sliding back into the glenoid fossa when the arm is returned to a neutral position. Occasionally, there will be tenderness along the anterior capsule margin.

Roentgenographic Evaluation

Regular anteroposterior and lateral roentgenographic views may be normal in this condition. A careful evaluation of the roentgenograms may reveal calcification at the inferior glenoid rim margin (Fig. 15–37).

This is probably evidence of a prior injury to the capsule and glenoid labrum with an attempt at repair. Owing to the difficulty of demonstrating the particular pathology, Rokous and co-workers described a modified axillary roentgenogram.[156] This roentgenographic technique was from West Point, and it has come to be known as the "West Point view."

The patient is placed in the prone position on the examining table. The shoulder is then built up approximately 3 inches from the examining table surface. The arm is abducted 90 degrees and rotated so that the forearm is resting over the edge of the table. The palm is facing down, and the head is turned away from the affected shoulder. The roentgenographic tube is positioned in such a manner that the central ray projects 25 degrees downward from the horizontal position and 25 degrees medially. The central ray is directed posteriorly approximately 12 to 14 cm inferior and 3 to 4 cm medial to the acromial edge.

Rokous and co-workers examined 63 patients with a history indicative of recurrent subluxation of the shoulder and were able to demonstrate an osseous abnormality of the glenoid rim in 53 patients. The typical

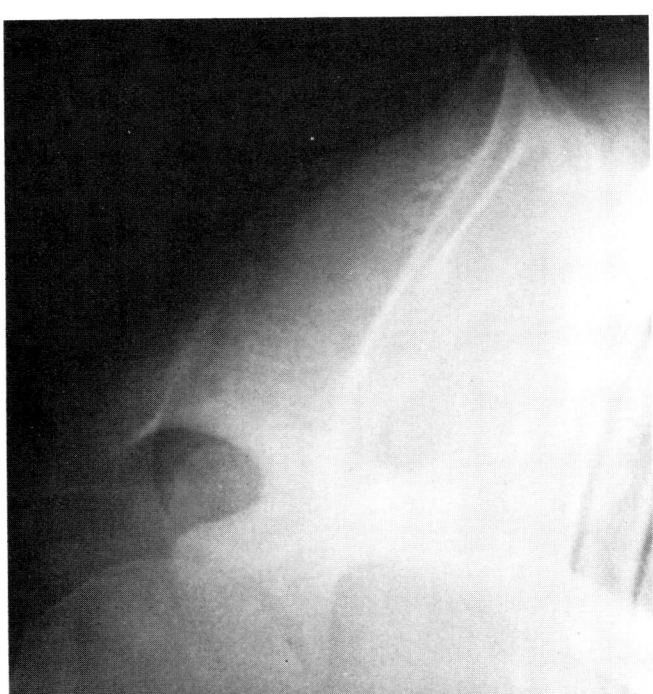

Figure 15–37   A "West Point" view.

osseous abnormality is a calcific process in the area of a probable Bankart lesion. These investigators believed the abnormality results from repeated episodes of instability and appears to be an abortive reparative process. It rarely represents a fracture. Biopsy of the abnormality reveals chondrification and ossification of the capsule and not ectopic calcification or fracture callus. Rokous and associates concluded that the changes are similar to those described on the medial aspect of a recurring dislocating patella.

An arthrogram of the shoulder may also be useful in diagnosis of this condition, and may reveal a redundant anterior capsule. Cineradiography may demonstrate the tendency of the shoulder to subluxate when the shoulder is placed in a position of external rotation.

Treatment

Rokous and associates found that a modified Putti-Platt type of repair was satisfactory in preventing episodes of recurrent subluxation.[156] It is probable that any type of repair that tightens the structures in the anterior aspect of the shoulder will maintain the humeral head in the glenoid fossa with external rotation motions. Therefore, the Magnuson-Stack or the Bristow repair is also probably indicated for treatment of this condition.

POSTERIOR DISLOCATION OF THE SHOULDER

Unfortunately, this particular entity is frequently "missed" in clinical practice. There appear to be three reasons for this situation. (1) It is a relatively rare injury, and most orthopedic surgeons have not had a great deal of experience with recognition and treatment of this condition. (2) For some peculiar reason a thorough physical examination of the shoulder is not always performed during the initial evaluation of patients presenting with a posterior dislocation. Every patient demonstrates a restriction of external rotation if this specific finding is properly evaluated. (3) Adequate

roentgenographic evaluation is not always obtained during the initial assessment of these patients.

In spite of these problems, posterior dislocation of the shoulder should be diagnosed without difficulty if an appropriate history is obtained and physical and roentgenographic examinations are performed. The true incidence of this lesion is probably less than 2 per cent. Rowe evaluated 394 shoulder dislocations, of which only 1.5 per cent were posterior dislocations.[159, 161] Since this is a relatively rare injury, most series on posterior dislocations do not have significant numbers in their total incidence and even fewer in their follow-up studies.

CLASSIFICATION

As outlined previously, there are three basic anatomical types of posterior dislocation. These are the subacromial, the subglenoid, and the subspinous. As with anterior shoulder dislocations, the position of the humeral head is governed by the force producing the lesion and the muscle balance about the shoulder.

By far the most common posterior dislocation is the subacromial type, which statistically accounts for 95 per cent or greater of the total. In this type, the humeral head is situated in a posterior position behind the glenoid and beneath the acromion, with the articular surface pointed in a posterior direction. It is common for a defect to be present in the humeral head, similar to the Hill-Sachs lesion in anterior dislocations except for being located in the anterior humeral head. This is due to direct pressure of the posterior glenoid rim against the anterior aspect of the humeral head with the posterior position.

The subglenoid type of dislocation is relatively rare. In this injury, the humeral head is displaced posteriorly and in an inferior position relative to the glenoid fossa.

The subspinous posterior dislocation also is seldom encountered. In this type, the humeral head is located in a posterior position in relationship to the glenoid fossa and is also inferior to the spine of the scapula.

Mechanism of Injury

Posterior dislocations of the shoulder may be the result of both direct and indirect forces. Direct injury is relatively rare and is due to a blow on the anterior aspect of the shoulder that drives the humeral head in a posterior direction. Indirect forces are much more common. Their effect is the exact opposite of an anterior dislocation, in that they involve internal rotation and adduction. The pathological changes produced are similar to those with an anterior dislocation, except that they are seen on the posterior aspect of the shoulder. There may be a redundancy or detachment of the posterior capsule. Associated fractures of the glenoid rim or the lesser tuberosity also may be present.

Physical Examination

The diagnosis of a posterior dislocation of the shoulder is not difficult if an adequate physical examination has been performed. The patient presents with very specific positive physical findings. In the subacromial variety the anterior contour of the shoulder is lost, and there is a prominence to the posterior aspect. Palpation along the anterior portion will frequently reveal a depression and in a thin individual, the humeral head may be palpated posteriorly. The involved extremity is characteristically held in a position of internal rotation and adduction. Any attempt at abduction or external rotation elicits significant pain.

In the rare subglenoid and subspinous dislocations the patient presents in a different manner. The involved extremity is held in approximately 20 to 30 degrees of abduction and internal rotation owing to the anatomical position of the humeral head. However, attempts at increasing the abduction or positioning the extremity in neutral or mild external rotation elicit significant pain.

Roentgenographic Evaluation

As outlined in the first portion of this chapter, Neer's trauma series is useful as a screening measure for fractures and dislocations about the shoulder. If this is combined with an axillary view the posterior

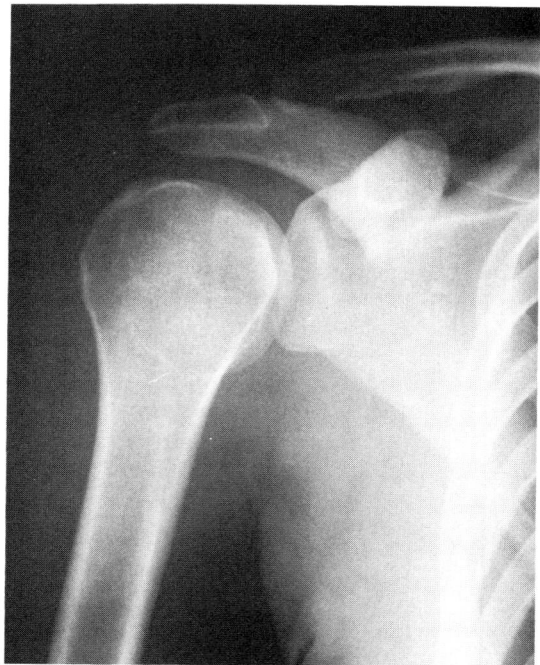

Figure 15–38   Anteroposterior view of the shoulder demonstrating a posterior dislocation. Note that both the lesser and greater tuberosities are in full view.

dislocation should be obvious. This view is also useful in demonstrating defects in the glenoid rim associated with the posterior dislocation (Figs. 15–38 to 15–40). Since the trauma series is taken perpendicular and parallel to the scapular plane, the dislocation will be evident. In the anteroposterior view there is normally a small amount of overlap of the posterior glenoid rim with the humeral head. In a posterior dislocation this normal small amount of overlap will be distorted. The proximal humerus will also be rotated in a posterior direction. The head itself may appear to be relatively hollow owing to the fact that the roentgenographic ray passes through both the lesser and the greater tuberosities secondary to the rotational deformity.

In the true lateral view the coracoid process, the spine of the scapula, and the body of the scapula will be noted to be in the form of a Y under normal circumstances. The head of the humerus is normally situated at the intersection of the limbs of the Y. In a posterior dislocation, it is quite

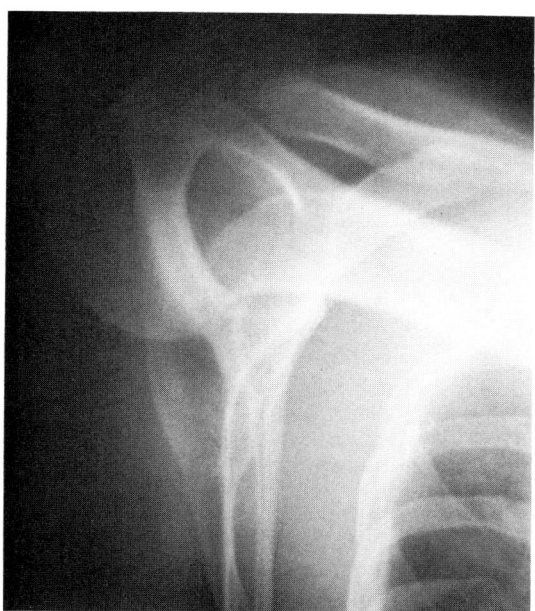

Figure 15–39 A scapular lateral view demonstrating the obvious posterior position of the humeral head.

A transthoracic lateral roentgenogram is also a useful technique to demonstrate the posterior dislocation. The advantage with this particular view, as with the trauma series, is that the patient does not have to move the upper extremity for appropriate positioning. Therefore, this view has become a popular screening procedure in many emergency rooms. A useful guide in interpreting these roentgenograms is the presence of Moloney's line. This line is similar to Shenton's line which demonstrates dislocation of the hip. Moloney's line is a smooth arch that is normally present in this view in the absence of a dislocation. The arch is formed by the shaft of the humerus, the inferior neck and head of the humerus, and the axillary border of the scapula. In the presence of a dislocation the normal smooth arch is altered so that it forms a sharp peak at the apex of the arch. This is a very useful sign in demonstrating a posterior dislocation.

obvious that the humeral head is situated in a posterior direction and is rotated posteriorly. The axillary view will also demonstrate the humeral head lying posterior to the glenoid rim. The compression fracture notch in the anterior humeral head is seen to best advantage in this view.

Treatment

The majority of these injuries may be treated by a closed reduction under appropriate anesthesia. One of the keys to reduction is obtaining adequate relaxation for reduction, and for this reason general anesthesia is preferred. The simplest method of reduction is to apply longitudinal downward traction to the involved extremity while at the same time applying direct pressure over the posterior aspect of the shoulder in an attempt to rotate the humeral head back into the glenoid fossa. This simple method will achieve reduction in a very high percentage of cases.

If this is not successful, then a form of reverse Kocher maneuver may be utilized. This involves applying gentle traction on the extremity with mild internal rotation followed by external rotation. The secret of success with this maneuver is applying slow gentle rotation to prevent fractures of the glenoid rim or the humerus.

RECURRENT POSTERIOR DISLOCATIONS

These are not very common problems. However, once the patient has been demonstrated to have had two episodes of

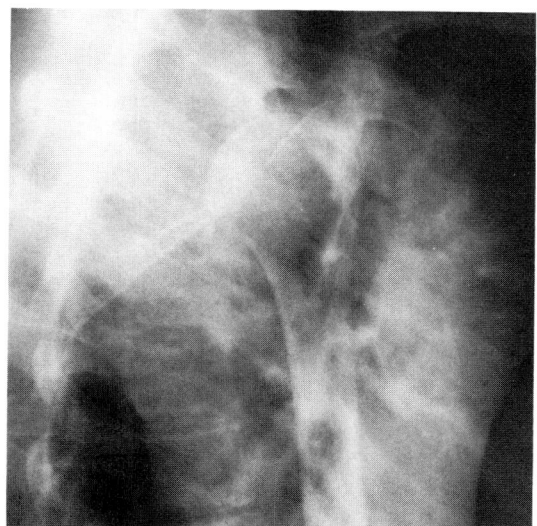

Figure 15–40 A transthoracic view demonstrating the obvious posterior position of the humeral head.

posterior dislocation, a surgical approach is warranted. As with recurrent anterior dislocations, the recurrent posterior dislocation may be easily reduced under appropriate parenteral analgesia. This will make the patient comfortable while a decision is made as to whether surgical correction is needed.

The procedures that are commonly employed for the surgical management of posterior dislocations include a reverse Bankart, a reverse Putti-Platt, a reverse Eden-Hybbinette, and a McLaughlin.

The McLaughlin technique is useful for the management of patients with a large defect in the anterior aspect of the humeral head and neck.[111] It involves the transfer of the subscapularis tendon into the defect within the humeral head. An anterior approach is utilized to expose the subscapularis muscle overlying the glenoid fossa. The subscapularis muscle is surgically detached from the lesser tuberosity, followed by reduction of the shoulder. The subscapularis tendon is then transferred directly into the defect within the anterior portion of the humeral head. The transferred tendon may be held in place by a serrated staple, sutured into the head through drill holes, or secured into the defect by a compression screw.

OLD POSTERIOR DISLOCATIONS

Unfortunately, although posterior dislocations of the shoulder are not common, the fact that they frequently go undetected is a definite problem. This results in the clinical presentation of an old "missed" dislocation of the shoulder. It is most frequent in the very elderly.

Physical Examination

Examination of the shoulder will reveal a depression in the normal anterior contour. The humeral head may be palpated in a posterior position in the thin patient. Unlike the acute posterior dislocation, a small functional range of motion of the shoulder may be present. Acute pain and spasm are usually absent. However, any attempt at forced external rotation and abduction will elicit discomfort.

Roentgenographic Findings

In addition to the findings described previously there is usually evidence of a large defect in the anterior humeral head. In fact, the longer the shoulder remains dislocated, the larger the defect present. This represents a compression fracture and is definitely a pressure phenomenon.

Treatment

As with anterior dislocations, a closed reduction may be attempted up to two or three weeks postinjury. After that time it is probably best to treat the patient with an open reduction because of the amount of scar formation that occurs, as well as the large defect that is usually present in the humeral head. Fortunately, problems with the vasculature are not prevalent in the posterior approach compared with the anterior approach for old anterior dislocations.

Postreduction. The immobilization time following reduction of a posterior dislocation is very similar to that outlined for the management of anterior dislocations. Young patients are managed with three to four weeks of immobilization. Older patients are immobilized for a maximum of one week, and then early motion is instituted. If the reduction is stable, the arm is held in a simple sling and swathe, or the patient is placed in a shoulder immobilizer. If there is some question as to the stability of the shoulder, it should be immobilized in a position of external rotation and slight abduction. This position may be maintained with the use of a modified shoulder spica.

A shoulder with definite instability following reduction may be managed with insertion of two smooth pins through the acromion down into the humeral head, as outlined by Wilson and McKeever.[191] The pins are removed at three weeks, and active therapy is begun.

INFERIOR DISLOCATION (LUXATIO ERECTA)

Although this is relatively uncommon, it is a distinct type of dislocation and deserves separate classification.

Mechanism of Injury

The specific mechanism of injury for this type of dislocation is hyperabduction of the shoulder. This type of forced maneuver results in the shaft of the humerus striking the acromion and levering the humeral head out of the glenoid fossa. This results in an inferior location of the humeral head, and the articular surface of the humeral head is pointed in a downward direction.

Physical Examination

The physical examination of the patient with this condition is very characteristic. The shaft of the humerus is pointing in an upward direction and is locked in this position. Owing to gravity the elbow falls into a flexed position. Any attempt at motion of the humerus elicits pain. If the patient is relatively thin, palpation of the lateral chest wall will usually reveal the presence of the humeral head. A careful documentation of the neurovascular status of the extremity should be performed.

Roentgenographic Evaulation

Standard roentgenographic anteroposterior and lateral views or the trauma series

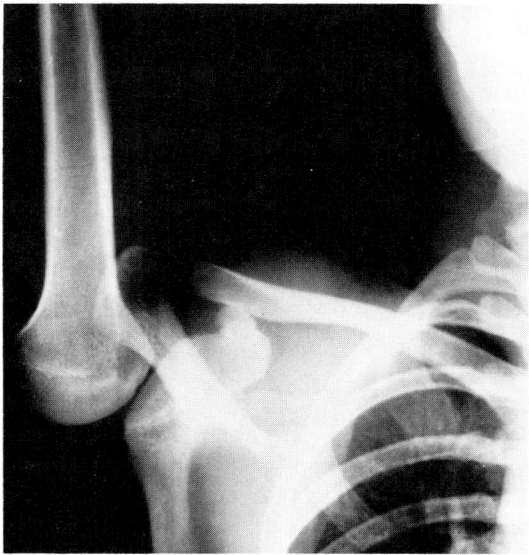

Figure 15–41 A patient with luxatio erecta. Note the inferior position of the humeral head with the arm pointed upward.

will reveal the inferior location of the humeral head. The shaft of the humerus will be noted to be pointing in an upward direction (Fig. 15–41). There may or may not be an associated fracture of the greater tuberosity.

Treatment

The simplest form of reduction is to apply longitudinal traction on the arm in an upward direction, gradually bringing the arm downward as traction is sustained. Countertraction is applied by an assistant's securing the trunk in a fixed position. The secret to the reduction is slow gentle traction; the humeral head must be disengaged from the inferior location before any attempt is made to slowly bring the arm down to the side. If forced manipulation is used, there is the danger that the humeral shaft will fracture owing to the leverage effect before the humeral head reaches the level of the glenoid fossa. The physician performing the reduction will frequently feel the humeral head slip upward back to the level of the glenoid fossa when longitudinal traction is applied. At this time the arm may be brought down to the side slowly with the traction maintained.

Rarely, the reduction cannot be performed under closed methods because the humeral head has buttonholed through the capsule. Under these circumstances it is best to perform an open reduction with a release of the capsule to allow the humeral head to assume its normal position.

Postreduction. The arm is maintained in a sling or shoulder immobilizer for four to five days for comfort. At the end of that time, gradual range-of-motion exercises are initiated.

SUPERIOR DISLOCATION

This is also a rare type of dislocation deserving a separate classification.

Mechanism of Injury

The injury is caused by a sudden force applied to the humerus in an upward and outward direction. The humerus is usually in adduction when the force is applied.

Physical Examination

Examination reveals acute swelling of the shoulder. There is tenderness to direct palpation over the acromion owing to an associated fracture. Motion of the shoulder elicits pain.

Roentgenographic Evaluation

This will usually reveal the humeral head to be located in a position superior to the glenoid fossa. The fractured acromion will also be displaced in a proximal direction. There may be a disruption of the acromioclavicular joint, and there may also be associated fractures of the clavicle.

Treatment

Treatment consists of a gentle closed reduction by applying a downard force with slight abduction.

ACROMIOCLAVICULAR DISLOCATIONS (A-C SEPARATIONS)

This is a very common injury, particularly among young athletic individuals. The recognition of the injury is not difficult, but the exact form of treatment remains controversial. In fact, at the present time support may be found in the literature for both closed and open management of these injuries. Therefore, to the young house staff the literature appears confusing. As more knowledge and clinical experience are obtained, a more rational approach to the problem will be taken.

MECHANISM OF INJURY

As stated, dislocation of the acromioclavicular joint is usually seen in young and middle-aged adults. In most series, the right shoulder is involved more frequently than the left. The reason for this right-sided predilection has never been completely explained. The current feeling is that since right-sided dominance is common, the right upper extremity is subjected to more violence in daily activities as well as in sports.

The exact mechanism of injury may be a direct or indirect force. The most common mechanism is a direct force, such as a fall on the point of the acromion, or a direct blow, as in football injuries, that drives the acromion and scapula downward and medially. The clavicular fibers of the trapezius and deltoid muscles tighten in an effort to resist this movement, resulting in a disruption of the ligamentous fibers. The continued downward thrust results in further disruption, splitting the trapezius into clavicular and scapular components and tearing the deltoid from the clavicle. The capsular structure covering the acromioclavicular joint tears, and frequently the meniscus between the acromioclavicular joint is torn. If the downward force is extensive, the first rib abuts the clavicle, producing a counterforce that may cause disruption of the coracoclavicular ligaments.

The other mechanism, indirect force, is a fall on an outstretched arm or flexed elbow with the arm in 90 degrees of flexion and a neutral lateral position. The humerus is driven against the glenoid fossa and acromion, causing backward displacement, with the clavicle remaining in a forward location, producing stress on the acromioclavicular and coracoclavicular ligaments.

CLASSIFICATION

The author has found the classification outlined by Allman to be very useful.[8] The injuries are graded according to the amount of disruption to the acromioclavicular and the coracoclavicular ligaments (Fig. 15–42). A grade 1 sprain results in a minor amount of capsular and ligamentous stretching without actual disruption. Grade 2 sprains rupture the capsule and acromioclavicular ligament. There is no associated disruption of the coracoclavicular ligaments. This injury produces a "subluxation." Grade 3 sprains are produced by severe force, resulting in a disruption of the acromioclavicular and coracoclavicular ligaments. This is also the injury that produces the severe disruption of the trapezius and deltoid muscles that is thought to play a role in the traumatic anatomical disruption of the injury. A true "dislocation" of the acromiocla-

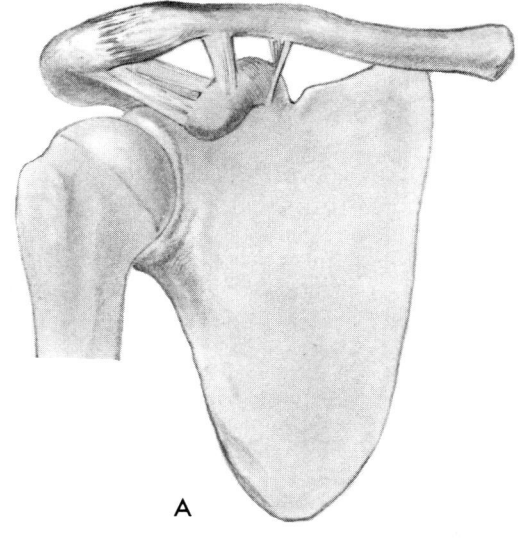

A

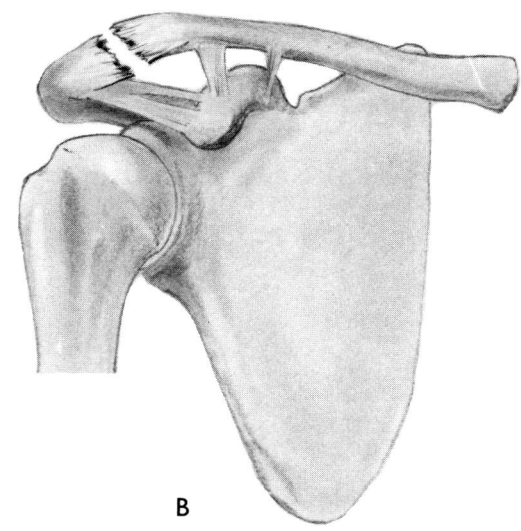

B

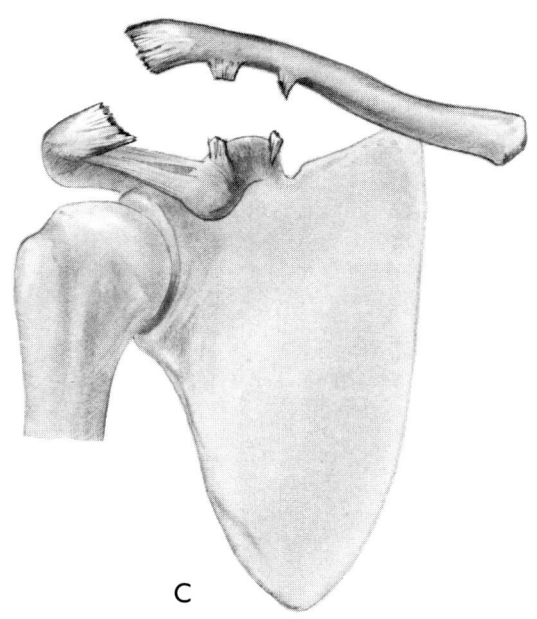

C

Figure 15–42 A Grade 1 sprain. B. Grade 2 sprain. C. Grade 3 sprain.

vicular joint is noted both clinically and roentgenographically.

PHYSICAL EXAMINATION

In a grade 1 injury there is mild swelling and localized tenderness directly over the acromioclavicular joint. However, there is no evidence of any subluxation or dislocation of the distal clavicle. Patients are able to complete a full range of motion, with mild discomfort over the acromioclavicular joint.

In a grade 2 injury, mild swelling and definite tenderness are present over the acromioclavicular joint. Patients are able to complete a full range of motion of the

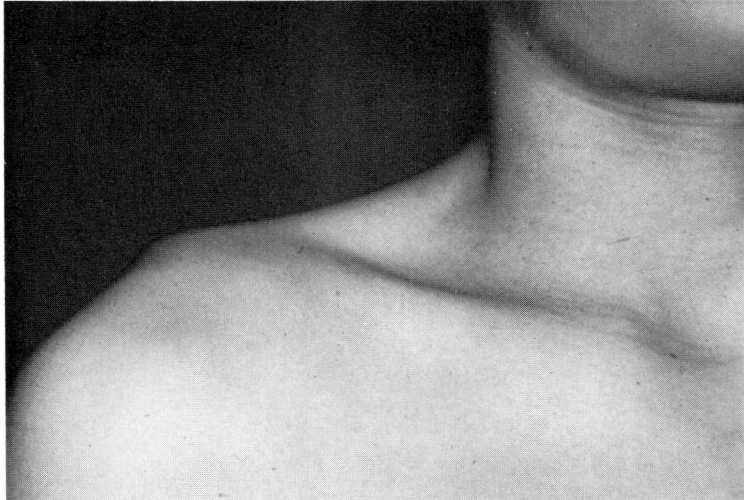

Figure 15–43 Clinical appearance of an obvious grade 3 separation. Note the elevation of the distal end of the clavicle.

shoulder, but there is significant pain associated with the extremes of motion. Occasionally, the distal portion of the clavicle is noted to be slightly elevated compared with the acromion. This is a subtle change and one that is not always evident clinically. However, the examiner may sense motion of the distal clavicle with application of slight downward pressure. Mild anteroposterior instability may also be evident.

A grade 3 injury is usually evident on gross physical examination. The distal end of the clavicle is noted to be elevated above the level of the acromion (Fig. 15–43).

There is an increased amount of swelling in this area compared with a grade 1 or a grade 2 injury. The examiner may be able to manually depress the distal end of the clavicle downward into its proper anatomical location. This will usually elicit significant pain. In contrast to grade 1 and grade 2 injuries, the patient normally will not move the shoulder. The arm is held at the side in a protective manner. Any attempt at motion of the shoulder results in significant pain in the vicinity of the acromioclavicular joint.

However, not all grade 3 injuries present with gross elevation of the clavicle. If the

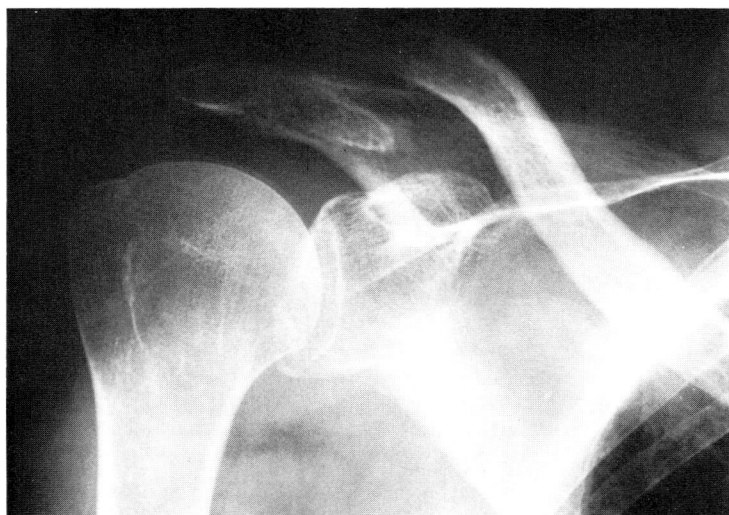

Figure 15–44 Anteroposterior view of a typical grade 3 injury.

patient is asked to hold a 10- to 15-lb weight in the hand of the involved extremity or if the examiner manually depresses the humerus, the distal clavicle may become more prominent.

ROENTGENOGRAPHIC EVALUATION

A routine anteroposterior view of the shoulder will not always document the type of injury present. If there is an obvious grade 3 injury with elevation of the distal end of the clavicle, the diagnosis is simple. However, there are examples of grade 2 and grade 3 injuries that are not evident on the routine anteroposterior view. A very important point to remember is that the contralateral uninjured shoulder must also be x-rayed for comparison purposes.

A useful roentgenographic view is obtained by directing the roentgenographic beam 15 degrees upward. This projection aids in determining whether there is mild elevation of the clavicle, as the acromioclavicular joint is not superimposed on the acromion process in this view.

The most useful roentgenographic aid is the so-called stress view, in which a regular anteroposterior view of the clavicle is obtained with the patient holding a 10-lb weight in the hand (Fig. 15–45). A second

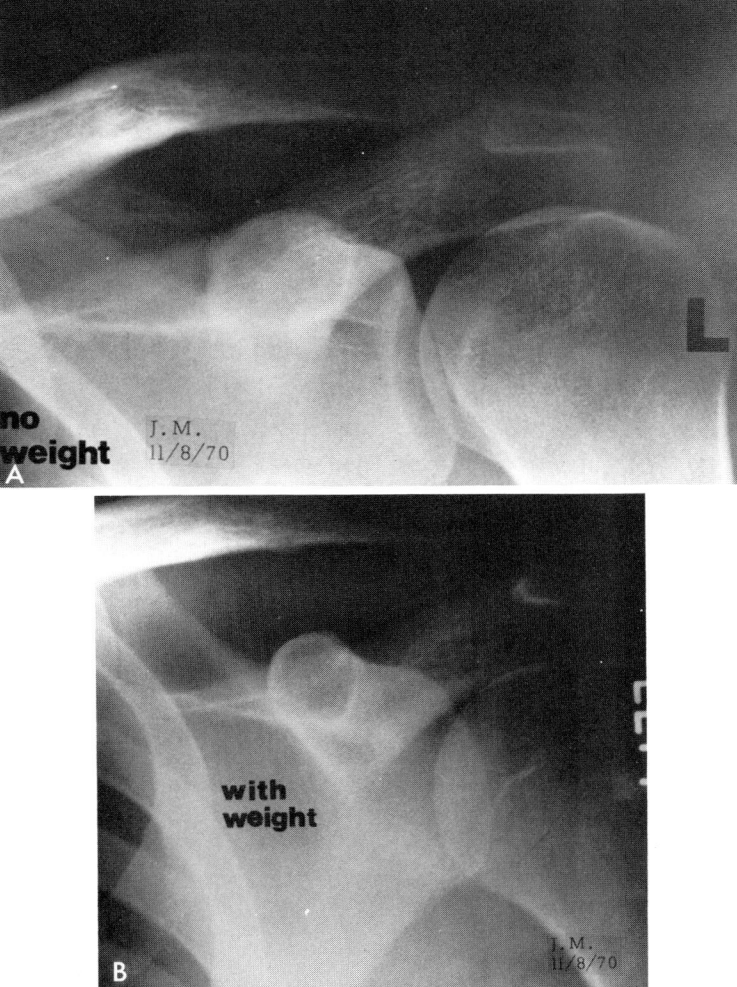

Figure 15–45 A. A grade 3 injury that is not entirely evident on the regular anteroposterior view. B. However, on the stress view the grade 3 injury is obvious.

anteroposterior roentgenogram is obtained and compared with the first. The downward stress will reveal coracoclavicular ligamentous damage reflected in an upward drift of the distal clavicle. If the clavicle does not elevate, one be relatively assured that the ligamentous structure is still intact. The differentiation is important, as it may well determine the method of treatment selected. Once again, the injured shoulder must be compared with the normal shoulder to ascertain the true extent of the injury. In a grade 1 injury there will be no evidence of subluxation or dislocation of the distal end of the clavicle. In a grade 2 injury, with a stress view, there may be evidence of slight subluxation of the distal end of the clavicle. In a grade 3 injury, with a stress view, there will be an obvious dislocation of the acromioclavicular joint.

TREATMENT

Grade 1 Injury

There is universal agreement that grade 1 injuries are treated conservatively. This consists of the application of ice to the acromioclavicular joint for the first 24 to 48 hours, followed by local moist heat. A simple sling is provided for three to four days until the acute reaction subsides, and then gradual graded range-of-motion exercises are encouraged.

Grade 2 Injury

Most series advocate conservative therapy for this type of injury. Since there is disruption of the acromioclavicular ligamentous complex, the shoulder must be partially protected to prevent progression to a complete grade 3 injury. Basically, there are three specific methods to accomplish this purpose. The first involves strapping or taping the acromioclavicular joint. Benzoin may be applied to the skin over the acromioclavicular joint. Regular tape may then be placed across the acromioclavicular joint with a definite downward force in order to hold the distal end of the clavicle in proper anatomical location. This is followed by placing the involved extremity in a regular sling to support the arm. In this manner the downward forces exerted on the shoulder

by gravity will be decreased. The author has never really been satisfied with this type of treatment. Not only is it difficult to obtain and maintain an appropriate reduction with this method, but definite skin problems are created. In short, the technique should probably be abandoned.

An alternative method is to apply a felt pad over the distal end of the clavicle and then loop a sling around the elbow and back over the pad. The sling is tightened to produce a downward force on the distal end of the clavicle and an upward force on the elbow. The wrist may then be suspended by a sling around the neck. This is a useful technique, but there is frequently difficulty in maintaining proper position of the sling around the elbow and the distal clavicle.

Third, various custom-made slings, such as the Kenny-Howard sling-halter, are very useful (Fig. 15–46). This device is designed with three separate components: a sling for the forearm, which keeps the acromion in an elevated positon; a shoulder strap applied over a piece of felt, applying a downward thrust to the distal clavicle; and a halter connected to the other components, which produces an adduction force pulling the shoulder strap and the sling inward. It has been the author's practice to maintain the sling-halter device for a three to four week period. It should be emphasized that the sling-halter must be worn constantly during this time. This will prevent further liagmentous strain and allow the reparative process to take place. Fibrous repair prevents future displacement at the acromioclavicular joint. Athletic activities are curtailed for an additional two to three weeks following removal of the device.

In the over–50-year-old group these injuries may be managed with a simple sling for two to three weeks for comfort. Active range-of-motion exercises are initiated at the end of this time. Residual pain and discomfort do not appear to be a problem in follow-up examination.

Grade 3 Injuries

Management of this injury is extremely controversial. Several articles report satisfactory results with closed measures, whereas others recommend an open method with equally satisfactory results. It

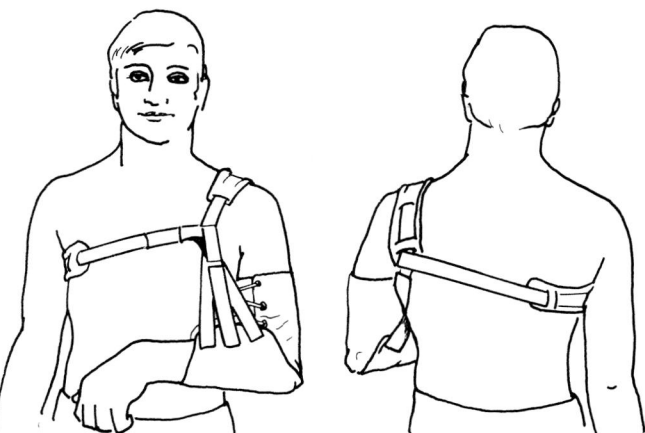

Figure 15–46 A pictorial representation of the Kenny-Howard sling-halter.

is the author's feeling that the patient's age and athletic activities must be taken into consideration before any type of treatment is initiated. In the elderly individual the injury may be managed with the use of a simple sling or a Kenny-Howard sling-halter device for four weeks. This is followed by gradual graded range-of-motion exercises.

The rationale of this treatment for this age group is that the majority of patients are satisfied with their results in follow-up examination. There may be a mild cosmetic "bump" over the acromioclavicular joint, and patients must be warned ahead of time that this may occur with this treatment. In spite of this deformity, patients by and large do not have significant discomfort. If they do have discomfort in follow-up, a simple resection of the distal portion of the clavicle will usually resolve the cosmetic deformity and abolish the pain.

In the middle-aged athletic individual the particular form of treatment is based more on the personal preference of the attending physician. The author believes that equally good results may be obtained with the use of a sling-halter device for four to six weeks and with open reduction and temporary internal fixation, as will be discussed. The advantage of conservative management is that operative intervention can be avoided. If pain and discomfort occur in the future owing to arthritis of the acromioclavicular joint, a simple resection of the distal clavicle, with or without ligamentous reconstruction, may be performed.

In the young athletic individual or the professional athlete, a more aggressive surgical approach with open reduction and temporary internal fixation is preferred by the author. Several specific techniques are available. In all the operative methods to be discussed, it is probably beneficial to excise any intraarticular disk remnants as part of the procedure. Definite damage to this anatomical structure is evident in almost all patients with a grade 3 injury. This probably predisposes to future arthritis and pain in the acromioclavicular joint and should be surgically excised. Four surgical procedures for the treatment of these injuries are widely used today. Each of these will be discussed separately.

Surgical Approach

OPEN REDUCTION AND PINNING. This technique, originally advocated by Phemister, involves a 3-inch incision along the distal aspect of the clavicular border, terminating at the lateral portion of the acromion process (Figs. 15–47 and 15–48).[150] The anterior deltoid and trapezius insertions into the clavicle and acromion are identified. These are reflected by subperiosteal dissection, exposing the distal clavicle and acromion. The joint is then inspected and intraarticular disk remnants are removed. Reduction is easily accomplished by downward pressure on the clavicle. One or two threaded wires (at least 5/64-inch in diameter) are inserted through the acromion into the clavicle for a distance of 3.5 cm. The tips of the wires are bent to prevent migration. The trapezius and deltoid are pulled distally and fixed with mattress sutures.

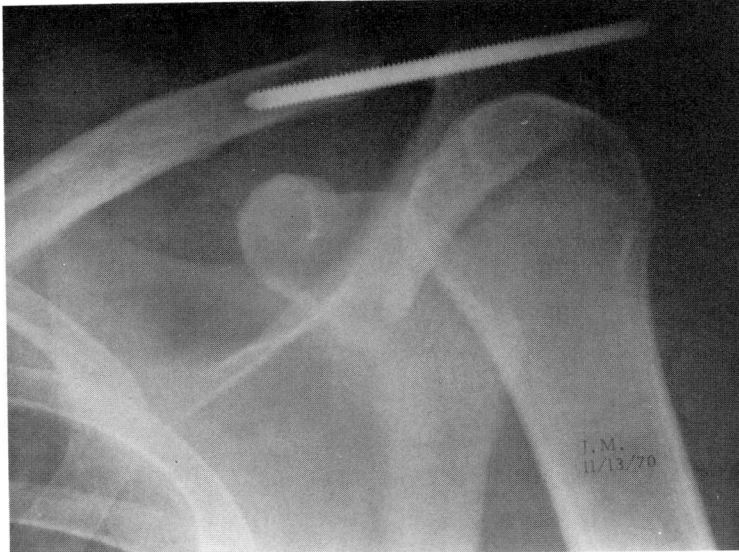

Figure 15–47 Open reduction and internal fixation with the use of a threaded wire.

Postoperatively, the arm is immobilized at the side of the trunk for a six week period. During this time, motion is restricted at the shoulder, as there is a distinct danger of breaking the internal fixation device if it is allowed. As mentioned in the beginning of this chapter, definite motion is present at the acromioclavicular joint which will stress the device. At the end of six weeks the patient is returned to the operating room, and the threaded wires are surgically removed. Graded range-of-motion exercises are then initiated.

This is a very useful technique in the management of the young athletic individual. Two points require emphasis. The first is that the internal fixation device should be bent to prevent migration; the second is that the fixation device should be buried under the skin rather than brought out through the skin. This will reduce the risk of infection.

BOSWORTH TECHNIQUE. As originally described by Bosworth, this technique involved fixation of the clavicle to the coracoid process (Fig. 15–49).[26, 27] The operative procedure was performed under local anesthesia without a formal arthrotomy of the acromioclavicular joint. The author believes the procedure should be performed under general anesthesia, and that the acromioclavicular joint should be inspected, with the removal of any intraarticular disk fragments. Kennedy has advocated the Bosworth technique with some personal modifications.[90]

The incision extends from the dislocation proper along the outer third of the clavicle over the medial fibers of the deltoid muscle to the palpable tip of the coracoid process in an S-shaped fashion. The deltoid is reflected from the outer aspect of the clavicle, but the

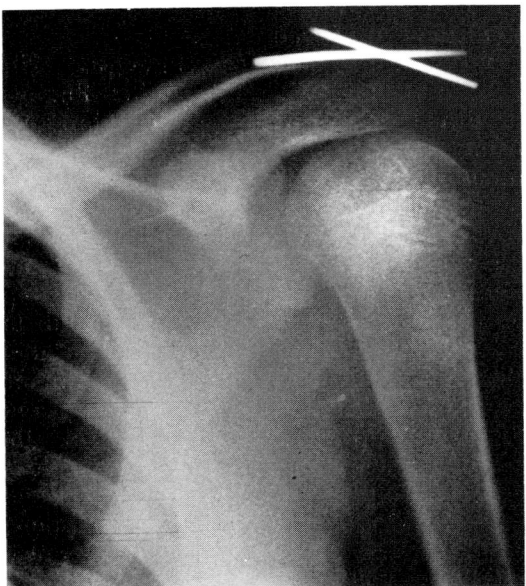

Figure 15–48 Open reduction and internal fixation with the use of two smooth Kirschner wires.

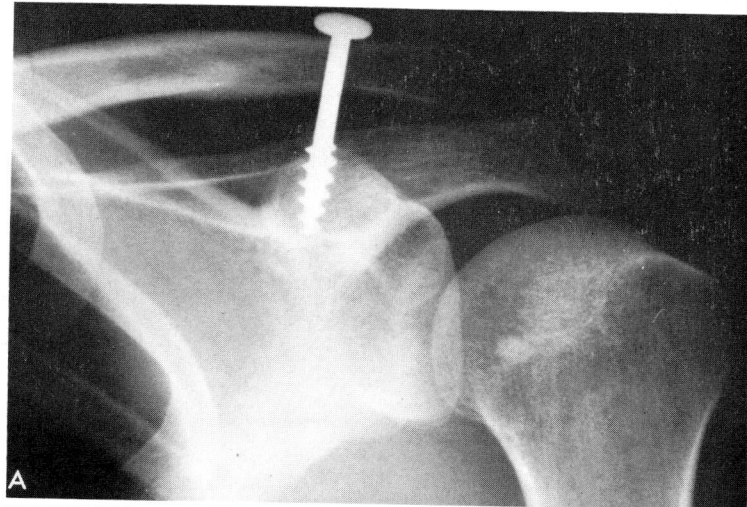

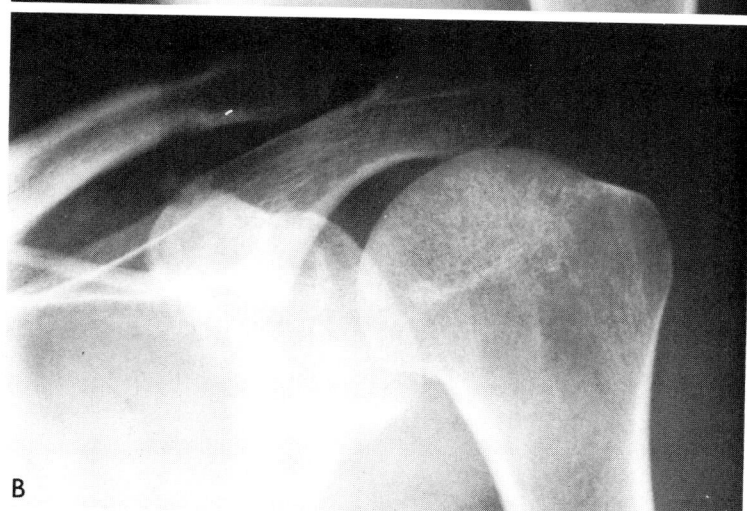

Figure 15–49 *A.* Bosworth screw technique. *B.* Following removal of the screw.

medial fibers are preserved. The coracoid process is then exposed. The conoid and trapezoid ligaments will be noted to be disrupted. The acromioclavicular joint is debrided.

A drill hole is then positioned through the clavicle directly over the base of the coracoid process. A smaller drill bit is utilized to drill the base of the coracoid process. A large lag screw is inserted through the clavicle and into the broad base of the coracoid process. The deltoid and trapezius muscles are then repaired.

Postoperative care does not include immobilization. Full abduction should be achieved at 7 to 14 days. Athletic activities are allowed at eight weeks. The author has not found this technique more effective than the others described, but does realize that good results may be obtained with it.

RESECTION. This method was popularized independently by Mumford and Gurd.[59, 60, 123] The lateral portion of the clavicle is exposed by a short curved incision. The deltoid muscle is reflected, and the distal portion of the clavicle is dissected subperiosteally (Fig. 15–50). The distal 3/4- to 1-inch of the clavicle is resected with the use of a power saw. The superior border of the remaining clavicle is then filed smooth to prevent any osseous prominence. The trapezius and deltoid muscles are repaired. Postoperatively, the shoulder is immobilized with a Velpeau dressing for

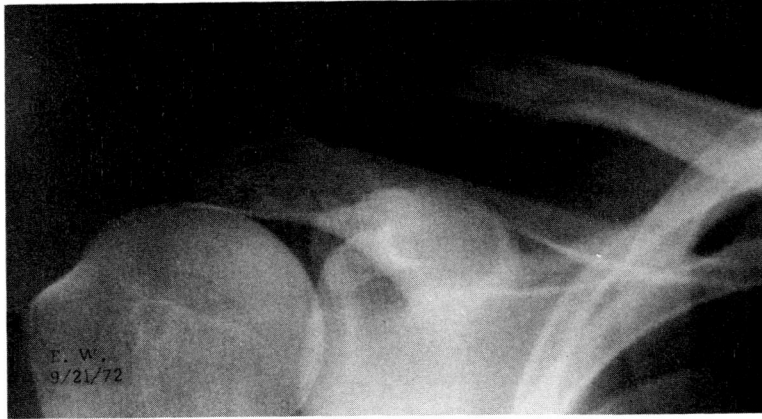

Figure 15–50 A simple excision of the outer portion of the clavicle for a third degree acromioclavicular separation. This is an example of having resected a little too much bone.

approximately one week. Active motion is then encouraged.

This is a useful technique provided there is not significant elevation of the clavicle. In other words, resecting the distal portion will not remove the prominence of the clavicle if it is high-riding at the beginning of treatment. This will result in a shorter high-riding clavicle. It is a useful technique to manage degenerative arthritis of the acromioclavicular joint which may develop following conservative treatment. Resection remains a popular technique for the management of these injuries. However, the author prefers the Weaver-Dunn technique, to be described.[187]

WEAVER-DUNN TECHNIQUE. The principle of this technique is an oblique resection of the distal portion of the clavicle and the transposition of the acromial portion of the coracoacromial ligament into the resected clavicle. This provides ligamentous support to hold the clavicle in normal position.

A curved incision, extending from the acromion medially along the lower border of the clavicle and curved gently over the coracoid, is utilized to expose the anterior portion of the origin of the deltoid and the insertion of the trapezius on the outer portion of the clavicle. The origin of the deltoid muscle is reflected laterally. The coracoacromial ligament is identified. The acromial portion of the coracoacromial ligament is then detached, and the ligament is dissected free to the coracoid process. The lateral 2 cm of the clavicle are resected in an oblique fashion, such that the inferior por-

tion of the oblique osteotomy overlies the coracoid process. The clavicle is held in its normal anatomical position, and the coracoacromial ligament is then approximated to the exposed surface of the clavicle. The excess portion of the ligament is excised. Two small drill holes are placed in the superior cortex of the clavicle, and the acromial portion of the ligament is transferred into the osteotomized portion of the clavicle and secured in position with heavy 0 silk sutures placed through the ligament and the prepared drill holes.

At the end of the procedure the clavicle should remain in anatomical position, held by the transferred coracoacromial ligament. Postoperatively, the arm is placed in a Velpeau bandage. Weaver and Dunn advocate circumduction exercises from the first day. The author prefers to immobilize the shoulder for three weeks and then allow circumduction exercises.

This is an excellent technique which may be employed for the management of acute as well as chronic grade 3 injuries. Physiologically it is appealing, as it excises the portion of the clavicle that may be involved in future degenerative arthritis, and it involves the transfer of a very useful ligament to hold the clavicle in proper position.

OLD DISLOCATIONS

Patients with old dislocations will usually present for treatment of pain and for the management of a cosmetic deformity. A simple resection of the distal 1 inch of the clavicle will relieve pain, but if the clavicle is situated in an elevated position a more appropriate procedure is the Weaver-Dunn technique. As a general procedure, this method produces excellent results in follow-up examination and is the technique preferred by the author.

STERNOCLAVICULAR DISLOCATIONS

This is not a common injury. It has been reported by Rowe to represent 3 per cent of shoulder girdle injuries.[160, 161] In other words, its incidence is comparable to that of posterior dislocations of the shoulder. Dislocations at the sternoclavicular joint may be anterior or posterior. By far the most common is the anterior type. Fortunately, the posterior type of dislocation is rare, as significant major complications may result from the posterior position of the proximal clavicle with compression on vital structures.

MECHANISM OF INJURY

This injury results only from significant force applied to the shoulder girdle. The applied forces may be direct or indirect. The former usually results from a motor vehicle accident, in which the anterior chest is suddenly thrust against a solid portion of the automobile. Direct force is exerted along the anteromedial aspect of the clavicle, producing a posterior dislocation of the sternoclavicular joint. However, the indirect force mechanism causes the majority of dislocations. This occurs by significant force transmitted from the anterolateral and posterolateral aspects of the shoulder. Athletic and industrial injuries account for most of these dislocations. An example of an athletic injury occurs in football when a player is lying on the football in the lateral decubitus position, and several opposing players pile on to insure the safety of the ball. Force is then transmitted along the lateral aspect of the shoulder girdle to the sternoclavicular joint proper. An example of an industrial injury occurs when a worker is pinned against a solid object by a moving piece of machinery, resulting in a lateral compression injury to both shoulders.

PHYSICAL EXAMINATION

This injury may occur as an isolated phenomenon or may be seen in association with the multiply injured patient. Careful examination of the shoulder girdle is required in the multiply injured patient if the dislocation is to be recognized. If it occurs as an isolated injury, pain will usually be localized to the area of the sternoclavicular joint. As with shoulder dislocations, the patient tends to hold the injured extremity by the chest and to support it with the uninjured extremity. In the presence of an anterior dislocation there is usually a significant prominence to the anterior aspect of the sternoclavicular joint. A significant amount of soft tissue hemorrhage occurs within this area, but the proximal portion of the clavicle can usually be palpated in a position anterior to the manubrium. In a posterior dislocation there may be a palpable defect along the anterior aspect of the sternoclavicular joint. A significant problem with a posterior dislocation is the fact that the patient may have respiratory difficulties secondary to airway compression. Dysphagia may also be present for the same reason.

In both types of dislocation any attempt at motion of the shoulder will elicit significant pain along the anterior shoulder girdle. The patient appears to be more comfortable either standing or seated, and experiences increased discomfort when positioned supine on the examining table.

ROENTGENOGRAPHIC EVALUATION

Routine anteroposterior views of the chest will usually reveal some asymmetry between the medial portions of the clavicle. However, this is not always evident, and this injury may easily be "missed" with routine roentgenographic evaluation. Certainly the physical findings are much more striking than the standard roentgenographic views. Tomograms are useful for further evaluation of the status of the sternoclavicular joint. Oblique views may occasionally be helpful. As the new scanning devices become available in radiology departments, they may become a standard technique to evaluate these injuries.

Anterior Dislocations

Many of these injuries may be managed with a closed reduction under general anesthesia. A general anesthetic is preferred, if at all possible, since it allows maximal muscle relaxation when manipulative reduction is being performed. The arm is abducted to the patient's side, and direct longitudinal traction is applied at 70 to 90 degrees of abduction. Countertraction is applied by an assistant through a sling around the chest wall, pulling in the opposite direction. The physician then places his fingers around the patient's clavicle in the midportion and applies a posteriorly directed force along the inner portion of the clavicle.

Alternatively, the physician may use the palm of his hand to apply direct posterior compression against the dislocated proximal portion of the clavicle. It is important to maintain the longitudinal traction on the patient's extremity while this manipulative reduction is performed. When the reduction is accomplished, adequate immobilization is obtained. Regardless of the type of immobilization employed, the shoulders must be held back in a "soldier position." A figure-of-eight harness or a plaster technique is usually sufficient. A sling for the extremity should also be provided to elevate the shoulder and counteract the downward pull of gravity. Six weeks is the accepted period of immobilization, after which exercises are initiated.

If the reduction is unstable, or if the initial attempt at reduction fails, open reduction and fixation are indicated. The sternoclavicular joint is exposed through a horizontal incision. The proximal end of the clavicle is identified and then repositioned in its proper anatomical location. A threaded pin may be inserted obliquely through the clavicle into the manubrium. The proximal portion of the pin is bent to prevent future migration. It is extremely important to bend the pin, as migration may well occur otherwise. Postoperatively, the patient is immobilized, as described previously, for six weeks. At the end of this time the patient is taken back to the operating room for surgical excision of the pin. Gentle range-of-motion exercises are then initiated. The older techniques of immobilization with the use of fascial slings have not been satisfactory in follow-up studies.

Posterior Dislocation

Almost all of these injuries may be managed with closed reduction techniques. The reduction is usually performed under general anesthesia. The arm is abducted with longitudinal traction applied, as in anterior dislocations. It is frequently useful to gradually extend the shoulder at the same time as the longitudinal traction is applied. The physician may then grasp the midportion of the clavicle between his fingers and apply direct upward force to lever the medial clavicle into proper position. If this does not accomplish reduction, a towel clip should be inserted into the clavicle under sterile conditions, followed by direct upward leverage through the towel clip. It is unusual for this technique to fail. Once the reduction is achieved, it is usually fairly stable. However, immobilization is maintained for four to six weeks, as described in the preceding section.

If closed reduction is unsuccessful, open reduction is indicated. The technique is similar to that described for anterior dislocations, and the same type of temporary pin fixation may be utilized.

Old Dislocations

The majority of these patients present with old anterior dislocations and are generally asymptomatic. In this group no specific treatment is required. However, if significant discomfort is present, an open reduction and reconstruction of the ligamentous structures with the use of temporary pin immobilization may be indicated. An alternative to this approach is to resect the medial portion of the clavicle. This may be performed with preservation of good function. It is important to remember that the clavicle may be resected up to the level of the coracoclavicular ligaments and not beyond.

REFERENCES

1. Abbott, L. C., and Lucas, D. B.: The function of the clavicle. Ann. Surg., *140*:583–599, 1954.
2. Adams, F. L.: The Genuine Works of Hippocrates. Vol. 2, pp. 553–654. London, Sydenham Society, 1849.
3. Adams, J. C.: Recurrent dislocation of the shoulder. J. Bone Joint Surg., *30B*:26–38, 1948.
4. Ahstrom, J. P., Jr.: Surgical repair of complete acromioclavicular separation. J.A.M.A., *217*: 785–789, 1971.
5. Albee, F. H.: Restoration of shoulder function in cases of loss of head and upper portion of the humerus. Surgery, *32*:1–19, 1921.
6. Alldred, A.: Subscapularis transplant for recurrent dislocation of the shoulder. J. Bone Joint Surg., *40B*:354, 1958.
7. Alldredge, R. H.: Surgical treatment of acromioclavicular dislocations. J. Bone Joint Surg., *47A*:1278, 1965.
8. Allman, F. L.: Fractures and ligamentous injuries of the clavicle and its articulation. J. Bone Joint Surg., *49A*:774–784, 1967.
9. Anderson, M. E.: Treatment of dislocations of the acromioclavicular and sternoclavicular joints. J. Bone Joint Surg., *45A*:657–658, 1963.
10. Arndt, J. H., and Sears, A. D.: Posterior dislocation of the shoulder. Am. J. Roentgenol., *94*:639–645, 1965.
11. Aston, J. W., and Gregory, C. F.: Dislocation of the shoulder with significant fracture of the glenoid. J. Bone Joint Surg., *55A*:1531–1533, 1973.
12. Badgley, C. E., and O'Connor, G. A.: Combined procedure for the repair of recurrent anterior dislocation of the shoulder. J. Bone Joint Surg., *47A*:1283, 1965.
13. Bankart, A. S. B.: Recurrent or habitual dislocation of the shoulder joint. Br. Med. J., *2*:1132–1133, 1923.
14. Bankart, A. S. B.: An operation for recurrent dislocation (subluxation) of the sternoclavicular joint. Br. J. Surg., *26*:320–323, 1938.
15. Bankart, A. S. B.: The pathology and treatment of recurrent dislocation of the shoulder joint. Br. J. Surg., *26*:23–29, 1939.
16. Basmajian, J. F.: Surgical anatomy and function of the arm trunk mechanism. Surg. Clin. North Am., *43*:1477, 1963.
17. Behling, F.: Treatment of acromioclavicular separations. Orthop. Clin. North Am., *4*:747–757, 1973.
18. Bennett, G. E.: Old dislocations of the shoulder. J. Bone Joint Surg., *18*:594–606, 1936.
19. Billington, R. W.: A new (plaster yoke) dressing for fracture of the clavicle. South. Med. J., *24*:667, 1931.
20. Blom, S., and Dahback, L. O.: Nerve injuries in dislocations of the shoulder joint and fractures of the neck of the humerus. Acta Chir. Scand., *136*:461–466, 1970.
21. Bloom, F. A.: Wire fixation in acromioclavicular dislocation. J. Bone Joint Surg., *27*:273–276, 1945.
22. Bloom, M. H., and Obata, W. G.: Diagnosis of posterior dislocation of the shoulder with use of Velpeau axillary and angle-up roentgenographic views. J. Bone Joint Surg., *49A*:943–949, 1967.
23. Böhler, L.: Die Behandlung von Verrenkungsbrüchen der Schulter. Dtsch. Z. Chir., *219*:238–245, 1929.
24. Bonnin, J. G.: Transplantation of the tip of the coracoid process for recurrent anterior dislocation of the shoulder. J. Bone Joint Surg., *51B*:579, 1969.
25. Bost, F., and Inman, V. T.: The pathologic changes in recurrent dislocation of the shoulder. A report of Bankart's operative procedure. J. Bone Joint Surg., *24*:595–613, 1942.
26. Bosworth, B. M.: Acromioclavicular separation. New method of repair. Surg. Gynecol. Obstet., *73*:866–871, 1941.
27. Bosworth, B. M.: Acromioclavicular dislocation: end results of screw suspension treatment. Ann. Surg., *127*:98–111, 1948.
28. Boyd, H. B.: Recurrent posterior dislocation of the shoulder. J. Bone Joint Surg., *54B*:379, 1972.
29. Boyd, H. B., and Hunt, H. L.: Recurrent dislocation of the shoulder. The staple capsulorrhaphy. J. Bone Joint Surg., *47A*:1514–1520, 1965.
30. Boyd, H. B., and Sisk, T. D.: Recurrent posterior dislocation of the shoulder. J. Bone Joint Surg., *54A*:779–786, 1972.
31. Brav, E. A.: An evaluation of Putti-Platt reconstruction procedure for recurrent dislocation of the shoulder. J. Bone Joint Surg., *37A*:731–741, 1955.
32. Brostrom, F.: Early mobilization of fractures of the upper end of the humerus. Arch. Surg., *46*:614, 1943.
33. Bryan, R. S., DiMichele, J. D., Ford, G. L., and Cary, G. R.: Anterior recurrent dislocation of the shoulder. Clin. Orthop., *63*:177–180, 1969.
34. Burrows, H. J.: Tenodesis of subclavius in the treatment of recurrent dislocation of the sternoclavicular joint. J. Bone Joint Surg., *33B*: 240–243, 1951.
35. Caldwell, J. A., and Smith, J.: Treatment of unimpacted fractures of the surgical neck of the humerus. Am. J. Surg., *31*:141–144, 1936.
36. Cave, A. J. E.: The nature and morphology of the costoclavicular ligament. J. Anat., *95*:170–179, 1961.
37. Codman, E. A.: The Shoulder. Boston, Thomas Todd, 1934.
38. Connolly, J.: X-ray defects in recurrent shoulder dislocations. J. Bone Joint Surg., *51A*:1235–1236, 1969.
39. Cubbins, W., Callahan, H., and Scuderi, C.: The reduction of old or irreducible shoulder dislocation. Surg. Gynecol. Obstet., *58*:129–135, 1934.

40. Curr, J. F.: Rupture of the axillary artery complicating dislocation of the shoulder. J. Bone Joint Surg., 52B:313–317, 1970.

41. DePalma, A. F.: Recurring dislocation of the shoulder. A symposium. J. Bone Joint Surg., 39B:9–58, 1948.

42. DePalma, A. F.: The role of the disks of the sternoclavicular and acromioclavicular joints. Clin. Orthop., 13:7–12, 1959.

43. DePalma, A. F.: Surgical anatomy of the acromioclavicular and sternoclavicular joints. Surg. Clin. North Am., 43:1540–1550, 1963.

44. DePalma, A. F., and Silberstein, C. E.: Results following a modified Magnuson procedure in recurrent dislocation of the shoulder. Surg. Clin. North Am., 43:1651–1653, 1963.

45. DePalma, A. F., Cooke, A. J., and Prabhakar, M.: The role of the subscapularis in recurrent anterior dislocations of the shoulder. Clin. Orthop., 54:35–49, 1967.

46. Dewar, F. P., and Barrington, T. W.: The treatment of chronic acromioclavicular dislocation. J. Bone Joint Surg., 47B:32–35, 1965.

47. Dickson, J. A., and O'Dell, H. W.: Phylogenetic study of recurrent anterior dislocation of the shoulder joint. Surg. Gynecol. Obstet., 93:357–365, 1952.

48. Dingley, A., and Denham, R.: Fracture-dislocation of the humeral head. A method of reduction. J. Bone Joint Surg., 55A:1299–1300, 1973.

49. Eden, R.: Zur Operation der habituellen Schulterluxation. Dtsch. Z. Chir., 144:269–280, 1918.

50. Einarsson, F.: Fractures of the upper end of the humerus. Discussion based on followup of 302 cases. Acta Orthop. Scand., (Suppl.) 32:10–209, 1958.

51. Elting, J. J.: Retrosternal dislocation of the clavicle. Arch. Surg., 104:35–37, 1972.

52. Eyre-Brook, A. L.: Recurrent dislocation of the shoulder. Lesions discovered in 17 cases, surgery employed, and intermediate report on results. J. Bone Joint Surg., 30B:39–46, 1948.

53. Fairbank, T. J.: Fracture subluxations of the shoulder. J. Bone Joint Surg., 30B:454–460, 1948.

54. Falkner, E. A.: Luxatio erecta of the shoulder joint. Med. J. Aust., 1:227–228, 1916.

55. Ferry, A., Rook, F. W., and Masterson, J. H.: Retrosternal dislocation of the clavicle. J. Bone Joint Surg., 39A:905–910, 1957.

56. Freedman, L., and Munro, R.: Abduction of the arm of the scapular plane. J. Bone Joint Surg., 48A:1503–1510, 1966.

57. Glessner, J. R.: Intrathoracic dislocation of the humeral head. J. Bone Joint Surg., 43A:428–430, 1961.

58. Gunther, W. A.: Posterior dislocation of the sternoclavicular joint. J. Bone Joint Surg., 31A:878–879, 1949.

59. Gurd, F. B.: A simple effective method for the treatment of fractures of the upper two-thirds of the humerus. Am. J. Surg., 47:443–453, 1940.

60. Gurd, F. B.: The treatment of complete dislocation of the outer end of the clavicle. A hitherto undescribed operation. Ann. Surg., 113:1094–1098, 1941.

61. Gurd, F. B.: Surplus parts of skeleton; recommendation for excision of certain portions as means of shortening period of disability following trauma. Am. J. Surg., 74:705–720, 1947.

62. Hall, M. C., and Rosser, M.: The structure of the upper end of the humerus with reference to osteoporotic changes in senescence leading to fractures. Can. Med. Assoc. J., 88:290–294, 1963.

63. Hall, R. H., Isaac, F., and Booth, C. R.: Dislocations of the shoulder with special reference to accompanying small fractures. J. Bone Joint Surg., 41A:489–494, 1959.

64. Harmon, P. H.: The posterior approach for arthrodesis and other operations on the shoulder. Surg. Gynecol. Obstet., 81:266–268, 1945.

65. Harmon, P. H., and Baker, D. R.: Fracture of scapula with displacement. J. Bone Joint Surg., 25:834–838, 1943.

66. Helfet, A. J.: Coracoid transplantation for recurring dislocation of the shoulder. J. Bone Joint Surg., 40B:198–202, 1958.

67. Heppenstall, R. B.: Fractures of the proximal humerus. Orthop. Clin. North Am., 6:467–476, 1975.

68. Heppenstall, R. B.: Fractures and dislocations of the distal clavicle. Orthop. Clin. North Am., 6:477–486, 1975.

69. Hermann, O. J.: Fractures of the shoulder joint with special reference to the correction of defects. A.A.O.S. Instructional Course Lectures, 2:359–370, 1944.

70. Hermodsson, I.: Rontgenologische Studien über die traumatischen und habituellen Schultergelenk-Verrenkungen. Acta Radiol. (Suppl.), 20:1–173, 1934.

71. Hermodsson, I.: Rontgenologische Studien uber die traumatischen und habituellen Schultergelenk-Verrenkungen nach unten. Translated by Moseley, H. and Overgaard, B. Montreal, McGill University Press, 1963.

72. Hill, H. A., and Sachs, M. D.: The grooved defect of the humeral head. A frequently unrecognized complication of dislocations of the shoulder joint. Radiology, 35:690–700, 1940.

73. Hill, N. A., and McLaughlin, H. L.: Locked posterior dislocation simulating a "frozen shoulder." J. Trauma, 3:225–234, 1963.

74. Hobbs, D. W.: Sternoclavicular joint: A new axial radiographic view. Radiology, 90:801–802, 1968.

75. Horn, J. S.: The traumatic anatomy and treatment of acute acromioclavicular dislocation. J. Bone Joint Surg., 36:194–201, 1954.

76. Howard, F. M., and Shafer, S. J.: Injuries to the clavicle with neurovascular complications. J. Bone Joint Surg., 47A:1335–1346, 1965.

77. Howard, N. J., and Eloesser, L.: Treatment of fractures of the upper end of the humerus; an experimental and clinical study. J. Bone Joint Surg., 16:1–29, 1934.

78. Hundley, J. M., and Stewart, M. J.: Fractures of

the humerus. A comparative study in methods of treatment. J. Bone Joint Surg., 37A:681–692, 1955.

79. Hybbinette, S.: De la transplantation d'un fragment osseux pour remedier aux luxations recidivantes de l'epaule; constations et resultats operatoires. Acta Chir. Scand., 71:411–445, 1932.

80. Imatani, R. J.: Fractures of the scapula: A review of 53 fractures. J. Trauma, 15:473–478, 1975.

81. Imatani, R. J., Hanlon, J. J., and Cady, G. W.: Acute, complete acromioclavicular separation. J. Bone Joint Surg., 57A:328–332, 1975.

82. Inman, V. T., Saunders, J. B. de C. M., and Abbott, L. D.: Observations on the function of the shoulder joint. J. Bone Joint Surg., 26:1–30, 1944.

83. Jacobs, B., and Wade, P. A.: Acromioclavicular joint injury. End result study. J. Bone Joint Surg., 48A:475–486, 1966.

84. Jens, J.: The role of the subscapularis muscle in recurring dislocation of the shoulder. J. Bone Joint Surg., 34B:780–781, 1964.

85. Joessel, D.: Ueber die Recidine der Humerus-Luxationem. Dtsch. Z. Chir., 13:167–184, 1880.

86. Johnston, G. W., and Lowry, J. H.: Rupture of the axillary artery complicating anterior dislocation of the shoulder. J. Bone Joint Surg., 44B:116–118, 1962.

87. Jones, L.: Reconstructive operation for non-reducible fractures of the head of the humerus. Ann. Surg., 97:217–225, 1933.

88. Jones, L.: The shoulder joint—observations on the anatomy and physiology of reconstructive operation following extensive injury. Surg. Gynecol. Obstet., 75:433–444, 1942.

89. Kelly, J. P.: Fractures complicating electroconvulsive therapy and epilepsy. J. Bone Joint Surg., 36B:70–79, 1954.

90. Kennedy, J. C., and Cameron, H.: Complete dislocation of the acromioclavicular joint. J. Bone Joint Surg., 36B:202–208, 1954.

91. Key, J. A., and Conwell, H. E.: Fractures, Dislocations, and Sprains. 5th ed. St. Louis, C. V. Mosby, 1951.

92. Knight, R. A., and Mayne, J. A.: Comminuted fractures and fracture-dislocations involving the articular surface of the humeral head. J. Bone Joint Surg., 39A:1343–1355, 1957.

93. Kocher, T.: Beitrage zur Kenntniss einiger paaraktisch wichtiger Fracture-neformen. Basel, Carl Sollman, 1896.

94. Kummel, B. M.: Fractures of the glenoid causing chronic dislocation of the shoulder. Clin. Orthop., 69:189–191, 1970.

95. LaFerti, A. D., and Nutter, P. D.: The treatment of fractures of the humerus by means of hanging plaster cast—"hanging cast." Ann. Surg., 114:919–930, 1955.

96. Laing, P. G.: The arterial blood supply of the adult humerus. J. Bone Joint Surg., 38A:1105–1116, 1956.

97. Lambdin, C. S., Young, S. B., and Unsicker, C. L.: A modified Bankart Putti-Platt shoulder capsulorrhaphy. J. Bone Joint Surg., 53A:1237, 1971.

98. Lazcano, M. A., Angel, S. H., and Kelly, P. J.: Complete dislocation and subluxation of the acromioclavicular joint. End results in 73 cases. J. Bone Joint Surg., 43A:379–391, 1961.

99. Lee, H. G.: Treatment of fracture of the clavicle by internal nail fixation. N. Engl. J. Med., 234:222–224, 1946.

100. Lester, C. W.: The treatment of fractures of the clavicle. Ann. Surg., 89:600, 1929.

101. Liberson, F.: The role of the coracoclavicular ligaments in affections of the shoulder girdle. Am. J. Surg., 44:145–157, 1939.

102. Lombardo, S. J., Kerlan, R. K., Jobe, F. W., Carter, V. S., Blazina, M. E., and Shields, C. L.: The modified Bristow procedure for recurrent dislocation of the shoulder. J. Bone Joint Surg., 58A:256–261, 1976.

103. Lowman, C. L.: Operative correction of old sternoclavicular dislocation. J. Bone Joint Surg., 10:740–741, 1928.

104. Lucas, G. L.: Retrosternal dislocation of the clavicle. J.A.M.A., 193:850–853, 1965.

105. Magnuson, P. B.: Treatment of recurrent dislocation of the shoulder. Surg. Clin. North Am., 25:14–20, 1945.

106. Magnuson, P. B., and Stack, J. K.: Bilateral habitual dislocation of the shoulders in twins, a familial tendency. J.A.M.A., 144:2103, 1940.

107. Magnuson, P. B.: Recurrent dislocation of the shoulder. J.A.M.A., 123:898–902, 1943.

108. May, V. R., Jr.: A modified Bristow operation for anterior recurrent dislocation of the shoulder. J. Bone Joint Surg., 52A:1010–1016, 1970.

109. Mazet, R.: Migration of a Kirschner wire from the shoulder region into the lung. Report of two cases. J. Bone Joint Surg., 25:477–483, 1943.

110. McLaughlin, H.: Trauma. Philadelphia, W. B. Saunders, 1959.

111. McLaughlin, H.: Posterior dislocation of the shoulder. J. Bone Joint Surg., 44A:1477, 1962.

112. McLaughlin, H. L., and Cavallaro, W. U.: Primary anterior dislocation of the shoulder. Am. J. Surg., 80:615–621, 1950.

113. McLaughlin, H. L., and MacLellan, D. I.: Recurrent anterior dislocation of the shoulder. J. Trauma, 7:191–201, 1967.

114. McMurray, T. B.: Recurrent dislocation of the shoulder. J. Bone Joint Surg., 43B:402, 1961.

115. Meyerding, H. W.: The treatment of acromioclavicular dislocations. Surg. Clin. North Am., 17:1199–1205, 1937.

116. Milch, H.: The treatment of recent dislocations and fracture-dislocations of the shoulder. J. Bone Joint Surg., 31A:173–180, 1949.

117. Moore, T. O.: Internal pin fixation for fracture of the clavicle. Am. Surg., 17:580–583, 1951.

118. Morrey, B. F., and Janes, J. M.: Recurrent anterior dislocation of the shoulder. Long-term followup of the Putti-Platt and Bankart procedures. J. Bone Joint Surg., 58A:252–256, 1976.

119. Moseley, H. F.: The clavicle: its anatomy and function. Clin. Orthop., 58:17–27, 1968.

120. Moseley, H. F.: Shoulder Lesions. 3rd ed. Edinburgh, E. & S. Livingstone, 1969.

121. Moseley, H. F., and Overgaard, B.: The anterior capsular mechanism in recurrent anterior dislocation of the shoulder. J. Bone Joint Surg., 44B:913–927, 1962.

122. Moshein, J., and Elconin, K. B.: Repair of acute

acromioclavicular dislocation, utilizing the coracoacromial ligament. J. Bone Joint Surg., *51A*:812, 1969.

123. Mumford, E. B.: Acromioclavicular dislocation. J. Bone Joint Surg., 23:799–802, 1941.
124. Murphy, I. D.: Sliding bone graft for connection of recurrent anterior dislocation of the shoulder. J. Bone Joint Surg., 50A:1270, 1968.
125. Neer, C. S., II.: Articular replacement for the humeral head. J. Bone Joint Surg., 37A:215–228, 1955.
126. Neer, C. S., II.: Prosthetic replacement of the humeral head — indications and operative technique. Surg. Clin. North Am., 43:1581–1597, 1963.
127. Neer, C. S., II.: Fracture of the distal clavicle with detachment of the coracoclavicular ligaments in adults. J. Trauma, 3:99–110, 1963.
128. Neer, C. S., II.: Fractures of the distal third of the clavicle. Clin. Orthop., 58:43–50, 1968.
129. Neer, C. S., II.: Displaced proximal humeral fractures; I. Classification and evaluation. J. Bone Joint Surg., 52A:1077–1089, 1970.
130. Neer, C. S., II.: Displaced proximal humeral fractures. II. Treatment of three-part and four-part displacement. J. Bone Joint Surg., 52A:1090–1103, 1970.
131. Neer, C. S., II.: Four-segment classification of displaced proximal humeral fractures. AAOS Instructional Course Lectures. Vol. XXIV, pp. 163–168. St. Louis, C. V. Mosby Co., 1975.
132. Nelson, C. L.: The use of arthrography in athletic injuries to the shoulder. Orthop. Clin. North Am., 4:775–785, 1973.
133. Nettles, J. L., and Linscheid, R.: Sternoclavicular dislocations. J. Trauma, 8:158–164, 1968.
134. Nettrour, L. F., Krufky, E. L., Mueller, R. E., and Raycroft, J. F.: Locked scapula: intrathoracic dislocation of the inferior angle. A case report. J. Bone Joint Surg., 54A:413–416, 1972.
135. Neviaser, J. S.: Acromioclavicular dislocation treated by transference of the coracoacromial ligament. Clin. Orthop., 58:57–68, 1968.
136. Nicholson, J. T.: Recurrent dislocation of the shoulder. J. Bone Joint Surg., 32B:510–511, 1950.
137. Nicola, T.: Recurrent anterior dislocation of the shoulder. J. Bone Joint Surg., 11:128–132, 1929.
138. Nicola, T.: Acute anterior dislocation of the shoulder. J. Bone Joint Surg., 31A:153–159, 1949.
139. Nutter, P. D.: Coracoclavicular articulations. J. Bone Joint Surg., 23:177–179, 1941.
140. Omer, G. E.: Osteotomy of the clavicle in surgical reduction of anterior sternoclavicular dislocation. J. Trauma, 7:584–590, 1967.
141. Osmond-Clarke, H.: Habitual dislocation of the shoulder. The Putti-Platt operation. J. Bone Joint Surg., 30B:19–25, 1948.
142. Osmond-Clarke, H.: Recurrent dislocation of the shoulder. J. Bone Joint Surg., 47B:194, 1965.
143. Oster, A.: Recurrent anterior dislocation of the shoulder treated by the Eden-Hybbinette operation. Follow-up on 76 cases. Acta Orthop. Scand., 40:43–52, 1969.
144. Palmer, I., and Widen, A.: The bone block

145. Patel, M. R., Pardee, M. L., and Singerman, R. C.: Intrathoracic dislocation of the head of the humerus. J. Bone Joint Surg., 45A:1712–1714, 1963.
146. Patterson, W. R.: Inferior dislocation of the distal end of the clavicle. J. Bone Joint Surg., 49A:1184–1186, 1967.
147. Pearson, G. R.: Radiographic technic for acromioclavicular dislocation. Radiology, 27:239, 1936.
148. Penn, I.: The vascular complications of fractures of the clavicle. J. Trauma, 4:819–831, 1964.
149. Perthes, G.: Über Operationen bei habitueller Schulterluxation. Dtsch. Z. Chir., 85:199–227, 1906.
150. Phemister, D. B.: The treatment of dislocation of the acromioclavicular joint by open reduction and threaded-wire fixation. J. Bone Joint Surg., 24:166–168, 1942.
151. Pilcher: Dislocation of the acromial end of the clavicle. N. Y. Med. J., 43:419–420, 1886.
152. Quigley, T. B.: Management of simple fractures of clavicle in adults. N. Engl. J. Med., 243:286–290, 1950.
153. Reeves, B.: Arthrography of the shoulder. J. Bone Joint Surg., 48B:424–435, 1966.
154. Roberts, S. M.: Fractures of the upper end of the humerus. An end result study which shows the advantage of early active motion. J.A.M.A., 98:367–373, 1932.
155. Rockwood, C. A., Jr.: The diagnosis of acute posterior dislocation of the shoulder. J. Bone Joint Surg., 48A:1220, 1966.
156. Rokous, J. R., Feagin, J. A., and Abbott, H. G.: Modified axillary roentgenogram. A useful adjunct in the diagnosis of recurrent instability of the shoulder. Clin. Orthop., 82:84–86, 1972.
157. Rothman, R. H., Marvel, J. P., and Heppenstall, R. B.: Anatomic considerations in the glenohumeral joint. Orthop. Clin. North Am., 6:341–352, 1975.
158. Rothman, R. H., Marvel, J. P., and Heppenstall, R. B.: Recurrent anterior dislocation of the shoulder. Orthop. Clin. North Am., 6:415–422, 1975.
159. Rowe, C. R.: Prognosis in dislocations of the shoulder. J. Bone Joint Surg., 38A:957–977, 1956.
160. Rowe, C. R.: Symposium on surgical lesions of the shoulder. J. Bone Joint Surg., 38A:977–1012, 1956.
161. Rowe, C. R.: Symposium on surgical lesions of the shoulder. Acute and recurrent dislocation of the shoulder. J. Bone Joint Surg., 44A:977–1012, 1962.
162. Rowe, C. R.: An atlas of anatomy and treatment of midclavicular fractures. Clin. Orthop., 58:29–42, 1968.
163. Rowe, C. R., Patel, D., and Southmayd, W. W.: The Bankart procedure. A long-term end-result study. J. Bone Joint Surg., 60A:1–16, 1978.
164. Rowe, C. R., Pierce, D. S., and Clark, J. G.: Voluntary dislocation of the shoulder. A preliminary report on a clinical, electromyogra-

method for recurrent dislocation of the shoulder joint. J. Bone Joint Surg., 30B:53–58, 1948.

phic, and psychiatric study of 26 patients. J. Bone Joint Surg., 55A:445–460, 1973.

165. Rowe, C. R., and Sakellarides, H. T.: Factors related to recurrences of anterior dislocations of the shoulder. Clin. Orthop., 20:40–47, 1961.

166. Rowe, C. R., and Ye, L. K.: A posterior approach to the shoulder joint. J. Bone Joint Surg., 26:580–584, 1944.

167. Rubin, S. A., Gray, R. L., and Green, W. R.: Scapular Y diagnostic aid in shoulder trauma. Radiology, 110:725–726, 1974.

168. Saha, A. K.: Dynamic stability of the glenohumeral joint. Acta Orthop. Scand., 42:491–505, 1971.

169. Samilson, R. L., and Miller, E.: Posterior dislocations of the shoulder. Clin. Orthop., 32:69–86, 1964.

170. Schulz, T. J., Jacobs, B., and Patterson, R. L.: Unrecognized dislocations of the shoulder. J. Trauma, 9:1009–1023, 1969.

171. Shaar, C. M.: Upward dislocation of acromial end of clavicle. Treatment by elastic traction splint. J.A.M.A., 92:2083–2085, 1929.

172. Skogland, L. B., and Sundt, P.: Recurrent anterior dislocation of the shoulder. The Eden-Hybbinette operation. Acta Orthop. Scand., 44:739–747, 1973.

173. Soule, A. B., Jr.: Ossification of the coracoclavicular ligament following dislocation of the acromioclavicular articulation. Am. J. Roentgenol., 56:607–615, 1946.

174. Speed, K.: Recurrent anterior dislocation of the shoulder; operative cure by bone graft. Surg. Gynecol. Obstet., 44:468–477, 1927.

175. Spigelman, L.: A harness for acromioclavicular separation. J. Bone Joint Surg., 51A:585–586, 1969.

176. Stimson, L. A.: An easy method of reducing dislocations of the shoulder and hip. Med. Record, 57:356–357, 1900.

177. Stimson, L. A.: Fractures and Dislocations. 3rd ed. Philadelphia, Lea Brothers, 1900.

178. Stimson, B. B.: A Manual of Fractures and Dislocations. 2nd ed. Philadelphia, Lea & Febiger, 1947.

179. Symeonides, P. P.: The significance of the subscapularis muscle in the pathogenesis of recurrent anterior dislocation of the shoulder. J. Bone Joint Surg., 54B:476–483, 1972.

180. Thompson, F. R., and Winant, E. M.: Unusual fracture subluxations of the shoulder joint. J. Bone Joint Surg., 32:575–582, 1950.

181. Townley, C. O.: The capsular mechanism in recurrent dislocation of the shoulder. J. Bone Joint Surg., 32A:370–380, 1950.

182. Townley, C. O.: Recurrent shoulder dislocations: pathogenesis and pathology. Clin. Orthop., 44:280, 1966.

183. Urist, M. R.: Complete dislocation of the acromioclavicular joint. The nature of the traumatic lesion and effective methods of treatment with an analysis of 41 cases. J. Bone Joint Surg., 28:813–837, 1946.

184. Urist, M. R.: Complete dislocation of the acromioclavicular joint. J. Bone Joint Surg., 45A:1750–1753, 1963.

185. Varney, J. H., Coker, J. K., and Cawley, J. J.: Treatment of acromioclavicular dislocation by means of a harness. J. Bone Joint Surg., 34A:232–233, 1952.

186. Viek, P., and Bell, B. T.: The Bankart shoulder reconstruction. J. Bone Joint Surg., 41A:236–242, 1959.

187. Weaver, J. K., and Dunn, H. K.: Treatment of acromioclavicular injuries, especially complete acromioclavicular separation. J. Bone Joint Surg., 54A:1187–1197, 1972.

188. Weitzman, G.: Treatment of acute acromioclavicular joint dislocation by a modified Bosworth method. J. Bone Joint Surg., 49A:1167–1178, 1967.

189. West, E. F.: Intrathoracic dislocation of the humerus. J. Bone Joint Surg., 31B:61–62, 1949.

190. Whitson, T. B.: Fractures of the surgical neck of the humerus. A study in reduction. J. Bone Joint Surg., 36B:423–427, 1954.

191. Wilson, J. C., and McKeever, F. M.: Traumatic posterior (retroglenoid) dislocation of the humerus. J. Bone Joint Surg., 31A:160–172, 1949.

192. Winfield, J. M., Miller, H., and LaFerte, A. D.: Evaluation of the hanging cast as a method of treating fractures of the humerus. Am. J. Surg., 55:228–249, 1942.

193. Young, C. S.: The mechanisms of ambulatory treatment of fractures of the clavicle. J. Bone Joint Surg., 13:299–310, 1931.

194. Zariczny, J. B.: Late reconstruction of the ligaments following acromioclavicular separation. J. Bone Joint Surg., 58A:792–795, 1976.

R. BRUCE HEPPENSTALL, M.D.

16 _____ *Fractures of the Humeral Shaft*

In general, fractures of the humerus are well tolerated by the individual and heal without serious problems with closed treatment. This injury is seen fairly frequently in an active orthopedic practice, and it is usually caused by significant trauma to the upper arm. Muscular forces play an active role in producing deformity of the humeral shaft, depending on the actual level of the fracture. The majority of malaligned fractures may, however, be handled satisfactorily by general simple closed means, and it is a rare occasion that requires open reduction and internal fixation to maintain control of the fracture itself. An additional factor in the closed management of these fractures is the fact that a significant amount of shortening or angulation or both will cause minimal functional loss or cosmetic deformity. There has been a recent wave of enthusiasm for managing these fractures with functional bracing techniques. The results to date with this form of treatment are very encouraging. This chapter deals with those fractures of the shaft of the humerus that occur distal to the humeral neck down to the condylar region. The supracondylar fracture itself is discussed in Chapter 17.

SURGICAL ANATOMY

As already mentioned, muscular forces play an important role in producing angular

deformities in fractures of the shaft of the humerus, and a thorough knowledge of the pertinent anatomy is essential for their management. The osseous structure of the humeral shaft is roughly cylindrical in the proximal portion. As the supracondylar region is approached, the width of the shaft increases and the surface itself tends to be flatter than in the cylindrical proximal portion. Anatomically, three distinct surfaces and two compartments exist. On the anterolateral surface of the humerus a mild enlargement known as the deltoid tuberosity is the site of insertion of the deltoid muscle. In the distal portion of the anterolateral aspect, the surface tends to merge with the anteromedial surface; here the brachialis muscle originates. The anteromedial surface does not have any specific osseous markings of note. A shallow groove commonly referred to as the spiral groove is present along the posterior surface and runs in a downward and lateral direction. The radial nerve is located in this anatomical groove.

Two distinct intermuscular septa divide the major portion of the arm into two separate compartments. The medial intermuscular septum takes origin from the lower border of the pectoralis and latissimus dorsi muscles and extends distally between the coracobrachialis and brachialis muscles anteriorly and the triceps muscle posteriorly to insert into the medial epicondyle. It is important to remember that

424

the ulnar nerve and the superior ulnar collateral artery pierce the medial intermuscular septum in its distal portion.

The lateral intermuscular septum takes origin at the insertion of the deltoid muscle and is firmly attached to the humerus as it extends distally to lie between the brachialis, the brachioradialis, and the extensor carpi radialis longus muscles anteriorly and the triceps muscle posteriorly. It is important to bear in mind that this intermuscular septum is pierced by the radial nerve and the radial collateral branch of the profunda brachii artery.

Collectively these intermuscular septa divide the major portion of the upper arm into two compartments. The anterior compartment contains the biceps, coracobrachialis, and brachialis muscles. The brachial artery and accompanying vein are located along the medial border of the biceps. The triceps and the radial nerve are located in the posterior compartment.

Blood is supplied to the humeral shaft through the nutrient branch of the brachial artery that originates at approximately the middle of the arm and then enters the anteromedial surface of the humerus. Additional blood supply is derived from the profunda brachii artery, which also provides a nutrient branch to the shaft of the humerus which enters the bone medial and slightly proximal to the spiral groove.

A relatively common variation in the distal portion of the humerus that the attending surgeon should be aware of is an anatomical structure known as the supracondylar process. This process is an osseous projection from the anteromedial surface of the humerus at a level approximately 2 inches proximal to the medial epicondyle. It varies in size and osseous structure. Its importance lies in a fibrous band that connects it with the medial epicondyle. When this band is present, the median nerve and the brachial artery may take an abnormal course in the distal portion of the humerus to pass behind the process and then forward between the fibrous band and the bone. This structure is estimated to be present in approximately 1 per cent of individuals.

The supraspinatus muscle inserts into the lateral portion of the proximal humerus and may produce a deforming force with fractures located just distal to its insertion. Fractures at this level present with a typical abduction deformity of the humeral head secondary to the pull of the rotator cuff mechanism. Fractures that occur just distal to the insertion of the pectoralis musculature present with a different anatomical configuration. The deltoid muscle is attached to the shaft of the humerus along the lateral aspect into the deltoid tuberosity. In a fracture between the distal portion of the pectoralis major insertion and the deltoid insertion, a typical adduction deformity of the proximal fragment occurs because of the inward pull of the pectoralis major on the proximal fragment and the outward pull of the deltoid on the distal fragment. This will frequently produce overriding of the fracture fragments. If a fracture occurs distal to the insertion of the deltoid musculature on the deltoid tuberosity, then the proximal shaft is pulled outward and abducted by the deltoid. The distal portion of the shaft of the humerus is then pulled in a proximal direction through the muscle action of the biceps, coracobrachialis, and triceps.

If these muscular insertions are borne in mind, the angulation and rotatory deformities produced by fractures at various levels in the humeral shaft are easily understood. These muscle actions must be taken into account in order to reduce the malalignment at the fracture site and to maintain the reduction.

MECHANISMS OF INJURY

Fractures of the shaft of the humerus are characteristically caused by direct injury. A rapid load impact concentrated in one portion of the shaft generates a force exceeding the modulus of elasticity and produces a typical fracture. In view of the direct violence producing the fracture, it is not difficult to understand why many present as open injuries. Many of them are also comminuted as a result of the violent trauma required to produce the fracture. Fortunately, there is a large amount of bulky muscle surrounding fractures of the shaft of the humerus, and it is felt that this is one of the reasons why nonunion is relatively uncommon in humeral shaft fractures treated by closed methods.

A smaller portion of these fractures may be produced by indirect trauma, such as that occurring from sudden violent muscle contraction or a fall on the outstretched arm. This type of mechanism frequently produces a spiral fracture of the midshaft of the humerus. Recently, spiral fractures of the humeral shaft have been reported following violent muscle activity — such as throwing a baseball overarm or performing gymnastics.

Pathological fractures may also be caused, through an indirect mechanism, by sudden muscular contraction. These fractures tend to occur in the proximal half of the humerus rather than at the junction of the middle and distal thirds — a common site for nonpathological fractures.

PHYSICAL EXAMINATION

Patients usually present with a history of direct trauma produced through a violent mechanism, such as an automobile collision or an industrial accident. The young athlete may present with a history of violent physical exertion in which he experienced sudden pain and discomfort in the humeral region. Gunshot wounds may also produce this type of injury; these are obvious at the time of physical examination. The pain is typically localized to the midportion of the humerus. Motion of the shoulder or elbow elicits pain secondary to muscle contraction, and a resultant deforming force is produced. The obvious deformity of the humeral area will depend in large measure on the level of the fracture, as discussed earlier in the section on surgical anatomy. These fractures usually produce an acute hematoma within the soft-tissue structures, and the result is an arm that is obviously enlarged compared with the contralateral normal one. Any stress on the humerus will elicit pain, and crepitus is usually palpable at the fracture site.

A careful neurovascular examination of the entire upper extremity is essential. This becomes extremely important in evaluating patients with fractures in the vicinity of the spiral groove, in which a neurological deficit secondary to radial nerve injury is not uncommon. Unfortunately, it is a common error to neglect this, and then it becomes difficult to determine whether the neurological deficit was present prior to the reduction or was secondary to the manipulation for reduction. This is, of course, very important prognostically and may also drastically affect the form of treatment outlined for the patient. Once the physical examination is completed, it is important to attempt to immobilize the upper extremity in order to make the patient comfortable during transit to the radiology department. This may be accomplished by a simple sling that will prevent excessive motion at the fracture site during transport.

ROENTGENOGRAPHIC EVALUATION

A thorough roentgenographic evaluation of the entire humeral shaft, including both the shoulder and elbow joints, is mandatory. It is customary to obtain both an anteroposterior and a lateral view. Oblique views are usually not necessary for diagnosis of the average humeral fracture. It is particularly important to obtain views of the shoulder and elbow joint, as the majority of these fractures are caused by severe direct trauma and there are frequently other associated injuries in the same extremity. The typical views may be obtained with the patient supine on a stretcher in order to cause as little discomfort as possible. It is also preferable to have the attending physician or house staff physician present to apply gentle traction on the extremity during positioning of the roentgenographic cassettes.

CLASSIFICATION

The classification of humeral shaft fractures should be kept as simple as possible. It should include information about whether the fracture is an open or closed injury. The level of the fracture is important, as several deforming forces are present, as outlined in the surgical anatomy section. The direction and degree of comminution of the fracture should be documented. Finally, at the time of the initial evaluation it is important to record any associated neurovascular insult.

TREATMENT OF HUMERAL SHAFT FRACTURES

The great majority of fractures of the humeral shaft may be treated by closed methods. It is only rarely that this type of fracture requires open reduction and internal fixation. In fact, in the author's experience, the large majority of patients presenting with nonunion of the humerus have undergone prior attempts at open reduction and internal fixation. All that is required in the management of these fractures by closed measures is contact of at least one third to one fourth of the bone at the fracture ends. Patients are able to tolerate a significant degree of angulation, and most authors feel that up to 30 degrees of angulation is satisfactory for both function and cosmetic appearance (Fig. 16–1).

Functional Bracing

As in many other areas of fracture management, Sarmiento and co-authors demonstrated the value of functional bracing in the management of fractures of the shaft of the humerus.[26] It was their feeling that closed methods were preferable because they required a shorter healing time, infection was uncommon, and nonunion was rare. The rate is low in these fractures, but nonunion has been variously reported to occur in from 1 to 12 per cent of patients.[4, 7, 9, 12, 23] Functional bracing provides a very adaptable method of treatment and one in which the patients appear more comfortable and are able to continue to perform activities of daily living. The patients are initially treated with a hanging cast or a coaptation U-splint prior to application of the functional brace. Once the acute reaction subsides, which is usually at one week after application, the cast is removed and a functional brace consisting of a well-molded Orthoplast sleeve is applied. The sleeve is maintained in position by Velcro straps, and as the edema subsides the sleeves may be tightened with these straps. The rationale for using this type of functional brace is that it provides for compression of the soft tissues as the edema subsides and allows for active functional contraction of the surrounding musculature, which is felt to have a beneficial effect on

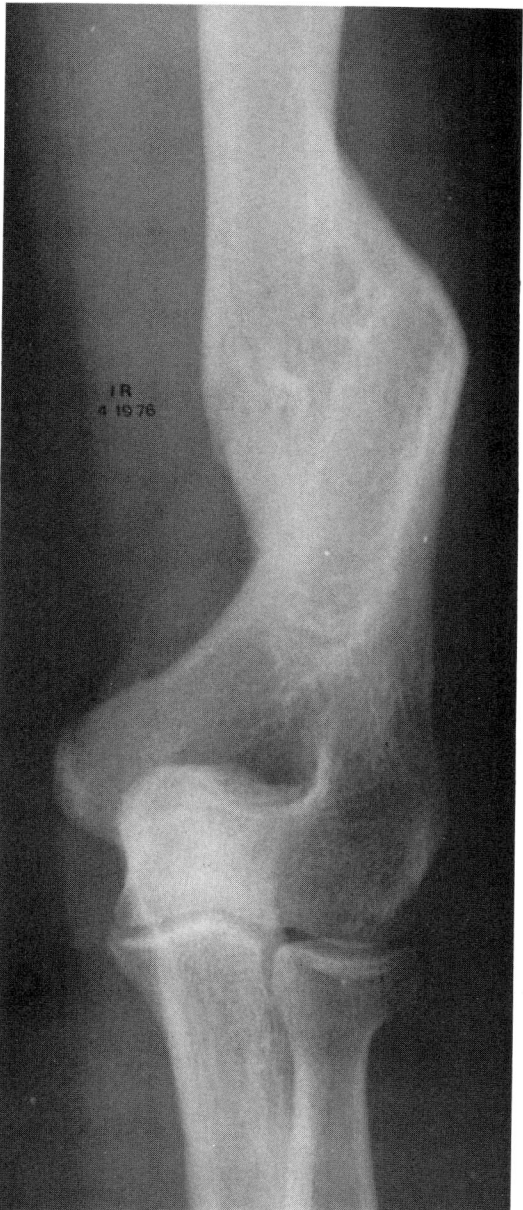

Figure 16–1 Anteroposterior view of a healed fracture of the distal third of the humerus. Note the degree of angulation at the healed fracture site. In spite of this degree of angulation the patient had almost no detectable clinical cosmetic deformity and had full function of the elbow. Angular deformities in humeral shaft fractures are well tolerated.

the fracture healing process proper. It has been demonstrated that this type of functional treatment stimulates development of a large bulky callus that is biomechanically stronger than the smaller callus produced by rigid immobilization.[26] The sleeve is maintained until there is demonstrated absence of pain and motion at the fracture site. The sleeve may be discontinued, on the average, at nine weeks postapplication.

This functional method of treatment is gaining widespread acceptance in present-day management of fractures in other areas and is well suited to fractures of the humeral shaft. The author has found it to be a very useful method and prefers either this method or the method that follows.

U-Shaped Coaptation Splint (Elephant Tongs)

This is another very useful method for management of fractures of the humeral shaft. It is similar in concept to "sugar-tongs" for the management of fractures in the region of the wrist. It is a much larger splint, however, which is applied under the axilla, extending around the elbow, and then back over the lateral aspect of the humerus to end over the shoulder proper. Because of the large size of this U-shaped splint compared with the sugar-tongs, the name "elephant tongs" has been coined for this device. This method allows for control of angulation at the fracture site while still permitting active flexion at the elbow joint and motion at the shoulder. Initially, a large stockinette is placed over the entire upper extremity to extend over the shoulder. Plaster slabs 4 to 6 inches wide and 8 to 10 slabs in depth are then applied to the arm, extending from just under the axilla along the medial aspect of the humeral area, around the elbow, and then back over the lateral aspect of the humerus and over the shoulder joint proper. The plaster slabs may then be molded in place with an Ace bandage or Kling. In this manner the angulation deformity tends to be corrected, and active motion at the shoulder and the elbow may be maintained. Following application of the elephant tongs, a simple sling is applied around the neck to suspend the forearm. After four or five days, when the acute reaction subsides, the sling around the neck is discontinued and active flexion range-of-motion exercises of the elbow are initiated. Mild pendulum exercises of the shoulder

may also be instituted one week following this maneuver (Fig. 16–2).

Another beneficial effect of this type of splint is that it does not permit distraction at the fracture site. Therefore, the fracture site proper has the benefit of active surrounding muscular contraction without separation of the fracture fragments. Mild degrees of angulation may occur with this functional treatment, but as stated previously, angulation is well tolerated with this type of fracture. The plaster tongs may be discontinued, on the average, at 9 to 10 weeks postapplication.

Hanging Cast

This type of treatment has been very popular in the past. It does allow for early active motion of the shoulder joint, and patients seem to be comfortable in this type of elbow joint immobilization. The author has two primary objections to the hanging cast. The first involves the possibility of distraction of the fracture fragments by the weight of the cast. For this reason, if this technique is selected the plaster must be light and must not distract the fracture surfaces. The basic premise is that with a light cast the mild traction that occurs will correct the angulatory deformity and will not cause overdistraction of the fracture fragments. The author has, however, seen cases in which too heavy a cast was applied and there was evidence of distraction at the fracture site, which may cause delayed union or nonunion.

The second criticism of this form of therapy is that the majority of fractures selected for this type of treatment occur in the midshaft of the humerus. It is not infrequent to find that the proximal border of a hanging cast applied here coincides with the level of the fracture. Therefore, any slight tilting of the cast will cause a fulcrum at the fracture site and may in itself cause angulation. Biomechanically, it is incorrect to place a possible fulcrum at a fracture site, as this will lead to excess motion and possible angulation (Fig. 16–3).

In spite of these two drawbacks, the author does not deny that various reports on the use of the hanging cast have provided adequate data showing that if this technique

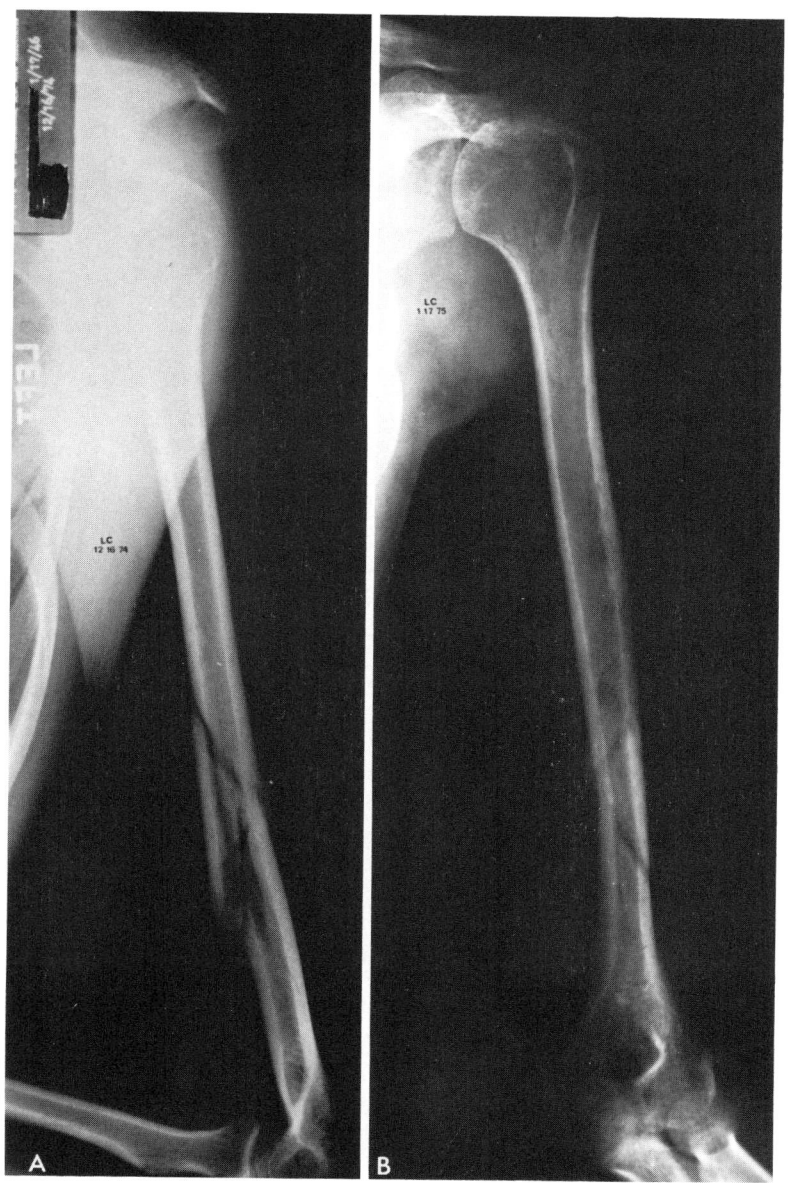

Figure 16–2 *A.* Comminuted fracture of the distal portion of the humerus with a large medial butterfly fragment. This was treated with elephant tongs. *B.* One month after treatment with elephant tongs there is evidence of beginning osseous consolidation.

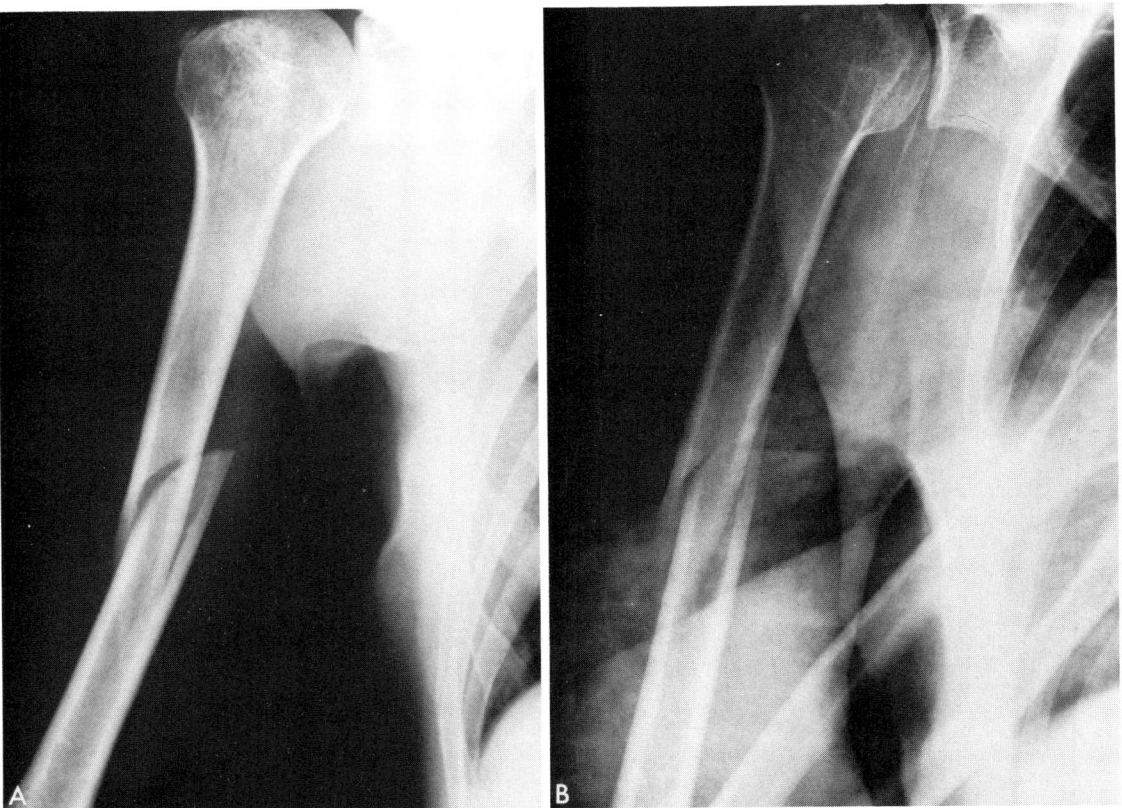

Figure 16-3   A. Fracture of the midshaft of the humerus with a broad surface. B. Following application of a hanging cast, the alignment of the fracture is improved. The proximal portion of the cast, however, is seen to lie directly over the fracture site proper. This produces a fulcrum at the fracture site.

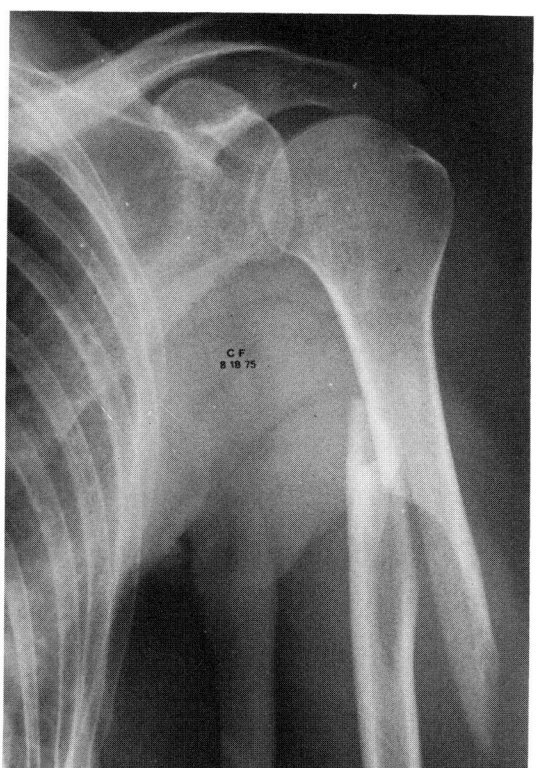

Figure 16–4 A long spiral fracture of the midshaft of the humerus. This is the type of fracture for which treatment with a hanging cast has been advocated. Note the long broad exposed surface for contact.

is properly applied a high percentage of patients will obtain union of their fractures.[3, 20, 23, 29]

A few technical points are in order. The patient should have his arm continuously dependent for proper management of this type of fracture with this technique. Proper application of a loop of plaster at the wrist is important in correcting angulation. If lateral angulation is present, the plaster loop must be placed on the dorsum of the wrist. This will tend to correct the lateral angulation spontaneously. If medial angulation is present, then the plaster loop must be placed on the volar aspect of the wrist.

In a 1959 study the Scientific Research Committee of the Pennsylvania Orthopaedic Society reported on the treatment of humeral shaft fractures from 1952 to 1956. Of 159 fractures of the humeral shaft, 54 per cent were treated with a hanging cast. This type of treatment produced union in 96 per cent of the patients so treated at an average of 10 weeks after application of the cast.[23] Similar studies have produced corresponding results. It is difficult to improve on these figures, but it is important to realize that proper attention to detail is necessary if this method is to produce satisfactory results. The technique appears to be best adapted to fractures with a broad exposed surface (Fig. 16–4) and least well adapted to simple transverse fractures of the shaft of the humerus.

Humeral Abduction Splints

This method has been advocated for severely comminuted fractures or fractures in which angulation of the shaft is difficult to control. It consists of splinting the arm and cast in a position of abduction that maintains proper alignment of the humerus. The problem with this type of treatment is that it does eliminate shoulder motion and severely restricts elbow motion. Therefore, it is not often used in modern medicine.

Shoulder Spica Cast

Use of this technique is limited in everyday practice. It is occasionally useful in children who will not cooperate in the management of these fractures with a brace, elephant tongs, or a hanging arm cast. It is also occasionally useful in the management of the patient with a highly unstable comminuted fracture in the early stages. It allows for good immobilization of the comminuted fragments, but consideration should be given to removing the spica as soon as possible once the fragments have become "sticky" in order to allow active motion of the shoulder and elbow. If this technique is selected, it is important to remember that the spica must be well molded around the iliac crest to prevent a pistoning effect that may occur with ambulation.

Skeletal Traction

This technique has very limited application. It has a place in the management of patients with severe open fractures in this area, as it does allow for easy access to the wound for adequate debridement and packing if necessary. It is also useful in patients with multiple injuries who require treatment in the recumbent position because of their other associated injuries.

The skeletal traction is supplied through insertion of a Steinmann pin (7/64-inch) through the olecranon process. The arm may then be maintained in a position horizontal to the bed with the arm held at 90 degrees of abduction. Lateral traction is then applied through a skeletal pin with a sling support under the humeral area suspended from the top of the bed. The forearm may also be suspended from above through a pulley system at the top of the bed. One of the disadvantages of this type of treatment is that it does limit the patient's

motion in bed, and if there is an associated pulmonary complication it does not permit adequate pulmonary toilet. Nevertheless, it may be useful in the management of patients with soft-tissue injuries associated with fractures of the humeral shaft.

Open Reduction

The indications for a primary open reduction of humeral shaft fractures are rare indeed. If there is significant difficulty in obtaining adequate reduction owing to the interposition of soft tissue between the fracture fragments, this may be an indication for primary open reduction (Fig. 16–5).

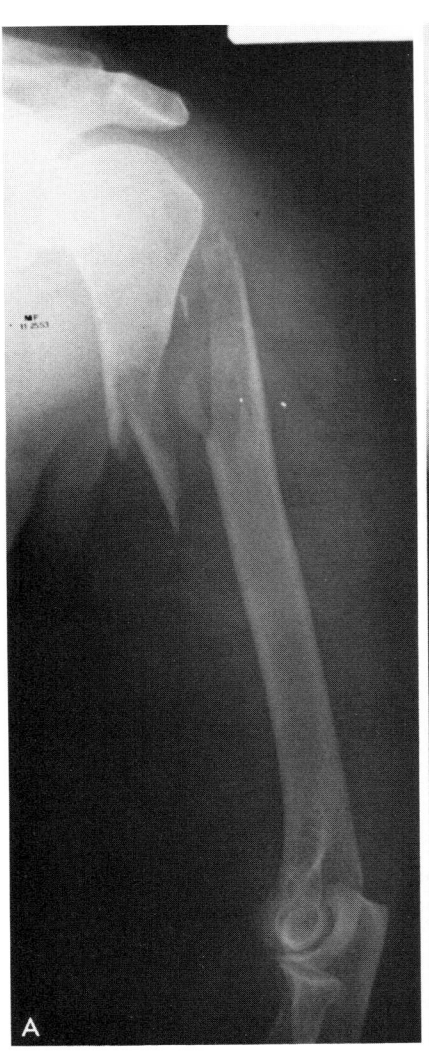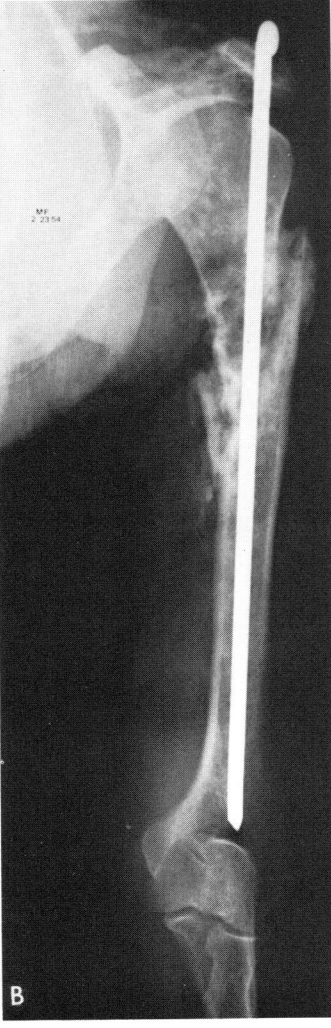

Figure 16–5 A. Anteroposterior view of a comminuted fracture of the proximal third of the humerus. There was extreme difficulty in obtaining adequate reduction of the fracture fragments. B. Following closed reduction and insertion of a Rush rod through the neck of the humerus down the humeral shaft. The fracture has healed three months postoperatively. This form of treatment is an alternative to open reduction.

The development of delayed union or nonunion may also be an indication for open reduction.

As stated previously, it has been the author's experience that the majority of nonunions of the shaft of the humerus encountered in everyday practice have been associated with prior attempts at open reduction and internal fixation. The results with functional bracing or with the use of elephant tongs or a hanging cast have been very good, the healing rate being greater than 90 per cent in the majority of reported series![3, 8, 16, 20, 23, 26] Therefore, in view of the

results of these conservative series, it is difficult to justify primary open reduction and internal fixation. One of the few indications for open reduction and internal fixation has been suggested by Holstein and Lewis.[17] This is a spiral type of fracture in the distal third of the humerus. The distal bone fragment is displaced proximally with its proximal end deviated radialward, and the radial nerve may be caught in the fracture site. It is the oblique surface of the distal end of the proximal fragment that may damage the nerve. The radial nerve is in direct contact with the humerus for a very

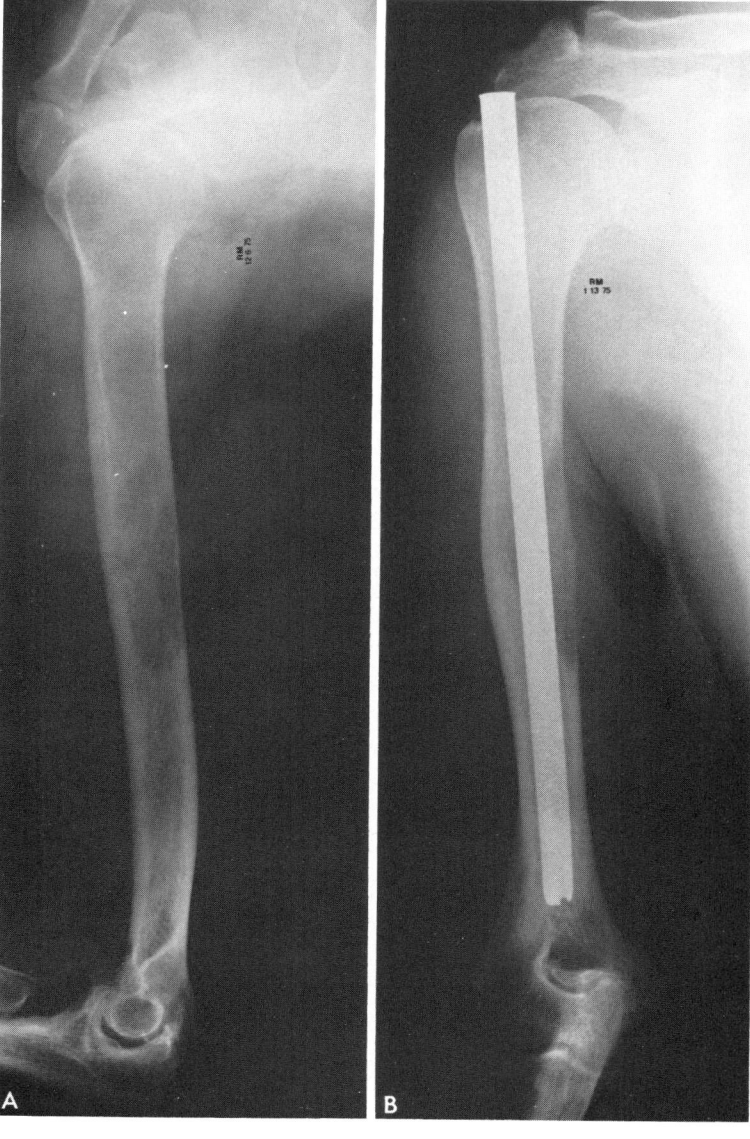

Figure 16–6 *A.* Pathological fracture of the midshaft of the humerus with disruption of the posterior medial surface. *B.* Following insertion of a Küntscher rod. Biopsy revealed metastatic adenocarcinoma.

short distance near the lateral supracondylar ridge, and it is in this area that the nerve pierces the lateral intermuscular septum before it passes on to the surface of the brachialis muscle. Since the nerve is the least mobile at this site it was the opinion of Holstein and Lewis that the lack of mobility was a prime factor in nerve injuries associated with fractures of the humerus at this level. Therefore, they felt that primary open reduction through an anterolateral approach was indicated with fractures of the distal third of the humerus with a demonstrable radial nerve paresis. The nerve is located, dissected free, and placed in a position lateral to the distal fragment. The fracture is then reduced, and the reduction is maintained either with screws or with plate fixation.

Pathological fractures secondary to malignant disease should also be considered for primary open reduction and internal fixation. It has been the author's experience that lesions at the junction of the proximal third and the middle third of the humerus may be managed by the insertion of an intramedullary rod through the neck of the humerus and down the shaft, maintaining reduction and allowing for early active functional use of the extremity (Figs. 16–6 and 16–7). In connection with this form of treatment the author has found it useful to perform a partial acromionectomy for ease of insertion of the intramedullary device. If this is not done, it is frequently difficult to insert the rod down the shaft of the humerus. The distal tip of the rod may impinge on the proximal medial surface of the humeral shaft because it cannot be inserted satisfactorily owing to the position of the acromion. There is little morbidity associated with a partial acromionectomy, and it greatly facilitates insertion of the rod. This type of procedure may be completed very quickly, and exposure of the pathological fracture site is not necessary, as curettings from the medullary shaft may be obtained for pathological evaluation. It is not uncommon to encounter a significant amount of bleeding with the use of this technique. For this reason the quick insertion of an intramedullary rod is beneficial, as it reduces the amount of hemorrhage, in comparison with open reduction of the fracture site and insertion of a compression plate device.

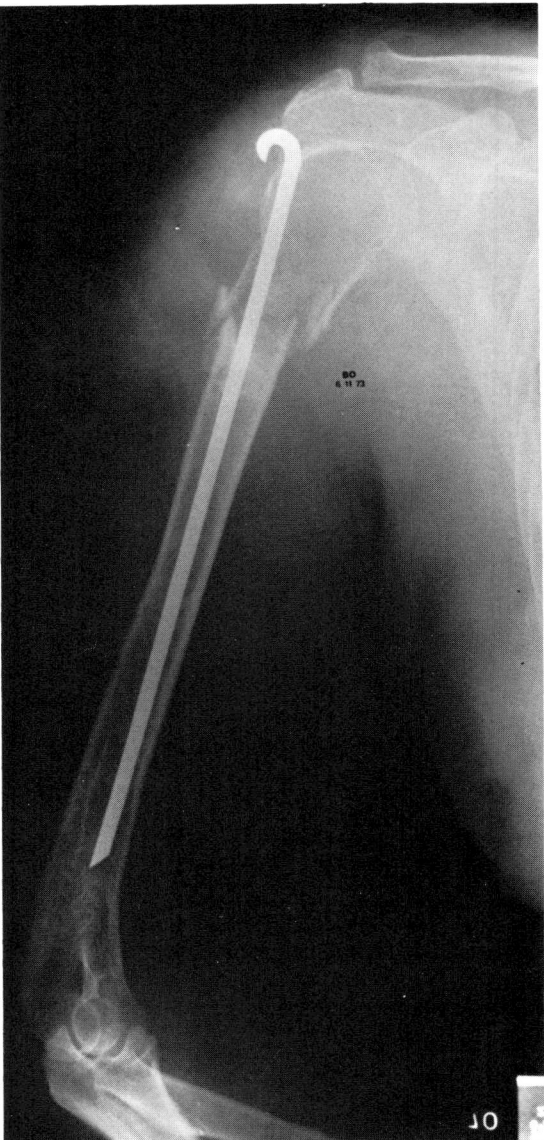

Figure 16–7 An alternative form of treatment for a pathological fracture of the proximal third of the humerus. A Rush rod has been inserted through the humeral neck and down the shaft of the humerus. This allows for early motion and has resulted in healing of the fracture following radiation.

A final indication for open reduction may be a humeral fracture in a patient with Parkinson's disease. In this patient it may be beneficial to obtain and maintain reduction through the use of an intramedullary device. The alternative to this type of internal fixation is to open the fracture site and insert a compression plate for stability.

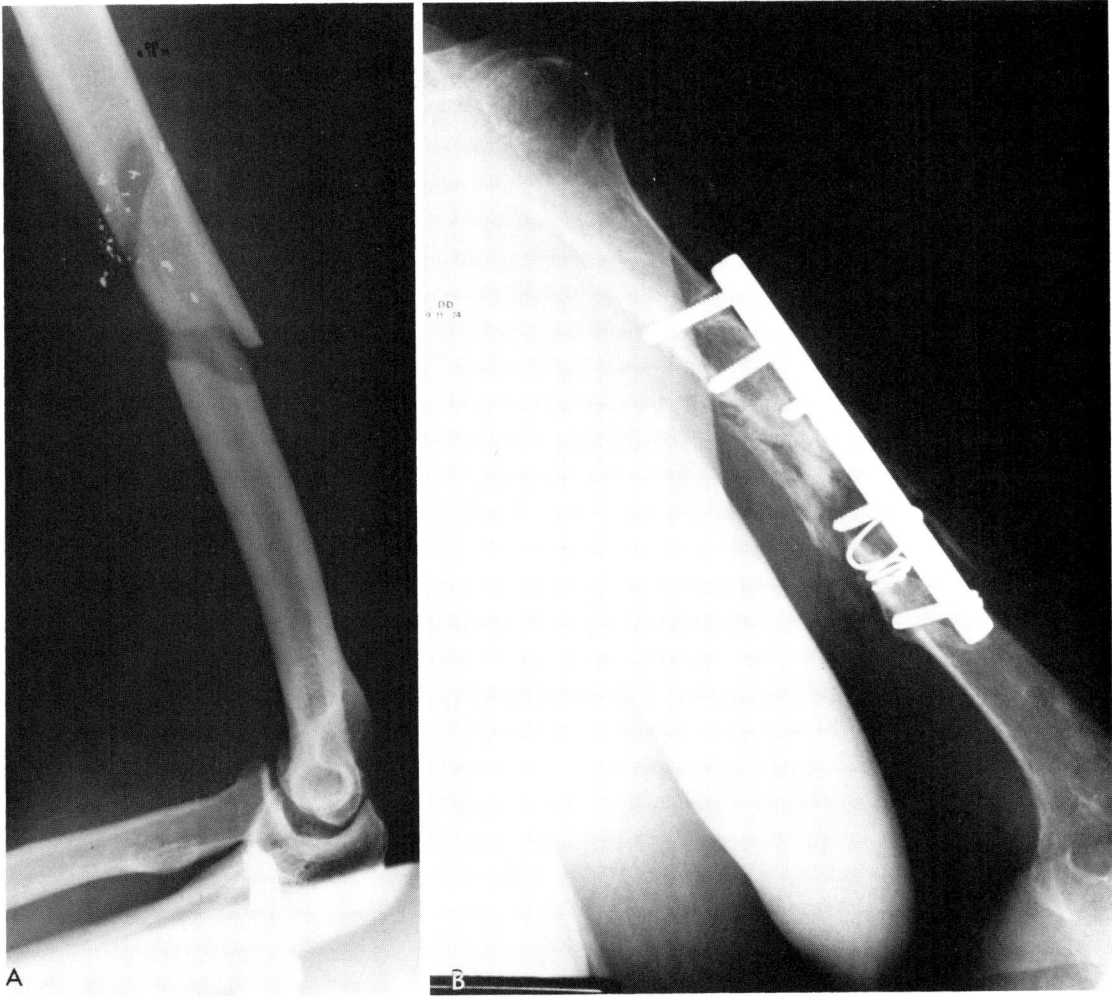

Figure 16–8 A. Lateral view of a comminuted fracture of the midshaft of the humerus caused by a gunshot. Note that skeletal traction is maintained through an olecranon pin. This injury was initially treated with debridement, irrigation, and packing open of the wound. The olecranon traction allowed for ease of dressing changes. *B*. Once the wound had been closed secondarily and there was no evidence of any infection it was decided to perform an open reduction and internal fixation with the use of a compression plate. This was an error in judgment and resulted in nonunion. This particular case could have been treated with a hanging arm cast or elephant tongs.

If comminution is present at the fracture site and a compression plate is selected as the form of treatment, then it is probably beneficial to add an iliac crest bone graft to increase the likelihood of healing (Fig. 16–8).

PROGNOSIS

As stated earlier, the majority of these fractures, more than 90 per cent, heal with conservative closed measures, including the use of a functional brace, coaptation-U-splint, or hanging cast. It is rare that primary open reduction and internal fixation are indicated in the everyday management of humeral shaft fractures. In almost all series, if the conservative approach is compared with an operative approach, there is a higher incidence of nonunion with primary open reduction and internal fixation than with closed management of these fractures.[23]

Neurovascular Compromise

An associated neurovascular compromise may alter the prognosis. The reader is referred to Chapter 34 for the overall management of nerve injuries and to Chapter 33 for the management of vascular injuries. Suffice it to state that if evidence of nerve impingement is present at the time of initial evaluation, the majority of patient series suggest that closed methods of treatment and continued observations for neurological recovery are indicated.[13, 19, 23, 28] If there is no evidence of spontaneous recovery within seven to eight weeks postinjury, exploration of the radial nerve may be indicated. At this time the fracture has usually progressed enough so that nerve exploration does not interfere with fracture healing. If a neurological deficit develops following an attempt at closed reduction, the majority of these injuries will prove to be associated with trauma to the nerve, but the nerve fibers will still be in continuity. Therefore, it is frequently advantageous to adopt a wait-and-see attitude. If at the end of seven to eight weeks there is no evidence of spontaneous recovery, then there is an indication for exploration of the nerve. It has, however, been demonstrated that delayed repair of the nerve may produce as good results as primary repair (Fig. 16–9).

It is important to remember to splint the wrist and fingers in an appropriate position until spontaneous recovery of the nerve

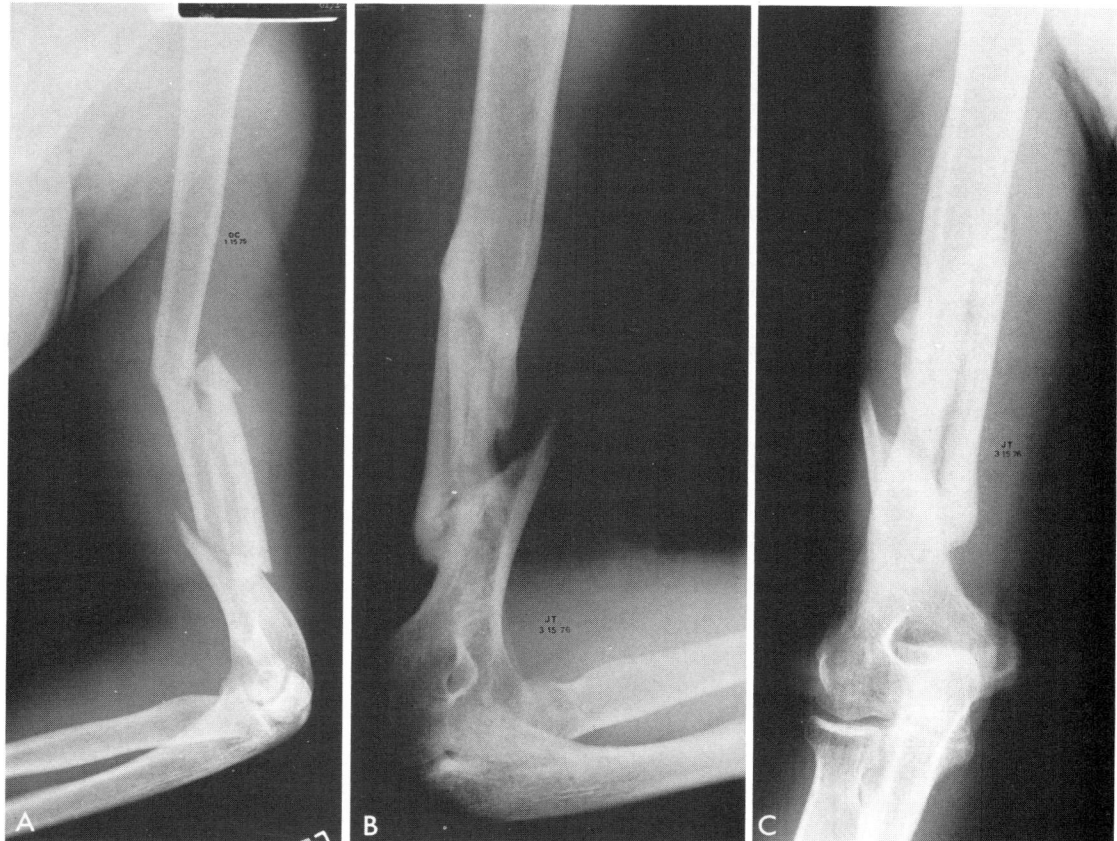

Figure 16–9   *A.* Severely comminuted fracture of the mid and distal shaft of the humerus resulting from a crush injury. There was definite radial nerve palsy immediately following this injury. The patient was treated with elephant tongs and a "cock-up" splint for the wrist. *B.* Lateral roentgenogram at 14 months postinjury. Note that there is definite evidence of healing of the severely comminuted fracture. The radial nerve had completely recovered function at three months. *C.* Anteroposterior view at 14 months postinjury reveals evidence of healing of the comminuted fracture.

occurs. If this is not performed, contractures and stiffness of the wrist and digits may result.

Vascular Injury

A vascular injury associated with a fracture of the humeral shaft should be primarily repaired. Whether or not internal fixation is required to protect the vascular repair is still a matter of controversy in some circles. The reader is referred to Chapter 33 for further considerations.

Nonunion

As stated earlier, it is the author's impression that the majority of nonunions of humeral shaft fractures are secondary to attempts at open reduction and internal fixation. The nonunion rate following closed management of fractures of the humerus is certainly less than 5 to 10 per cent in the majority of series. Once nonunion is established, it requires aggressive surgical treatment in an attempt to obtain union—usually open reduction and internal fixation with a compression plate if possible. If comminution is present, it is the author's feeling that an iliac crest bone graft should be added. It is important to protect the radial nerve during open reduction and internal fixation for nonunion in the midshaft region. One of the precautions to avoid injury to the radial nerve is not to utilize lion-jaw forceps to keep the bone fragments reduced while applying a compression plate. If this type of clamp is placed around the humerus to maintain reduction, it is quite possible for the clamp itself to damage the radial nerve in the posterior aspect, where it is in very close proximity to the bone. For this reason the author prefers to obtain an open reduction by manual methods and have the assistant hold the bone fragments in proper alignment during insertion of the initial screws to fix the plate to the humerus. An alternative method is to employ large pointed bone-holding forceps that grasp the humerus along the medial and lateral aspects for reduction but do not violate the posterior aspect of the humerus, thereby avoiding injury to the radial nerve. Nonunion in general is discussed further in Chapter 4.

REFERENCES

1. Bennett, G. E.: Fracture of the humerus with particular reference to nonunion and its treatment. Ann. Surg., 103:994, 1936.
2. Blum, L.: Double pulley traction in the treatment of humeral shaft fractures. Surg. Gynecol. Obstet., 65:812, 1937.
3. Caldwell, J. A.: Treatment of fractures of the shaft of the humerus by hanging cast. Surg. Gynecol. Obstet., 70:421, 1940.
4. Campbell, W. C.: Ununited fractures of the shaft of the humerus. Ann. Surg., 105:135, 1937.
5. Cartner, M. J.: Immobilization of fractures of the shaft of the humerus. Injury, 5:175–179, 1973.
6. Charnley, J.: The Closed Treatment of Common Fractures. Baltimore, Williams & Wilkins, 1961.
7. Christensen, S.: Humeral shaft fractures, operative and conservative treatment. Acta Chir. Scand., 133:455–460, 1967.
8. Comfort, T. H.: The sugar-tong splint in humeral shaft fractures. Minn. Med., 56:363–366, 1973.
9. Coventry, M. B., and Laurnen, E. L.: Ununited fractures of the middle and upper humerus. Special problems in treatment. Clin. Orthop., 69:192–198, 1970.
10. Doran, F. S. A.: The problems and principles of the restoration of limb function following injury as demonstrated by humeral shaft fractures. Br. J. Surg., 31:351, 1944.
11. Duthie, H. L.: Radial nerve in osseous tunnel at humeral fracture site diagnosed radiographically. J. Bone Joint Surg., 39B:746, 1957.
12. Fenyo, G.: On fractures of the shaft of the humerus. A review covering a 12-year period with special consideration of the surgically treated cases. Acta Chir. Scand., 137:221–226, 1971.
13. Garcia, A., Jr., and Maeck, B. H.: Radial nerve injuries in fractures of the shaft of the humerus. Am. J. Surg., 99:625, 1960.
14. Gilchrist, D. K.: A stockinette-Velpeau for immobilization of the shoulder girdle. J. Bone Joint Surg., 49A:750–751, 1967.
15. Gregersen, H. N.: Fractures of the humerus from muscular violence. Acta Orthop. Scand., 42:506, 1971.
16. Holm, C. L.: Management of humeral shaft fractures. Fundamentals of nonoperative techniques. Clin. Orthop., 71:132–139, 1970.
17. Holstein, A., and Lewis, G. B.: Fractures of the humerus with radial nerve paralysis. J. Bone Joint Surg., 45A:1382–1388, 1963.
18. Kennedy, J. C., and Wyatt, J. J.: An evaluation of the management of fractures through the middle third of the humerus. Can. J. Surg. 1:26–33, 1957.
19. Klenerman, L.: Fractures of the shaft of the humerus. J. Bone Joint Surg., 48B:105–111, 1966.
20. Laferte, A. D., and Rosenbaum, M. G.: The "hanging cast" in the treatment of fractures of the humerus. Surg. Gynecol. Obstet., 65:230, 1937.
21. Laing, P. G.: The arterial blood supply of the adult humerus. J. Bone Joint Surg., 38A:1105, 1956.
22. Newman, A.: The supracondylar process and its fracture. Am. J. Roentgenol., 105:844, 1969.

23. Pennsylvania Orthopaedic Society, Scientific Research Committe: Fresh midshaft fractures of the humerus in adults. Evaluation of treatment during 1952–56. Pa. Med. J., *62*:848, 1959.

24. Ruedi, T., Moshfegh, A., Pfeiffer, K. M., and Allgower, M.: Fresh fractures of the shaft of the humerus. Conservative or operative treatment? Reconstr. Surg. Traumatol., *14*:65–74, 1974.

25. Rush, L. V., and Rush, H. L.: Intramedullary fixation of fractures of the humerus by the longitudinal pin. Surgery, *27*:268, 1950.

26. Sarmiento, A., Kinman, P. B., Galvin, E. G., Schmitt, R. H., and Phillips, J. G.: Functional bracing of fractures of the shaft of the humerus. J. Bone Joint Surg., *59A*:596–601, 1977.

27. Seddon, H. J.: Nerve lesions complicating certain closed bone injuries. J.A.M.A., *135*:691, 1947.

28. Shaw, J. L., and Sakellarides, H.: Radial nerve paralysis associated with fractures of the humerus: A review of forty-five cases. J. Bone Joint Surg., *49A*:899, 1967.

29. Stewart, M. J., and Hundley, J. M.: Fractures of the humerus. A comparative study in methods of treatment. J. Bone Joint Surg., *37A*:681, 1955.

30. Whitson, R. O.: Relation of the radial nerve to the shaft of the humerus. J. Bone Joint Surg., *36A*:85, 1954.

R. BRUCE HEPPENSTALL, M.D.

Injuries ———————————————— 17
of the
Elbow

A discussion of elbow injuries must include fractures in the supra- and intercondylar areas as well as olecranon and radial–ulnar fractures. It must also include dislocations, both of the elbow proper and of the radial–ulnar articulation. Ligamentous injuries also occur in this joint and produce significant disabilities.

Elbow injuries occur in all age groups. They are frequently encountered in pediatric patients, in whom supracondylar fractures may produce significant deformities and disability if they are not properly managed. In the adult, several varieties of condylar fractures often are seen secondary to hyperextension injuries or direct trauma. These include supra-, trans-, and intercondylar fractures. Isolated fractures of the condyles and epicondyles occur, and fractures of the articular surface of the elbow joint are occasionally encountered. These injuries frequently cause significant deformity and restricted range of motion of the elbow.

Stability of the elbow joint is provided by osseous structures together with surrounding soft tissue, muscles, and ligaments. However, if there is a break in the continuity of either the osseous structure or the surrounding ligamentous structures, instability may result. The elbow joint is similar to the knee in that ligamentous injuries must be treated aggressively and properly. If they are not correctly managed, gross instability may result, with a significant decrease in functional ability. The same is true of various types of fractures and dislocations of the elbow.

For this reason there has been a trend toward aggressive operative intervention in many elbow injuries. Intrinsic stability may be obtained by proper internal fixation of the injured part, which will then permit early protective range-of-motion exercises. If this approach is followed, the severe contractures that have been seen in the past following prolonged conservative immobilization of elbow injuries can be avoided. In other words, the return of the injured elbow to functional activity will help to insure continued mobility and decreased morbidity. However, indiscriminate surgical procedures may in themselves result in postoperative adhesions and calcification of the surrounding ligamentous structures. Therefore, it is extremely important to make a thorough evaluation of patients with elbow injuries regarding definitive treatment in order to avoid secondary complications.

SURGICAL ANATOMY

The elbow joint is formed from the articulations of the distal portion of the humerus with the radius and ulna. The distal portion of the humerus presents two important articulating surfaces. On the lateral aspect, the rounded capitellum surface articulates with the head of the radius which has a normal concave articular surface. On the medial aspect, the rounded

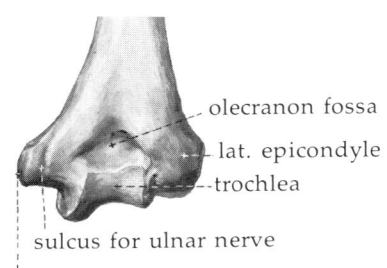

A.   Posterior view of the distal part (condyle) of the right humerus.

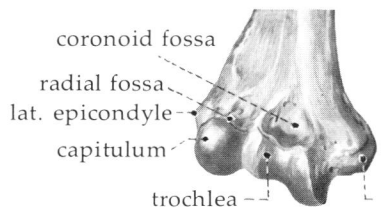

B.   Anterior aspect of the distal part (condyle) of the right humerus.

Figure 17–1 A. Anterior view of the humerus demonstrating the relationship of the capitellum to the trochlea at the distal humeral surface. B. Posterior view of the humerus revealing the olecranon fossa and the trochlea for articulation of the ulna. (Courtesy of M. Langman and M. W. Woerdeman and W. B. Saunders Co., Philadelphia. Atlas of Medical Anatomy, 1978.)

surface of the trochlea articulates with the ulna through the trochlear notch of the ulna (Fig. 17–1). The trochlear notch of the ulna does provide for some gliding stability of the elbow joint, as it extends from the tip of the olecranon to the coronoid process. The anatomical configuration of the proximal portion of the ulna allows for a proper arc of flexion and extension. In the flexed position, the coronoid process of the proximal ulna glides into the coronoid fossa at the anterior aspect of the distal humerus. In extension, the olecranon glides into the olecranon fossa, located at the posterior aspect of the distal humerus.

The anatomical configuration of the distal portion of the humerus and the radial–ulnar articulations provide for a normal carrying angle. A normal valgus angulation of the forearm in relation to the upper arm occurs

with extension of the elbow. As the elbow is gradually extended, the hand assumes a position lateral to the thigh, which allows for ease of carrying various objects. The normal carrying angle varies from 5 to 28 degrees, with an average of 15 degrees in adults. Extreme care must be taken in the management of fractures of the humeral condyles or an alteration of the normal carrying angle may result. This is particularly true of supracondylar fractures in the pediatric age group.

The common deformity resulting from improper management of this fracture is a varus angulation of the forearm in relation to the distal humerus. This produces a reversal of the normal carrying angle and has been described as a "gunstock" deformity. This deformity clearly limits the functional capacity of the forearm, as it is difficult to carry objects in the hand with the elbow in the extended position because the hand tends to abut against the lateral aspect of the thigh.

The articulation of the radial head with the proximal ulna and the distal humerus enables pronation and supination of the forearm (Fig. 17–2). This allows for manual dexterity with placement of the hand in the appropriate position for function. The radial head appears as a disk-like anatomical structure. It is larger in size than the remaining portion of the proximal radius and is united with this portion by the anatomical neck of the radius. The articular cartilage extends over the peripheral portion of the head, enabling motion between the radial head and the ulna through the radial notch and the surrounding annular ligament. This articulation is commonly referred to as the proximal radioulnar joint.

The distal portion of the humerus is divided into two major components known as the condyles. Anatomically, these structures differ in size, the medial condyle being definitely smaller on cross section than the lateral condyle. The distal articulating surface of the medial condyle is known as the trochlea, and the articulating surface of the lateral condyle is known as the capitellum. The articular surfaces of the humeral condyles are not directly in line with the remainder of the shaft of the humerus. They project in a forward and

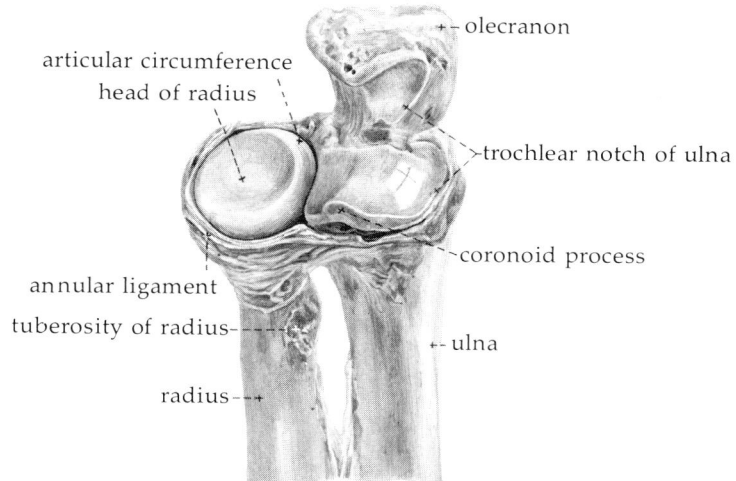

Figure 17-2 Relationship of the radial head to the proximal ulna. (Courtesy of M. Langman and M. W. Woerdeman and W. B. Saunders Co., Philadelphia. Atlas of Medical Anatomy, 1978)

Right proximal radioulnar joint.

downward position of approximately 45 degrees.

Any malalignment of the articular surface of the condyle produced by improper positioning of a fracture through the condyle will alter the gliding surface of the distal end of the humerus, thereby limiting flexion and extension. This is another reason for an aggressive surgical approach to insure proper alignment of the condylar surfaces following various types of condylar fractures.

Each condyle has a specific anatomical structure located along the peripheral aspect, at the side of the condyle proper. These structures are known as the medial and lateral epicondyles. The medial epicondyle is slightly larger than the lateral epicondyle and is the site of origin for the flexor group of muscles of the forearm. The lateral epicondyle is the site of origin for the superficial extensor muscles of the forearm. Each epicondyle has significant anatomical structures originating from its surface, and fractures of the epicondyles may present with displacement of the epicondylar fragment secondary to a deforming muscular force.

The olecranon process is a large curved osseous structure which forms the proximal portion of the ulna. The articulating surface of the olecranon extends from the proximal tip of the olecranon through a definite arc to the coronoid process. A definite articular notch, known as the sigmoid or semilunar notch of the ulna, produces a distinct depression of the olecranon process, which articulates directly with the trochlea of the humerus. This anatomical configuration of the olecranon articulating surface aids in obtaining stability of the elbow joint. If fractures occur through the olecranon process, they extend into the intraarticular portion and may produce instability of the elbow joint. Therefore, strict anatomical restoration of the olecranon process is necessary to provide added stability. However, in the elderly, the olecranon may occasionally be sacrificed in significant comminuted fractures without complete sacrifice of stability of the joint.

This brief review of the gross osseous structure of the elbow joint allows the reader to see how superficial these osseous structures are and how each is involved in determining the gross integrity of the elbow joint. If the elbow joint is flexed to 90 degrees, three distinct osseous structures are readily palpable. In this position the epicondyles and the olecranon process form an equilateral triangle in a plane parallel to the posterior surface of the humerus. This relationship is altered in full extension, when the epicondyles and the olecranon process are located in the same horizontal plane along the posterior aspect of the elbow. Thus, the examiner can readily determine if the gross osseous integrity of the elbow joint has been maintained following an injury.

SOFT TISSUE STRUCTURES

The capsular attachments to the distal humerus and radioulnar articulations are as follows: The anterior portion of the capsule is attached to the anterior aspect of the humerus directly above the radial and coronoid fossae. It extends distally to the anterior aspect of the coronoid process of the ulna and also to the anterior portion of the annular ligament surrounding the proximal radius. The posterior portion of the capsule is attached proximally to the upper aspect and peripheral portions of the olecranon fossa. Distally, it extends to the upper and lateral portions of the trochlear notch of the ulna and to the annular ligament of the radius.

Four distinct ligamentous structures are found in the elbow joint. These are the radial and ulnar collateral ligaments, the quadrate ligament, and the annular ligament. The radial collateral ligament is attached to the lateral epicondyle just under the common extensor tendon, which also originates from this structure. It then extends from the lateral epicondyle in a distal direction to insert into the annular ligament of the radius.

The ulnar collateral ligament has been described as three separate bands. However, these bands are continuous and form a definite structure along the medial aspect of the elbow joint. The ulnar collateral ligament originates from the medial epicondyle and extends distally, forming a triangular structure as a result of the divergence of the distal portions of the ligament. The anterior and posterior portions of the distal aspect are thicker and stronger than the weaker central portion. The anterior band extends distally to attach along the medial portion of the coronoid process. The middle band extends distally to blend in with the oblique ligament of Cooper which spans the interval between the olecranon and the coronoid process. The posterior band extends in a slightly backward direction to attach along the medial aspect of the olecranon.

The quadrate ligament is a thin structure which spans the distance from the medial aspect of the neck of the radius to the distal portion of the radial notch of the ulna.

The annular ligament is a structure that comprises approximately four fifths of a circle and is attached anteriorly and posteriorly to the margins of the radial notch of the humerus. It contains the radial head in the radial notch and also receives the major part of the attachment of the radial collateral ligament.

Part I ——————— **FRACTURES OF THE ELBOW** ———————

CLASSIFICATION OF ELBOW FRACTURES

Fractures of the elbow may be classified as supracondylar fractures (extension and flexion types), transcondylar fractures, intercondylar fractures (T or Y), fractures of the medial and lateral condyles, fractures of the medial and lateral epicondyles, humeral articular surface fractures, proximal ulnar (olecranon) fractures, and fractures of the proximal radius (radial head).

SUPRACONDYLAR FRACTURES

This is probably the most frequent elbow fracture in children and is relatively rare in adults. It has characteristically been divided into two types, depending on the position of the distal fragment. In the extension type of supracondylar fracture, the distal fragment is located posterior to the proximal humeral shaft. In the flexion type, the distal fragment is located along the anterior aspect of the humeral shaft. The extension fracture is the one most frequently encountered in everyday practice. The flexion type is not as common and is more difficult to treat. The discussion that follows pertains to adult supracondylar fractures. The reader is referred to Chapter 9 for the treatment of the more common pediatric supracondylar fractures.

EXTENSION FRACTURE

This type of injury is not often seen in the adult, and the mechanism of injury is not as straightforward as in the child. These injuries are seen following a direct fall on the upper extremity with the elbow in extension. The force is transmitted to the supracondylar area, and if the force is great enough it may produce a supracondylar fracture. However, in the adult, the usual injury produced by a fall with the arm in this position is a Colles' fracture of the wrist. Occasionally, however, the bone fatigues in the supracondylar area instead of in the wrist. A direct blow to the distal humerus may produce a hyperextension fracture. This may occur secondary to a patient's sustaining a direct injury in a fall in which a solid object strikes the distal humeral portion, breaking the fall.

Physical Examination

On physical examination the patient with this injury presents with a swollen elbow. It is important to differentiate a supracondylar fracture from a dislocated elbow, which is more common in adults. The differentiation is aided by the fact that the normal elbow presents three specific osseous structures for examination. The medial and lateral epicondyles and the tip of the olecranon normally form an equilateral triangle. With a supracondylar fracture this relationship is usually not disturbed. If a posterior dislocation of the elbow is present, this relationship will be altered because the tip of the olecranon will be situated in a more posterior position than normal. It is important to bear this distinction in mind in the examination of patients presenting with this injury. The neurovascular status of the upper extremity should be carefully documented. A supracondylar fracture may produce a compromise of the neurovascular bundle secondary to swelling in the antecubital space.

There is also the possibility of a direct injury produced by the jagged edge of the distal humeral shaft fragment, similar to the injury seen in the pediatric patient. Fortunately, this complication is very rare in adults. It is extremely important to avoid the fully flexed position in the early management of these patients, as this may impair circulation to the distal portion of the upper extremity secondary to increased swelling in the antecubital space with increased interstitial pressure. This may of itself decrease or obliterate the blood flow across the elbow and into the forearm.

Roentgenographic Examination

This fracture is visible on routine anteroposterior and lateral roentgenograms of the elbow. On the anteroposterior view, the usual supracondylar fracture will present as a relatively transverse fracture line just proximal to the origin of the articular capsule. There may be evidence of malalignment of the distal fragment secondary to a lateral or medial deviation of the distal fragment in relation to the proximal humeral shaft. On the lateral view, the distal fragment will be seen to be slightly posterior to the humeral shaft fragment (Fig. 17–3). The fracture line itself usually extends obliquely, with the distal portion of the fracture line located along the anterior surface of the humerus and the proximal portion associated with the posterior aspect of the humerus. In the adult, there is usually little displacement present. This is in contrast to the child, in whom there is frequently significant displacement on initial evaluation.

Treatment

The main complication to be avoided is damage to the neurovascular bundle. Since there is usually a significant amount of swelling about the elbow with this fracture, it is advantageous to obtain reduction as soon as possible. This will restore normal alignment and reduce the interstitial pressure secondary to increased swelling. The

EXTENSION

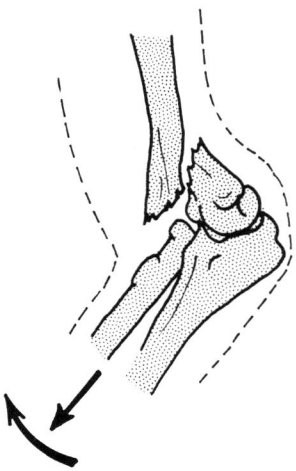

Figure 17–3 Extension type of supracondylar fracture. Note that the distal humeral fragment is situated posterior to the humeral shaft.

patient will instinctively guard the elbow and it is usually necessary to administer a brachial block or a general anesthetic to obtain reduction. Once satisfactory anesthesia has been obtained, an assistant immobilizes the proximal humeral shaft while the operator applies direct traction to the forearm and elbow in a longitudinal axis to the shaft of the humerus. It is occasionally beneficial to apply a slightly posterior axial force to disengage the fracture fragments.

No attempt should be made to flex the elbow and bring the distal humeral fragment into proper apposition until satisfactory traction has been applied to disengage the fracture fragments. If traction has not been applied prior to attempted reduction, there is the possibility of damaging the brachial artery. The elbow is then flexed to bring the distal fragment in line with the proximal humeral shaft, and the flexion is increased to 90 degrees or greater, provided the status of the pulses at the wrist is satisfactory. If pulse pressure at the wrist is decreased or obliterated, the amount of flexion must be reduced.

The author has found that the application of a long arm cast, with the forearm held in slight pronation, provides satisfactory maintenance of the reduction. The entire anterior aspect of the cast as well as the soft dressing about the antecubital fossa is then removed to allow for mild swelling in this area. A long arm cast should not be applied without this provision. A satisfactory alternative is to apply a posterior splint to maintain the reduction and then to convert this to a long arm cast once the swelling in the antecubital area has subsided. The cast is then maintained for an eight-week period. At this time there is satisfactory healing, and a posterior splint can be applied. The arm may be removed from the splint for daily, very gentle range-of-motion exercises. The fracture itself is usually completely healed by 8 to 12 weeks.

Traction. If there has been significant swelling in the antecubital area, it is advantageous to attempt Dunlop's traction or overhead skeletal traction. This allows for reduction in the swelling in the antecubital area without endangering the vascular supply to the forearm. Dunlop's traction is applied by having the patient lie supine with the involved upper extremity at 90 degrees of abduction at the shoulder joint and the humerus extended out over the bed. A weight is then attached through a sling over the distal humeral area. Skin traction is applied to the forearm with the elbow at approximately 30 to 50 degrees of flexion.[30] This will tend to realign the distal humeral fragment with the humeral shaft.

Overhead skeletal traction is also useful in managing patients with severe swelling of the antecubital area and a possible compromise of the vascular supply to the forearm (Fig. 17–4). With the patient supine, a medium-sized Kirschner wire is inserted through the olecranon at right angles to the humeral shaft. A traction bow is then applied to the Kirschner wire, and the forearm is placed in the overhead position. The traction device is then suspended in a position straight up from the bed. A sling is placed around the forearm and is suspended by a small weight through a pulley system from the overhead frame. The elbow is therefore maintained at approximately 90 degrees of flexion, and the forearm will fall naturally into the pronated position. D'Ambrosia has demonstrated that this type of traction apparatus will aid in the prevention of a cubitus varus deformity of the elbow.[26] The pronated position of the forearm places tension on the medial col-

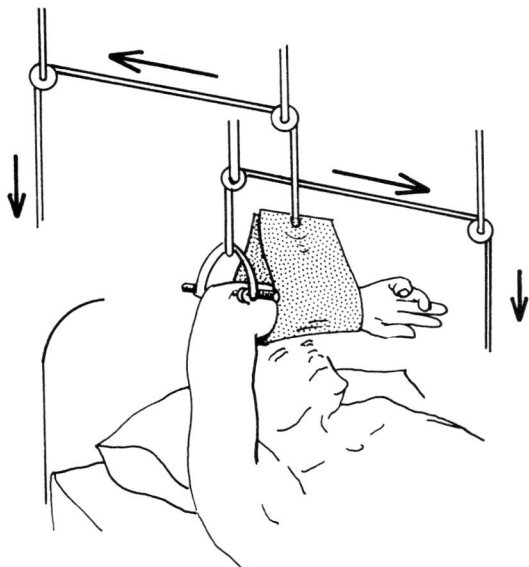

Figure 17–4 Overhead skeletal traction. The forearm tends to assume a pronated position, which aids in reduction of the fracture.

lateral ligament, which then pulls the fragments into proper position and corrects any varus angulation of the distal fragment.

Once the swelling has subsided from the elbow joint and the risk of vascular compromise has decreased, the upper extremity may be placed in a long arm cast with the elbow at 90 to 110 degrees of flexion. The disadvantage of the Dunlop and overhead skeletal traction methods is that they require hospitalization for varying lengths of time. It must be emphasized that if there is any question of vascular status or swelling of the elbow when a posterior plaster splint or a long arm cast has been applied as initial definitive treatment, the patient should be admitted for observation.

An alternative form of treatment involves appropriate reduction under anesthesia, followed by crossed Kirschner wire fixation of the fragment. A Kirschner wire is passed from the lateral condyle across the fracture site and into the medial portion of the humeral shaft. A similar wire is passed from the medial condyle into the lateral humeral shaft. The wires may be buried and a posterior plaster slab applied. The advantage of this method is that it allows for early elbow motion and a shorter hospital stay.

FLEXION FRACTURE

This is an extremely rare fracture in the adult. The mechanism of injury may be a backward fall with the arm held at 90 degrees of flexion. If the force is suddenly broken by a solid object striking the posterior aspect of the distal humerus, it is possible that a flexion type of supracondylar fracture may result.

Physical Examination

On physical examination it should be relatively simple to differentiate this injury from a dislocated elbow because the equilateral triangle secondary to the three main osseous prominences of the elbow joint is not disrupted. Swelling may occur secondary to this fracture, and safeguards must be taken to prevent vascular insufficiency to the forearm.

Roentgenographic Examination

On roentgenographic examination the fracture line will be seen to be located just above the origin of the articular capsule, as in the hyperextension injury. The lateral view will show the distal humeral fragment to be located in a slightly anterior position to the long axis of the humeral shaft (Fig. 17–5). The fracture line itself is the reverse of that in a hyperextension injury. With a

FLEXION

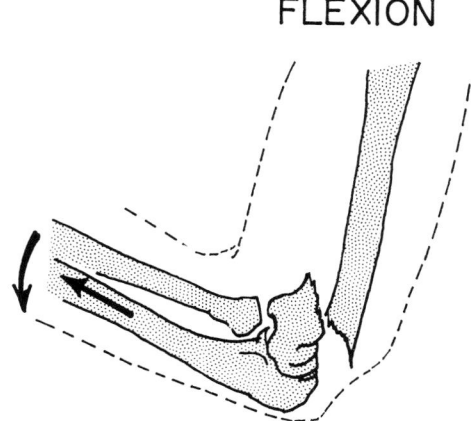

Figure 17–5 A flexion type of supracondylar fracture. Note that the distal humeral fragment is situated anterior to the humeral shaft fragment.

flexion injury, the distal portion of the fracture line is located along the posterior aspect of the humeral shaft, while the proximal portion is located along the anterior aspect of the humeral shaft.

Treatment

If there is significant displacement of the fracture fragments, an appropriate anesthetic is usually required for reduction. As with a hyperextension injury, it is important to apply traction to the forearm and elbow in the long axis of the humeral shaft. This will help to disengage the fracture fragments prior to reduction by gentle manipulation of the distal fragment in a posterior direction relative to the humeral shaft. The arm is then usually immobilized in a position of slight extension. If the arm is placed in a position of hyperflexion, the fracture may displace. As with hyperextension fractures, care must be taken to avoid excess swelling. If there is evidence of excess swelling and possible vascular insufficiency, Dunlop's traction, overhead skeletal traction, or cross Kirschner wire fixation may be appropriate.

TRANSCONDYLAR FRACTURES

This type of fracture, also called a dicondylar fracture, occurs at the level of the epicondyles and extends through the olecranon fossa. The difference between a supracondylar and a transcondylar fracture lies in the fact that a transcondylar fracture is situated within the joint capsule, while a supracondylar fracture is located proximal to the joint capsule. Fortunately, the majority of these fractures in adults are relatively nondisplaced.

Treatment is with a posterior plaster splint with the elbow at 90 degrees or with a long arm cast with the anterior portion along the antecubital area removed.

INTERCONDYLAR FRACTURES (T OR Y)

This type of fracture, fortunately not a common one, is difficult in terms of management because the condylar surfaces must be realigned with each other to prevent any incongruity at the joint surface. Besides this major undertaking, the condyles themselves must be realigned to the proximal shaft of the humerus. It is essential that the condylar surfaces be realigned with each other in order to prevent future arthritis and restriction of motion. The majority of intercondylar fractures occur in older patients in whom the injury is secondary to osteoporosis.

MECHANISM OF INJURY

The mechanism of injury is secondary to a direct blow on the proximal ulna, which tends to drive the wedge-shaped olecranon upward into the distal humeral surface, producing a splitting of the humeral condyles. In the author's experience, the majority of these injuries are associated with motor vehicular accidents and are the result of a significant force applied to the proximal ulnar area. However, this fracture is occasionally seen secondary to a fall with the elbow in the semiflexed position. In the elderly patient the force does not have to be severe because osteoporosis may have significantly weakened the structural integrity of the distal humeral area. In patients who have sustained significant trauma to the elbow joint, the problem is frequently compounded by associated soft tissue injuries, which may lead to an open fracture.

PHYSICAL EXAMINATION

Physical examination will usually reveal a grossly swollen elbow with pain associated with any type of motion. The normal triangular configuration of the bony prominences may be disrupted secondary to separation and displacement of the condyles. The examiner is usually aware of the fact that the condyles appear to have independent motion with mild stress. Associated lacerations may well be present, and a frank open fracture is not uncommon with an injury secondary to severe trauma. It is important to document the neurovascular status relative to the forearm and hand, as there may be significant impairment associated with these fractures. This complication is increased if there is significant displacement of the condylar fragments.

ROENTGENOGRAPHIC EXAMINATION

The roentgenographic evaluation reveals a Y-or T-shaped intercondylar fracture. In simple terms, the fracture extends up through the intercondylar area. It may then spread out in a Y shape to affect both the lateral and medial aspects of the distal humerus. Or a T-shaped fracture may be produced secondary to a transverse pattern of the fracture line proximal to the intercondylar area.

In an attempt to better describe intercondylar fractures, Riseborough and Radin classified them into four identifiable types.[92] Type 1 involves an undisplaced intercondylar fracture extending between the capitellum and the trochlea. In a type 2 injury, the fracture line separates the capitellum and trochlea, but there is no appreciable rotation of the osseous fragments. Type 3 is a type 2 fracture in which there is a significant rotatory deformity. Type 4 is a fracture with evidence of significant comminution of the articular surfaces and widespread separation of the humeral condyles. This is a useful working classification and should be followed as an aid in the management and ultimate prognosis of intercondylar fractures.

TREATMENT

In recent years there has been a more aggressive surgical approach to the management of intercondylar fractures. If the fragments can be openly reduced and adequate internal fixation obtained, range-of-motion exercises can be instituted immediately after surgery. The rationale for this form of treatment is that it is best to return the limb to early functional use. However, it is not always an easy task to obtain adequate internal fixation with these fractures because only very large fragments are suitable for internal fixation. If there are severely comminuted fragments without major osseous stock, this form of treatment is not applicable. We have all seen patients with terrible-appearing roentgenograms who still have adequate function of the elbow.

Conversely, we have seen patients who have satisfactory reduction of the fragments through internal fixation, but limited range of motion of the elbow. Therefore, it can be appreciated that there is no specific treatment for this injury that "guarantees" good results.

The author has found the classification proposed by Riseborough and Radin very helpful in deciding which form of treatment should be selected for a specific injury.

Type 1

Type 1 fractures present with a fracture line through the intercondylar area extending between the capitellum and trochlea. There is no significant displacement of the fragments. This fracture may be managed with a posterior splint or a long arm cast, with the portion over the antecubital fossa removed to allow for swelling.

Gentle range-of-motion exercises may be initiated at four weeks postinjury. If a long arm cast is used initially, it can be removed and replaced with a posterior plaster splint. The extremity can then be removed from the posterior plaster splint two to three times per day for gradual range-of-motion exercises. The splint is then reapplied by the patient between the exercise periods to protect the elbow from reinjury. Motion should not be forced at this stage, and the patient should be instructed to start out with gentle motion exercises. The uninjured extremity may be utilized to aid in motion of the injured extremity. Once the patient is comfortable and regains 30 to 40 degrees of motion, active musculature contraction may be initiated to aid range of motion of the injured extremity.

A careful follow-up is required in the management of these patients, as it is important to obtain a satisfactory range of motion by two to three weeks following the initiation of active exercise. If motion is not satisfactory at that time, supervised physical therapy should be undertaken in an attempt to increase function. The goal of such therapy is not to force range of motion, as this will not produce satisfactory results, but to provide instruction and assistance in gentle range-of-motion exercises along with continued encouragement to the patient. Whirlpool therapy is also beneficial in attempting to regain a satisfactory arc of motion. In summary, the majority of type 1 fractures may be handled by conservative measures.

Type 2

In type 2 fractures the injury separates the capitellum from the trochlea, but there is no significant rotation of the osseous fragments (Fig. 17–6). The main goal in the management of this fracture is to restore the proper alignment of the condyles in relation to each other. It is extremely important to reduce any gap between the condylar fragments in order to achieve anatomical restoration of the articular surface of the capitellum and trochlea. This goal may be accomplished by one of the five following methods.

Overhead Traction. A Kirschner wire may be placed through the olecranon at right angles to the humeral shaft. Frequently the separated humeral condyles will gradually realign under continuous overhead traction.

The advantage of this approach is that gradual range-of-motion exercises may be initiated while active traction is holding the fracture fragments in proper alignment. The disadvantage is that the patient must be maintained in the hospital for a period of two to three weeks until the fragments become stable enough to place the extremity in a long arm cast with the elbow at 90 degrees of flexion.

This method is frequently employed by the author in patients who present with open intercondylar fractures. It is important that this fracture be adequately debrided and irrigated following the initial injury and then placed in overhead traction. This will allow for frequent inspection of the open wound. Overhead traction is extremely useful in the management of these injuries as it provides ease of access for frequent dressing changes and allows for early range-of-motion exercises during the man-

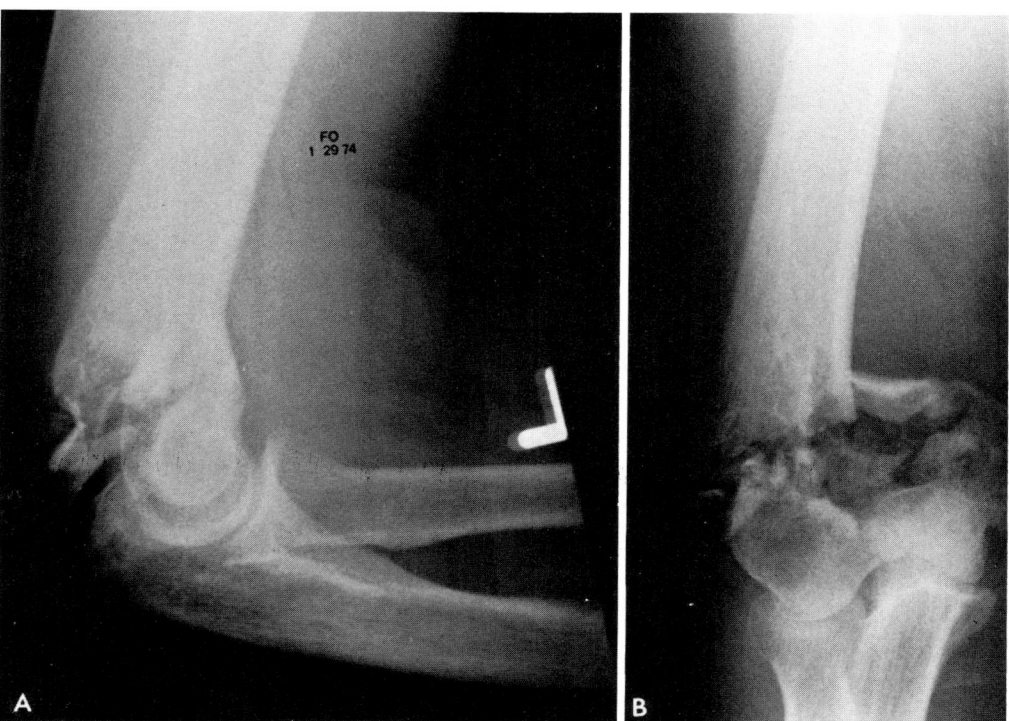

Figure 17–6 *A.* Lateral roentgenogram of a type 2 fracture. Note that there is no significant rotation of the condylar fragment. *B.* Anteroposterior view of a type 2 intercondylar fracture. Comminution is present, and there is slight separation of the capitellum from the trochlea. There is no significant rotation of the humeral condyles.

agement of the wound. Once the wound has healed satisfactorily the extremity may be placed in an appropriate long arm cast.

Pins in Plaster. A pins in plaster technique is also applicable to this type of injury. In this form of treatment, a Kirschner wire is placed through the olecranon at right angles to the humeral shaft. This allows for appropriate traction to aid in realigning the humeral condylar fragments. A second Kirschner wire is then driven through both humeral condyles in an alignment parallel to the olecranon wire. This maneuver stabilizes the humeral condyles and prevents any gross displacement. A third Kirschner wire is placed through the remaining humeral shaft fragment in a direction parallel to the first two wires. A long arm cast is then applied which incorporates all three wires.

This method provides for adequate stabilization of the fracture fragments, but it does not allow for early range-of-motion exercises of the elbow. The Kirschner wires are removed at six to eight weeks, and gentle range-of-motion exercises are initiated, provided there is roentgenographic evidence of beginning osseous union. Although this method is occasionally useful, it is not frequently employed in the management of these injuries.

Open Reduction and Internal Fixation (Posterolateral Approach). Another form of treatment is open reduction with adequate internal fixation to provide stability for early range of motion. In general, a posterolateral approach, as originally described by Campbell, is best.[17] In this technique, the skin incision extends from a point about 4 inches proximal to the elbow joint on the posterolateral aspect of the humeral area to 1 inch distal to the posterior aspect of the elbow joint. The triceps is then identified, and an inverted V-shaped incision is placed into the distal portion of the triceps, producing a tongue of the triceps aponeurosis which is then freed and reflected distally. Once this maneuver is completed, the posterior aspect of the humeral condyles and the tip of the olecranon process are easily visualized. The condyles may then be manipulated back into proper alignment, and direct visualization will insure proper anatomical reduction of the articular surface. A compression screw may then be inserted through the lateral con-

dyle, extending across the fracture site and into medial humeral condyles. A second compression screw may be inserted in a similar fashion. This will usually provide significant stability at the fracture site proper.

With this approach the olecranon fossa in the distal humerus can be directly visualized, and insertion of a compression screw which will limit extension by blocking full excursion of the olecranon can be avoided. This complication may develop during an attempt to make a small incision over the lateral humeral condyle to insert a compression screw without visualizing the posterior aspect of the elbow. A third compression screw may then be inserted from the lateral condyle extending proximally across the fracture site into the proximal shaft of the humerus.

In this manner, firm internal fixation, which will allow for early range of motion, may be obtained. The tongue of the triceps aponeurosis is then relocated and sutured to the main body of the triceps. Graded motion may be initiated one to two weeks postoperatively.

Open Reduction and Internal Fixation (Transolecranon Approach). A similar form of open reduction and internal fixation may be employed with the use of a transolecranon approach. This technique limits the amount of soft tissue dissection, but it has the disadvantage of an osteotomy of the olecranon which requires additional internal fixation. A second drawback is that it does not provide adequate exposure in the supracondylar area. However, one specific advantage of this approach is that it offers improved visualization of the articular surface, particularly along the anterior aspect. Although this technique does have merit, the author prefers the posterolateral approach of Campbell for internal fixation.

Conservative Management. Occasionally, a more conservative approach may be beneficial. With this treatment, perfect anatomical restoration is sacrificed in favor of early motion. A posterior plaster slab is applied for approximately one week until the acute reaction subsides. The splint is then removed during the day for selected periods of gentle motion of the elbow. The posterior splint is reapplied between exercises as a protective mechanism. This form of therapy is frequently useful in elderly patients in whom internal fixation is not attempted owing to their general medical condition. Under these circumstances, it is not uncommon to achieve a reasonable functional range of motion of the elbow in the presence of a poor anatomical alignment on roentgenograms.

Type 3

Like type 2 fractures, type 3 fractures involve the separation of the capitellum and trochlea, with the added features of appreciable rotation of the osseous fragments. This fracture frequently requires operative reduction and internal fixation. Since there is a rotatory component in the fracture deformity, there is gross incongruity of the articular surface. For this reason, the author has treated the majority of these fractures by primary open reduction with adequate internal fixation (Fig. 17–7). The alternate methods described for the treatment of type 2 fractures may also be employed, but open reduction and internal

fixation are decidedly preferable. The posterolateral approach of Campbell is favored by the author. This allows for adequate inspection of the articular surface and the supracondylar area.

A satisfactory reduction of the condyles in relation to each other is performed initially. This requires manipulative reduction, as the condylar surfaces may be significantly rotated in this type of injury. Internal fixation is then performed as described earlier, with two compression screws extending from the lateral condyle into the medial humeral condyle. A third compression screw may be inserted through the lateral humeral condyle in a proximal direction across the fracture site into the humeral shaft fragment.

An alternative form of treatment is to apply a small 4-holed compression plate along the lateral aspect of the distal humerus. It is important to realize that the compression plate must be bent to conform to the normal curvature of the lateral humeral condyle in relation to the distal humeral shaft. This type of internal fixation may be

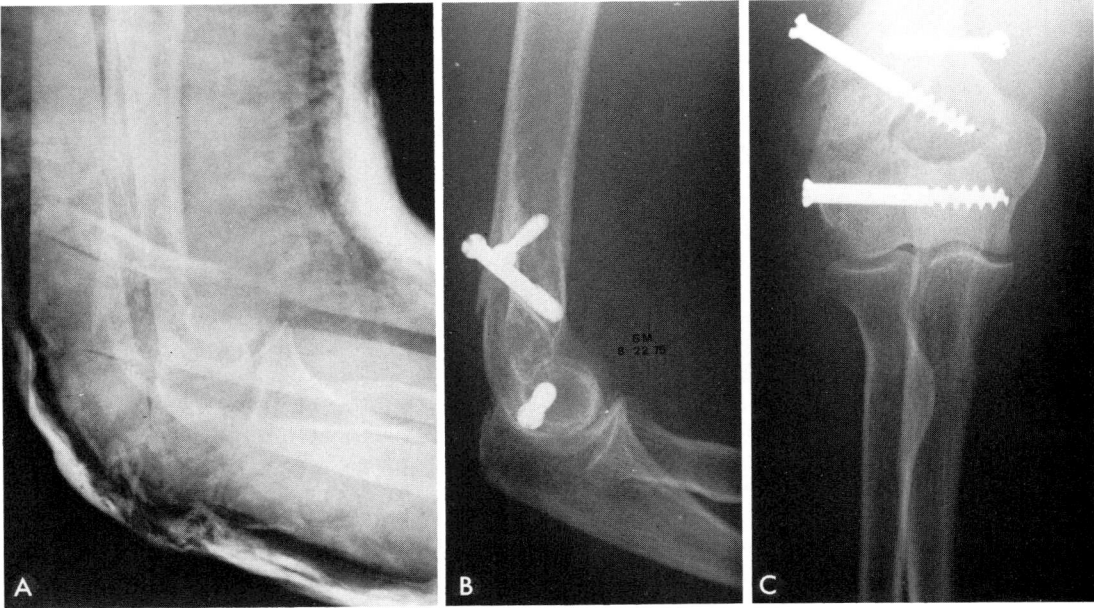

Figure 17–7 A. Lateral roentgenogram of a type 3 intercondylar fracture. Note the rotation of the humeral condylar fragment. B. Lateral roentgenogram of the same fracture two months after open reduction and internal fixation with compression screws. Note that the rotatory deformity of the humeral condyle has been corrected, and gross alignment has been restored. C. Anteroposterior view demonstrating satisfactory alignment of the fracture fragments with evidence of healing. The middle screw tended to back out a little, but the fracture went on to uneventful healing.

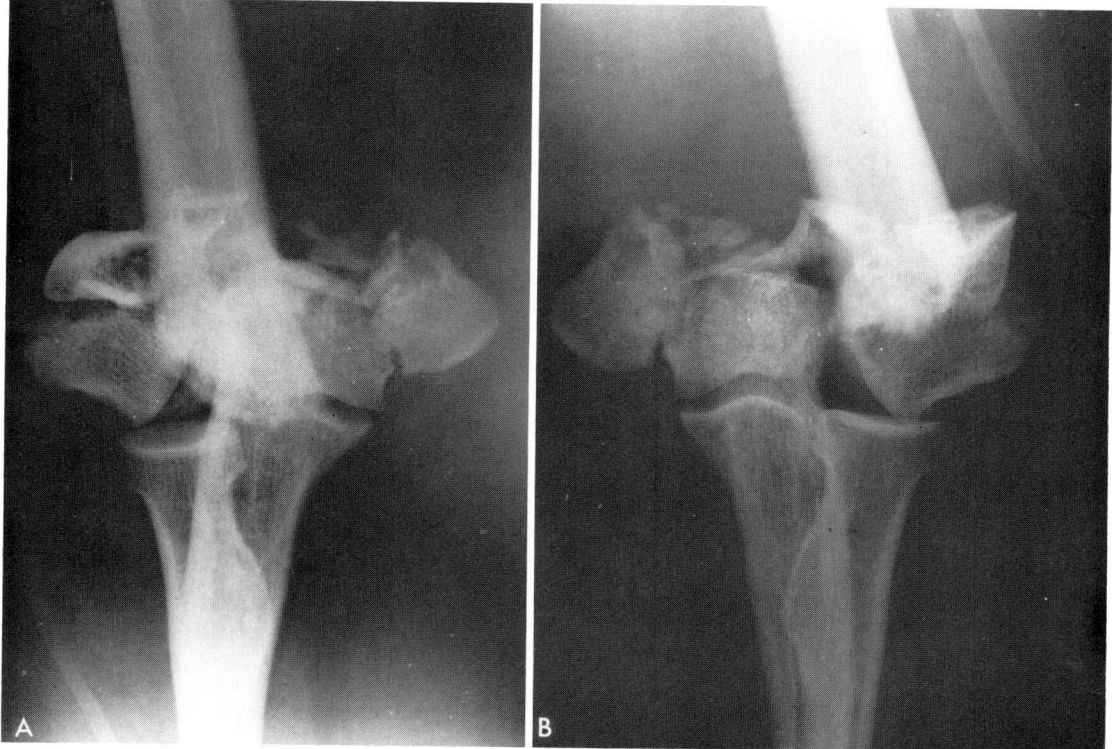

Figure 17–8   A and B. Anteroposterior view of a type 4 intercondylar fracture.

supplemented with a compression screw, if required, to obtain firm fixation of the osseous fragments.

If there is significant comminution of the distal humeral fragment in association with two or three large condylar fragments, it is frequently beneficial to first obtain satisfactory internal fixation of the condylar fragments with compression screws. The extremity is then placed in overhead skeletal traction to maintain proper alignment of the distal humeral area. In this way the articular surface of the distal humerus will be reconstructed, and the olecranon pin traction will allow for gradual range-of-motion exercises as proper alignment of the condyles to the humeral shaft fragment is maintained.

At the end of two to three weeks, the patient may be removed from the olecranon pin traction and placed in a posterior plaster splint. If there is satisfactory evidence of beginning osseous union at six to eight weeks postinjury, range-of-motion exercises may be undertaken.

As with type 2 fractures in the elderly, a conservative approach is occasionally useful. The elbow is positioned in a posterior plaster slab until the acute reaction has subsided, and then early range-of-motion exercises are initiated in spite of the unreduced roentgenographic appearance of the fracture. This form of treatment is not quite as successful in type 3 fractures as it is in type 2 fractures. In general, the rotatory deformity associated with this type of intercondylar fracture limits the effectiveness of this therapy. However, it is occasionally useful in an elderly patient for whom internal fixation is contraindicated because of the primary medical condition.

Type 4

In type 4 fractures there is evidence of significant comminution of the articular surfaces associated with widespread separation of the humeral condyles (Fig. 17–8). It is the widespread comminution of the articular surface that significantly alters the prognosis. For this reason the author prefers to treat this injury with overhead olecranon traction. The objective of this form of therapy is to obtain early range of motion in spite of the gross anatomical disruption of the articular surfaces. It has the disadvantage of requiring the patient to be hospitalized for two to four weeks until the beginning of osseous stability allows removal of traction and institution of gentle range-of-motion exercises. It has been the author's experience with this injury that in spite of a discouraging roentgenographic picture, relatively useful functional motion may be regained.

If this form of treatment does not provide satisfactory range of motion of the involved elbow, an arthroplasty or prosthetic replacement of the elbow may be performed as a delayed procedure. If an obvious osseous block is present, preventing satisfactory motion, an arthroplasty may be performed with excision of the osseous fragment. Total-joint elbow replacements are still undergoing therapeutic trials, and the results with the existing devices require further follow-up. However, this does seem to be a reasonable approach if an arthroplasty does not produce satisfactory motion. With improved implants in the future, this treatment may play a significant role in the delayed approach to these severe injuries.

LATERAL CONDYLAR FRACTURES

It is important to recognize this type of injury as it may lead to instability of the elbow joint. Fortunately, fractures of the humeral condyles are uncommon, constituting less than 5 per cent of all fractures of the distal humerus. However, lateral condylar fractures are more common than medial condylar fractures.

MECHANISM OF INJURY

The mechanism of injury may be either a direct or an indirect force. Direct forces usually occur through the posterior aspect of the elbow in flexion. The prominent lateral condyle may be fractured by such a force. Another mechanism of direct trauma

is force applied to the proximal ulna. A force in a longitudinal direction may produce an intercondylar fracture. However, if the force is not longitudinal, it may result in a fracture of the lateral condyle. Indirect trauma results from an abduction force directed to the forearm with the elbow in extension and then transmitted to the lateral condyle, which may fracture. If the force is severe enough, an unstable fracture of the lateral condyle may result, with disruption of the medial collateral ligament.

PHYSICAL EXAMINATION

Physical examination will usually reveal a grossly swollen elbow along the lateral aspect. The examiner is generally able to appreciate independent motion of the lateral condyle compared with the distal humerus. Crepitus is frequently present. In a severe fracture of the lateral condyle, instability of the elbow may be present, particularly with an abduction stress of the forearm. If the injury is severe enough, the medial collateral ligament may also be ruptured, and this will result in an increase in the normal carrying angle.

ROENTGENOGRAPHIC EXAMINATION

Standard anteroposterior and lateral roentgenograms of the elbow will reveal this type of fracture. In general, two types of fracture lines are produced (Fig. 17–9). In the first, the fracture line is located in the lateral aspect of the joint, extending from a point lateral to the radial ridge of the trochlea proximally into the supracondylar ridge. In the second type, the fracture line occurs in the midportion of the joint at a location medial to the radial ridge of the trochlea and extending proximally into the supracondylar ridge. The distinction between these two types of fracture lines is extremely important. In the first type the elbow joint itself is stable. In the second type the elbow joint may be unstable, and there may be an associated rupture of the medial collateral ligament with an increase in the valgus carrying angle at the elbow.

STABLE
I

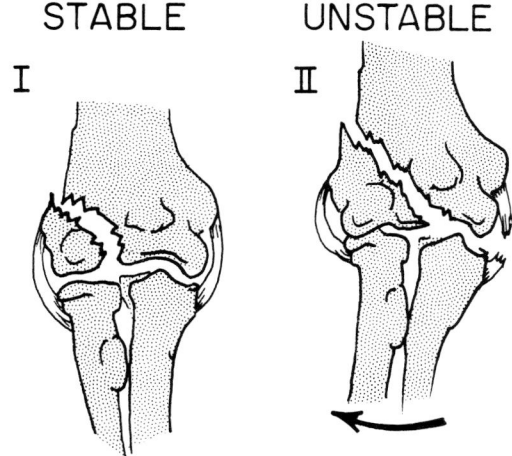

UNSTABLE
II

Figure 17–9 Two basic types of lateral condylar fractures. Type 1 is considered stable. Type 2 is considered unstable. There is a tendency toward a valgus deformity at the elbow with a mild abduction force applied to the forearm. There may be an associated rupture of the medial collateral ligament.

TREATMENT

In a type 1 fracture that is nondisplaced, treatment is with a long arm cast in flexion for three to four weeks, followed by gradual graded range-of-motion exercises. If there is significant displacement of a type 1 fracture, a closed reduction should be performed. This is usually accomplished with the elbow in extension and a slight adduction force applied to the forearm. The operator's thumb can then be applied to the lateral condylar fragment, and direct pressure may relocate the fragment into proper anatomical position. The author prefers to insert a compression screw across the lateral condyle into the distal humerus. With this method, early range of motion may be instituted. If internal fixation is not employed, a three to four week interval is required until the fracture becomes "sticky" enough to begin motion exercises.

In the treatment of type 2 fractures, open reduction and internal fixation are preferred. This injury occurs medial to the radial ridge of the trochlea and may produce lateral instability (Fig. 17–10). A direct lateral approach will expose the lateral condylar fragment, and manipulative reduction may be performed. One or two cancellous compression screws are then inserted through the lateral condyle into the distal humerus to provide stability. As with

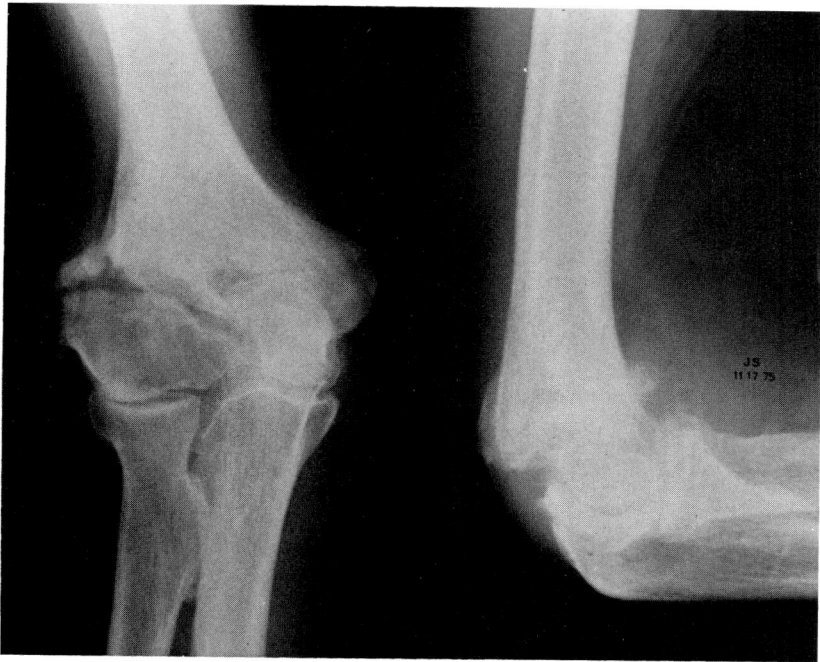

Figure 17–10 An anteroposterior and lateral view of a type 2 fracture of the lateral condyle.

intercondylar fractures, it is important not to place the compression screw into the olecranon fossa, since this may act as a block to extension. If there was gross instability of the elbow joint prior to open reduction, operative repair of the torn medial collateral ligament should be performed at the same time. If adequate internal fixation has been obtained, early range-of-motion exercises may be started at one to two weeks postoperatively.

MEDIAL CONDYLAR FRACTURES

As stated earlier, fractures of the medial condyle are less common than those of the lateral condyle. Both may result from direct or indirect forces. Direct forces occur in an injury to the medial aspect of the elbow and usually result in a fracture of the more prominent medial epicondyle, although they may also produce a fracture of the medial condyle proper. An indirect mechanism may be an adduction force applied to the forearm with the elbow in extension. This concentrates the forces along the medial aspect of the elbow and may cause a medial condylar fracture.

PHYSICAL EXAMINATION

Physical examination will usually reveal a grossly swollen elbow along the medial aspect. These fractures do not produce instability. The examiner can usually appreciate independent motion of the medial condyle compared with the distal humerus. Crepitus is usually present.

ROENTGENOGRAPHIC EXAMINATION

The roentgenographic findings usually reveal a fracture extending from the trochlear groove in a proximal direction up to the supracondylar ridge. The anteroposterior view will demonstrate the fracture, and the lateral view will aid in determining the amount of displacement.

TREATMENT

Conservative treatment is usually indicated for undisplaced fractures of the me-

dial condyle. It includes the application of a long arm cast or posterior splint, with the elbow in flexion and the hand in slight pronation. The plaster immobilization is maintained for three to four weeks until the fracture becomes "sticky," at which time gradual gentle range-of-motion exercise may be initiated.

Displaced medial condylar fractures, like displaced lateral condylar fractures, are treated more aggressively. The reduction may be accomplished with the elbow in extension by applying a slight abduction force. Pressure against the medial condyle will usually result in a reduction.

The author prefers to treat all of these fractures with internal fixation because displacement is quite common. The medial condyle may be approached through a direct medial incision. It must be remembered that the ulnar nerve lies in close proximity to this fracture fragment. It is important to directly expose the nerve and transpose it anteriorly to prevent injury. The medial condylar fragment may then be firmly fixed to the distal humerus with a compression screw. A point to bear in mind is that the cross-sectional area of the medial condyle is smaller than in the lateral condyle, sometimes making it difficult to insert a compression screw for firm fixation. An alternate form of internal fixation is to insert two small smooth Kirschner wires. After adequate fixation has been obtained, early gentle range-of-motion exercises may be initiated.

EPICONDYLAR FRACTURES

Epicondylar fractures are rare in the adult. Fractures of the medial epicondyle are more common than those of the lateral epicondyle (the reverse is true of fractures of the condyles proper). Lateral epicondylar fractures are very rare. The treatment consists of simple immobilization until the pain subsides, after which active early motion can be initiated.

Fractures of the medial epicondyle are also uncommon. If they occur, they may include a small segment of the medial condyle as well. The usual mechanism of injury is a direct blow. Because the medial epicondyle is more prominent, it is susceptible to trauma from a direct blow. Treatment of a nondisplaced fracture involves one week of immobilization in a posterior plaster splint, with the elbow and wrist in slight flexion and the forearm in slight pronation. Motion is then initiated with the objective of obtaining early full range of motion. It is very unusual for displacement of the medial epicondyle to cause symptoms. The fracture usually heals with a fibrous union and is in general painless. If pain or ulnar nerve symptoms do occur, the small osseous fragment can be excised at a later date with a good functional result.

ARTICULAR SURFACE FRACTURES

CAPITELLUM

Fortunately, fractures of the capitellum are very rare, constituting less than 1 per cent of elbow fractures. As with other intraarticular fractures, no soft tissue attachment is involved. For this reason it is not uncommon to find significant displacement of the intraarticular fracture, since it is relatively free to move within the joint. It is extremely important to differentiate fractures of the capitellum from fractures of the lateral condyle.

Mechanism of Injury

The mechanism of injury is thought to be a transmitted force. This is particularly applicable when the elbow is in slight flexion with the wrist in pronation, as is frequently seen in an attempt to break a fall.

Physical Examination

On physical examination a hemarthrosis is normally palpable. There is pain associated with motion of the joint. If the intraarticular fragment is displaced in an anterior direction, there may be a block to flexion produced by the position of the fragments in the coronoid or radial fossa. Occasionally crepitus may accompany motion of the elbow. Pronation and supination of the forearm also may produce pain in the elbow.

Roentgenographic Examination

Two types of capitellar fractures may be seen on roentgenographic evaluation. Type 1 is a complete fracture involving a significant portion of the osseous structure of the capitellum (Fig. 17–11). This is known as the Hahn-Steinthal type. Type 2 involves

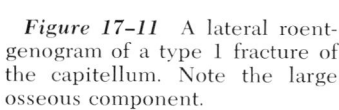

Figure 17–11 A lateral roentgenogram of a type 1 fracture of the capitellum. Note the large osseous component.

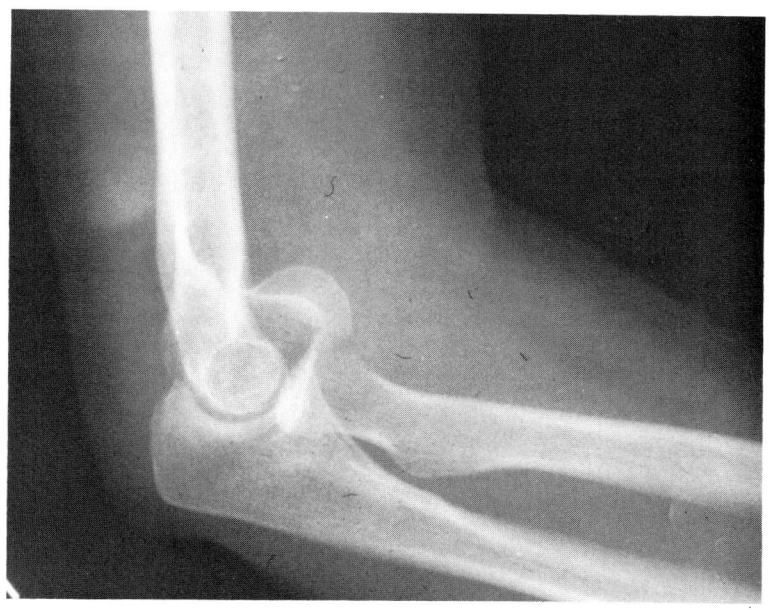

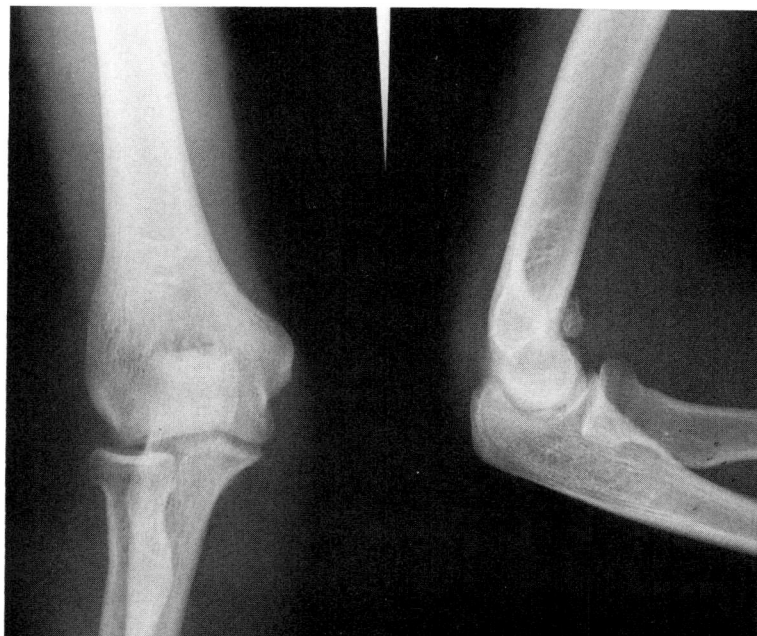

Figure 17–12 A type 2 fracture of the capitellum. The slight irregularity of the articular surface of the capitellum is best seen in the lateral view.

mainly articular cartilage with minimal bone attached (Fig. 17–12). This is known as the Kocher-Lorenz type. The fragment may not be visualized on the regular anteroposterior view but is usually demonstrated on the lateral view. The fragment is most often located anterior and proximal to the main body of the capitellum. For this reason it is best demonstrated in the lateral view. Occasionally, combined fractures of the radial head and capitellum are observed. If an associated radial head fracture is present, it is usually relatively nondisplaced.

Treatment

The majority of these fractures have a small portion of the subchondral bone attached to the articular surface fragment. Therefore, if these fractures can be replaced in proper alignment it is not uncommon for them to unite. The articular surface is not altered, as it receives its nutrition primarily from the synovial fluid. There are definite proponents to closed reduction by manipulation with the elbow in full extension. Longitudinal traction on the forearm is attempted in order to produce an adduction force of the forearm, which tends to open

the lateral aspect of the elbow. Direct pressure may then be placed on the articular surface fragment by the operator's thumb. If the elbow is then placed in the position of flexion, the radial head may hold the fragment in proper position. The problem with this treatment is that it requires immobilization, with the elbow in flexion for a period of four to six weeks, prior to active motion of the elbow joint.

The author prefers operative management of these fractures. The elbow may be explored through a posterolateral anconeus splitting incision, which gives access to the radial head and the articular surface of the capitellum. If the fragment is comminuted, the author prefers operative excision combined with early motion of the elbow. If there is a single large fragment, it is frequently beneficial to provide internal fixation of the articular surface fragment. This may be obtained with the use of small pins, similar to Smillie pins, which are utilized occasionally for osteochondritis dissecans of the knee.

The alternative to this treatment is to secure internal fixation with a small compression screw. The screw should be inserted in the posterior portion of the condyle, with the tip of the screw protruding through the defect and engaging the osseous portion of the articular surface fragment. As in the management of osteochondritis dissecans of the knee, the articular surface is not penetrated. If it is not possible to obtain internal fixation in this manner, it may be appropriate to reduce the fragment under direct visualization and then place the elbow in flexion, locking the radial head against the fragment to maintain the reduction.

However, the author's experience has been that excision of the fragment, particularly if it is comminuted, combined with early active motion of the elbow, results in very little disability. Recently Alvarez and his colleagues suggested operative excision for the majority of capitellar fractures.[6] They found that patients demonstrated increased motion and less pain with active excision of the fragment.

TROCHLEA

This type of fracture is very rare indeed. Suffice it to state that a small fracture of the trochlea is probably best managed with operative excision. A large fragment is probably best treated with operative reduction. If the fragment is large enough, internal fixation as in fractures of the capitellum, may be indicated. However, a relatively large and comminuted fragment is probably best treated with operative excision. If the fragment is excised, it is extremely important to provide for early motion of the elbow.

RADIAL HEAD FRACTURES

The management of this type of fracture has changed in recent years. In the past, it was felt that if a third of the radial head was involved in a fracture, primary excision of the radial head was probably the treatment of choice. However, recent management has centered on trying to preserve the radial head and regain early motion. There is still not universal agreement as to exactly how all radial head fractures should be managed.

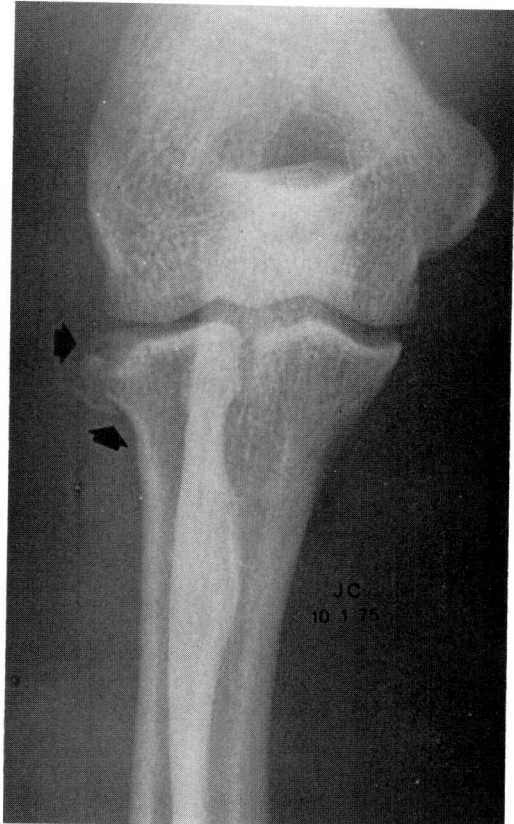

Figure 17–13 A type 2 marginal fracture of the radial head with some displacement.

CLASSIFICATION

A useful working classification of the three basic types of radial head fractures was proposed by Mason. Type 1 includes undisplaced fractures, type 2 marginal fractures with displacement (Fig. 17–13), and type 3 comminuted fractures. This classification aids in distinguishing the various types of radial head fractures and may be useful in regard to prognosis.

MECHANISM OF INJURY

The mechanism of injury in radial head fractures may be direct or indirect trauma. Direct trauma occurs as result of a blow against the lateral aspect of the elbow joint proper. This may produce a nondisplaced or a displaced fracture of the radial head. Indirect trauma results from a fall on the outstretched upper extremity, with the force transmitted along the forearm to the radial head which abuts against the capitellar surface. This also may produce a nondisplaced or displaced fracture of the radial head. The author has found that there is a slightly increased incidence of radial head fractures secondary to indirect trauma as compared with direct trauma.

PHYSICAL EXAMINATION

Patients presenting with radial head fractures usually demonstrate some restriction of motion of the forearm or elbow. In general, pronation and supination produce pain along the anterolateral aspect of the elbow joint. Flexion–extension is usually limited by an accompanying hemarthrosis within the joint. There is almost always acute tenderness to deep palpation directly over the radial head. This may be accentuated by applying direct pressure over the radial head while attempting pronation and supination of the forearm. A "fullness" is noted along the lateral aspect of the elbow and is secondary to hemarthrosis. If there is widespread separation of the fracture fragments, occasionally a fragment of the radial head may be palpable in the soft tissues along the anterolateral aspect of the elbow.

ROENTGENOGRAPHIC EXAMINATION

Nondisplaced fractures of the radial head are famous for not being evident on the initial routine anteroposterior and lateral views. For this reason oblique views may be necessary to aid in ruling out a radial head fracture. Occasionally patients will present with pain in the elbow unassociated with a demonstrable radial head fracture, even with special oblique views. In this case, it is

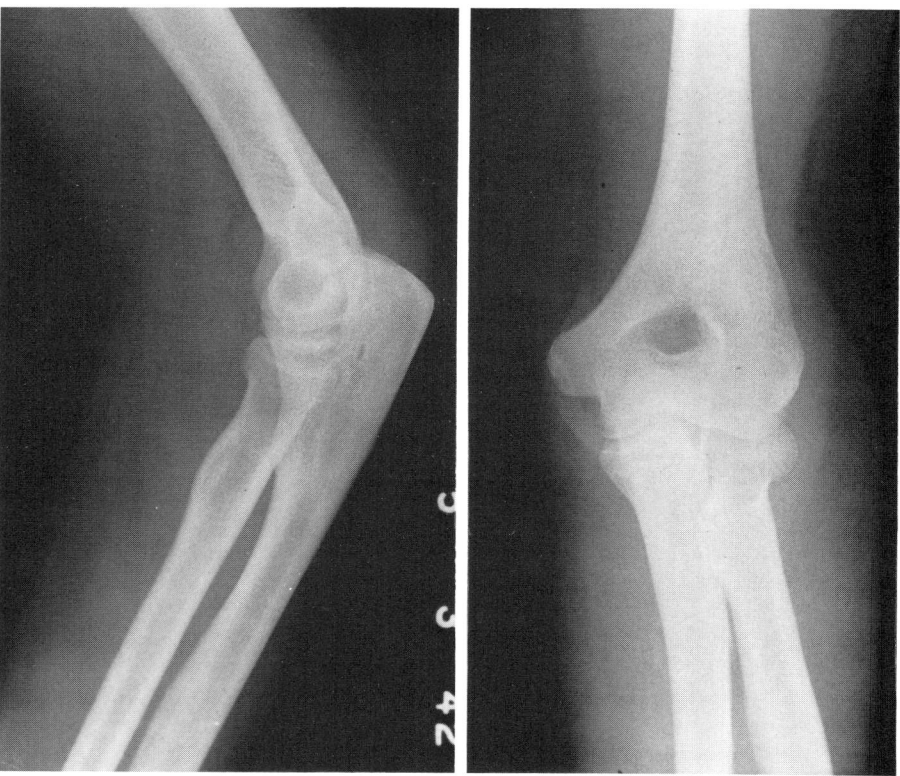

Figure 17–14 A hidden radial head fracture with evidence of positive anterior and posterior fat pad sign.

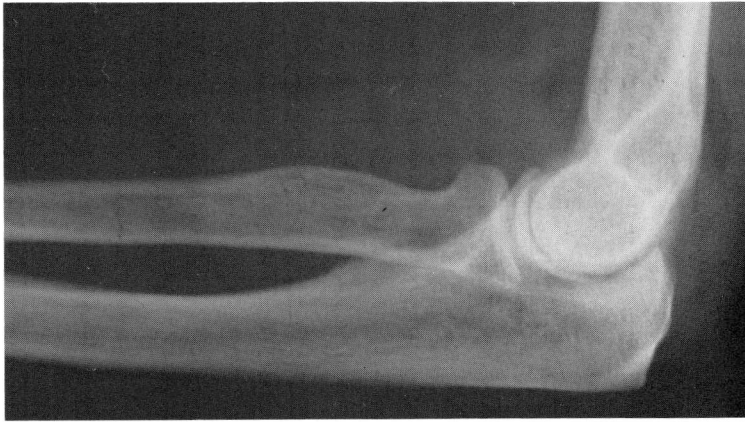

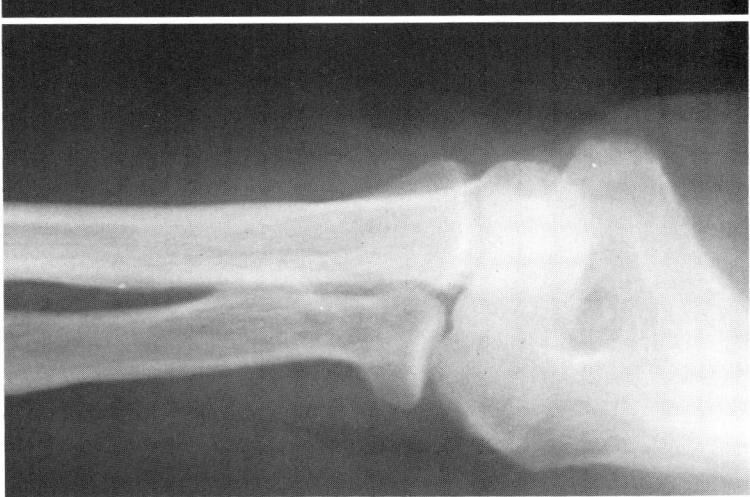

Figure 17–15 A suggestion of a marginal fracture of the radial head with definite anterior and posterior fat pad signs.

customary to reevaluate the situation at approximately one week with new roentgenograms. At this time the fracture of the radial head may be demonstrated.

A very helpful sign in regard to hidden radial head fractures is known as a positive fat pad sign (Fig. 17–14). Anatomically, there are two fat pads present at the elbow joint. An anterior fat pad is located between the synovial and fibrous capsules in the coronoid fossa, and a posterior fat pad is found within the olecranon fossa. Under normal conditions the anterior fat pad is visible on a lateral roentgenogram; the posterior fat pad is not normally visualized. However, in the presence of a hemarthrosis within the elbow joint, the fat pads may be displaced. In this circumstance, the anterior fat pad appears in a more anterior aspect of the elbow joint than normal, and the posterior fat pad becomes visible.

This is a very important diagnostic sign, and the author feels that its presence should be evaluated in all elbows that have sustained trauma. If the fat pads are prominent, the attending physician should consider a radial head fracture to be present until it is ruled otherwise. It is true that an effusion from any cause will produce prominent fat pads. However, the usual reason for the presence of the fat pad sign following trauma to an elbow is a fracture of the radial head (Fig. 17–15).

The anteroposterior roentgenogram will normally demonstrate the articular surface of the radial head, and a fracture line may be visible on this view. The lateral roentgenographic view will aid in determining the amount of displacement or impaction owing to the fracture. It is also helpful in ruling out an associated fracture of the articular surface of the capitellum.

TREATMENT

As stated earlier, there has been a definite trend toward conservative management of these fractures. It has been the author's experience that if the elbow joint is aspirated shortly after trauma is sustained, patients will obtain significant relief of pain. Early initiation of motion will frequently produce excellent results even in the presence of mild-to-moderate displacement of radial head fractures.

There is almost universal agreement on treating type 1 undisplaced fractures conservatively. Patients are given a sling to wear for comfort during the day but are encouraged to remove the sling for 15- to 20-minute intervals in order to obtain a reasonable range of motion of the elbow joint. Occasionally an undisplaced fracture may be slightly displaced with early range-of-motion therapy, but this does not seem to be detrimental to the final results. It is extremely important to try to return the elbow to functional activity following this type of fracture, using the methods outlined throughout this book.

The management of type 2 marginal fractures with displacement has been more controversial (Fig. 17–16). McLaughlin's recommendations have been followed by many practitioners.[72] He felt that if there was depression greater than 3 mm or angulation greater than 30 degrees, the radial head should be primarily excised. The author prefers the method of Charnley, in which early motion is initiated following the injury, and careful observation of the progression of motion is performed over a two-week period.[20] If at the end of this time there is no evidence of good functional recovery of elbow motion, the radial head is excised. It has never been definitely documented in a well-controlled study that delayed excision of the radial head contributes to a higher incidence of myositis ossificans.

Surgical management of type 3 comminuted fractures of the radial head tends to be more aggressive. The author feels that the radial head should be excised within the first two to three days postinjury if at all possible. This approach has been adopted because severe comminution of the radial head definitely alters its articular surface and may produce secondary changes in the

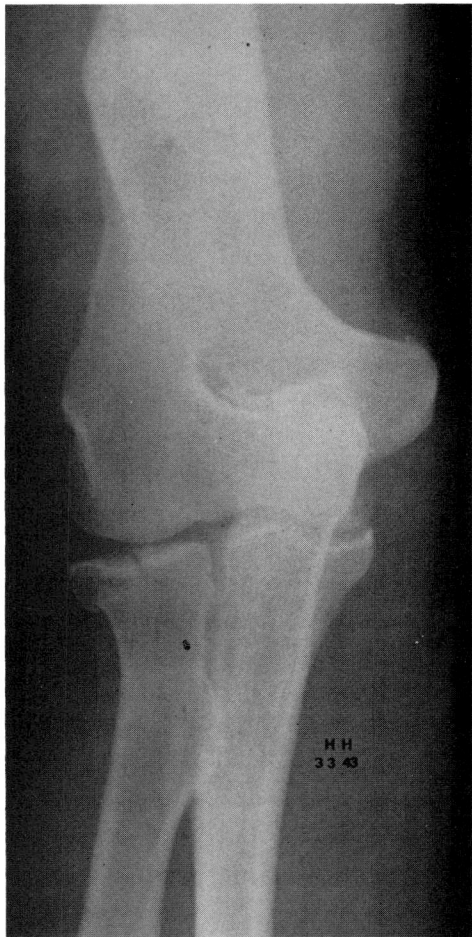

Figure 17–16 A type 2 marginal fracture with some slight displacement and involvement of more than one third of the radial head. In the past this injury was treated with radial head excision. This patient was treated with aspiration of the joint and early motion with a very satisfactory result.

capitellum if it is not removed. This is particularly true if there is any displacement of the comminuted fragments. The displacement may produce an effect similar to that seen with shaving a block of wood. In other words, the exposed sharp surface of the bone may act as an abrasive area that "shaves off" the articular surface of the capitellum with motion of the elbow. This effect has also been noted in displaced fractures of the patella.

In most cases, function is satisfactory following radial head excision in comminuted fractures. Excision of the radial head is best accomplished through an anconeus splitting incision, which avoids damage to the radial nerve. It must be kept in mind that the radial nerve is located just anterior to the radial head; in an anterolateral approach, it is very easy to damage the radial nerve. Once the radial head has been excised, patients are encouraged to regain motion as soon as possible. That is not to say that manipulation is attempted, but that gentle encouragement regarding range-of-motion exercises is essential. Radial head excision does not lead to instability of the elbow joint under these conditions. It has been pointed out in several series that subluxation of the distal radioulnar joint may occur following excision of the radial head. Although this is true, it is also true that very few patients are symptomatic in this regard.

Prosthetic replacement of the radial head following excision has been advocated in some centers. However, it does not seem to make sense to apply a plastic surface to articulate with relatively normal articular cartilage on the opposite apposing surface. Other studies on joint replacement have demonstrated that articular cartilage changes occur if a plastic surface is supplied for articulation. Since there is very little morbidity associated with radial head excision, it does not make much physiological sense to attempt prosthetic replacement of the radial head. Perhaps with future development of improved materials this may be a reasonable approach, but it is very controversial at the present time.

Radial head fractures also occur in association with dislocations about the elbow. This injury is discussed in the section on fracture–dislocations of the elbow.

OLECRANON FRACTURES

This type of fracture is relatively common in a busy orthopedic practice. The olecranon process is subcutaneous and is exposed to direct trauma. Adults are particularly susceptible to this fracture, which is relatively rare in children. Most authors feel that in the child the olecranon process is relatively strong compared with the distal end of the humerus. It is important not to confuse a fracture of the olecranon with one of the patella cubiti, which is an accessory ossicle located within the triceps tendon

just as it inserts into the tip of the olecranon.

MECHANISM OF INJURY

Like other injuries, olecranon fractures may be caused by direct and indirect forces. The usual fracture is produced by a direct fall on the tip of the olecranon, with all the forces concentrated in this area. This may well result in a comminuted fracture because of the high energy absorbed at the time of injury. An indirect force resulting from a fall on the outstretched upper extremity with the elbow in slight flexion may also produce a fracture. Under these conditions a fracture may be caused by a sudden violent contraction of the triceps mechanism in an attempt to break the fall. This indirect force may result in an oblique or transverse avulsion fracture of the olecranon. If the fracture has been caused by a direct force, there is frequently evidence of comminution, with marked displacement of the main olecranon fragment in a proximal direction. The fragment is displaced proximally by the contraction of the triceps mechanism. If the injury is due to an indirect force, producing an oblique or transverse fracture, there may be minimal displacement at the fracture site since the triceps aponeurosis may be relatively intact. This will aid in preventing displacement of the olecranon fragment. A final mechanism may cause a hyperextension injury which occurs with dislocation of the elbow joint.

PHYSICAL EXAMINATION

The diagnosis is usually fairly evident on physical examination. There is tenderness over the olecranon on direct palpation. There may also be a definite palpable gap secondary to the displacement of the proximal portion of the ulna. Crepitus is usually present. Since this is an intraarticular fracture, significant hemarthrosis is present within the elbow joint. The patient will usually hold the forearm in a position of slight flexion. Active extension against gravity is abolished owing to the separation of the fragments. The combination of lack of extension, localized swelling over the olecranon with a palpable defect in the olecranon process, and tenderness to direct palpation confirm the diagnosis.

ROENTGENOGRAPHIC EXAMINATION

Roentgenographic evaluation includes a typical anteroposterior and lateral view. The fracture is usually evident on the anteroposterior view, but the most important view is the true lateral because it demonstrates the amount of displacement of the olecranon from the parent ulna (Fig. 17–17). The amount of displacement of the proximal fragment is extremely important in determining the type of treatment. If there is evidence of gross comminution of the olecranon process, then there is usually evidence of direct trauma to the olecranon. If an oblique or transverse fracture with minimal displacement is evident, this usually indicates an avulsion injury sec-ondary to active contraction of the triceps mechanism.

TREATMENT

This fracture has enjoyed a wide variety of treatment approaches. It was not until 1884 that Lister attempted open reduction and internal fixation of an olecranon fracture, utilizing his new method of antisepsis. He took this approach because of his dissatisfaction with conservative methods. Lister performed internal fixation with a wire loop which has been modified in recent years. The surgical management was further expanded in the United States by McKeever and Buck when they advocated excision of the proximal osseous fragment and repair of the triceps mechanism.[71] Intramedullary screw fixation for the man-

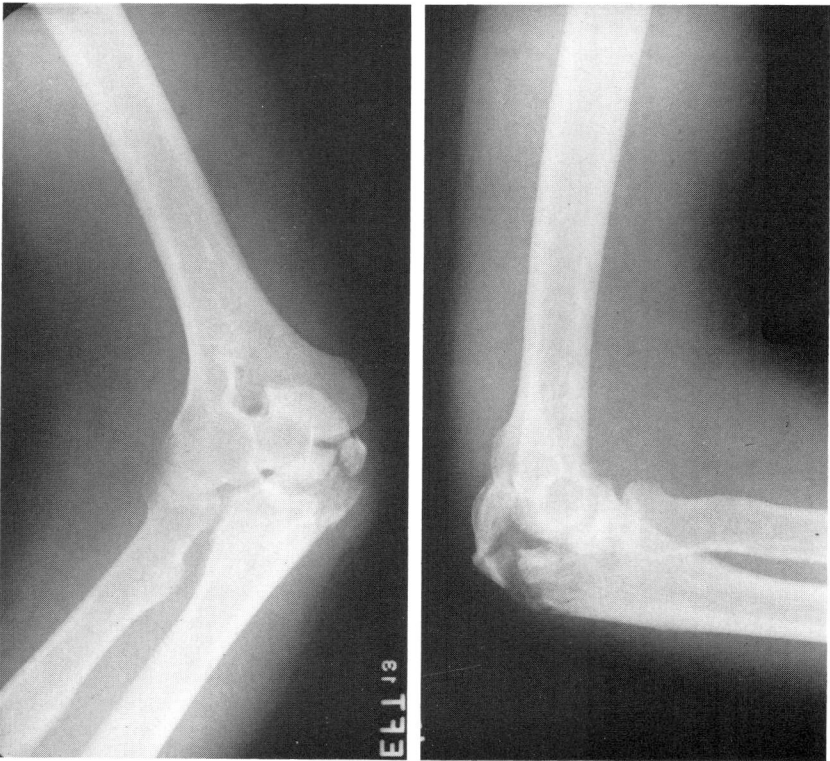

Figure 17–17   A comminuted olecranon fracture with evidence of displacement of the proximal fragments. This was treated with excision of the comminuted proximal fragments and reattachment of the triceps mechanism to the proximal ulna.

agement of these fractures was advocated by MacAusland.[66]

The author has adopted a relatively aggressive surgical approach for the management of most of these fractures. If there is no displacement of the fracture fragment, it is conceivable that the injury may be managed by application of a long arm cast with the elbow held at 45 degrees of flexion for four weeks. At the end of that time, active gentle range-of-motion exercises up to 90 degrees of flexion may be instituted. At the end of six weeks, the flexion may be increased to 100 to 110 degrees. The fracture should not be immobilized in full extension since this may make it very difficult to obtain motion later on.

However, as stated, it is the author's opinion that the majority of olecranon fractures should be treated by open reduction and internal fixation. This allows early range-of-motion exercises to prevent the complications of elbow stiffness and lack of power of extension. Several methods of internal fixation are available.

Internal Fixation Techniques

Tension band wiring, a method developed by the AO group,[77] provides significant stability to the fracture site (Fig. 17–18). Basically, this type of fixation converts tensile forces occurring across the fracture site into active compressive forces. This is an excellent technique and one highly recommended by the author. It is particularly applicable to the management of transverse and oblique fractures. The fracture site is exposed through a posterolateral incision. The proximal fragment is then mobilized distally and reduced. Two small Kirschner wires are inserted parallel through the olecranon process, across the fracture site, and into the ulna. The proximal portions of the wires are bent in an upward direction. A wire suture is then

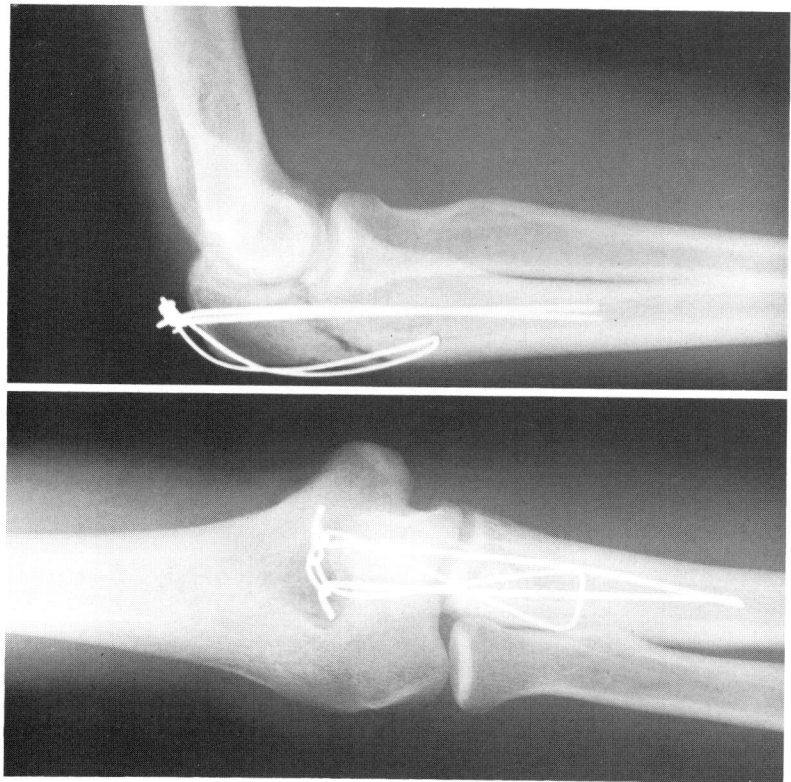

Figure 17–18 Tension band technique for an olecranon fracture. Motion was initiated one week following internal fixation. Uneventful healing ensued.

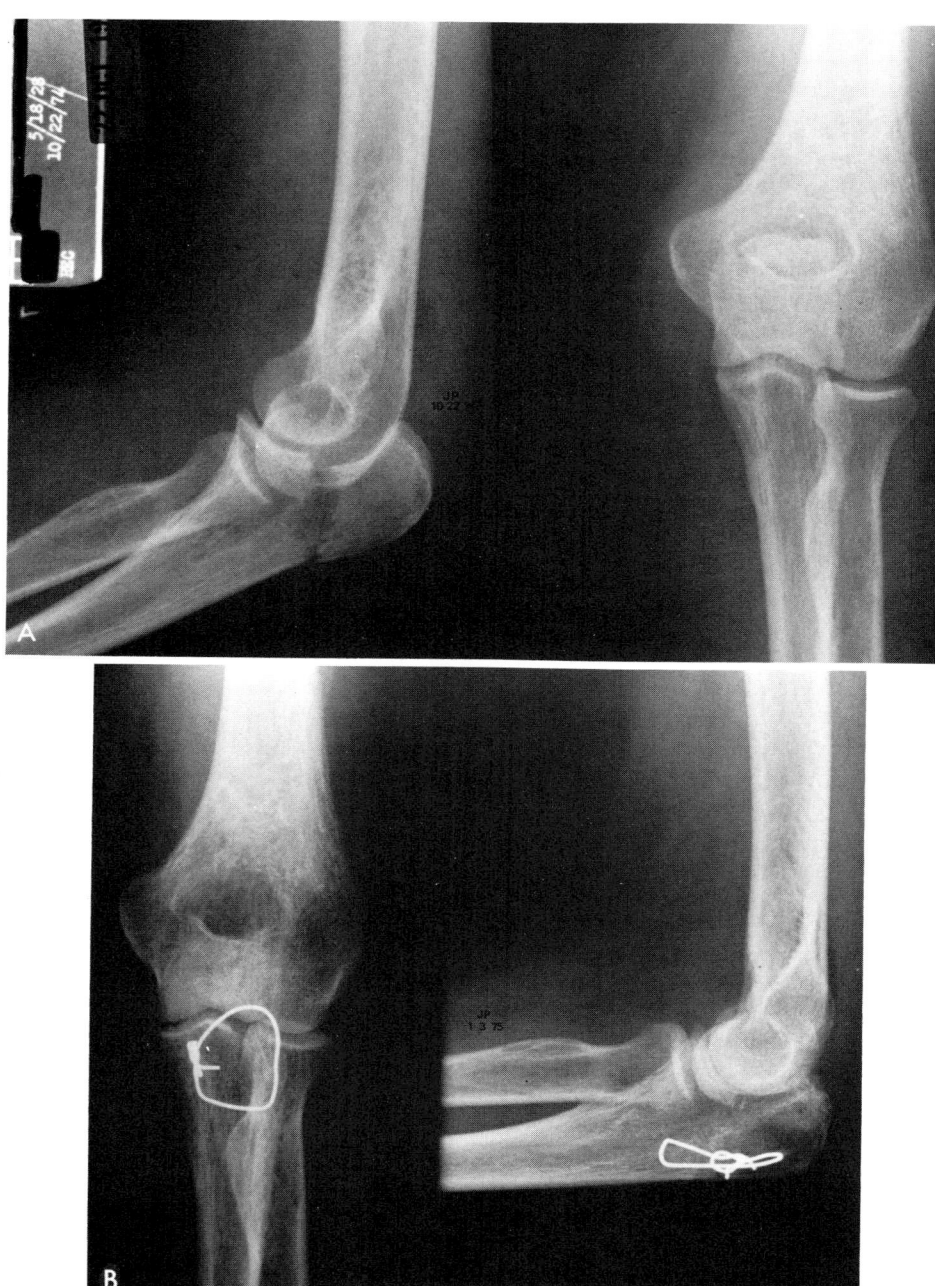

Figure 17–19   *A.* A mildly displaced olecranon fracture. *B.* Treatment included open reduction and internal fixation with the use of circular wire. Complete healing is evident three months postinjury.

passed behind the triceps mechanism to engage on the anterior aspect of the Kirschner wires. The suture is brought through in a typical figure-of-eight configuration along the superficial portion of the olecranon and passed through a drill hole distal to the fracture site in the parent ulna along the superficial border. In this manner, the figure-of-eight suture extends from the tip of the olecranon process over the olecranon process proper, across the fracture site, and into the parent subcutaneous border of the ulna.

It appears at first that this type of fixation will cause the fracture site to separate at the articular surface. However, with the active pull of the triceps mechanism, the fracture site is closed by virtue of the tension band effect. The reader is referred to the AO Manual for further details.

A second technique is to apply a circular wire for internal fixation (Fig. 17–19). This is not as effective an internal fixation method as the tension band.

A third operative method that is very useful involves the insertion of an oblique compression screw that traverses the fracture site in a bicortical fashion.[117] The compression screw is placed in the tip of the olecranon, extending across the fracture site at right angles to emerge at the anterior cortex of the coronoid process (Fig. 17–20). This type of fixation is particularly applicable to oblique fractures of the olecranon. A special lag screw is necessary so that compression is applied across the fracture site. If a completely threaded screw is utilized, it may prevent active compression across the fracture site. The reduction is performed through a standard posterolateral surgical approach. It is important to select a screw that not only has a lag effect but also has fairly large screw threads to afford adequate purchase. It is also necessary for the tip of the screw to penetrate the anterior cortex of the ulna, as this provides additional stability.

If this technique is used, it is important to

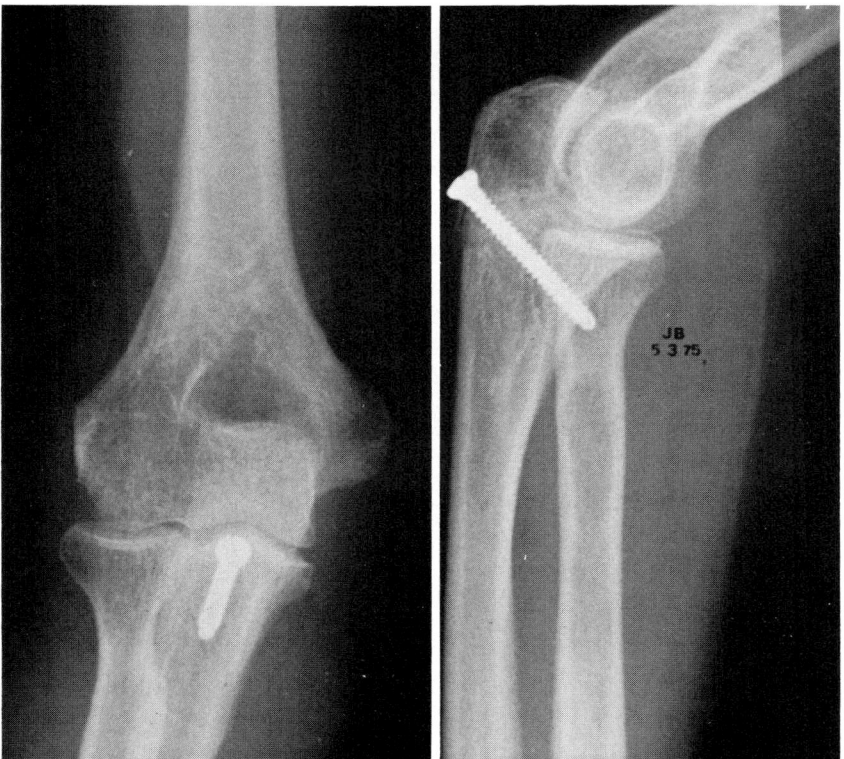

Figure 17–20 An olecranon fracture treated with an oblique bicortical screw. It would have been better to insert a lag compression screw in this type of fracture. However, the fracture healed uneventfully.

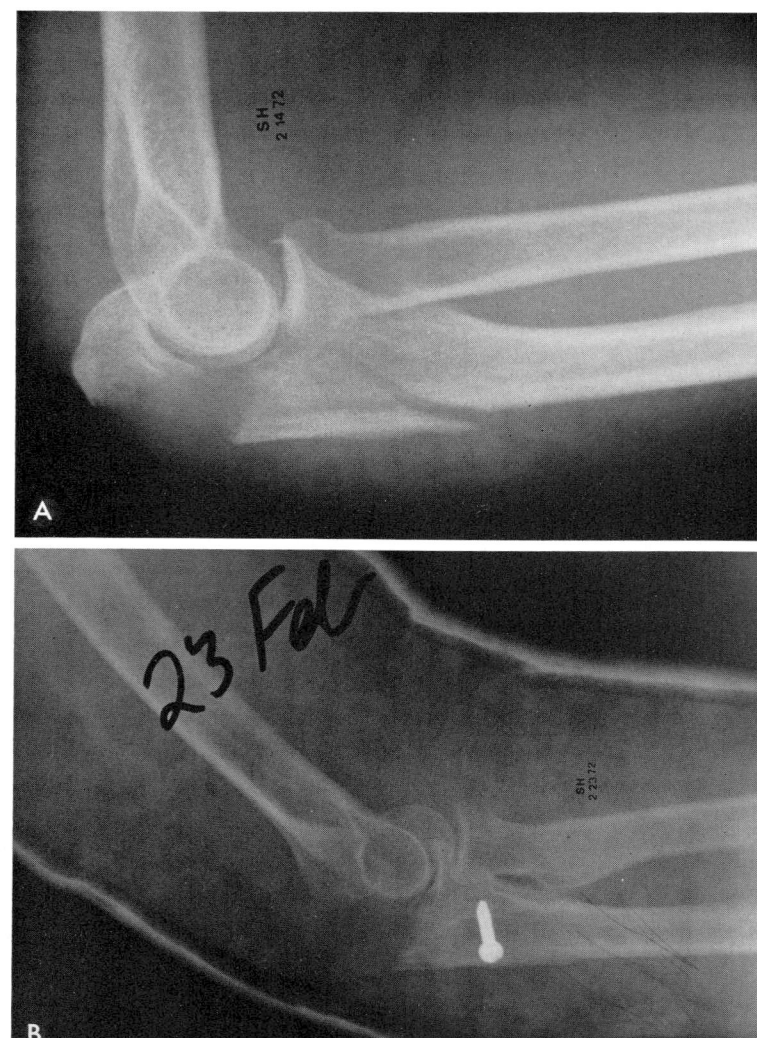

Figure 17-21   *A.* A comminuted displaced olecranon fracture. *B.* Management included open reduction and internal fixation of the distal fragment to the parent ulna. The proximal displaced fragment was then excised, and the triceps mechanism was attached to the proximal ulna. Uneventful healing resulted.

remember two specific details. The correct screw must be selected, and the screw must not be placed within the joint surface. The screw must be located just under the articular surface, extending in an oblique manner.

A fourth operative method is to excise the comminuted fragments and reattach the triceps tendon to the ulna. In this method a small portion of the articular surface of the ulna and coronoid process must be intact, or dislocation will result. This is a useful procedure in the face of significant comminution or in the elderly (Fig. 17–21).

Part II ———————— **DISLOCATIONS OF THE ELBOW** ————————

Dislocations of the elbow are not rare. They are encountered at least once or twice a year in an average orthopedic practice and are surpassed in frequency only by shoulder dislocations. As with other types of dislocations, this injury must be reduced as soon as possible. This is especially important in elbow injuries because the longer the elbow remains dislocated, the greater the amount of swelling and limited motion. The immediate danger with persistent swelling at the elbow joint is a decrease in circulation to the forearm, resulting in a possible impending Volkmann's ischemic contracture of the forearm and hand. If these injuries are not managed correctly, it is not uncommon to end up with a painful, severely restricted range of motion of the elbow. Even with aggressive proper treatment, full range of motion does not always return following dislocation.

CLASSIFICATION

Several classifications of elbow dislocations have been proposed. However, in all classifications the distal end of the humerus is the fixed point, and the dislocations are described in relation to the amount of displacement of the radius and ulna from the distal humerus. The author prefers to include dislocations without fractures in a single category and to consider fracture–dislocations of the elbow as a separate entity. Therefore, a discussion of elbow dislocations includes the following:

1. Dislocations of the proximal portion of the radius and ulna (posterior, lateral, medial, anterior, and divergent).
2. Isolated ulnar dislocations.
3. Recurrent dislocations.
4. Old dislocations.

DISLOCATIONS OF THE PROXIMAL RADIUS AND ULNA

POSTERIOR DISLOCATIONS

Posterior dislocations of the elbow are the most frequent primary elbow dislocations. It is interesting that although a significant force is required to produce this type of dislocation, it is not unusual to encounter a pure posterior dislocation unassociated with a fracture. The deformity is usually quite obvious following the injury, and the patient presents with restricted motion.

Mechanism of Injury

The usual mechanism of injury is direct trauma from a fall on an outstretched forearm which is held in extension. With the arm in extension, the buttressing effects of the coronoid process and the radial head are not as strong as they are with the elbow in a position of flexion. For this reason the force is transmitted down the radius and ulna in a proximal direction, resulting in the olecranon levering the ulna and the radius posteriorly and the distal humerus anteriorly. A significant amount of soft tissue disruption occurs with this injury. The anterior capsule of the elbow joint is torn. The brachialis is frequently also torn or completely avulsed from the coronoid process during the injury. By virtue of the significant displacement there is also definite damage to the collateral ligaments. If there has been significant posterior displacement, there may be damage to the median or radial nerves secondary to a stretching mechanism.

Physical Examination

On physical examination the diagnosis is not difficult. The patient usually presents with significant swelling about the elbow joint secondary to the soft tissue disruption and displacement. The normal equilateral triangle configuration along the posterior aspect of the elbow is altered. The tip of the olecranon is noted to be in a much more posterior direction than normal. The forearm is usually held in a semiflexed position. If flexion or extension of the elbow is attempted, severe restriction of motion is noted, and the limited motion that is present is very painful. It is extremely important to document the neurovascular status of the forearm and hand. If this is not done, it may be difficult to ascertain whether any residual neurovascular deficit existed prior to the reduction or resulted from the maneuver to reduce the elbow.

Roentgenographic Examination

Regular anteroposterior and lateral roentgenographic views are essential in regard to treatment. If there is extensive delay in obtaining roentgenographic views and the typical physical findings are present, the author feels that an attempt at mild reduc-

tion should be performed. The danger in leaving the elbow dislocated for a prolonged period owing to such a delay is not justified, as increasing swelling about the elbow will occur, with the ever-present danger of a Volkmann's contracture. Therefore, the attending physician must insist upon roentgenograms as soon as possible. Even if the elbow is reduced prior to obtaining roentgenograms, they are essential postreduction in order to rule out any associated fractures.

Regular anteroposterior views in the presence of dislocation will reveal posterior displacement of the olecranon and the radial head. There will be superimposition of the overlying distal end of the humerus. A normal joint line will therefore not be present. Lateral roentgenograms will reveal posterior displacement of the olecranon and the radial head (Fig. 17–22). The tip of the coronoid process will be located within the olecranon fossa or will be compressed into the distal portion of the humerus. The radial head will appear under the humeral condyle.

Treatment

As previously stated, the elbow should be reduced as soon as possible and the neurovascular status determined. If there is any indication of absence of the peripheral pulses or of severe delay in capillary filling of the fingers, it is mandatory to obtain immediate reduction, followed by careful

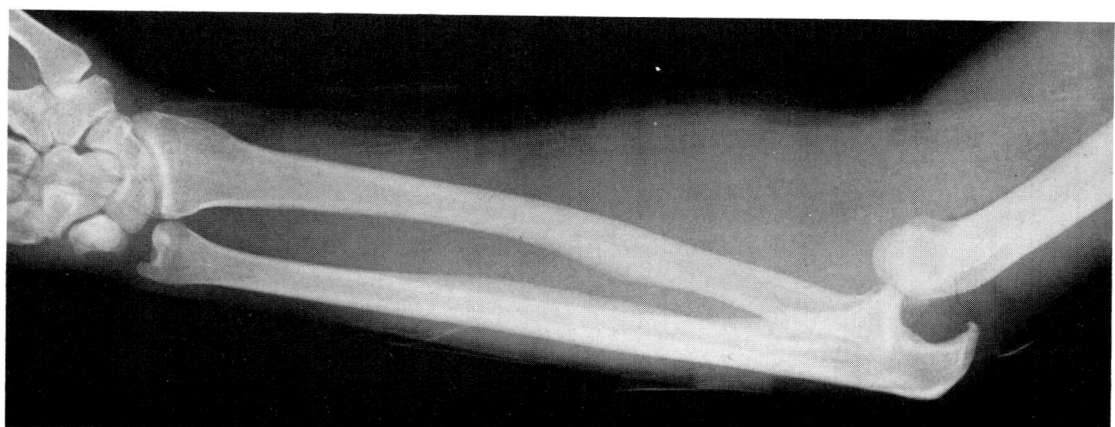

Figure 17–22 Lateral roentgenogram of typical posterior dislocation without evidence of fracture. Note the posterior position of the olecranon and radial head.

reassessment of the vascular status. If there is still no evidence of return of adequate peripheral pulses or capillary filling, an arteriogram should be obtained. It is the author's feeling that an attempt at gentle closed reduction may be performed without the aid of a general anesthetic or regional block.

The reduction is performed as follows: An assistant applies gentle countertraction on the distal humerus by placing his hands around the anterior portion of the distal humeral shaft. Following appropriate countertraction, the attending physician applies downward traction to the proximal portion of the forearm, which brings the coronoid out of the olecranon fossa. With gentle downward traction continuously applied, the entire forearm is brought into a position of flexion at the elbow. In most instances the physician will feel the elbow reduce with this maneuver. Once the reduction has been obtained, the elbow is placed through a gentle range of motion to determine its stability.

If the patient resists any attempt at reduction, a regional block anesthesia should be employed, as described in Chapter 8, or a general anesthetic must be administered. The author has found that a reduction may be achieved with closed methods. If reduction cannot be achieved by a simple closed method, it is best to attempt an open reduction rather than repeated forceful attempts at closed reduction. Roentgenograms are again obtained following the reduction in order to determine the presence of any small fracture fragments. The reduction is maintained with a posterior plaster splint or with a collar and cuff sling holding the elbow in 100 to 110 degrees of flexion.

The author recommends admitting these patients for overnight observation to keep a close check on the neurovascular status of the extremity. Ice is applied to the elbow to decrease the edema. Repeat roentgenograms are obtained the next morning prior to discharging the patient from the hospital, in order to insure that the elbow has remained in the reduced position. The patient is reevaluated four days later, and at that time gentle motion may be instituted. Most authors agree that attempts at manipulation are contraindicated. The patient should be encouraged to perform gentle range-of-motion exercises of the involved elbow, but forced passive range-of-motion exercises are contraindicated. If the latter is attempted, a further restriction of motion may result, and this may also lead to an increased likelihood of traumatic myositis ossificans.

If at the time of the initial reduction the patient was noted to be unstable with attempted gentle motion at the elbow, it is appropriate to maintain the immobilization for 10 to 14 days. However, an extended period of immobilization beyond this time is not indicated. If motion is not reinstated at the end of two weeks, it usually indicates severe restriction of motion with elbow contractures. Since the joint capsule was torn at the time of injury, it may heal in a scarred, shortened position. This in itself will produce thick contractures.

It has been the author's experience that even with early reduction and early range-of-motion exercises, many patients are left with a 10 to 15 degree flexion contracture of the elbow. Serial roentgenographic evaluations should be made at 4 and 14 days postreduction so that a recurrent dislocation will not go undetected.

LATERAL DISLOCATIONS

True lateral dislocations of the elbow are relatively rare. In these injuries it is not uncommon to have an associated fracture of the lateral condyle.

Physical Examination

Diagnosis is established by the disruption of the normal equilateral posterior osseous triangle. The tip of the olecranon is noted to lie in a more lateral position than normal. The prominent medial condyle may be palpable, and a gap may be felt which represents the articular surface of the medial condyle of the humerus. The radial head may also lie in a more lateral position, and a step-off may be present between the lateral humeral condyle and the lateral prominence of the radial head.

Roentgenographic Examination

The anteroposterior roentgenogram will reveal the radial head and the proximal ulna

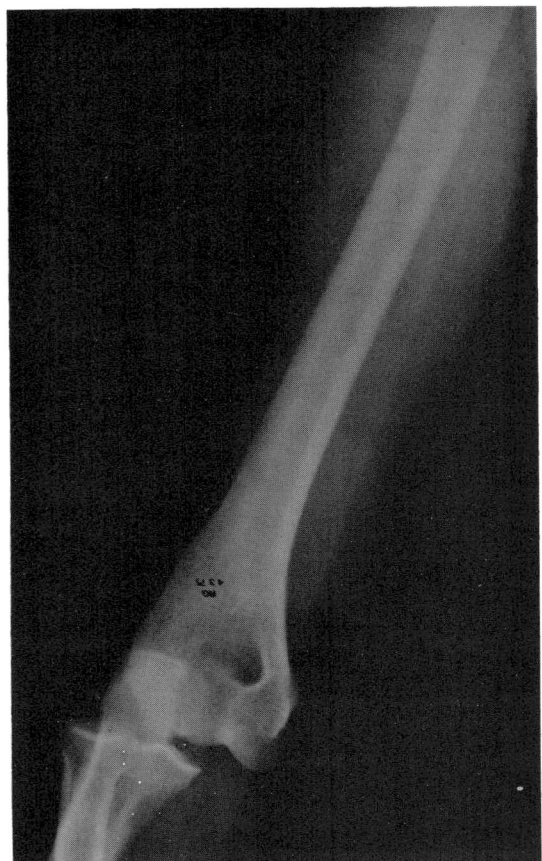

Figure 17–23   An anteroposterior view of a posterolateral elbow dislocation.

to be situated in a more lateral position than normal (Fig. 17–23). The two osseous structures tend to dislocate as a unit owing to the intact inter-osseous membrane. The lateral roentgenogram may reveal the sigmoid notch articulating in the sulcus between the capitellum and trochlea rather than in its normal trochlear position.

Treatment

Reduction is normally easily accomplished by exerting a downward force on the proximal forearm bones, and then applying a direct pressure against the radial head or the lateral aspect of the olecranon. Again, the range of motion of the elbow is assessed following the reduction. Most of these dislocations are relatively stable after they are reduced. As with a posterior dislocation, motion is initiated early in the treatment.

MEDIAL DISLOCATIONS

A medial dislocation is extremely rare. The routine anteroposterior roentgenographic view will usually reveal the sigmoid notch of the olecranon to be situated in a more medial position than normal. On lateral roentgenographic evaluation, a gap will be seen between the radial head and the articular surface of the humerus. There may also be a gap between the olecranon and the trochlea.

Treatment

Reduction is easily obtained by downward traction on the proximal forearm bones along with a lateral force directed against the medial olecranon. Range of motion is then evaluated in the reduced position. As with other dislocations, early motion is encouraged.

ANTERIOR DISLOCATIONS

A pure anterior dislocation in the absence of an associated olecranon fracture is extremely rare. The usual mechanism of injury has been described as a fall on the flexed elbow with the force transmitted to the olecranon. In most instances there is an associated fracture of the olecranon, although cases without an associated fracture of the olecranon have been reported.

Physical Examination

On physical examination the diagnosis is fairly straightforward. The normal equilateral osseous posterior triangle is disrupted. The olecranon is noted to be lying in a more proximal position along the anterior aspect of the humerus. The articular surface of the distal humeral condyles may be palpable. The forearm is usually maintained in a position of extension.

The great danger in this type of injury is compromise of the soft tissue structures along the anterior aspect of the elbow. A traumatic injury to the brachial artery or the median nerve also may occur.

Roentgenographic Examination

A standard anteroposterior roentgenogram will reveal that the olecranon process and the radial head are situated in a more proximal direction than normal. A lateral roentgenogram will show the tip of the olecranon to be lying against the anterior aspect of the distal humerus.

Treatment

Reduction is relatively simple, with traction applied to the forearm distally as a direct downward force is applied against the proximal forearm. Once reduction is obtained, the stable range of motion is determined. The neurovascular status of the forearm is then carefully evaluated. If there is any evidence of compromise of the vascular supply to the forearm, an arteriogram should be obtained. It is also important to determine whether or not the triceps mechanism is still intact.

Postoperatively, the elbow is maintained at 90 degrees of flexion with a posterior plaster splint. Motion is actively started at 10 to 14 days postreduction. It is important to obtain serial roentgenograms to check for the development of myositis ossificans in the brachial muscle, which may occur following this injury. Myositis ossificans may significantly limit future range of motion. If this complication does develop, surgical excision should be delayed for at least one year postinjury.

DIVERGENT DISLOCATION

This is another rare injury in which both the radius and ulna are dislocated but in diverging directions, with the lower end of the humerus located between the two structures. Two types are described for the sake of completeness. In the anteroposterior type, the proximal portion of the ulna is located posterior to the distal aspect of the humerus, and the radial head is located in the anterior aspect of the distal humerus. The lateral type is an extremely rare injury, in which the proximal portion of the ulna is displaced medially and the radius is displaced laterally. The injury is thought to be due to a forced pronation mechanism of the forearm in the extended position.

Physical Examination

On physical examination of the anteroposterior type of fracture, the examiner may be able to palpate the tip of the olecranon in a more posterior position than normal, and the radial head may also be palpable along the anterior aspect of the distal humerus. In the lateral type, the elbow joint proper is grossly widened. The radial head may be palpated in a more lateral direction than normal, and the olecranon will be noted to be medially displaced. The equilateral triangle will also be disrupted.

Treatment

In the anteroposterior type of dislocation, reduction is obtained by applying distal traction to the forearm associated with a downward force to the proximal forearm bone, as in reduction of a regular posterior dislocation. The radial head may then be directly levered into appropriate position. The reduction is maintained by placing the forearm in flexion and supination.

In the lateral type, reduction is accomplished by distal traction on the forearm associated with a vise-like action against the radius and ulna. Reduction is maintained in flexion and supination. Immobilization is achieved with the use of a posterior plaster splint for three weeks, at which time motion is gradually initiated.

ISOLATED ULNAR DISLOCATION

This is a very uncommon injury. It is described as classically occurring in an anterior or posterior direction. Although the posterior dislocation is rare enough, the anterior dislocation is extremely rare. Mechanism of injury of the posterior dislocation is felt to be forced hyperextension and adduction of the elbow. Under these conditions, the radius remains in its normal position, while the ulna dislocates in a posterior direction. In this injury, the medial collateral ligament is torn, but the lateral collateral ligament is intact. There may also be an associated fracture of the coronoid process. The forearm is maintained in almost complete extension. The tip of the olecranon is palpated posterior to the elbow joint, and flexion is markedly restricted. In an anterior dislocation, the patient maintains the elbow in a flexed position. There is also an increase in the normal carrying angle.

TREATMENT

In a posterior dislocation, reduction is accomplished by applying distal traction with the forearm in extension and supination. The forearm is then brought into the flexed position.

Reduction of an anterior dislocation is achieved by applying distal traction on the forearm and direct downward pressure over the proximal ulna, with the forearm in pronation. Immobilization is maintained with the use of a posterior splint in the flexed position for the posterior dislocation and at 90 degrees of flexion for the anterior dislocation. Motion is initiated at two to three weeks postinjury.

RECURRENT DISLOCATIONS

Recurrent dislocations of the elbow are relatively rare. Several theories have been advanced for the mechanism of recurrent injury. In separate studies, King and Reichenheim both concluded that it was due to insufficiency of the trochlear notch.[60, 90] They contended that the biceps tendon should be transplanted to the coronoid process in order to provide a block to recurrent dislocations. On the other hand, Osborne and Cotterill felt that the essential lesion responsible for this problem was attenuation of the posterolateral ligament and capsular structures.[81] It was their contention that a lateral "pocket" developed in the capsule and led to recurrent dislocations.

In a more recent study, Hassmann and his colleagues also concluded that recurrent dislocations resulted from laxity of the lateral capsule and collateral ligament.[43] They did not feel that extensive surgical procedures, such as bone blocks or tendon transfers, were indicated, believing that the capsular repair outlined by Osborne and Cotterill was sufficient treatment. In general, repair of the lateral side of the elbow joint is usually all that is required.

OLD DISLOCATIONS

Old dislocations of the elbow are occasionally encountered, usually following posterior dislocations. The incidence of this serious problem may be decreased by serial roentgenographic evaluation and careful physical evaluation of patients, sequentially following reduction of a posterior dislocation. The rule of thumb is to attempt closed reduction under a general anesthetic up to 21 days after the injury.

Allende and Freytes reviewed the treatment of a series of old dislocations of the elbow and concluded that reduction by closed methods failed after a period of three weeks. Open reduction has been advocated until six months postinjury. After that time it is generally agreed that significant changes occurring within the joint prevent a good result. Arthrodesis will provide a stable, painless elbow under these conditions, but this severely limits function. It is possible that total joint replacement has a place in the management of these patients, particularly in the elderly.

Part III ———————— **FRACTURE–DISLOCATIONS** ————————

RADIAL HEAD FRACTURE AND POSTERIOR DISLOCATION

The radial head fracture may be seen in association with a posterior dislocation of the elbow (Fig. 17–24). The mechanism of injury is thought to be a fall on the outstretched elbow in the presence of mild pronation of the forearm.

ROENTGENOGRAPHIC EXAMINATION

On routine anteroposterior roentgenographic evaluation the olecranon will be seen to lie in a more proximal direction than normal. The radial head will also be noted to be in a more proximal position. On the lateral view, a portion of the radial head frequently remains within the joint in close

proximity to the capitellum. The remainder of the radial head may be still attached to the radial neck and lie posterior to the humeral condyle.

TREATMENT

Treatment includes reduction of the dislocation, preferably performed under a general anesthetic or regional block. The reduction is accomplished by longitudinal traction on the forearm with direct downward pressure over the proximal forearm bones, followed by gradual flexion of the elbow while the traction is being maintained. Once the reduction has been performed, repeat roentgenograms will reveal the position of the radial head fragment. If

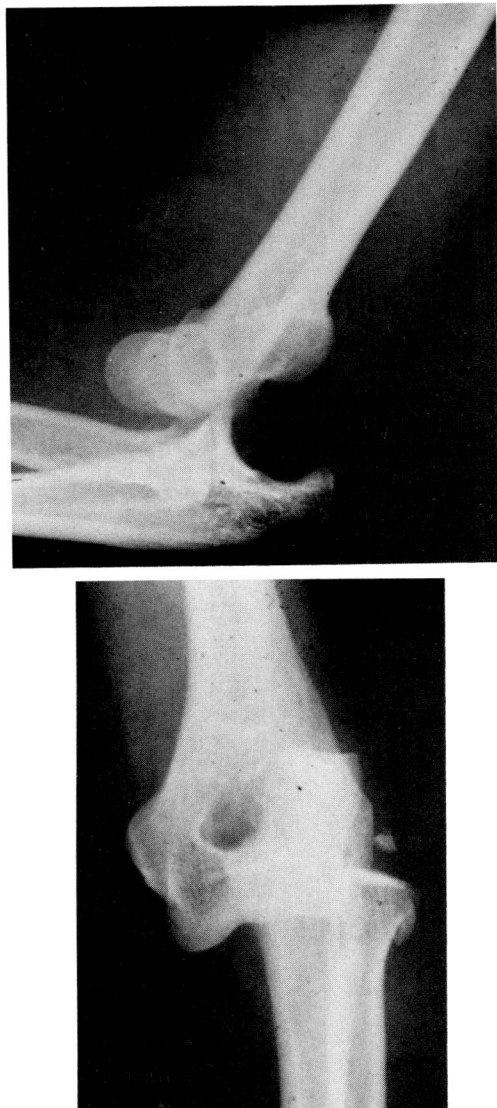

Figure 17–24   Posterolateral dislocation of the elbow with a chip fracture of the radial head.

the position of the fragment is satisfactory and if no more than one half of the radial head is involved, consideration should be given to leaving the radial head in position and instituting early motion at one week postinjury. If motion is not satisfactory at two to three weeks following initiation of motion, the radial head may be removed.

CORONOID PROCESS FRACTURES AND POSTERIOR DISLOCATION

This type of injury is encountered fairly frequently. The mechanism is again a fall on the outstretched extended elbow. The brachial muscle avulses the coronoid process at its insertion.

ROENTGENOGRAPHIC EXAMINATION

Anteroposterior roentgenograms will demonstrate the olecranon process and radial head to be in a more proximal position than normal. Lateral roentgenographic evaluation will reveal the posterior location of the olecranon and radial head. The coronoid process will be avulsed and may be lying in the front of the joint.

TREATMENT

Treatment consists of performing a closed reduction of the posterior dislocation. This is accomplished under a general anesthetic or regional block. Longitudinal traction is applied to the forearm, and a direct downward force is applied to the proximal forearm bone. The forearm is then brought up into flexion while traction is maintained. Roentgenograms are next obtained in the operating room.

If the coronoid process fragment is small and in relatively close proximity to its normal position, operative intervention is not indicated. The elbow is maintained in flexion with the use of a posterior splint for one week, when gradual motion is initiated. If the fragment is large and significantly displaced, it may have to be operatively repaired. This may be performed by a direct anterior approach to the elbow, with the fragment maintained in position by two small crossed Kirschner wires.

This is a serious injury, as the presence of a free fragment of bone along the brachialis may stimulate the onset of myositis ossificans. Therefore, it is not uncommon for patients with this type of injury to end up with a flexion contracture of the elbow.

COMBINED RADIAL HEAD AND CORONOID PROCESS FRACTURE WITH POSTERIOR DISLOCATIONS

This is a very serious injury which may lead to gross instability of the elbow joint. The author has found this a difficult problem in management. Patients should be informed at the outset that it is not uncommon to end up with severe limitation of motion after treatment of this injury. The mechanism of this injury is felt to be a fall with the elbow in extension and the forearm in some degree of pronation.

ROENTGENOGRAPHIC EXAMINATION

Roentgenographic evaluation in an anteroposterior plane will reveal the proximal location of the olecranon, the radial neck, and the radial shaft (Fig. 17–25). A lateral roentgenographic view will reveal the posterior displacement of the olecranon and radial neck situated posterior to the humeral condyles. The coronoid process will be noted to lie in front of the humeral condyle, and a portion of the radial head may also be located here.

TREATMENT

Treatment of this injury is by routine closed reduction under a general or regional anesthetic, as outlined for a posterior dislocation of the elbow. The elbow is then gradually passed through a range of motion, and any tendency to redislocate is noted.

It is the author's feeling that excision of the radial head, even in the presence of a mild step-off deformity, is not indicated in the initial management of these injuries because it may lead to further instability with recurrent dislocation. The remaining intact portion of the radial head may be brought up into contact with the humeral condyle by placing the forearm usually in a

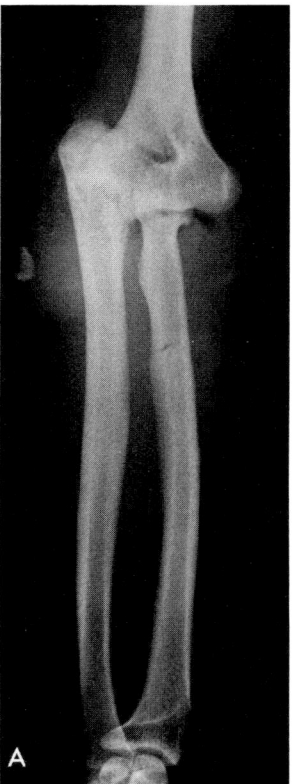

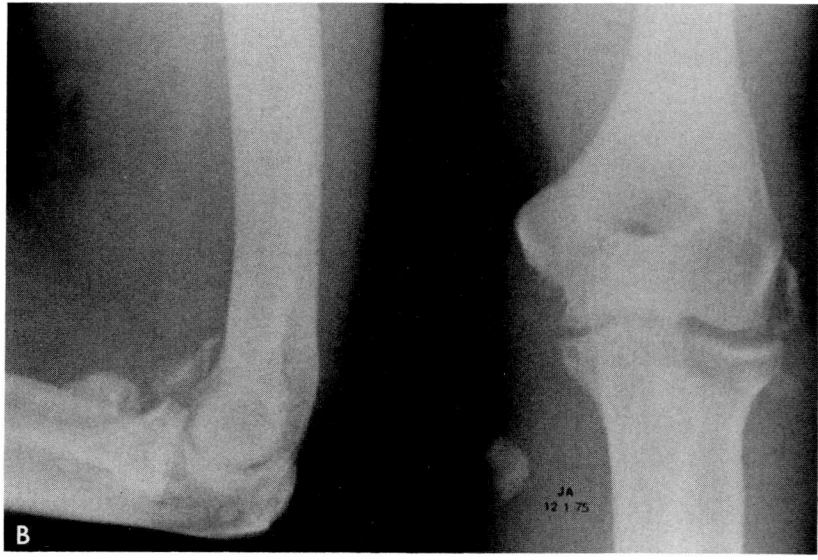

Figure 17–25   A. Anteroposterior view of a posterior dislocation of the elbow with a fracture of the radial head and coronoid process. *B.* Two months following closed reduction. Note the displacement of the coronoid process and calcification of the lateral ligament of the elbow. The result was a 30 degree flexion contracture of the elbow.

position of supination. The purpose of this maneuver is to swing the remaining portion of the radial head to abut against the humeral condyle. This maneuver may provide some stability to prevent redislocation in the presence of a coronoid fracture.

If stability is not achieved with the elbow in 90 to 100 degrees of flexion, then the author has found that the insertion of a smooth Steinmann pin through the olecranon, across the elbow joint, and into the distal humerus is required to maintain reduction. The pin is then incorporated in a long arm cast, with the entire anterior portion of the cast removed over the antecubital fossa. The pin is removed at the end of two weeks, and gradual motion is initiated. Forced manipulation in an attempt to increase range of motion is definitely contraindicated. The author's experience with this maneuver shows that, although the majority of patients end up with restricted motion, the elbow will at least remain in the reduced position.

If an attempt is made to initially excise the radial head, recurrent dislocation is a definite problem. The only alternative is to excise the radial head and insert a fixation pin across the olecranon into the humerus for stabilization.

If the coronoid process fragment is large, an attempt may be made to openly reduce this fragment back into position and hold it with crossed Kirschner wire fixation. This fixation may add a little stability to the elbow joint.

In any event, these injuries are extremely difficult in regard to management, and elbow disability is a frequent consequence.

LATERAL CONDYLAR FRACTURE WITH POSTERIOR DISLOCATION

This type of injury is encountered occasionally. The mechanism of injury is a fall on the extended elbow. The anteroposterior roentgenographic view will demonstrate the proximal location of the olecranon and radial head. The lateral roentgenographic view will frequently reveal the posterior position of the radial head and olecranon, with the capitellum in close proximity to the radial head.

Treatment consists of reducing the posterior elbow dislocation in a standard fashion.

Roentgenograms are then obtained in the operating room. If the fragment is large enough, internal fixation should be considered. If the fragment is comminuted, consideration should be given to excising the fragment and beginning early motion at one week. If internal fixation is provided for the separated fragment, motion may be initiated at one to two weeks if the fixation is secure. The elbow is maintained in flexion until mobilization is initiated.

OLECRANON FRACTURE WITH ANTERIOR DISLOCATION

This injury is not infrequent in a busy orthopedic practice. The mechanism of injury is a fall on the semiflexed elbow with direct trauma to the olecranon. The force produces a fracture of the olecranon and an anterior dislocation of the elbow. As with any type of anterior dislocation, the danger of neurovascular compromise must be ruled out.

ROENTGENOGRAPHIC EXAMINATION

A standard anteroposterior view of the elbow will reveal a fracture of the olecranon process associated with proximal displacement of the remainder of the ulna and the radial head. The lateral roentgenographic view will demonstrate the radial head in a position anterior to the distal portion of the humerus in association with the remainder of the ulna. The olecranon fragment will lie in a posterior direction.

TREATMENT

Treatment involves standard reduction of the anterior dislocation. The neurovascular status of the upper extremity is determined. If there is good evidence of peripheral pulses, roentgenograms are obtained and the status of the olecranon fracture evaluated. The author believes that the best form of treatment is firm internal fixation of the olecranon fragment with the tension band method, followed by the initiation of early motion. Postoperatively, the elbow is maintained in 90 to 100 degrees of flexion with the use of a posterior splint. A careful check should be maintained on the neurovascular status of the forearm. Motion is initiated at one to two weeks postinjury, since the tension band technique provides enough stability for early motion.

ULNAR FRACTURES WITH DISLOCATION OF RADIAL HEAD (MONTEGGIA'S FRACTURE)

This injury is discussed in Chapter 18.

REFERENCES

1. Adler, J. B., and Shaftan, G. W.: Radial head fractures; is excision necessary? J. Trauma, 4:115–136, 1964.
2. Adler, S., Fay, G. F., and MacAusland, W. R., Jr.: Treatment of olecranon fractures. Indication for excision of the olecranon fragment and repair of the triceps tendon. J. Trauma, 2:597–602, 1962.
3. Aitken, A. P., and Childress, H. M.: Intraarticular displacement of the internal epicondyle following dislocation. J. Bone Joint Surg., 20:161, 1938.
4. Aldredge, G. N., Jr., and Gregory, C. F.: Triceps advancement in olecranon fractures. J. Bone Joint Surg., 51A:816, 1969.
5. Allende, G., and Freytes, M.: Old dislocations of the elbow. J. Bone Joint Surg., 26:691–706, 1944.
6. Alvarez, E., Patel, M. R., Nimberg, G., and Pearlman, H. S.: Fracture of the capitulum humeri. J. Bone Joint Surg., 57A:1093–1096, 1975.
7. Arnold, J. A., Nasca, R. J., and Nelson, C. L.: Supracondylar fractures of the humerus. The role of dynamic factors in prevention of deformity. J. Bone Joint Surg., 59A:589–595, 1977.
8. Ashurst, A. P. C.: An anatomical and surgical study of fractures of the lower end of the humerus. Philadelphia, Lea & Febiger, 1910.
9. Aufranc, O. E., Jones, W. N., and Bierbaum, B. E.: Open supracondylar fracture of the humerus. J.A.M.A., 208:682–685, 1969.
10. Bakalim, G.: Fractures of radial head and their treatment. Acta Orthop. Scand., 41:320–331, 1970.
11. Balchandani, R. H.: Unreduced dislocations of the elbow. J. Bone Joint Surg., 51B:781, 1969.
12. Barr, J. S., and Eaton, R. G.: Elbow reconstruction with a new prosthesis to replace the distal end of the humerus. J. Bone Joint Surg., 47A:1408–1413, 1965.
13. Bickel, W. H., and Perry, R. E.: Comminuted fractures of the distal humerus. J.A.M.A., 184:553–557, 1963.
14. Brown, R. F., and Morgan, R. G.: Intercondylar T-shaped fractures of the humerus. J. Bone Joint Surg., 53B:425–428, 1971.
15. Bryan, R. S., and Bickel, W. H.: "T" condylar fractures of distal fractures of distal humerus. J. Trauma, 11:835, 1971.
16. Bush, L. F., and McClain, E. J., Jr.: Operative treatment of fractures of the elbow in adults. AAOS Instructional Course Lectures, 16:265–277, 1959.
17. Campbell, W. C.: Malunited fractures and unreduced dislocations about the elbow. J.A.M.A., 92:122–128, 1929.
18. Caravias, D. E.: Forward dislocation of the elbow without fracture of the olecranon. J. Bone Joint Surg., 39B:334, 1957.
19. Cassebaum, W. H.: Open reduction "T" and "Y" fractures of the lower end of the humerus. J. Trauma, 9:915–925, 1969.
20. Charnley, J.: The Closed Treatment of Common Fractures. Edinburgh, E. & S. Livingstone, 1950.
21. Christopher, F., and Bushnell, L. F.: Conservative treatment of fracture of the capitellum. J. Bone Joint Surg., 17:489–492, 1935.
22. Colton, C. L.: Fractures of the olecranon in adults: classification and management. Injury, 5:121–129, 1973.
23. Conn, J., and Wade, P. A.: Injuries of the elbow (a ten year review). J. Trauma, 1:248–268, 1961.
24. Coonrad, B. W.: A review of severe elbow injuries. J. Bone Joint Surg., 38A:1396, 1956.
25. Daland, E. M.: Fractures of the olecranon. J. Bone Joint Surg., 15:601–607, 1933.
26. D'Ambrosia, R. D.: Supracondylar fractures of the humerus—prevention of cubitus varus. J. Bone Joint Surg., 54A:60–66, 1972.
27. Darrach, W.: Open reduction of fractured external condyle of humerus. Ann. Surg., 63:486–487, 1916.
28. Darrach, W.: Open reduction of fractures of the capitellum. Ann. Surg., 63:487–488, 1916.
29. Dunlop, J.: Traumatic separation of the medial epicondyle of the humerus in adolescence. J. Bone Joint Surg., 17:577–587, 1935.
30. Dunlop, J.: Transcondylar fractures of the humerus in childhood. J. Bone Joint Surg., 21:59–73, 1939.
31. Dunn, A. W.: A distal humeral prosthesis. Clin. Orthop., 77:199–202, 1971.
32. Eastwood, W. J.: The T-shaped fracture of the lower end of the humerus. J. Bone Joint Surg., 19:364–369, 1937.
33. Edman, P., and Lohr, G.: Supracondylar fractures of the humerus treated with olecranon traction. Acta Chir. Scand., 126:505–516, 1963.
34. Eriksson, E., Sahlen, O., and Sandohl, U.: Late results of conservative and surgical treatment of fracture of the olecranon. Acta Chir. Scand., 113:153–166, 1957.
35. Evans, E. M.: Pronation injuries of the forearm, with special reference to the anterior Monteggia lesion. J. Bone Joint Surg., 31B:578–588, 1949.
36. Evans, E. M.: Supracondylar Y-fractures of the humerus. J. Bone Joint Surg., 35B:381–385, 1953.
37. Fairbank, H. A. T.: Discussion of two cases of disability at the wrist joint following excision of the head of the radius. Proc. R. Soc. Med., 24:904–905, 1930.

38. Fitts, W. T., Jr.: Fractures of the upper extremity (a review of experience in World War II). Am. J. Surg., 72:393–403, 1946.

39. Garceau, G. J.: Fractures of the lower end of the humerus. J.A.M.A., 112:623–626, 1939.

40. Gejrot, W.: On intra-articular fractures of the capitellum and trochlea of humerus with special reference of treatment. Acta Chir. Scand., 71:253, 1932.

41. Gosman, J. A.: Recurrent dislocation of the ulna at the elbow. J. Bone Joint Surg., 25:448–449, 1943.

42. Harmon, P. H.: Treatment of fractures of the olecranon by fixation with stainless steel screws. J. Bone Joint Surg., 27:328–329, 1945.

43. Hassman, G. C., Brunn, F., and Neer, C. S.: Recurrent dislocation of the elbow. J. Bone Joint Surg., 57A:1080–1084, 1975.

44. Hasner, E., and Husby, J.: Fracture of the epicondyle and condyle of the humerus. Acta Chir. Scand., 101:195, 1951.

45. Henderson, R. S., and Robertson, I. M.: Open dislocation of the elbow with rupture of the brachial artery. J. Bone Joint Surg., 34B:636–637, 1952.

46. Highsmith, L. S., and Phalen, G. S.: Sideswipe fractures. Arch. Surg., 52:513–522, 1946.

47. Ho, K. C., and Marmor, L.: Entrapment of the ulnar nerve at the elbow. Am. J. Surg., 121: 355–356, 1971.

48. Howard, J. L., and Urist, M. R.: Fracture–dislocation of the radius and ulna at the elbow joint. Clin. Orthop., 12:276–284, 1958.

49. Hoyer, A.: Treatment of supracondylar fractures of the humerus by skeletal traction in an abduction splint. J. Bone Joint Surg., 34A:623–637, 1952.

50. Jackman, R. J., and Pugh, D. G.: The positive elbow fat pad sign in rheumatoid arthritis. Am. J. Roentgenol., 108:812–818, 1970.

51. Jacobs, J. C., and Kernodle, H. B.: Fractures of the head of the radius. J. Bone Joint Surg., 28:616–622, 1946.

52. Johansson, H., and Olerud, S.: Operative treatment of intercondylar fractures of the humerus. J. Trauma, 11:836–843, 1971.

53. Jones, K. G.: Percutaneous pin fixation of fractures of the lower end of the humerus. Clin. Orthop., 50:53–69, 1967.

54. Kapel, O.: Operation for habitual dislocation of the elbow. J. Bone Joint Surg., 33A:707–714, 1951.

55. Keon-Cohen, B. T.: Fractures at the elbow. J. Bone Joint Surg., 48A:1623–1639, 1966.

56. Kerin, R.: Elbow dislocations and its association with vascular disruption. J. Bone Joint Surg., 51A:756–758, 1969.

57. Kilburn, P., Sweeney, J. G., and Silk, F. E.: Three cases of compound posterior dislocation of the elbow with rupture of the brachial artery. J. Bone Joint Surg., 44B:119–121, 1962.

58. King, B. B.: Resection of the radial head and neck (an end-result study of thirteen cases). J. Bone Joint Surg., 21:839–857, 1939.

59. King, D., and Secor, C.: Bow elbow (cubitus varus). J. Bone Joint Surg., 33A:572–576, 1951.

60. King, T.: Recurrent dislocation of the elbow. J. Bone Joint Surg., 35B:30–54, 1953.

61. Kini, M. G.: Dislocation of the elbow and its complications. J. Bone Joint Surg., 22:107–117, 1940.

62. Knight, R. A.: Management of fractures about the elbow in adults. AAOS Instructional Course Lectures, 14:123–141, 1957.

63. Kohn, A. M.: Soft tissue alterations in elbow trauma. Am. J. Roentgenol., 82:867–874, 1959.

64. Linscheid, R. L., and Wheeler, D. K.: Elbow dislocations. J.A.M.A., 194:1171–1176, 1965.

65. Loomis, L. K.: Reduction and after-treatment of posterior dislocation of the elbow. Am. J. Surg., 63:56–60, 1944.

66. MacAusland, W. R.: The treatment of fractures of the olecranon by longitudinal screw or nail fixation. Ann. Surg., 116:293–296, 1942.

67. Mann, T. S.: Prognosis in supracondylar fractures. J. Bone Joint Surg., 45B:516–522, 1963.

68. Mason, M. L.: Some observations on fractures of the head of the radius with a review of one hundred cases. Br. J. Surg., 42:123–132, 1954.

69. Mazel, M. S.: Fracture of the capitellum. J. Bone Joint Surg., 17:483–488, 1935.

70. McDougall, A. M., and White, J.: Subluxation of the inferior radio-ulnar joint complicating fracture of the radial head. J. Bone Joint Surg., 39B:278–287, 1957.

71. McKeever F. M., and Buck, R. M.: Fracture of the olecranon process of the ulna. J.A.M.A., 135:1–5, 1947.

72. McLaughlin, H. L.: Trauma. Philadelphia, W. B. Saunders, 1959.

73. Milch, H.: Dislocation of the inferior end of the ulna; suggestions for a new operative procedure. Am. J. Surg., 1:141–146, 1926.

74. Milch, H.: Unusual fractures of the capitulum humeri and the capitulum radii. J. Bone Joint Surg., 13:882, 1931.

75. Milch, H.: Fractures and fracture dislocations of the humeral condyles. J. Trauma, 4:592–607, 1964.

76. Miller, W. A.: Comminuted fractures of the distal end of the humerus in the adult. J. Bone Joint Surg., 46A:644–657, 1964.

77. Müller, M. E., Allgower, M., and Willenegger, H.: Manual of Internal Fixation. New York, Springer-Verlag, 1970.

78. Nicholson, J. T.: Compound comminuted fractures involving the elbow joint; treatment by resection of fragments. J. Bone Joint Surg., 38:565, 1946.

79. Norell, H. G.: Roentgenologic visualization of extra-capsular fat; its importance in the diagnosis of traumatic injuries to the elbow. Acta Radiol., 42:205–210, 1954.

80. O'Connor, B. T., and Taylor, T. K. F.: The conservative approach to radial head fractures. J. Bone Joint Surg., 44B:743, 1962.

81. Osborne, G., and Cotterill, P.: Recurrent dislocation of the elbow. J. Bone Joint Surg., 48B:340–346, 1966.

82. Patrick, J.: Fracture of the medial epicondyle with displacement into the elbow joint. J. Bone Joint Surg., 28:143–147, 1946.

83. Patterson, R. F.: A method of applying traction in T- and Y-fractures of the humerus. J. Bone Joint Surg., 17:476–477, 1935.

84. Pike, W.: Fracture of the head of the radius. J. Bone Joint Surg., 51B:198, 1969.

85. Pinder, I. M.: Fracture of the head of the radius in adults. J. Bone Joint Surg., *51B*:386, 1969.

86. Pollack, W. J., and Parkes, J. C., II.: Early reconstruction of the elbow following severe trauma. J. Trauma, *10*:839–852, 1970.

87. Quigley, T. B.: Aspiration of the elbow joint in treatment of fractures of the head of the radius. N. Engl. J. Med., *240*:915–916, 1949.

88. Radin, E. L., and Riseborough, E. J.: Fractures of the radial head. (A review of eighty-eight cases and analysis of the indications for excision of the radial head and non-operative treatment). J. Bone Joint Surg., *48A*:1055–1064, 1966.

89. Reich, R. S.: Treatment of intercondylar fractures of the elbow by means of traction. J. Bone Joint Surg., *18*:997–1004, 1936.

90. Reichenheim, P. P.: Transplantation of the biceps tendon as a treatment for recurrent dislocation of the elbow. Br. J. Surg., *35*:201, 1947.

91. Rhodin, R.: On the treatment of fracture of the capitellum. Acta Chir. Scand., *86*:475–486, 1942.

92. Riseborough, E. J., and Radin, E. L.: Intercondylar T-fractures of the humerus in the adult (a comparison of operative and non-operative treatment in twenty-nine cases). J. Bone Joint Surg., *51A*:130–141, 1969.

93. Roberts, N. W.: Displacement of the internal condyle into the elbow joint. Lancet, 2:78–79, 1934.

94. Roberts, P. H.: Dislocation of the elbow. Br. J. Surg., *56*:806–815, 1969.

95. Robertson, R. C., and Bogart, F. B.: Fracture of the capitellum and trochlea, combined with fracture of the external humeral condyle. J. Bone Joint Surg., *15*:206–213, 1933.

96. Rombold, C.: A new operative treatment for fractures of the olecranon. J. Bone Joint Surg., *16*:947–949, 1934.

97. Rush, L. V., and Rush, H. L.: A reconstruction operation for comminuted fractures of upper third of the ulna. Am. J. Surg., *38*:332–333, 1937.

98. Smith, F. M.: Displacement of the medial epicondyle of the humerus into the elbow joint. Ann. Surg., *124*:410–425, 1946.

99. Smith, F. M.: Kirschner wire traction in elbow and upper arm injuries. Am. J. Surg., *74*:770–787, 1947.

100. Smith, F. M.: Medial epicondyle injuries. J.A.M.A., *142*:396–402, 1950.

101. Smith, L.: Deformity following supracondylar fracture of the humerus. J. Bone Joint Surg., *42*:235–252, 1960.

102. Smith, L.: Supracondylar fractures of the humerus treated by direct observation. Clin. Orthop., *50*:37–42, 1967.

103. Spear, H. C., and Jones, J. M.: Rupture of the brachial artery accompanying dislocation of the elbow or supracondylar fracture. J. Bone Joint Surg., *33A*:889–894, 1951.

104. Speed, J. S.: Surgical treatment of condylar fractures of the humerus. AAOS Instructional Course Lectures, 7:187–194, 1950.

105. Speed, J. S.: Treatment of fractures of ulna with dislocation of head of radius (Monteggia fracture). J.A.M.A., *115*:1699–1705, 1940.

106. Spinner, M., and Kaplan, E. B.: The quadrate ligament of the elbow—its relationship to the stability of the proximal radio–ulnar joint. Acta Orthop. Scand., *41*:632–647, 1970.

107. Strachan, J. C. H., and Ellis, B. W.: Vulnerability of the posterior interosseous nerve during radial head excision. J. Bone Joint Surg., *53B*:320–323, 1971.

108. Strug, L. H.: Anterior dislocation of the elbow with fracture of the olecranon. Am. J. Surg., 75:700–703, 1948.

109. Swenson, A. L.: The treatment of supracondylar fractures of the humerus by Kirschner-wire transfixion. J. Bone Joint Surg., *30A*:933–997, 1948.

110. Taylor, T. K. F., and O'Connor, B. T.: The effect upon the inferior radio–ulnar joint of excision of the head of the radius in adults. J. Bone Joint Surg., *46B*:83–88, 1964.

111. Thompson, H. C., III, and Garcia, A.: Myositis ossificans (aftermath of elbow injuries). Clin. Orthop., *50*:129–134, 1967.

112. Thornton, L.: Fractures of the humerus treated by means of the Hoke plaster traction apparatus. J. Bone Joint Surg., *12*:911–917, 1930.

113. Trynin, A. H.: Intercondylar T-fracture of elbow. J. Bone Joint Surg., *23*:709–711, 1941.

114. Van Gorder, G. W.: Surgical approach in supracondylar T-fractures of the humerus requiring open reduction. J. Bone Joint Surg., *22*:278–292, 1940.

115. Villagrana, J. C.: Advantages of operative treatment of fractures of the elbow. J. Bone Joint Surg., *14*:65–72, 1932.

116. Wade, F. V., and Batdorf, J.: Supracondylar fractures of the humerus (a twelve year review with followup). J. Trauma, *1*:269–278, 1961.

117. Wadsworth, T. G.: Screw fixation of the olecranon after fracture or osteotomy. Clin. Orthop., *119*:197–201, 1976.

118. Wheeler, D. K., and Linscheid, R. L.: Fracture–dislocations of the elbow. Clin. Orthop., *50*:95–106, 1967.

119. Wickstrom, J., and Myer, P. R., Jr.: Fractures of the distal humerus in adults. Clin. Orthop., *50*:43–51, 1967.

120. Wiley, J. J., Pegington, J., and Horwich, J.: Traumatic dislocation of the radius at the elbow. J. Bone Joint Surg., *54B*:501–507, 1974.

121. Wilson, J. N.: The treatment of fractures of the medial epicondyle of the humerus. J. Bone Joint Surg., *42B*:778–781, 1960.

122. Yelton, C. L.: Injuries about the elbow. J. Bone Joint Surg., *37A*:650, 1955.

123. Zeitlin, A.: The traumatic origin of accessory bones at the elbow. J. Bone Joint Surg., *17*:933–938, 1935.

R. BRUCE HEPPENSTALL, M.D.

Fractures _____ 18
of the
Forearm

Fractures of the forearm occur in all age groups. They are usually the result of direct trauma and therefore may present as open or closed injuries. It is extremely important to obtain anatomical restoration of the osseous structures involved, or severe limitation of supination and pronation of the forearm may result. It is also important to pay strict attention to both the elbow and the wrist joints in the assessment forearm fractures. If these structures are not carefully evaluated in the management of forearm fractures, a Monteggia or Galeazzi fracture may be overlooked.

In recent years there has been a definite trend toward open reduction and internal fixation with the use of compression plates for fractures of both bones of the forearm. This provides for restoration of the osseous architecture and also allows for early functional activity. The management of single-bone forearm fractures is still relatively controversial, but there is a current trend toward early functional bracing of these injuries.

SURGICAL ANATOMY

A thorough appreciation of the anatomy of the forearm structures is required for proper management of forearm fractures. The radius and ulna are long, thin, rather tubular structures that have contact only at their extremities (Fig. 18–1). Sage has performed detailed anatomical studies of both the radius and the ulna.[38] He found that the radius, which is a relatively straight structure, demonstrated a radial bowing of approximately 9.3 degrees and a dorsal bowing of approximately 6.4 degrees. If the forearm is placed in full supination, the radius demonstrates a lateral bow and the ulna a slight medial bow. An abnormal rotation or malalignment of the forearm bones will result in a definite decrease in pronation and supination.

The articulation of the radial head with the proximal ulna allows for rotatory motion of the forearm. If the forearm is placed in full supination, the radius and ulna assume an almost parallel alignment. Pronation of the forearm produces a rotatory movement of the radius around the ulna so that the distal portion of the radius is swung around medially, crossing over the ulna. This motion is aided by the interosseous ligament and the distal radioulnar joint. The interosseous membrane spans the radius and ulna. The fibers of the interosseous membrane are oriented obliquely extending from the proximal origin on the radius to the distal insertion on the ulna. The interosseous membrane is a strong structure, occupying an important space. If the interosseous space is reduced by a surrounding callus or malalignment of the forearm bones, rotatory motion of the forearm will be restricted. There are three major muscular structures connecting the radius and ulna in the forearm. These are the pronator teres, the pronator quadratus and the supinator.

481

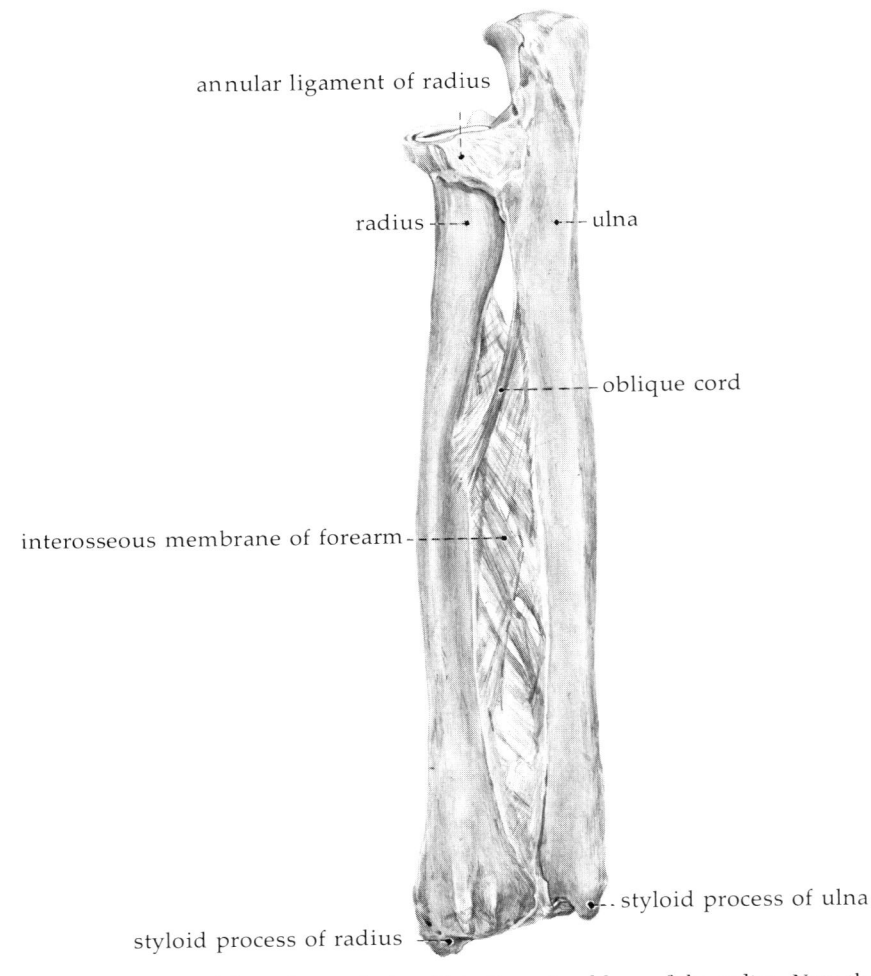

annular ligament of radius

radius

ulna

oblique cord

interosseous membrane of forearm

styloid process of ulna

styloid process of radius

Figure 18–1   Gross anatomy of the radius and ulna. Note the natural bow of the radius. Note the interosseous space between the forearm bones with full supination. (Courtesy of J. Langman and M. W. Woerdeman and W. B. Saunders Co., Philadelphia, Pa. Atlas of Medical Anatomy, 1978.)

Pronation

Pronation is achieved through the action of the pronator teres and quadratus muscles and as a function of the median nerve. The pronator teres arises from two heads. The humeral head originates from the medial aspect of the distal humerus, and the smaller ulnar head originates from the coronoid process of the ulna. Both heads join in the proximal portion of the forearm and then have a common insertion into the shaft of the radius at approximately the midportion along the lateral aspect.

The pronator quadratus is a quadrilateral muscle originating from the distal quarter of the shaft of the ulna along the anterior aspect. Its fibers are arranged in an almost transverse direction to insert into the anterior aspect of the radius at about the distal quarter. This muscle receives its nerve supply from the anterior interosseous branch of the median nerve.

Spinner described a syndrome secondary to malfunction of the anterior interosseous nerve.[46] In this syndrome, the patient is unable to flex the distal interphalangeal joints of the index finger and thumb. Hyperflexion of the proximal interphalangeal joints of the index finger and the metacarpal phalangeal joint of the thumb occurs. There is a paralysis of the pronator quadratus function and hyperextension of the distal interphalangeal joint of the index finger and the interphalangeal joint of the thumb.

Supination

Supination of the forearm is performed by the supinator and the biceps muscles (Fig. 18–2). The supinator, the primary muscle involved in supination, is more effective with the forearm in a position of slight extension. The biceps is more functional when the forearm is in a position of slight flexion. Supination is primarily a function of the radial nerve which supplies the supinator, and the musculocutaneous nerve which supplies the biceps.

The supinator originates from the lateral

Figure 18–2 The supinator and pronator muscles of the right forearm in the supine position in a front view. Note the relationship of the supinator and pronator teres muscles on the radius. These muscles produce deforming forces, depending on the level of the fracture. (Courtesy of J. Langman and M. W. Woerdeman and W. B. Saunders Co., Philadelphia, Pa. Atlas of Medical Anatomy, 1978.)

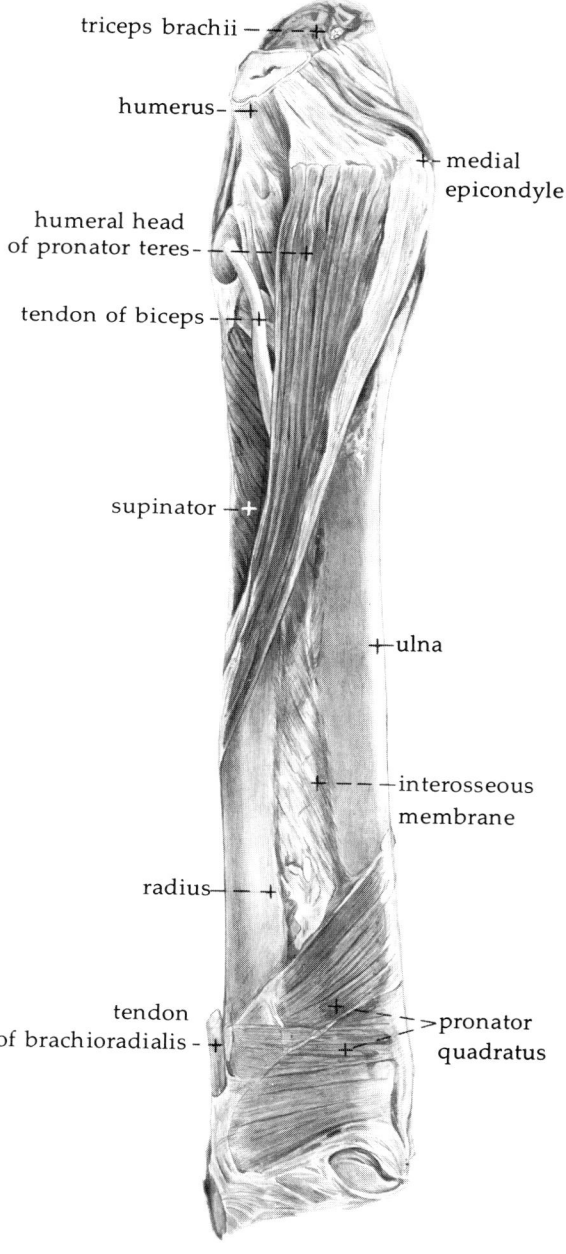

aspect of the distal humerus and the radial collateral and annular ligaments. It inserts into the lateral aspect of the proximal radius, extending from an area in proximity to the radial tuberosity distally to the attachment of the pronator teres.

If the anatomy of the forearm is borne in mind, it is not difficult to understand the deforming forces involved in a fracture depending on the level of fracture. If a fracture occurs distal to the insertion of the supinator and just proximal to the insertion of the pronator teres, the supinator will exert a strong force on the proximal radial fragment, causing it to lie in a position of maximum supination. The pronator will exert a force on the distal radius, so that it will come to lie in a position of pronation. If the fracture occurs distal to the pronator teres, the deforming forces are not quite as strong, since the supinator and biceps forces tend to equalize each other.

It may be easily appreciated that it is important not only to achieve gross alignment of forearm fractures but also to take rotation into account in the management of these injuries.

FRACTURES OF BOTH BONES OF THE FOREARM

This injury is relatively common in the pediatric age group and seen less often in the adult. Proper management is essential with these injuries if patients are to regain functional use of the forearm.

MECHANISM OF INJURY

This fracture may be produced by direct or indirect trauma. Direct trauma results from striking the forearm directly against a solid object. This is seen in injuries associated with automobile accidents and falls from a height. Another direct mechanism of injury that is being encountered with increasing frequency is the so-called night-stick fracture. The name is derived from a citizen's attempt to protect himself from a police officer's nightstick. The forearm is raised over the head to protect the skull from a direct blow, and the forearm receives the direct trauma from the nightstick. This

may result in a single forearm fracture or a fracture of both bones of the forearm.

The indirect mechanism of injury is a fall on the outstretched arm. This is the most frequent mechanism of injury in children.

PHYSICAL EXAMINATION

The diagnosis in patients presenting with fractures of both bones of the forearm is usually obvious. Regardless of the level at which the fracture occurs, there is a tendency for overriding of the fracture fragments and gross shortening of the upper extremity secondary to muscle contraction. In addition to the obvious shortening, there is usually a definite palpable and visible swelling at the site of the fracture. Patients present with exquisite pain. The forearm and arm are held immobile in order to prevent motion at the fracture site which increases pain. Gentle examination of the forearm will reveal crepitus at the fracture site. There is usually an associated large hematoma within the forearm, producing tense soft tissue structures. A careful neurovascular examination is essential at the time the patient is first evaluated. Neurological deficits are not common but do exist with this type of fracture.

ROENTGENOGRAPHIC EXAMINATION

This fracture can usually be evaluated with routine anteroposterior and lateral views, although oblique views are occasionally helpful. It is extremely important to include roentgenographic examination of the elbow and the wrist in forearm fractures. If this is not done, Monteggia or Galeazzi fractures may be overlooked. There may also be significant fractures of the distal humerus or wrist as a result of significant trauma to the upper extremity. In the routine anteroposterior view of the forearm, the level of the fractures can be evaluated and the degree of comminution and medial or lateral displacement determined (Fig. 18–3). The lateral roentgenogram will reveal the degree of shortening present and the amount of dorsal or volar overlap. The degree of comminution may also be determined from this view.

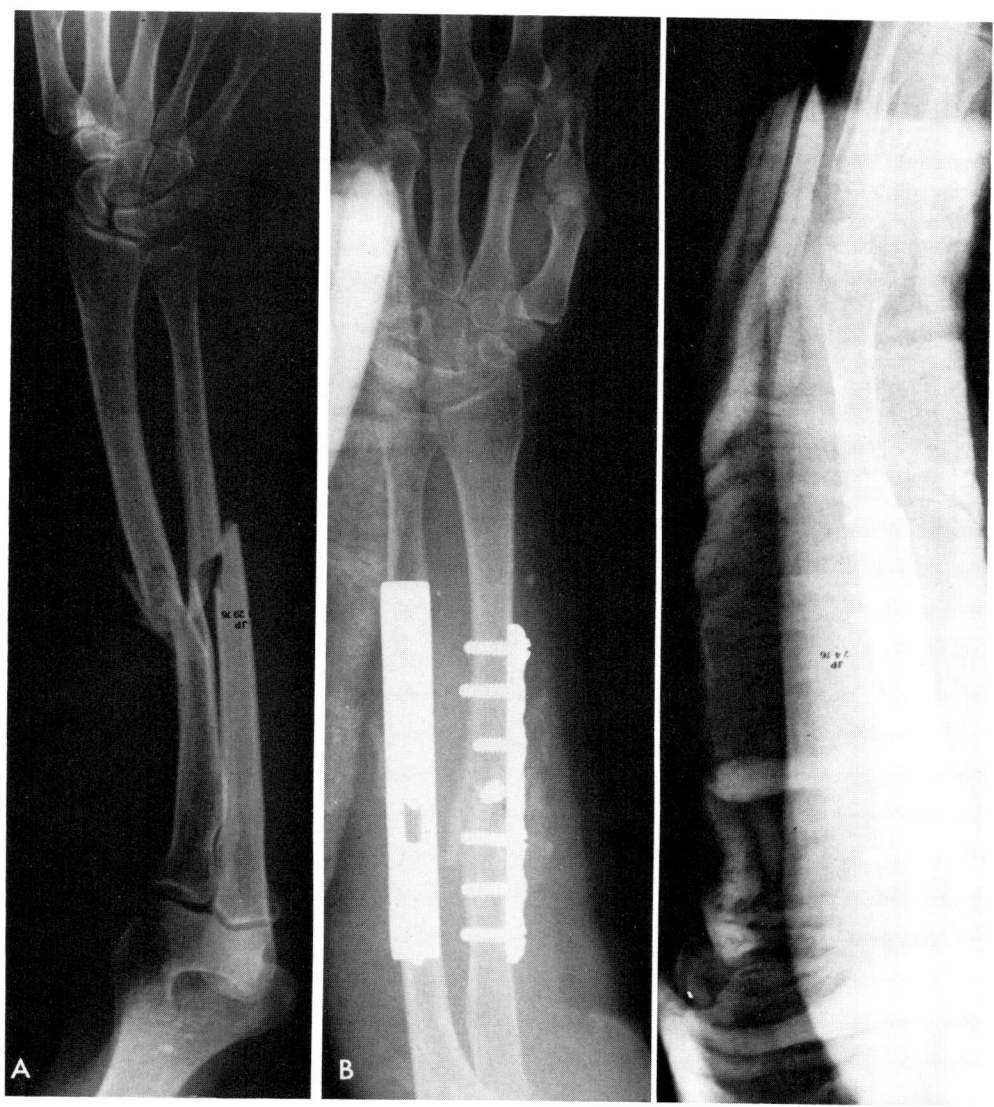

Figure 18–3   A. An anteroposterior view of a fracture of both bones of the forearm. Note the comminution of the radial fracture. B. It was treated with open reduction and internal fixation with the use of compression plates and iliac crest bone graft owing to the comminution. Uneventful healing resulted.

In 1945, Evans described a special roentgenographic view known as the "tuberosity view" that determines the amount of rotation of the fracture fragments.[18] This view is taken with the forearm placed parallel to the x-ray film. The humeral condyles are placed equidistant from the roentgenographic cassette. The roentgenographic tube is then placed above the forearm and rotated 20 degrees toward the olecranon. This angle will determine the prominence of the bicipital tuberosity of the radius.

Standard roentgenographic texts illustrate the prominence of the bicipital tuberosity with various degrees of pronation and supination. If these charts are then compared to the roentgenogram obtained from the patient, the degree of rotation of the proximal radial fragment may be determined. In full pronation, the bicipital tuberosity is noted to face in a direct lateral position. In full supination, the tuberosity faces directly medially or toward the ulna. If the forearm is placed in neutral rotation, the tuberosity is seen to face in a mid- or neutral position.

This view is helpful in determining the amount of rotation of the proximal fragment. This becomes important if closed reduction is selected as the form of treatment because it will allow the surgeon to determine in what degree of rotation the forearm must be placed to match the rotation of the proximal fragment.

TREATMENT

In recent years there has been a definite trend toward open reduction and internal fixation of fractures of both bones of the forearm with the use of compression plates.[2, 14] The majority of these fractures present with significant initial displacement. Although it is unusual for a patient to present with an undisplaced fracture of both bones of the forearm, the appropriate treatment for this injury is a long arm cast with the hand held in neutral position and the elbow flexed to 90 degrees. If this type of therapy is selected, frequent roentgenographic evaluation will be required to determine if future displacement of the fracture occurs. This will require weekly roentgenographic evaluation for a total of three weeks. At the end of that time the cast will probably have to be changed owing to decreased edema and the fact that the cast may have become loose. A new, snugly fitted long arm cast is applied, and weekly roentgenograms are obtained for an additional three weeks. At that point a decision should be made as to whether to apply a functional forearm brace or to continue with a long arm cast for an additional six weeks.

Nonoperative Treatment

If open reduction and internal fixation are not suitable because of the patient's medical condition, a closed reduction and plaster immobilization may be selected as treatment. A brachial block is preferred for anesthesia. Following administration of the block, the patient's extremity is positioned over the edge of the stretcher with the elbow flexed to 90 degrees. The fingers are then suspended with the use of a Chinese finger cot traction apparatus. Countertraction is applied to the distal humeral area with the use of a muslin bandage around the distal humerus. A weight of 15 lb is attached to the bandage to provide the necessary countertraction force. Rotational deformity is corrected by positioning the distal fragments in the appropriate amount of supination. Roentgenograms are then obtained, and if reduction is not satisfactory a closed manipulation is performed. Repeat roentgenograms are taken, and if the findings are satisfactory a long arm cast is applied. Additional roentgenograms are obtained after the application of the cast. Special care is taken not to overdistract the fracture fragments, as this will interfere with fracture healing. Roentgenograms are obtained every two weeks until six weeks later when the cast is usually changed. If loosening occurs prior to this time, the cast must be changed sooner. If at six weeks the roentgenograms reveal early healing with callus, a functional brace may be put on for an additional four to six weeks or a new long arm cast may be applied. The protective measures are continued until clinical evaluation and roentgenograms reveal satisfactory healing. This may vary from 10 to 20 weeks postinjury in most cases.

Operative Treatment

Displaced fractures must be treated much more aggressively than undisplaced ones. As already stated, this is by far the most common type of presentation (Fig. 18–4). The author has treated the majority of these patients with open reduction and internal

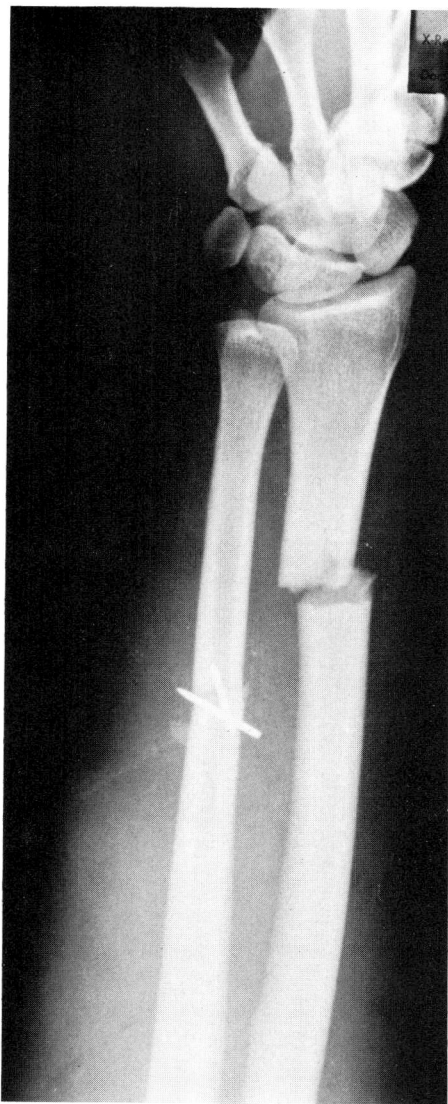

Figure 18–4 This is an example of how *not* to treat a fracture of both bones of the forearm. An open reduction was attempted, and minimal internal fixation of the ulna with crossed Kirschner wires was performed. The patient presented with evidence of nonunion six months postinjury. If internal fixation is selected as a method, adequate secure fixation must be obtained.

fixation with the use of compression plates. It has been demonstrated in several series that treatment by closed reduction and external fixation does not produce a high percentage of satisfactory results.[6, 8, 25] In contrast, several series have demonstrated markedly improved results with the use of the open reduction and internal fixation technique.[2, 10, 12, 14, 22, 32]

If these fractures occur as an isolated injury, the author prefers to perform open reduction and internal fixation within the first two to three days postinjury. If, however, these fractures are associated with other major skeletal injuries, it is preferable to splint the fractures and perform an open reduction and internal fixation at five to seven days postinjury when the gross metabolic deficits have been corrected.

The author has demonstrated that there is a definite decrease in oxygen delivery to a standardized wound for at least four to five days postinjury in patients who have suffered multiple injuries.[21] It is also well known that hypoxia increases the susceptibility of soft tissue wounds to infection. For this reason the author prefers a delay of five to seven days before performing internal fixation in patients who have received multiple trauma. In this manner the incidence of wound infections following the operative internal fixation should be decreased.

Several compression plates are currently on the market for the treatment of these fractures. Initially, the ASIF (Association for the Study of Internal Fixation) type of compression plate, which included an outrigger device to provide active compression, was utilized. However, a dynamic compression plate developed by the AO group has received recent enthusiasm.[31] The reader is referred to Chapter 7 for further details. This type of plate allows for active compression at the fracture site, which provides for rigid internal fixation (Fig. 18–5). The plates are applied in a specific location, depending on the site of the fracture. In fractures of the proximal half of the radius, the compression plate is placed along the dorsal aspect of the radius, through a Thompson approach. In fractures of the distal half of the radius, the plate is placed along the volar surface of the radius, through a lateral approach.

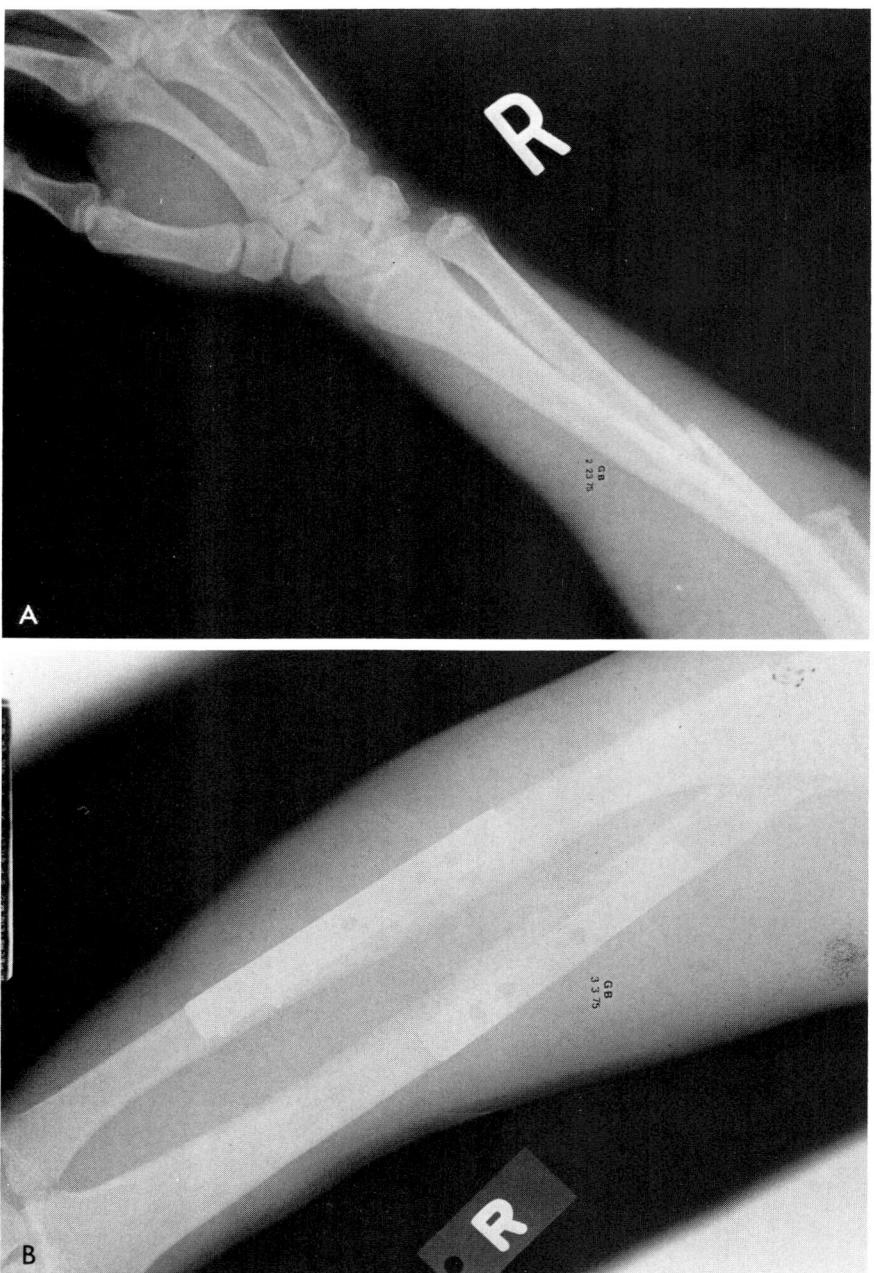

Figure 18–5 *A.* Roentgenographic evaluation is inadequate because the elbow is not included. This is a comminuted fracture of both bones of the forearm. *B.* Anteroposterior view of the same fracture treated with open reduction and internal fixation with the use of a compression plate and an iliac crest bone graft. Uneventful healing occurred at three months.

In an ulnar fracture, the plate may be placed on the volar or the dorsal surface. It is advisable to select a 5- or 6-holed plate for the management of these fractures.

In the past it was claimed that these compression plates should be inserted with the least amount of stripping of the periosteum as possible. It was felt that there was less disruption of the blood supply if the muscle was dissected free of the periosteum and the plate was placed directly on top of the periosteum. However, Whiteside has recently demonstrated that there is an increased disruption of the blood supply to the surrounding musculature if this technique is followed.[51, 52] His studies revealed that there was less disruption of the blood supply if the periosteum was stripped over the fracture site than if the muscle was dissected free of the periosteum. This is an important new concept. It has been the author's practice to apply the compression plate through a subperiosteal approach with care to disrupt the surrounding musculature as little as possible during the procedure. As in other uses of compression plating, it is important to prebend the plate slightly so that proper compression of the opposite cortex may be obtained.

If comminution is present at the fracture site, it has been the author's practice to include a bone grafting procedure from the iliac crest. A butterfly fragment is managed by obtaining interfragmentary compression with the use of AO compression screws. The compression plate may then be applied as the standard buttress plate. Cancellous bone obtained from the iliac crest is placed across the fracture site. It is customary to arbitrarily place a bone graft on the other fractured forearm bone as well, even if there is no evidence of comminution in this bone. If this practice is adopted, the incidence of nonunion following comminuted fractures of the forearm will be decreased.[2]

Postoperative Management. The postoperative management of these fractures depends to a great extent on the amount of fixation obtained at the time of the operative procedure. If the surgeon feels that he obtained satisfactory internal fixation, the patient may be managed without external fixation postoperatively, and early functional range-of-motion exercises of the elbow and wrist may be started. The alternative to this therapy is to apply a posterior gutter splint to the extremity and have the patient remove the splint for selected periods during the day for active motion of the elbow and wrist. If the degree of fixation obtained is questionable, the patient is placed in a posterior plaster splint for the immediate postoperative period. This splint is converted to a long arm cast three days postoperatively. The time of removal of the cast will depend on the degree of fixation achieved and the sequential roentgenographic evaluation of the fracture healing process.

Alternative Operative Methods

INTRAMEDULLARY NAILS. The concept of intramedullary nailing is not new. As described in the chapter on femoral fractures, Küntscher introduced his device for intramedullary fixation in the late 1940's. The problem with many intramedullary nail designs is that the concept of a round nail within the round medullary canal is not sound in terms of control of rotation. In other words, this type of design does not provide significant control of rotation of the fracture fragments. Therefore, in 1959 Sage introduced two new designs for an intramedullary nail for the treatment of forearm fractures.[38]

A straight nail was designed for use in the ulna, and a prebent nail, which conformed to the natural bow of the radius, was designed for radial fractures. The ulnar nail is inserted in a retrograde manner and is not difficult to manipulate. The reader is referred to Sage's original article for further description of the ulnar nail. The radial nail is inserted through the radial styloid and then advanced down the intramedullary canal toward the radial neck. Since the purpose of these nails is to provide relatively firm internal fixation, their use in fractures of the distal third of the radius is limited. This is due to the fact that the medullary canal expands in this area and rigid fixation is not possible.

Sage also recommended iliac crest bone grafting for the majority of cases. The problem with this approach is that inserting the nail down the intramedullary canal would certainly disrupt the blood supply to the endosteum. If this is coupled with periosteal stripping in an attempt to apply an iliac crest bone graft, there is no doubt

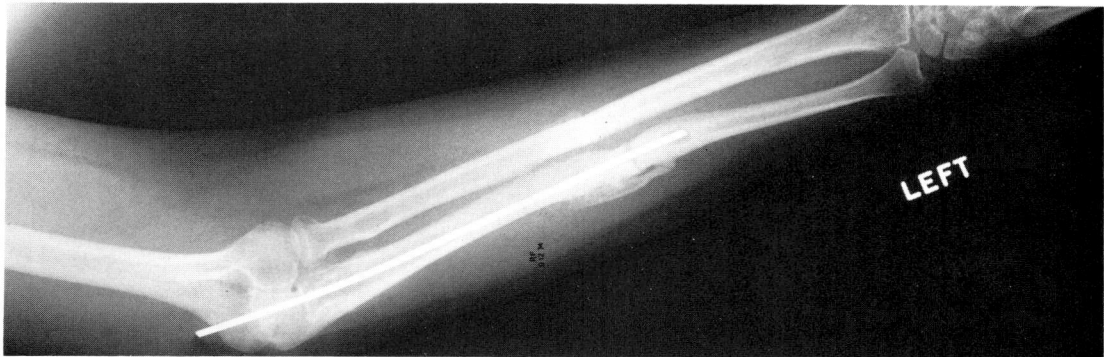

Figure 18–6 A forearm fracture treated with a Rush rod. This is not adequate fixation, as evidenced by this nonunion.

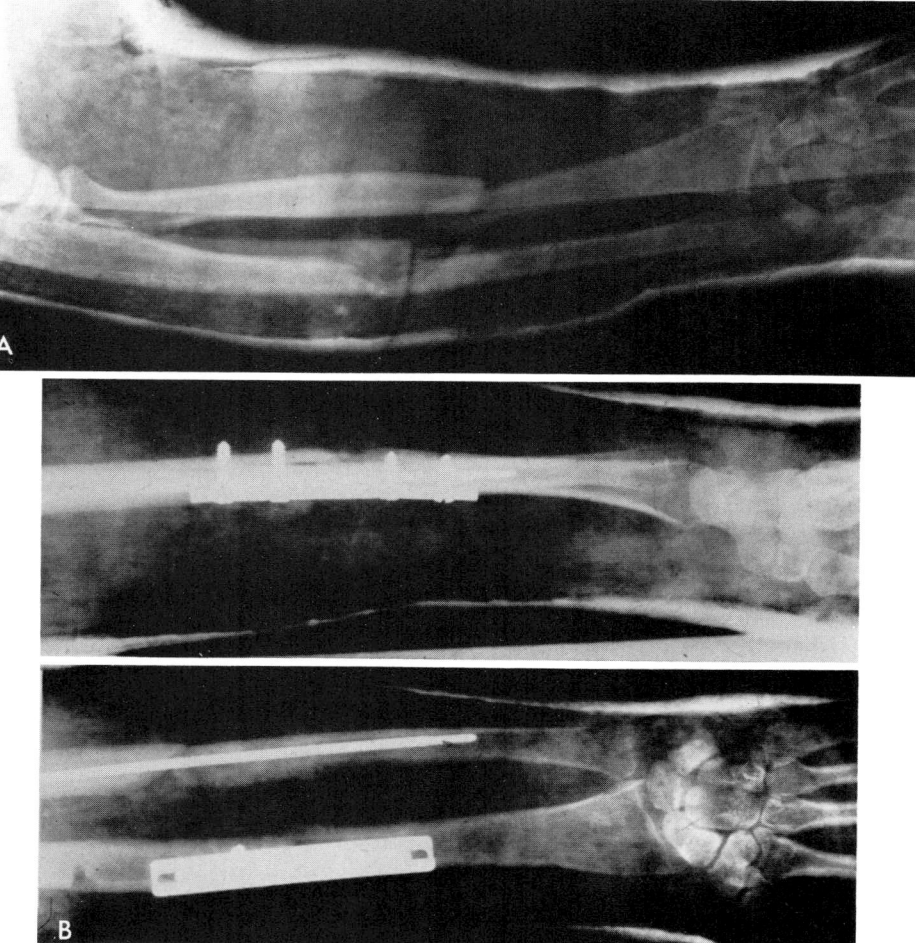

Figure 18–7 *A.* An open fracture of both bones of the forearm treated with initial debridement and plaster fixation. *B.* At 10 days postinjury the wound had healed, and the fractures were managed with open reduction and internal fixation with the use of a compression plate for the radius and a Rush rod for the ulna. This does not provide adequate fixation. The radius healed, but the ulna went on to nonunion.

that the bone would be devitalized in the vicinity of the fracture. However, the author certainly cannot argue with the good results reported by Sage, with a nonunion rate of only 6.2 per cent.[38]

RUSH RODS. Rush rods have also been advocated for the management of fractures of both forearm bones. The problem with this device is that its round design does not provide for rigid internal fixation of these fractures (Fig. 18–6). It has been the author's experience that a large percentage of fractures treated with Rush rods result in nonunion. This outcome is probably secondary to a lack of satisfactory immobilization.

COMPRESSION PLATE AND INTRAMEDULLARY ROD. Another approach is to insert a compression plate for one of the forearm fractures and supplement this with a Rush rod for the other forearm bone fracture. The author's experience with this technique has been that the forearm bone treated with the compression plate may go on to union, but the fracture treated with the Rush rod will frequently go on to nonunion (Fig. 18–7). Again, this is probably related to a lack of rigid internal fixation associated with the Rush rod. For this reason the author does not advocate this method. Physiologically, if the forearm is to be opened for the insertion of a compression plate it is a relatively simple matter to utilize the second incision for the application of the second compression plate. It adds very little morbidity to the procedure, and it certainly will increase the incidence of union.

PINS IN PLASTER. This method is more applicable to the management of Colles' fractures and tibial fractures. However, it has been recommended occasionally for the management of forearm fractures. The patient is taken to the operating room and administered a brachial block or an appropriate general anesthetic. Once anesthesia has been accomplished, the upper extremity is placed in the Chinese finger trap traction apparatus. Countertraction is then applied to the distal humeral area, and the forearm bones are manipulated into appropriate alignment. Roentgenograms are obtained in the operating room.

Once acceptable position has been achieved, two smooth Steinmann pins are inserted into the distal forearm bones, and

two are inserted through the proximal forearm in parallel fashion. The pins are then incorporated in a long arm plaster cast. The pins are usually maintained in position for a total of six to eight weeks, when they are removed and a new long arm cast is applied. This cast remains in place until there is roentgenographic evidence of healing.

EXTERNAL FIXATION DEVICES. Recently a new external fixation device has been designed. This is known as the Hoffman external fixating device, and it is frequently employed for the management of severe tibial fractures. It could also conceivably be used in the management of forearm fractures. The author has had no experience with this technique for forearm fractures, but it may have applicability in the future. The concept of rigid external fixation associated with active functional use of the extremity certainly is appealing.

FRACTURES OF A SINGLE BONE OF THE FOREARM

RADIAL FRACTURES

Isolated fractures of the shaft of the radius are relatively uncommon compared with the typical Colles' fracture of the distal radius. A physiological reason for this is the fact that the bone within the shaft of the radius is thoroughly compact and resistant to fracture. The bone at the distal end of the radius has a large cancellous component and is not as resistant to fracture (Fig. 18–8). Two types of radial shaft fractures will be discussed. The first type involves a fracture of the proximal two-thirds of the radius. The second type occurs at the junction of the middle and distal thirds of the radius and is frequently associated with a dislocation or subluxation of the distal radioulnar joint. It is known as the Galeazzi fracture.[19]

Type 1 (Proximal Radius)

Mechanism of Injury. The mechanism of injury in the proximal radial fracture (type 1) is direct or indirect trauma. The former is secondary to a direct blow to the proximal forearm, such as that produced in a nightstick injury. The incidence of this

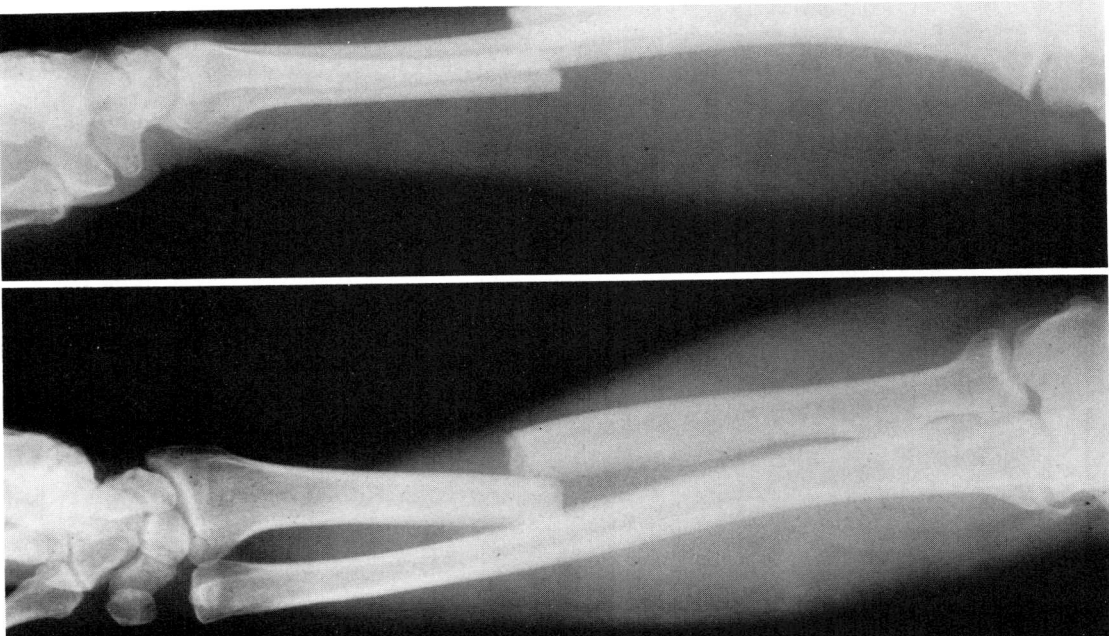

Figure 18–8 A simple fracture of the radius with displacement. There is no associated fracture of the ulna. This type of injury may be treated with open reduction and internal fixation with the use of a compression plate or may be managed with a functional brace technique following reduction.

fracture is decreased because it is usually the relatively superficial ulna that is fractured in this injury. Indirect trauma is usually produced by a fall on the outstretched forearm. This is similar to the mechanism that produces a fracture of both bones of the forearm, but a single radial fracture unassociated with an ulnar fracture results.

Treatment. Undisplaced fractures of the proximal radius may be treated with a long arm cast. The amount of supination of the forearm in the cast will depend on the level of the fracture. If the fracture is in the proximal portion of the radius just distal to the insertion of the supinator, the forearm should be placed in full or almost full supination. If, on the other hand, the fracture is in the midportion of the radius, the forearm does not have to be placed in significant supination. Displaced fractures of the proximal radius are best treated by open reduction and internal fixation with the use of a compression plate.

Type 2 (Galeazzi Fracture)

This is a fracture of the junction of the middle and distal thirds of the radius,

unassociated with a fracture of the ulna. If there is an associated subluxation or dislocation of the distal radioulnar joint, it is known as a Galeazzi fracture (Fig. 18–9). This type of fracture has been frequently overlooked in the past. In 1934, Galeazzi stated that the subluxation of the distal radioulnar joint is often present at the time of initial evaluation, and if it is not present then, it may well occur during the course of treatment.[19]

In 1957, Hughston reported a series of 41 cases of Galeazzi fractures and pointed out the high incidence of failure of closed treatment.[23] Of the cases managed without surgery, 92 per cent were failures. He then went on to describe several factors that he felt were responsible for the loss of reduction (the reader is referred to his original article).

Mechanism of Injury. As with fractures in the proximal two-thirds of the radius, the mechanism of injury in distal radial shaft fractures is direct trauma to the lateral aspect of the distal radius and indirect trauma as a result of a fall on the outstretched forearm. This type of injury has been referred to as a reverse Monteggia fracture.

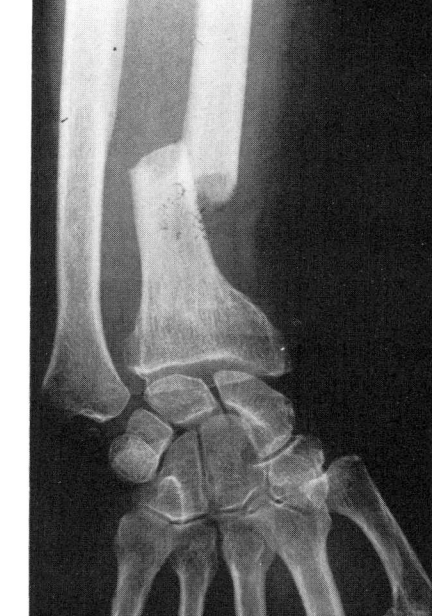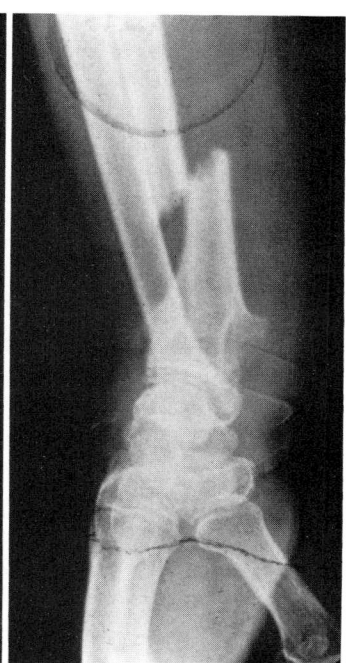

Figure 18–9 A Galeazzi fracture. Note the shortening and displacement of the radius. If this occurs without an associated fracture of the ulna, the distal radioulnar articulation must be altered. This was treated with open reduction and internal fixation with the use of a compression plate for the radial fracture.

Physical Examination. Patients present with pain and tenderness to direct palpation along the distal third of the radius. There is frequently pain and discomfort along the distal radioulnar joint as well, and there may be a prominence secondary to subluxation or dislocation of the distal aspect of the ulna. The examiner may have the impression that the distal aspect of the ulna can be reduced through a mechanism of direct pressure against the distal aspect of the ulna. Motion of the wrist will produce pain, and pronation or supination of the forearm is usually painful.

Roentgenographic Examination. As with other forearm fractures, it is extremely important to obtain roentgenographic views of the entire forearm, including the elbow and the wrist joint. Standard anteroposterior and lateral views will usually reveal this type of fracture. On the routine anteroposterior view the fracture of the radius is seen to be located at the junction of the middle and distal thirds. It is frequently transversely oriented. If there is significant displacement of the radial fracture, the examiner should be alert to the possibility of a problem with the proximal or distal radius. This is due to the fact that if one of the forearm bones fractures with significant displacement, there is usually an associated "give" to the other forearm bone. If this does not fracture within its substance, the proximal portion may be sprung at the elbow, or the distal portion may be sprung at the wrist. For this reason careful evaluation of the elbow and wrist are mandatory. The distal radioulnar articulation may appear to be "sprung." On the lateral view there is usually some evidence of dorsal displacement, and the distal ulna may be noted to lie in a more dorsal position than normal.

Treatment. The closed management of these injuries is usually not satisfactory (Fig. 18–10). This is an extremely unstable type of fracture, and even if satisfactory reduction has been obtained with initial reduction it is common to find a loss of reduction during the course of treatment. Mikić recently described the management of 125 patients with this type of injury.[29] It was his belief that children should be treated with closed methods and that adults should be treated with open reduction and internal fixation.

The best form of treatment is probably open reduction and internal fixation of the radial shaft fracture with application of a compression plate. If the distal end of the

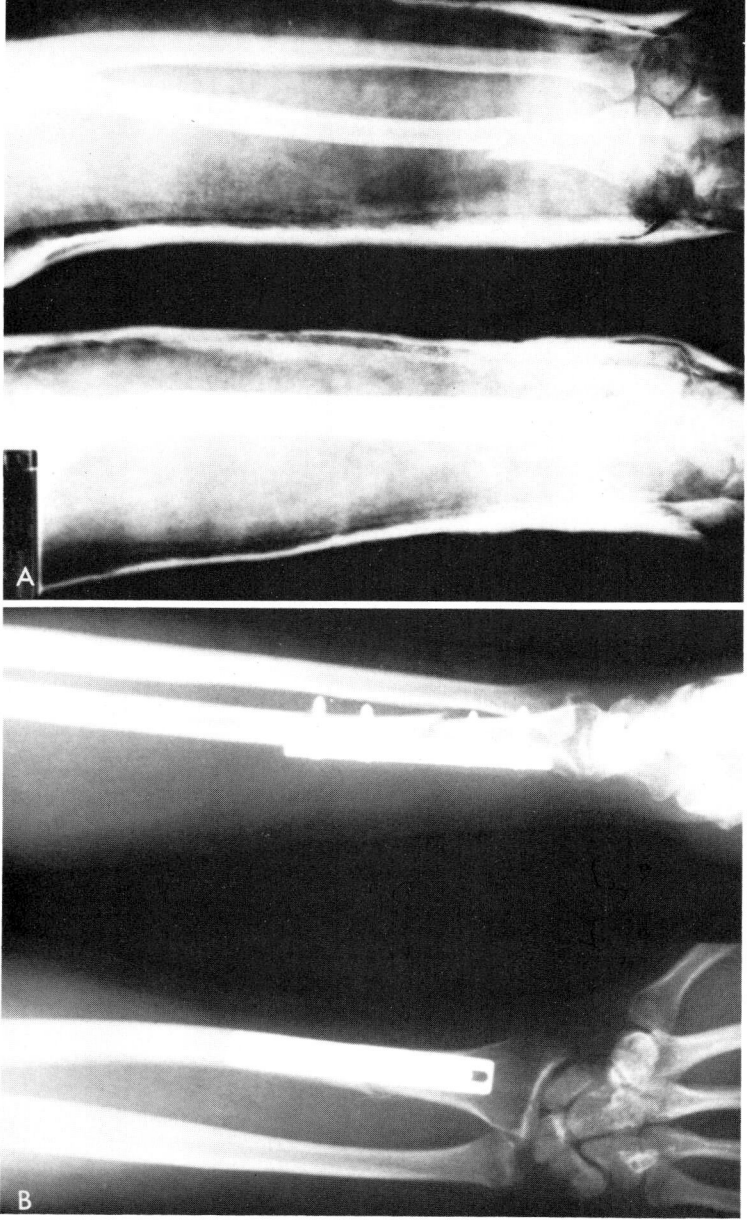

Figure 18-10 A. A Galeazzi fracture treated with initial closed reduction and plaster immobilization. *B.* The injury was ultimately managed with open reduction and internal fixation with a compression plate for the radial fracture. The ulnar subluxation was in satisfactory position, and the fracture went on to uneventful healing.

ulna appears to be relocated and stable, the extremity may be treated with a long arm cast. If, however, the distal end of the ulna appears to be unstable in spite of internal fixation of the radius, it is probably best to reduce the distal end of the ulna and transfix it with two crossed Kirschner wires. This will allow the ruptured triangular fibrocartilage to heal in appropriate position. At the end of four weeks the plaster

immobilization is discarded, and the crossed Kirschner wires are removed. Functional activity of the extremity is then initiated.

It is best not to consider resection of the distal ulna unless significant discomfort occurs in the future. Excising the distal ulna at the time of internal fixation of the radial fracture also is probably contraindicated. If at a later date the patient is symptomatic because of a recurrent subluxation or dislocation of the distal ulna, a Darrach type of resection of the distal ulna may be performed.

ULNAR FRACTURES

In general, two types of ulnar fractures are encountered in practice today. The first type is a fracture of the shaft of the ulna unassociated with any other osseous injury. The second is known as the Monteggia fracture. It is a fracture of the proximal third of the ulna associated with an anterior dislocation of the radial head.

Type 1 (Nightstick Fracture)

The majority of these fractures are closed injuries. They may occur at any age but are more frequent in the young to middle-aged group.

Mechanism of Injury. This type of fracture may be produced by direct trauma, such as that associated with a nightstick, or by indirect trauma as a result of a fall on the outstretched arm. Injury due to direct trauma is being seen with increasing frequency in today's society. It is produced when an individual lifts the upper extremity over the head in an attempt to ward off a blow from a police officer's nightstick. The full force of the blow is usually transmitted

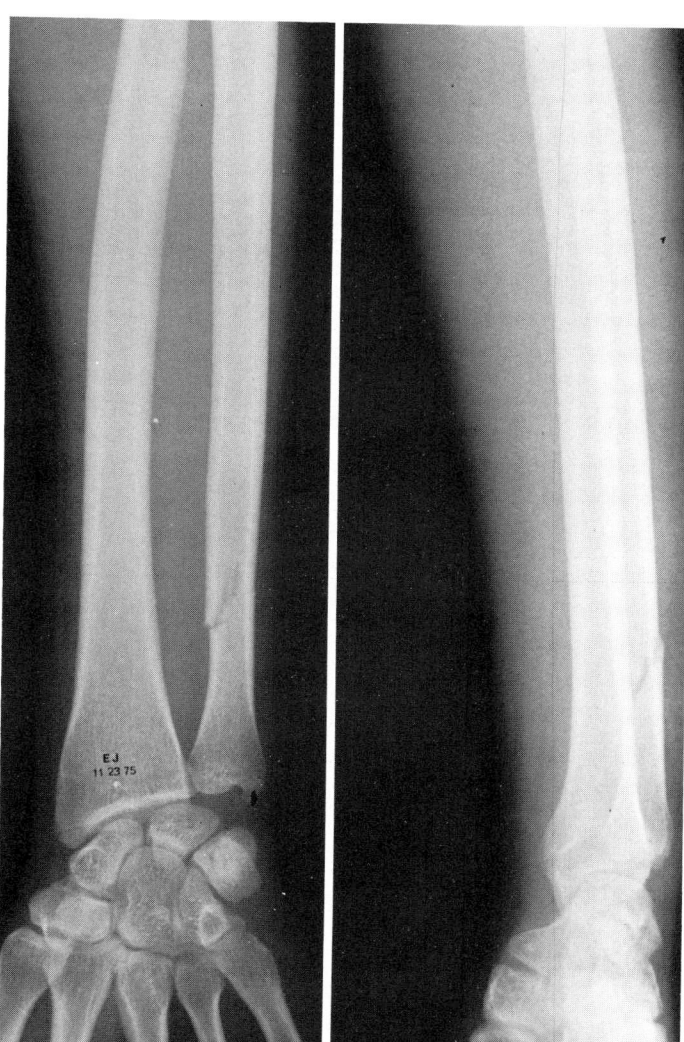

Figure 18–11 A nondisplaced fracture of the ulna treated with a functional brace.

to the ulna which lies in a superficial location. The fracture may be simple or comminuted. If the force of the blow is excessive, it may fracture the radius as well as produce a fracture of both bones of the forearm. However, the single ulnar fracture is the injury most commonly encountered.

Treatment. Recently, Sarmiento and his colleagues demonstrated that these patients may be treated with the use of functional bracing techniques (Fig. 18–11).[41] Their results showed that in 72 cases of functional bracing for isolated ulnar fractures there were no instances of nonunion, and there was very little loss of pronation or supina-

tion. It was their feeling that the results compared favorably with methods of open reduction and internal fixation. At the beginning of their series, they applied orthoplast forearm braces with supracondylar extensions and a plastic wrist joint. In the second half of their series, they applied only circumferential sleeves with Velcro straps. All patients were treated with initial application of a long arm cast for a median time of 12 days prior to application of the brace. The average healing time was 9.9 weeks following injury.

This functional method of treatment has been discussed in other chapters of this text,

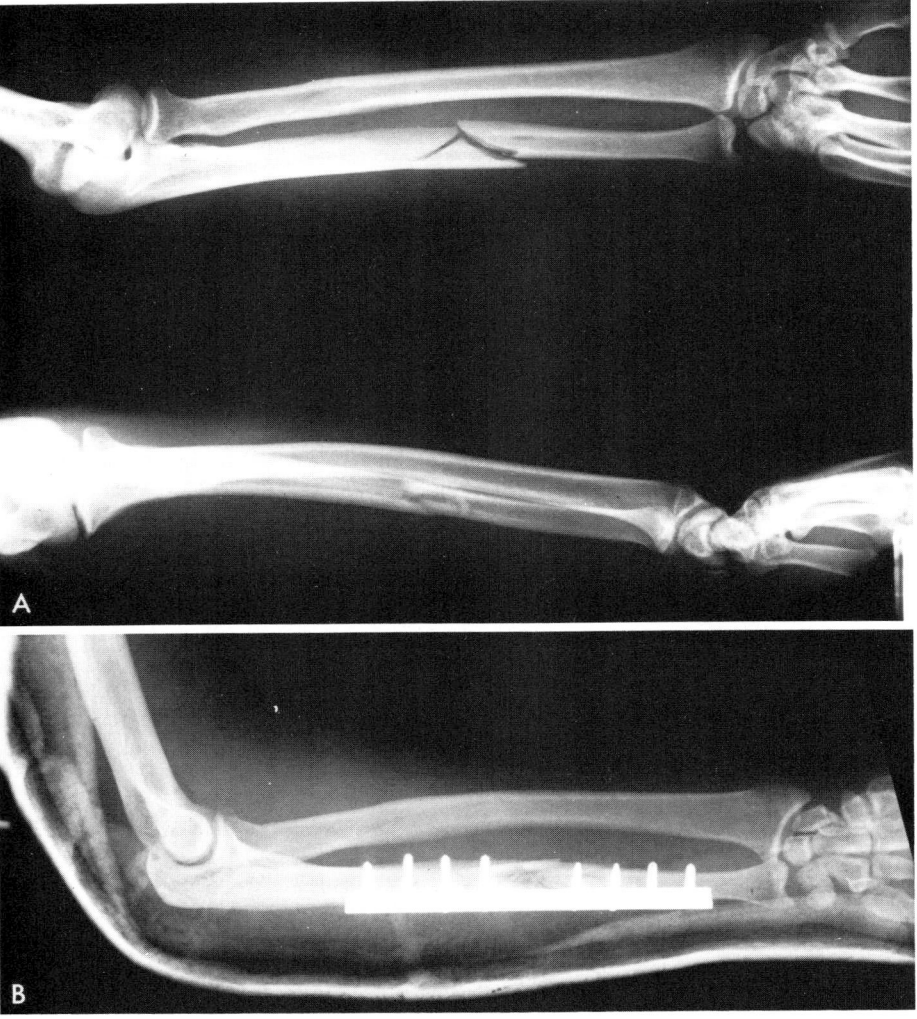

Figure 18–12   A. A comminuted fracture of the ulna. B. Treatment included open reduction and internal fixation with the use of a compression plate and an iliac crest bone graft because of the comminution.

and it certainly has physiological appeal. It is true that an increased amount of callus is produced by functional bracing compared with that produced by internal fixation with compression plates (Fig. 18–12). However, it has been demonstrated that the larger build-up of callus imparts additional strength to the healed bone compared with that obtained with a compression plate. We also must remember that in an active individual the compression plate must be electively removed at a later date.

Prior to Sarmiento's report,[41] the author had been accustomed to performing open reduction and internal fixation with a compression plate for this type of injury. Since that time, the functional bracing technique has been used and appears to produce satisfactory results.

Type 2 (Monteggia Fracture)

A fracture of the proximal third of the ulna associated with an anterior dislocation of the radial head has generally been known as a Monteggia fracture.[30] However, in 1967 Bado reported a spectrum of these injuries and combined them all under the term "Monteggia lesion."[3] His classification is helpful in bringing the various types under a single heading.

Type 1 is a fracture of the middle or upper third of the ulna with anterior angulation of the ulna associated with an anterior dislocation of the radial head. It accounts for 60 per cent of the total number. Type 2 (15 per cent) is a similar ulnar fracture but with posterior angulation associated with a posterior dislocation and frequently a fracture of the radial head (Fig. 18–13). Type 3 (20 per cent) is an ulnar fracture just distal to the coronoid process associated with a lateral dislocation of the radial head. Type 4 (5 per cent) is an ulnar fracture in the upper or middle third associated with an anterior dislocation of the radial head and a fracture of the proximal third of the radius distal to the bicipital tuberosity.

A recent review conducted by Bruce and his associates included a survey of 310 Monteggia fractures.[10] It was noted that type 1 fractures occurred in 65 per cent of cases, type 2 in 18 per cent, type 3 in 16 per cent and type 4 in 1 per cent. It was quite clear from their findings that type 1 is the most common variety of Monteggia fracture.

Mechanism of Injury. Although controversy still exists as to the precise mechanism of injury in Monteggia lesions, two specific causes have been suggested. The first a direct blow over the posterior aspect of the ulna, such as that produced by a nightstick. The second is a fall on the outstretched upper extremity with the forearm in marked pronation. In support of the latter mechanism, Evans was able to produce this fracture in cadavers through a mechanism of pronation of the forearm.[17]

Therefore, it is likely that the type 1 Monteggia lesion may be caused by either a

ANTERIOR   POSTERIOR

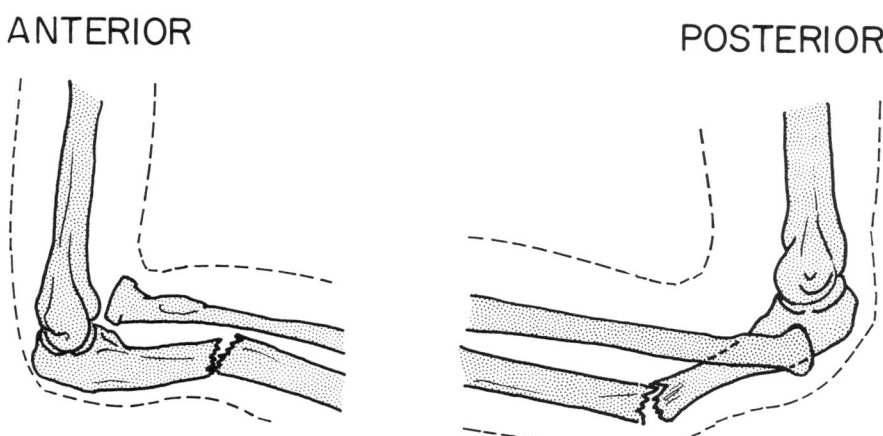

Figure 18–13 The two most commonly encountered Monteggia fractures. On the left, a type 1 fracture with anterior dislocation of the radial head and anterior bowing of the ulnar fracture. On the right, a type 2 fracture with posterior dislocation of the radial head and posterior angulation of the ulnar fracture.

direct blow or an indirect force associated with marked pronation of the forearm. The exact mechanism of injury of types 2, 3, and 4 lesions is still being debated. The reader is referred to the articles of Bado and Bruce and his co-workers.[3, 10]

Physical Examination. The physical findings vary according to the lesion. However, an obvious deformity is usually present. In type 1 lesions there is anterior angulation of the fractured ulna, and the anteriorly dislocated radial head may be palpated in the antecubital fossa. In type 2 lesions there is posterior angulation of the ulna, and the posteriorly dislocated radial head may be palpated in a superficial location along the posterior aspect of the elbow. In type 3 lesions there is lateral angulation of the ulna, and the radial head may be palpated in a lateral position. In type 4 lesions there are obvious radial and ulnar shaft fractures, and the dislocated radial head may be palpated in an anterior location.

In all these lesions there is significant pain in the vicinity of the elbow with attempted motion. Associated nerve lesions include the radial and posterior interosseous nerve, but these are usually transient and function is recovered.

Roentgenographic Examination. This type of lesion is frequently overlooked on routine roentgenograms (Fig. 18–14). Part of the problem may be the attending physician's lack of understanding of the specific lesion. A second reason is inadequate initial roentgenographic evaluation. As stated before, it is extremely important to include the elbow and wrist in the evaluation of any injury to the forearm. The type of roentgenographic picture depends on the particular type of Monteggia fracture. Bado's classification is a good working guide and should be followed.[3]

Treatment. Controversy still exists as to the exact form of treatment of Monteggia lesions in adults. Closed treatment has been recommended for children, and the results of the recent study by Bruce and his colleagues seem to favor this approach.[10]

It appears that the appropriate treatment of the adult Monteggia lesion is by open reduction and internal fixation. The ulnar fracture is internally fixed with the use of a compression plate, and the radial head is reduced by a closed manipulation. If the closed manipulation is unsuccessful in reducing the radial head, open reduction will have to be performed. Type 2 lesions associated with significant fracture of the radial head may require operative fixation of the ulnar fracture with the use of a com-

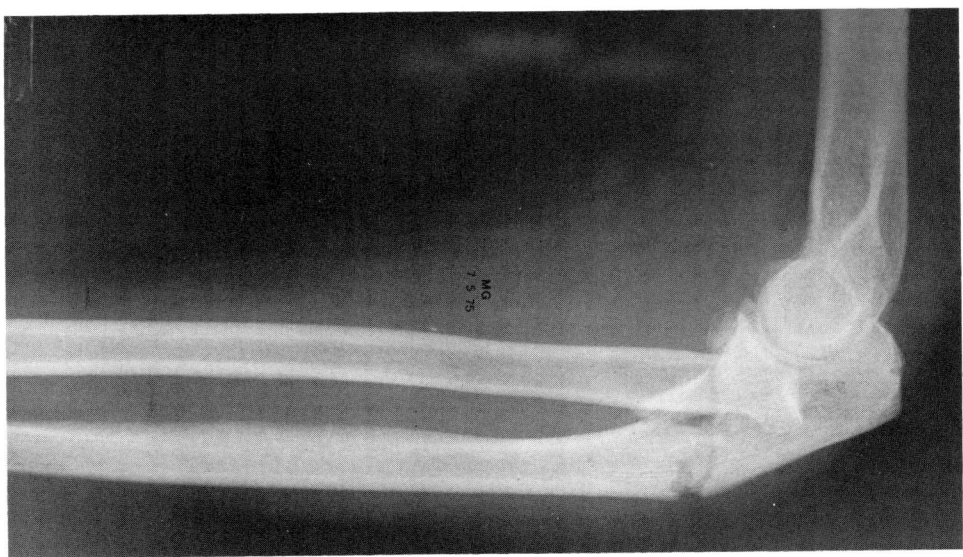

Figure 18–14   A type 2 Monteggia fracture with a fracture of the radial head, posterior dislocation, and posterior angulation of the ulnar fracture. It was treated by open reduction and internal fixation with the use of a small compression plate for the ulnar fracture and a closed manipulation of the radial dislocation.

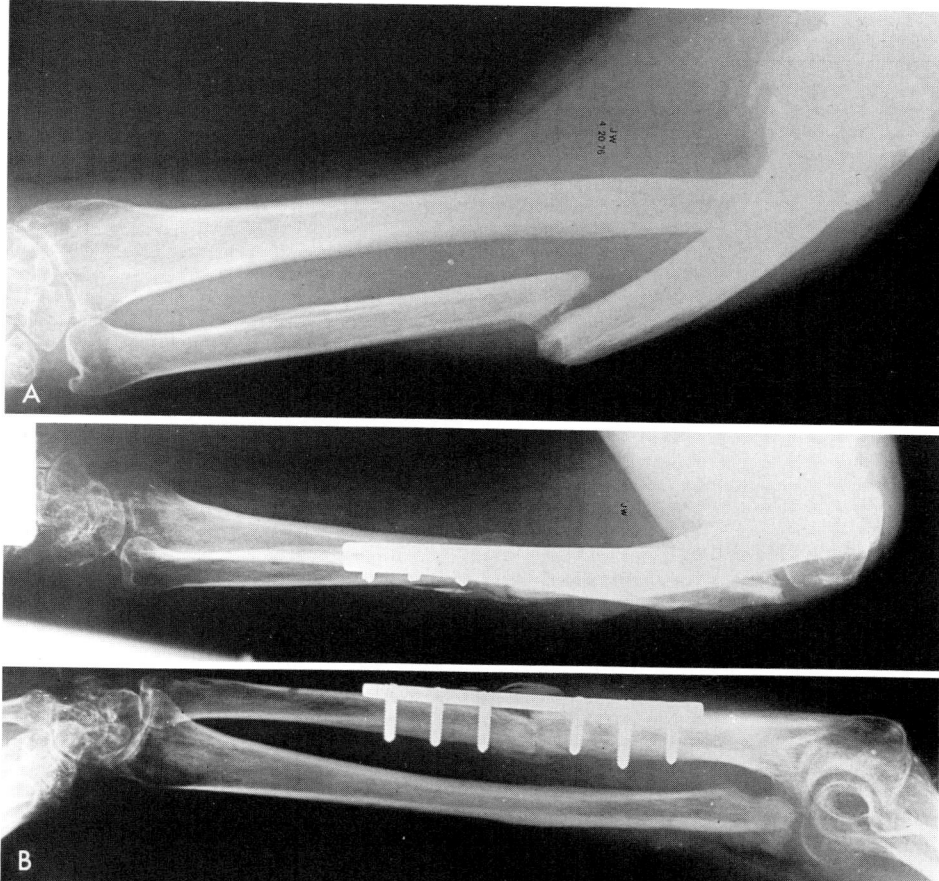

Figure 18–15 *A*. A neglected type 2 Monteggia fracture with nonunion of the ulnar fracture. *B*. Treatment was by open reduction and internal fixation of the ulnar fracture with application of a compression plate and an iliac crest bone graft. The posterior fracture–dislocation of the radial head was managed with excision of a loose fragment of the radial head and repositioning of the radial shaft. The ulnar fracture eventually healed, and the patient demonstrated 80 per cent range of motion of the elbow.

pression plate and excision of the radial head at the same time. The type 3 lesion may also be treated by internal fixation of the fractured proximal ulna and a closed reduction of the lateral dislocation of the radial head. Type 4 lesions are probably best treated by operative internal fixation of both bones of the forearm with the use of compression plates and closed manipulation of the radial head dislocation. If there is significant comminution associated with any of the fractures, it is probably appropriate to apply an iliac crest bone graft at the time of internal fixation (Fig. 18–15).

The position of the upper extremity following operative treatment is important. The most appropriate position of the elbow following internal fixation is with the elbow held in 110 degrees of flexion. This position is maintained for at least six weeks. At the end of that time, gradual mobilization is initiated. Sequential roentgenograms at two-week intervals are indicated to insure that displacement has not occurred.

Even with appropriate aggressive treatment of a Monteggia fracture, the results in follow-up are not always good. It was Watson-Jones' feeling that 95 per cent of patients with this type of fracture may have some permanent disability.[50] In the review by Bruce and his associates, only 24 per cent of adult Monteggia fractures had acceptable results.[10] Therefore, it can be easily appreciated that this type of injury is very severe and carries a guarded prognosis even with the best treatment.

OPEN FOREARM FRACTURES

Open fractures of the forearm are treated by initial aggressive irrigation and debridement in the operating room. If the wound is large and appears to be grossly contaminated, it is best to treat it by open packing with Betadine-soaked sponges, followed by elective secondary closure at five to seven days, or by allowing healing by granulation tissue after removal of the packing. The patient is at risk if primary closure is attempted as the initial procedure, even following appropriate irrigation and debridement. Some form of drainage must be supplied to prevent a catastrophe.

Once the wound has healed and the patient is responding systemically, definitive treatment of the forearm fractures may be initiated. If a fracture of both bones of the forearm is present and the wound has healed satisfactorily after seven to ten days, it may be appropriate to consider open reduction and internal fixation with the use of compression plates as a definitive procedure. As discussed in Chapter 30, it is important to obtain cultures and to initiate appropriate intravenous antibiotics at the time of initial treatment of these open wounds.

Nonunion of Forearm Fractures

The incidence of nonunion of forearm fractures has certainly decreased since the development of compression plates. The rigid immobilization provided by compression plates appears to stimulate healing (Fig. 18–16). Most cases of nonunion encountered in modern practice are secondary to closed methods of treatment or to inadequate internal fixation. A closed reduction with remaining displacement of the fracture fragments will end in nonunion in a high percentage of cases.

The author continues to see several examples of nonunion of forearm fractures secondary to initial treatment with Rush rods as the internal fixation device. The standard Rush rod does not provide adequate fixation for these fractures and its use

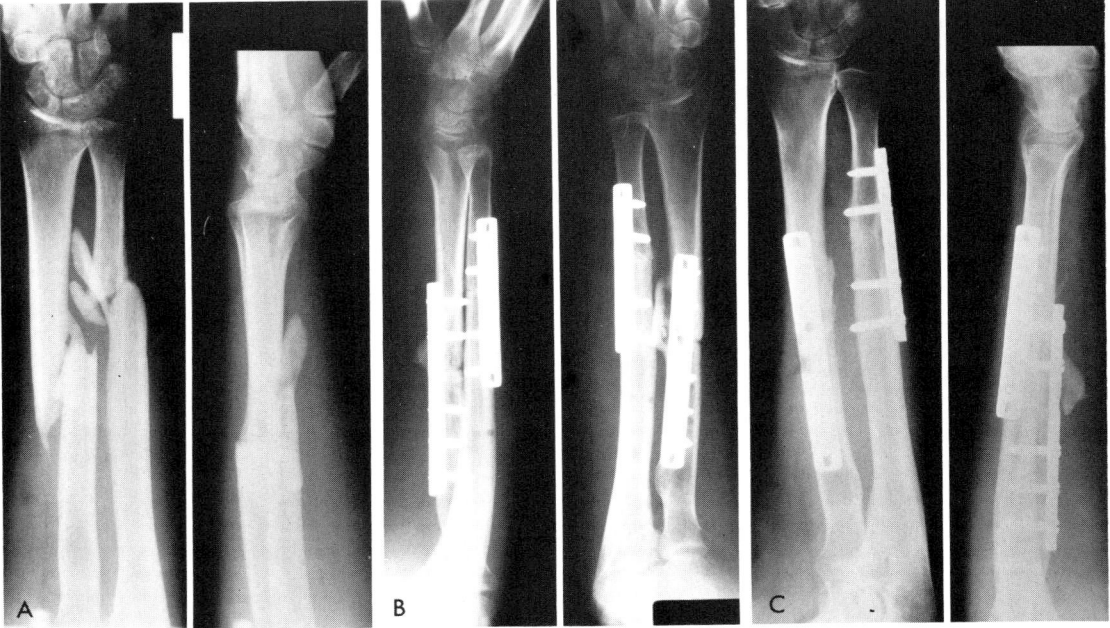

Figure 18–16 *A.* Nonunion of a fracture of both bones of the forearm. *B.* Open reduction and internal fixation with compression plates and an iliac crest bone graft. Note the improvement in alignment of the fractures. Active compression at the fracture site also stimulated healing. *C.* The fractures went on to uneventful healing at three months postoperatively.

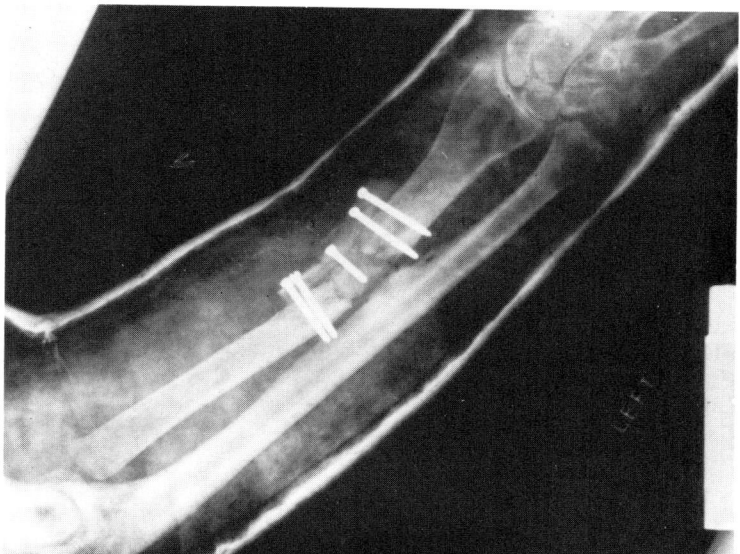

Figure 18–17 An alternate way to treat nonunion. This is a comminuted fracture of the midshaft of the radius treated with a large iliac crest onlay bone graft.

may result in nonunion. Likewise, forearm fractures treated with a compression plate for one bone and a Rush rod for the other bone will frequently result in nonunion of the bone that was treated with the Rush rod. Once again, this appears to be due to inadequate fixation, since the forearm bone treated with the compression plate will often heal.

The incidence of nonunion of comminuted fractures of the forearm can certainly be decreased by the addition of an iliac crest bone graft at the time of open reduction and internal fixation with compression plates (Fig. 18–17). It is a good rule of thumb to apply a bone graft in the presence of comminution.

As in other operative procedures, there is no room for inadequate surgical technique during open reduction and internal fixation. An improperly applied compression plate not only increases the incidence of nonunion but also exposes the patient to the risk of infection. There is no substitute for good surgical technique during the insertion of compression plates. This is particularly true of forearm fractures, since compression plating is frequently employed in the management of these injuries.

Nonunion associated with a significant loss of bone in the forearm is a very difficult problem to treat. If infection has been ruled out, a useful technique is to insert a piece of the fibula or a large portion of the iliac crest in the bone defect and then apply a compression plate to span the bone graft, with fixation to the proximal and distal portions of the remaining bone. A lengthy time interval is required for incorporation of these large portions of bone, but this technique does have merit. In all likelihood, it probably takes one to one-and-a-half years for the incorporation of a large bone graft spanning an osseous defect. An alternative form of treatment for nonunion with a large osseous defect is to apply dual onlay bone grafts to bridge the defect.

If attempts to span a large radial defect fail, it is sometimes best to consider a fusion of the distal ulna to the carpal bones in order to provide some stability to the forearm. A functional extremity may be salvaged by this procedure.

CROSS UNION OF FOREARM FRACTURES

Fortunately, this complication is not frequent if adequate compression plating techniques are utilized. During the insertion of compression plates it is important to limit the soft tissue dissection as much as possible, or cross union of the forearm bones may result. This complication has been seen in closed management of forearm fractures with inappropriate reduction. Significant displacement of the fracture fragments and a narrowing of the interosseous space may act as a stimulus to cross union.

It is fair to state that once this complication develops it is extremely difficult to manage. If the position of the hand is satsifactory, then the treatment of choice is often to refrain from any further operative procedures. However, this is not true if the hand is not in a good position of function. Under these conditions an osteotomy of the forearm bones may be indicated in order to place the hand in a more functional position.

Very occasionally a synostosis of the forearm bones may be treated successfully if the interposing bone is resected and a Silastic membrane is inserted between the bones. However, patients must be advised that the success rate of this procedure is very low.

REFERENCES

1. Anderson, L. D.: Compression plate fixation and the effect of different types of internal fixation on fracture healing. J. Bone Joint Surg., *47A*:191–208, 1965.
2. Anderson, L. D., Sisk, T. D., Tooms, R. E., and Park, W. I.: Compression-plate fixation in acute diaphyseal fractures of the radius and ulna. J. Bone Joint Surg., *57A*:287–297, 1975.
3. Bado, J. L.: The Monteggia lesion. Clin. Orthop., *50*:71–76, 1967.
4. Boyd, H. B.: Surgical approaches. *In* Crenshaw, A. H. (ed.): Campbell's Operative Orthopaedics, Vol. 1, 5th Ed. St. Louis, C. V. Mosby, 1971.
5. Boyd, H. B.: Surgical exposure of the ulna and proximal third of the radius through one incision. Surg. Gynecol. Obstet., *71*:86–88, 1940.
6. Boyd, H. B., Lipinski, S. W., and Wiley, J. H.: Observations on non-union of the shafts of the long bones, with a statistical analysis of 842 patients. J. Bone Joint Surg., *43A*:159–167, 1961.
7. Boyd, H. B., and Boals, J. C.: The Monteggia lesion. A review of 150 cases. Clin. Orthop., *66*:94–100, 1969.
8. Bradford, C. H., Adams, R. W., and Kilfoyle, R. M.: Fractures of both bones of the forearm in adults. Surg. Gynecol. Obstet., *96*:240–244, 1953.
9. Brav, E. A.: Further evaluation of the use of intramedullary nailing in the treatment of gunshot fractures of the extremities. J. Bone Joint Surg., *39A*:513–520, 1957.
10. Bruce, H. E., Harvey, J. P., and Wilson, J. C.: Monteggia fractures. J. Bone Joint Surg., *56A*:1563–1576, 1974.
11. Burwell, H. N., and Charnley, A. D.: Treatment of forearm fractures in adults with particular reference to plate fixation. J. Bone Joint Surg., *46B*:404–424, 1964.
12. Caden, J. G.: Internal fixation of fractures of the forearm. J. Bone Joint Surg., *43A*:1115–1121, 1961.
13. Campbell, W. C., and Boyd, H. B.: Fixation of onlay bone grafts by means of Vitallium screws in the treatment of unusual fractures. Am. J. Surg., *51*:748–756, 1941.
14. Dodge, H. S., and Cady, G. W.: Treatment of fractures of the radius and ulna with compression plates: a retrospective study of one hundred and nineteen fractures in seventy-eight patients. J. Bone Joint Surg., *54A*:1167–1176, 1972.
15. Eggers, G. W. N.: Internal contact splint. J. Bone Joint Surg., *30A*:40–51, 1948.
16. Eggers, G. W. M., Shindler, T. O., and Pomerat, C. M.: The influence of the contact–compression factor on osteogenesis in surgical fractures. J. Bone Joint Surg., *31A*:693–716, 1949.
17. Evans, E. M.: Pronation injuries of forearm with special reference to anterior Monteggia fracture. J. Bone Joint Surg., *31B*:578–588, 1949.
18. Evans, E. M.: Rotational deformity in the treatment of fractures of both bones of the forearm. J. Bone Joint Surg., 27:373–379, 1945.
19. Galeazzi, R.: Arch. Orthop. Unfallchir., *35*:557–562, 1934.
20. Henry, A. K.: Extensile Exposure. 2nd Ed. Baltimore, Williams & Wilkins, 1957.
21. Heppenstall, R. B., Littooy, F. N., Fuchs, R., Sheldon, G. F., and Hunt, T. K.: Gas tensions in healing tissues of traumatized patients. Surgery, 75:874–880, 1974.
22. Hicks, J. H.: Fracture forearm treatment by rigid fixation. J. Bone Joint Surg., *43B*:680–687, 1961.
23. Hughston, J. C.: Fracture of the distal radial shaft. Mistakes in management. J. Bone Joint Surg., *39A*:249–264, 1957.
24. Jinkins, W. J., Lockhart, L. D., and Eggers, G. W. N.: Fractures of the forearm in adults. South. Med. J.,53:669–679,1960.
25. Knight, R. A., and Purvis, G. D.: Fractures of both bones of the forearm in adults. J. Bone Joint Surg., *31A*:755–764, 1949.
26. Lam, S. J. S.: Delayed internal fixation for fractures of the radial shaft. Guy's Hosp. Rep., *114*:391–400, 1965.
27. Lam, S. J. S.: The place of delayed internal fixation in the treatment of fractures of the long bones. J. Bone Joint Surg., *46B*:393–397, 1964.
28. Marek, F. M.: Axial fixation of forearm fractures. J. Bone Joint Surg., *43A*:1099–1114, 1961.
29. Mickić, Z.: Galeazzi fracture–dislocations. J. Bone Joint Surg., *57A*:1071–1079, 1975.
30. Monteggia, G. B.: Instituzioni Chirurgiche. Vol. 5. Milan, Maspero, 1814.
31. Müller, M. E., Allgower, M., and Willenegger, H.: Technique of internal fixation of fractures. New York, Springer-Verlag, 1965.
32. Naiman, P. T., Schein, A. J., and Seiffert, R. S.: Use of ASIF compression plates in selected shaft fractures of the upper extremity. Clin. Orthop., *71*:208–217, 1970.
33. Patrick, J.: A study of supination and pronation, with special reference to the treatment of forearm fractures. J. Bone Joint Surg., 28:737–748, 1946.

34. Peiro, A., Andres, F., and Fernandez-Esteve, F.: Acute Monteggia lesions in children. J. Bone Joint Surg., *59A*:92–97, 1977.
35. Penrose, J. H.: The Monteggia fracture with posterior dislocation of radial head. J. Bone Joint Surg., *33B*:65–73, 1951.
36. Reckling, F. W., and Cordell, L. D.: Unstable fracture–dislocations of the forearm. The Monteggia and Galeazzi lesions. Arch. Surg., *96*:999–1007, 1968.
37. Ritchie, S. J., Richardson, J. P., and Thompson, M. S.: Rigid medullary fixation of forearm fractures. South. Med. J., *51*:852–856, 1958.
38. Sage, F. P.: Medullary fixation of fractures of the forearm. A study of the medullary canal of the radius and a report of fifty fractures of the radius treated with a prebent triangular nail. J. Bone Joint Surg., *41A*:1489–1516, 1959.
39. Sargent, J. P., and Teipner, W. A.: Treatment of forearm shaft fractures by double plating. A preliminary report. J. Bone Joint Surg., *47A*:1475–1490, 1965.
40. Sarmiento, A., Cooper, J., and Sinclair, W. F.: Forearm fractures–early functional bracing. A preliminary report. J. Bone Joint Surg., *57A*:297–304, 1975.
41. Sarmiento, A., Kinman, P. B., Murphy, R. B., and Phillips, J. G.: Treatment of ulnar fractures by functional bracing. J. Bone Joint Surg., *58A*:1104–1107, 1976.
42. Smith, F. M.: Monteggia fractures; analysis of 25 consecutive fresh injuries. Surg. Gynecol. Obstet., *85*:630–640, 1947.
43. Smith, H., and Sage, F. P.: Medullary fixation of forearm fractures. J. Bone Joint Surg., *39A*:91–98, 1957.
44. Smith, J. E. M.: Internal fixation in the treatment of fractures of the shaft of the radius and ulna in adults. J. Bone Joint Surg., *41B*:122–131, 1959.
45. Speed, J. S., and Boyd, H. B.: Treatment of fractures of the ulna with dislocation of head of radius (Monteggia fracture). J.A.M.A., *115*:1699–1704, 1940.
46. Spinner, M.: The anterior interosseous nerve syndrome. J. Bone Joint Surg., *52A*:84–94, 1970.
47. Thompson, J. E.: Anatomical methods of approach in operations on the long bones of the extremities. Ann. Surg., *68*:309–329, 1918.
48. Valande, M.: Luxation en arriere du cubitus avec fracture de la diaphyse radiale. Bull. Mem. Soc. Chir. Paris, *55*:435–437, 1929.
49. Venable, C. S.: An impacting bone plate to attain close apposition. Ann. Surg., *133*:808–812, 1951.
50. Watson-Jones, R.: Fractures and Joint Injuries, Vol. 2, 4th Ed. Edinburgh, E & S Livingstone, 1955.
51. Whiteside, L., and Lesker, P. A.: The effects of extraperiosteal and subperiosteal dissection. I. On blood flow in muscle. J. Bone Joint Surg., *60A*:23–25, 1978.
52. Whiteside, L., and Lesker, P. A.: The effects of extraperiosteal and subperiosteal dissection II. On fracture healing. J. Bone Joint Surg., *60A*:26–30, 1978.

A. LEE OSTERMAN, M.D.

and

F. WILLIAM BORA, JR., M.D.

19 _____ Injuries of the Wrist

INTRODUCTION

The wrist is the foundation of the hand and, as such, injuries can disable its basic function. Finger stiffness and weakness of grip following fractures of the distal radius, the painful grip of an ununited navicular, and persistent symptoms after a trivial wrist sprain are all common occurrences. Kaplan[11] defines the wrist as extending from the radial metaphysis to the metacarpal, and Flatt[9] emphasizes its importance as the essential link of the forearm to the hand. Like a universal joint, the wrist has the mobility to place the hand in multiple spatial orientations. Such positioning, by altering the functional length of the extrinsic flexor and extensor tendons that cross the wrist, helps control and coordinate digital sweep and power. Once positioned, the bones, ligaments, and primary motors of the wrist provide the stable base necessary to support the functional forces generated, as in power grip. The consequences, therefore, of any wrist injury ultimately affect hand function and explain the finding of Bacorn and Kurtzke[23] in their follow-up study of wrist injury of a 24 per cent incidence of hand disability in a working population.

Wrist injuries are common, representing 14 per cent of all extremity injuries seen in our emergency room. They present difficulties not only in treatment but in diagnosis. The latter problem relates to the complexity of the wrist with its kaleidoscopic radiographic appearance and its 21 separate articulations with their network of ligamentous connections. Thus, the functional anatomy and dynamics of the wrist must precede any discussion of pathology.

RADIOCARPAL AND DISTAL RADIOULNAR JOINTS

SURGICAL ANATOMY

The wrist is subdivided into the following anatomical units (Fig. 19–1): radius and radiocarpal joint, ulna and distal radioulnar joint, carpal mechanism, and carpometacarpal articulations. For comprehensive anatomy the reader is referred to other texts;[11, 15, 17] this discussion will be directed to clinical situations.

The radius, which plays a secondary role at the elbow, becomes the dominant bone at the wrist, being responsible for the entire bony articulation between the forearm and the hand and thus subject to the major forces in falls on the outstretched hand. This shock-absorbing role is compromised by the cancellous structure and thin cortical veneer of the flared distal radius. Four surfaces as well as the radiocarpal joint are present at this level (Fig. 19–2). The posterior surface is slightly convex, with grooves locating the extensor tendons. This close apposition of tendon and bone is especially

504

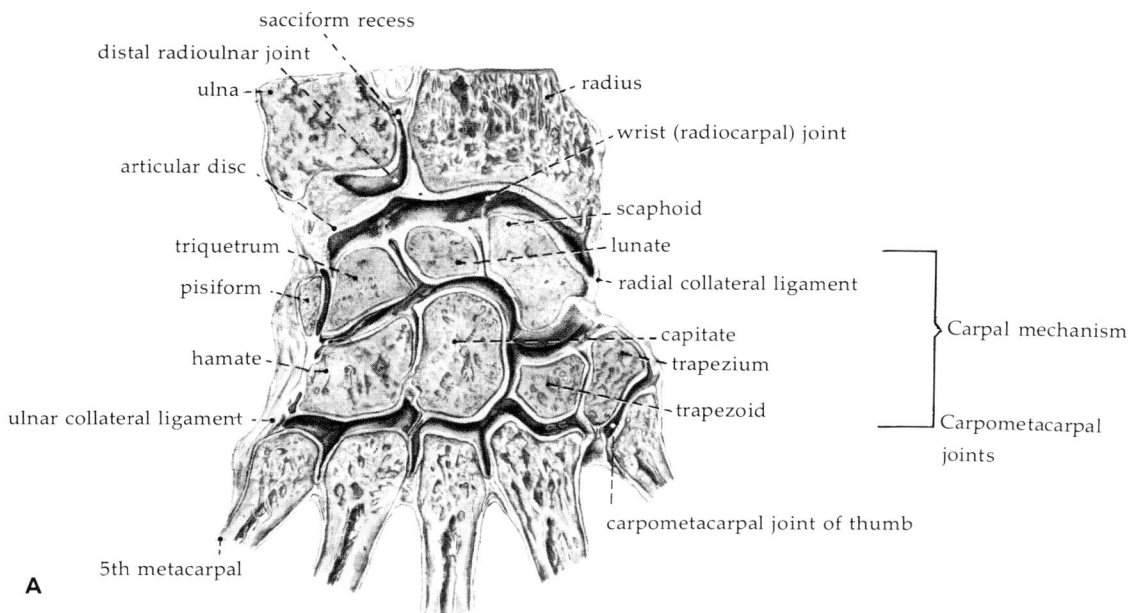

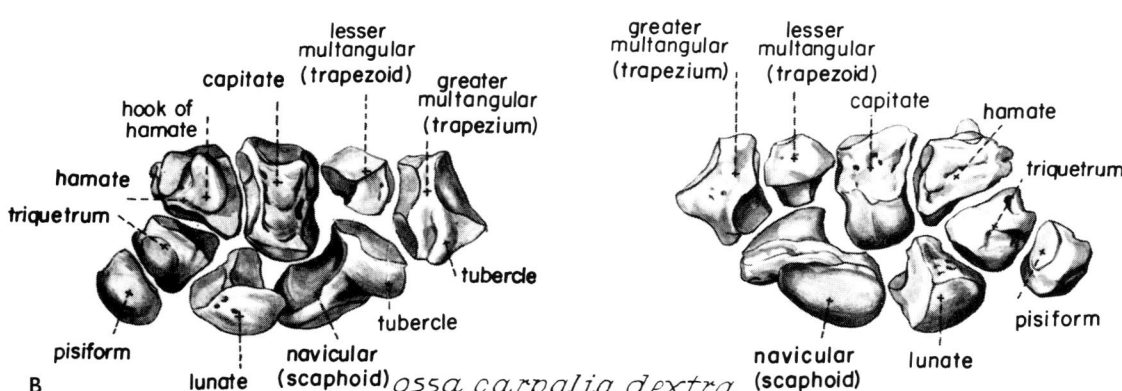

Figure 19-1   A. Frontal section of the wrist showing the elbow-shaped distal radioulnar joint, the radiocarpal joint, the carpal mechanism, and the carpometacarpal joints. *B*. Gross anatomy of the carpal bones. (Courtesy of J. Langman and M. W. Woerdeman and the W. B. Saunders Company. Atlas of Medical Anatomy, 1978.)

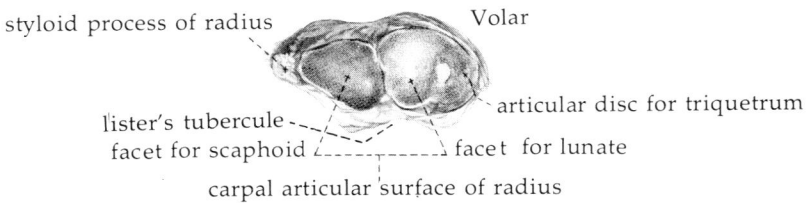

styloid process of radius | Volar
lister's tubercule
facet for scaphoid | articular disc for triquetrum
facet for lunate
carpal articular surface of radius

A. Articular surface of right radius and ulna for carpal bones.

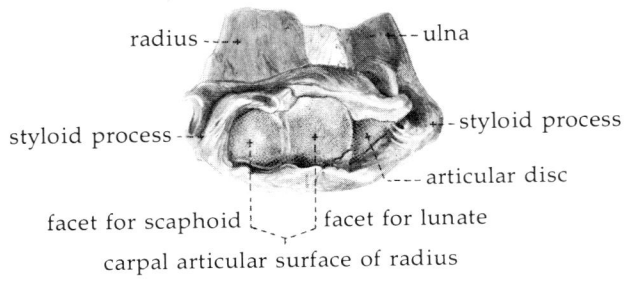

radius — ulna
styloid process — styloid process
— articular disc
facet for scaphoid | facet for lunate
carpal articular surface of radius

B. Proximal articular surface of right radius and ulna for carpal bones.

Figure 19–2 End-on view of the articular surface of the radius, showing the individual facets of the navicular and the lunate as well as the triangular fibrocartilage. Note Lister's tubercle on the dorsum of the radius, a frequent site of extensor tendon rupture following Colles' fracture. (Courtesy of J. Langman and M. W. Woerdeman and the W. B. Saunders Company. Atlas of Medical Anatomy, 1978.)

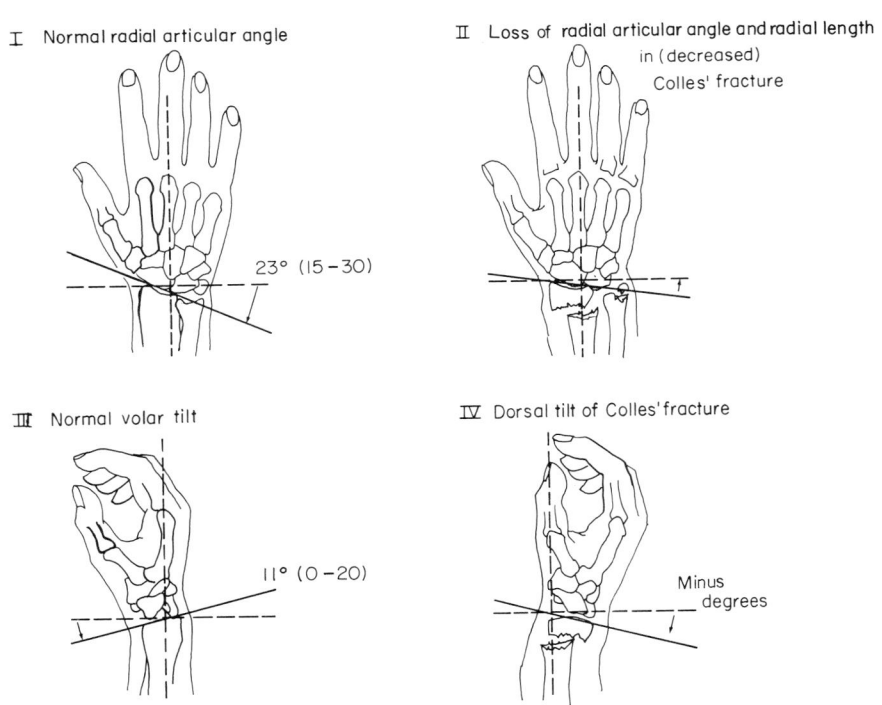

I Normal radial articular angle   23° (15–30)

II Loss of radial articular angle and radial length in (decreased) Colles' fracture

III Normal volar tilt   11° (0–20)

IV Dorsal tilt of Colles' fracture   Minus degrees

Figure 19–3 Measurements of the distal radius in normal wrists and in those with Colles' fracture. On the antero-posterior film the normal radius has an articular tilt, measured from the tip of the radial styloid to its medial border, of 23 degrees, with a range of 15 to 30 degrees. The radial styloid extends an average of 12 mm distal to the medial articular surface. In Colles' fracture both radial articular angle and radial length are decreased, as seen in Figure 19–2. On the lateral film the radius has a normal volar tilt of 11 degrees, with a range of 0 to 20 degrees. In Colles' fracture, the distal radius is angulated dorsally (see Fig. 19–4). Restoration of normal volar tilt is almost never seen following Colles' fracture.

true of the extensor pollicis longus, which crosses a dorsal prominence known as Lister's tubercle, and is a frequent site of posttraumatic rupture. Laterally, the bone projects to the radial styloid, site of both the brachioradialis insertion and the radial collateral ligament attachment. The tip of the styloid projects beyond the distal radioulnar joint an average of 12 mm, and from it the radial articular surface slopes ulnarward an average of 23 degrees (Fig. 19–3).[32] These measurements, made from an anteroposterior x-ray, are useful in determining the degree of radial shortening following radial fracture. Medially, the radius has an articular cartilage–lined concavity that articulates with ulna (see Fig. 19–1). The anterior surface is also concave and covered by the pronator quadratus, over which the flexor tendons and median nerve pass as they enter the carpal canal.

The radiocarpal joint is the synovial lined articulation between the forearm and the hand. Its joint surface tilts volarly as well as ulnarward and has two concave facets that articulate with the navicular and lunate (see Fig. 19–2). This volar tilt, seen in the lateral x-ray, averages 12 degrees and is used as a measure of dorsal radial displacement (Fig. 19–3). In fractures of the distal radius, the medial third of the radiocarpal joint is formed by the articulation of the triangular fibrocartilage (articular disk) and the triquetrum (Fig. 19–4). This fibrocartilage originates from the medial aspect of

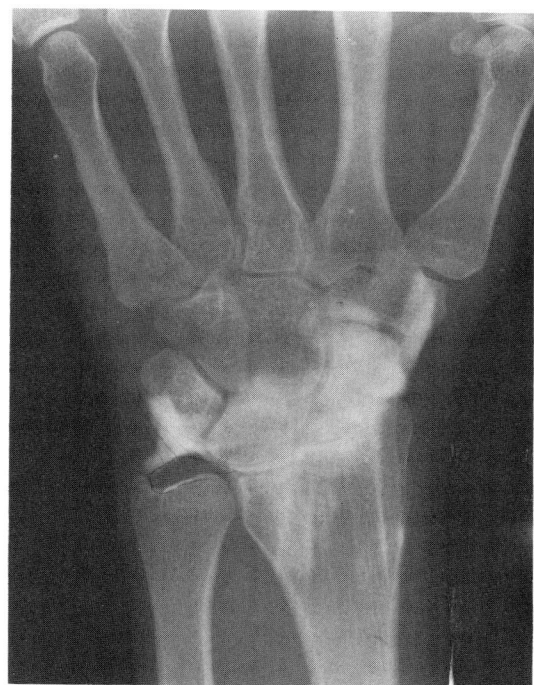

Figure 19–5 Normal arthrogram. Dye has been injected into the radiocarpal joint. The intact triangular fibrocartilage prevents dye from entering the distal radioulnar joint. The prestyloid recess is also clearly seen as a diverticulum on the left side of the arthrogram.

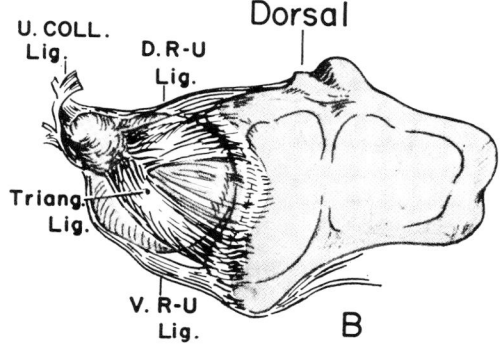

Figure 19–4 Triangular fibrocartilage. The triangular fibrocartilage stands out from its insertion on the ulnar aspect of the radius just medial to the lunate facet and inserts at the base of the ulnar styloid. It is reinforced both dorsally and volarly by radioulnar ligaments. The ulnar collateral ligament can also be seen arising from the medial aspect of the base of the ulnar styloid. (Courtesy of D. G. Vesely and *Clinical Orthopaedics and Related Research. Clin. Orthop. Rel. Res., 51:75, 1967.)*

the radius and inserts at the base of the ulnar styloid, separating the radiocarpal from the distal radioulnar joint and isolating the ulna from direct articulation with the carpal bones (Fig. 19–5). In 30 to 60 per cent of cases, however, this cartilage is perforated, allowing communication between the two joints.[17, 21, 79] Such perforations can be seen on arthrograms but also may occur as asymptomatic age-related degeneration. The radiocarpal joint may also communicate with the midcarpal joints through defects in the carpal interosseous ligaments.

Motion at the wrist joint consists of volar flexion and dorsiflexion (extension) and radial and ulnar deviation. Pronation and supination are forearm motions involving the radioulnar joints. The standard normal values of these ranges of motion are as follows.

Wrist

Dorsiflexion: 0 to 80 degrees
Volar flexion: 0 to 85 degrees

Ulnar deviation: 0 to 35 degrees
Radial deviation: 0 to 20 degrees
Forearm
Pronation: 0 to 90 degrees
Supination: 0 to 90 degrees

Controversy arises when attempts are made to separate these motions into precise joint contributions. The classic argument is that the radiocarpal joint participates primarily in volar flexion and ulnar deviation, while dorsiflexion and radial deviation are midcarpal motions.[11, 94] However, some have claimed that the reverse is true.[87, 95, 96] These differing interpretations serve to emphasize that movement occurs simultaneously at the radiocarpal and the midcarpal joints throughout wrist motion. This will be discussed fully in the section dealing with the carpal mechanism. The origin of pronation and supination at the wrist in relationship to the distal radioulnar joint is clear.

At its distal end the ulnar shaft expands into a bulbous head and styloid process. The lateral two thirds of the head is articular cartilage, which forms the corresponding gliding surface around which the radius rotates through an arc of 150 degrees.[84] The phylogenetic history of the ulna is one of progressive retreat from the carpus,[17] and this leads to a variable relationship between the radial articular surface and the ulnar head. In approximately 60 per cent of cases they are equal, while in 15 per cent the ulna is longer, and in 25 per cent it is shorter.[97, 130] The last-named type, called negative ulnar variance or simply ulna minus, is associated with an increased incidence of aseptic necrosis of the lunate (Kienböck's disease).

Likewise, the styloid process has a variable extension beyond the head, although it usually terminates about 1 cm proximal to the radial styloid. The extensor carpi ulnaris tendon lies in a fixed fibro-osseous sheath on the posterior aspect of the ulna, lateral to the styloid. With the ulna's adjustment to full pronation, its functional pull is that of an ulnar deviator rather than a wrist extensor.[20] The ulnar styloid lies within a synovial diverticulum, the prestyloid recess. This cavity communicates with the radiocarpal joint and is bounded proximally by triangular fibrocartilage, medially by the ulnar collateral ligament, and distally by the ulnotriquetral ligament, a meniscoid-type

structure first emphasized by Lewis.[17] It can be clearly seen in arthrograms of the wrist (Fig. 19–5), isolated in this synovial lined recess and often one of the earliest target sites of rheumatoid arthritis. The neck and tip of the ulnar styloid have no direct ligamentous attachments. Such attachments are at the base, with the thickened insertion of the triangular fibrocartilage laterally and the ulnar collateral ligament medially. As such, most styloid fractures represent avulsion fractures and occur at this basal level.

As mentioned, the triangular fibrocartilage divides the radiocarpal joint from the L-shaped distal radioulnar joint. The vertical limb of the joint lies between the ulnar head and the radial notch, and the horizontal limb between the ulnar head and the triangular fibrocartilage. The capsule is lax in order to accommodate the 150 degree radial arc of motion. The restraints of this considerable range of motion are both intrinsic and extrinsic to the joint. The intrinsic stability derives from the triangular fibrocartilage, which blends with the volar and dorsal radioulnar ligaments (see Fig. 19–4). These thickened bands are taut in phase with rotation, the volar being tight in supination and the dorsal in pronation.[68, 73, 79, 84] The depth and bony configuration of the articulation is an additional element in intrinsic stability.

Extrinsic stabilizers are related to the rotational position of the joint and include the checkrein effect of the extensor carpi ulnaris,[20] the pronator quadratus,[16] the crossed radial and ulnar shafts in pronation,[18] and the interosseous membrane. The oblique fibers of the last-named structure tighten as a fist is made and thus protect the distal radioulnar joint from diastasis. Lastly, it should be pointed out that any shortening of one of the forearm bones or loss of elbow biomechanics alters the function of the distal radioulnar joint. Subluxations of this joint have been described as an aftereffect of both radial head fracture[71] and radial head excision.[83]

The 180 degree arc of pronation and supination available at the wrist requires several adjustments. The radius rotates 150 degrees about a relatively fixed ulnar head such that their shafts are completely crossed. Proximal radial head rotation within its orbicular ligament and the corresponding bowing of both the radial and the ulnar shafts are essential for full movement.

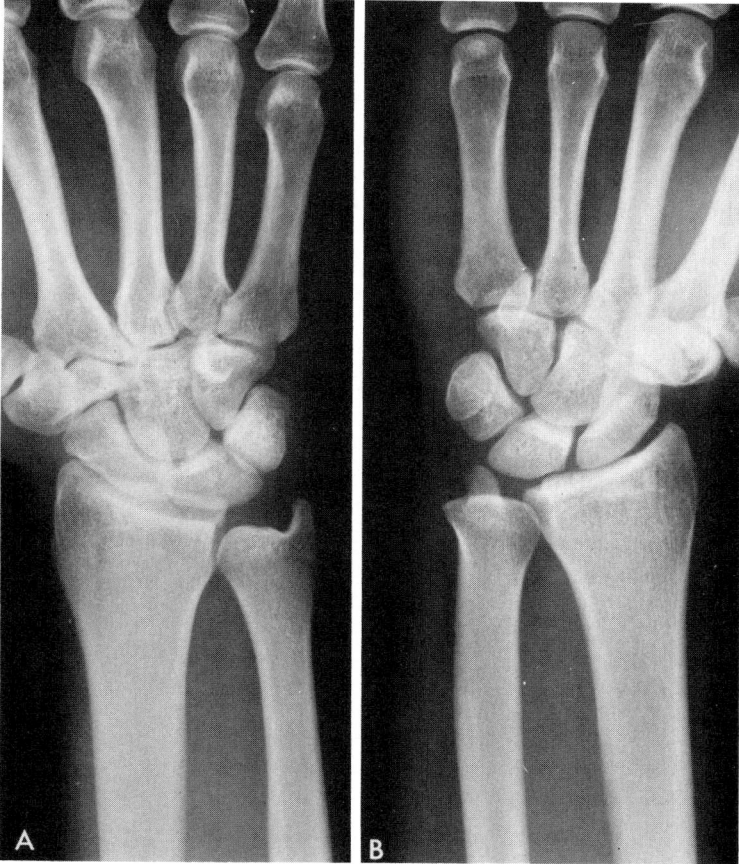

Figure 19–6 *A* and *B* Normal right wrist in pronation and supination. It is well to remember that the radius rotates around the relatively fixed ulna. The ulnar styloid does seem to change position during this motion, however, so that it is medial and anterior in full pronation (*A*). In full supination it is central and posterior (*B*). In injury to the distal radioulnar joint, loss of this ulnar styloid positioning may be seen.

The ulnar head also shifts through a smaller arc, moving dorsally in pronation and volarly in supination. In pronation the ulnar styloid lies medially, moving to a central and volar position in supination. This anatomical relationship between the distal ulna and radius is a useful guideline on anteroposteror roentgenograms (Fig. 19–6); when disturbed, it suggests injury to the distal radioulnar joint.

MECHANISMS OF INJURY

The wrist is the major shock absorber in a fall on the outstretched hand. The factors that determine the specific injury that results are the position of the wrist at impact, the physical properties of the bones and ligaments, the magnitude of the injuring force, and the rate at which the stress is applied.

A force directed against the palm of a dorsiflexed wrist displaces fragments differently from a similar force against the dorsum of a volar flexed wrist. In fractures of the distal radius, the former results in the common dorsal angulation of the Colles fracture, the latter in the rarer volar displacement of a Smith fracture. In the original 1847 description of his eponymic fracture, Smith noted that the mechanism of his patient's injury was a fall on the back of the hand "in endeavoring to save himself from being run over."[63] Yet this simple mechanism does not explain the variety of lesions resulting from falls on the outstretched wrist: distal radial fractures with or without ulnar fractures, navicular fractures, and other carpal fractures and dislocations.

As early as 1908[39] investigations were begun on loading the dorsiflexed wrist. By strapping cadaver arms to his body and then falling on them, Lilienfeldt noted that distal radial fractures resulted when the wrist was dorsiflexed between 60 and 90 degrees. Dorsiflexion of greater than 90 degrees produced carpal injury. He also noted that if these dynamically loaded wrists were in ulnar deviation, an associated fracture of the radial styloid was present, and conversely that radial deviation impact produced a fracture of the ulnar styloid. Frykman,[33] in his excellent thesis, reported similar findings and consistent fracture types with both static and dynamic loading of cadaver limbs. Interestingly, the greater the dorsiflexion, the greater was the force required to fracture the distal radius and the more likely were navicular and other carpal injuries. Weber and Chao[121] confirmed the extreme of dorsiflexion necessary for navicular fracture by consistently creating navicular waist fractures in wrists loaded in 95 degrees of dorsiflexion and 10 degrees of radial deviation. This radial deviation assured the thenar impact of the load and concentrated the force across the navicular waist.

All bones fail initially in tension. The aforementioned loading conditions producing specific injuries correlate with the combination of tensile loads transmitted at the wrist ligaments and the compressive contact loads of the opposed bony surfaces. In the dorsally angulated Colles fracture, therefore, these compound loads initiate failure on the volar cortex of the radius and, as the force proceeds, compression of the dorsal cortex. In the navicular waist fracture, the proximal pole is tethered by the taut radionavicular and naviculolunate ligaments besides being wedged between the radius and the capitate. The distal pole, being the site of applied load and lacking such stabilizers, continues to dorsiflex. When this dorsiflexion exceeds 95 degrees the bending moment is magnified and concentrated in the critical waist area. The fracture begins on the volar surface of the navicular waist at the junction between the fixed proximal pole and the unsupported distal pole.[121]

Rotational stresses add a further dimension to the pathomechanics of injury. Forearm pronation and supination are clearly primary loading forces in dislocations of the distal radioulnar joint, but they are also complicating forces in other wrist injuries. Pronation has been implicated as a primary force in the majority of Smith's

fractures.[60] In this mechanism the fall is broken by the supinated palm, while the forearm and body weight pivot around it as a fixed axis.

Aside from the direction of the force, both the magnitude and the rate of loading determine the type of injury produced. Both these factors must exceed a certain critical value that is dependent on the physical properties of the bone and soft tissue prior to fracture. Given the age-related changes in these structures, the degree of trauma needed to produce a distal radial fracture varies inversely with age.[1] The equivalent fracture in a child or older adult following a simple fall requires a fall from a height or a traffic accident in a young adult. Such age-related differences might also be expected to apply to the rate of applied load, with a more slowly applied stress causing fracture in the older age group. Little specific information, however, is available on the rate of applied load to wrist injury. From similar areas of investigation, however, one would predict that more rapidly applied stress would result in ligamentous or dislocation injuries.

While proportional to both the amount and the rate of the applied load, the extent and nature of the injury are also related to certain endogenous factors. First is the anatomical peculiarity of the region — for example, the contact surface of the distal radius with the carpus and the lack of such contact by the ulna. Second, there is a progressive change in the resistance of bone to fracture, which is both age- and sex-dependent. The fragility of the distal radius seen in epiphyseal separation injuries of children peaks in the 5- to 15-year-old group. Here the cartilaginous growth plate is the weakest link, and this determines the site of injury.[57, 62, 65] Interestingly, in children under five, whose bones are relatively elastic, torus fractures and other nonepiphyseal injuries are most common.

There is a dramatic rise in distal wrist fractures in postmenopausal women that parallels the decreased severity of the traumatic mechanism.[1] It is tempting to attribute this increased fragility of the bone to the corresponding increase in osteoporosis. Although no direct evidence of this link is forthcoming, several observations suggest its relevance. The tensile strength required to break the distal radius is 50 per cent greater in the male skeleton.[1] According to Reifenstein,[13] osteoporosis is five times more prevalent in aging women than in men and develops rapidly at menopause. Lastly, while the nature of trauma is less severe, the greatest fracture displacement occurs in the aging population[1] and the incidence of secondary radial collapse is higher. This suggests inherent metaphyseal weakness in this group. In fact, some authors[1, 10] have suggested distal radial fracture as an index of osteoporosis.

The frequent cluster of distal radial fractures, fractures of the proximal femur, and vertebral body compression fractures is a pattern usually seen in postmenopausal women. The incidence of distal radial fractures in this group actually increases the risk of a subsequent fracture threefold. However, in the individual patient, overt evidence of generalized osteoporosis requiring treatment is a rarity, and identification of the conclusive defect in the increased fragility of bone awaits a better understanding of skeletal metabolism. It is safe to conclude, however, that the endogenous quality of the skeletal and ligamentous structures is the dominant factor in most fractures of the distal radius.

DISTAL RADIAL FRACTURES

Fractures of the distal radius, defined as those occurring within 3 cm of the radiocarpal joint, are one of the most common fractures in humans. They account for 10 per cent of all fractures seen in our adult emergency room and over 12 per cent of all fractures seen in the Children's Hospital of Philadelphia. They constitute over 80 per cent of all radial fractures seen. In an unselected population, the annual rate of incidence is difficult to ascertain. Data from defined populations in Scandinavia suggest that the annual fracture rate is in the neighborhood of 1 per 1,000.[1, 38] Such data are misleading, however, as they neglect age and sex statistics in regard to the incidence of this fracture. Postmenopausal women show a dramatic rise to an annual incidence of 54 per 10,000 because of the endogenous reasons already cited. It should be noted that this is four times the occurrence of hip fractures in the same group. Men do not show this dramatic increase,

and thus after age 50 the ratio of distal radial fractures in women to men is approximately seven or eight to one. An earlier peak incidence of these fractures occurs in children with open epiphyses, but here the sex distribution is equal.

Despite this frequency and the narrowly defined anatomical localization, distal radial fractures display infinite variety, behaving individually enough to lead some authors to conclude that no two distal radial fractures are alike. On the other hand, many loosely refer to any fracture of the distal radius as a Colles fracture. To avoid such confusion, many attempts have been made to categorize distal radius fractures into specific types. Most such classifications, however, have found no practical application. For example Ehalt's[38] detailed system describes 34 different groups. However, several classifications, including that of Destot,[7] have been adopted and recommended by later authors. Destot distinguished two main groups of distal radial fracture—anterior and posterior. He further divided them according to the line of fracture, differentiating extraarticular fractures, such as the classic Colles and Smith fractures, from those that are intraarticular, such as Barton's and radial styloid fractures. Most textbooks[5, 8, 12, 14] and articles[3, 33] have adopted this system.

With reference to the more common dorsally displaced distal radial fracture, two classifications have won recognition. In the first, that of Gartland and Werley,[34] three groups are differentiated:

1. Simple fractures not involving the joint surface.
2. Fractures involving the joint surface but without displacement of the fragment.
3. Comminuted fractures with the line of displaced fragments running into the joint surface.

DePalma,[29] Dowling,[30] and others have employed this system. Frykman[33] suggested eight categories, depending on the involvement of the articular surfaces of either the radiocarpal or the distal radioulnar joint and the presence or absence of a distal ulnar fracture. Articular damage and distal ulnar fracture carry a worse prognosis. Dobyns and Linscheid consider this the most logical outline.[8]

To be workable, any classification must contain several points.

1. It must be simple in order to be easily remembered.
2. It must organize the fracture pattern such that it may be easily recognized and in turn properly treated.
3. Given these implications for treatment, it should underline those factors that affect the functional end result.

The classification we have chosen together with the prognosis factors (Table 19–1) should fulfill these criteria. Although such simplification is an aid in diagnosis and treatment, it is not feasible for comparison of treatment results; a more detailed classification, such as Frykman's, should be used for this purpose.[33] A word should be added concerning the prognosis factors. In general, the greater the degree of articular surface involvement, the greater the initial displacement, the more comminuted the fracture site, and the more involved the ulnar side of the wrist, the worse the prognosis. It should also be noted that these factors possess parallel relationships, such that the more closely the degree of initial displacement coincides with the degree of comminution and the degree of shortening,

TABLE 19–1   Classification of Distal Radial Fractures

Type of Fracture
   I. Dorsal displacement
      A. Colles' fracture
         1. Extraarticular
         2. Intraarticular
            a. Dorsal rim fracture (dorsal Barton's)
  II. Volar displacement
      A. Smith's fracture
         1. Extraarticular
         2. Intraarticular
            a. Volar rim fracture (volar Barton's)
 III. Styloid fractures
      A. Radial (chauffeur's)
      B. Ulnar
 IV. Epiphyseal fractures

Prognosis Factors
   Articular surface involvement
   Initial displacement
   Degree of comminution
   Involvement of the ulnar side of the wrist, either as a styloid fracture or as damage to the distal radioulnar joint

the greater the disturbance in the normal distal radioulnar relationships. Most reports in the literature agree as to the prognostic value of these factors but differ on their relative importance. Our purpose is to alert the physician to the possibly complicated nature of the injury he may be treating.

It is common knowledge that fractures across joint surfaces that heal with imperfect anatomical surfaces and subsequent incongruity predispose the joint to arthritic changes. The distinction between articular and nonarticular fractures, however, is not always obvious. In Barton's fractures or in chauffeur's fracture, in which the fracture lines outline several major articular fragments, the extension into the radiocarpal joint is clear. However, in the older patient with a comminuted distal radial fracture, the injury to the distal articular cartilage is more difficult to define. With estimates of articular damage running from 33 per cent[33] to 88 per cent,[34] the discrepancy arises in determining its severity. Sevitt,[50] in a histological evaluation of classic healing Colles' fractures in an older population, found that 75 per cent of those fractures without marked x-ray evidence of surface damage had fissure fractures extending into the joint surface. We have used arthroscopy on several distal radial fractures and have noted similar fissure fractures not visible on roentgenograms. While such data tend to support those who find greater articular involvement in the comminuted distal radial fractures of the elderly, such damage is minor and usually heals uneventfully. The incidence of severe articular damage is therefore closer to the 20 to 30 per cent range.

The degree of initial displacement is a second prognostic factor. Fissure fractures and fracture-dislocations constitute clearly definable groups. Such simple fractures of the distal radius constitute approximately 12 to 15 per cent of radial fractures in most series, and there is little disagreement about treatment or final outcome. Fracture-dislocations, on the other hand, are rare, complicated injuries that have a guarded prognosis.[56] In Colles' fractures, the distinction has been made between fractures with dorsal angulation and those with more pronounced displacement of the fragments.[7, 25, 34, 38] Although some authors have questioned the significance of the initial displacement on the functional end results,[24, 33] such displacement correlates with either the severity of the injuring force in younger patients or the degree of comminution in older ones. Both of these influence the result.

When considering the factor of comminution, one must recall that the collapse of the fracture of the distal radius is really produced by the cancellous structure of the bone, similar to that in fractures of the calcaneus, vertebral body, and tibial plateau. As we shall see, anatomical reduction is often possible, but the cavities that remain from this compression of spongy bone do not become primarily filled with new bone but with clots of blood. These are thus unstable fractures, and settling of the fracture fragments is common despite adequate immobilization. In fact, this led Marsh[41] and others to conclude that the comminuted fracture regresses to a deformity practically identical to the one that was present initially. Where there exists a good buttress of bone against which the reduction can be maintained, shortening and collapse may be prevented. Fractures in the older age group, however, are almost by definition comminuted and predisposed to some degree of malunion.

Although most authors agree that the more anatomical the result the better the prognosis, there is less agreement on the primary question of whether the severely comminuted fracture, healing with a predictable malunion, has a markedly less favorable prognosis. We agree with those authors[22, 25, 26, 29, 32-35, 49] who claim a definite relationship between the degree of comminution of the fracture and the functional end results. In our series, approximately 20 per cent of distal radial fractures had enough comminution or intraarticular involvement or both to warrant more complicated treatment in order to avoid radial shortening, arthritis, and subsequent problems with the radioulnar joint.

The importance of the ulnar side of the wrist is emphasized in Frykman's classification[33] and in general throughout the Scandinavian literature. This involvement can take several forms: ulnar styloid fracture, injuries of the triangular fibrocartilage, instability of the distal radioulnar joint, and intraarticular fractures of this joint with late joint incongruity. Taylor and Parsons[82] clas-

sified distal radial fractures into two main groups, injury to the triangular disk being the determining factor. In their opinion, prognosis is governed to a great extent by the presence of these injuries. The incidence of ulnar injuries associated with distal radial fractures is quite high. Ulnar styloid avulsion fractures accompany radial fractures in approximately 60 per cent of cases.[23, 32, 38] Frank radial ulnar dislocation is quite rare, but in Weigl's series,[21] injuries of the triangular fibrocartilage were present in over 50 per cent of the fractures that were demonstrated arthrographically or operated on. Persistent ulnar joint problems affect the functional result in approximately 15 per cent of cases in most series.

Although not mentioned as a prognostic factor, age may have some influence on the functional results. As stated, there are three common ages for certain types of distal radial fractures: children under 16, young adults, and the middle-aged and elderly. In the older age group, in whom comminution and settling of the fragments are more frequent, the anatomical result is less exact but the functional result is often satisfactory. This may be because fewer demands are made on the wrist in this group.[38] In cases of residual deformity in young adults, however, increased symptomatology is noted. Also, we have found the greatest disability and the poorest results in fractures in young adults that are comminuted or intraarticular or both. These injuries, usually secondary to severe trauma and often resembling a typical Colles fracture, usually have marked soft tissue damage and a very guarded prognosis.

Colles' Fracture

In 1814, in a paper remarkable for its wealth of detail and accurate description, the Irish surgeon Abraham Colles described the dorsally displaced distal radial fracture that bears his name.[27] His description of a nonarticular fracture occurring 1½ inches proximal to the radiocarpal joint was meant to counteract the then prevalent belief that all injuries to the wrist were dislocations. The term has since been generalized to include any dorsally displaced fracture, regardless of joint involvement or comminution, that results from a fall on the extended wrist. The Colles fracture represents well over 90 per cent of all distal radial fractures.

The classic deformity in Colles' fracture has three components: (1) dorsal angulation of the distal radial articular cartilage; (2) loss of the normal ulnar slope of the radius with radial position of the hand; and (3) shortening and loss of radial length. The radial articular cartilage has a normal volar tilt of 12 degrees, with extremes of 4 degrees dorsal and 21 degrees volar (see Fig. 19–3). The hallmark of a dorsal fracture is the backward displacement and loss of volar tilt. The normal radial angle is 23 degrees, with a range of 15 to 30 degrees (see Fig. 19–3). Gartland[34] has pointed out that such radial deviation is often associated with a supination deformity of this distal fragment secondary to the deforming force of the brachioradialis.[47] Normally, the radial styloid projects 13 mm beyond the distal radioulnar surface, with an average of 8 to 18 mm; this is shortened in Colles' fracture. The reversal of the volar angle is the most difficult of the three deformities to correct, but fortunately it is the least disabling. Radial shortening with radial displacement of the hand is the most disabling and must be corrected by treatment. Earlier attempts,

however, to indict a single element of this classic displacement as the cause of poor functional results are misleading, and most failures in therapy of Colles' fracture show inferior restoration of all deformed parts.

These deformities explain the typical clinical appearance of a Colles fracture, which has been called the dinner fork deformity. Associated findings include marked swelling of the dorsal aspect of the wrist, point tenderness across the dorsum, and painful motion. On palpation of the ulnar side of the joint one may discover not only point tenderness but also a dorsal prominence of the ulna.

Roentgenograms should be obtained in at least two planes and preferably in three — anterior, lateral, and oblique. The anterior view shows radial shortening and loss of the radial slope (Fig. 19–7A). Articular involvement and bony comminution and any styloid fractures can also be observed. Oblique projections help in determining articular surface involvement. The lateral view (Fig. 19–7B) shows the degree of dorsal displacement. Disruption of the distal radioulnar joint also is apparent in the lateral view with either dorsal or volar displacement of the ulnar head. In

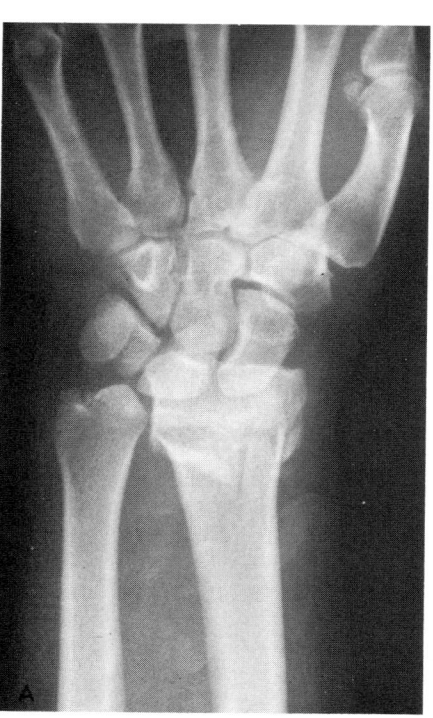
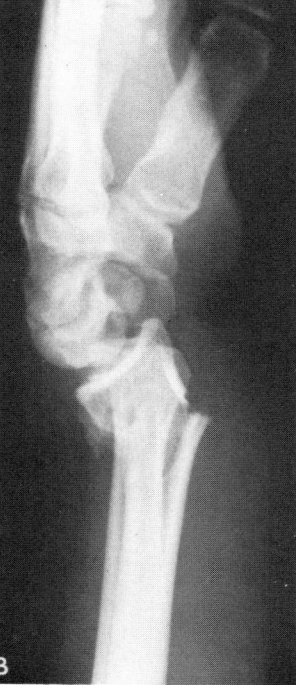

Figure 19–7 A. Anteroposterior roentgenogram of a classic Colles fracture. Note the radial shortening and loss of radial articular angle. *B.* Lateral view. The dorsal tilting of the articular surface is obvious.

cases that are anatomically confusing it is often helpful to obtain x-rays of the normal uninjured wrist. The films should be scanned for the presence of other injuries, such as carpal fracture or carpal displacement.

Treatment. The considerable controversy that surrounds the treatment of Colles' fracture centers on the following points: (1) method of reduction; (2) type of anesthesia used for reduction; (3) criteria for acceptable reduction; (4) position, type, and duration of immobilization; and (5) treatment of the severely comminuted intraarticular fracture. There is general agreement on the treatment of the fissure fracture, the nondisplaced fracture, and the fracture with minimal dorsal angulation: immobilization in a short arm cast for three to four weeks.

Over 85 per cent of Colles' fractures, however, require some reduction. Although it has been stated that there are as many methods of reduction as there are fracture surgeons, several basic maneuvers are involved in all methods. Two fundamental techniques are active manipulation and passive gravity traction. Jones and Charnley[4] popularized the former method of manipulative reduction of the fragment by dorsiflexion of the distal fragment followed by immediate volar flexion and then pronation to "lock" the fracture fragments in place. Throughout this procedure an assistant applies countertraction at the elbow.

The more popular method, especially when there is marked displacement or comminution, is a variation of the one first recommended by Böhler.[2] The patient is placed on the treatment table with the affected arm extending over the edge of the table at a 90 degree angle to the body. Finger trap traction is applied to the thumb and index and middle fingers, using either the web wire Japanese-type trap or the Weinberger apparatus. Countertraction is provided by a padded sling with 10 to 15 lb of weight placed over the humerus. Adequate anesthetization must be achieved prior to hanging in the finger traps. After 15 minutes of uninterrupted traction, radial length will be restored. Occasionally, some gentle manipulation of the fracture fragments is helpful.

Local, extremity block, and general anesthesia all have their place in the reduction of these fractures. The type used should be decided by the patient's general health, recent food intake, associated injury, anesthetic risk, and obesity and by the swelling and severity of the fracture. Local anesthesia is quick, simple, and adequate for most reductions. The technique involves the insertion of a 20-gauge needle under aseptic conditions into the fracture hematoma, aspiration of the hematoma, and injection of 10 to 20 ml of 1 per cent Xylocaine or 0.5 per cent Marcaine. With strict precautions we have not experienced sepsis as a complication of this method.

The argument that this converts a closed fracture to a potentially open one is probably overrated. If a patient has an ulnar styloid fracture or pain on the ulnar aspect of the wrist, it is often useful to inject this area as well prior to reduction. The patient may be given supplemental systemic medications, such as Valium, Demerol, or morphine. Extremity block and general anesthesia are used for displaced fractures when more complete muscular relaxation is needed or when operative intervention, such as pins in plaster, is planned.

The criteria for an acceptable reduction are not well established, owing to divergent opinion concerning the correlation between anatomical and functional results. Although good functional results are sometimes seen with poor anatomical results, it is a mistake to accept the poor reduction in the confidence that serious disability is a rare sequela, especially in the older patient. The general principle that the closer the fracture is to a joint the greater is the need to restore its exact anatomical relationships applies to the Colles fracture. We feel that radial shortening is the least acceptable deformity, because hand mobility and power are severely compromised if this length is not restored.[33, 34] DePalma felt that shortening of more than 4 mm contributes to an unsatisfactory result because of distal radioulnar problems.[29] Twenty-five degrees of dorsal tilt has been reported to be compatible with acceptable hand and wrist function. Follow-up studies have shown measurable volar tilt in as much as 70 to 80 per cent of Colles' fractures reported.[25, 29, 30, 33, 34, 36, 38, 48, 53] An articular surface that is perpendicular to the shaft, radial shortening of 2 mm or less, and good apposition of bony surfaces are the reduction objectives. Once these are accomplished, weekly x-ray studies for the subsequent three weeks are needed to be sure the reduction is maintained.

Immobilization of the Colles fracture is far from standardized, suggesting that none of the methods has afforded completely satisfactory results. This dissatisfaction is related to the recurrence of the original deformity. It is not surprising that the fractures that most often collapse are those with severe comminution, intraarticular involvement, or both. Owing to the cancellous structure of the distal radius, the injury produces a triangular zone of compression of the dorsal and radial aspects, which become cavities when the fracture is anatomically reduced. This gap is initially filled with hemorrhage, which is only gradually replaced by fibrous and cartilaginous tissue, finally changing to spongy bone that bridges the fragments.[50] The incidence of such secondary displacement ranges from 40 to 70 per cent.[25, 38]

Colles, in his initial article,[27] described using both a volar and a dorsal wooden splint. In the succeeding 150 years, immobilization techniques have included dorsal splints, volar splints, sugar tong splints, long arm casts, and short arm casts. The yardstick of the efficiency of any form of immobilization is the number of secondary displacements, and as yet no convincing data exist for choosing one method over another. Recent work by Sarmiento[48] utilized a functional brace that preserved early motion and obtained satisfactory results. As might be expected, the brace was no better than other treatments in preventing collapse. In displaced fractures, we prefer to use a long arm cast for the first few weeks, followed by a short arm cast for further immobilization.

Concerning casting, three principles are inviolate. No cast for a Colles fracture should extend beyond the metacarpophalangeal joint (knuckles) dorsally or the distal palmar crease volarly. This is in order to permit full digital motion. Second, any significant degree of edema or neurological symptoms following cast application necessitate splitting of the cast. Third, the best method to prevent disabling shortening in the wake of distal radial fracture is awareness of the problem and frequent clinical

follow-up. Most studies show that the displacement occurs within the first 10 days,[25, 33] and thus the patient should be closely observed during this time. Our protocol includes follow-up x-rays on days 3, 10, and 21. Any significant loss of position on these roentgenograms is an indication for rereduction of the fracture.

Certain positions of immobilization have been advocated for minimizing the collapse in Colles' fractures. Initially, a reversal of the supposed mechanism of injury was thought to be helpful in preventing collapse. This is the classic Cotton-Loder position of forced full palmar flexion, ulnar deviation, and pronation.[28] This extreme position should be avoided, as it is deleterious to regaining either wrist or digital motion in addition to its association with median nerve compression.[40] Most authors now subscribe to moderate ulnar deviation and moderate palmar flexion. Both pronation[24, 41] and supination[31, 47, 48, 53] have their advocates. The reasons for using supination in the treatment of Colles' fractures are as follows. (1) The forearm bones are parallel and not crossed as in pronation, permitting effective immobilization as well as easy radiological evaluation; (2) the brachioradialis muscle inserting on the radial styloid is rendered ineffective as a distorting force;[47] (3) dorsal ulnar subluxations are reduced in supination; (4) rehabilitation is easier, since gravity rotates the supinated forearm and each useful motion of the hand tends to pull it into pronation; and (5) any ultimate loss of forearm rotation is a loss of pronation which is easily compensated by humeral adduction, whereas no such compensation is possible for a loss of supination. At present, we immobilize fractures in the position of neutral to slight supination: 20 to 30 degrees of palmar flexion and 15 to 30 degrees of ulnar deviation. As to the length of immobilization, most authors feel that six weeks is the minimum for a comminuted Colles fracture.[34] Present data on severely comminuted fractures suggest that slipping can occur up to eight weeks, and therefore immobilization is recommended for this period.[48]

Given the relative ineffectiveness of plaster alone to prevent shortening in comminuted Colles' fractures, attention has been increasingly focused on the use of pin fixation or external skeletal traction for those injuries that are considered unstable because of dorsal comminution and intraarticular involvement. Böhler[2] is credited with the first description of pins in plaster technique for self-contained skeletal traction. Many variations of this distal and proximal pin fixation through the metacarpals and proximal forearm bones have been described,[26, 35, 41] and these are referred to in Green's article.[35] In each of these techniques, the basic principle is the same—self-contained traction to prevent shortening of the radius at the fracture site. Many centers use this technique routinely in comminuted Colles' fracture. We reserve the use of pins in plaster for the more comminuted and displaced intraarticular fractures, which represent about 15 to 20 per cent of distal radial fractures (Fig. 19–8A). We also feel the technique is indicated in patients who show unacceptable loss of position during the first two weeks of routine plaster immobilization.

Although the procedure is simple, it requires asepsis and some form of regional or general anesthesia. Following reduction, smooth Kirschner wires, usually 3/16 of an inch, are passed through the bases of the second and third metacarpals and through the radius at least 2 inches proximal to the fracture site (Fig. 19–8B). A short arm cast is applied with the wrist in neutral position. It is important that the cast as well as the pins allow unrestricted finger and elbow motion. Also, traction should be reduced prior to incorporation of the pins in plaster to prevent overdistraction of the fragments. As pointed out by several authors,[26, 35] the period of immobilization is eight weeks, because radial shortening can occur with earlier pin removal and such shortening is the most debilitating residual effect of Colles' fractures. Green[35] reported good functional results in over 80 per cent of patients using this method. Its advantages are a short arm cast and free digits, which prevent elbow and finger joint stiffness. Its disadvantages include pin breakage, pin tract infection, and overzealous distraction.

Other stabilization procedures have been suggested. Pin placement obliquely through the ulna into the distal radial fragment was recommended by DePalma.[29] Dowling has reported that fixation by crossed Kirschner wires[30] showed satisfactory results and was an improvement over plaster treatment alone; a similar technique was introduced by Rush,[45] who treated fractures of the distal radius by his specially designed pin. Some authors[53] have advocated primary resection of the distal end of the ulna in severely comminuted fractures of the radius, because they observed that rapid healing occurred in the compressed radial fragments, permitting earlier mobilization and better functional results. While we have had little experience with these methods, we feel that improved anatomical results do follow such stabilization treatments (Fig. 19–8C); more data are needed to determine whether their use significantly improves the functional result.

Postreduction Care. Patients should be followed closely with serial x-rays taken at one and two weeks after the initial postreduction study, as this represents the crucial period when loss of reduction may occur. In most series, finger stiffness is a major cause of subsequent disability,[23] and it is important to make the patient understand that early motion of the fingers is critical to the functional result. Exercises should include full flexion and extension of the fingers for sustained periods of 10 to 20 seconds as well as some functional activities. One of our favorites is to have the patient crumple up a piece of newspaper singlehandedly with the casted arm. This activity requires the use of all the digital motors. Active range of motion of the proximal joints of the shoulder and elbow should also be emphasized. We have our patients raise their casted arm over and behind their heads daily. Reactive swelling and edema in the hand are minimized with this program. Slings are discouraged, as they encourage the dependent position of the extremity and minimal use of the shoulder.

We do not routinely use a formalized physical therapy program following discontinuance of immobilization but rely on active functional exercises. We reserve physical therapy for those patients with poor motivation who require constant supervision and encouragement and for those in whom appropriate functional progress is absent in the early postreduction period. Physical therapy does not counteract ne-

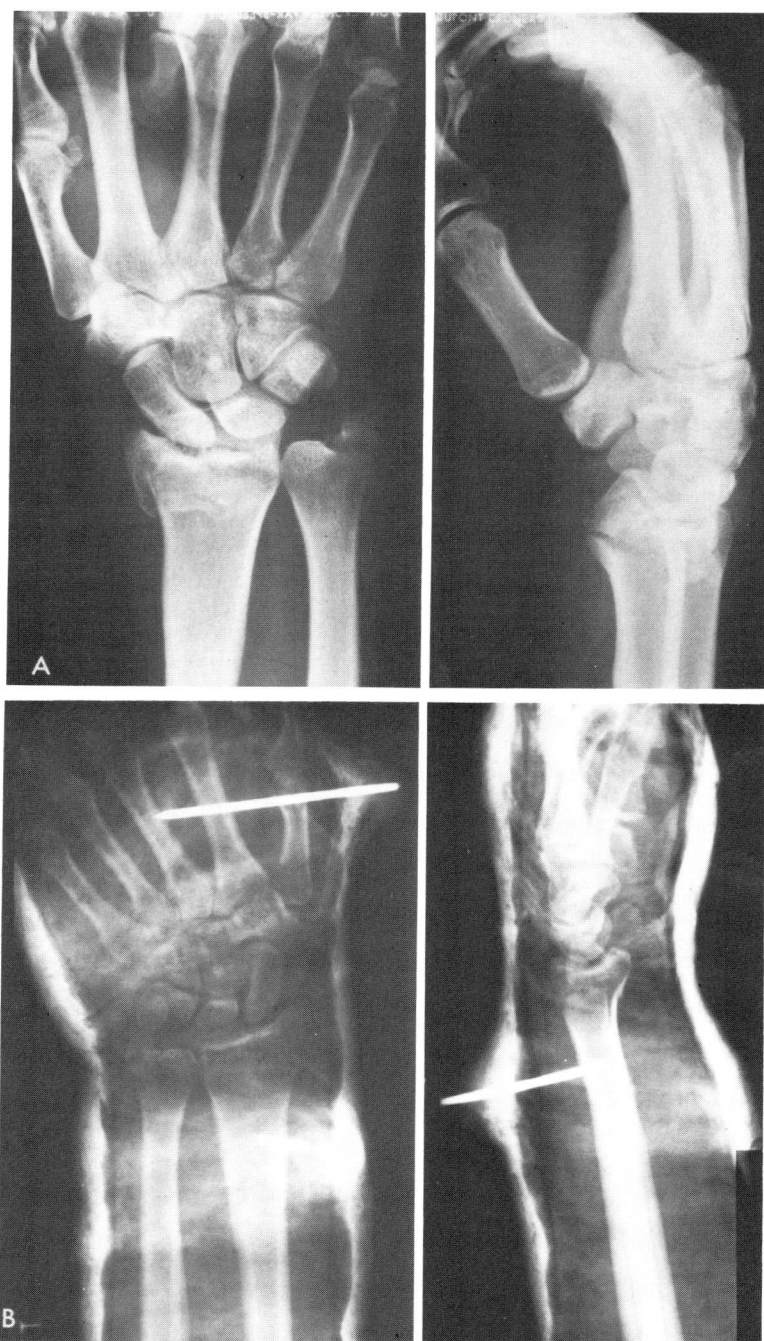

Figure 19–8   *A.* Comminuted intraarticular fracture in anteroposterior and lateral views. *B.* Postreduction x-rays with pins and plaster. Note that the distal pin transverses only the second and third metacarpal, while the proximal pin is in the distal radius proximal to the fracture site. Postreduction x-rays show good restoration of radial articular angle and radial length; radial tilt is restored at neutral. *C.* Four-month follow-up of this Colles fracture. Note the maintenance of good radial articular length and tilt and radial articular angle. The radial articular tilt remains at neutral. The sites of the pinholes can be clearly seen in the second metacarpal and the proximal radius. At this time, patient had full range of digital motion and was functionally normal and back at work.

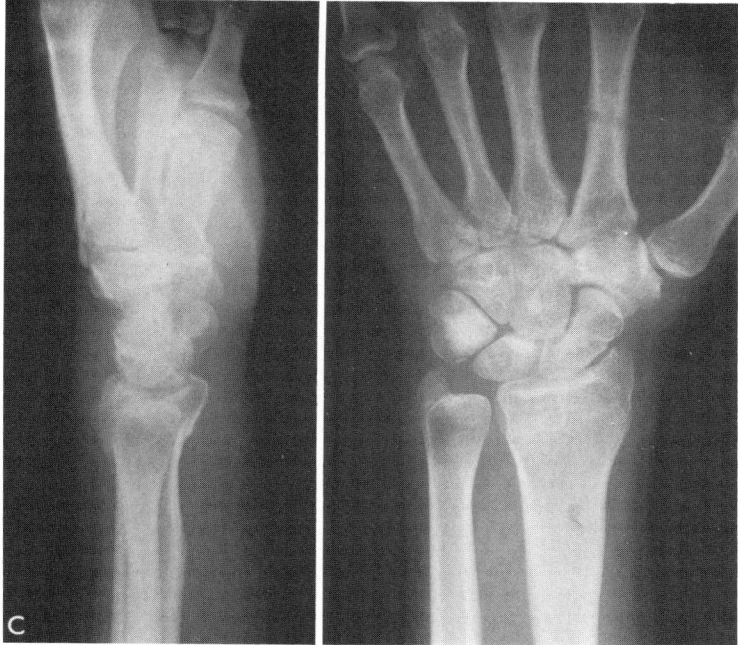

Figure 19–8   Continued

glect of early active functional exercises. The most common pitfalls in the management of Colles' fractures are listed in Table 19–2.

End Results and Complications. The period of disability following Colles' fracture will necessarily be influenced by such factors as age, severity of fracture, the relationship to a compensation injury, and the activities expected of the wrist. In general, however, a period of three and one-half to four months can be regarded as a reasonable time before full activity can be resumed. Even then, however, many pa-

tients will complain of weather ache or pain with certain activities, such as wringing clothes or pronating and supinating to turn a doorknob. Most surgeons would agree with Lidstrom[38] that residual symptoms persist in approximately 20 per cent of all Colles' fractures, although significant functional impairment occurs in only about 10 per cent and is related to complications of the injury.

Few surgeons share the experience of Watson-Jones,[14] who concluded that after suitable treatment "it should be impossible to know which wrist was fractured." As already stated, some degree of residual deformity is the rule, but such malunion does not always reflect a poor functional result. Colles[27] stated that "one consolation only remains, that the limb will at some remote period again enjoy perfect freedom in all its motions, and be completely exempt from pain; the deformity, however, will remain undiminished through life." Although some authors concur,[24, 51] the majority feel that the forgiveness of the wrist joint is not inevitable.[26, 29, 30, 33, 38, 45, 48, 49] These divergent views arise from the differing requisites used in the studies of end results.

TABLE 19–2   Common Pitfalls in Managing Distal Radial Fractures

1. Inadequate follow-up with serial x-rays and loss of reduction
2. Cast extending beyond metacarpophalangeal joints
3. Neglect of early active motion of the digits
4. Neglect of elbow and shoulder exercises
5. Neglect of initial elevation
6. Ignoring patient's complaint of pain or failure to gain early pain-free digital motion
7. Failure to split any tight compressive cast or wrapping
8. Overlooking of an associated nerve injury, especially of the median nerve

Table 19–3   Complications and Sequelae of Colles' Fractures

Malunion
Radiocarpal arthritis
Distal radioulnar joint problems
Finger and shoulder stiffness
Tendon injuries; extensor pollicis longus rupture
Nerve problems, especially of median nerve
Posttraumatic reflex sympathetic dystrophy

Complications and sequelae of Colles' fracture (Table 19–3) include loss of the volar distal articular tilt and the radial length. As has been stated, there is a general matching of the cosmetic and anatomical results. With this deformity, then, specific wrist motions are limited. Volar flexion and ulnar deviation are usually more restricted than dorsiflexion and radial deviation, but only 3 per cent of patients with such loss of mobility consider it detrimental to their

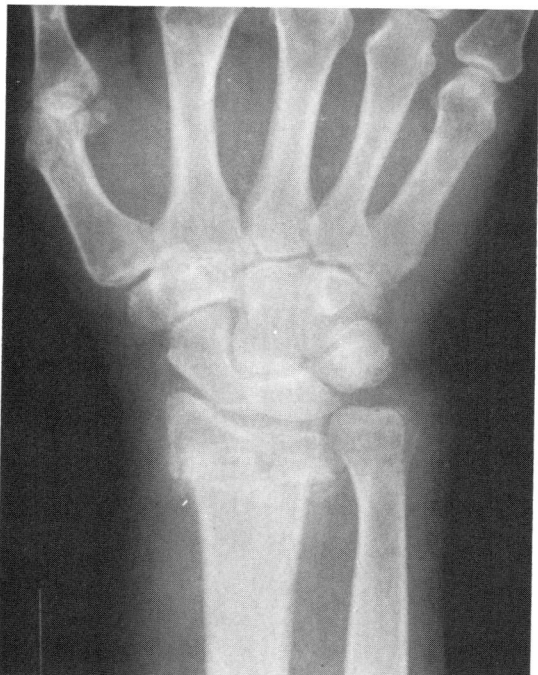

Figure 19–9 Malunion of Colles' fracture. Note that the fracture was allowed to heal in marked shortening. The radial styloid is now at the level of the ulnar head with consequent disruption of the radioulnar joint. Also note the small avulsion fracture of the ulnar styloid which has not healed. Symptomatically, this patient had pain and was limited in all motions of the wrist.

functional outcome.[33] Loss of radial length can be severe (Fig. 19–9), and when it occurs many patients complain of excessive fatigability and weakness of the hand and wrist. Several studies using the Jamar dynamometer have confirmed weakness of grip strength in about 25 to 30 per cent of patients.[33, 38, 48] While such complaints are seldom severe, there are malunions that interfere significantly with wrist and hand function. A variety of operative techniques have been recommended for the correction of this residual deformity.[6, 38] We prefer a corrective biplanar osteotomy with an iliac bone graft inserted into the dorsal and radial side of the deformity to restore the radius to its normal length. Our indications for this procedure are rare; it is used in young patients or in those with skilled jobs when the deformity precludes employment.

The importance of the ulnar side of the wrist in the disability following Colles' fracture has made the name of Darrach nearly as famous as that of Colles himself. Involvement of the ulnar side of the wrist occurs in the majority of Colles' fractures, either as an injury to the triangular fibrocartilage or as an avulsion fracture of the ulnar styloid. Most authors feel ulnar involvement worsens the prognosis.[8, 30, 33, 38, 82] Dysfunction of the distal radioulnar joint is also a complication of Colles' fracture caused by radial shortening (Fig. 19–9) or by direct extension of the fracture into the joint (Fig. 19–10). Symptoms include persistent tenderness over the ulna, weakness and pain on using the hand in pronation or supination functions, decrease in pronation and supination motions, and prominence of the distal ulna. Resection of the distal ulna, first described by Darrach,[69] helps improve forearm rotation. It is important to resect no more bone than is necessary—an inch is all that is usually required. Dingman[70] and others[74] reported good results with this method. Ulnar deviation of the hand can be prevented if less than 1 inch of ulna is resected, and distal ulnar instability can be prevented by surgically tethering the distal ulna to the extensor carpi ulnaris. Swanson[81] has recommended the use of a silicone rubber ulnar head implant to prevent ulnar shortening complications. We prefer to resect only the dorsal prominence and the lateral aspect of the ulna, leaving intact the majority of the

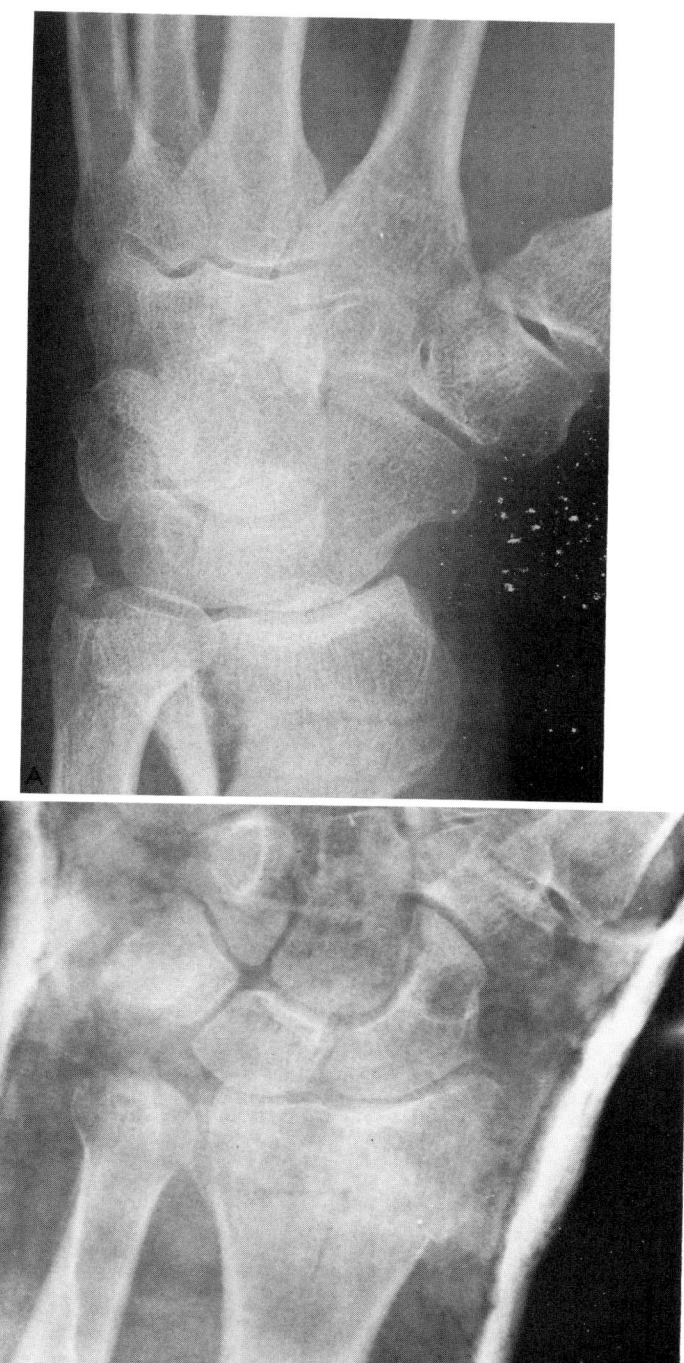

Figure 19–10   Fracture involving the distal radioulnar joint. *A.* This fracture represents an avulsion of the radial joint surface by the triangular fibrocartilage. *B.* Postreduction films. The patient healed with asymptomatic and unlimited pronation and supination.

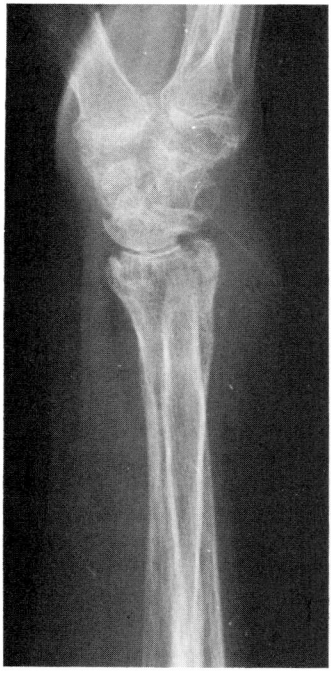
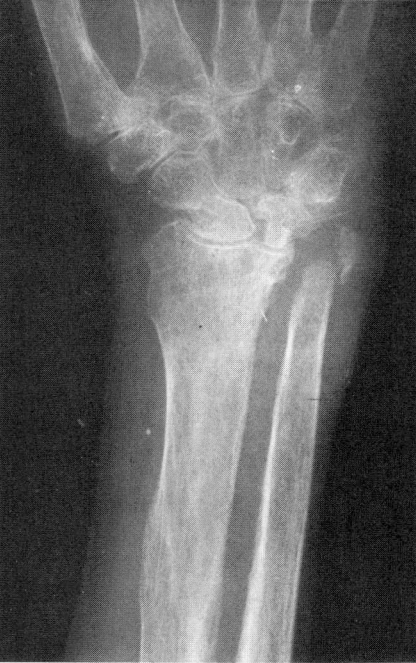

Figure 19–11 Modified Darrach resection of the distal ulna. Darrach described resecting 1 inch of the distal ulna to improve pronation and supination. To prevent complications, such as excessive ulnar deviation of the hand or painful and excessively volar remainder of the distal ulna, we have been using a modified Darrach procedure shown here, in which only the radial ulnar articulation and the dorsal bump are removed. This leaves the base of the ulnar styloid and its ligamentous stabilization intact, while providing good symptomatic relief.

ulnar head and ulnar styloid with its ligamentous insertions (Fig. 19–11).

Other forms of treatment have included a Milch[12] shortening osteotomy of the ulna, a fusion of the distal radioulnar joint, and lastly, if instability of the ulna and not the radioulnar joint is the major problem, various forms of tendon and fascia reconstruction.[75, 76]

Avulsion fractures of the radial styloid

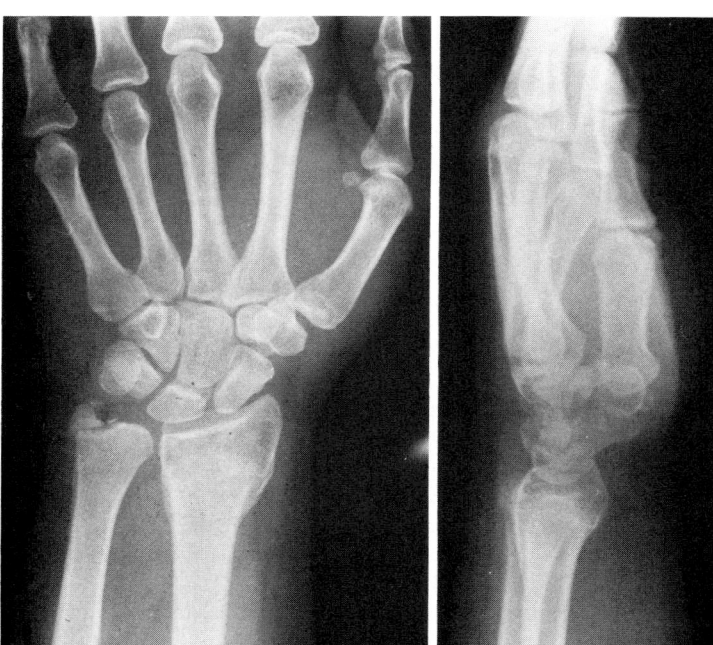

Figure 19–12 Ulnar styloid nonunion two years following Colles' fracture. The nonunion of this patient was completely asymptomatic.

are evident on x-ray in about 60 per cent of Colles' fractures.[33, 38] Approximately 20 per cent fail to show bony union (Fig. 19–12). Nonunions, however, are for the most part asymptomatic, and when tenderness and other symptoms occur they are probably related more to the underlying soft tissue damage of the triangular fibrocartilage and ulnar collateral ligament than to the styloid fracture itself. We have excised the ulnar styloid fragment in some cases with good symptomatic relief, but this is not widely performed.

Nerve injuries do occur with Colles' fractures. Their incidence ranges from 0.5 per cent to 3 per cent,[33, 40, 43, 44, 54] and the majority of these involve the median nerve. Median nerve injuries are of two types, primary and delayed. The former includes any median nerve injury presenting in the first six weeks, both those that are present initially and those that develop during immobilization secondary to the Cotton-Loder position[40] or to excessive callus formation. Transient median nerve symptoms are common and usually caused by hemorrhage and swelling; they respond to elevation and reduction of the fracture. However, if the median nerve loss is complete or occurs postreduction, we feel immediate exploration and release of the transverse retinaculum ligament is indicated. Delayed median nerve injury or "tardy median nerve palsy," as it was labeled by Phalen,[43] refers to the late onset of median nerve symptoms following a fracture that has healed either in malunion or with secondary degenerative disease. Such trauma, however, was a definite etiology in only 5 per cent of carpal tunnel syndromes in his series. Injuries to the ulnar nerve have also been reported,[33, 54] but these are extremely rare.

Failure of the dorsal cortex of the distal radius subjects the extensor pollicis longus to uneven bony fragments over Lister's tubercle; rupture has been reported in approximately 0.7 per cent of Colles' fractures.[52] When this occurs the patient is unable to extend the distal phalanx of the thumb against resistance or to raise the thumb metacarpal away from the hand. Early treatment is tenorrhaphy, but late injuries require tendon grafting or tendon transfer.

The incidence of reflex sympathetic dystrophy in Colles' fracture varies from 1 to 16 per cent.[33, 37, 38] The term encompasses a wide clinical spectrum and is known by many different names: causalgia, hand-shoulder syndrome, and Sudeck's atrophy. The reader is referred to Lankford's[37] excellent review of this complex problem. Early recognition is the keystone of treatment. The following associations should increase the physician's index of suspicion: pain disproportionate to the degree of fracture and pain away from the site of the injury, especially in the shoulder and fingers; intolerance to finger joint motions; hyperesthesia and hyperhidrosis in the hand; and vascular reactivity consisting of either mottle cyanosis or erythema. Although the basic cause of these syndromes remains an enigma, the effect of the sympathetic overactivity is well established—hence the use of sympathetic blockade in treatment. Adjuncts to therapy include analgesics, tranquilizers, occupational therapy, nerve stimulators, and surgery to relieve inciting causes, such as carpal tunnel.

Posttraumatic arthritis after Colles' fracture ranges from less than 5 per cent to over 40 per cent. This discrepancy arises from the various methods of evaluation used by different authors. In the rare cases in which severe functional disability correlates with marked degenerative changes and incapacitating pain we have resorted to wrist fusion with good results. Wrist arthroplasty, including joint replacement, has been used in selected cases.

Finally, it is worth noting the common association between hip and wrist fracture in elderly women. Nearly one quarter of those who have one fracture subsequently have the other. Often they occur during the same fall, and if the radial fracture is not severe it may be missed. The complications listed earlier can occur with any fracture of the distal radius, but it should be pointed out that median nerve injury is more frequently associated with Smith's fracture than with Colles' fracture. Arthritis is more common after the intraarticular fractures of the Barton or the chauffeur type.

Dorsal Rim Fracture (Barton's Fracture)

This dorsal rim articular fracture is often included with Colles' fracture because of the dorsal displacement of the fracture fragment. Moreover, its mechanism of injury and clinical appearance mimic those of the classic Colles fracture. Yet its treatment and prognosis justify giving it separate consideration. The tendency of the carpal bones to displace dorsally with the radial fragment underlines the true diagnosis of this injury as a fracture-dislocation. In 1838, John Rhea Barton[55] described the volar and dorsal fracture-dislocation of the wrist. Some confusion exists as to the specific lesions in his cases, but his clinical descriptions were precise and clear: these are articular fracture-dislocations. In that paper, Barton emphasized the dorsal rim fracture and only briefly referred to its volar counterpart. Thus, lovers of eponyms have considered it logical to confine "Barton's" to dorsal rim articular fracture and "reverse Barton's" to its volar counterpart.

The injury is more common in the younger age group but generally rare, representing only 1.5 per cent of Böhler's large series.[2] Roentgenographic studies and an awareness of the fracture are the keys to diagnosis. Oblique x-rays are very helpful in delineating the portion of intact volar radius. Often the radial fragment is a large piece suitable for fracture fixation (Fig. 19–13A).

Management of this fracture is a subject almost as controversial as its proper eponymic nomenclature. Barton recommended the use of two splints, which were to be changed every four to five days to allow early motion, in treating both the dorsal and the volar margin articular fractures. He also advocated early motion to prevent adhesions and joint stiffness. In an era when rest and rigid immobilization were widely practiced, Barton foresaw the benefit of early motion to preserve joint function.

The minimally displaced dorsal rim fracture should not be mistaken for a Colles fracture, as it must be reduced and immobilized in dorsiflexion rather than in the standard volar flexion of a Colles fracture. Immobilizing the wrist in volar flexion allows the lunate to press against the unstable dorsal fragment and thus renders it vulnerable to upward and backward subluxation. Instead, one must manipulate the wrist so that the lunate is placed against the nonfractured portion of the volar radius, usually a wrist position of 35 degrees of dorsiflexion (Fig. 19–13B). If an acceptable reduction cannot be maintained, we favor either external skeletal immobilization, such as pins in plaster or, in some cases, direct internal fixation of the fracture fragment using Kirschner wires or a small buttress plate, as has been advocated for the volarly displaced Barton fracture.[59, 60]

Dorsal Barton's Fracture

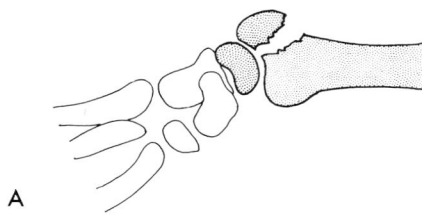

A

Reduction in Dorsiflexion

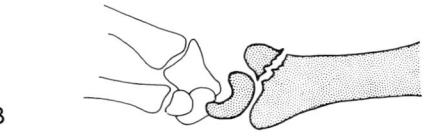

B

Figure 19–13 Dorsal rim fracture. Dorsal Barton's fracture. A. Schematic rendering of the dorsal Barton fracture showing the tendency of the lunate to displace the dorsal articular fragment. B. Reduction is the opposite of that in Colles' fracture and requires 30 degrees of dorsiflexion to place the lunate against the intact volar articular surface of the radius.

Distal Radial Fractures with Volar Displacement (Smith's and Volar Barton's Fractures)

In 1847, another Irish surgeon, Robert William Smith, described "a fracture of the lower end of the radius, from half an inch to an inch above the articulation, with displacement of the lower fragment forwards."[63] The inferior radioulnar joint is disrupted, or the ulnar styloid is avulsed. The volar displacement and deformity he described are often referred to as a reversed Colles fracture. It has been likened to a garden spade, since there is a dorsal prominence over the distal end of the upper fragment and fullness of the wrist on the volar aspect due to the displaced distal fragment. The head of the ulna is prominent on the dorsum of the wrist. Such fractures represent between 5 and 10 per cent of

Smith's Fracture

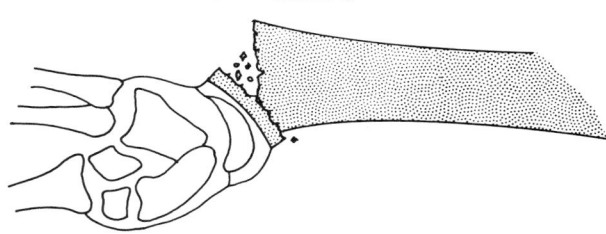

Figure 19–14 Schematic representation of Smith's fracture. Here the radius is displaced volarly. Median nerve injury is more common than in Colles' fracture.

distal radial fractures, tend to occur in a younger age group, and have a slightly worse prognosis than Colles' fracture.

Given the variation of the lines of fracture, the impaction, and the intraarticular involvement, the definition of Smith's fracture, like that of Colles' fracture, rests on more clinical grounds. Thomas[64] separated such volarly displaced fractures into three distinct types defined by the obliquity of the fracture line. Type I is a nonarticular fracture extending across the cancellous portion of the radius, often comminuted and often accompanied by a fracture of the ulnar styloid, and seen in older patients (Fig. 19–14). Type 2 is the anterior marginal fracture associated with anterior subluxation of the carpus (see Fig. 19–17). This type, as mentioned earlier, had been first described by Barton nine years earlier and is often referred to as a reverse Barton fracture. The third type of fracture in Thomas's group is a nonarticular fracture occurring in younger patients with severe trauma. The fracture line is transverse, and there is little comminution. While conceding some difficulties with this classification, Ellis and others[60] have accepted its use. Contrary to this and in agreement with DeOliveira,[58] we feel there are important reasons for not considering the Smith fracture and the anterior fracture-dislocation of Barton (Ellis's type 2) as similar injuries. We think that like dorsal marginal fractures and the classic Colles fractures, the tendency toward carpal displacement and the different position of immobilization required in the anterior marginal fracture warrant its distinction from the classic Smith fracture. Woodyard[66] confirmed the worst prognosis for such intraarticular fractures.

In his original description, Smith implicated a fall on the dorsum of the wrist as the mechanism of injury. This has been debated, and other mechanisms have been proposed, including a fall on the supinated wrist followed by pronation of the upper limb,[64, 66] and a direct blow to the dorsa of the knuckles of the hand as it grips the handlebar in motorcycle accidents.[64] In many of these injuries, however, the exact mechanism of injury is unknown. The patient presents with a garden spade deformity and a tenderness of the distal radius. X-ray views similar to those for Colles' fracture show the variable degree of volar displacement of the distal radial fracture, usually with comminution (Fig. 19–15). Again, oblique projections are helpful in determining the presence of an anterior marginal fracture. The lateral film is necessary to determine any carpal displacement.

In those fractures requiring reduction, the technique we use is very similar to that described for Colles' fracture in the use of anesthesia, finger traps, and countertraction. Manual manipulation of the fracture, when required, differs from that in dorsally displaced fractures in that the pressure is applied volarly and the reduction is completed by twisting the hand into supination. In the century following the description of these fractures, virtually all reports recommended plaster cast immobilization in the position of dorsiflexion.[2, 4, 6, 14] Thomas and others[8, 60, 64] have, however, advocated supination and slight palmar flexion. Our preference is for a neutral position with supination. We initially use a long arm cast, which is reduced to a short arm cast at three weeks; weekly x-rays are taken to rule out early loss of position. As in the case of Colles' fracture, when severe comminution exists or loss of position occurs, pins in plaster immobilization is used. Median nerve injury is slightly more common in Smith's fracture, and the prognosis for

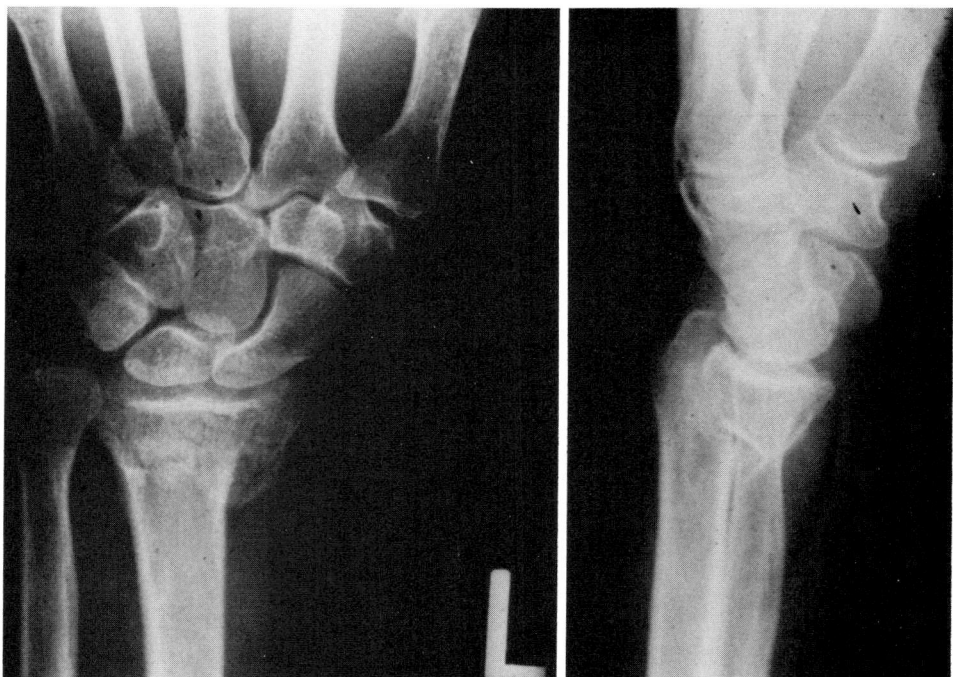

Figure 19-15   Anteroposterior and lateral roentgenograms of classic Smith's fracture. The loss of radial articular angle and radial lengths are similar to that of Colles' fracture, but the displacement as seen on the lateral view of the distal fragment is volar rather than dorsal. Associated avulsion fracture of the ulnar styloid occurs in approximately 40 per cent of cases.

Volar Barton's Fracture

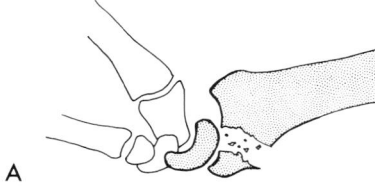

A

Reduction in Volar Flexion

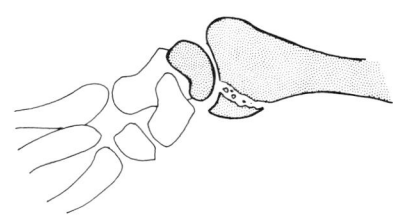

B

Figure 19-16   *A.* Schematic drawing of a volar Barton fracture (also called type 2 Smith's fracture). The key here is the instability of the fracture if it is placed in dorsiflexion, as the lunate will subluxate against the unstable volar articular fragment. *B.* Reduction is accomplished in volar flexion by keying the lunate against the intact dorsal articular surface.

return to full function is slightly worse than that for Colles' fracture. In general, however, the complications are the same as those for Colles' fracture.

This is not true, however, for the volar marginal articular fracture of the distal radius, or volar Barton's fracture. As noted in the discussion of dorsal Barton's fracture, this injury had been described nine years prior to Smith's description by John Rhea Barton. As Smith's is often referred to as a reversed Colles', so this injury is referred to as a reverse Barton fracture (Fig. 19–16). With fracture of the volar lip of the articular surface of the radius and its volar displacement, the lunate loses its normal carpal relationships and tends to displace with the radial fragment (Fig. 19–17). As in dorsal Barton's fractures, the lunate must be keyed into the intact radial surface; thus, this requires immobilization in volar flexion (see Fig. 19–16), not dorsiflexion as in a classic Smith fracture. Again, this fracture should not be thought of as a Smith fracture, since in general the latter require dorsiflexion, a position that in volar marginal fractures is unstable and to be avoided.

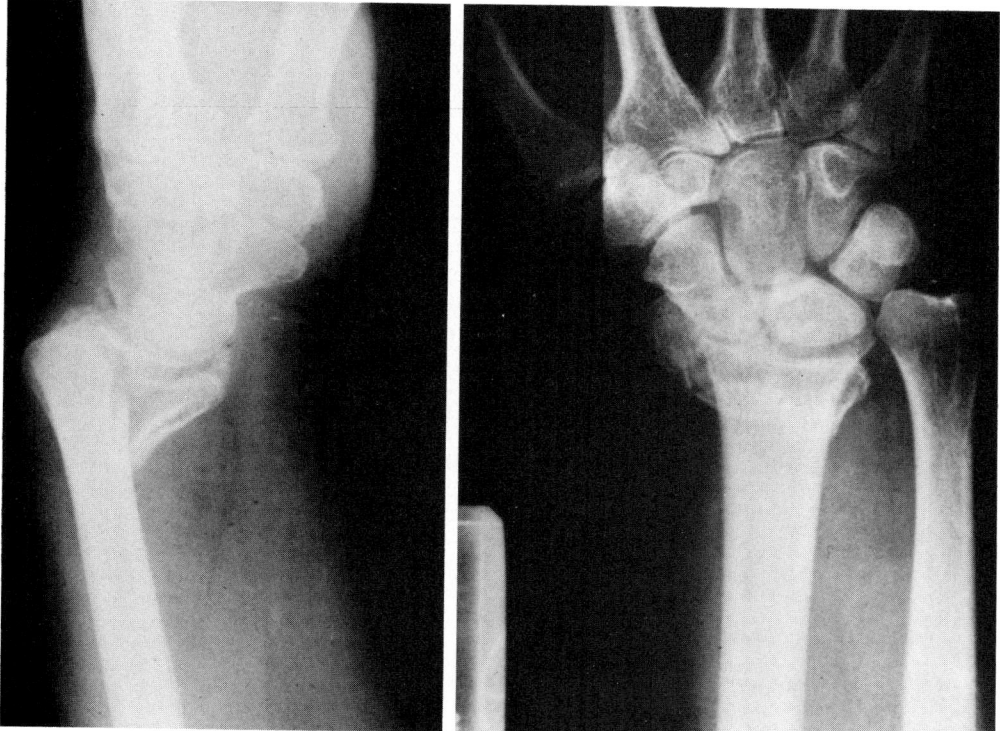

Figure 19–17 Anteroposterior and lateral roentgenograms of a typical volar Barton fracture. Note the subluxation of the carpus with the volar articular fragment. This fracture was treated by pins in plaster.

With significant displacement, several authors have advocated internal fixation,[58, 60] and we agree. This can be done using K-wire fixation or a small plate following reduction of the fragment. This is our preferred method of treatment when the wedge-shaped volar fragment composes 30 per cent or more of the articular surface of the distal radius on the lateral view. Despite the size of the volar fragment on x-ray, it is not uncommon to find small free fragments of bone and cartilage in the radiocarpal joint. This may explain the generally poorer prognosis of these fracture-dislocations.[58]

FRACTURES OF THE RADIAL AND ULNAR STYLOIDS

Fractures of the radial styloid may occur as isolated injuries or in association with many types of wrist fractures. They have often been referred to as chauffeur's, backfire, or Model-T fractures[59, 61] and were noted in the first two decades of this century with the advent of the automobile. The majority of such injuries occurred prior to the introduction of the self-starter, when the individual had to start the vehicle using a crank or handle to create the spark. Chauffeur's fracture still occurs, although rarely, and now the injury is associated more with steering wheel and handlebar injuries. Another mechanism is a fall on the radially deviated wrist, in which the forces are transmitted through the scaphoid to the articular surface of the radius.

The fracture line starts within the articular surface of the radius and runs vertically upward and outward to the lateral border of the radius (Fig. 19–18). The fracture is best seen on the anteroposterior view (Fig. 19–19). It is rarely displaced, but when a large fragment is sheared it may have the potential for radiocarpal displacement and may be thought of as a lateral fracture-dislocation analogous to the volar and dorsal Barton fractures (Fig. 19–20). In general, we immobilize this fracture in a long arm cast in supination with 15 degrees of ulnar

Chauffeur's Fracture

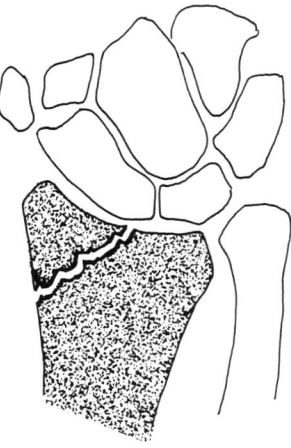

Figure 19–18 Schematic representation of a fracture of the radial styloid, or chauffeur's fracture. Like Barton's fracture, it is an intraarticular fracture of the radius.

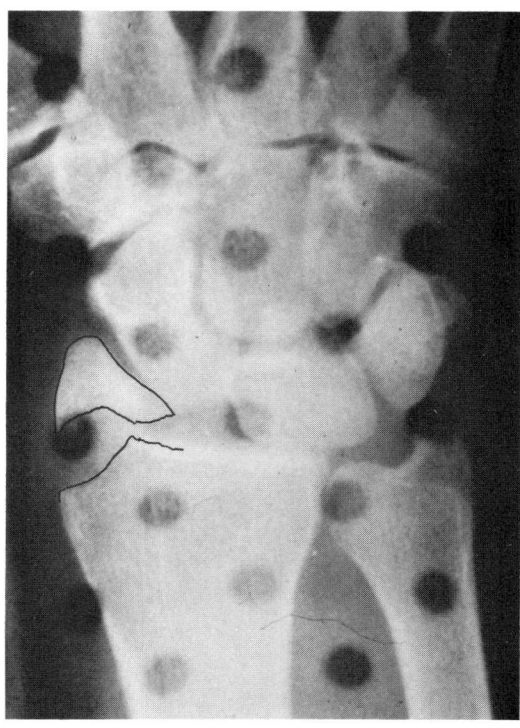

Figure 19–20 A displaced radial styloid fracture, in which carpal subluxation or dislocation can occur. This fracture must be reduced anatomically like any intraarticular fracture.

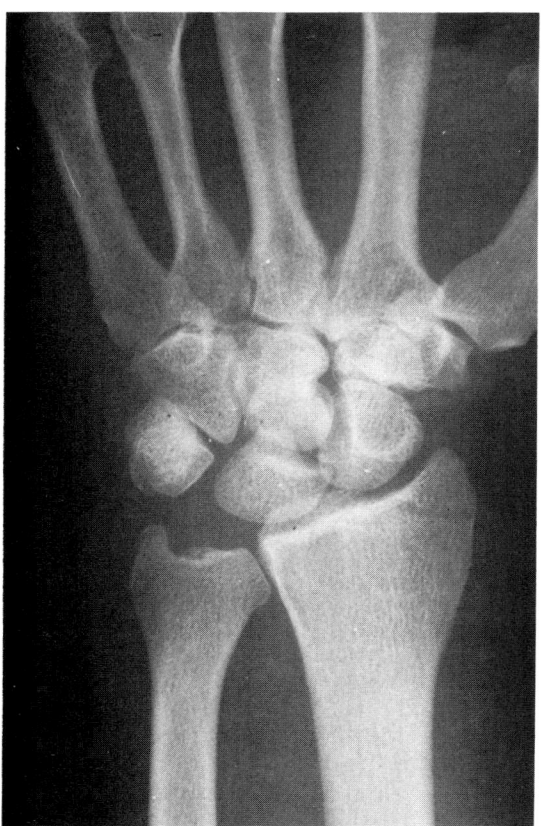

Figure 19–19 Nondisplaced radial styloid fracture. Such a fracture is treated in a long arm cast for three weeks, then in a short arm cast for two weeks.

deviation. The position of supination helps to overcome the deforming pull of the brachioradialis, as noted by Sarmiento.[47] If a large fragment is present with or without carpal subluxation, we prefer accurate reduction and internal fixation of the fragment (Fig. 19–20).

Fractures of the styloid process of the ulna are most frequently associated with distal radial fractures. They are present in between 50 and 60 per cent of these cases and are the result of avulsion injuries at the insertion of the triangular fibrocartilage (see Fig. 19–9). Occasionally, fractures of the styloid may occur as a separate injury from indirect violence due to a sudden forceful radial twist of the wrist or a direct blow. The clinical signs and symptoms of the isolated ulnar fracture differ from those of fractures seen elsewhere in that there is relatively little pain. The feeling is rather an annoying discomfort, and there is only slight limitation of function. These injuries are usually visible on a routine anteroposterior radiograph. Differential diagnosis includes non-union of an ulnar styloid following a distal radial fracture, which occurs in 10 to 20 per cent of cases (see Fig. 19–12). Another condition is anomalous carpal bone, such as an os styloides or os triangulare.[17] Associated distal radioulnar joint disruption should be ruled out by appropriate x-rays. Our treatment is a short arm cast for six weeks, as healing frequently occurs by fibrous union. Painless wrist motion is the usual outcome.

Distal Radial Fractures in Children

The growth plates of the distal radius and ulna fuse between the ages of 14 and 18, and falls on the outstretched hand commonly result in one of several injuries in children. Younger children usually sustain a bone fracture, frequently greenstick in type, proximal to the growth plates. The adolescent sustains a fracture proximal to the growth plate with some displacement. The fragments may be displaced either volarly or dorsally, as in Colles' or Smith's fractures, and their mechanisms of injury are similar. Articular surface involvement and fracture-dislocations of the wrist are extremely rare in children.

In younger children, with their relatively elastic bone and thick periosteum, a torus fracture is common.[57, 62, 65] This is a complete transverse fracture in which there is a buckling of the bone much in the manner that a crushed beer can collapses on one side and bulges on the opposite side. It is usually best seen in the anteroposterior view but is often missed. The second type of injury is the greenstick fracture, in which the fracture seems to be bent but one cortex and the periosteum appear intact. In general, the treatment of a torus fracture, usually of the distal radius, requires only plaster immobilization for three weeks. There is some controversy concerning greenstick fractures, in that many surgeons[57] advocate a forceful completion of the fracture as part of the initial manipulation. In general, unless there is marked angulation we do not complete the fracture.

A displaced fracture of both bones of the distal radius and ulna (Fig. 19–21) is treated by manipulation in the manner described by Rang[62] and Charnley.[4] In the common dorsally displaced fracture, we favor palmar flexion, ulnar deviation, and pronation maintained by a long arm, well-molded cast. In younger children we usually extend the cast distally to the knuckles for the first several days, as their fingers do not become stiff. Bayonet apposition is acceptable, and healing usually is complete by six weeks. As Blount has stated,[57] the younger the child and the nearer the fracture is to the growth plate, the more angulation one can accept. In general, we accept 30 degrees or less of dorsal angulation in a child over six (Fig. 19–22). It has been noted that the potential for growth and remodeling in children is such that at a year it is often difficult to tell which wrist had been fractured.

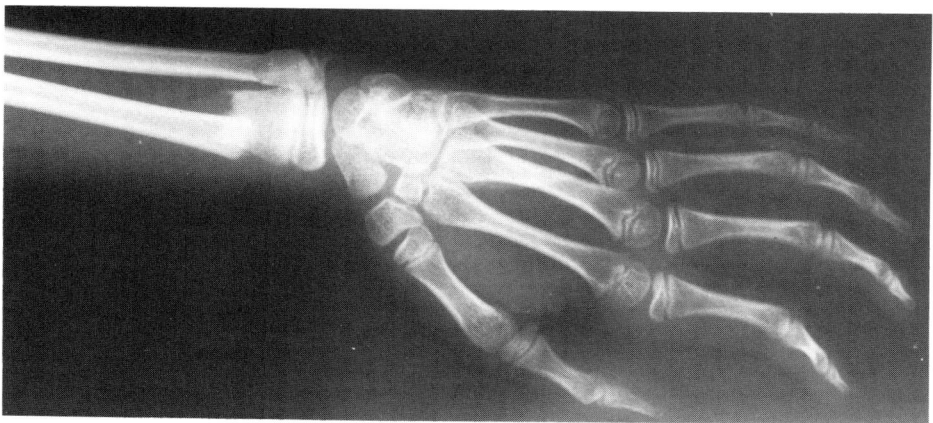

Figure 19–21 Displaced fracture of both bones in a six-year-old boy following a fall on the outstretched hand. Once bayonet apposition is obtained, these fractures usually heal uneventfully within six weeks and remodel to a completely normal roentgenographic appearance.

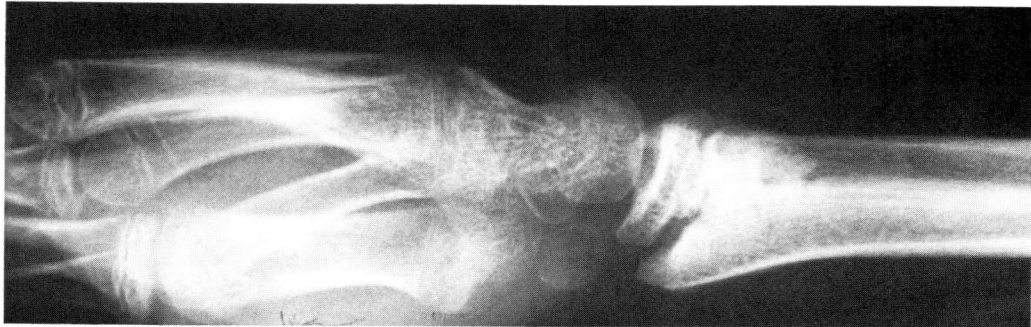

Figure 19–22 Epiphyseal fracture of a distal radius. This is analogous to a Colles fracture in a child, in which the fracture occurs through the growth plate, the weakest portion of the child's bone. Salter and Harris described five variations of epiphyseal injuries, characterizing them by the course of the fracture line through the epiphyseal growth plate and metaphysis.

Salter and Harris classified epiphyseal injuries into several types.[5, 62] At the distal radial level, their type 2 injury, in which a triangular fragment of the dorsal margin of the metaphysis is avulsed, is the most common (Fig. 19–23). The signs and symptoms are similar to those of an adult Colles

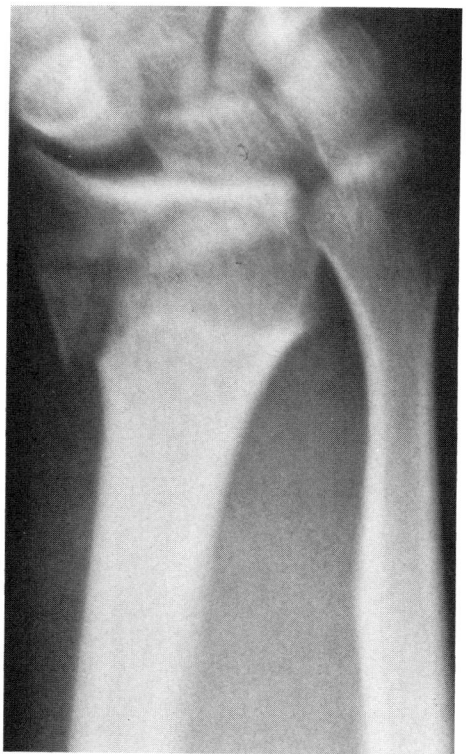

Figure 19–23 The classic epiphyseal fracture of the distal radius occurs through the growth plate and exits with a triangular metaphyseal fragment—the Salter 2 fracture. These fractures usually have a good prognosis.

fracture, and x-rays reveal the typical dorsal displacement through the growth plate. In type 1 Salter injuries, in which the fracture extends across the growth plate, short arm immobilization for six weeks is recommended. The manipulative reduction and immobilization of displaced fractures are the same as those used in the adult Colles fracture. It is important to secure an accurate reduction of the epiphysis, but repeated or overzealous manipulative efforts are to be avoided in order to minimize damage to the growth plate. Even though the reduction is perfect or the initial displacement minimal, there is always the possibility that the subsequent growth of the epiphysis may be arrested. The child's parents should always be informed of this complication. The child is usually immobilized for three weeks in a long arm cast, which is reduced to a short arm cast for another three weeks, and then followed at regular intervals until complete remodeling has occurred.

RADIOCARPAL AND RADIOULNAR DISLOCATIONS

As we have seen, displacement of the proximal carpal row on the radius is often seen in association with marginal articular fractures, such as volar and dorsal Barton's and radial styloid fractures. The isolated radiocarpal dislocation without fracture is so rare that it is not mentioned in most textbooks. The direction of the dislocation may be volar or dorsal, and each case represents a loss of integrity of the radiocarpal ligaments. As might be expected, loose-ligamented individuals are most prone to this rare injury. Clinically and symptomatically the wrist injury appears similar to any distal radial fracture. The lateral x-ray is the most useful in diagnosing the direction of the dislocation. The reduction should be done immediately and is usually easily accomplished with traction alone. Wrist immobilization is maintained in a neutral position. Postreduction x-rays should be carefully scanned to rule out the presence of any articular fractures, which must be accurately reduced. Immobilization is continued for six weeks; no cases of recurrent radiocarpal dislocation have been reported with this treatment.

Traumatic dislocations of the distal radioulnar joint are more common injuries. We have already noted the seriousness and frequent incidence of this injury. Distal radial fractures with several other injuries should lead one to suspect distal radioulnar problems. These injuries are: fracture of the distal third of the radial shaft; the Galeazzi fracture with radioulnar dislocation (Fig. 19–24);[78] radial head fractures, known as the Essex-Lopresti lesion;[71] and isolated fractures of the ulnar styloid in which the styloid is held in its normal relationship to the radiocarpal mass by the ulnar collateral ligament and avulsed by the displaced ulnar shaft. Much attention, however, has been focused on the isolated dislocation of the radioulnar joint (Fig. 19–25). Such dislocations are universally referred to[68, 73, 79, 80, 84, 85] as either ulnar-dorsal or ulnar-volar to the radius. They are more correctly described as dislocations of the mobile radiocarpal mass around the fixed ulna. However, volar and dorsal dislocations of the distal ulna are accepted in this discussion because of the clinical appearance and the common usage. Dorsal dislocations are more common than volar ones, especially if those dislocations resulting from an altered relative length of the radius and ulna are included. The predominant mechanism of injury is torsional stress. The dorsal ulnar dislocation is caused by a hyperpronation force, whereas the volar ulnar dislocation results

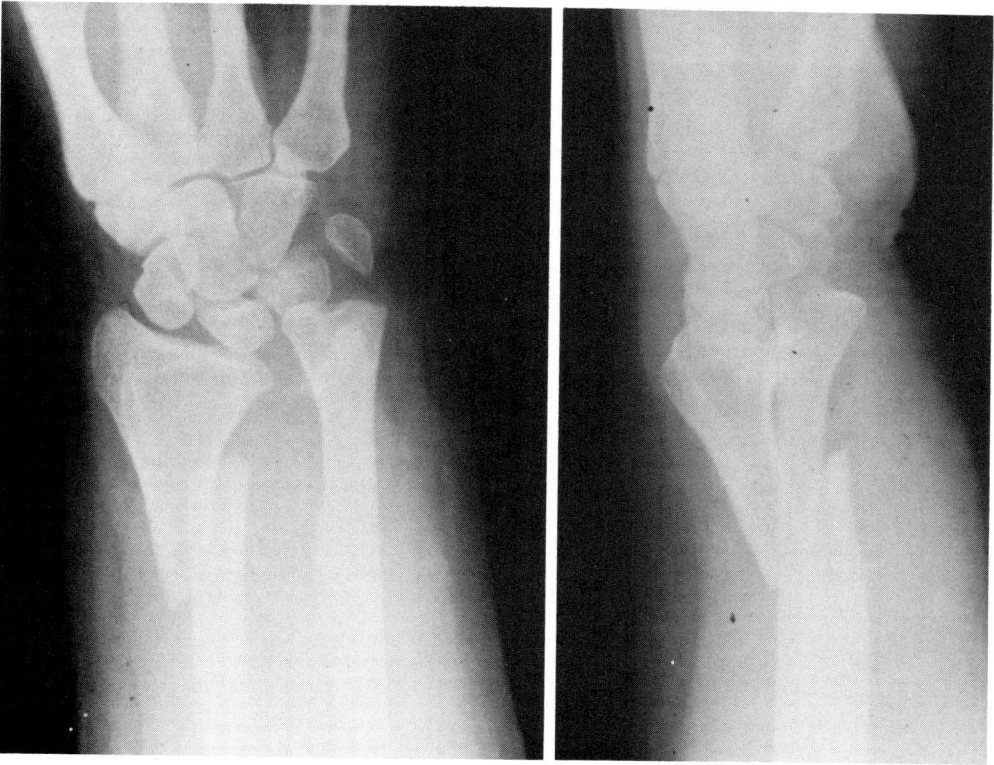

Figure 19–24 Galeazzi fracture-dislocation of the distal radius and ulna. The dislocation of the radioulnar joint is obvious on both the anteroposterior and the lateral films.

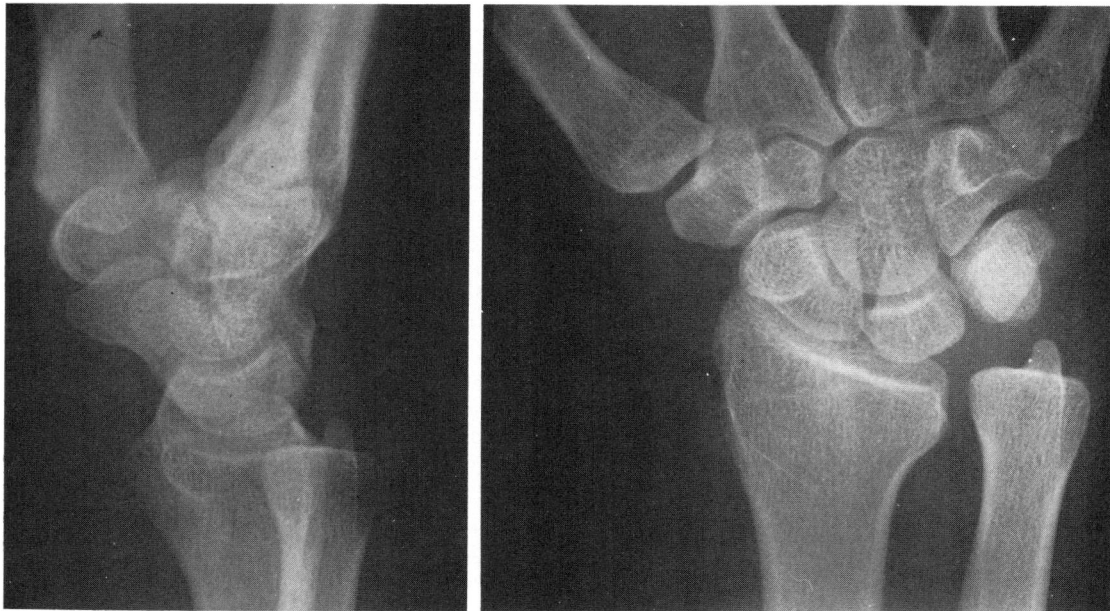

Figure 19–25 Isolated dorsal dislocations of the distal radioulnar joint. The lateral view shows the ulna riding dorsally to the radius. The pronated view (right) shows the central position of the ulnar styloid instead of its normal medial position in pronation, also indicating a disruption of a distal radioulnar joint. See Figure 19–6.

from a hypersupination injury. The stabilizing elements of the distal radioulnar joint were discussed in the section on surgical anatomy. It should be recalled that such dislocation involves a disruption of either the volar or the dorsal radioulnar ligament (see Fig. 19–4), depending on the direction of dislocation and the extent of damage to the triangular fibrocartilage.

The diagnosis is often overlooked. The dorsal or volar prominence of the displaced ulna is often obscured by soft tissue swelling, and x-rays are often read as negative for fracture. Point tenderness over the distal ulna as well as marked restriction of pronation and supination should alert the examiner to this injury. After anesthetizing the joint with Xylocaine one may observe an asymmetrical gross piano key–like instability of the ulna. Heiple[73] noted the difficulties associated with a radiographic diagnosis of this lesion. A true lateral view is mandatory, because oblique projections are confusing owing to the variable overlap of the distal radius and ulna. Comparison views of the uninjured wrist may be useful. Lastly, anteroposterior x-rays taken in full pronation and supination should show the normal migration of the ulnar styloid from a

medial location on the pronation film to a central location on the supination film (see Fig. 19–6). If the forearm is pronated and the styloid process appears to be over the center of the distal ulna, displacement of the distal radioulnar joint is present.[80] Arthrography can also be helpful in delineating tears of the triangular fibrocartilage in questionable cases of subluxation (Fig. 19–26). In the acute isolated dislocation, the reduction usually can be carried out simply by rotating the volar dislocation in pronation and the dorsal dislocation in supination under local anesthesia. If the dislocation is unstable, as in a Galeazzi fracture-dislocation, the reduced distal radioulnar joint can be pinned by percutaneous Kirschner wires. The reduction should be maintained in a long arm cast for six weeks to allow for ligamentous healing.

In the treatment of recurrent or chronic dislocations of this joint, over 26 different operations have been described; these are well catalogued by Veseley.[84] They follow the two basic types: soft tissue stabilizations and bone resections. The former[75, 84] involve the use of fascia lata or local tendon material for the re-creation of the radial and ulnar ligaments. In general, however, soft

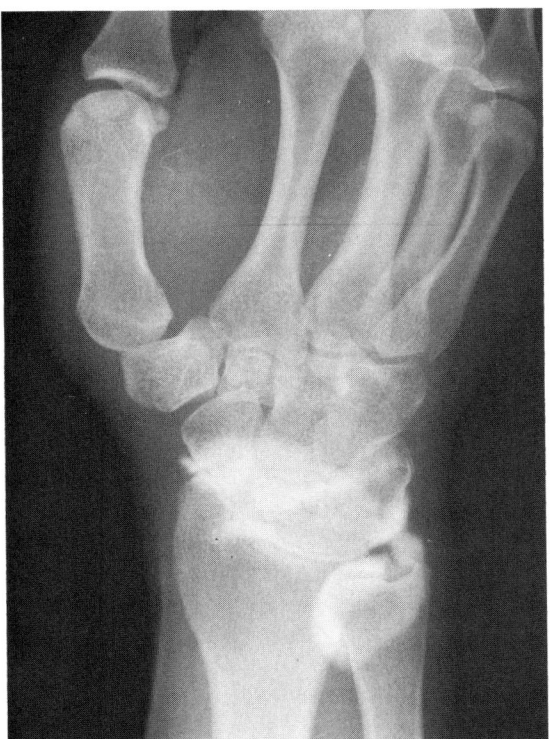

Figure 19–26 Arthrogram of a injured radioulnar joint. Note that the dye injected in the radiocarpal joint has gone through a tear in the triangular fibrocartilage into the distal radioulnar joint. Such perforations of the triangular fibrocartilage can occur in up to 30 per cent of the population as an age-related phenomenon. In a younger symptomatic person, however, such tears manifest acute disruption of the triangular fibrocartilage.

tissue procedures are unpredictable and result in either excessive limitation of rotation or recurrence of deformity. To treat such limitation of rotation, Darrach[69] advocated resection of the distal ulna. This is by far the most commonly used procedure, and there have been several excellent follow-up reports on this method.[70, 74] The type of resection we prefer was described in the section on complications of distal radial fractures. It should be restated that the goal should be to preserve the ulnar styloid process and its attachments.

THE CARPAL MECHANISM

Traditional descriptions of the anatomy of the carpal area are confusing, often conflicting, and surprisingly inadequate in de-

lineating the cause and, more critically, the treatment of carpal injuries. As the complex anatomical and kinematic relationships of the carpal bones have become appreciated, a more logical approach to carpal injuries has become possible. In this regard, the investigative efforts of Flatt,[9] Dobyns and Linscheid,[8, 155, 163] Taleisnik,[96] and Mayfield[94] have been instrumental in identifying the salient functional features.

The carpus consists of eight bones, organized into two distinct rows. The proximal row contains the navicular, lunate, triquetrum, and the sesamoidlike pisiform bone; the distal row contains the greater multangular, lesser multangular, capitate, and hamate (see Fig. 19–1). However, this concept of two clearly defined rows of bones sticking together through thick and thin fails to conform to the dynamics of wrist function. The first clarification was based on the recognition by Landsmeer[91] and Fisk[104] of the unique position of the navicular as an intercalated segment between the two rows. Their concept was a multilinked structure formed by the hand and distal carpal row, proximal carpal row, and forearm bones, these links being bridged by the navicular bone. Under axial loading the tendency of this multilinked structure to collapse in a zigzag or, as Fisk put it, the "concertina" (accordionlike), deformity was resisted by the navicular. Hence, in navicular waist fractures in which this stabilizing role is compromised, the wrist tends to collapse on itself. A second concept, that of the fixed carpometacarpal unit, was first postulated by Wood-Jones[15] and later experimentally verified by Flatt.[92] This states that the second and third metacarpals together with the capitate and the lesser multangular move as one unit throughout the range of carpal motions.

However, the columnar theory advocated by Taleisnik[96] best fits the dynamics of wrist function and the carpal response to injury. These columns are: a central column consisting of the lunate and the fixed unit; a radial column consisting of the navicular and the thumb axis; and an ulnar column consisting of the triquetrum and the ulnar border rays. These columns are coupled and interdependent.[90, 91] For example, the capitate articulates with both the navicular and the lunate. Hence, as its motion is conveyed to the proximal row, mutual displacements occur in both these bones. The function of the triquetrum in these interactions remains enigmatic, but since it is a major site for the attachment of both the volar and the dorsal ligaments, one can predict that its role, once clarified, will be prominent.

Wrist motion occurs in multiple planes: volar flexion and dorsiflexion (extension), radial and ulnar deviation, and pronation and supination. The relative contributions of the radiocarpal and the midcarpal to each of the motions have been studied by many investigators[86, 87, 90, 92, 94-96, 98] not only to provide a functional organization of wrist kinematics but also to implement treatment modalities, such as ligament reconstruction, arthrodeses, and prosthetic designs. Most authors agree with Flatt's proofs[92] that the center of all wrist motion lies within the head of the capitate and that radial deviation is essentially midcarpal and ulnar deviation is radiocarpal. The most heated controversy surrounds volar flexion and dorsiflexion (extension). Our studies agree with those[95, 96] that assign the greater portion of dorsiflexion (60 per cent) to the radiocarpal joint and, conversely, 60 per cent of volar flexion to the midcarpal joint. Individual patient variations as well as different methods of study may explain the discrepant data of other authors. The aspect that deserves the greater emphasis, however, is the simultaneous movement and reciprocal adjustment of the radiocarpal and midcarpal joints throughout the flexion-extension arc.

No tendons insert on the carpal bones, and thus all carpal motions are reactive to metacarpal and forearm motion. The motion of the hand is carried out through the fixed unit of the metacarpals and capitate to the proximal carpal row, which adjusts by mutual displacement of the lunate and the navicular. This continuous adaptive interplay of the proximal row and the fixed unit is controlled by the geometrical contours of the individual carpal bones and the carpal ligaments.[90] These structural characteristics allow for a loosely fitting arrangement of the carpal bones in volar flexion. As the wrist is dorsiflexed, the carpal bones abut in a progressively tighter packing, such that in maximum dorsiflexion the lunate and the navicular are locked against the radius by the distal carpal row. MacConaill[93] labeled this progressive locking of the carpal bones in dorsiflexion the screw-vise phenomenon, in which all the carpal bones are tightly screwed together as in a vise. This phenomenon helps explain the susceptibility of the carpal structures to injury through falls on the dorsiflexed wrist.

As important as the geometrical surfaces of the bones is the complex arrangement of wrist ligaments that maintains these intimate intercarpal relationships and controls the highly sophisticated intercarpal motion. In traditional anatomical descriptions, little attempt was made to identify specific ligaments in the fibrous capsule that encompasses the wrist joint. Lewis[17] was the first to emphasize that this capsule had specific reinforcing ligaments, which he identified as the dorsal and palmar radiocarpal ligaments. Other investigators[94, 96] further refined this work.

The concept of radial and ulnar collateral

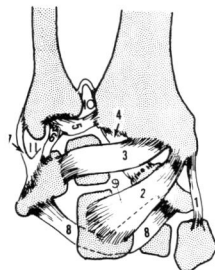

1	RADIAL COLLATERAL		7	ULNAR COLLATERAL
2	RADIO- (NAVICULO)-CAPITATE		8	ARCUATE (Henle)
3	RADIO-LUNATE-TRIQUETRUM		9	SPACE OF POIRIER
4	RADIO- NAVICULAR		10	DISTAL-RADIO-ULNAR JOINT
5	TRIANGULAR FIBROCARTILAGE		11	PRESTYLOID RECESS
6	ULNO-TRIQUETRAL			

Figure 19-27 Schematic representation of the volar wrist ligaments. The majority of these volar intracapsular ligaments originate from the radius and insert on varying carpal bones. 1. The radial collateral ligament is volar on the radius and inserts in the distal tubercle of the navicular and into the trapezium. 2 and 3. The radiocapitate and radiolunate triquetrum ligaments are strong volar ligaments. 4. The radionavicular ligament inserts on the interosseous ligament and part of the proximal pole of the navicular. 5. The triangular fibrocartilage is seen originating on the medial radius and inserts on the base of the ulnar styloid. The ulnar complex of ligaments arises from the triangular fibrocartilage and inserts on the triquetrum. The distal radioulnar joint is labeled 10. The prestyloid recess, a synovial recess that is frequently the first site of involvement in rheumatoid arthritis, surrounds the unattached tip of the ulnar styloid. The space shown in 9 is a potential weak spot supporting this volar ligamentous apparatus, through which the lunate may subluxate or dislocate.

ligaments as dominant lateral and medial stabilizers like those of the finger or knee joints is no longer valid. Instead, the radial collateral ligament is best seen as a thickened band extending volarly from the radial styloid to the navicular tuberosity and the trapezium (Fig. 19–27). The ulnar collateral ligament runs from a broad attachment at the base of the ulnar styloid to a roughened area on the ulnar aspect of the triquetrum and pisotriquetral ligament. This volar and ulnar collateral ligament is reinforced by intraarticular merging with the triangular fibrocartilage, which arises from the radius and attaches to the inner aspect of the styloid base. These two basal insertions are responsible for the ulnar styloid avulsion fracture that accompanies distal radial fractures. The ulnar styloid tip has no ligamentous attachments and lies within the prestyloid recess.

Except for the ulnar collateral ligament, the volar carpal ligaments arise from the radius and the triangular fibrocartilage, thus suspending the carpus from those structures. Fibers of the volar radiocarpal ligament can be dissected into several discrete, thickened ligaments (Fig. 19–27). Just ulnarward from the radial collateral is the radiocapite ligament that grooves the navicular waist as it passes from the radial styloid to insert on the capitate. The navicular rotates around this ligament, extending vertically in wrist volar flexion and horizontally in dorsiflexion (Fig. 19–28). A third strong arcade of fibers passes from the radius, inserting in both the lunate and the triquetrum. In between these two strong areas are weaker fibers that are particularly vulnerable to injury when the wrist is stressed. It is through this interligamentous area, known as the space of Poirier (see Fig.

19–27), that the lunate is dislocated into the carpal canal in lunate dislocations.

Although thinner and less distinct than the capsule, the dorsal radiocarpal ligament possesses several bands, the major one extending from the dorsal radius to the dorsal pole of the lunate, finally inserting firmly into the dorsal ridge of the triquetrum. On the ulnar side of the carpus, the triquetrum is a stronghold of ligamentous insertions. It shares with the navicular the region of the arcuate ligament of Henle, a V-shaped intrinsic structure centered on the capitate near the center of wrist rotation (see Fig. 19–27).

Strong intraarticular ligaments connect the eight carpal bones together and further stabilize the fixed unit of the distal carpal row and the second and third metacarpals. These intraosseous ligaments blend both volarly and dorsally with the radiocarpal ligaments and are frequently involved in severe wrist injuries. In this regard, the naviculolunate intraosseous ligament deserves particular emphasis. The dorsal fibers are short relative to the length of the volar fibers,[90, 91, 94] allowing mutual displacements of the navicular and the lunate similar to the opening and closing of a scissors (Fig. 19–29). Such a coupled shift must occur in dorsiflexion as these two bones adjust to the axial loading of the capitate. The naviculolunate ligament thus coordinates this motion while resisting any excessive distraction. A second reinforcing ligament, the radionavicular ligament, inserts variably on either the navicular or the lunate to reinforce this connection. When excessive axial and rotatory forces disrupt these ligaments,[94, 151, 155] naviculolunate dissociation occurs with symptoms of weakness, pain, and clicking in the wrist.

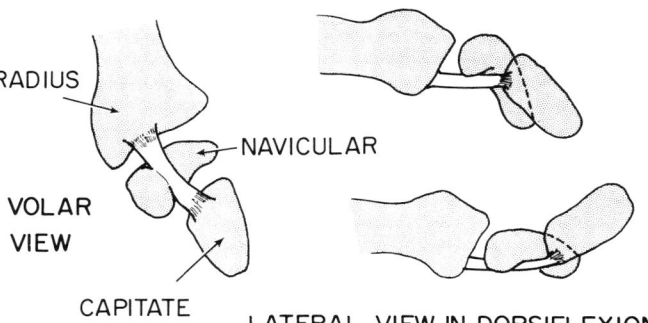

LATERAL VIEW IN VOLAR FLEXION

Figure 19–28 Schematic representation of the rotation of the navicular around the volar radiocapitate ligament. This can be seen in the lateral view with volar flexion and dorsiflexion of the wrist. The navicular accommodates this motion by becoming vertical in volar flexion and horizontal in dorsiflexion.

RADIUS

NAVICULAR

VOLAR VIEW

CAPITATE

LATERAL VIEW IN DORSIFLEXION

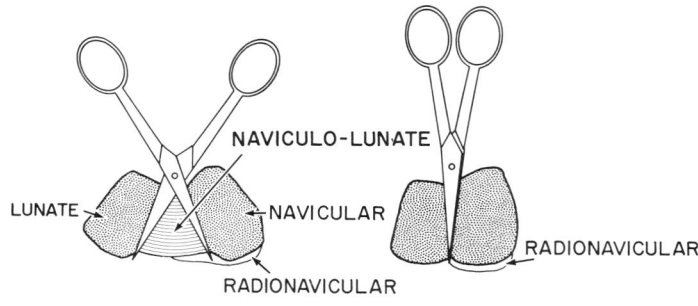

Figure 19-29 Schematic rendering of the naviculolunate interosseous ligament and the radionavicular ligament. The naviculolunate interosseous ligament is a strong ligament connecting the lunate to the navicular. Dorsally, its fibers are shorter than its volar fibers, and thus this ligament acts like the hinge of a scissors. In a dorsiflexed position, the capitate moves proximally against the lunate and the navicular, which separates to accommodate the proximal portion of the capitate. In volar flexion, the carpal bones are loosely packed, and the navicular and lunate approximate each other. A second ligament, the radionavicular ligament, attaches volarly to both the interosseous ligament and the proximal pole of the navicular. Both the interosseous ligament and the volar radionavicular ligament must be torn for naviculolunate dissociation to occur.

Thus, carpal stability derives from the bony architecture of the individual carpal articulations and their respective ligamentous restraints. Carpal motion is a response to distally based musculotendinous activity and represents synchronous and simultaneous adjustments of each carpal bone within the limits of its ligamentous stabilization. When these limits are exceeded, the ensuing disruption, whether a carpal fracture, a carpal dislocation, or a combination of both, must be carefully analyzed in order to best restore the balance of the carpal mechanism. The specific nature of any injury will of course depend on the position of the hand on impact, the mechanical properties of the bones and ligaments, and the magnitude of the injuring force.

CARPAL FRACTURES

Isolated carpal fractures are approximately one-tenth as frequent as distal radial fractures but, as can be seen in Table 19-4,

they are by no means uncommon. Given the irregular geometrical contours of the carpal bones and their degree of overlapping on multiple radiographic projections, these fractures are often missed. Whenever point tenderness and limited range of motion are present following a fall on the outstretched hand, the physician should be suspicious of a carpal injury and exhaust all efforts to identify a specific lesion. The diagnosis of wrist sprain should not be used to dismiss a suspicious injury as trivial. Many carpal injuries are not evident on initial x-rays and may require several weeks for resorption to make fracture lines distinct. Any significant wrist injury, even in the face of negative x-rays, should be immobilized for several weeks and then x-rayed again.

FRACTURES OF THE NAVICULAR

As can be seen in Table 19-4, the navicular or scaphoid bone accounts for over 60 per cent of all carpal injuries. The navicular occupies a particularly vulnerable anatomical position in the wrist. It spans both the distal and the proximal carpal rows and acts as a link communicating the motion of the distal row to that of the proximal row. It is a curved, elongated bone with four of its six surfaces being articular. Proximally it articulates with the radius, distally with the trapezium and the trapezoid, and medially with the lunate and the capitate. This large articular area leaves only dorsal and lateral ridges through which the nutrient blood supply can enter.

Understanding the blood supply of the navicular is important in terms of treatment and prognosis. The classic work of Taleisnik

TABLE 19-4 Incidence and Distribution of 453 Isolated Carpal Bone Fractures

Carpal Bone	Number	Percentage
Navicular	278	61.2
Lunate	32	7.0
Triquetrum	62	13.6
Pisiform	6	1.4
Trapezium	24	5.4
Trapezoid	14	3.1
Capitate	19	4.3
Hamate	18	4.0
Total	453	100.0

and Kelly[118] describes the extraosseous and intraosseous blood supply. The extraosseous supply consists of the dorsal, laterovolar, and distal blood vessel groups. These arise from the radial artery or the radial artery in its superficial palmar branch. All arterial groups penetrate the waist of the navicular except for the distal group, which enters at the tuberosity. The laterovolar group is the largest of the three arteries and enters volar and lateral to the radionavicular articular surface. In approximately one third of navicular bones, all arterial supply enters distal to the navicular waist. This precarious arrangement makes the proximal navicular fragment susceptible to avascular necrosis in fractures of the waist. Unfortunately, given present methods, it is impossible to distinguish the navicular at risk because of this variation in its blood supply.

Study of the interosseous blood supply reveals that the lateral, volar, and dorsal groups anastomose, while the distal group supplies only the tuberosity.[14, 118] The lateral volar group, the main source of blood, breaks up into two to four main branches that supply the proximal two thirds of the bone and terminate in an arcade system. Advocates of both the volar and the dorsal surgical approaches to the navicular have each claimed the merit of vascular protection to justify their methods. Injection studies favor neither approach, and we prefer the Russe volar approach for the greater exposure it provides.[115]

The biomechanical role of the navicular as a stabilizing link indispensable to the normal reciprocal motions of the carpal mechanism has been previously discussed. As Landsmeer and others[91, 93, 104, 107] have shown, with navicular failure the carpus collapses in a zigzag deformity in which the distal carpal row crumples into the proximal carpus. The stabilizing effect of the navicular is lost either by fracture of the navicular waist or by disruption of its proximal ligamentous support.

Incidence and Mechanism of Injury

Fractures of the navicular are primarily an injury of young males in their second through fourth decades and usually result from athletic or work-related injuries. In some series, the number of males is as high as 85 per cent. This injury is caused by a fall on the outstretched hand similar to the mechanism of distal radial fractures in the elderly. With forced dorsiflexion, the navicular and other carpal bones lie in a tightly packed arrangement and are tethered by the taut volar ligaments. Radial deviation pins the navicular waist against the dorsal lip of the radius, which then acts as a fulcrum. Recently, Weber and Chao[121] have demonstrated experimentally that greater than 95 degrees of dorsiflexion (slight radial deviation) predictably causes waist fractures. In this mechanism, the distal end of the navicular is driven over the radial lip while the proximal portion of the navicular remains secured by its ligamentous attachments.

Types of Navicular Fractures

The easiest and most prognostically significant classification of navicular fractures divides them by location. Watson-Jones[14] classically divides the navicular into thirds; however, we identify four separate locations (Fig. 19–30): tubercle, distal pole, waist, and proximal pole. Approximately 70 per

Fractures of the Navicular

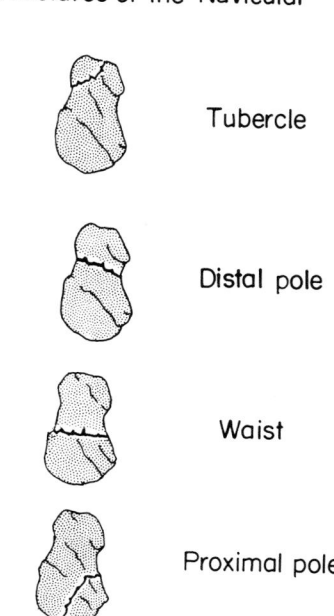

Tubercle

Distal pole

Waist

Proximal pole

Figure 19–30 Classification of navicular fractures. Tubercle fractures are avulsion fractures of the radial collateral ligament. Distal pole and waist fractures make up the bulk of navicular fractures. Proximal pole fractures may represent an avulsion fracture of the radionavicular ligament and are extremely susceptible to avascular necrosis.

cent of the fractures occur at the waist or middle third, 10 per cent in the distal pole, and the remaining 20 per cent in the proximal pole. In the uncomplicated nondisplaced navicular fracture, fractures of the tubercle, distal pole, and waist heal in an average of eight weeks.[115, 120] Fractures of the proximal pole require approximately 12 weeks to heal. The orientation of the fracture line is, according to Russe,[115] also of practical significance. The more horizontal the line in relation to the long axis of the navicular, the more quickly healing will occur. He postulates that this is related to the compressive forces exerted across such a fracture line. Fracture healing time, therefore, is proportional to the distance from the distal navicular pole, the orientation of the fracture line, and the time that elapses from injury to initial treatment.

Diagnosis

The patient usually reports a fall on the dorsiflexed wrist. On examination, tenderness in the anatomical snuffbox should be considered pathognomonic. This finding should alert the physician to the possibility of navicular fracture even in the face of negative roentgenographic studies. Other findings may include tenderness on the

radial volar aspect in the area of the proximal wrist crease, painful grip, and decreased and painful wrist motion. There may also be swelling of the wrist joint.

Recommended radiological studies include anteroposterior, lateral, and oblique projections as well as an anteroposterior view in ulnar deviation in an attempt to open any fracture line present. It must be remembered that many nondisplaced navicular fractures are difficult or impossible to diagnose on the initial x-rays (Fig. 19–31A). Such fractures are stable, since they are surrounded by an intact or almost intact cartilaginous shell. McLaughlin[108] advocates aspiration of the wrist when a navicular fracture is suspected. If the fluid is clear or slightly tinged with blood, a nondisplaced fracture of the navicular is highly probable. It should be remembered that in such fractures several weeks may be required for bone resorption and widening of the fracture line, rendering it more visible. If a frank hemarthrosis is found, the diagnosis of navicular fracture is usually obvious radiologically.

Emphasizing the fact that initial x-rays (Fig. 19–31A) are often negative in these injuries, we recommend that any patient who presents with a suspected nondisplaced navicular fracture be immobilized in

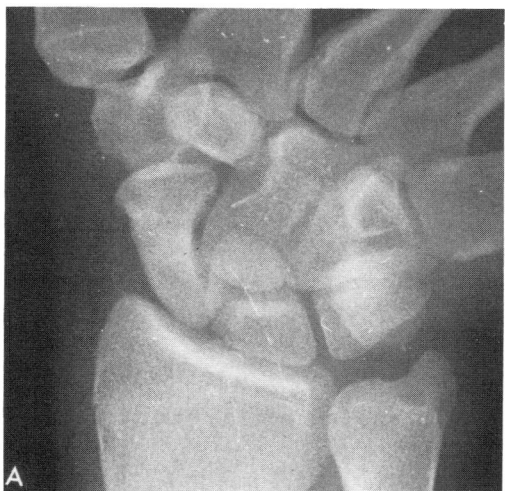 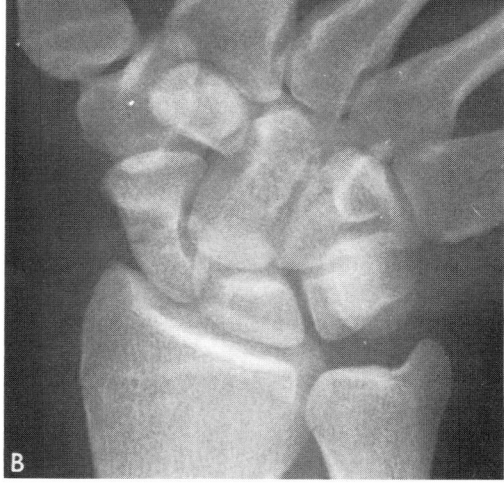

Figure 19–31 The importance of clinical suspicion in treating navicular fractures. *A.* The patient fell on his dorsiflexed wrist. On examination he had pain in the anatomical snuffbox associated with limitation of motion. The view was negative for navicular fracture. *B.* Because of clinical suspicion, however, the patient was splinted and x-rayed two weeks later. Here, the nondisplaced fracture of the waist is obvious. Immobilization was continued for seven more weeks, and the fracture progressed to uneventful union.

a cast for several weeks and then x-rayed again (Fig. 19–31B). If at that time the wrist is not tender and has a full range of motion with x-rays still negative, immobilization may be discontinued. If, however, x-rays are still negative but the tenderness persists, further immobilization for several weeks is recommended. If x-rays after a four-week interval are again negative, immobilization may be discontinued. Although it is often claimed that the navicular fracture heals poorly, it should be emphasized that over 90 per cent heal without any complication. With early diagnosis and appropriate treatment, the prognosis is excellent.

A fracture of the tubercle is an avulsion injury in which the radial collateral ligament pulls off its bony attachment. Treatment consists of a short arm cast for approximately six weeks, and the course is usually uneventful.

Once diagnosed, acute body fractures

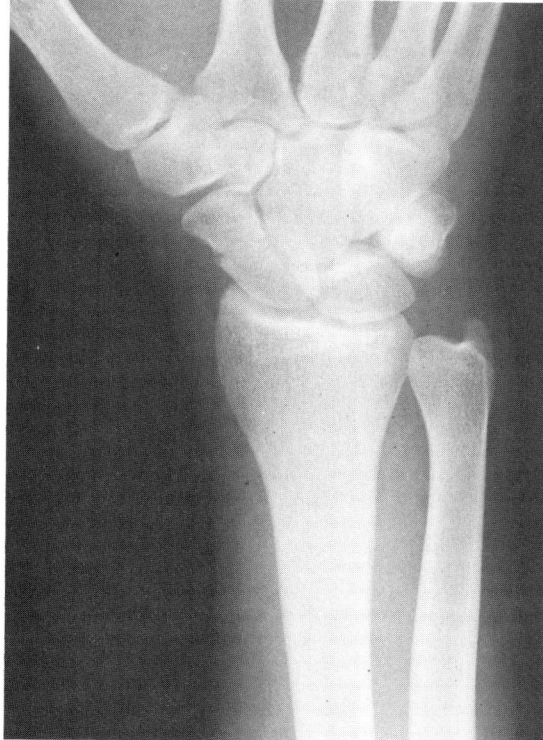

Figure 19–32 Navicular fracture of the waist. The patient was immobilized for six weeks initially in a long arm cast brought out to the level of the thumb. This was cut down to a short arm cast at four weeks, and the fracture went on to uneventful union at ten weeks.

(Fig. 19–32) without displacement require immobilization. No universally accepted position of immobilization exists. Dorsiflexion and radial deviation are most commonly used,[2, 101, 105, 108, 110] but some authors recommend ulnar deviation or slight volar flexion.[121] Friedenberg,[105] in a classic study on experimentally produced horizontal fractures at all levels of the navicular, found that the fracture fragments are firmly apposed when the wrist is dorsiflexed at least 30 degrees and radially deviated. Another controversial issue is the inclusion of the thumb or elbow in the cast.

Thomaidis,[119] studying anatomical specimens, found that supination and pronation caused motion across experimentally produced waist fractures. Such motion might be expected because of the ligamentous attachments of the proximal navicular pole to the distal radius. Likewise, motion of the thumb and first metacarpal result in some movement of the distal fragment of the fractured navicular transmitted through the articulation of the trapezium. We have observed motion at the fracture site with thumb and elbow movement under cineradiography. Based on such observations, our standard treatment includes a long arm cast with the elbow at 90 degrees, the wrist extended 30 degrees in 15 degrees of radial deviation, and the thumb included to the base of the proximal phalanx. The fingers are excluded.

The duration of immobilization can be stated as the time required for radiographic union. Unfortunately, this simple yardstick is often lacking or lags behind the clinical picture, and thus the tendency is to overimmobilize these fractures. By six weeks, the patient is usually clinically asymptomatic and thus can offer little help in judging bony union. In general, we subscribe to those healing times mentioned earlier; that is, distal pole and waist fractures require 8 to 12 weeks of immobilization, and proximal pole fractures require 12 to 16 weeks of immobilization. In doubtful cases, we resort to motion views of the wrist, including ulnar deviation, to see if gapping occurs as well as to tomography or arthrography. Bone scanning and arthroscopy of the wrist have proved of very little benefit in diagnosing union. Depending on the age of the patient, long arm immobilization is discontinued at four to six weeks and replaced by a prona-

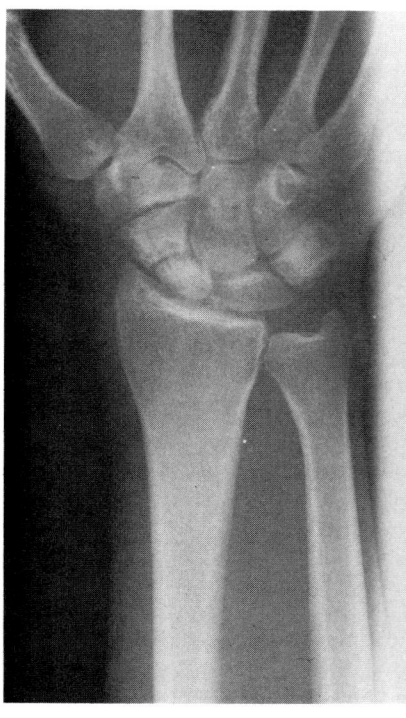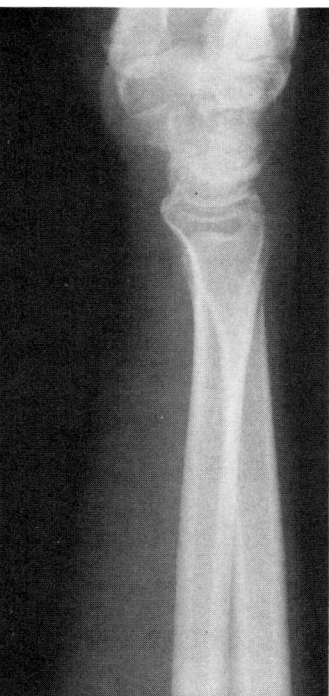

Figure 19–33 Fracture of the proximal pole of the navicular. These fractures have an increased incidence of avascular necrosis, and nonunion as shown here in this two-year-old fracture.

tion-supination lock that allows flexion-extension of the elbow or simply by a short arm cast. Following removal of immobilization, the patient is protected by a short arm splint until full active wrist motion is obtained. Acute fractures of the proximal pole are similarly treated, with the recognition that the incidence of nonunion and avascular necrosis is increased in this fracture (Fig. 19–33).

A special dilemma in treating the nondisplaced navicular fracture is posed by the congenital bipartite navicular. In this condition, the separation usually occurs at the waist or middle portion of the navicular. While many authors feel it is a traumatic condition, others[116] believe it has a true incidence of approximately 1 in 1000 individuals. Several theories have been suggested, including the presence of more than one ossification center or the persistence of an enlarged sesamoid bone. Radiographic criteria that may be helpful include the rounded and smooth edges of the defect, the absence of cyst formation, and the lack of motion on cineradiography. There is also a tendency toward bilaterality.

In fractures of the body with displacement, a closed reduction with the wrist in dorsiflexion and radial deviation is attempted. If anteroposterior and lateral x-rays confirm the anatomical reduction, the fracture is casted like fractures without displacement. Once displacement occurs, however, closed reduction is extremely difficult, as the navicular fragments tend to assume a 90-90 position with the distal untethered fragment hyperflexed 90 degrees on the proximal fragment (Fig. 19–34). Such a position is unacceptable, and open reduction and internal fixation are recommended if closed reduction fails. We prefer the Matte-Russe[115] approach, reducing the fragments and stabilizing them with a large iliac bone graft; others have resorted to cancellous screws or Kirschner wires.[106, 109] Such displaced navicular fractures often accompany carpal instability patterns, such as perilunate dislocations. In this case, reduction and treatment of carpal instability are performed in addition to open reduction of the navicular fragments. In either case, the principle is the same: anatomical reduction and stabilization of the navicular axis.

Navicular Nonunion

The difficulty lies in the definition of navicular nonunion. Although widening of

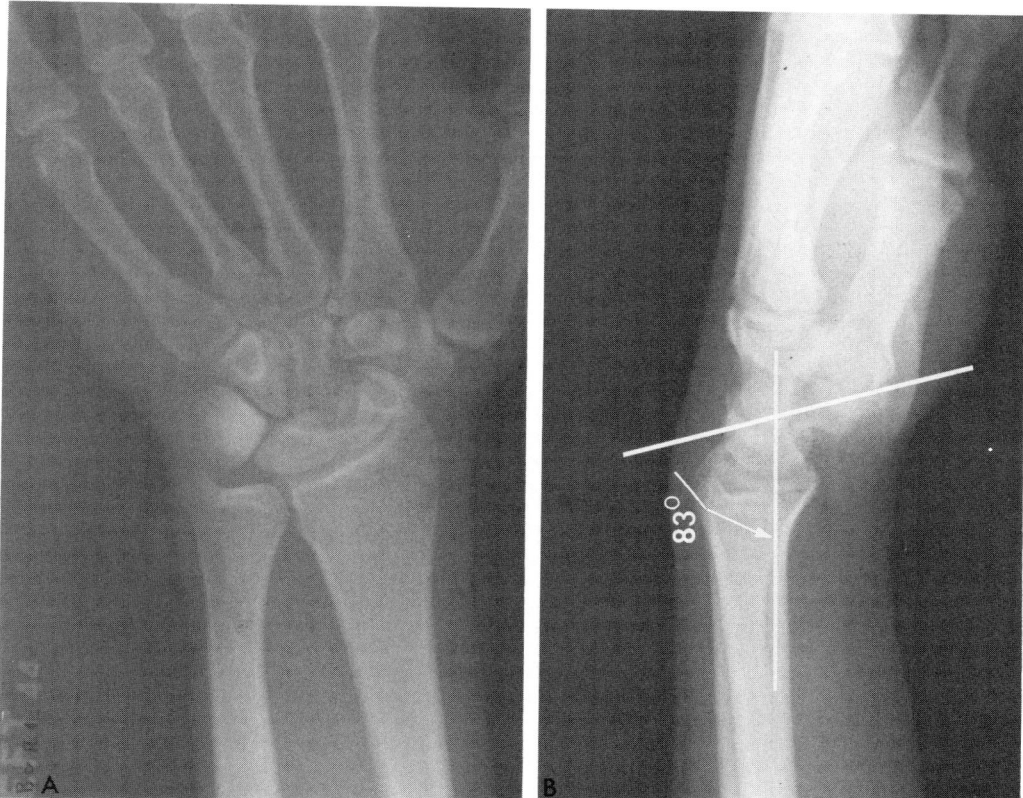

Figure 19–34 *A* and *B*. Navicular fracture showing collapse deformity. The anteroposterior view shows a displaced navicular fracture seen as a cortical ring outline over the body of the navicular. When the navicular lunate angle is measured (Fig. 19–41) it is shown to be increased, suggesting a more vertical than normal position of the distal fragment of the navicular. Here, the navicular lost its stabilizing function of spanning both the proximal and the distal row and instead has collapsed on itself. Stress is generated by this collapsed position and may be one of the factors in the high incidence of nonunion in navicular waist fractures.

the fracture cleft, cyst formation, and sclerosis of the fracture ends have been used in the past (see Fig. 19–33), the latter changes may not occur for several months or years. Proximal pole sclerosis has been observed in up to 30 per cent of fresh fractures,[115] and while this may suggest delayed union it is not an absolute sign of nonunion (Fig. 19–35). Perhaps a more reasonable definition is a fracture that shows no evidence of radiographic healing on three separate examinations one month apart.

Etiology of the nonunion includes the biomechanical forces placed across the navicular linking mechanism, the interference of synovial fluid, the lack of periosteal callus with only endosteal consolidation, the precarious navicular blood supply in some patients, the failure to obtain an anatomical reduction, and most importantly, the failure

to make the initial correct diagnosis, with absent, delayed, or inadequate immobilization.

Historically, nonunions have been treated by myriad techniques. These include prolonged immobilization,[14] excision of one or both fragments,[8] proximal row carpectomy,[153] internal screw fixation,[106, 109] prosthetic replacment,[141] drilling of the fracture fragments,[5, 110] limited intercarpal arthrodesis,[131, 138] radiocarpal arthrodesis,[6] bone grafting,[103, 111, 112] styloidectomy,[100, 117] or combinations of these. The presence of a nonunion, however, does not necessarily indicate that one of the aforementioned treatments should be undertaken. Decisions about surgery must be based on the patient's disability, occupation, age, and motivation. We differentiate delayed union or nonunion into four types: delayed union;

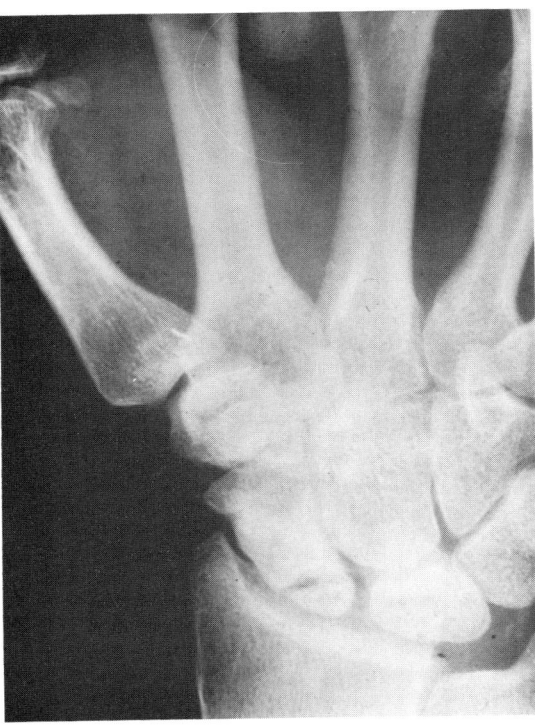

Figure 19–35 Navicular nonunion. This patient presented with pain on motion of the wrist two years following a trivial wrist injury. The anteroposterior view shows sclerosis, cyst formation, and persistence of the fracture cleft. Lateral views show the collapsed deformity associated with such fractures. Treatment was by Matte-Russe bone grafting. The fracture healed uneventfully, and the wrist was asymptomatic.

nonunion without wrist arthritis; nonunion with avascular necrosis without wrist arthritis; and nonunion with or without avascular necrosis but with wrist arthritis.

If, on serial films taken in the course of three to four months, no evidence of progressive healing is noted, operative intervention is recommended. At this stage, we favor the technique of Matte-Russe.[115] Thirty years ago, the Swiss surgeon Matte described the resection through the dorsal approach of the fibrotic tissue, filling the fracture gap with autogenous cancellous bone. To Matte's technique Russe added the volar approach, bridging the fragments not only with cancellous bone but with a corticocancellous graft. Using the volar approach, the navicular fracture is exposed and reduced. In those fractures that have collapsed in a 90-90 position, such reduction can be extremely difficult. Because of the cartilaginous shell of the navicular, the fracture line is not always apparent but can usually be localized with the use of a Kirschner wire. All abnormal fibrous tissue is excised at the level of pseudarthrosis, and both fragments are curetted out (Fig. 19–36) using a Hall drill. The corticocancellous graft obtained from the iliac crest is fitted snugly in this excavated groove, with care taken not to distract the bony fragments. A long arm cast is worn until there is radiological union. With this technique, Russe[115] obtained union in 20 of 22 patients; others have achieved union in greater than 95 per cent of cases.[111, 120] Using this technique, we have obtained union in all but 2 of 67 patients. One of these nonunions occurred when the patient removed her cast two weeks postsurgery. Over 85 per cent of patients have been pleased with their results and have returned to their regular activities. We have noted no correlation between the duration of the nonunion and the time of bone graft consolidation.

Recently, we have begun to investigate a newer technique using the percutaneous insertion of battery-powered electrodes, as described by Brighton (see Chapter 3). One or two 20-μA cathodes are drilled into the fracture site under local anesthesia, and the patient is casted in our routine manner (Fig. 19–37). These cathodes are removed at between eight to twelve weeks, at which time union has been completely solid in five of the six patients in whom this

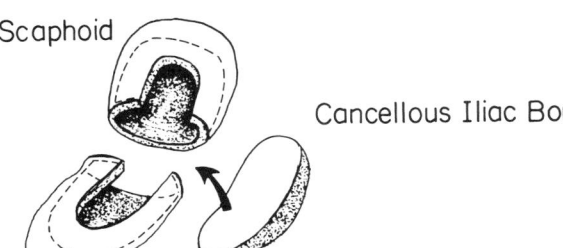

Scaphoid

Cancellous Iliac Bone Graft

Figure 19–36 Procedure used in Matte-Russe bone grafting. The cancellous iliac bone graft is slotted in the cartilaginous navicular shell, which has first been reduced. Care should be taken not to distract the fracture fragment. Such grafts heal on an average of 14 to 16 weeks.

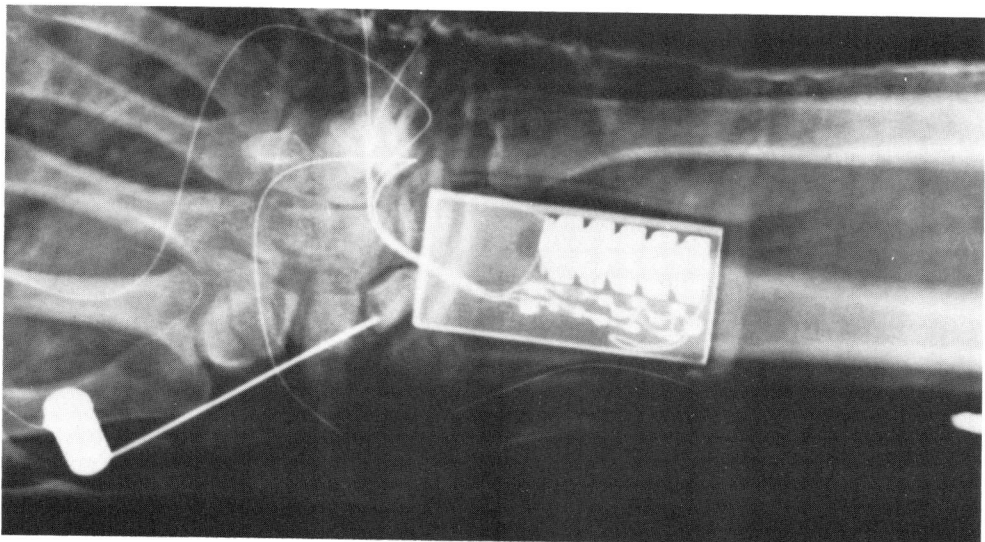

Figure 19–37 Electrical treatment of navicular nonunion. The electrode tip is at the fracture site in the waist of the navicular. The battery pack is seen as the box overlying the patient's radius. This fracture healed after eight weeks of electrode therapy.

technique has been used. Given this low degree of morbidity, we are now considering the use of this technique in those navicular fractures at risk for nonunion, such as the displaced fracture-dislocation, in which operating time and donor bone graft morbidity problems should be minimized.

In those nonunions with avascular necrosis of the proximal fragment (Preiser's disease)[114] or without evidence of wrist arthritis, our approach is tailored not only to the patient's symptoms but also to the size of the articular fragment. Minimal symptoms may require no treatment or simply intermittent immobilization. If aseptic necrosis involves a major fragment, the Matte-Russe procedure, limited intracarpal arthrodesis, and prosthetic replacement of the navicular have been performed equally often. If the avascular segment is less than 20 per cent, we prefer excision of this piece and insertion of a collagenous spacer, such as the palmaris longus tendon rolled up on itself like an anchovy.

If degenerative changes have already occurred in the radiocarpal joint we employ a styloidectomy with or without excision of the fibrous tissue and iliac bone grafting. In the younger patient with arthritic changes and severe symptoms, we rely on radio-carpal fusion. Despite some glowing re-

ports,[153] we reserve proximal carpectomy for those patients who do not make strenuous demands on the wrist. Such individualization of treatment reminds us that nonunion of the carpal navicular is a very complex problem that will not be solved by any one surgical procedure.

FRACTURES OF THE TRIQUETRUM

The second most common carpal bone fracture occurs in the triquetrum. The triquetrum is the most ulnar of the proximal row carpal bones and is a stronghold of ligamentous attachments both volarly and dorsally (see Fig. 19–27). The avulsion fractures occurring at these ligamentous insertions therefore account for the majority of triquetral fractures. The mechanism of injury is excessive volar flexion or dorsiflexion of the wrist. Symptoms, as with all wrist injuries, include pain, swelling, restricted motion, and point tenderness usually located on the dorsal aspect.

Bartone and others[124, 143] have distinguished two types of fracture. Type 1 is a bony avulsion fracture, and type 2 is the rarer fracture of the body. Dorsal avulsion fractures can be seen only in the lateral or oblique view (Fig. 19–38). These fragments may be single or multiple and usually have

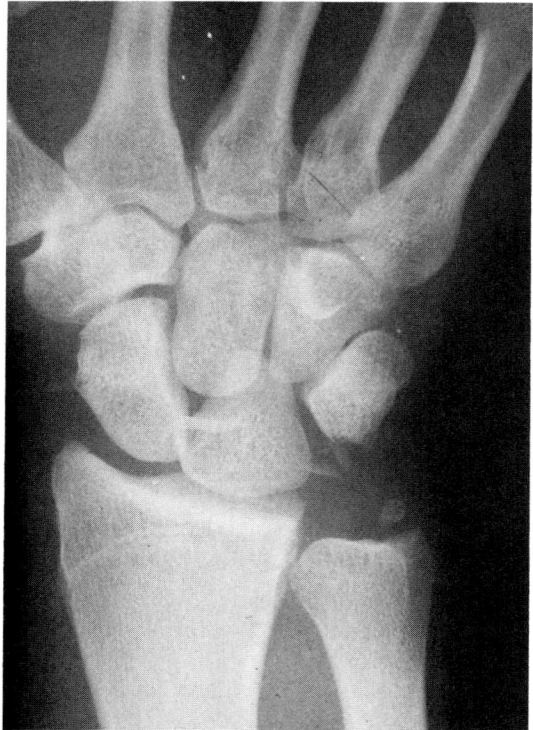

Figure 19–38 Fracture of the triquetrum. This patient had a rotatory injury of the wrist with an avulsion of the ulna styloid as well as several avulsion fragments from the proximal portion of the triquetrum. Most of these fragments, however, are from the dorsal aspects and are best seen on a lateral view.

a slight separation from the bone. Treatment is guided by ligamentous rather than bony healing, and thus a short arm plaster cast with the wrist in 30 degrees of dorsiflexion is worn for three to six weeks. Symptoms following such immobilization, rather than serial x-rays, should be the guide to continued immobilization. The rarer body fracture is best seen on the standard anteroposterior film of the wrist and usually heals satisfactorily with six weeks of cast immobilization.

LUNATE FRACTURES AND KIENBÖCK'S DISEASE

Injuries of the lunate constitute 7 per cent of isolated carpal injuries (Table 19–4). Given the significant overlap of the centrally placed lunate in all plain film projections, these data underestimate the frequency of the most common lunate fracture, the longitudinal compression fracture. Experimental work[133] has shown that such a fracture occurs as the lunate is wedged between the proximal capitate and the radius when the wrist is placed in forced dorsiflexion and ulnar deviation. As in all carpal bone injuries, swelling and painful, limited wrist motion are present, but gross deformity and crepitus are rare. Again, the advisability of short-term immobilization and repeated x-ray examination for any wrist injury should be emphasized. If, after such a period of immobilization, point tenderness persists over the lunate, lateral tomography and high-resolution bone scan may be useful in confirming a lunate compression fracture. Our management of this fracture includes six weeks of immobilization as well as a prognostic discussion with the patient concerning the nature of avascular necrosis. Avulsion fractures of the lunate, either dorsally or volarly, do occur and can be diagnosed on the oblique films. As with triquetral avulsion fractures, complications and late sequelae are minimal. Treatment involves wrist immobilization for a period of six weeks.

The most common complication of lunate injuries is avascular necrosis. The pathogenesis is still unknown. Kienböck[134] described the progressive collapse of the lunate as lunatomalacia. He believed the condition was caused by an interruption of the volar and dorsal blood supply as a primary circulatory disorder with secondary fragmentation. Modern opinion cites the compression fracture, with interruption of the volar and dorsal blood supply, as the primary cause. The significant association of Kienböck's disease with negative ulnar variance,[127, 130] which places abnormal loading stress on the lunate, reinforces this thesis. Ulnar variance refers to the relationship of the distal articular surface of the radius to that of the distal ulna. Neutral variance is present when these articular surfaces are at the same level (in approximately 60 per cent of cases), while negative ulnar variance (occurring in 25 per cent) means that the distal radius extends 1 mm or more beyond the distal ulnar surface. Seventy-five per cent of patients with Kienböck's disease demonstrate negative ulnar variance. Given the relatively low

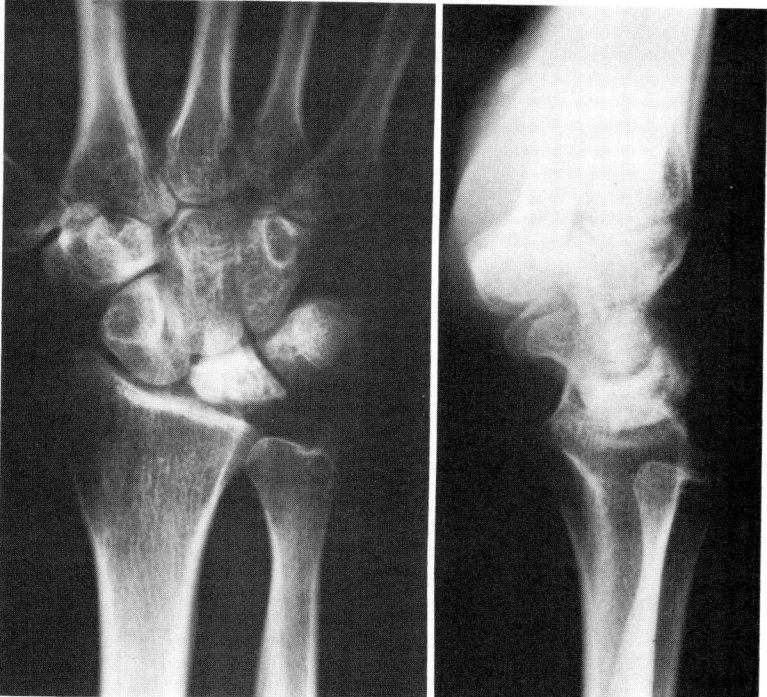

Figure 19-39 Avascular necrosis of the lunate, or Kienböck's disease. Shown here is a stage 1 Kienböck's disease with marked density of the lunate bone. This patient had symptoms of aching in the wrist with repetitive and strenuous use.

incidence of avascular necrosis in the general population, however, such negative ulnar variance is best seen as a predisposing rather than a sole cause, to which trauma and hereditary influences must be added. Kienböck's disease is found most commonly in males in the second to fourth decades and in the dominant hand. It bears no relationship to other forms of osteochondritis or avascular necrosis, such as Legg-Calvé-Perthes disease.

Three radiographic stages of Kienböck's disease can be recognized.[135] In stage 1 (Fig. 19–39) the architecture of the lunate in relation to the other carpal bones is preserved, but definite osteosclerotic density changes are evident on the regular films of the lunate. In questionable cases, cast immobilization for several weeks may accentuate the increased density of the lunate relative to the other carpal bones. Clinical symptoms at this time are aching when using the wrist and painful but full range of motion. Stage 2 shows progressive collapse and fragmentation of the lunate, with proximal migration of the capitate and disturbance of other intracarpal relationships. At this stage, pain is usually a predominant symptom as well as diminished grip

strength and wrist motion. In stage 3, the lunate collapse has progressed to generalized radiocarpal osteoarthritis, with joint space narrowing and osteocyte formation. The symptoms are those of degenerative joint disease, with variable pain but usually severely limited wrist motion.

Whenever treatment results are inadequate, procedures abound and the treatment of Kienböck's disease is no exception. There are over 18 procedures described in the literature, including: prolonged cast immobilization;[129, 135] lunate drilling and grafting;[129] ulnar lengthening or, conversely, radial shortening;[8, 127] lunate excision;[139] lunate arthroplasty either with a silicone prosthesis[135, 141] or soft tissue interposition;[137] proximal row carpectomy;[152, 153] limited intracarpal arthrodesis;[131, 138] and radiocarpal fusion.[144] The symptoms of stage 1 are those of reactive synovitis. We treat these with intermittent cast immobilization and an organized wrist and grip therapy program.

It should be noted that no cure of established Kienböck's disease with such conservative splinting has been reported. At this stage ulnar lengthening to correct negative ulnar variance also may play a role.

Our experience, although limited to several anecdotal cases, has been encouraging. In stage 2, when collapse is occurring or has occurred but no significant intercarpal changes or arthritis have yet developed, we prefer silicone lunate arthroplasty. Limited intracarpal fusion may also have a role, especially before collapse is complete. In stage 3, we prefer radiocarpal fusion in the symptomatic wrist of a young manual laborer, whereas proximal row carpectomy is a reasonable alternative in a wrist with less strenuous demands.

OTHER CARPAL FRACTURES

Other isolated carpal fractures occur (Table 19–4) and present difficulties in radiographic diagnosis similar to those of the lunate or triquetrum. Fractures of the trapezium are usually associated with fracture-dislocations of the first metacarpal (Bennett's fractures) and are discussed in Chapter 20. Two other entities should be briefly mentioned: capitate fractures and hamate fractures.

As the center of wrist rotation, the capitate is surrounded and protected by the meta-carpals and other carpal bones. Most fractures occur through the body of the capitate and are often associated with fracture-dislocations of the carpus.[122] Isolated body fractures are nondisplaced and heal uneventfully in a short arm cast for six weeks. With these fractures it is important to exclude any other carpal abnormality.

Fractures of the hamate, and specifically the hook of the hamate, have gained increasing attention because of the frequency with which the diagnosis is missed.[125, 128, 140, 143] From the body of the hamate, the hook projects volarly and may be palpated just distal to the pisiform on the ulnar aspect of the wrist. The pisohamate ligament, the hypothenar muscles, and the transverse carpal ligament attach to its tip. Radially, the hook of the hamate helps define Guyon's canal, through which the ulnar nerve passes and which is susceptible to concurrent injury. The most common mechanism of injury is a direct blow, usually by a tennis or other racket striking the volar ulnar aspect of the hand. The correct diagnosis is best made on a carpal tunnel view (Fig. 19–40). If the diagnosis is made initially, cast immobilization for several weeks is indicated. The ulnar nerve

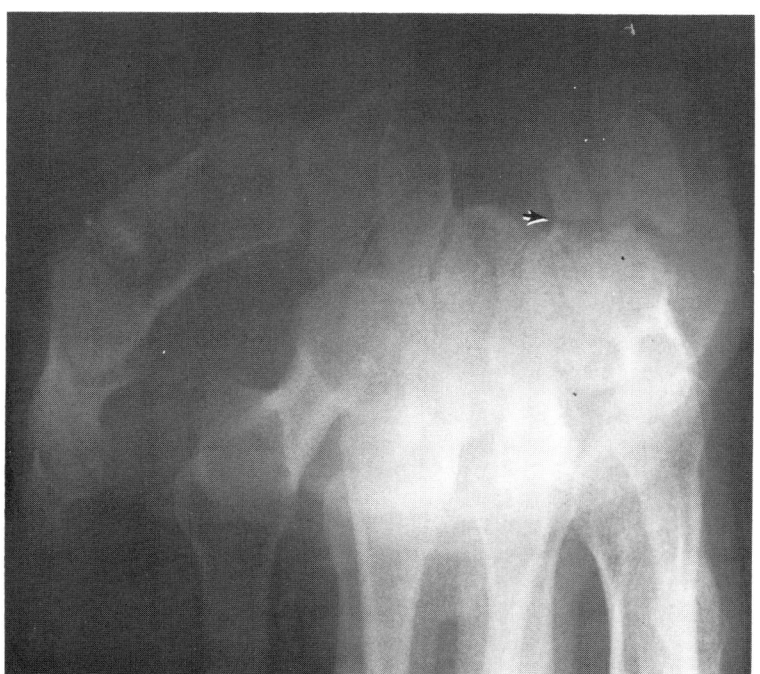

Figure 19–40 Fracture of the hook of the hamate. This carpal tunnel view shows the thumb metacarpal off to the left, and the carpal tunnel, the trapezium, and the proximal pole of the navicular on the left. On the right the pisiform is seen laterally and the hamate with the fracture at its hook (*arrow*). This fracture was missed for several months in this professional golfer. Treatment involved excision of the ununited fragment.

should be specifically examined, as its proximity renders it vulnerable to direct contusion, hemorrhage, or late fibrosis.[123, 132] Another common complication of this fracture is nonunion.[128, 140] If such an ununited fracture remains painful, good relief of symptoms can be obtained by excision of the ununited fragment.

CARPAL DISLOCATIONS AND FRACTURE-DISLOCATIONS

Carpal dislocations and fracture-dislocations are challenging problems not only in diagnosis but in treatment. Analyzing the complex intracarpal relationships can be simplified by remembering several salient points. On the posteroanterior projection of the wrist, the space between all the carpal bones should be equal. The silhouette of the lunate should be quadrilateral and that of the navicular should be canoe-shaped, as opposed to a double cortical ring or end-on appearance. The lateral x-ray is the most important film in establishing the relationships of the carpal bones. The distal radius, the lunate, and the capitate are identified on the lateral view as forming three c's: the c of the proximal capitate, the c of the distal and proximal lunate, and the c of the radial articular surface. These three c's should lie in the same axis (Fig. 19–41). If there is any doubt, x-rays should be taken of the uninjured wrist. Recently the Mayo Clinic group[163] has pointed out the importance of the lunate navicular angle seen on the lateral view (Fig. 19–41). The angle is drawn by bisecting the lunate in its midplane between the dorsal and the volar poles; a second line is drawn bisecting the navicular through the midpoints of its proximal and distal poles. The navicular lunate angle formed by the wrist in neutral position or slight dorsiflexion averages 47 degrees, with a range of 30 to 60 degrees. Navicular lunate angles of greater than 60 degrees suggest a disruption of the normal carpal architecture, such as a vertical position of the navicular or a dorsal position of the lunate. Such deformities can occur with disruption of the navicular lunate ligaments or with navicular fracture (see Fig. 19–34). Thus, by looking at the silhouette patterns of the carpal bones on the posteroanterior x-ray and by identifying the three c's and

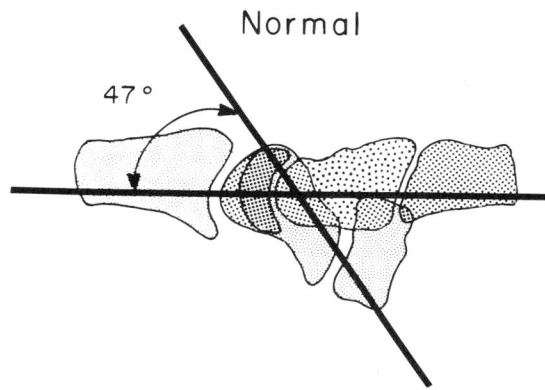

Figure 19–41 Normal navicular lunate angle of 47 degrees, with a range of 30 to 60 degrees. This angle, first popularized by Dobyns and Linscheid,[163] is drawn in the following manner. The navicular is bisected in its longitudinal axis by a line drawn through the proximal and distal poles, midpoint between the volar and the dorsal surfaces. This axis is then joined by a line bisecting the lunate between its volar and dorsal surfaces. The intersection of these lines forms the navicular lunate angle. When the lunate articular surface is facing dorsally or the navicular is more vertical, as in navicular lunate dissociation or navicular fracture, this angle is increased. It is important that the angle be measured on a lateral film taken in neutral to slight dorsiflexion. Another important relationship, the axis of the "three c's," can also be appreciated. The most distal c is the proximal pole of the capitate. The lunate forms the second c and the distal articular surface of the radius the third c. All should lie on the same axis.

the navicular lunate angle on the lateral films, the examiner can identify any significant intercarpal disruptions. Given the fact of seven major carpal bones, the permutations of injury are incalculable, but several distinct patterns can be recognized.

GROUP 1 (Fig. 19–42)

Perilunar Dislocation

A fall from a height or a moving activity is responsible for perilunar dislocations. The patient complains of pain with motion and weakness of power grip. Median nerve paresthesias are occasionally present. Lateral x-rays show the capitate dorsal and proximal to the lunate, which remains in its normal relationship to the distal radial articular surface (Fig. 19–43). The remain-

GROUP I

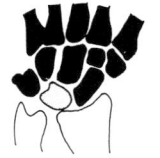
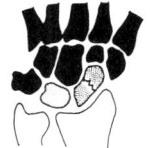
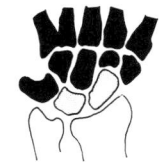

Perilunar Dislocation

A

Perilunar Dislocation
and
Navicular Fracture

B

Perilunar- Navicular
Dislocation

C

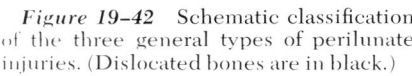

Figure 19–42 Schematic classification of the three general types of perilunate injuries. (Dislocated bones are in black.)

ing carpal bones dislocate with the capitate but retain a normal relationship to each other. Adequate muscle relaxation by general or extremity block anesthesia is necessary when closed reduction of an acute injury is attempted. Traction is applied to the hand in the longitudinal axis of the forearm against a counterforce exerted on the arm with the elbow flexed to 90 degrees. Digital pressure is applied dorsally over the capitate as a counterforce is exerted volarly to the distal radius and the lunate. If reduction is appreciated, x-rays are taken in the operating room. If the reduction is successful, a short arm cast with the wrist in 20 degrees of extension is applied for six to

eight weeks; if it is not successful, open reduction is performed using a transverse dorsal incision. After reduction by direct vision is obtained, the capitate is secured to the lunate and the radius by pins. Perilunar dislocations seen two weeks or more after injury require open reduction.[146, 148] Acute injuries treated by closed reduction have a better prognosis than those that require open reduction.[145, 148, 160]

Perilunar Dislocation and Navicular Fracture

Acute perilunar dislocation with navicular fracture seen early is treated by closed

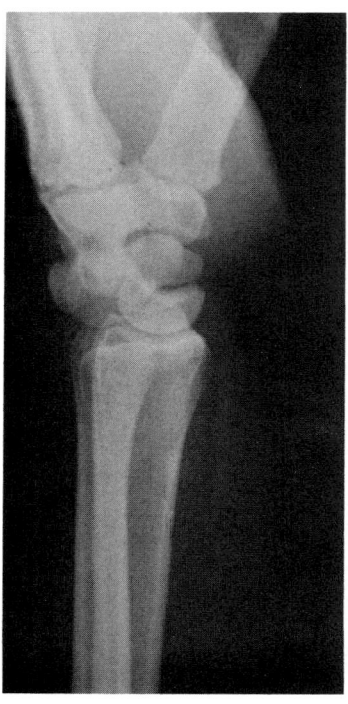
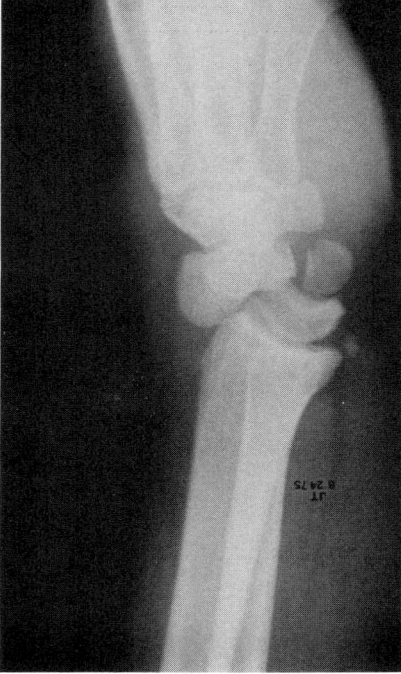

Figure 19–43 A lateral and oblique film of a 28-year-old man who fell 18 feet off a ladder landing onto his dorsiflexed right wrist. The wrist was generally swollen on all motions and painful. Lateral x-rays showed a disruption of the three c's. The capitate c is lying dorsal to the lunate and the distal radial c. This is a type A simple perilunar dislocation. The dislocation was reduced. The patient was held in a long arm cast for eight weeks and at a four-year follow-up had an asymptomatic wrist.

reduction using the same maneuver as that for perilunar section. The reduction is acceptable if the lunate and the capitate are properly aligned, if the navicular fragments are in direct contact with proper rotation, and if a line through the long axis of the navicular fragments and the two fracture fragments as a unit forms a 45 degree angle with the long axis of the radius. If the acute injury is not satisfactorily reduced or is more than two weeks old, open reduction is needed.[8, 148, 156] Open reduction requires both dorsal and volar incisions, with pins placed between the lunate and the capitate after reduction. A bone graft from the ilium is placed in the navicular following reduction. The wrist is held in 20 degrees of extension following either open or closed treatment until the fracture has healed. Because a navicular fracture may take six months or longer to heal, normal wrist motion is rarely obtained and the prognosis is guarded.

Perilunar-Navicular Dislocation

Perilunar-navicular dislocation is a rare injury caused by a fall on the extended wrist. The lunate and the navicular remain in normal relationship to the radius, and the remaining carpal bones dislocate dorsally, as demonstrated on the lateral x-ray. Closed reduction of acute injuries may be achieved by applying digital pressure dorsally to the capitate and volarly to the navicular and the lunate, with traction applied to the long axis of the radius. If reduction is demonstrated roentgenographically, a cast is applied to the wrist in 20 degrees of extension and the wrist is so held for eight weeks. Failure to obtain reduction requires open reduction through a dorsal incision, with pinning of the carpal bones after reduction. Repair of intercarpal ligament ruptures may be performed depending upon their appearance at surgery.[148, 155]

GROUP 2 (Fig. 19–44)

Lunate Dislocation

A fall from a height or a moving activity is usually responsible for lunate dislocation. The patient complains of pain with motion and weakness of power grip and pinch. The injured wrist is swollen, and ecchymoses may be present volarly. Median nerve paresthesias can be caused by nerve stretch from pressure of the dislocated lunate bone or from bleeding around the nerve in the carpal canal area. An anteroposterior x-ray projects the dislocated lunate as a triangular bone rather than its usual normal quadrilateral shape. A space can be seen on the x-ray between the navicular and the triquetrum. The important true lateral x-ray shows the lunate volar to the distal radial articular surface with the capitate positioned in direct line with the distal radius (Fig. 19–45).

General or extremity block anesthesia may be used to reduce the acute injury. Traction is exerted on the wrist by pulling the hand against a counterforce applied to the arm with the elbow in 90 degrees of flexion. With the wrist in extension, digital pressure is exerted over the dislocated lunate. If relocation of the lunate is appreciated, the wrist is brought into volar flexion to hold the reduction. A lateral x-ray in

GROUP II

Figure 19–44 A schematic representation of lunate-associated dislocations. (Dislocated bones are in black.)

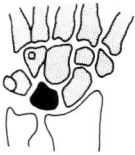

Lunate Dislocation

A

Lunate Dislocation
and
Navicular Fracture

B

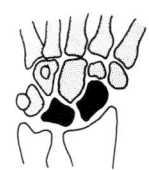

Lunate – Navicular
Dislocation

C

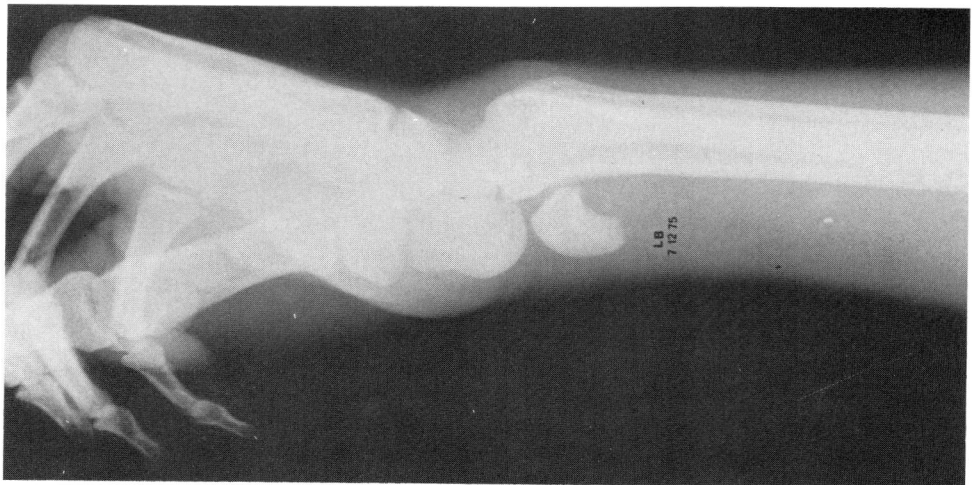

Figure 19–45   Lateral view of a classic lunate dislocation with the lunate resting in the carpal canal, causing median nerve symptoms in this patient. The lunate is seen underlying the volar aspect of the radius. The injury was opened volarly and a carpal tunnel release performed. The lunate and carpal bones were reduced, and the patient went on to have an asymptomatic but stiff wrist.

the operating room documents the reduction. If closed reduction fails, open reduction is needed and is always required if the injury is more than two weeks old.[145, 146, 148] Open reduction and surgical relocation of the lunate has been reported by using either a volar or a dorsal approach. The authors recommend the volar approach because it permits repair of the volar radiocarpal ligament. If the lunate sags volar to the radius on the lateral x-ray, its position should be corrected prior to wound closure by digital pressure and pinning of the lunate to the radius. After reduction the wrist is immobilized in neutral position for one month, when exercises are begun. Early reduction of an acute lunate dislocation has a good prognosis; old dislocations requiring open reduction have a guarded prognosis. Avascular necrosis, redislocation of the lunate, and wrist arthritis are the most common complications.

Lunate Dislocation and Navicular Fracture

A fall from a height or a moving activity is usually the cause of this injury. The wrist is swollen, and motion is painful on physical examination. Median nerve involvement should be ruled out initially. X-rays in the true anteroposterior and lateral planes show dislocation of the lunate (usually volar) with fracture of the navicular. The proximal fragment of the navicular may dislocate with the lunate.

The acute injury requires general or extremity block anesthesia. Traction is exerted on the wrist in the longitudinal plane of the forearm by pulling the hand against a counterforce applied to the arm with the elbow flexed at 90 degrees. Digital pressure is exerted on the volar surface of the wrist at the level of the dislocated bones with the wrist in extension. If relocation is appreciated, the wrist is placed in flexion to hold the reduction. Anteroposterior and lateral roentgenograms are taken in the operating room to confirm the reduction. If the lunate is not in its normal relationship to the radius or if the navicular fragments are not in contact and positioned in correct rotation and alignment, open reduction is necessary. A volar approach is recommended, with a lunate-to-radius pin and a navicular bone graft from the ilium. The wrist is held in neutral position until the navicular fracture unites.

Lunate-Navicular Dislocation

This rare injury is caused by a force with the wrist in dorsiflexion. Roentgenograms show a gap between the greater multangular and the triangular bone on the anteroposterior view; the lateral projection demonstrates volar displacement of the lunate and the navicular in relation to the

Lunate Dorsiflexion Instability

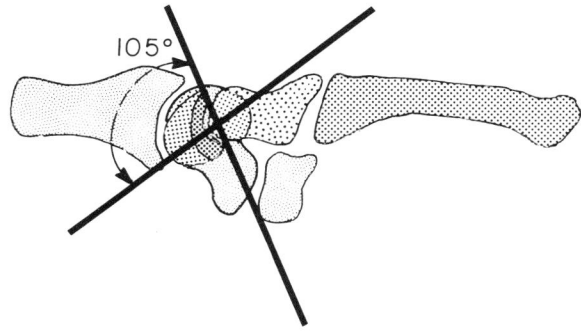

Figure 19–46   Lunate dorsiflexion instability pattern. This is a more common carpal subluxation, in which the navicular lunate angle as drawn in Figure 19–41 is found to be increased. The articular surface of the lunate faces dorsally. The instability patterns were popularized by Dobyns and Linscheid.[163]

radius, with the capitate engaging the distal radius. If closed reduction fails, open reduction is required, with pinning of the navicular and lunate to the radius. Exercises are started after six weeks of immobilization.

CARPAL SUBLUXATIONS

NAVICULAR-LUNATE DISASSOCIATIONS

On a lateral x-ray of the wrist, lines drawn between the long axes of the navicular and the lunate form an angle of about 47 degrees, with a range of 30 to 60 degrees (see Fig. 19–41). If, following a wrist injury, lines drawn between these points are in the range of 100 degrees, *lunate dorsiflexion instability* has occurred (Fig. 19–46).[163] Patients with this intracarpal injury com-

plain of pain with hand functions. A lateral x-ray of the wrist shows the lunate facing more dorsally than normal, increasing its angle relationship to the navicular. Some patients do not require any treatment, and wrist splinting for a month is successful in most cases. If symptoms persist in a patient whose job requires power grip, surgical reconstruction of the scapholunate ligament should be considered.[155] The replacement of the scapholunate ligament is performed through a dorsal approach, using a tendon graft or slip of an extensor tendon in the area. Patients may present with a history of a wrist sprain; the lateral x-ray will show that lines drawn between the middle of the long axis of the navicular and the lunate have an angle of 27 degrees. This intercarpal ligamentous injury, *lunate palmar flexion instability* (Fig. 19–47),[163] shows the lunate facing volarly compared with the

Lunate Palmar Flexion Instability

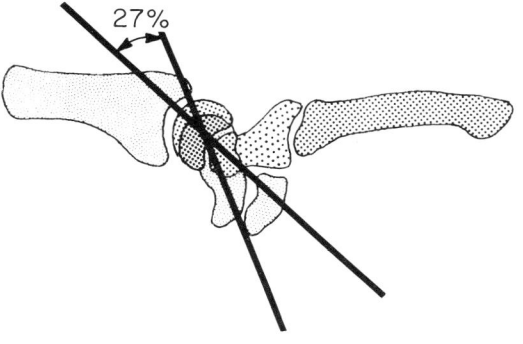

Figure 19–47   Lunate palmar flexion instability. Here the lunate navicular angle is decreased as the lunate faces volarly and distally. (After Dobyns and Linscheid)

Navicular Rotary Subluxation

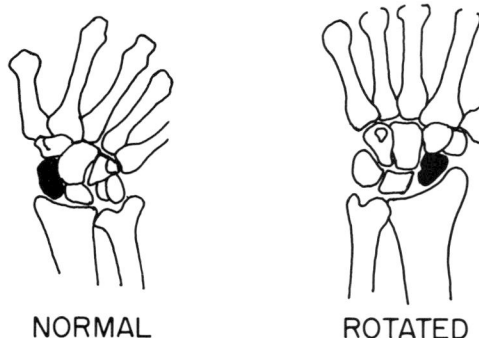

NORMAL   ROTATED

Figure 19–48 Schematic rendering of navicular rotatory subluxation. On the anteroposterior film note that the interim between the navicular (*dark*) and the lunate (*white*) is seen to be increased. The normal contour of the navicular becomes more oval and does not project the usual canoe-silhouette.

normal position, decreasing its angle relationship to the navicular. Wrist pain usually subsides with splinting for a month.

NAVICULAR ROTARY SUBLUXATION

After wrist injury, patients with localized tenderness over the navicular area should be suspected of and treated for navicular fracture. If repeat x-rays at follow-up visits show no fracture and wrist pain persists, the possibility of navicular rotary subluxation should be considered.[150, 155, 159] The anteroposterior x-ray of a navicular with a rotary subluxation injury shows an oval contour rather than the normal canoe-shaped outline (Fig. 19–48) and a gap of 3 mm or greater between the navicular and the lunate (with the wrist in ulnar deviation).

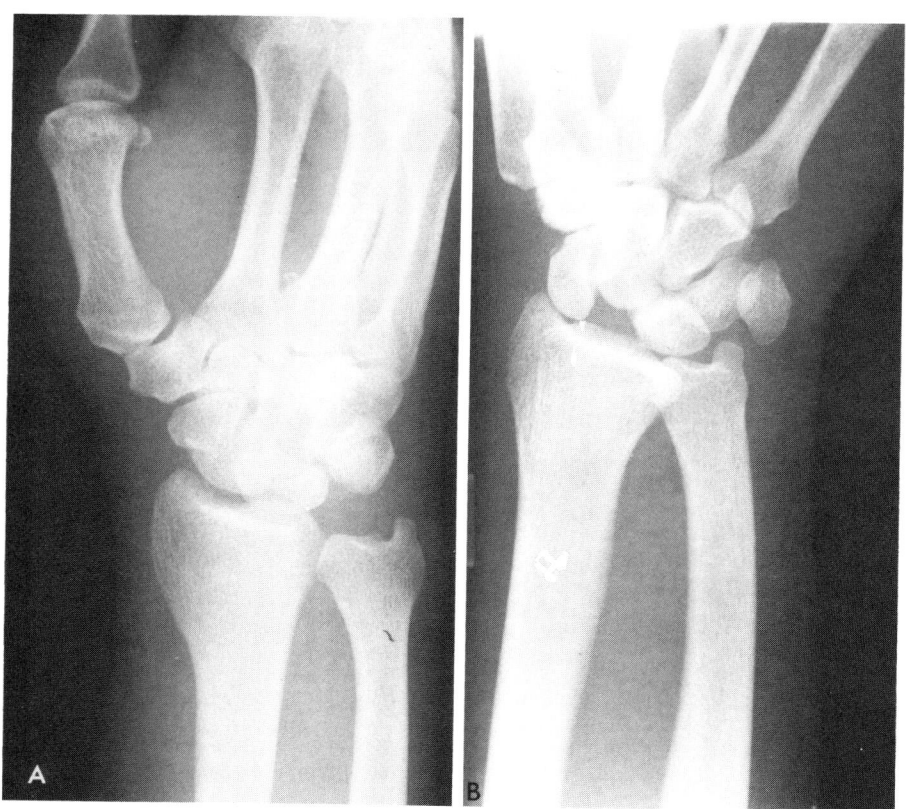

Figure 19–49 *A* and *B*. X-ray of a navicular rotary subluxation. This patient complained of clicking as well as of wrist pain associated with use. An anteroposterior film (*B*) taken in ulnar deviation exaggerates the gap between the navicular and the lunate. This gap has been called the Terry Thomas sign (for the British actor with the gaptoothed smile.) Note that the separation of the navicular and the lunate is greater than 3 mm.

(This is the so-called Terry Thomas sign, for the English actor with a large gap between his front teeth) (Fig. 19–49). A line drawn between the long axis of the radius and the navicular in the normal wrist measures an angle of 47 degrees, but in a wrist with rotary subluxation of the navicular, the angle approaches 90 degrees and is classified as a lunate dorsiflexion instability. Wrist motion elicits a clicking sensation as the navicular rotates on its long axis. Patients with this injury have a rupture of the scapholunate ligament, and the clicking abnormality is frequently their most serious concern. If the patient's occupation requires power grip and if working causes wrist pain, the surgical relocation of the navicular and replacement of the scapholunate ligament should be considered. The ligament is reconstructed using a tendon graft or a slip of extensor tendon from the dorsal aspect of the wrist. The reconstructed ligament is passed through drill holes in the dorsum of the lunate and the navicular. Following open reduction, six weeks of immobilization are required for soft tissue healing.[155] We and others have also done several lunate-navicular wrist fusions with good results.[145]

REFERENCES

General

1. Alffram, P.-A., and Bauer, G. C. H.: Epidemiology of fractures of the forearm: a biomechanical investigation of bone strength. J. Bone Joint Surg., 44A:105, 1962.
2. Böhler, L.: The Treatment of Fractures. 5th Ed. New York, Grune & Stratton, 1956.
3. Cautilli, R. A., Joyce, M. F., Gordon, E., and Juarez, R.: Classifications of fractures of the distal radius. Jefferson Orthop. J., 3:46, 1973.
4. Charnley, J.: The Closed Treatment of Common Fractures. 3rd Ed. Baltimore, Williams & Wilkins, 1961.
5. Conwell, H. E., and Reynolds, F. C.: Key and Conwell's Management of Fractures, Dislocations, and Sprains. 7th Ed. St. Louis, C. V. Mosby, 1961.
6. Crenshaw, A. H.: Campbell's Operative Orthopaedics. 5th Ed. St. Louis, C. V. Mosby, 1971.
7. Destot, E.: Injuries of the Wrist. London, Ernest Benn, 1925.
8. Dobyns, J. H., and Linscheid, R. L.: Fractures and dislocations of the wrist. In: Rockwood, A. A., and Green, D. P. (eds.): Fractures. Philadelphia, J. B. Lippincott, 1975, p. 345.
9. Flatt, A. E.: Kinesiology of the hand. AAOS Instructional Course Lectures. Vol. 18. St. Louis, C. V. Mosby, 1961, p. 266.
10. Gay, J. D. L.: Radial fracture as an index of osteoporosis. Can. Med. Assoc. J., 3:156, 1974.
11. Kaplan, E. B.: Functional and Surgical Anatomy of the Hand. 2nd Ed. Philadelphia, J. B. Lippincott, 1965.
12. Milch, H., and Milch, R. A.: Fracture Surgery. New York, Hoeber-Harper, 1959.
13. Reifenstein, E. C., Jr.: Relationships of steroid hormones to the development of osteoporosis in aging people. Clin. Orthop. Rel. Res., 10:206, 1957.
14. Watson-Jones, R.: Fractures and Joint Injuries. Vol. 2. 4th Ed. Baltimore, Williams & Wilkins, 1955.
15. Wood-Jones, F.: Principles of Anatomy as Seen in the Hand. Baltimore, Williams & Wilkins, 1942.

Anatomy of the Radius and Distal Radioulnar Joint

16. Johnson, R. K., and Shrewsbury, M. M.: Pronator quadratus in motions and stabilization of radius and ulna at the distal radioulnar joint. J. Hand Surg., 1:205, 1976.
17. Lewis, O. J., Hamshere, R. J., and Bucknill, T. M.: Anatomy of the wrist joint. J. Anat., 106:539, 1970.
18. Patrick, J.: A study of supination and pronation. J. Bone Joint Surg., 28:737, 1946.
19. Salter, N., and Darcus, H. D.: Amplitude of forearm and humeral rotation. J. Anat., 87:407, 1953.
20. Spinner, M., and Kaplan, E. B.: Extensor carpi ulnaris: its relationship to the stability of the distal radioulnar joint. Clin. Orthop. Rel. Res., 68:124, 1970.
21. Weigl, K., and Spira, E.: The triangular fibrocartilage of the wrist joint. Reconstr. Surg. Traumatol., 11:139, 1969.

Colles' Fracture

22. Anderson, R., and O'Neil, G.: Comminuted fractures of the distal end of the radius. Surg. Gynecol. Obstet., 78:434, 1944.
23. Bacorn, R. W., and Kurtzke, J. R.: Colles' fractures: a study of two thousand cases from the New York State Workmen's Compensation Board. J. Bone Joint Surg., 35A:643, 1953.
24. Cassebaum, W. H.: Colles' fracture: a study of end results. J.A.M.A., 143:963, 1950.
25. Castaing, J.: Revue de chirurgie orthopedique et reparatrice de l'appareil moteur. Tome 50, No. 5, 1964.
26. Cole, J. M., and Obletz, B. E.: Comminuted fractures of the distal end of the radius treated by skeletal transfixion in plaster cast: an end-result study of 33 cases. J. Bone Joint Surg., 48A:931, 1966.
27. Colles, A.: On the fracture of the carpal extremity of the radius. Edinb. Med. Surg. J., 10:182, 1814. [Reprinted in Clin. Orthop. Rel. Res., 83:3, 1972.]
28. Cotton, F. J.: The pathology of fracture of the lower extremity of the radius. Ann. Surg., 32:194, 388, 1900.
29. DePalma, A. F.: Comminuted fractures of the distal end of the radius treated by ulnar pinning. J. Bone Joint Surg., 34A:651, 1952.

30. Dowling, J. J., and Sawyer, B., Jr.: Comminuted Colles' fractures: evaluation of a method of treatment. J. Bone Joint Surg., *43A*:657, 1961.

31. Fahey, J. H.: Fractures and dislocations about the wrist. Surg. Clin. North Am., 37:19, 1957.

32. Freiberg, S., and Lundström, B.: Radiographic measurements of the radiocarpal joint in normal adults. Acta Radiol. Diagn., *17*:249, 1976.

33. Frykman, G.: Fracture of the distal radius including sequelae—shoulder-hand-finger syndrome, disturbance in the distal radioulnar joint, and impairment of nerve function: a clinical and experimental study. Acta Orthop. Scand., (Suppl.) *108*:1, 1967.

34. Gartland, J. J., Jr., and Werley, C. W.: Evaluation of healed Colles' fractures. J. Bone Joint Surg., *43B*:245, 1961.

35. Green, D. P.: Pins and plaster treatment of comminuted fractures of the distal end of the radius. J. Bone Joint Surg., *57A*:304, 1975.

36. Hinding, E.: Fractures of the distal end of the forearm. Acta Orthop. Scand., *43*:357, 1972.

37. Lankford, L. L., and Thompson, J. E.: Reflex sympathetic dystrophy, upper and lower extremity: diagnosis and management. AAOS Instructional Course Lectures, 26:163, 1977.

38. Lidstrom, A.: Fractures of the distal end of the radius: a clinical and statistical study of end-results. Acta Orthop. Scand. (Suppl.):*41*, 1–118, 1959.

39. Lilienfeldt, A.: Über die Erzeugung der typischen Verletzungen der Hand Wurzelknowchenind des Radiusburckes. Z. Orthop. Chir., 20:437, 1908.

40. Lynch, A. C., and Lipscomb, P. R.: The carpal tunnel syndrome and Colles' fractures. J.A.M.A., *185*:363, 1963.

41. Marsh, H. O., and Teal, S. W.: Treatment of comminuted fractures of the distal radius with self-contained skeletal traction. Am. J. Surg., *124*:715, 1972.

42. Mayer, J. H.: Colles' fracture. Br. J. Surg., 27:629, 1940.

43. Phalen, G. S.: Reflections on 21 years' experience with the carpal tunnel syndrome. J.A.M.A., *212*:365, 1970.

44. Robbins, H.: Anatomical study of the median nerve in the carpal tunnel and etiologies of carpal tunnel syndrome. J. Bone Joint Surg., *45A*:953, 1963.

45. Rush, L. V., and Rush, M. L.: Evolution of medullary fixation of fractures by longitudinal pins. Am. J. Surg., 78:324, 1949.

46. Rychak, J. S., and Kalenak, A.: Injury to the median and ulnar nerves secondary to fracture of the radius. J. Bone Joint Surg., 59A:414, 1977.

47. Sarmiento, A.: The brachioradialis as a deforming force in Colles' fracture. Clin. Orthop. Rel. Res., 38:86, 1965.

48. Sarmiento, A., Pratt, G. W., Berry, N. C., and Sinclair, W. F.: Colles' fracture, functional bracing in supination. J. Bone Joint Surg., *57A*:311, 1975.

49. Scheck, M.: Long-term followup of treatment of comminuted fractures of the distal end of the radius by transfixation with Kirchner wires and cast. J. Bone Joint Surg., *44A*:337, 1962.

50. Sevitt, S.: Healing of fractures of the lower end of

the radius: histologic and angiographic study. J. Bone Joint Surg., *53B*:519, 1971.

51. Smaill, G. B.: Long-term followup of Colles' fracture. J. Bone Joint Surg., *47B*:80, 1965.

52. Smith, F. M.: Late rupture of extensor pollicis longus tendon following Colles' fracture. J. Bone Joint Surg., 38:49, 1946.

53. Spira, E., and Weigl, L.: Comminuted fracture of the distal end of the radius. Reconstr. Surg. Traumatol., *11*:128, 1969.

54. Zoega, M.: Fractures of the lower end of the radius with ulnar nerve palsy. J. Bone Joint Surg., *48B*:514, 1966.

Other Radiocarpal Injuries

55. Barton, J. R.: Views and treatment of an important injury to the wrist. Med. Examiner, *1*:365, 1838.

56. Bilos, Z. J., Pankovich, A., and Velda, S.: Fracture-dislocation of the radiocarpal joint. J. Bone Joint Surg., *59A*:198, 1977.

57. Blount, W. F.: Fractures in Children. Baltimore, Williams & Wilkins, 1955.

58. DeOliveira, J. C.: Barton's fractures. J. Bone Joint Surg., *55A*:586, 1973.

59. Edwards, H. C.: Mechanism and treatment of backfire fracture. J. Bone Joint Surg., 8:701, 1926.

60. Ellis, J.: Smith's and Barton's fractures: a method of treatment. J. Bone Joint Surg., *47B*:724, 1965.

61. Fitzsimons, R. A.: Colles' fracture and chauffeur's fracture. Br. Med. J., 2:357, 1938.

62. Rang, M.: Children's Fractures. Philadelphia, J. B. Lippincott, 1974.

62a. Salter, R. B., and Harris, W. R.: Injuries involving the epiphyseal plate. J. Bone Joint Surg., *45A*:587, 1963.

63. Smith, R. W.: A Treatise on Fractures in the Vicinity of Joints, and on Certain Forms of Accidental and Congenital Dislocations. Dublin, Hodges and Smith, 1854.

64. Thomas, F. B.: Reduction of Smith's fracture. J. Bone Joint Surg., *39B*:463, 1957.

65. VanHerpe, L. B.: Fractures of forearm and wrist in children. Orthop. Clin. North Am., 7:543, 1976.

66. Woodyard, J. E.: Review of Smith's fractures. J. Bone Joint Surg., *51B*:324, 1969.

Distal Radioulnar Joint Injuries

67. Coleman, H. M.: Injuries of the articular disc at the wrist. J. Bone Joint Surg., *42B*:522, 1960.

68. Dameron, T. B., Jr.: Traumatic dislocation of the distal radioulnar joint. Clin. Orthop. Rel. Res., 83:55, 1972.

69. Darrach, W.: Partial excision of lower shaft of ulna for deformity following Colles' fracture. Ann. Surg., 57:764, 1913.

70. Dingman, P. V. C.: Resection of the distal end of the ulna (Darrach operation): an end-result study of 24 cases. J. Bone Joint Surg., *34A*:893, 1952.

71. Essex-Lopresti, P.: Fractures of radial head with distal radioulnar dislocation. J. Bone Joint Surg., *33B*:244, 1951.

72. Freundlich, B. D., and Spinner, M.: Nerve compression syndrome in derangements of the

proximal and distal radioulnar joints. Bull. Hosp. Joint Dis., 29:38, 1968.

73. Heiple, K. G., Freehafer, A. A., and Van't Hof, A.: Isolated traumatic dislocation of the distal end of the ulna or distal radioulnar joint. J. Bone Joint Surg., 44A:1387, 1962.

74. Kessler, I., and Hecht, O.: Present application of the Darrach procedure. Clin. Orthop. Rel. Res., 72:254, 1970.

75. Liebolt, F. L.: A new method for repair of the distal radioulnar joint. N. Y. State J. Med., 50:2817, 1950.

76. Lippman, R. K.: Laxity of the radioulnar joint following Colles' fracture. Arch. Surg., 35:772, 1937.

77. McDougall, A., and White, J.: Subluxation of the inferior radioulnar joint complicating fractures of the radial head. J. Bone Joint Surg., 124:715, 1972.

78. Mikic, Z. D.: Galeazzi fracture dislocations. J. Bone Joint Surg., 57A:1071, 1975.

79. Rose-Innes, A. P.: Anterior dislocation of the ulna at the inferior radioulnar joint: case reports, with a discussion of the anatomy of rotation of the forearm. J. Bone Joint Surg., 42B:515, 1960.

80. Snook, G. A., Chrisman, O. D., Wilson, T. C., and Wietsma, R. D.: Subluxation of the distal radioulnar joint by hyperpronation. J. Bone Joint Surg., 51A:1315, 1969.

81. Swanson, A. B.: Implant arthroplasty for disabilities of the distal radioulnar joint. Orthop. Clin. North Am., 4:373, 1973.

82. Taylor, G. W., and Parsons, C. L.: Role of discus articularis in Colles' fracture. J. Bone Joint Surg., 20:149, 1938.

83. Taylor, T. K. F., and O'Connor, B. T.: The effect upon inferior radioulnar joint of excision of the head of the radius in adults. J. Bone Joint Surg., 46B:83, 1964.

84. Vesely, D. G.: The distal radioulnar joint. Clin. Orthop. Rel. Res. 51:75, 1967.

85. Weseley, M. S., Barenfeld, P. A., and Bruno, J.: Volar dislocation of the distal radioulnar joint. J. Trauma, 12:1083, 1972.

The Carpal Mechanism: Anatomy and Biomechanics

86. Andrews, J. G., and Youm, Y.: Biomechanical investigation of wrist kinematics. J. Biomech., 12:83, 1979.

87. Arkless, R.: Cineradiography in normal and abnormal wrists. Am. J. Roentgenol., 96:837, 1966.

88. Boyes, J. H.: Bunnell's Surgery of the Hand. 5th Ed. Philadelphia, J. B. Lippincott, 1970.

89. Beckenbaugh, R. D., and Linscheid, R. L.: Total wrist arthroplasty: Preliminary report. J. Hand Surg., 2:337, 1977.

90. Kauer, J. M. G.: The interdependence of carpal articulation chains. Acta Anat., 88:481, 1974.

91. Landsmeer, J. M. F.: Atlas of Hand Anatomy. Edinburgh, Churchill Livingstone, 1976.

92. McMartry, R. Y., Youm, Y., Flatt, A. E., and Gillespie, T. E.: Kinematics of the wrist. I. Experimental study of radial-ulnar deviation and flexion-extension. J. Bone Joint Surg., 60A:423, 1978.

93. MacConaill, M. A.: The mechanical anatomy of

the carpus and its bearing on some surgical problems. J. Anat., 75:166, 1941.

94. Mayfield, J. K., Johnson, R. P., and Kilcoyne, R. F.: The ligaments of the wrist and their functional significance. Anat. Rec., 186:417, 1976.

95. Sarrafran, S. K., Melaned, J. L., and Goshgarian, G. M.: Study of wrist motion in flexion and extension. Clin. Orthop. Rel. Res., 126:153, 1977.

96. Taleisnik, J.: Ligaments of the wrist. J. Hand Surg., 1:110, 1976.

97. Viernstein, K., and Weigert, M.: New methods for treatment of lunate malacia. Reconstr. Surg. Traumatol., 11:154, 1969.

98. Volz, R. G.: The development of a total wrist arthroplasty. Clin. Orthop. Rel. Res., 116:209, 1976.

99. Waugh, R. L., and Sullivan, R. F.: Anomalies of the carpus. J. Bone Joint Surg., 32A:682, 1950.

Navicular Fracture

100. Barnard, L., and Stubbins, S. G.: Styloidectomy of the radius in the treatment of nonunion of the carpal navicular. J. Bone Joint Surg., 30A:98, 1948.

101. Barr, J. S.: Fracture of the carpal navicular bone. An end result study in military personnel. J. Bone Joint Surg., 35A:609, 1953.

102. Bentzon, P. G. K., and Randlov-Modsen, A.: On fracture of the carpal scaphoid. Acta Orthop. Scand., 16:30, 1946.

102a. Brighton, C. T., Friedenberg, Z. B., Mitchell, E. J., and Booth, R. E.: Treatment of nonunion with constant direct current. Clin. Orthop. Rel Res., 124:106, 1977.

103. Dooley, B. J.: Inlay bone grafting for nonunion of the scaphoid by the anterior approach. J. Bone Joint Surg., 50B:102, 1968.

104. Fisk, G. R.: Carpal instability and the fractured scaphoid. Ann. R. Coll. Surg. Engl., 46:63, 1970.

105. Friedenberg, Z. B.: Anatomic considerations in the treatment of carpal navicular fractures. Am. J. Surg., 78:379, 1949.

106. Gasser, H.: Delayed union and pseudarthrosis of the carpal navicular: treatment by compression screw osteosynthesis. J. Bone Joint Surg., 47A:249, 1965.

107. Gilford, W. W., Bolton, R. H., and Lambrinudi, C.: The mechanism of the wrist joint with special references to fracture of the navicular. Guy's Hosp. Rep., 92:52, 1943.

108. McLaughlin, H. L., and Parkes, J. C.: Fracture of the carpal navicular bone: gradations in therapy based upon pathology. J. Trauma, 1:311, 1969.

109. Maudsley, R. H., Ascot, R., and Chen, S. C.: Screw fixation in the management of the fractured carpal scaphoid. J. Bone Joint Surg., 54B:432, 1972.

110. Mazet, R., and Hohl, M.: Fractures of the carpal navicular. J. Bone Joint Surg., 45A:82, 1963.

111. Mulder, J. D.: The results of 100 cases of pseudarthrosis in the scaphoid bone treated by the Matti-Russe operation. J. Bone Joint Surg., 50B:110, 1968.

112. Murray, G.: End results of bone grafting for

nonunion of the carpal navicular. J. Bone Joint Surg., 28:749, 1946.

113. Pennsylvania Orthopaedic Society: Evaluation of treatment for nonunion of the carpal navicular. 44A:169, 1962.

114. Preiser, G.: Über eine typische post-traumatische und meist zur spontan Fraktur Fuhendre Ostitis Naviculous Carp. Zb. Chir., 37:929, 1910.

115. Russe, O.: Fracture of the carpal navicular. J. Bone Joint Surg., 42A:759, 1960.

116. Sherwin, J. M., Nagel, D. A., and Southwick, W. O.: Bipartite carpal navicular and the diagnostic problem of bone partition. J. Trauma, 11:440, 1971.

117. Smith, L., and Friedman, B.: Treatment of ununited fracture of the carpal navicular by styloidectomy of the radius. J. Bone Joint Surg., 38A:368, 1956.

118. Taleisnik, J., and Kelly, P. J.: The extraosseous and intraosseous blood supply of the scaphoid bone. J. Bone Joint Surg., 48A:1126, 1966.

119. Thomaidis, V. T.: Elbow-wrist-thumb immobilization in the treatment of fractures of the carpal scaphoid. Acta Orthop. Scand., 44:679, 1973.

120. Verdan, C., and Narakas, A.: Fractures and pseudarthroses of the scaphoid. Surg. Clin. North Am., 48:1083, 1968.

121. Weber, E. R., and Chao, E. Y.: An experimental approach to the mechanism of scaphoid waist fractures. J. Hand Surg., 3:142, 1978.

Other Carpal Fractures and Kienböck's Disease

122. Adler, J. B., and Shaftan, G. W.: Fractures of the capitate. J. Bone Joint Surg., 44A:1537, 1962.

123. Baird, D. B., and Friedenberg, Z. B.: Delayed ulnar nerve palsy following a fracture of the hamate. J. Bone Joint Surg., 50A:570, 1968.

124. Bartone, N. F., and Grieco, R. V.: Fractures of the triquetrum. J. Bone Joint Surg., 38A:353, 1956.

125. Bowen, T. L.: Injuries of the hamate. Hand, 5:235, 1973.

126. Borgeskov, S., Christiansen, B., Kjaer, A., and Balsyev, I.: Fracture of the carpal bones. Acta Orthop. Scand., 37:276, 1966.

127. Brolin, I.: Post-traumatic lesions of the lunate bone. Acta Orthop. Scand., 34:167, 1964.

128. Carter, P. R., Eaton, R. G., and Littler, J. W.: Ununited fracture of the hook of the hamate. J. Bone Joint Surg., 59A:583, 1977.

129. Dornan, A.: The results of treatment in Kienböck's disease. J. Bone Joint Surg., 31B:518, 1949.

130. Gelberman, R. M., Salamn, P. B., Janst, J. M., and Posch, J. L.: Ulnar variance in Kienböck's disease. J. Bone Joint Surg., 57A:674, 1975.

131. Graner, O., Lopes, E. I., Carvalho, B. C., and Atlas, S.: Arthrodesis of the carpal bones in the treatment of Kienböck's disease. Painful ununited fractures of the navicular and lunate bones with avascular necrosis and old fracture-dislocations of carpal bones. J. Bone Joint Surg., 48A:767, 1966.

132. Howard, F. M.: Ulnar nerve palsy in wrist fractures. J. Bone Joint Surg., 43A:1197, 1961.

133. Kashiwaji, D., Fujiwara, A., Inoue, T., et al.: An experimental and clinical study on lunatomalacia. Proceedings of the American Society for Surgery of the Hand, Las Vegas, 1977.

134. Kienböck, R.: Über traumatische Malazie des Mondbeins und ihre Folgzustände. Fortschr. Rontgenstr., B16:77, 1910.

135. Lichtman, D. M., Mack, G. R., MacDonald, R. T., Gunther, S. F., and Wilson, J. N.: Kienböck's disease: role of silicone arthroplasty. J. Bone Joint Surg., 59A:899, 1977.

136. McClain, E. J., and Boyes, J. H.: Missed fractures of the greater multangular. J. Bone Joint Surg., 48A:1525, 1966.

137. Nahigian, S. H., Li, C. S., Richey, D. G., and Shae, D. T.: The dorsal flap arthroplasty in the treatment of Kienböck's disease. J. Bone Joint Surg., 52A:245, 1970.

138. Schwartz, S.: Localized fusion at the wrist joint. J. Bone Joint Surg., 49A:1591, 1967.

139. Stack, J. K.: End results of excision of the carpal bones. Arch. Surg., 57:245, 1948.

140. Stark, H. F., Jobe, F. W., Boyes, J. H., and Ashworth, C. R.: Fracture of the hook of the hamate in athletes. J. Bone Joint Surg., 59A:575, 1977.

141. Swanson, A. B.: Silicone rubber implants for the replacement of the carpal scaphoid and lunate bones. Orthop. Clin. North Am., 1:299, 1970.

142. Watson, H. Kirk, John, T. R., Hempton, R. F., and Jones, D. S.: Limited wrist arthrodesis. Proceedings of the American Society for Surgery of the Hand, San Francisco, 1979.

143. Wiot, J. F., and Dorst, J. P.: Less common fractures and dislocations of the wrist. Radiol. Clin. North Am., 4:261, 1966.

Carpal Dislocations

144. Campbell, C. J., and Keskain, T.: Total and subtotal arthrodesis of the wrist inlay technique. J. Bone Joint Surg., 46A:1520, 1964.

145. Campbell, R. D., Jr., Lance, E. M., and Yeoh, C. B.: Lunate and perilunar dislocations. J. Bone Joint Surg., 46B:55, 1964.

146. Campbell, R. D., Jr., Thompson, T. C., Lance, E. M., and Adler, J. B.: Indications for open reduction of lunate and perilunate dislocations of the carpal bones. J. Bone Joint Surg., 47A:915, 1965.

147. Dunn, A. W.: Fractures and dislocations of the carpus. Surg. Clin. North Am., 52:1513, 1972.

148. Green, D. P., and O'Brien, E. T.: Open reduction of carpal dislocations: indications and operative techniques. J. Hand Surg., 3:250, 1978.

149. Hill, N. A.: Fractures and dislocations of the carpus. Orthop. Clin. North Am., 1:275, 1970.

150. Howard, F. M., Fahey, T., and Wojcik, E.: Rotatory subluxation of the navicular. Clin. Orthop. Rel. Res., 104:134, 1974.

151. Hudson, T. M., Carajol, W. J., and Kaye, J. J.: Isolated rotatory sublux of the carpal navicular. Am. J. Roentgenol. Radium Ther. Nucl. Med., 126:601, 1976.

152. Jorgensen, E.: Proximal row carpectomy. J. Bone Joint Surg., 51A:1104, 1969.

153. Inglis, A. E., and Jones, E. C.: Proximal row carpectomy for diseases of the proximal row. J. Bone Joint Surg., 59A:460, 1977.

154. Meyers, M. H., Wells, R., and Harvey, J. P.: Naviculocapitate fracture syndrome. J. Bone Joint Surg., 53A:1383, 1971.

155. Palmer, A. K., Dobyns, J. H., and Linscheid, R. L.: Management of post-traumatic instability of the wrist secondary to ligament rupture. J. Hand Surg., 3:507, 1978.

156. Russel, T. B.: Intercarpal dislocations and fracture-dislocations. A review of 59 cases. J. Bone Joint Surg., 31B:524, 1949.

157. Stein, A. H.: Dorsal dislocation of the lesser multangular bone. J. Bone Joint Surg., 53A: 377, 1971.

158. Tanz, S.: Perilunar dislocations. Clin. Orthop. Rel. Res., 57:147, 1968.

159. Vaughan-Jackson, O. J.: Case of recurrent subluxation of the carpal scaphoid. J. Bone Joint Surg., 31B:532, 1949.

160. Wagner, C. J.: Perilunar dislocations. J. Bone Joint Surg., 38A:1198, 1956.

161. Wagner, C. J.: Fracture-dislocations of the wrist. Clin. Orthop. Rel. Res., 15:181, 1959.

162. Worland, R. L., and Dick, H. M.: Transnavicular perilunate dislocations. J. Trauma, 15:407, 1975.

163. Linscheid, R. L., Dobyns, J. H., Beabout, J. W., and Bryan, R. S.: Traumatic instability of the wrist: diagnosis, classification, and pathomechanics. J. Bone Joint Surg., 54A:1612, 1972. Follow-up review article in American Academy of Orthopedic Surgeons: Instructional Course Lectures Vol. XXIV. St. Louis, C. V. Mosby, 1975, p. 182.

F. WILLIAM BORA, JR., M.D.
and
A. LEE OSTERMAN, M.D.

20 _____ Injuries of the Hand

It has been estimated in many studies, including those by the Departments of Labor of the State of New York[10] and the Commonwealth of Pennsylvania,[2] that approximately one third of all reported injuries occur to the hand. The ultimate prognosis of such injuries is related to the injury itself, the primary treatment, and the secondary treatment if later reconstruction is necessary.

ANATOMY AND BIOMECHANICS OF THE DIGIT

A complete review of the anatomy of the hand is beyond the scope of this chapter, but the reader is referred to the classic works of Wood-Jones[21] and Kaplan.[17] A brief review of the anatomy and biomechanics of the digits, including the forces that control the motion of and the stress on the metacarpophalangeal and interphalangeal joints, will be presented.

ANATOMICAL CONSIDERATIONS

The bony architecture of the hand consists of five rays, each composed of a metacarpal and its respective phalanges (Fig. 20–1). Wood-Jones[21] has functionally partitioned the hand into a fixed stable unit consisting of the second and third metacarpals, around which move the mobile

units — the radial thumb and the ulnar fourth and fifth metacarpals. The second and third metacarpals achieve their stability from the countersinking of their bases into the distal carpal row and from the insertion of the primary wrist-stabilizing muscles onto their shafts. Likewise, the articulations of the mobile metacarpals are smooth-faceted joints with multiple planes of motion. The stability of the fixed unit must be maintained, or both the function and the strength of the mobile borders will be lost.

A second structural concept inherent in the bony architecture is the presence of three arches in the hand. These include a fixed transverse arch through the distal carpal row, a mobile transverse arch through the metacarpal heads, and a linking longitudinal arch formed by each ray, the apex being at the MCP joint level (Fig. 20–2). Both Littler[20] and Flatt[4] have graphically defined the importance of these arches for digital sweep and power.

As highlighted by Kuczynski in his excellent review,[18] structural considerations are also important in understanding joint function at both the metacarpophalangeal (MCP) and the interphalangeal levels (PIP, DIP). Both joints rely on passive ligamentous as well as dynamic muscular stability. The former consists of a joint capsule, a volar plate with a loose membranous proximal origin and a less mobile fibrous distal attachment, and a collateral ligament complex. These are, however, individualized to

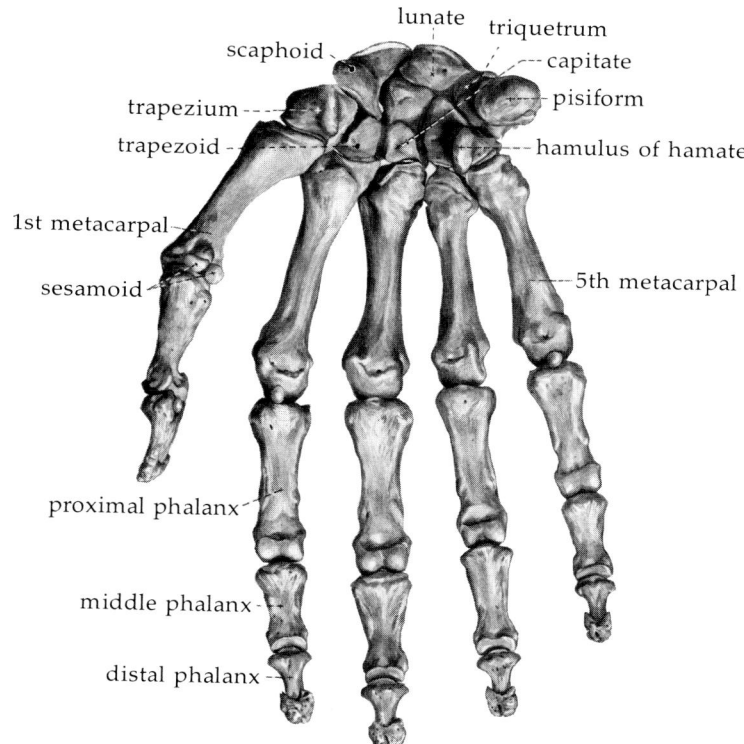

Figure 20-1 Bones of the hand. Fixed unit of the hand (*shaded*). (Courtesy of J. Langman and M. W. Woerdeman and the W. B. Saunders Co., Philadelphia. *Atlas of Medical Anatomy*, 1978.)

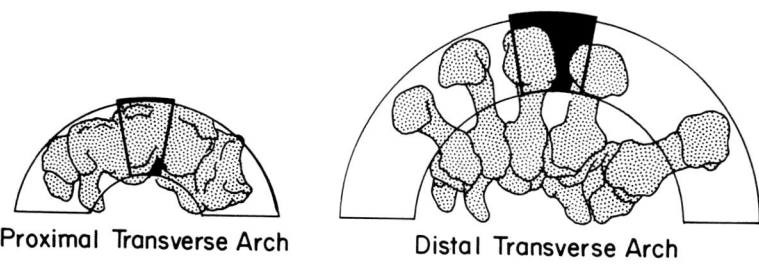

Proximal Transverse Arch   Distal Transverse Arch

Figure 20-2 Arches of the hand (after Flatt).

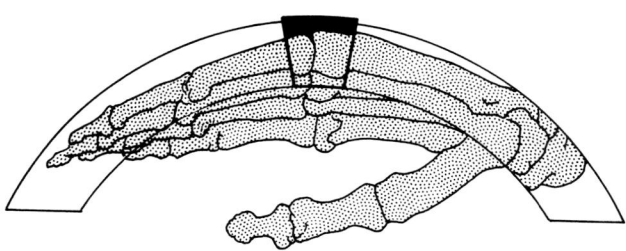

Longitudinal Arch

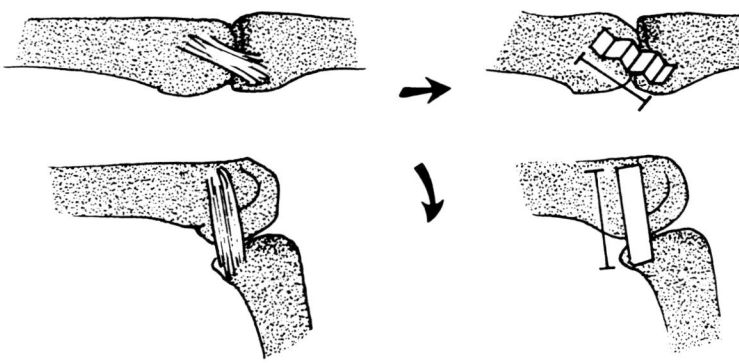

Figure 20–3 Effect of positioning on collateral ligament length.

the particular joint configuration. The MCP joint is a ball-and-socket articulation with multiple planes of motion and collateral ligaments that are relatively short and slack in extension and taut in flexion (Fig. 20–3). Hence, prolonged immobilization of this joint in extension will result in limited flexion secondary to ligament contracture. The proximal interphalangeal joint (PIP) is usually considered to be a hinge joint. This implies a similarity to a door hinge or box lid in which only one kind of movement is permitted, namely, a swing around the stationary pin of a hinge (Fig. 20–4). When examined more closely, however, the middle phalanx glides around the head of the proximal phalanx with joint motion. Its collateral ligament complex is subject to less cam effect, and when immobilized it should ideally be positioned in only slight flexion (less than 40 degrees) to avoid residual flexion contracture.

The finger is controlled by two groups of muscles, the extrinsics and the intrinsics (Fig. 20–5). The extrinsic muscles are the primary forces for the isometric functions of power grip and precision handling (pinch). The intrinsic muscles provide the delicate modulations and balance necessary to the articular system. The action of these muscles is mediated through the tendons, which create counterbalancing constant forces at the joint surfaces and the surrounding ligamentous structures, thus providing dynamic stability as well as joint motion.

In flexion movements, the distal interphalangeal (DIP) joint is flexed by the flexor digitorum profundus, the PIP joint by the flexor digitorum sublimis, and the MCP joint primarily by the intrinsics and secondarily by both flexor digitorum muscles. Extension of the interphalangeal joints is mediated by a dual system of the extensor digitorum and the dorsal expansion of the interossei, whereas MCP extension is an extrinsic function. The refinement of this complex system exceeds our scope, but the reader is referred to the works of Milford[31] and Smith.[32]

BIOMECHANICS

The forces acting at any given joint are the result of the constraints imposed by the articular surfaces and ligaments and the tension developed in the tendons and muscles.[7] These forces include both the agonistic and the antagonistic muscles. The inclusion of the antagonistic elements is particularly important in isometric function of the finger, since the joint is believed to

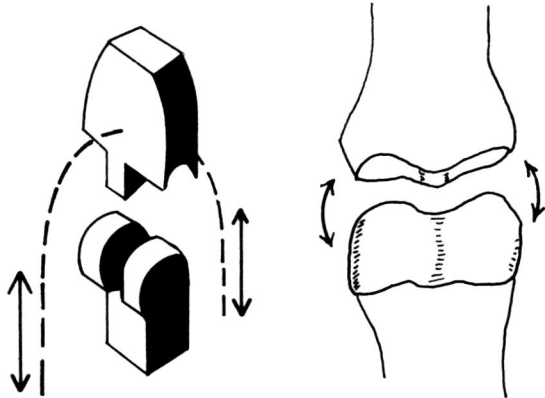

Figure 20–4 The proximal interphalangeal joint is bicondylar with an intercondylar ridge and groove.

DORSAL VIEW

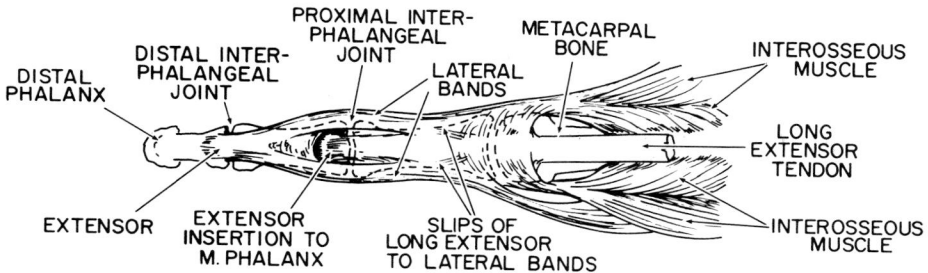

LATERAL VIEW

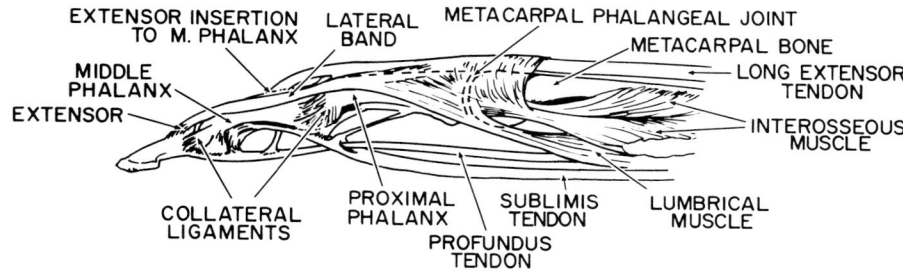

Figure 20–5 Muscle-tendon anatomy of the digit.

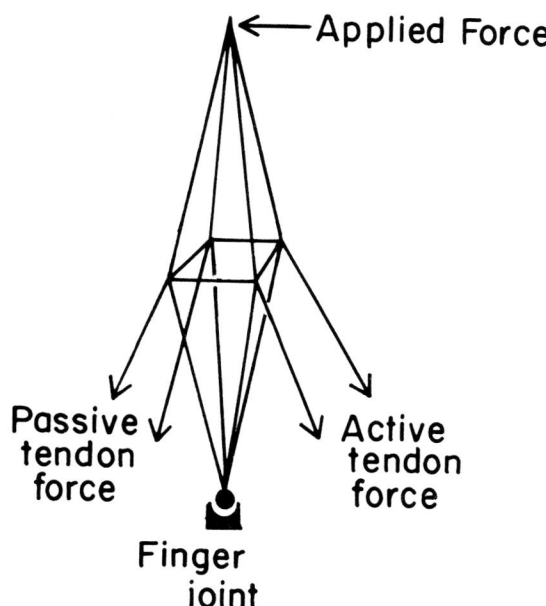

Figure 20–6 Normal forces applied to the metacarpophalangeal joint resemble a pylon. Chao, E., Opgrande, J. Axmeer, F. "Three Dimensional force-analysis of finger joints in selected isometric functions." Biomech 9, 387, 1976.

react in a manner similar to a pylon (Fig. 20–6).[13] The antagonistic tendons produce counterbalancing tension for the purpose of reducing the subluxation forces at the joint. Under this condition, the compressive force at the joint is increased, which also enhances stability. Normal joint surfaces are capable of bearing large compressive loads, but the ligamentous capsules are relatively tenuous under excessive tension.

As previously stated, the proximal interphalangeal (PIP) joint is considered to be a hinge joint. It is known that the axis of movement in the PIP joint changes, shifting in the palmar direction during flexion.

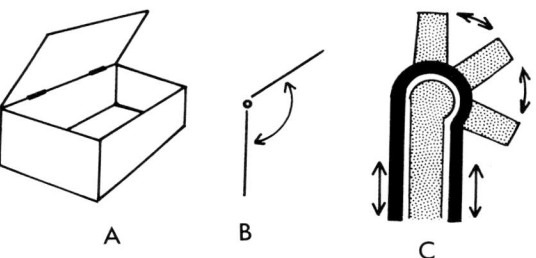

Figure 20–7 Proximal interphalangeal joint motion.

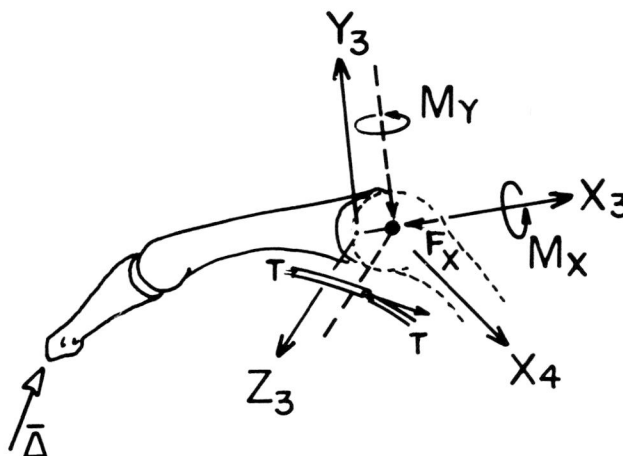

Figure 20–8 The orientation of constraint forces applied to the metacarpophalangeal joint. (*From:* Chao, E., Opgrande, J., Axmeer, F. "Three dimensional face analysis of finger joints in selected isometric functions." Biomech. 9, 387, 1976. $\bar{A}$ = applied force, Z_3 = volar force, M_x = rotatory force.

Superficially, the joint has the appearance of a pulley, with the middle phalanx sliding on the head of the proximal phalanx and a part of a loop completed by the flexor and extensor tendons (Fig. 20–7).[19] The loop-and-pulley system could be made quite stable, allowing only flexion and extension. However, this is not the case in the PIP joint, which is bicondylar with an intercondylar ridge and groove, that are not fully congruous, permitting other movements to take place in the joint. Some provisions seem to exist for passive displacements at these joints for gripping irregular objects and for making a fist or using a power grip.

The range of motion at the PIP joint averages 115 degrees of palmar flexion and 10 degrees of hyperextension. At the DIP joint there is virtually no hyperextension and between 45 degrees and 90 degrees of flexion. The diarthrodial MCP joints permit a wide range of movement. Virtually no stability is offered by the configuration of the joint surfaces, but support is provided by the joint capsule and especially by the collateral ligaments and the volar plate. Because of the great complexity of its movements, it is subjected to a broader range of controls and consequent stress (Fig. 20–8). Flexion is limited by the dorsal capsule and extension by the tough fibrous volar plate. Medial and lateral movements are limited chiefly by the collateral ligaments and to a lesser degree by the capsule and the volar plate. Motion of the MCP joint is 90 degrees of palmar flexion and 20 degrees of

hyperextension, on the average. During flexion the collateral ligaments become taut as they are displaced over the volar tubercles of the metacarpal head.

Radial and ulnar deviation is greatest when the MCP joint is in mild flexion (0 to 45 degrees), a position in which the ligaments are the loosest. Ulnar deviation is considerably greater than radial, and is least prominent in the ring finger. The average passive angulations are given for the four fingers in Table 20–1.

The normal index and long fingers do not bear straight-line relationships to their respective metacarpals. The shape of the articular condyles and the arrangement of the ligaments are such that there is a mean ulnarward angulation at the MCP joint of 14.7 degrees and 13.2 degrees, respectively, from the projected longitudinal metacarpal axis (Fig. 20–9). There is some evidence that the hand normally functions with the fingers angulated in an ulnar attitude with respect to the metacarpals. It seems unlikely that the deviation results from use or wear, because the disposition to passive ulnar drift is noted in normal infant hands. Some maneuvers clearly exert an ulnar-ward-directed force on the index and long fingers. It has been suggested that in some forms of power grip, such as grasping a doorknob or holding a full saucepan by the handle, an ulnar stress is placed on the index and successive fingers. The findings that the radial collateral ligament is stronger than the ulnar indicate, however, that the hand can normally resist such stresses.

TABLE 20-1   Average Passive Angulations at the Metacarpophalangeal Joints

	Index	*Long*	*Ring*	*Little*
Maximum radial deviation	13.3°	8.2°	14.2°	19.4°
Maximum ulnar deviation	42.7°	34.5°	20.2°	33.1°
Mean normal angulation (ulnar)	14.7°	13.2°	3.1°	6.9°
Lateral collateral ligament (abs. length)	18.0°	17.0°	14.5°	15.0°
Medial collateral ligament (abs. length)	15.1°	15.0°	14.0°	13.1°

When considering the mechanics of the MCP system, it may be noted that the proximal phalanx will tend to rotate on a transverse axis, the base having considerable volar (and potentially dislocating) force, and the distal end having dorsal force. Since the proximal end should be the stable base of the finger, the effect of this disturbance of balance will be of major importance. Under normal circumstances, the collateral ligaments, together with the proximal phalangeal insertion of the extensor tendon, effectively counteract this dislocating influence. It has been shown that lengthening of the collateral ligaments, combined with the force of the powerful flexor tendons in metacarpophalangeal joint problems, will inevitably lead to volar subluxation.[12] Although ulnar drift at the MCP joints attracts more attention, volar subluxation is more disabling.[22]

PRIMARY TREATMENT

A proper history, which includes the age, handedness, and occupation of the patient, should be obtained. A thorough physical examination, including neurological testing and routine x-rays, is necessary. The primary treatment of hand injuries includes elevation, immobilization and debridement for open injuries, as well as antibiotics when indicated. Tetanus prophylaxis should be considered for any open wound. Excellent monographs on primary care are available, such as those by Flatt[4] and Weckesser.[9] Certain points should be emphasized.

Before examining the obvious injury, an overall check of associated injuries and vital functions should be made. Any upper extremity hemorrhage can and should be controlled by direct pressure. These priorities observed, examination of the hand may proceed.

The most common error in treating hand injuries is the failure to diagnose. This is a greater pitfall when an open wound or fracture exists. The human tendency is to concentrate on the obvious, and thus tendon, nerve, or vascular injuries may go unrecognized. Such errors can be avoided by systematic functional testing distal to the level of the injury. Furthermore, localized tenderness, either with a chip fracture or without, should alert the physician to the presence of ligamentous or tendinous damage.

Cleansing and debridement are primary principles in the treatment of any open wound. The degree of debridement remains controversial. Radical debridement has such a mutilating effect on subsequent hand function that its use is seldom warranted.

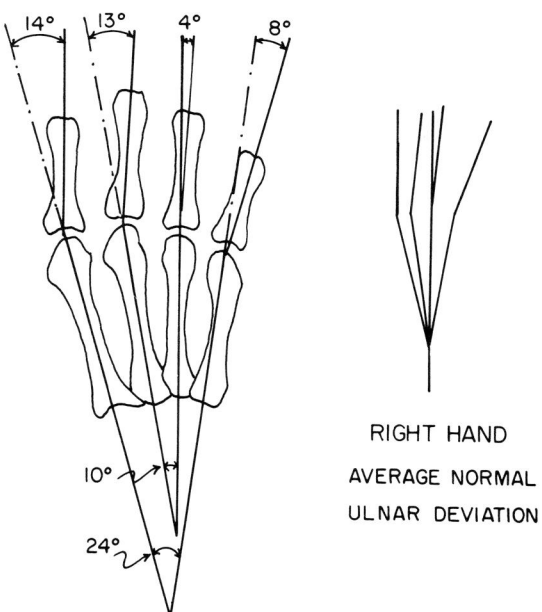

RIGHT HAND

AVERAGE NORMAL

ULNAR DEVIATION

Figure 20-9   Average ulnar deviation of the digits at the metacarpophalangeal joints.

We favor a cautious debridement, removing obviously devitalized tissue but preserving essential structures. Further debridement is performed as necessary. In hands with severe soft tissue loss, this often occurs at the time of wound coverage, several days after the initial debridement. In most cases, adequate debridement of open fractures of the distal phalanx can be performed under local anesthesia in the emergency room.

The necessity for extensive debridement finds its most heated arguments in gunshot wounds of the hand. Most bullet wounds in our civilian practice are termed low-velocity injury, e.g., 22-caliber with bullet speed of less than 1800 feet per second. While these do cause destruction of tissue in the bullet's path, this area is smaller than that of the high-velocity war wound. Given the exuberant blood supply of the hand and our desire to protect uninjured structures, we do not routinely explore these low-velocity bullet tracks or retrieve metallic fragments that do not interfere with neurovascular or joint function. Following cleaning and local debridement, which usually includes excision and culturing of the entry wound, the hand is splinted and elevated. A broad-spectrum antibiotic may be administered. In injuries caused by larger caliber bullets, such as .38-caliber, or whenever vital functional structures are involved, the patient is hospitalized for a period of observation and treatment.

It is common to see nonprogressive neural dysfunction away from the direct path of the bullet. This is usually a neurapraxia with a favorable prognosis. Worsening of neural function or nerve injury related to the bullet track requires exploration. Other factors influencing a decision for major debridement and exploration include severe initial contamination and vascular compromise. Whatever primary management is chosen, the entry and exit wounds should initially be left open.

The presence of a fracture caused by a bullet does not alter our approach unless there is marked loss of bony substance. Such loss is always accompanied by extensive soft tissue injury. Following the initial debridement, the challenge of these cases is to prevent shortening and maintain skeletal stability. This stabilization should be done initially and usually requires cross pinning to an intact metacarpal, or the use of wire spacers, as advocated by Brown.[71] Recently, we have used the minature Hoffman apparatus for this purpose. Once wound healing has occurred, the defect can be bone grafted. Neglecting early stabilization of such injuries can frustrate later attempts at functional rehabilitation.

The principle of nonclosure of gunshot wounds applies to any hand wound with extensive contamination, to wounds seen later than eight hours post injury, and to those inflicted by bites, either human or animal. It is well to remember the bacterial spectrum of the human mouth.[70, 76, 79] Neglect of such oral contamination can lead to serious complications. Conventional management of human bites includes irrigation, debridement, immobilization, elevation, close observation (often in the hospital), and empirical use of a broad-spectrum, penicillinase-resistant antibiotic.[72] Recent literature has suggested that penicillin be added to the drug regimen because of its particular effectiveness against anaerobic flora and *Eikenella corrodens*, a gram-negative organism common in normal mouth flora.[73] Appropriate cultures, including aerobic, anaerobic, and 10 per cent carbon dioxide atmospheres, should be taken prior to antibiotic therapy. Any clenched fist fracture (most commonly seen in the fourth and fifth metacarpal heads) associated with an open wound should be considered to be caused by the opponent's incisor and treated as a human bite wound.

Elevation is another keystone of treatment. This helps minimize the edema fluid which is implicated in increasing the collagen content, and hence scarring, in the healing wound. Subsequent joint stiffness, tendon adhesions, and delayed recovery are the result. The classic example of such an injury response is the dorsal crush injury without fracture. The swelling is usually impressive and, if neglected, will prolong the recovery time. Elevation and splinting are necessary to hasten recovery. We do not routinely use slings, which often insure that the injured hand remains dependent at the side and also have an inhibiting effect on proximal joint use. Instead, we emphasize the Statue of Liberty position during ambulation and the pillow or stockinette elevation when at rest.

Short-term immobilization is our final recommendation for all hand injuries, regardless of fracture. This is related to the importance of the soft tissue injury. The soft tissue injury and its subsequent reaction are often more important in terms of eventual disability than the bony injury. Immobilization minimizes the inflammatory response of the injured soft tissue and allows the repair process to proceed without interruption.

The immobilization period should be long enough to allow healing, but short enough to avoid stiffness. For soft tissue contusions this is approximately one week, while most fractures and tendon injuries require three to six weeks. The tendency to treat the radiograph and prolong immobilization until there is complete obliteration of the fracture line is unnecessary and should be avoided. Since the powerful extrinsic muscles originate proximally, the wrist should be included in any hand immobilization.

The position of splinting an injured hand is classically described with 30 degrees of wrist dorsiflexion and the fingers held as if gripping a soft ball. This concept originated in an era when little more than stability in this grasping position was expected of hand treatment. Given current rehabilitation techniques, the optimal position is 30 degrees of dorsiflexion of the wrist, 60 to 70 degrees of flexion at the metacarpophalangeal joints, and slight flexion at the interphalangeal joints (Fig. 20–10). This safe position maintains ligament length for the

reasons cited in the anatomy section, while the metacarpophalangeal flexion has the added benefit of controlling rotatory deformity. By protecting collateral ligament length and the skeletal arches, this "intrinsic plus" position affords a quicker restoration of joint mobility and digital power.

Most fractures of the metacarpals and phalanges can be treated by closed reduction and external immobilization as described. Some difficult fractures however, are displaced, with soft tissue between the fragments, or have segmental bone loss and require internal fixation. Likewise, many fractures involving significant articular surface demand anatomical reduction and internal fixation. Lastly, chip fractures are the telltale sign of ligament or tendon injuries, and these, rather than the fracture, represent the disabling lesion. The following section on specific injuries includes these tendon and ligament injuries as well as dislocations and fractures.

TENDON INJURIES

EXTENSOR MECHANISM

In recent years the problems of flexor tendon injury have dominated the stage, resulting in neglect of the more common and equally difficult problems inherent in extensor tendon injury. The anatomical complexities (Fig. 20–5) and dynamics of the extensor mechanism must be appreciated; these have received ample coverage

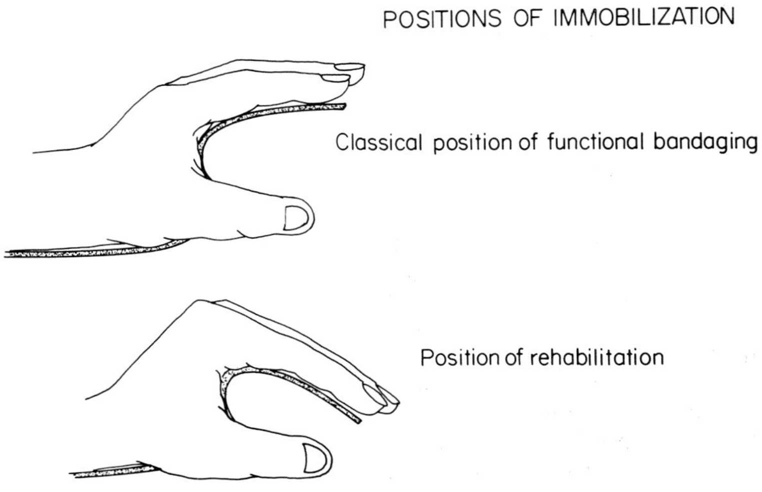

POSITIONS OF IMMOBILIZATION

Figure 20–10 Positions of immobilization.

Classical position of functional bandaging

Position of rehabilitation

MALLET FINGER

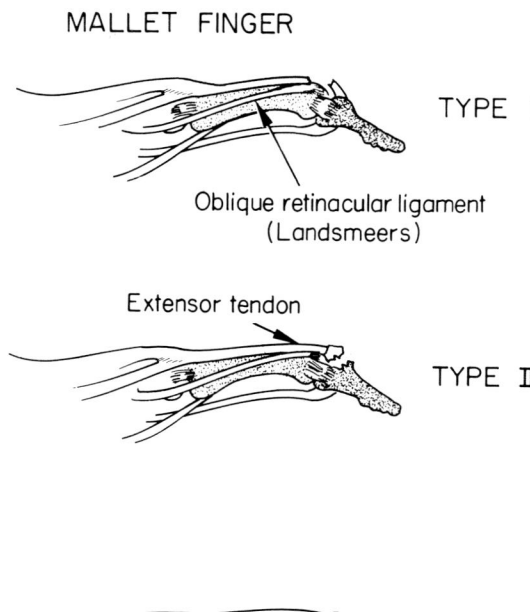

TYPE I

Oblique retinacular ligament
(Landsmeers)

Extensor tendon

TYPE II

TYPE III

Figure 20–11   Types of mallet finger.

in the literature.[27, 36] The act of finger extension is far more complex than that of flexion, since it requires an orchestration of the extrinsic extensor tendons, the intrinsic muscles, and the retinacular system besides the synergistic role of the flexor tendons.[28, 31, 32] The relative strength of the opposing finger flexors must be considered, as it may extend the treatment time for extensor injuries. The extensor mechanism is most frequently injured at the joint level, and each joint level has its own peculiar problems.

Mallet Finger—Distal Interphalangeal Joint

The mallet, baseball, or drop finger results from the loss of extensor tendon continuity to the distal phalanx at or near its insertion into the dorsal articulating lip. The injury can be caused by the end of the finger being forcibly flexed with the extensor tendon taut, or by laceration of the tendon and/or Landsmeer's ligaments at the level of the DIP joint. Stretch of the tendon fibers without complete division results in

mild distal drop with lack of extension of between 5 and 20 degrees. Some weak active extension is maintained. Extensor tendon rupture or tear of the tendon from its distal insertion results in a 40 to 45 degree extension lag and complete loss of active extension of the distal joint. A small fragment of distal phalanx (dorsal articulating lip) may be avulsed with the extensor tendon. Laceration at the level of the DIP joint may produce an extension lag of up to 90 degrees owing to laceration of the tendon insertion, Landsmeer's ligament, the dorsal capsule, and the skin. Hyperextension of the PIP joint may occur because the extensor force to the DIP joint moves proximally and is directed to the PIP joint. It is most commonly seen in patients with lax volar plates.

The three types of mallet finger injuries include: type 1, injury to the tendon only; type 2, avulsion of the tendon from the dorsal cortex with a small piece of distal phalanx attached to the tendon; and type 3, fracture of the dorsal cortex of the distal phalanx with the tendon attached to a large piece of the distal phalanx. The pull of the profundus tendon may cause volar subluxation of the distal fragment of the distal phalanx in the type 3 (Fig. 20–11).

There are nearly as many treatments recommended as there are patients.[24, 25, 28, 34, 35] If the mallet finger is open, surgical repair is indicated. We usually combine internal fixation, with the distal joint in extension, with repair of the lacerated structures. The majority of type 1 and type 2 injuries are closed and should remain so (Fig. 20–12A). Treatment consists of splinting the distal joint in extension for a minimum of six weeks. Some authors have advocated casting of the PIP joint in 60 degrees of flexion in this injury. We do not routinely immobilize the PIP joint because of stiffness, but prefer a simple extension splint, as illustrated in Figure 20–12B and C. The need for constant splinting must be emphasized repeatedly to the patient, for any removal of the splint and drooping of the finger will defeat the therapeutic purpose. One can achieve a satisfactory result in well over 60 per cent of the cases that are properly splinted. Our standard routine is six to eight weeks of constant splinting, followed by four weeks of splinting at night. During the latter four weeks, active PIP flexion exercises are begun.

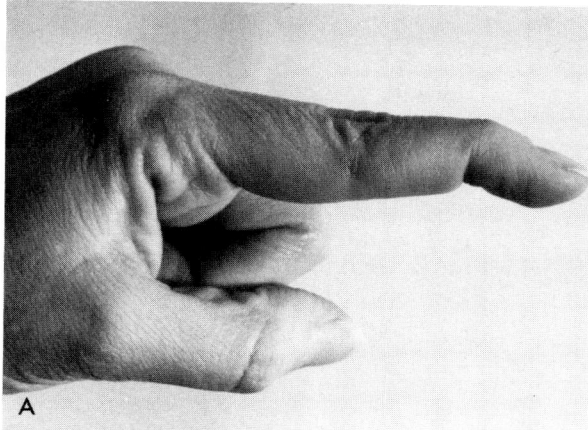

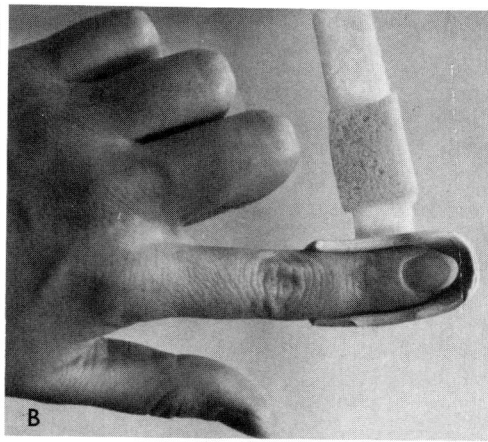

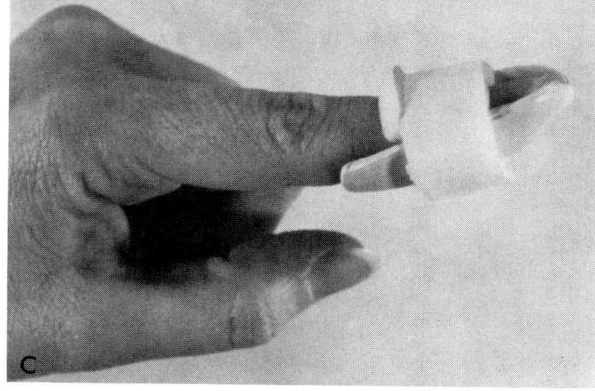

Figure 20–12 A. Mallet finger. B and C. Conservative treatment of mallet finger–splint with distal interphalangeal joint held straight.

Because of bone-to-bone healing, a type 2 injury has a more favorable prognosis. Occasionally, however, the fracture may be displaced, as in Figure 20–13, and this may be an indication for operative repair. In this case, the small bone fragment may be ignored and the tendon repaired using the technique of a pull-out wire. In the type 3 injury, the pull of the profundus tendon may cause volar subluxation of the distal fragment and subluxation of the distal joint. Open reduction and internal fixation of the fracture and relocation of the subluxation are indicated in this injury.

Mallet fingers seen up to eight weeks following injury can benefit from extension splinting. Injuries seen after this time are probably best left untreated. Follow-up

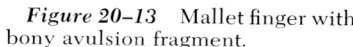

Figure 20–13 Mallet finger with bony avulsion fragment.

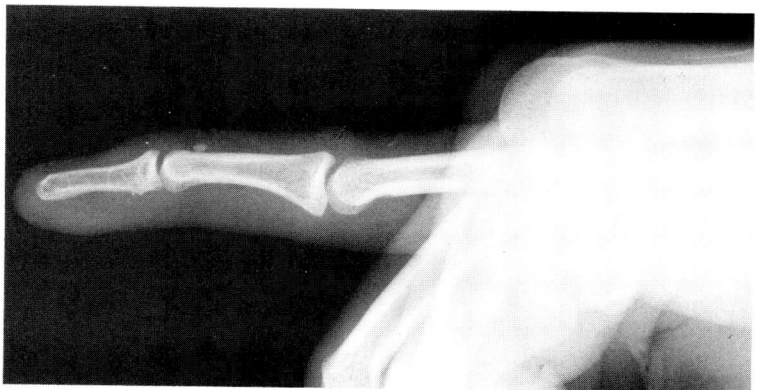

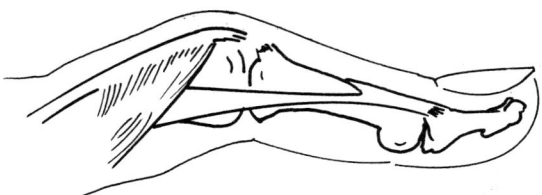

Figure 20–14 Boutonnière deformity.

studies have shown little functional deficit or residual arthritis from type 1 or type 2 mallet fingers.[96] Stark[34] found that only 20 per cent of the mallet fingers treated in his series had an extension loss of more than 30 degrees. PIP joint motion, distal joint flexion, and grip strength were normal. When treatment of a chronic mallet finger is indicated, DIP fusion gives a more predictable result than tendon reconstruction.

Boutonnière Deformity — Proximal Interphalangeal Joint

The next most common closed extensor injury is the boutonnière or buttonhole deformity. The clinical attitude of a digit with a boutonnière deformity is a flexion of the proximal interphalangeal joint and a hyperextension of the distal interphalangeal joint (Fig. 20–14). It results from the disruption of the central slip of the extensor tendon combined with a tearing of the triangular ligament that joins the lateral bands. This allows the lateral bands to slip below the axis of motion of the PIP joint, with a subsequent extensor pull at the distal interphalangeal joint. Both the central slip disruption and the lateral band migration are important components of this injury. The cause is a laceration, direct blunt force, or anterior dislocation of the PIP joint, or a sudden forced flexion of the PIP joint with the central slip maximally taut.

The diagnosis is difficult to make immediately after injury because the lateral bands, which also extend the proximal interphalangeal joint, are still dorsal to the axis of motion of this joint and therefore provide extension for it. With time, however, the lateral bands migrate volar to the axis of the PIP joint. This has two effects: Their original extensor force becomes a flexor force at the PIP joint, and because this position increases the length of their route there is

increased tension at the insertion, causing distal interphalangeal joint hyperextension. The reader is referred to Souter's excellent article.[33]

Central slip ruptures are as common as the jammed or dislocated finger and are often misdiagnosed. The swollen PIP joint is a complex diagnostic problem, but an effort should be made to localize the lesion. Maximal tenderness located dorsally over the insertion of the central slip should lead one to suspect this injury. If tenderness is more lateral over the collateral ligaments, or more volar, one should suspect lateral ligament injury or volar plate injury. A lateral x-ray should be taken of any swollen PIP joint. Bony avulsion injury is uncommon in central slip rupture, but often in severe injuries a volar subluxation of the middle phalanx will be noted. Acute central slip injuries without boutonnière deformity should be splinted in extension at the PIP joint for a minimum of four weeks. The DIP joint should be left free for both active and passive range of motion. If a boutonnière attitude is present or if volar subluxation of the PIP joint has occurred, this may require pinning and operative repair. Central slip ruptures older than six weeks require surgery consisting of dorsal replacement of the lateral bands or tendon graft reconstruction of the central slip. Many procedures have been described.[23, 24, 26, 29, 30, 33, 37] It should be noted that the primary functional complaint of patients with a chronic boutonnière deformity is the lack of terminal joint flexion. If this can be corrected by occupational therapy or sometimes by operative repair, the flexion deformity of the PIP joint may not be disabling enough to require surgery.

FLEXOR MECHANISM

Open injuries to the flexor tendons are common, but are outside the focus of this chapter. The interested reader is referred to several articles listed in the references.[41-45] A very common complicating factor of open flexor tendon injuries is that of concomitant digital nerve laceration, present in approximately 50 per cent of cases. Associated middle or proximal phalangeal fractures are relatively uncommon, occurring in only 5 to

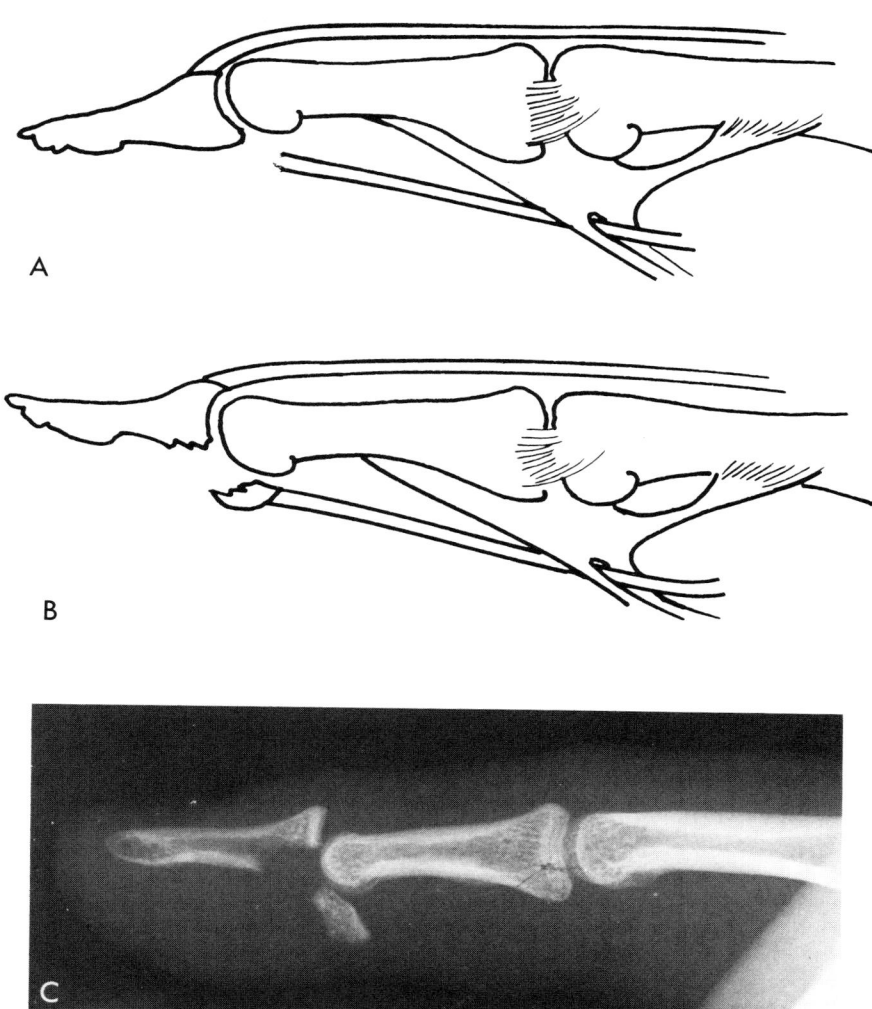

Figure 20–15 Rupture of profundus insertion. *A.* Tendon insertion avulsion. *B.* Tendon insertion avulsion with bone attached. *C.* X-ray of tendon insertion avulsion with bone attached and dorsal dislocation of distal phalanx.

6 per cent of patients with such injuries.[43] Such fractures, when they do occur, should be accurately reduced and firmly immobilized. They often require internal fixation. Severely comminuted or contaminated fractures may preclude primary tendon repair.

Avulsion of the Profundus Tendon Insertion

Avulsion of the profundus insertion into the base of the distal phalanx at the volar

articulating lip occurs frequently in football players.[38-40, 46] The mechanism of injury is a sudden digital hyperextension of the DIP joint as the flexor digitorum profundus is actively contracting. While any finger can be affected, the ring finger is most often avulsed because it lacks independent extension and because it is biomechanically the center of the grasping digits. As in mallet fingers, there are basically three types of avulsion. The tendon may rupture from its insertion cleanly (Fig. 20–15A), or with a small bone fragment from the volar aspect of the distal phalanx (Fig. 20–15B), or, very rarely, with a large fragment from the volar cortex. The last type may be associated with a dorsal subluxation of the DIP joint (Fig. 20–15C).

Another complicating factor of this injury, given the peculiarities of the flexor tendons, is the level to which the avulsed tendons retract. These levels are (1) the chiasm of the flexor superficialis, causing a flexion contracture of the PIP joint, (2) the base of the finger, or (3) the palm at the lumbrical origin. These levels also bear a relationship to the remaining blood supply of the avulsed tendon. The profundus tendon receives its blood supply in part from its insertion into the distal phalanx, the long and short vincula, and the intratendinous vessels. Retraction into the palm represents a rupture of both vincula and hence a substantial loss of blood supply. In retractions to the flexor chiasm or the base of the finger, the long vincula often remains intact thus preserving greater blood supply. There is no obvious deformity associated with the injury, but inability to flex the DIP joint of the injured digit is noted on physical examination as well as tenderness at the level where the retracted tendon comes to rest. A lateral x-ray of the injured digit is helpful in making the diagnosis if bone has been avulsed with the tendon.

Along with these factors, the time interval from injury is an important consideration in treatment. If the injury is seen within the first two weeks, the tendon or tendon-bone unit may be reattached. This is done regardless of the level of retraction. A standard pull-out wire technique is used. To avoid flexure contraction of the PIP joint, the postoperative immobilization is done with the wrist and MCP joints in flexion, but the PIP and DIP joints in minimal flexion. Beyond three weeks in tendons retracted into the palm, reattachment is risky because normal sublimis function may be compromised. If the tendon is retracted only to the level of the PIP joint, the reinsertion may be done at an even later date. While tendon grafting through an intact sublimis has its advocates for late injuries,[40] many patients may not need treatment. If, however, the patient's occupation requires terminal joint fixation, an arthrodesis or tenodesis will provide satisfactory terminal joint stabilization.

LIGAMENTOUS INJURIES

VOLAR PLATE

The volar plate is a fibrocartilaginous structure present on the volar aspect of each joint. The structure of the volar plate is such that the more compliant proximal membranous portion adjusts as a forming force, and the thickened distal fibrocartilage portion tears or avulses with a fragment of bone from the volar aspect of the middle phalanx. At the metacarpophalangeal joint level, the volar plates are connected by a deep transverse metacarpal ligament. A volar plate rupture can occur at any of the three joints of a digit, but is seen most frequently at the proximal interphalangeal joint level. Volar plate injuries are typically caused by a blow on the end of the finger producing a hyperextension force and often a dorsal dislocation of the joint. A PIP volar plate usually pulls away at the middle phalangeal attachment (Fig. 20–16). The distal fibrocartilaginous attachment often avulses with a chip of bone, and this is evident on a lateral x-ray of a digit. Together with central slip ruptures and collateral ligament injuries, volar plate injury should be suspected in any swollen joint. In this injury, the maximum tenderness will be exhibited over the volar aspect of the involved joint. When the acute swelling has subsided, pain may be present on the volar aspect of the joint on extension of the finger, and often there are symptoms of catching or locking of the joint with flexion. Instability of the involved joint occurs with either active or passive extension, because of the loss of the normal volar checkrein effect of the volar plate. In a chronic volar plate injury, this instability presents as a classic swan neck deformity.

The recommended treatment for an acute volar plate injury, seen before four weeks, is

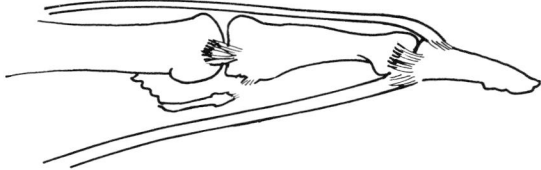

Figure 20–16   Volar plate avulsion at proximal interphalangeal joint.

placement of the PIP joint at 30 degrees of flexion.[53] The early removal of the volar aspect of the cast after the injured digit has been placed in flexion is a modification of this treatment.[51] This provides an extension block and permits flexion while scar tissue repairs the volar plate injury. Old volar plate injuries that are symptomatic require added tissue to stabilize the volar aspect of the joint. This can be accomplished by a sublimis slip from the involved finger or by a free tendon graft.[1, 6]

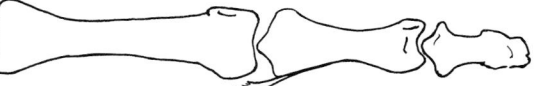

Figure 20-17   Collateral ligament avulsion at proximal interphalangeal joint.

COLLATERAL LIGAMENT INJURIES EXCLUSIVE OF THE THUMB

The anatomical structures of the interphalangeal and metacarpophalangeal ligaments are similar, with a cordlike collateral ligament originating at the tuberosity of the proximal joint component and a lower fanlike accessory ligament inserting into the volar plate. They differ in that the tension of the PIP collateral ligament is essentially the same in extension and flexion, while the MCP joint ligaments are tight in flexion and relaxed in extension[18] (as mentioned earlier). This difference is due to the eccentric dorsal origin of the collateral ligament from the metacarpal head, relaxing the ligament on extension and stretching the ligament when the joint is flexed. The placement of metacarpophalangeal joints in flexion is therefore necessary following hand injuries, or extension contractures may occur.

Collateral ligament injury is usually caused by an abduction or adduction force exerted on the finger when the joint is in an extended position. While it may occur at any joint, the PIP rather than the DIP joint is usually involved owing to its longer lever arm (Fig. 20-17). The injury is frequently sports-related and involves the radial collateral ligament more often than the ulnar collateral ligament. With the exception of the thumb, the border digits — the index and small fingers — are the collateral ligaments that are most frequently injured.

At surgery, the most common defect found in total ligament rupture is separation of the ligament from its proximal attachment. In approximately one half of the cases retracted portions of the ligament are observed to be folded into the joint. The injury

is frequently associated with a partial tear of the volar plate.

This is the third entity to be considered in the examination of the swollen joint. Clinically, the patient will exhibit localized tenderness on the sides of the joint and pain on attempts at stress testing. Plane anteroposterior x-rays will often reveal a small bony avulsion from the lateral side of the joint. Occasionally, stress x-rays using local anesthesia are helpful in documenting complete ligamentous instability. Such instability exists with complete rupture. In untreated injuries seen late, a swollen tender mass, which has been labeled a ligamentous callus,[50] is often seen with associated joint laxity.

Most collateral ligament injuries are partial tears and may be satisfactorily treated by immobilization for three weeks with the interphalangeal joint in 30 degrees of flexion. A complete rupture that is acute and has demonstrable lateral instability is best treated by early suture.[50] Late ruptures that are symptomatic may be treated by a tendon graft placed through holes in the lateral aspect of the phalanges at the level of the injured joint.[50, 53]

COLLATERAL LIGAMENT INJURIES – THE THUMB

The critical functional importance of the thumb in pinch and power grip makes collateral ligament injuries to the thumb extremely disabling. This is most commonly seen at the level of the metacarpophalangeal joint. Cooney[14] and others have calculated the magnitude of the forces active at the metacarpophalangeal joint to be four or five times the applied force at the fingertip. For example, in normal pinch, these applied forces can be 4 or 5 kg and rise to 20 to 30 kg in power grip. These forces are resisted by the constraining collateral ligaments, the intrinsic musculature insertions,

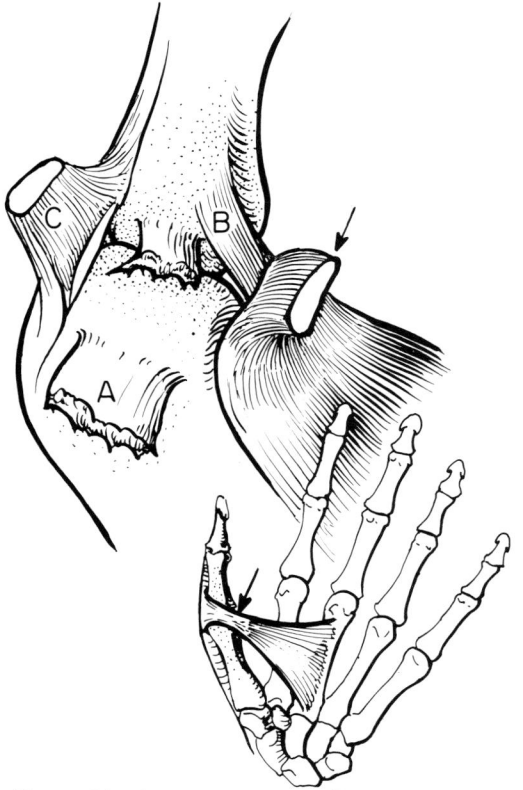

Figure 20–18   Injury to: *A.* collateral ligament. *B.* adductor insertion to proximal phalanx. *C.* adductor aponeurosis to extensor tendon, ulnar aspect of metacarpophalangeal joint of thumb.

and the extrinsic muscular tendons. In addition to the injury to the collateral ligament itself, the volar plate, the adductor insertion into the proximal phalanx, or the attachment of the adductor aponeurosis into the extensor tendon of the thumb may be injured (Fig. 20–18).

Ulnar instability of the metacarpophalangeal joint occurs three times more frequently than radial instability. Most patients describe a hyperextension force as the cause of injury, and recently the ski pole has been indicated as a frequent culprit.[67] The patient presents with a swollen metacarpophalangeal joint of the thumb, pain and weakness of pinch, and tenderness localized over the injured collateral ligament. When lateral stress is applied to the ulnar collateral ligament, pain will be increased and instability may be demonstrated (Fig. 20–19). If significant instability is noted, stress roentgenograms may be obtained (Fig. 20–20). For a complete examination, local anesthesia is often required. In the acute injury, angulation of more than 45 degrees suggests that total disruption of the collateral ligament has occurred. Another sign that may be useful has been described by Smith.[67] This is volar subluxation of the proximal phalanx on the metacarpal head. He reported that greater

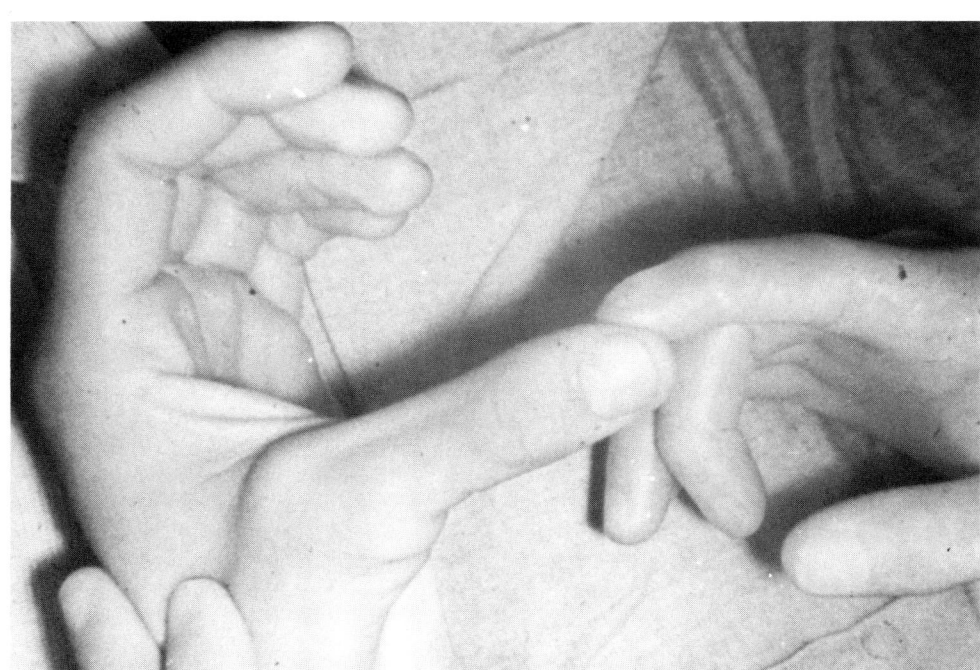

Figure 20–19   Stress test for gamekeeper's thumb.

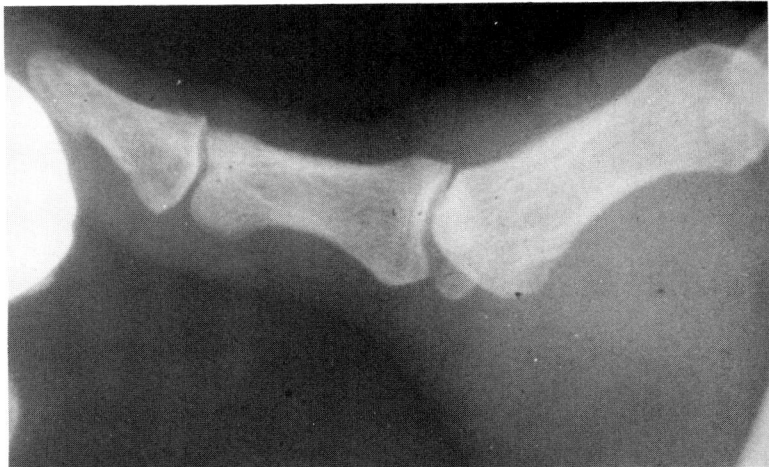

Figure 20-20 X-ray of ulnar collateral ligament with instability greater than 45 degrees.

than 3 mm of subluxation is indicative of complete collateral disruption. X-rays will also reveal an avulsed portion of bone, usually the proximal phalanx, in approximately 25 per cent of cases.

Treatment of this injury depends on the time lapse since injury, the degree of instability, and the patient's occupation and symptoms. Acute injuries, with less than 45 degrees of instability, represent partial tears and may be treated satisfactorily with a thumb spica holding the metacarpophalangeal joint in slight flexion for a period of 4 to 6 weeks. Depending on the ruthlessness with which the instability is sought, such immobilization has a failure rate of 5 to 10 per cent. In Smith's series, 40 per cent of his patients with posttraumatic instability had received prior casting. Stener[68] was the first to emphasize this point. He attributed such failures to complete collateral ligament rupture with a retraction and eversion of the proximal portion of the ligament beneath an intact adductor aponeurosis, which effectively isolated it from the reparative process. Recently, Bowers[61] documented the usefulness of a metacarpophalangeal joint arthrogram in the diagnosis of an everted ligament, in order to identify those patients who require surgery.

Acute injuries with greater than 45 degrees of instability require direct collateral ligament repair, and this provides a satisfactory result (Fig. 20–21). Significant volar subluxation of the proximal phalanx is another indication for primary operative repair. In approximately one quarter of cases

a bony avulsion fragment is present (Fig. 20–22A) and acts as a diagnostic marker. If the fragment is small and non-displaced, a cast immobilization is performed. If, how-

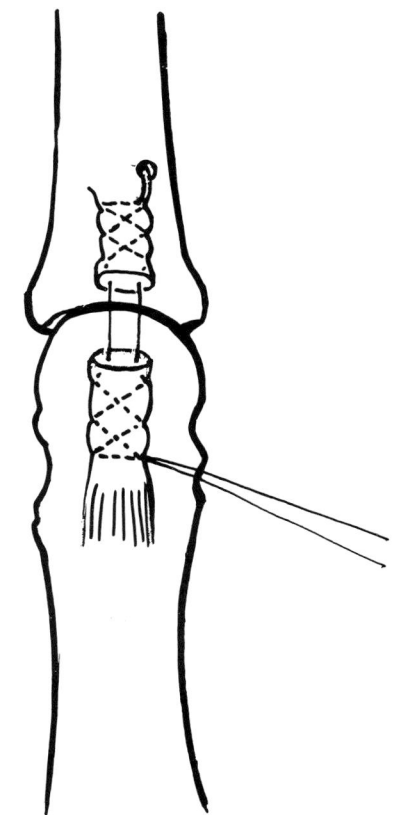

Figure 20-21 Repair of an acute rupture of the ulnar collateral ligament of the thumb.

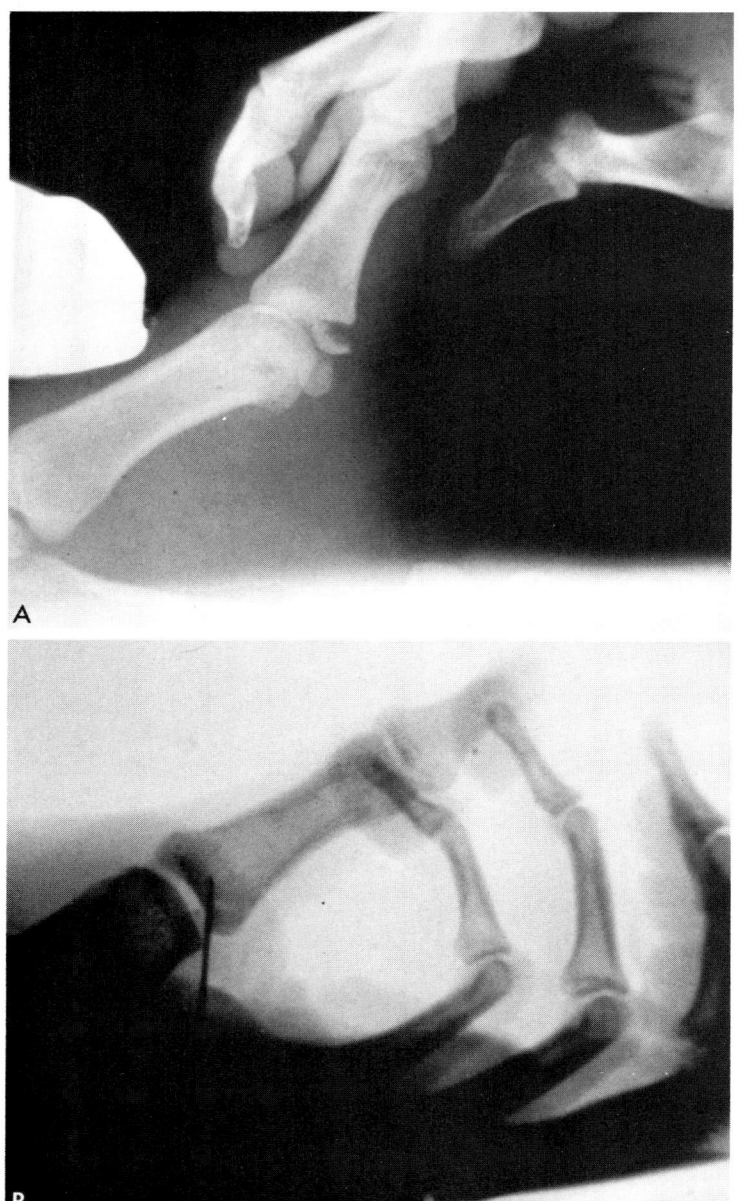

Figure 20–22 A. Rupture of the ulnar collateral ligament of the thumb, with bone attached. B. Open replacement of the fragment with pin fixation.

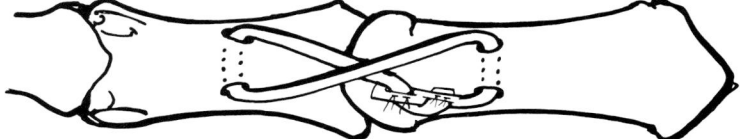

Figure 20-23 Replacement of the ulnar collateral ligament with a tendon graft.

ever, it is displaced or represents greater than 20 per cent of the articular surface, replacement and fixation of the fragment with pins or wire are indicated (Fig. 20-22B).

Given the nature of ligamentous healing, primary operative repair of collateral ligament injuries is less predictable in patients seen more than three weeks postinjury. Patients with disabling pain, weakness of pinch, and demonstrable joint instability may be treated with collateral ligament reconstruction. Reconstruction of the ligament with a flexor tendon graft placed through drill holes in the bone gives a satisfactory result (Fig. 20-23). Advancement of the phalangeal insertion of the adductor has also been recommended (Fig. 20-24).[65] In our series, while the latter procedure resulted in slightly greater pinch strength and less bulk directly over the repair site, the former provided a more normal range of metacarpophalangeal joint motion. Coonrad[63] in his study of over 1000 thumbs, noted the great variability in metacarpophalangeal and intraphalangeal motion of the thumb. Interestingly, however, in any one patient, the total arc of motion at these two joints approaches a constant average. Thus, those with marked flexibility of the interphalangeal joint had less flexibility at the metacarpophalangeal joint and vice versa. In patients with limited interphalangeal motion the loss of metacarpophalangeal joint motion may be troublesome. We routinely use the palmaris longus tendon, if present, for tendon graft reconstructions, because of the predictable stability attained and the lessened restriction of joint motion.

Campbell in 1955,[62] initially described this chronic instability of the ulnar collateral ligament in Scottish gamekeepers, whose injury resulted from the repetitive stretching force of wringing the necks of their catches. It is not an acute injury. While

gamekeeping is declining, there are occupations, such as industrial cutting with heavy shears or professional sports, in which such repetitive stress occurs. Patients with metacarpophalangeal joint instability whose work requires power grip and pinch have been satisfactorily treated with a combination of adductor advancement and a tendon graft to replace the injured ulnar structures (Fig. 20-25A), as in this professional baseball pitcher (Fig. 20-25B). Patients with painful metacarpophalangeal joints and roentgenographic evidence of arthritis are best treated with arthrodesis.

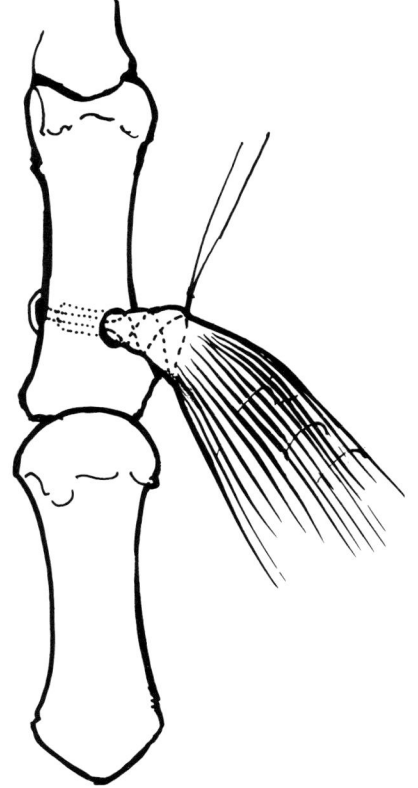

Figure 20-24 Adductor advancement for old rupture of the ulnar collateral ligament of the thumb.

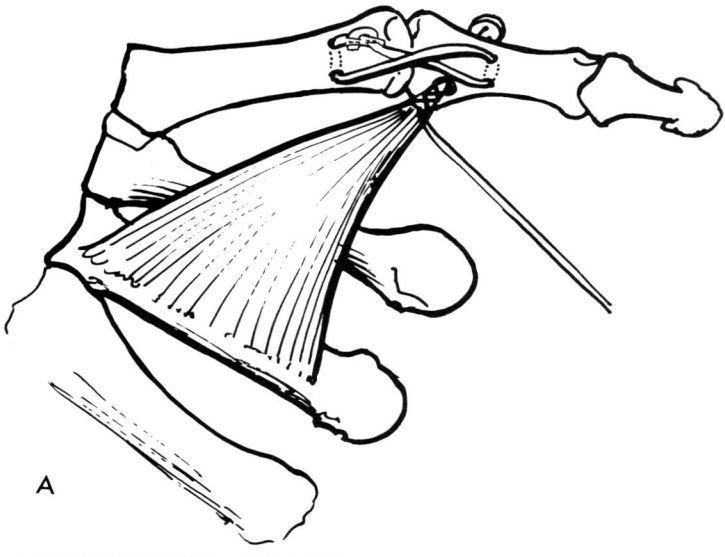

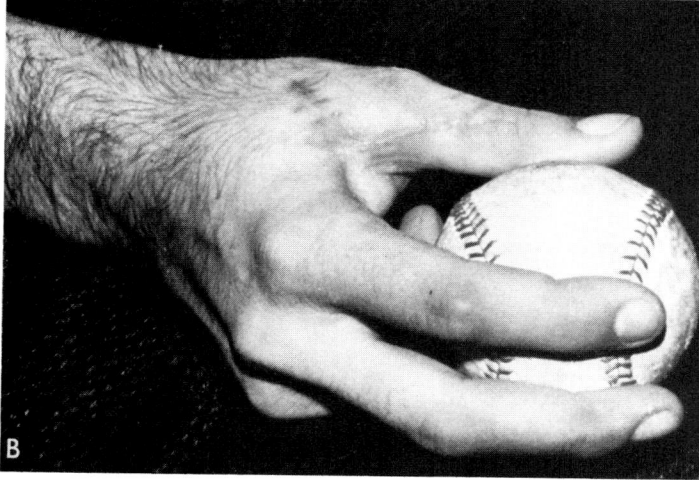

Figure 20–25 *A.* The use of both a tendon graft and the adductor advancement for chronic ulnar instability in young, active patients (i.e., athletes). *B.* Satisfactory ulnar stability in a baseball pitcher one year after the combined procedures.

FINGER DISLOCATIONS

Acute dislocations of the finger joints are common. The proximal interphalangeal joint is the most frequently injured, but dislocations of all the joints in the hand, including the carpometacarpal joints, have been reported. An awareness of the intricate anatomy of the joint structures is essential to appreciate the significance of these injuries. Except for the carpometacarpal joint, each finger joint consists of a joint capsule, primary and accessory collateral ligaments, a volar plate and contiguous cartilaginous surfaces, and extrinsic flexor and extensor insertions. As Moberg[53] has stated, any dislocation represents a total disruption of one of these structures. Once the dislocation has been reduced, the specific injury is diagnosed and treatment is carried out as outlined in the previous section.

Several other points are worth emphasizing. Dislocations are produced by severe trauma. It is not unusual, however, for the injury to present as merely a painful swollen finger, having gone back into place spontaneously or through the efforts of the patient or a friend. Thus, the initial presentation of the acute injury may appear quite innocuous to the patient and the treating

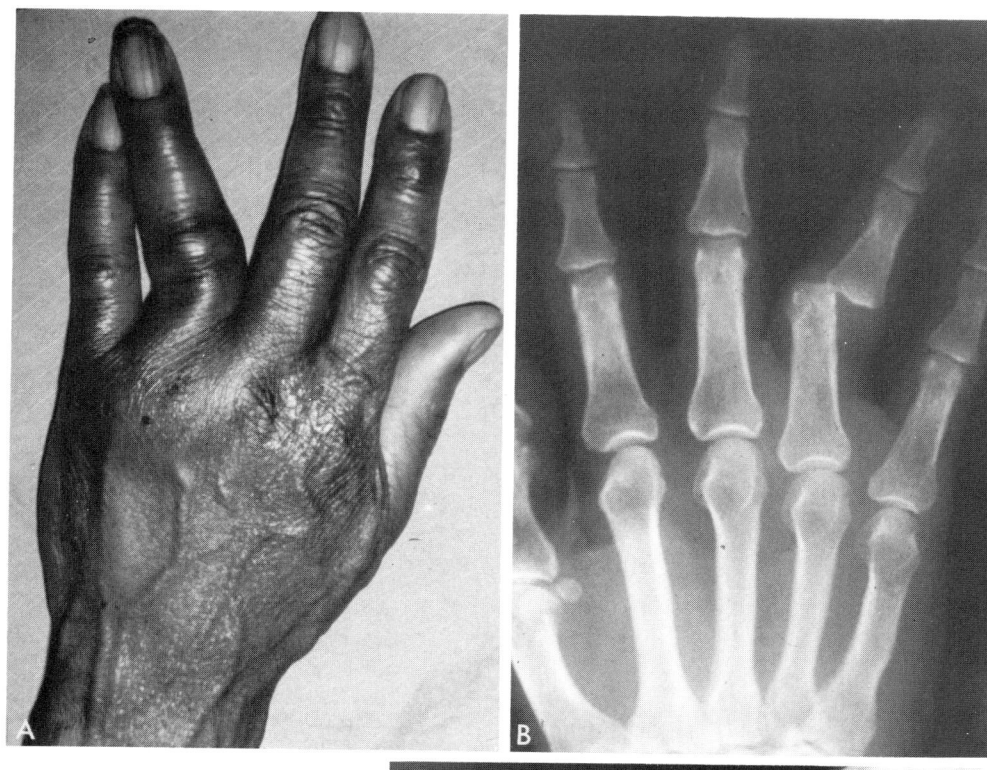

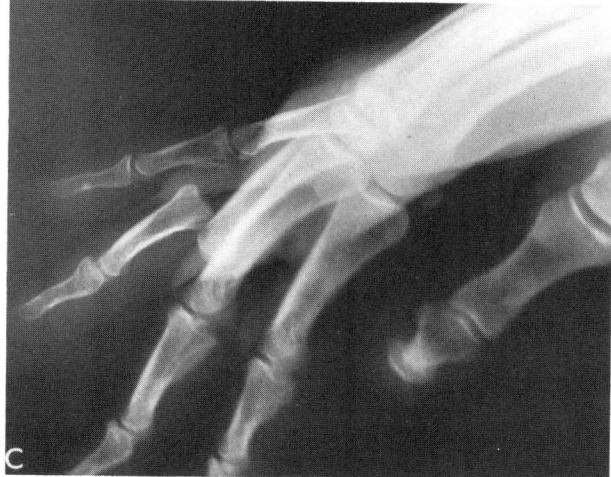

Figure 20–26 *A* to *C*. Acute dislocation of proximal interphalangeal joint of ring finger. *A*. Clinical appearance. *B* and *C*. Anteroposterior and lateral x-rays. Treatment was closed reduction and immobilization in 40 degrees of flexion for three weeks.

physician. Consequently, many of these injuries are undertreated or neglected, and the result can be significant, late physical disability. As with dislocations elsewhere, pre- and postreduction x-rays are helpful. The latter are especially needed as a precaution to assure the accuracy of the reduction as well as to identify small bony avulsion fragments. Stability should be gently tested postreduction and an attempt made to identify the specific injured structures. Although every direction of dislocation has been reported, the majority are dorsal, with an occasional rotatory or lateral component (Fig. 20–26). Dorsal dislocations are the result of hyperextension injuries of the fingers and are usually easily reduced with longitudinal traction alone.

Distal interphalangeal joint dislocation is uncommon because of the inherent stability of the joint and the short lever arm against which the force must act. The skin and its fibrous septa further stabilize the joint. In fact, many dislocations of the distal interphalangeal joint are open injuries. Irreducible dislocations have been reported.[55] These have resulted from entrapment either of the volar plate or of the flexor tendon insertion. Once reduced, the distal interphalangeal joint should be held in 10 to 15 degrees of flexion for a period of 3 weeks. This may be facilitated by Kirschner wire fixation. Open dislocations, like any open injury, should be cleaned and debrided. If contamination is minimal, the skin may be loosely approximated.

Proximal interphalangeal joint dislocations are the most frequent of all dislocations of the upper extremity. These are essentially of three types, classified according to initial displacement and postreduction stability. They are dorsal dislocation without major fracture, unstable dorsal fracture-dislocation, and volar dislocation. To each of these injuries a lateral component or collateral ligament injury may be added. As mentioned, the deformities are often reduced or at least partially reduced when initially seen, and therefore localized tenderness, stress testing, x-rays, and patient history are often required to document the initial injury.

Dorsal dislocations are primarily volar plate injuries with or without associated collateral ligament injury. In those injuries in which a fracture of the distal volar plate or a small avulsion fracture is present, the reduction is easily accomplished by longitudinal traction. Immobilization in 20 to 30 degrees of flexion for 3 weeks is followed by a program of gentle active range-of-motion exercises. If the volar fracture fragment of the middle phalanx is large, the reduction is considered unstable and subsequent treatment is difficult. There is a tendency to recurrent joint subluxation, and some degree of joint stiffness is inevitable. For these unstable fractures many treatments have been advocated but few consistent successes have been seen. Treatments include immobilization of the joint in an advanced degree of flexion, extension block splinting,[51] open reduction and internal fixation,[59] tridirectional traction in a banjo frame,[56] and force-coupling immobilization.[47] Eaton[3]

prefers to excise a comminuted base of the middle phalanx, regaining a stable joint reduction by volar plate reattachment. We generally utilize extensor block splinting or volar plate reattachment.

The third type of PIP dislocation is the rare volar dislocation. As described by Spinner and Choi,[57] this injury is invariably associated with avulsion of the central slip of the extensor tendon from its insertion into the dorsal base of the middle phalanx. The cause of this injury is (1) a varus or valgus force producing a rupture of the collateral ligament or volar plate; and (2) an anterior-directed force that displaces the base of the middle phalanx forward, rupturing the central slip of the extensor mechanism. These authors advocated primary repair of the central slip to avoid the inevitable boutonnière deformity and primary repair of the other injured structures along with pinning of the joint in extension. However, we would agree with Eaton[38] that if the extension lag is less than 30 degrees, extension splinting of the PIP joint is a reasonable alternative.

Irreducible dislocations of the PIP joint have been reported. In dorsal dislocations this is usually an interposition of the volar plate, while for anterior dislocations it is a buttonholing of the phalangeal head between the central slip and the lateral band. Open dislocations are usually of the dorsal type and usually stable. The open wound is handled similarly to open DIP dislocations.

Metacarpophalangeal joint dislocations of the fingers are rare and virtually always involve the border digits—the index and small fingers. They are basically of two types: the simple, in which closed reduction is possible and casting with the metacarophalangeal joints in 60 degrees of flexion for a period of 3 weeks is followed by gentle active motion; the second is the complex type that is irreducible in a closed manner. The mechanism of both injuries is usually a fall on the outstretched hand which forces the metacarpophalangeal joint into hyperextension. In an irreducible injury, the volar plate is torn from its metacarpal membranous attachment, causing the proximal phalanx to be displaced dorsally. The metacarpal head is prominently displaced into the palm, where it is buttonholed. Kaplan's classic study[49] de-

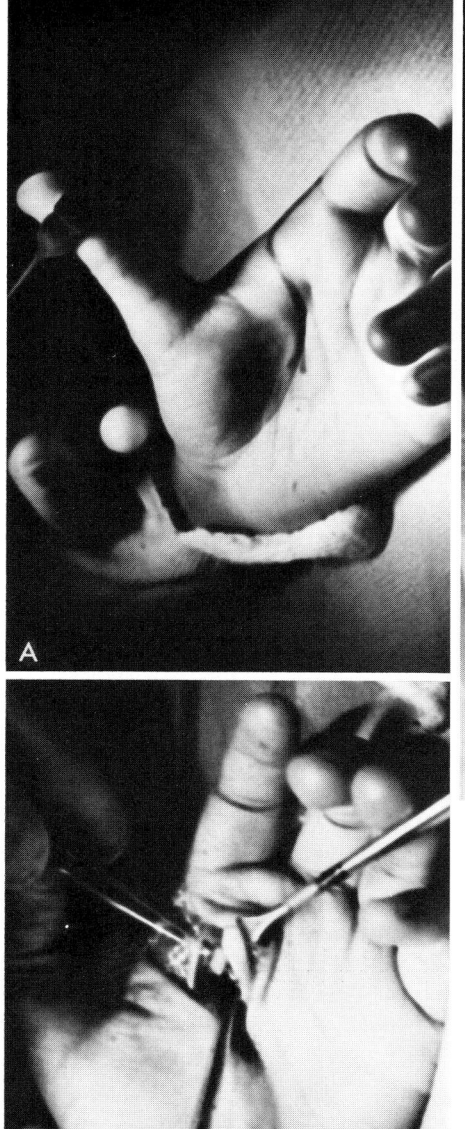

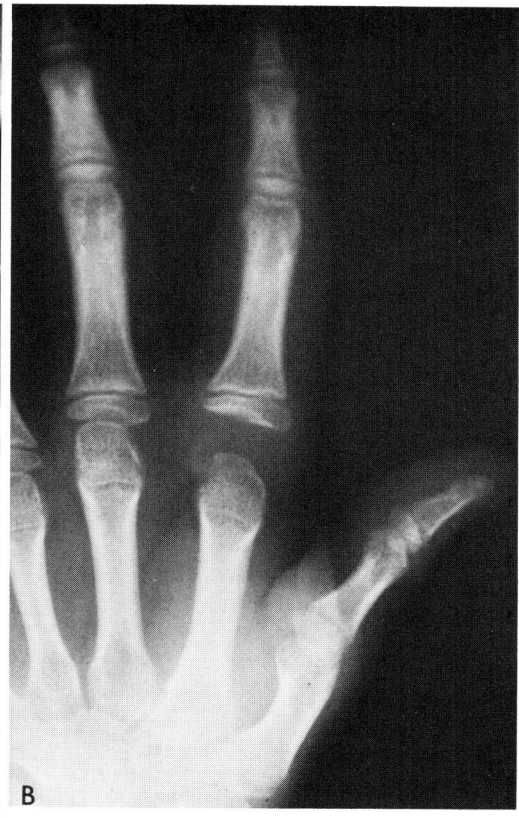

Figure 20–27 Complex dislocation of the index metacarpophalangeal joint. *A*. Pathognomonic skin dimpling. *B*. Widened joint space on x-ray. *C*. Surgical exposure showing vulnerability of digital nerves.

scribed the pathogenesis of this trapping as follows: The metacarpal head is held between the volar plate and natatory ligament distally, by the superficial transverse ligament proximally, by the flexor tendon on the ulnar side, and by the lumbrical and neurovascular structures on the radial side. The clinical pathognomonic sign of a com-

plex dislocation is puckering of the skin caused by the vertical fibers that anchor the dermis and palmar fascia (Fig. 20–27A). A widened joint space, frequently indicative of the interpositioned volar plate, is seen on radiographs (Fig. 20–27B). Despite these definitive signs of complex dislocation, one gentle attempt at reduction, using longi-

tudinal traction, is advisable. If it is unsuccessful, a volar approach is used and the
interposed volar plate is surgically removed. One must be extremely cautious in
the exposure to prevent neurovascular injury to the radial digital artery and nerve,
which are directly beneath the skin (Fig.
20–27C). Postoperatively, we splint the
metacarpophalangeal joint for three weeks
in a position of moderate flexion. Protected
early motion may be begun after that time.
Late complex dislocations that have been
inadequately treated may require a dorsal
incision to reduce the joint.

Dislocations of the metacarpal bases
at the carpometacarpal joint do occur
and are frequently misdiagnosed. The majority of these injuries are dorsal and involve the mobile fourth and fifth metacarpal
bases, but volar and central metacarpal
dislocations have been reported.[104-106, 111, 112]
A true lateral x-ray of the metacarpal bases
is essential for diagnosis. Although reduction of the dorsal subluxation or dislocation
is usually quite simple by longitudinal
traction and closed manipulation, the degree of ligamentous damage makes these
dislocations quite unstable. Internal fixation with a Kirschner wire is therefore
recommended, followed by immobilization
of the repair for four to six weeks. Recurrent
dorsal subluxation or instability can
seriously compromise grasp because of
persistent pain. When the injury is seen at a
late date, arthrodesis of the affected joints is
the best treatment. Care must be taken to
insure the normal curvature of the transverse metacarpal arch. One complicating
injury that has received recent attention in
the literature is damage to the ulnar nerve
in the rare volar dislocation of the fourth
and fifth metacarpal bases.[104] Open reduction should include exploration of the ulnar
nerve at this level.

THUMB DISLOCATIONS

As a border digit intimately involved in
all phases of hand function, the thumb is
particularly susceptible to dislocation. As in
the fingers, these dislocations may occur at
the inter-phalangeal joint, the metacarpophalangeal joint, or the carpometacarpal
joint. Like distal interphalangeal joint dis-

locations of the fingers, dislocations of the
inter-phalangeal joint of the thumb are
usually dorsal and are usually associated
with an open injury. Unlike the distal joint
finger dislocations, however, in which
avulsion fractures of the extrinsic tendon
insertions are common, the continuity of the
extensor and flexor tendon insertions is
maintained. Reduction is usually easily
accomplished, and the joint is immobilized
in 10 to 15 degrees of flexion for approximately 3 weeks.

Dislocations of the thumb metacarpophalangeal joint may be dorsal, volar, lateral, or
any combination of these. Collateral ligament injury is present in all lateral and volar
dislocations and in many dorsal dislocations. The treatment of this injury is discussed in the section on collateral joint
injuries of the thumb; the reader should
recall that if, after reduction, radial or ulnar
instability of greater than 45 degrees is
demonstrated, operative intervention is
recommended. Pure dorsal dislocations,
however, may not have collateral instability
(Fig. 20–28). The mechanism of injury is
forcible hyperextension, which results in
tearing of the volar plate. The collateral
ligaments may remain intact as the proximal
phalanx slides dorsally, like a visor on a cap,
over the metacarpal head. In one retrospective study, 7 per cent of complete dorsal
dislocations treated with immobilization
alone had residual instability.[60] As in metacarpophalangeal joint dislocations of the
finger, thumb dislocations at this level may
be described as simple or complex, depending on their reducibility.[69] An interposed volar plate, the flexor tendons, and
the intrinsic muscles are the structures that
often make closed relocation difficult. Once
reduced, simple dislocations are treated in a
thumb spica with 15 degrees of flexion at
the metacarpophalangeal joint for 4 weeks.
Complex dislocations are explored through
a midlateral incision centered over the collateral ligament. Once reduced, they are
immobilized as in the simple dislocation.

Pure dislocations of the thumb metacarpal
from the trapezium are rare because of the
strong volar ligamentous support of this
joint. More commonly, one sees a Bennett's
fracture. Dislocation of this joint is always
dorsal; that is, the metacarpal overrides the
saddle of the trapezium dorsally (Fig. 20–

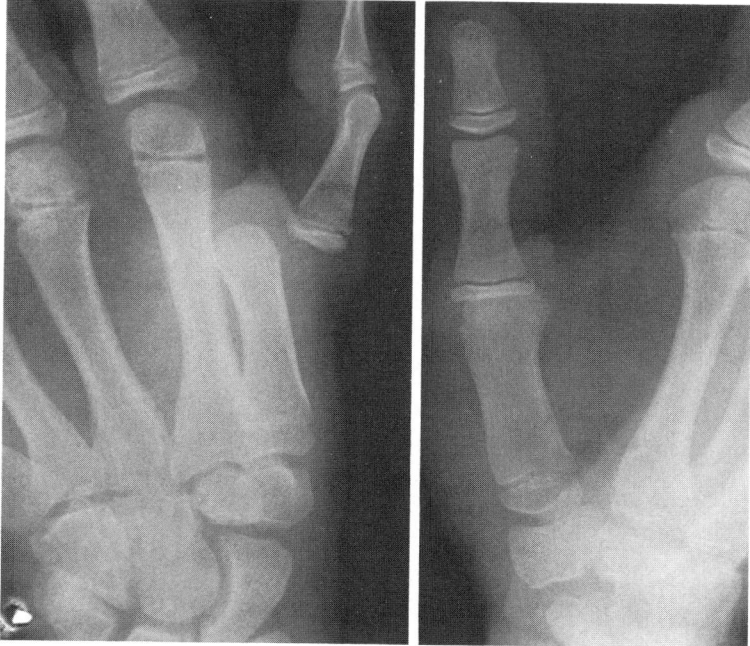

Figure 20–28 Acute dislocation of the metacarpophalangeal joint of the thumb, requiring open reduction and thumb spica fixation in 40 degrees of flexion for 3 weeks.

29). Anatomical reduction is usually readily accomplished and can be maintained by casting the thumb in abduction or by internal fixation.[66] True anteroposterior radiographs of the metacarpophalangeal joint must be obtained to insure the accuracy of reduction. The major problem of this injury, however, is late instability.[64] Eaton and Littler have described an operation for late reconstruction of the volar ligament using a slip of the flexor carpi radialis tendon.[3] If, however, arthritic changes are present either at surgery or on the x-ray, arthroplasty or arthrodesis of the joint is the preferred treatment.

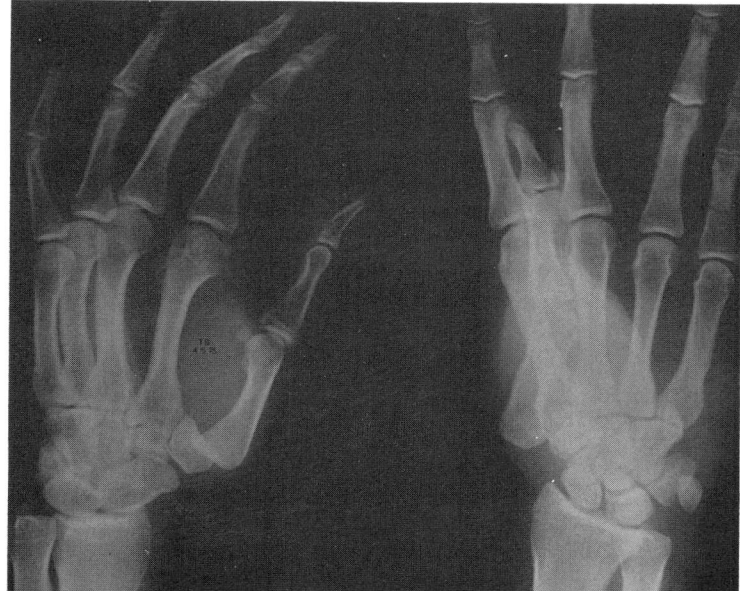

Figure 20–29 Acute dislocation of the carpometacarpal joint of the thumb, treated by closed reduction.

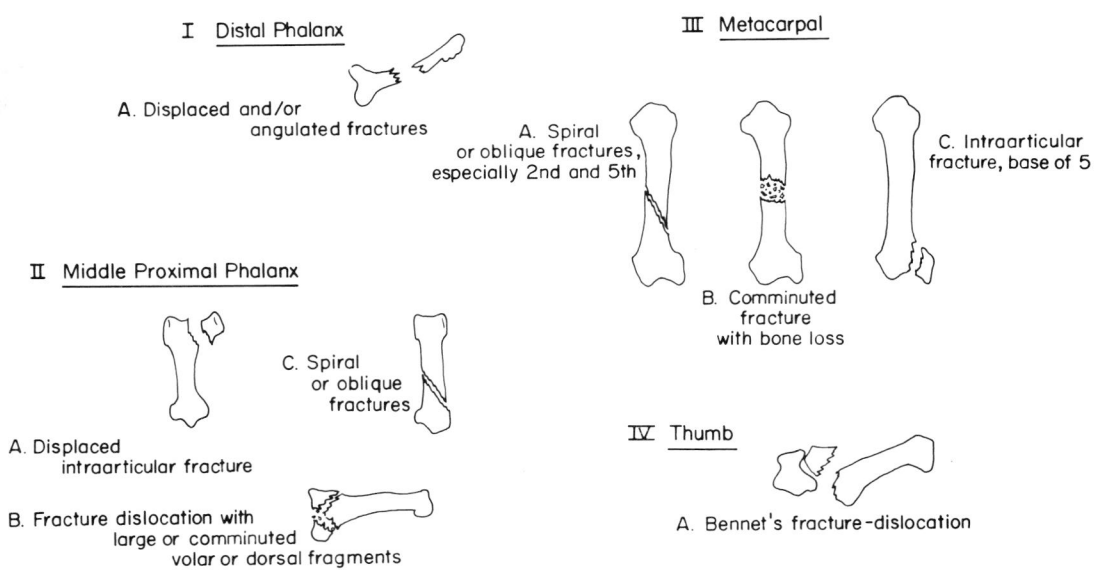

I Distal Phalanx

A. Displaced and/or
   angulated fractures

II Middle Proximal Phalanx

C. Spiral
   or oblique
   fractures

A. Displaced
   intraarticular fracture

B. Fracture dislocation with
   large or comminuted
   volar or dorsal fragments

III Metacarpal

A. Spiral
or oblique fractures,
especially 2nd and 5th

C. Intraarticular
   fracture, base of 5

B. Comminuted
   fracture
   with bone loss

IV Thumb

A. Bennet's fracture-dislocation

Figure 20–30 Classification of unstable fractures.

FRACTURES

Fractures involving the digits of the hand are the most frequent of all fractures. As noted in the initial remarks, treatment of any fracture requires a system of priorities. The whole patient and the complete upper extremity must be considered first. The degree of soft tissue injury and the pathomechanics of the fracture, including its stability, must then be analyzed. During treatment, all motion not interfering with healing should be encouraged, and once fracture healing has occurred, functional rehabilitation is begun. A successful result not only achieves fracture union but also avoids disabling complications, such as stiffness, malunion, and arthritis. Most digital fractures can and should be treated by closed reduction and external immobilization. Our preferred method of external immobilization and the reasons for it have been discussed previously (Fig. 20–10). Several bone and joint injuries of the hand are classified as unstable, in that they do not respond to closed methods of treatment and tend to redisplace or angulate following closed reduction. Figure 20–30 illustrates the injuries that we consider unstable. Specific treatment of these unstable fractures is discussed in the appropriate sections. In

general, however, treatment of these fractures is troublesome and the result often unpredictable. Recognition of the injury as unstable and early referral will often save much frustration.

FRACTURES OF THE DISTAL PHALANX

Fractures of the distal phalanx account for more than half of all hand fractures, the distal portion of the hand being most exposed to injury. There are three types of extraarticular fractures of the distal phalanx. These are longitudinal, transverse, and comminuted. The comminuted type is the most common. It usually involves the distal tuft of the phalanx and is, in general, associated with the greatest amount of soft tissue damage. Significant displacement is rare owing to the fibrous tissue septa radiating from the bone into the soft tissue. Crush injuries are the most common cause, and clinically severe swelling and subungual hematoma formation are usually evident. Acutely, these hematomas can be drained using the tip of a heated paper clip with a resulting marked relief of pain. In most cases, the nail should be left in place, as it acts as a splint for the fracture.

Often there is damage to the nail or a laceration of the nailbed in fractures to the distal phalanx, and its deformity is worrisome to the patient. It is important to remember that the nail root or germinal bed, the source of nail growth, is located at the proximal base of the nail. Damage to this germinal center will result in deformity or even permanent loss of the nail. As the nail grows, it migrates distally across the nailbed proper. Lacerations of the nailbed are common and should be accurately aligned and repaired with 6-0 or finer absorbable suture.[92] Complete re-growth of the nail normally takes four to five months.

Treatment of the closed, nondisplaced distal phalanx fracture requires protection for several weeks. Depending on the soft tissue damage, a volar splint with inclusion of the fingers and wrist is sometimes recommended. Transverse fractures can occur near the base and frequently demonstrate angulation. This angulation is often dorsal because of the profundus tendon insertion flexing the distal fragment. Once reduced, these fractures may best be treated with a smooth Kirschner wire pinning. Similar internal fixation may be needed in open fractures in which there are large fragments with marked displacement (Fig. 20–31). It should be noted that many fractures of the distal phalanx will attain a fibrous rather than a bony union, and radiographic healing may require several months. Also, hypersensitivity and soreness of the tip may persist. In some patients, this may require either sensory retraining or desensitization, as discussed under complications. A final word of caution: One should always check for intraarticular fragments, which suggest either an extensor tendon or a flexor tendon avulsion injury.

Open fracture of the distal phalanx is, as mentioned, often associated with skin loss and should be regarded as a complicated soft tissue injury. These fingertip avulsions

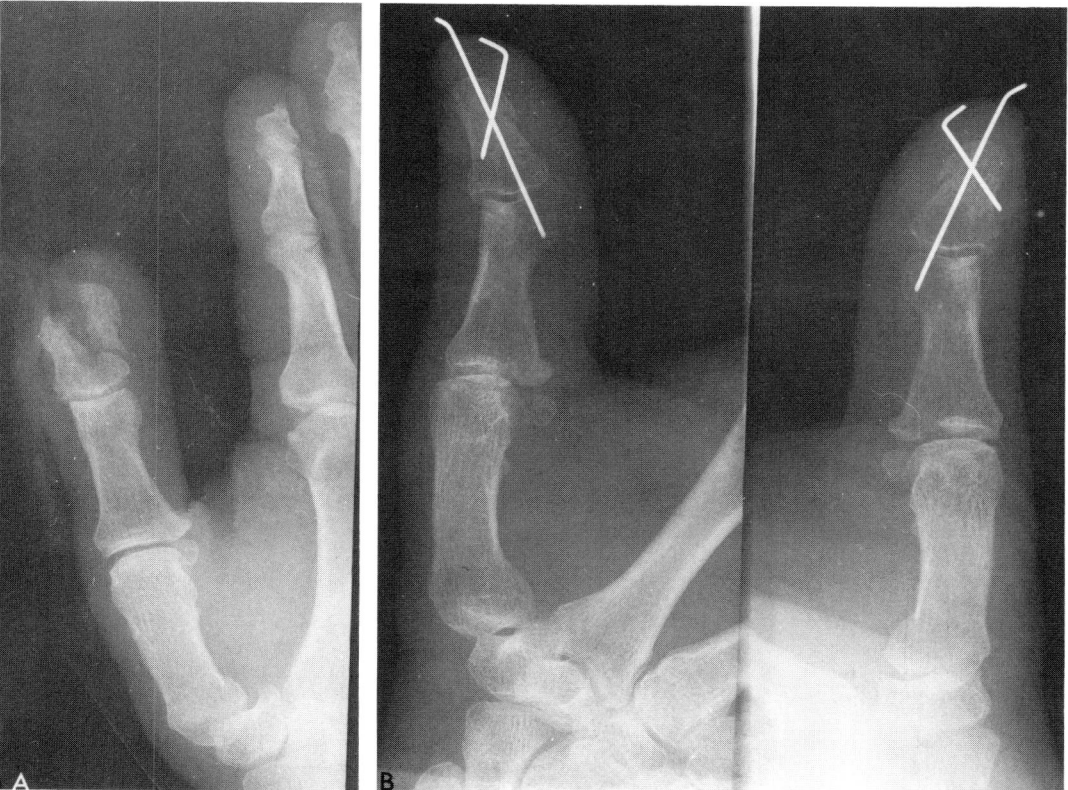

Figure 20–31 *A.* Open displaced fracture of the distal phalanx of the thumb. *B.* Satisfactory healing after open reduction with pin fixation one month postinjury.

distal to the DIP joint are as common as the car door and the kitchen knife and, if treated incorrectly, can result in severe disability. The goal is to maintain digital length and provide bone coverage with nontender, well-padded skin that has good sensation. It is not surprising that many techniques have been proposed for the care of this injury. They are listed in Table 20–2 and range from benign neglect to microvascular replantation. No one method is universally acceptable. We agree with those who argue for the individualization of these injuries. The personal profile of the patient, the physical characteristics of the wound, and the time interval from injury together with the surgeon's expertise are involved in any therapeutic decision. The pros and cons of each method are listed in Table 20–2.

FRACTURES OF THE MIDDLE PHALANX

Fractures of the middle phalanx occur less frequently than those of the proximal phalanx, but their mechanisms of injury are similar, as are their usual anatomical levels of injury. Similar principles of treatment are thus applicable; these will be discussed under Fractures of the Proximal Phalanx.

One major difference, however, is the extensive sublimis tendon insertion to the base and volar shaft area of the middle phalanx. Thus, minimal angulation and displacement will occur with fractures through the region of this sublimis insertion. For these nondisplaced fractures, simpler methods, such as buddy taping[50] or casting for three weeks, may apply. However, fractures outside the sublimis insertion, such as those through the volar cortex at the base, may angulate dorsally or those at the neck may angulate in a volar direction (Fig. 20–32A). The overall collapsing forces of the more distally inserted flexor profundus and the extensor hood tend to produce overriding of these unstable fractures. Once reduced, they are best treated by internal fixation (Fig. 20–32B). Intracondylar fractures are also potentially unstable,

TABLE 20–2   Fingertip Injuries with Skin Loss

Procedure	Advantages	Disadvantages
Benign Neglect Nonadherent dressing coverage	Only in children	Slow healing, 4–12 weeks Excessive granulation Tender scar
Shortening Bone and soft tissue for closure Usually removal of nail matrix Keep scar dorsal	Simple	Loss of length and cosmesis Hypersensitivity

Free Graft Coverage
Split or full-thickness
The thinner the graft, the more rapid the take
Thin split over exposed bone but not over
   volar plate
	Simple
	Good if soft tissue bed is
	   adequate
		Donor site needed
		Hypersensitivity

Local Flaps, Same Finger Bilateral V-Y (Kutler) Single V-Y flap (Atasoy) Volar flap advancement Rotational flap	Best if bone and soft tissue are of equal length	Tip scarring Hypersensitivity
Hand Pedicle Flaps Palmar pedicle, thenar flap Cross finger pedicle Neurovascular island pedicle	Sensation and pulp restored	Joint stiffness Second procedure Donor site numbness

Remote Pedicle Flaps
Abdominal, iliac, pectoral, cross arm
	Only in extreme cases with
	   multiple and large areas
	   of tissue loss
		Donor site
		Second procedure

Replantation
Possibly for thumb
	Limited value for injuries
	   distal to DIP joint
		Microvascular surgery
		   needed

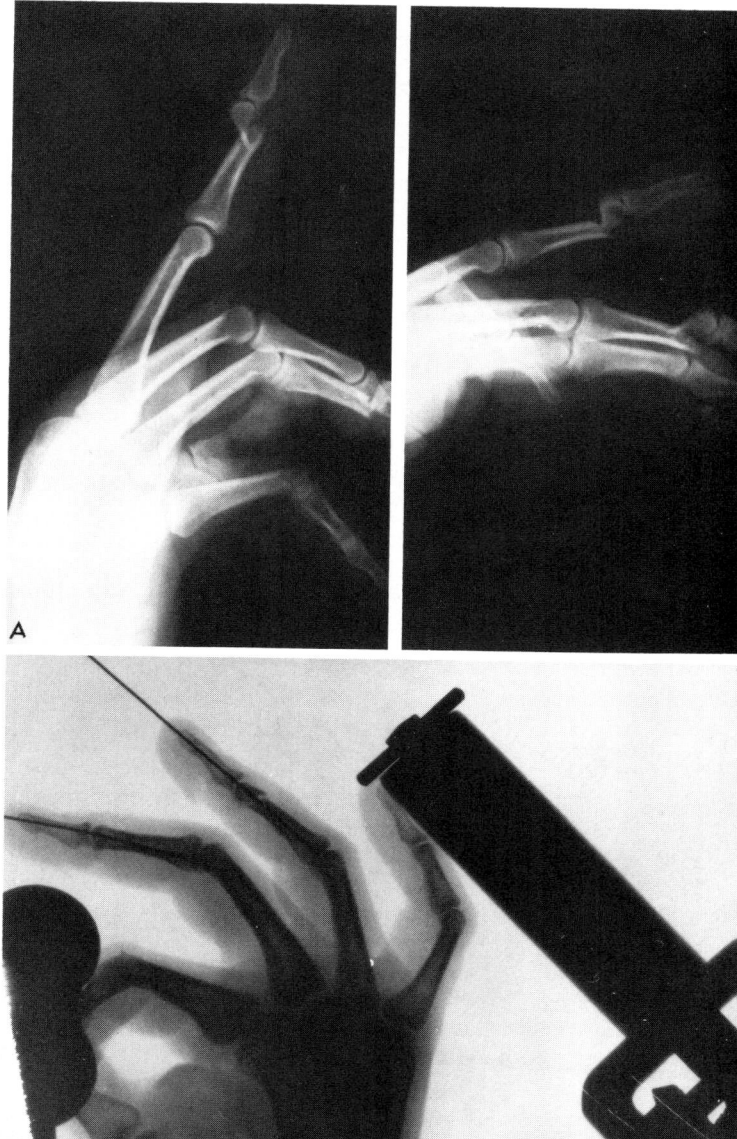

Figure 20–32 *A.* Displaced fractures of the neck of the middle phalanges in the long and ring fingers in the same patient. *B.* Treatment by open reduction with pin fixation.

as are those of the proximal phalanx, and may require internal fixation. Lastly, it is important to recognize the intraarticular fractures of the base of the middle phalanx, such as those associated with central slip avulsion and volar plate injury. As mentioned previously, large fragments (greater than 30 per cent) or those associated with dislocation require anatomical reduction and often internal fixation. Severe comminution of an intraarticular fracture may not be amenable to internal fixation and may best be treated by early guarded motion.

FRACTURES OF THE PROXIMAL PHALANX

Fractures of the proximal phalanx are common digital injuries. Shortening, angulation, and rotation are the major deformities that must be corrected. The four common types of fractures of the proximal phalanges are at the level of the neck, shaft, base, and condyles (Fig. 20–33). Although there are no large tendon insertions on the proximal phalanx, the collapsing force of the more distally inserted tendons is even greater there than in the middle phalanges.

NECK

SHAFT

BASE

CONDYLE

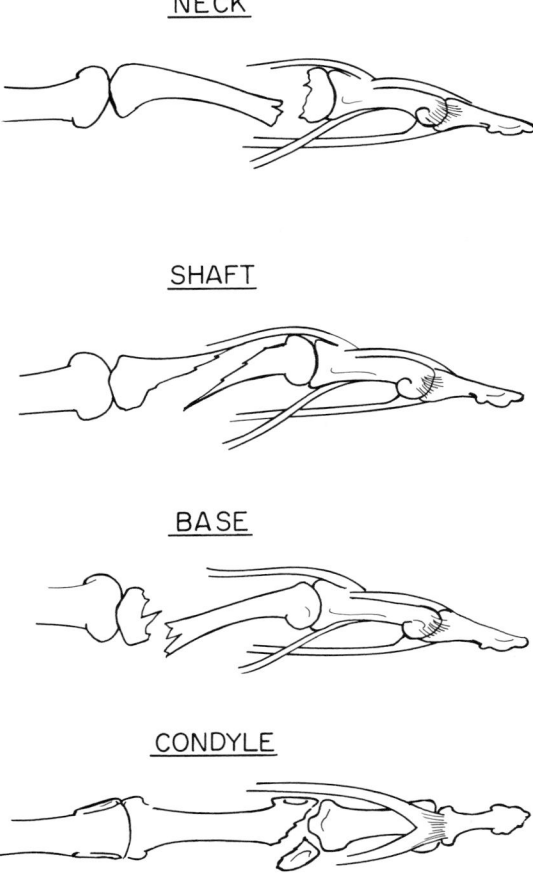

Figure 20–33　Four common types of fracture of the middle and proximal phalanx.

Hence, there is a greater tendency toward displacement. Also, the closeness of the flexor and extensor tendons to the bone increases the risk of subsequent tendon adherence and restriction of motion of both interphalangeal joints. Extraarticular fractures at the base and neck are usually transverse, while fractures of the shaft are either oblique or transverse, depending on the direction and magnitude of the injuring force. Direct or shear forces tend to produce transverse fractures, while rotatory forces produce oblique and spiral fractures. The location and amount of force creating the fracture determine the resultant deformity.

Extraarticular fractures of the base of the proximal phalanx are the most common epiphyseal injuries in children. They often present with lateral or volar angulation. A rotatory component may also be present.

Fractures in this area account for approximately 25 per cent of all proximal phalanx fractures and are most frequent in the small and ring digits. Reduction of these fractures is usually easily obtainable and can be maintained by metacarpal joint flexion of 70 degrees. As noted by Mansoor and others,[87, 96] many of these fractures are impacted and hence stable. In young children, significant angulation of the volar dorsal plane may be accepted, as motion in the plane of the joint will correct with time. In adults or older children, angulation of more than 20 degrees should not be accepted, as it results in loss of both flexion and extension at the proximal interphalangeal joint. Lateral angulation of up to 15 degrees can be accepted. As mentioned, such fractures of the proximal phalanx should be immobilized with the wrist in 30 degrees of extension, the metacarpophalangeal joint flexed to 70 degrees, and the proximal interphalangeal joints slightly flexed, as noted in Figure 20–11.

Such immobilization will also help to control the rotatory deformities that are often seen with such proximal fractures and may cause disability to the patient. It is important to remember in all hand fractures, whether proximal phalanx, middle phalanx, or metacarpal, that rotation significant enough to cause finger overlap is not readily visible on an x-ray or by inspection when the fingers are extended. The deformity becomes obvious only when the fingers are flexed. The plane of the fingernails may give some indication of the deformity, but the easiest way to observe it is with finger flexion. As stated, metacarpophalangeal joint flexion helps prevent the overlap that might complicate such injuries.

Fractures of the shaft represent about 50 per cent of fractures of the proximal phalanx. They are basically of two types: the long oblique spiral and the transverse midshaft fracture (Fig. 20–34). Because of the tendon forces, the oblique fracture tends to shorten as well as rotate. If such shortening is less than 3 mm[80] external immobilization and frequent follow-up may be indicated. However, given the potential instability of these fractures, we favor internal fixation. Furthermore, anatomical reduction may produce less callus to interfere with the adjacent tendons. The Swiss AO group has a small screw-and-plate set, but we prefer

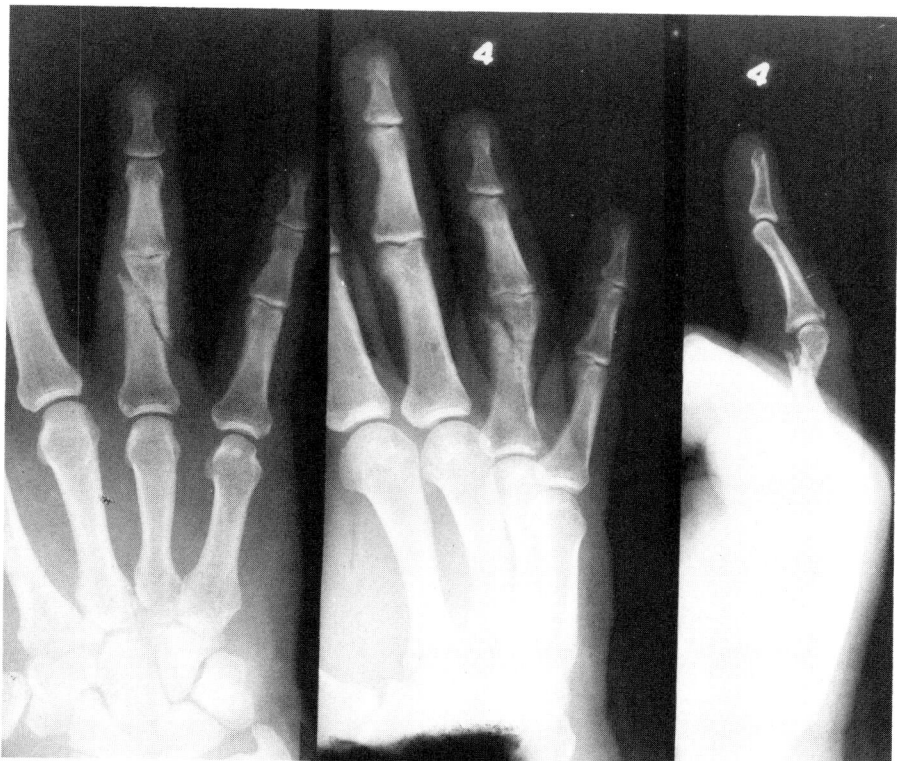

Figure 20-34   Oblique fracture of the proximal phalanx.

pinning with a Kirschner wire placed at 90 degrees to the fracture site as the most versatile means of fixing these fractures (Fig. 20–35).[78, 82] If the fracture is undisplaced, this fixation is done percutaneously. If open reduction is required, the approach is through a longitudinal tendon-splitting exposure. The other type of shaft fracture is the transverse fracture, which usually presents with volar angulation. The proximal fragment is usually flexed, while the distal fragment tends to hyperextend. This produces an extensor lag at the PIP joint. Further buckling is produced by the overpull of the extrinsic flexor system. These fractures are usually easy to reduce and, once reduced, stable. Hence, they can be mobilized in our position of functional bandaging. Severely comminuted fractures, however, are unstable and may require percutaneous pinning.

A third type of extraarticular fracture is the distal transverse fracture just proximal to the PIP joint. As in the middle phalanx, such fractures are usually associated with volar angulation at the fracture site. Reduc-

tion is usually feasible, but marked flexion of the PIP joint is required to maintain stability. Since the PIP joint tolerates such immobilization poorly, internal fixation may be recommended so that early guarded motion may be begun. Accurate reduction is important, because with dorsal angulation greater than 15 degrees the proximal fragment may impinge on PIP flexion as a volar bony block.

The most common intraarticular fractures, those associated with ligamentous or tendinous damage, have been discussed previously. Condylar fractures occur at the head of the metacarpal, proximal, or middle phalanx and are intraarticular. They represent about 5 per cent of proximal phalangeal fractures. All but the undisplaced are associated with angular deformity. When angulation occurs, the phalanx distal to the fracture deviates in the direction in which its bony support has been lost. The mechanism of injury is most commonly indirect trauma or lateral movement of the base of the phalanx, which impacts the condyle of the more proximal bone. Anatomical reduc-

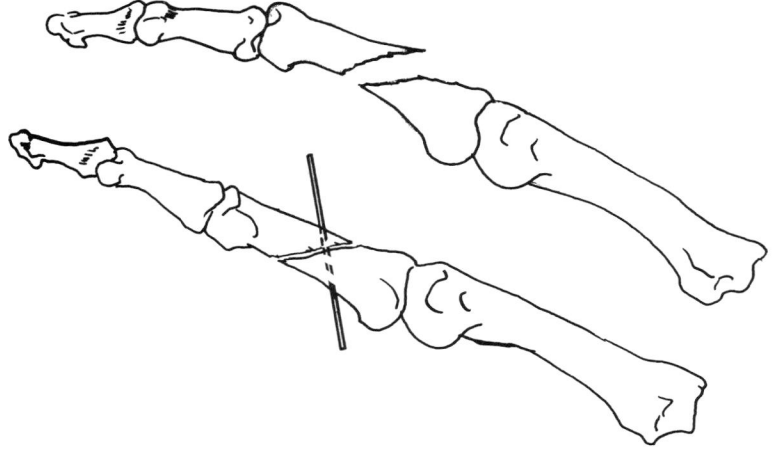

Figure 20–35 Drawing of closed reduction with pin fixation of the oblique fracture.

tion is essential, and thus internal fixation is recommended. In undisplaced fractures this is done percutaneously, while open reduction is reserved for displaced fractures. Again, a dorsal exposure is most commonly used. Once good fixation is obtained, early motion is begun.

In our series of phalangeal fractures, about 75 per cent can easily be treated with external immobilization in the position of functional bandaging, as described. The average time of immobilization is three weeks, though it may be longer with open or comminuted fractures. Unstable fractures are treated with internal fixation which, in our hands, is usually Kirschner wire fixation. For the sake of completeness, the use of traction in treating such fractures must be mentioned. Numerous methods, such as skeletal, fingernail, pulp, or skin traction, have been advocated.[5] In some hands, traction may produce effective results, but we feel its general use is not indicated.

FRACTURES OF THE METACARPAL EXCLUSIVE OF THE THUMB

For fractures of the finger metacarpals, the general principles associated with phalangeal fractures apply. Consequently, fractures of the metacarpal are best classified according to their anatomical location as those of the head, neck, shaft, or base. Several anatomical points should be borne in mind. The metacarpals have a gentle dorsal curve and thus contribute to the

longitudinal arch of the hand (Fig. 20–2). Their bases are involved in the proximal transverse arch, while their heads are involved in the distal transverse arch. The intrinsic muscles of the hand originate on the shaft of the metacarpals. The index and long finger metacarpals are part of the fixed unit of the hand; they therefore lack the mobility to accommodate to malunion that is seen in the ulnar digits. Given the intervening soft tissue and the tethering effect of the deep transverse metacarpal ligament connecting their heads, metacarpal fractures present less displacement than those of the phalanges.

Fractures of the head are distal to the origin of the collateral ligament and are usually the result of crush or missile injuries. They are often open injuries with marked comminution. They also may be seen as the extension of either shaft or neck fractures. If several large fragments are present, an attempt at open reduction and internal fixation may be made. More commonly, however, the metacarpal head is so shattered that any attempt at fixation is as successful as nailing scrambled eggs to the wall. These injuries are best treated with early motion beginning at one to two weeks or at the first indication of joint stiffness. If the fracture is seen late, and limitation of motion or pain predominants, arthroplasty is the treatment of choice.

Fractures of the neck are the most common metacarpal injury and are the result of striking an unyielding object, usually in an altercation. For this reason they have been named "boxer" fractures and are most commonly seen in the small and ring metacarpals. However, as Brown[71] has pointed out, professional boxers most frequently fracture the long, index, or thumb metacarpal, which is a more direct extension of their thrusting forces. Classically, the injuring force is parallel to the long axis of the metacarpal; the fractures are usually transverse, with comminution of the volar cortex and volar angulation. The latter results from overpull of the interossei and the bowstringing effect of the flexor tendons. The patient presents with a shortened, angular deformity. In addition, the normal knuckle contour is lost when the fist is clenched, and there is swelling and pain on digital pressure at the injury site. As discussed in the general care section, any clenched fist injury associated with an open wound should be considered grossly contaminated by the opponent's oral flora. It is well to remember that many patients presenting with this fracture will be embarrassed to volunteer the true mechanism of injury and the treating physican should have a high index of suspicion.

As in most common fractures, numerous approaches to treatment have been advocated, running the gamut from "grin and bear it" to open reduction and internal fixation.[103] We would agree with most authors, who feel that the majority of these injuries can be treated closed in a simple short arm splint or cast. In one study of a compensation population, Hunter[105] found little disability associated with such fractures, even when significant volar angulation was present. The problem of a painful palmar lump, which represents the displaced metacarpal head, and consequent limitation of power grip did not materialize in his study. The amount of acceptable volar angulation varies with the metacarpal head involved. As mentioned earlier, fractures of the index and long metacarpals, because of their intimate relation to the fixed unit of the hand and their lack of mobility, tolerate a lesser degree of volar angulation. The ring finger metacarpal has moderate mobility and can accommodate as much as 20 degrees of angulation, but greater deformity requires reduction and cast or pin fixation. The small finger metacarpal is the most mobile digital metacarpal and can adjust to a fracture with 30 to 40 degrees of angula-

tion (Fig. 20–36). A fracture with greater than 40 degrees of angulation or any fracture with a significant rotatory deformity causing small finger overlap or ulnar spread must be reduced and fixed with a cast or pin, or rotatory deformity may persist (Fig. 20–37).

When reduction is required, we prefer the method introduced by Jahss, the so-called 90–90 method.[106] Following local or block anesthesia, the MCP joint is flexed as much as possible, and the PIP joint of the same finger is flexed to 90 degrees. While the collateral ligaments of the MCP joint are holding the displaced head in this position, proximal pressure is placed at the PIP joint with simultaneous counterpressure placed against the metacarpal shaft. Immediate reduction is usually satisfactory, but given the amount of volar comminution, reangulation of the distal metacarpal fragment is common. For this reason, Jahss advocated immobilizing the proximal phalanx in 90 degrees at the PIP joint, thus using it to maintain the reduction. This

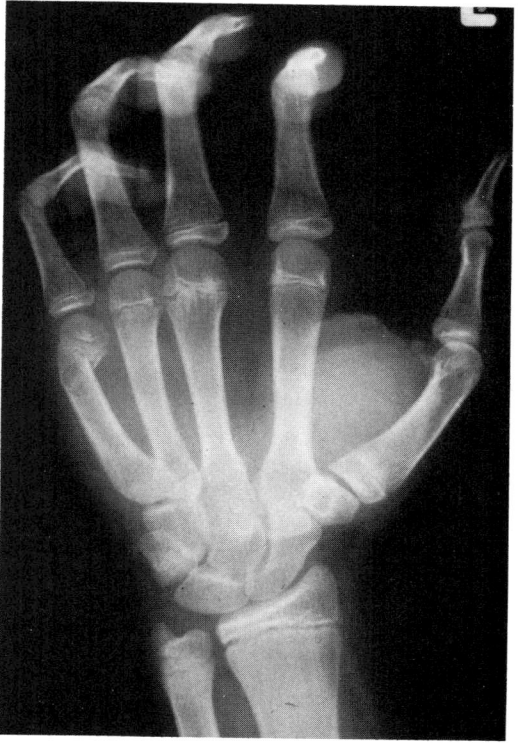

Figure 20–36 Boxer's fractures with minimal rotation and angulation, treated satisfactorily with a volar splint.

MALROTATION BOXER'S FRACTURE

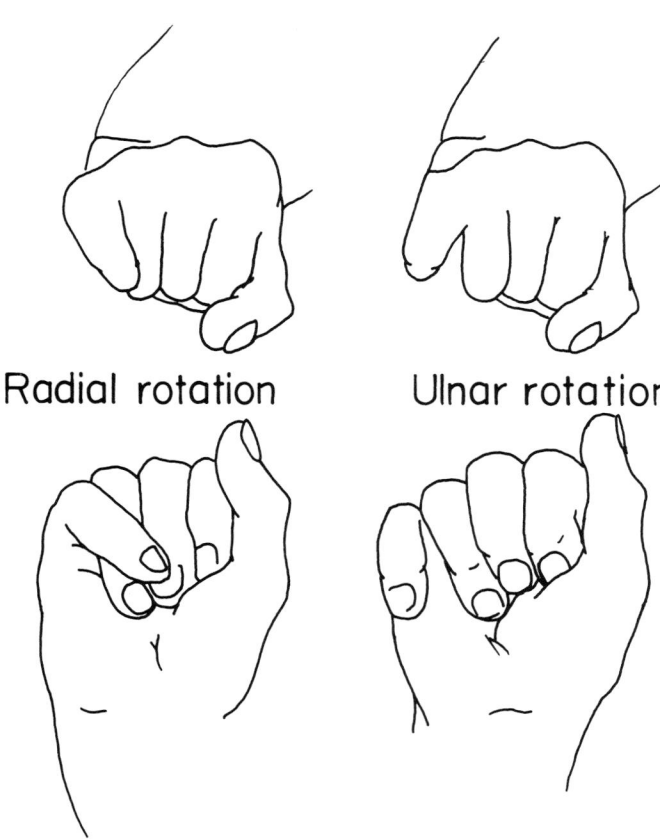

Radial rotation   Ulnar rotation

Figure 20–37 Boxer's fractures with malrotation. Angulation and rotation cause either radial overlap or ulnar spread.

method should be discouraged, as it causes significant PIP stiffness as well as pressure problems over the dorsal skin of the PIP joint. Both the involved finger and the adjacent finger are immobilized in our standard position of rehabilitation for a period of usually three to four weeks. If unacceptable angulation recurs, reduction arc pin fixation is recommended. Unless there is significant disruption of metacarpophalangeal joint motion, fractures seen later than two weeks are best treated by benign neglect.

Fractures of the metacarpal shaft are usually transverse or oblique. Transverse fractures occur with direct trauma or sudden forcible angulation. Oblique fractures result from a torque force applied to the finger as a distal lever. Transverse fractures tend to angulate dorsally owing to the action of the intrinsic muscles pointing across the fracture site. Again, the common presentation is that of a palpable angulatory deformity with

pain and soft tissue swelling over the involved metacarpal. Depending on the amount of angular deformity there is some loss of contour of the knuckle, but not as much as is seen with metacarpal neck fractures. Oblique fractures of the shaft of metacarpals tend not to angulate, but rather to shorten and rotate. The long and ring metacarpals shorten least because of the tethering effect of the deep transverse metacarpal ligament. The index and small finger metacarpals are stabilized unilaterally, so the degree of shortening and malrotation is more severe. Most of these fractures can be treated closed for a period of four to five weeks in our standard shortarm cast. It is often wise to internally stabilize fractures of the index finger, because of its importance in hand function (Fig. 20–38), and also short oblique fractures of the other metacarpals. This is mandatory if there is any rotatory deformity.

As discussed in the introductory section,

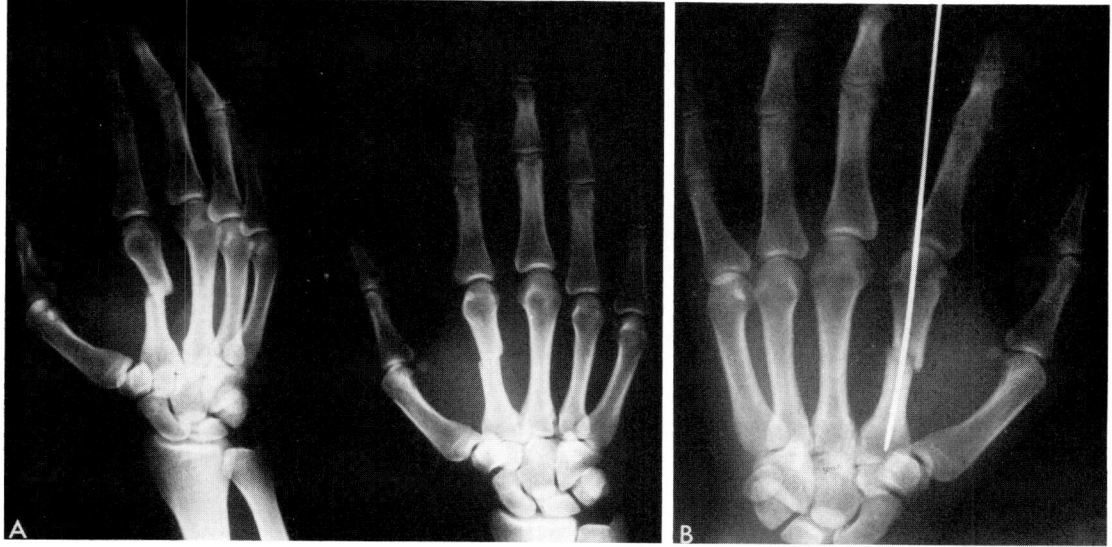

Figure 20–38 A. Transverse displaced fracture of the shaft of the index metacarpal. B. Closed anteroposterior reduction and pinning.

some metacarpal shaft fractures are associated with severe comminution or significant bony loss. These are most commonly the result of explosive bullet injuries or severe crushing forces. Soft tissue injury is severe. The inherent instability of such a metacarpal fracture requires internal fixation. This is usually done by cross pinning to an adjacent metacarpal, by using Kirschner wire spacers as recommended by Brown, or by using a Hoffmann apparatus. While the soft tissue wounds heal, tissue relationships of the hand are maintained, and bone grafting can be performed at a later date.

Fractures of the base of the metacarpals, with the exception of the thumb and little finger, are typically the result of crush injuries. They are often impacted and, given their firm ligamentous attachments proximally, tend to be quite stable. A true lateral x-ray of the base of the metacarpal or oblique x-rays of the metacarpal may be needed to diagnose this injury. These x-ray views are mandatory when clinical suspicion is aroused by swelling and point tenderness at the base of the metacarpals. As noted previously, dislocations are often associated with these fractures, and such dislocations, owing to their disruption of this ligamentous support, are unstable and require internal fixation.

Fractures of the base of the fifth metacarpal are special cases. The stability of the carpometacarpal joint of the little finger depends on the articular surfaces of the bones and on the ligaments and muscles attached to them. The bones involved are the hamate, the base of the metacarpal of the little finger, and the base of the metacarpal of the ring finger. The hypothenar muscles also contribute to the stability and motion of this joint. The extensor carpi ulnaris tendon inserts at the dorsoulnar aspect of the base of the little finger metacarpal and may cause ulnar and proximal displacement of the metacarpal following an injury to the stabilizing structures of the joint; this injury simulates Bennett's fracture (Fig. 20–39). The fifth metacarpal has a wide range of motion at the carpometacarpal joint articulation, averaging 30 degrees of flexion-extension. Rotatory movements, which contribute to the normal cupping of the palm in grasp and in opposition of the small finger to the thumb, are also present. The mobile hypothenar unit rotates toward the rest of the hand, and an injury resulting in the dislocation of the metacarpal over the hamate compromises the metacarpohamate motion and therefore weakens power of grip.

A force transmitted along the longitudinal axis of the metacarpal or applied directly over the metacarpohamate joint causes the injury. The degree of displacement of the metacarpal is determined by the magnitude and angle of the force causing the injury.

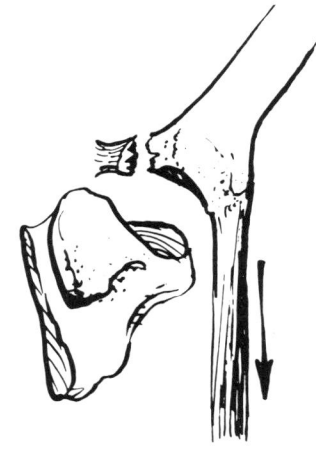

Figure 20-39 Fracture-dislocation of the carpometacarpal joint of the small finger metacarpal simulates Bennett's fracture.

The actions of the extensor carpi ulnaris and the hypothenar muscles contribute to the deformity (Fig. 20-40). The carpometacarpal joint of the little finger is obscured in routine roentgenograms by overlap of the hamate on the base of the metacarpal of the little finger. As a result, undisplaced fractures as well as fractures with dislocation may easily be overlooked. A clear profile of the articular surfaces of the metacarpal and the hamate and the relationship of these two bones will be seen on a roentgenogram taken with the forearm pronated 30 degrees from the routine anteroposterior position.

Patients with an injury to the carpometacarpal joint of the little finger comprise three groups.[100] Group 1 patients have an intraarticular fracture of the metacarpal without displacement. In group 2, there is an intraarticular fracture with minimum ulnar displacement of the fifth metacarpal, but the articular surfaces of the bones remain engaged. Group 3 patients have an acute fracture with dislocation.

The method of treatment is similar for groups 1 and 2: a molded cast or plaster splint is applied for four weeks without manipulation. Patients in group 3, in whom the joint surfaces are not in apposition, require open operation and pin fixations (Fig. 20-41). A cast is applied for five weeks, after which time the pins are removed.

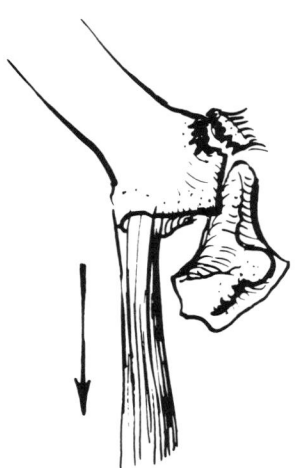

Direction of pull by Hypothenar muscles

Direction of pull by Extensor carpi ulnaris

Figure 20-40 The hypothenar muscles and the extensor carpi ulnaris pull, producing the deformity after fracture of the basal joint of the small finger metacarpal.

FRACTURES OF THE THUMB METACARPAL

The thumb is essential to hand function, as it participates in every hand activity. Its unique ability depends upon free movement at the carpometacarpal joint. It is this saddle joint that allows the arcs of abduction-adduction, flexion-extension, and opposition. It is thus important to divide fractures of the base of the first metacarpal into those that involve this joint and those that are extraarticular.

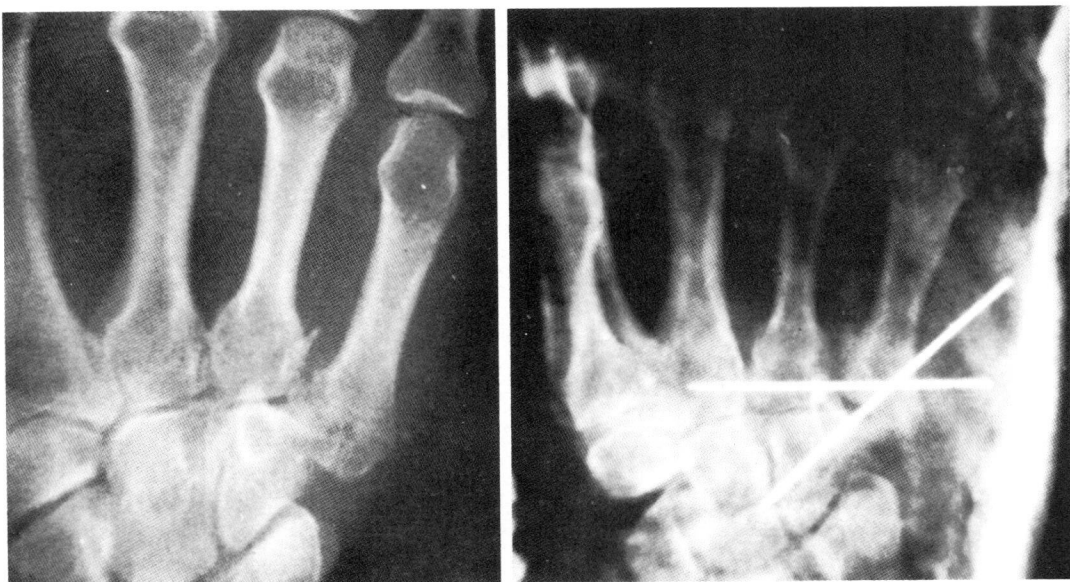

Figure 20–41   On the left, an old displaced fracture of the carpometacarpal joint of the small finger metacarpal. On the right, open reduction and pin fixation of the injury.

Extraarticular fractures of the thumb metacarpal (Fig. 20–42A) are usually caused by a direct blow.[115] The complex deforming forces in these fractures involve the abductor pollicis longus abducting the proximal fragment while the distal fragment is adducted by the thenar musculature and supinated by the extrinsic extensors. Angulation of less than 35 degrees is well tolerated because of the mobility of the basal joint, but greater deformity may require pin fixation. Following reduction the metacarpal should be placed in radial abduction.

In 1882, Bennett described the intraarticular fracture-dislocation of the base of the first metacarpal that bears his name.[111] The mechanism of injury is usually actual compression with the metacarpal partially flexed. In reality, this is an avulsion fracture in which the volar ulnar lip of the trapezium remains in its normal anatomical relationship to the greater multangular, while the metacarpal shaft and the dorsal radial articular surface are displaced by the abductor pollicis longus. The clinical deformity may be indistinguishable from that of a shaft fracture. Three types have been described (Fig. 20–42B and C).

Type 1 Bennett's fracture is a dislocation of the metacarpal and the greater multangular with a wafer of bone attached to the ulnar carpometacarpal ligament. The injury requires open reduction and pin fixation of the metacarpal to the greater multangular.[112] Repair of the ulnar carpometacarpal ligament is also necessary. We follow the techniques originally described by Moberg and Gedda.[113] Type 2 Bennett's fracture is a dislocation of the metacarpal to the radial side of the greater multangular with a large piece of bone attached to the ulnar carpometacarpal ligament. This can usually be treated by closed reduction and percutaneous pinning between the metacarpal and greater multangular. An image intensifier is helpful in this procedure. If the ulnar fragment at the base of the metacarpal cannot be aligned to the metacarpal with closed reduction, open reduction with pin or wire fixation between the metacarpal fragments may be necessary.

It should be noted that in the treatment of both types of Bennett's fractures there are those who recommend benign neglect or who feel that casting alone may provide functional results.[118] More frequently, the natural history of an untreated or missed Bennett's fracture-dislocation is one of progressive traumatic arthritis, increasing pain, and diminished pinch strength. Type 3 Bennett's fracture (Fig. 20–42D), originally described by Silvio Rolando[117] in 1910, is a comminuted intraarticular metacarpal base

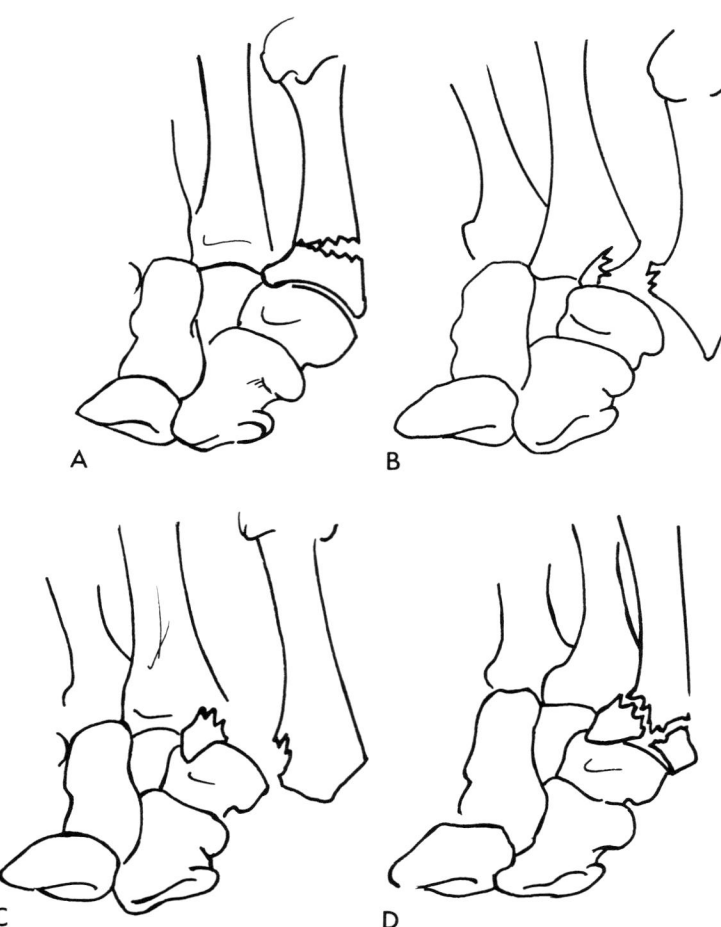

Figure 20–42 *A.* Fracture of the base of the shaft of the thumb metacarpal, not including the joint. *B.* Bennett's fracture with a wafer of bone attached to the ulnar carpometacarpal ligament. *C.* Bennett's fracture with a moderate-sized bone fragment attached to the ulnar carpometacarpal ligament. *D.* Rolando fracture — comminuted intraarticular fracture of the basal joint of the thumb.

fracture. These fractures differ from the classic Bennett's fracture, which were described by him as having major Y or T components; more often the shattering is so complete that internal fixation is impossible. Attempts at open reduction are unduly meddlesome; our treatment is a thumb spica for four weeks followed by active motion exercises.

For the Bennett's fracture-dislocation seen late (after three weeks) the treatment is tailored to the degree of pain, weakness of pinch, and the degree of joint instability. Arthroplasty or arthrodesis is the treatment of choice if arthritic joint changes are present.

HAND FRACTURES IN CHILDREN

Most pediatric orthopedic texts state that hand fractures are uncommon in children,

and several statistical analyses have tended to confirm an incidence of between 7 and 10 per cent.[124] Leonard and Dubravcik were able to collect 276 fractures over a 10-year period in a general orthopedic practice.[125] This represented 0.5 per cent of all their diagnoses. A prospective two-year study was made of hand fractures seen in children at the Children's Hospital of Philadelphia. Tuft fractures were excluded. The study included 268 consecutive hand fractures, which represented 21 per cent of all fractures seen during that time. The hand fracture was by far the most common pediatric fracture, surpassing fractures of the distal forearm (14 per cent) and the tibia and ankle (12 per cent).

Over 70 per cent of these injuries were epiphyseal fractures. The proper treatment of this injury requires knowledge of the pathological anatomy, the physiological process of healing, and the proper hand

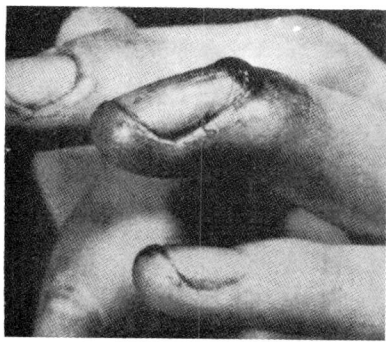
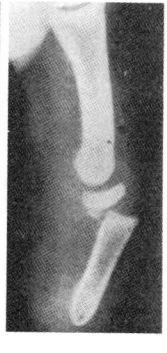

Figure 20-43 Epiphyseal fracture of the distal phalanx simulating a mallet finger. (Courtesy of N. Seymour and the *Journal of Bone and Joint Surgery.* J. Bone Joint Surg., *48B*:348, 1966.)

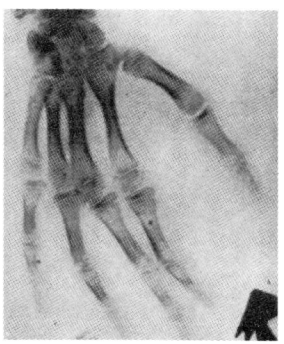
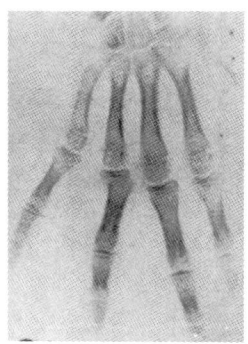

Figure 20-44 Simple closed epiphyseal fracture. (Courtesy of F. W. Bora, Jr., M.D., Nissenbaum, M.D., and P. Ignatius, M.D., and *Orthopedics Digest.* Orthop. Dig., *11*:11, 1976.)

position for bony alignment during the postreduction period. An epiphysis is located at the proximal end of each phalanx. Metacarpal epiphyses are distal except for the thumb, which is proximal. All of the epiphyses in the hand are of the primary or pressure type, contributing to longitudinal bone growth.

Classically, the epiphyseal plate is divided into several layers: the zone of resting cartilage cells; the zone of proliferating cells; and the zone of cell columns, which can be subdivided into the hypertrophic cell zone and the zone of provisional calcification. Specific biochemical processes occur in each zone. As described in

Salter and Harris'[126] classic work on injuries to the epiphyseal plate, fractures through the plate were originally believed to go through the juncture of the hypertrophic cell zone and the zone of provisional calcification. More recent work by Bright[121] and others has shown, however, that most fractures follow an undulating course, going through all zones. Despite this, the majority of these fractures rarely involve the cellular layer of growth, and little disturbance of growth should be expected. Epiphyseal fractures are common injuries in the growing end, because the joint ligaments and tendons and their attachments to bone are stronger than the epiphyseal plate.

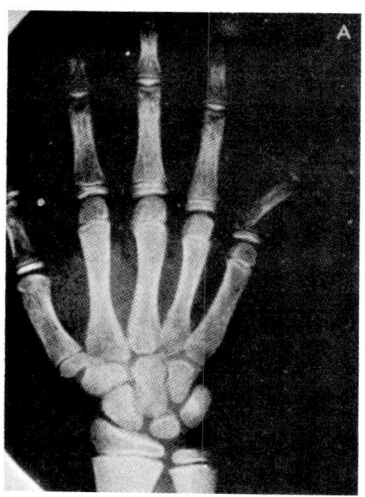
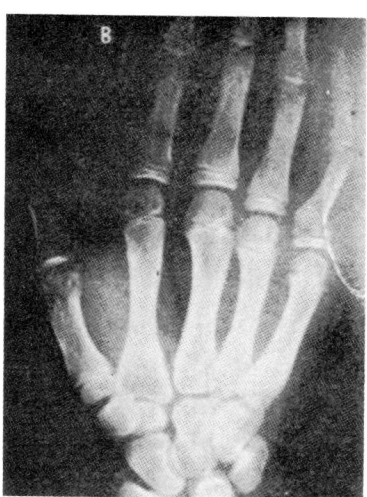
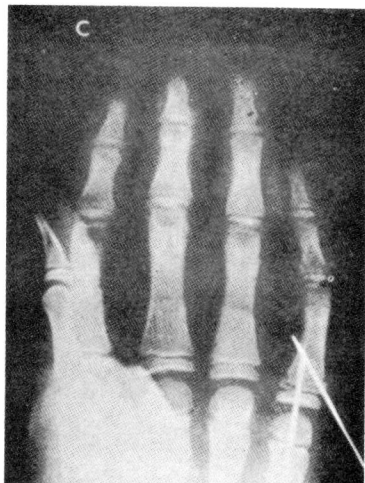

Figure 20-45 Closed, displaced epiphyseal fracture requiring closed reduction and percutaneous pinning. (Courtesy of F. W. Bora Jr., M.D., M. Nissenbaum, M.D., and P. Ignatius, M.D., and *Orthopedics Digest.* Orthop. Dig., *11*:11, 1976.)

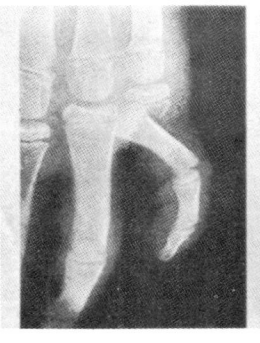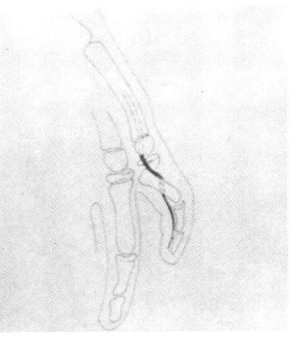

Figure 20–46 Open epiphyseal fracture with soft tissue interposition between the fragments. Open reduction with pin fixation was required. (Courtesy of F. W. Bora, Jr., M.D., M. Nissenbaum, M.D., and P. Ignatius, M.D., and *Orthopedics Digest*. Orthop. Dig., *11*:11, 1976.)

Some specific injuries should be mentioned. The mallet finger of children represents not a loss of extensor tendon continuity, but rather an epiphyseal fracture (Fig. 20–43). The extensor tendon attaches on the epiphysis, while the flexor profundus inserts on the metaphysis, thus forceful flexion causes a Salter type 2 fracture. It is treated by immobilization in extension for four weeks. Eighty per cent of epiphyseal injuries in children occur at the base of the proximal phalanx and are Salter type 2 in nature. As shown in Figure 20–44, the majority are easily reduced without anesthesia and immobilized in the position of rehabilitation for a period of three weeks.

Proximal phalanx fractures of the small finger may show marked ulnar angulation and have been fondly termed the extra-octave fracture. An initial attempt at gentle reduction over a pencil placed in the web space should be tried. Often, however, the reduction is unstable, and percutaneous pin fixation is required to prevent reangulation (Fig. 20–45). In rare instances, such a fracture may be completely irreducible, and open reduction and pin fixation are necessary (Fig. 20–46). In this injury the flexor tendons are interposed between the fragments, preventing reduction.

The base of the proximal phalanx and the base of the metacarpal are common sites of epiphyseal fractures of the thumb. A closed injury at the metacarpophalangeal joint level, resulting in ulnar or radial instability of the proximal phalanx on the metacarpal,

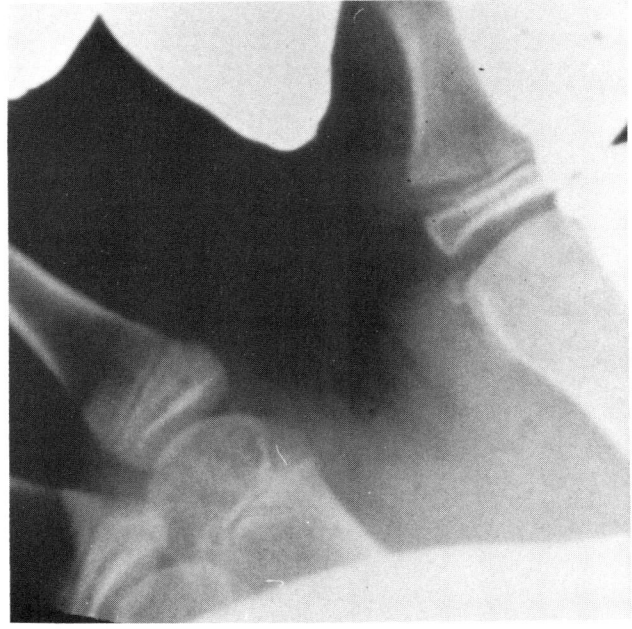

Figure 20–47 Epiphyseal fracture of the proximal phalanx of the thumb, simulating ulnar collateral ligament injury with ulnar instability by stress x-ray.

is probably an epiphyseal fracture of the proximal phalanx rather than a collateral ligamentous injury (Fig. 20–47). Treatment is by closed reduction and thumb spica immobilization for three weeks. Bennett's fractures are extremely rare in children under 13 years of age.

COMPLICATIONS OF HAND FRACTURES

As in any fracture, complications of finger fractures may include infection and nonunion. Stiffness, malunion, sensory problems, and arthritis, however, are the major causes of morbidity following hand fractures.[127]

Stiffness is the most common sequela of hand fractures and is an expected treatment complication. Every effort should be made to minimize this disability by correct positioning of the hand, a short period of immobilization, and emphasis on early active motion.

As mentioned earlier, the optimal functional position of casting is with the wrist in 30 to 40 degrees of dorsiflexion, the MCP joints at 60 to 70 degrees of flexion, and the IP joints at 5 to 10 degrees of flexion. This position helps to maintain the arches of the hand, control digital rotation, and preserve collateral ligament length. Any stiffness that does develop will be easier to rehabilitate. Second, in any initial treatment positioning, elevation of the injured part is critical. This helps to reduce the injury edema that subsequently organizes into fibrosis. If a sling is used, it should be adjusted to avoid dependency of the injured part, and intermittent sling-free periods should be prescribed.

Immobilization without injury is, however, sufficient to cause contracture. Peacock,[131] using experimental evidence, showed that this stiffness resulted from soft tissue adherence to bone in areas normally meant to be freely gliding and from shortening of the periarticular tissues by new collagen synthesis. Hence, any immobilization should be for the shortest possible time, usually three to four weeks for most hand fractures. Clinical examination rather than radiological evidence of union should determine the duration of immobilization.

Lastly, early motion of the whole upper extremity is an essential preventive measure. By preventing stasis, motion helps to reduce edema and maintain a physiological environment for all the involved tissues. The use of internal fixation for certain fractures and of less restrictive casting has advanced this concept. Early motion should include the elbow and shoulder joints, as this will prevent development of most sympathetic dystrophy syndromes.

Any injury can aggravate disease states that are already present, such as rheumatoid arthritis or Dupuytren's contracture. In the former, it is common to find advanced osteoporosis after the injury and its treatment.

Numerous papers have dealt with the difficult problem of the established joint contracture.[18, 127, 129, 132, 133, 135] As stated, all treated fractures develop stiffness which diminishes with active use within a few weeks postimmobilization. If improved joint motion does not occur or persistent joint contracture develops, its cause can be divided into two categories: articular and extraarticular. The former includes basic joint surface damage from cartilage loss, bony deformity, or capsular and collateral ligament injury. Extraarticular pathology includes tissue adhesions found in the skin, intrinsic and extrinsic tendons, or palmar fascia. The prognosis is more favorable in the extraarticular contracture.

Distinguishing between articular and extraarticular pathology is difficult, and often the contracture is a combination of both elements. If the passive range of motion at the joint is greater than its active range, extraarticular pathology predominates. The tests for intrinsic tightness described by Bunnell, Doherty, and Curtis[128] further distinguish the offending structures. A true lateral x-ray is mandatory to visualize the joint surfaces.

Nonoperative management follows the protocol listed in Table 20–3. Since hand function depends more on MCP than on PIP flexion, and 45 degrees of flexion at the latter joint can be compatible with good use; hence, any extension contracture of the metacarpophalangeal joint requires earnest attention. We do use dynamic splinting of all types, but find that contractures of severe magnitude require outrigger traction. These measures are especially useful in the flexion contractures of the PIP joint. The course of all hand rehabilitation must be intense, supervised at least triweekly, and have

TABLE 20–3 Protocol for Rehabilitation Treatment of Stiff Fingers—S/P Fracture

Active Range of Motion—usually at 3 weeks
1. Gross finger flexion and extension
2. Flexion/extension of individual joints with proximal joints stabilized
3. Activities involving wrist extension to facilitate finger flexion
4. Nonresistive or minimally resistive exercises and activity necessitating grip and opposition

Resistive Range of Motion—usually at 4–5 weeks
1. Resistive exercise and activity, i.e., Theraplast, Play-doh, rubber band exercise boards for finger flexion/extension, pinch, and opposition activities
2. Activities and exercise involving wrist extension and providing resistance to finger flexion

Passive Range of Motion—usually at 5–6 weeks; limited value
1. Gentle → aggressive passive range of motion
2. Activities and exercises providing passive extension (rolling Theraplast) and passive flexion (strapping fingers around sanding handles)

Splinting—usually at 5–6 weeks
1. Dynamic splinting to ↑ extension of all joints
   a. Outriggers with rubber band pull
   b. Three-point pressure splints
2. Dynamic splinting to ↑ flexion of all joints
   a. Flexion straps
   b. Flexion gloves or gauntlets
   c. Flexion via rubber bands and hooks on fingernails
   d. Outriggers with rubber band pull

Edema Control
1. Massage
2. Elevation—avoid warm dependent soaks
3. String-wrapping
4. Wearing of rubber gloves

Heat
1. Warm soaks
2. Paraffin baths
3. Hot pack
All often used prior to exercise. May be contraindicated if swelling is a problem.

Medications
1. Judicious use of analgesia and narcotics
2. Antiinflammatory drugs
3. Intraarticular steroid injection 0.5 ml dexamethasone

the full cooperation and motivation of the patient. Wynn Parry's excellent book is highly recommended.[137]

In recalcitrant joints with good joint surfaces on lateral x-ray, surgical release is considered. Curtis[128] popularized the surgical treatment of joint stiffness by capsulectomy. This procedure may require a simultaneous extrinsic tenolysis. Other authors[130] have modified his techniques and some have questioned whether the early motion obtained is lasting. Harrison,[130] in a one-year follow-up study, concluded that the motion is maintained. Extension contractures fared better than flexion contractures, regaining over 40 degrees of flexion in most

joints, while the average later extension gain averaged only 25 degrees, and several joints lost motion. If joint destruction is advanced, arthroplasty should be considered and resection arthroplasty or the interpositional joint prosthesis as popularized by Swanson[134] may be used.

BONY PROBLEMS

Whereas nonunion is unusual in hand fractures, malunion is common. Nonunion most frequently occurs with infection, soft tissue interposition, or major bony loss, as found in high-velocity missile injuries.

Symptomatic malunion, however, may result from the most trivial fracture. The deformity may be one of angulation, shortening, or rotation.

Angulation is seen most commonly in the dorsal-volar plane in midshaft fractures and in the radial-ulnar plane in articular fractures. Thus, displaced fractures in these areas usually require internal stabilization. Shortening occurs with extensive comminution or bone loss, and in oblique diaphyseal fractures of the metacarpal or proximal phalanx. If such bony collapse appears imminent, internal fixation should be used to preserve bony length. The amount of shortening that can be tolerated varies and is most detrimental to the fixed unit metacarpals (index and long fingers) and the proximal and middle phalanges. Thumb function is remarkably resistant to residual deformities of both types. Both angulation and shortening are evident on x-ray examination.

Malrotation, however, demands attention to the clinical attitude of the finger. Concentration on the x-ray may blind the surgeon to the obvious malposition. Malrotation can be especially disabling, as the fingers become entangled when making a fist. The hand should be checked in several planes, including (a) an end-on view of the tips of the extended fingers, and (b) a frontal view with the metacarpophalangeal joints flexed. In the extended position all fingernails should lie in the same plane. When flexed, the fingertips converge on the thenar eminence. Immobilizing the hand in the previously described functional position usually prevents rotatory deformity.

While children will remodel angular deformities in the plane of joint motion, lateral angulation (and any angulation in an adult) and rotational deformity will not spontaneously correct. When a malunion is severe enough to disturb function, only osteotomy will correct it. Several types have been described;[132, 135] the approach may be made either through the original fracture site or at a more proximal metaphyseal site where rapid union can be expected.

NERVE PROBLEMS

Following any hand fracture, but especially after crush injuries of the distal phalanx, one can see disturbances of sensation. These may be localized to the injured finger or diffusely spread throughout the upper extremity. Reflex sympathetic dystrophy or hand-shoulder syndrome occurs most frequently after wrist fracture, but can also be seen with hand fractures. As mentioned in Chapter 19, the best management is anticipation of the problem and early active motion not only of the injured hand but also of the more proximal joints.

More often, a hyperreactive state is present in the distal pulp area, with the patient complaining of erythema, swelling, and hypersensitivity. Most cases will spontaneously resolve with use, but in recalcitrant fingers we employ desensitization techniques to the sensitive areas. These are done by the hand therapist and include tactile stimuli using different textures, pressures, a local tapping, and vibration as well as graded resistance activities. In the hypersensitive hand following crush fracture injury, the sensory reeducation techniques described by Dellon and Curtis may be helpful.[129]

TRAUMATIC ARTHRITIS

Intraarticular fractures, fracture-dislocations, and crush injuries frequently result in traumatic arthritis. The proximal interphalangeal joint is a frequent site of such residual disability. Aching and stiffness are common complaints, but pain severe enough to interrupt sleep is rare. Physical examination reveals a chronic thickening of the joint and a limitation of motion varying from mild to rigid. (A lateral x-ray will reveal the degree of joint destruction.) In most cases, symptoms can be controlled by a judicious use of exercises, splinting, and antiinflammatory drugs. When instability, stiffness, or severe pain predominates, arthroplasty or fusion is warranted.

In the thumb, traumatic arthritis can result in severe functional impairment. This can occur at either the metacarpophalangeal or the trapiziometacarpal (basal) joint. In the latter, such joint destruction is a sequela of Bennett's fracture. The forces generated at the thumb and the constant participation of the thumb joints in grasp and pinch activities make any arthritis of these joints particularly disabling. Often the joints are unstable and tend to sublux with use. Pain is usually localized to the involved joint. Axial compression of the thumb may produce both pain and palpable crepitus. Instability can often be demonstrated. Pinch and grip strengths are reduced. In basal joint disease, x-rays will often reveal arthritic changes of the trapezioscaphoid and trapeziotrapezoid articulations as well.

In mild cases, conservative therapy, as outlined previously, is beneficial, but progressive joint deterioration is the rule. For the metacarpophalangeal joint we favor fusion in 15 degrees of flexion. In isolated basal joint arthritis, either arthroplasty or fusion is successful.

REPLANTATION

Upper extremity amputations are not only dramatic but frequent. The development of microsurgical techniques, however, has made the replantation of devascularized parts feasible (Fig. 20–48). (To clarify any misconception, a replantation is the reattachment of a totally separated part, whereas in revascularization the part may be physiologically amputated but retains some link to its owner, such as a skin bridge.) In the 10 years since Komatsu and Tamai[148] first reported the successful replantation of a thumb and with the reports of the Chinese experience, microvascular surgery has advanced to the rational point at which results are measured in terms of useful function and not mere survival. In any busy replantation center, replantations, as opposed to revascularizations, average 60 to 70 per cent of the total surgery (Table 20–4). Several other points are immediately evident from Table 20–4. Revascularizations enjoy higher success rates than replants. Avulsed and severely crushed parts are poor candidates, averaging only 20 to 40 per cent viability. Reattachments in clean guillotine injuries, however, approach 85 to 90 per cent in all centers, and the proportionally larger vessels of proximal wrist and forearm replants have even higher patency rates. Lastly, Kleinert's[147] data point out the importance of experience in determining survival rates.

These established results stand on the shoulders of the experimental work of the late 1960's. Jacobson and Suarez[146] first emphasized the value of the operating scope. Refinements in technique progressed with the independent efforts of Buncke,[139] Daniel,[142] Kleinert,[147] Ikuta,[145] O'Brien,[153] and others. All this required simultaneous instrumentation development, such as vessel clamps, microneedles, and suture materials. For example, in 1967 the smallest needle available was 0.2 mm in diameter and limited vessel anastomosis to calibers of about 3 mm. Currently, 10-0 monofilament nylon swedged onto needles of less than 100 μ is used to repair vessels with diameters of less than 1 mm. Thus, while Malt[151] in 1962 could pioneer replantation of the arm in a 12-year-old boy, digital replantation had to await a size reduction. With this accomplishment, together with the pioneering successes of the late 1960's, initial viability became secondary to end functional result. A rational approach matured with defined indications, refined techniques, and recognized complications. Controversies always remain and follow-up evaluations still depend over-much on survival data. The following outline is meant to underline management principles; for specific detail the reader is referred to several excellent reviews and books.[138, 141, 144, 151, 152]

INDICATIONS

The misguided replantation is an essay in frustration in which failure may be a blessing. The time, energy, and money invested to save a working man's index finger which in the end remains stiff and bypassed is a hard lesson. The patient has read *Reader's Digest* and knows that fingers can be replanted. His desire is naturally for normality, and the immediacy of the loss blurs understanding. It is in this emotionally charged situation that a logical decision about replantation must be made. When replantation is inadvisable or unfeasible, the surgeon must orient the patient's expectations and aim the discussion toward a reasonable therapeutic decision. Proper patient selection is the difficulty as well as the cornerstone of any functional replantation.

General factors to be considered in replantation are patient age, handedness, vocation, other injuries or preexistent systemic conditions, psychological state, and skill of the surgeon. Best results are found

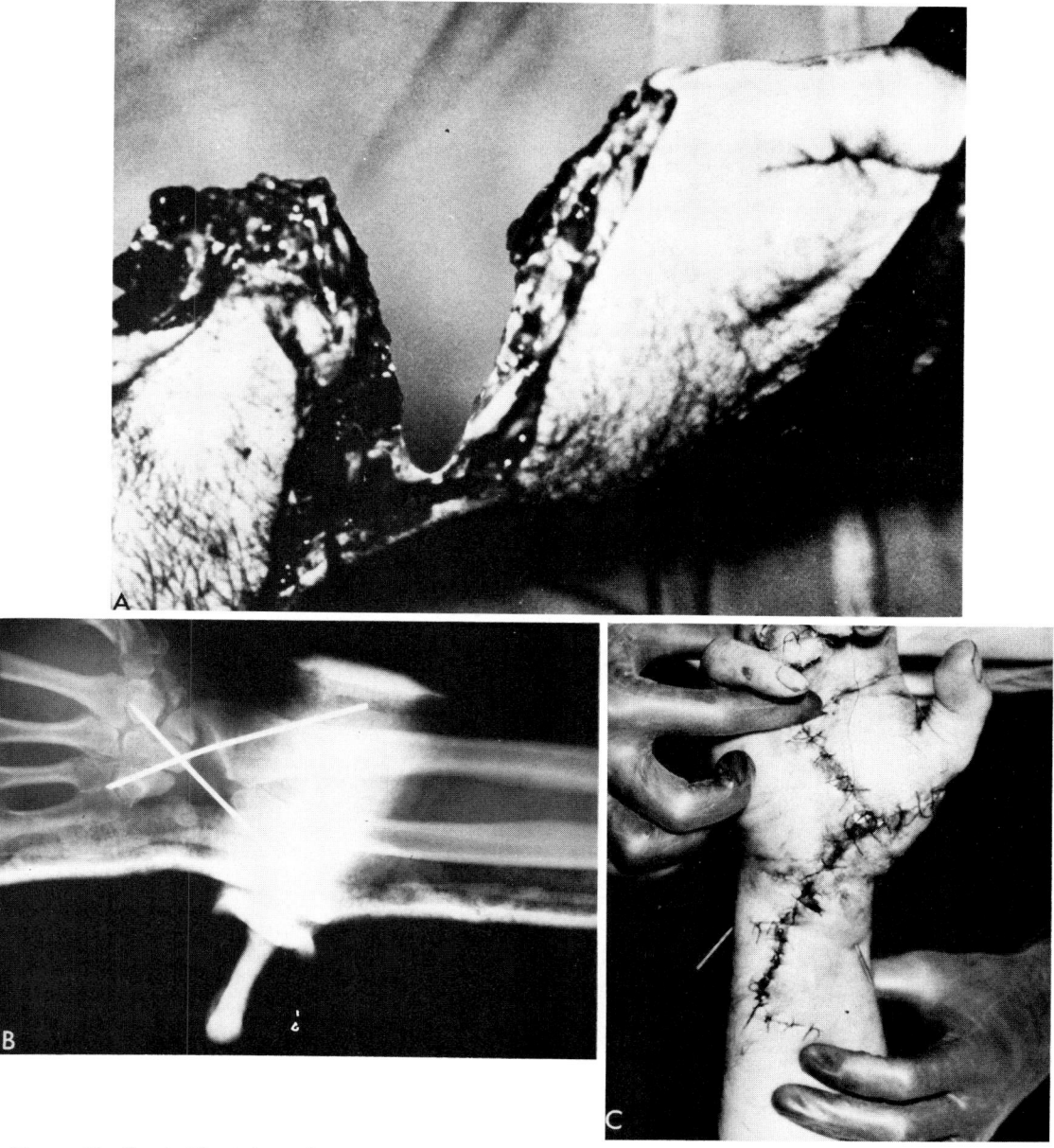

Figure 20-48 A. Physiological amputation of the wrist. B. Bony stabilization of the replant. C. Successful replant two weeks later.

in the second through fourth decades; surprisingly, children under 10 and adults over 70 fare the worst.[157] In the former case this is due to technical problems of the anastomoses; it is one of the few instances in which a child's tadpole response to injury is unavailing. Despite this, repairs of any injury in a child, at any level, should be attempted. There is some empirical evi-

dence that diabetics, moderate hypertensives, and those with atherosclerotic vascular disease may do poorly. Any other injury that jeopardizes the patient or precludes the necessary prolonged operating time is a contraindication. From a functional viewpoint, the musician will have different demands from the truck driver, and replantation must be individualized accordingly.

TABLE 20-4   Survival Data from Major Replant Centers

Author	Reported Number	Degree and Type	% Survival
Kleinert (USA)	>150	All replants 41 (1974)	27
		(1975)	69
		50 (1976)	90
		If severe crush	40
Ikuta (Japan)	>120	All replants proximal to wrist	88
		Digits	75
Millesi (Austria)	181	Both types	86
O'Brien (Australia)	130	Replant	74
		Revascularization	82
		Guillotine, local crush	88
		Avulsion, severe crush	42
Tamai (Japan)	>179	At wrist level 11	100
		Digits 168	89
Urbaniak (USA)	121	Replant	80
		Revascularization	93

Cosmesis may be so vital to some that even "fingers without sensation are better than being without fingers." Finally, microvascular anastomosis is a skill acquired by repetition, preferably in a microvascular laboratory. It is here, on animals, that experience with microscope use and basic anastomotic techniques can amplify surgical skill. Those not familiar with the techniques would be best advised to refer their patients to a microsurgical center.

The type, level of injury, and ischemia time are also important factors. The three basic types defined by mechanism of injury are the guillotine, the crush, and the avulsion. While the sharp clean-cut guillotine injury is the most suitable for replantation, it is unfortunately the rarest. Moderate crush amputations, such as those produced by the power saw, represent the majority of replantation candidates. Severe crushing, marked contamination, and avulsion are relative contraindications. Multiple-level injuries to the stump or amputated part usually preclude reattachment. All amputations proximal to the midmetacarpals should be attempted, with the proviso that bulk ischemic muscle mass subjects the patient to the hazard of muscle necrosis, including myoglobinuric renal failure, severe acidosis, hyperkalemia, and shock. Normothermic (often called warm) ischemia time of greater than ten hours to any amputation containing significant muscle bulk is a definite contraindication.

Ischemia time refers to the interval from

TABLE 20-5   Anatomical Indications for Replantation

Digit	Site	Replantation Comment
Thumb	Proximal to IP joint	Always, even if avulsed
Single digit, especially index or small finger	Proximal to sublimis insertion	Rarely; pollicization or ray resection better
Multiple digits	Proximal to sublimis insertion	Least damaged part to best site; later, salvage parts of useless fingers
Single or multiple	Distal to IP joint; sublimis intact	Probably. Most centers report good results, but controversial
Any transverse amputation proximal to metacarpophalangeal joint and below elbow		Yes, provided minimal ischemia time if large muscle bulk
Any amputation in a child		Yes

time of injury until replantation and correlates with replant viability. Any amputated part should be cooled immediately, as this significantly prolongs part survival. When experimentally cooled to an optimal 4° C, monkey replants have survived devascular intervals of 24 hours, and human digits have remained viable for up to 12 hours. For cooling, amputated parts should be wrapped in a sterile saline-soaked dressing and placed in a plastic bag immersed in iced water. At all costs, freezing of the amputated part should be avoided.

Aside from these general indications, specific anatomical recommendations for replantation have been made (Table 20–5).[148, 152, 156, 157] Because the thumb is essential to hand function, replantation should always be attempted, even in avulsion injuries.

MANAGEMENT: PREOPERATIVE, INTRAOPERATIVE, AND POSTOPERATIVE

Once a decision for replantation is reached, technical steps become crucial. This is most obvious in the microsurgery itself but pre- and postoperative care should not be underestimated, as they may be just as critical.

Emergency Room

Initial management is aimed at shortening ischemia time. As previously described, cooling of the amputated part is critical. The patient is stabilized and given both an antitetanus injection and antibiotics. Laboratory studies should include a coagulation profile as well as radiographs of both stump and amputated part. Under no circumstances should any connecting tissue, such as a skin bridge, be divided. Any vascular perfusion should be avoided, as this further damages vessel walls. Any damaged part should be protected to avoid further vascular insult.

Operating Room

The length of microsurgical operations, the exacting nature of the repairs, and the microscopic visual concentration all predispose the surgeon to fatigue and often

misguided decisions. A team approach not only avoids exhaustion but shortens ischemia time. Ideally, while the first team prepares the stump, a second team identifies and tags the key structures in the amputated part. Regional anesthesia, such as an axillary or supraclavicular block, is preferred because it avoids prolonged general anesthesia and also increases peripheral blood flow secondary to its sympathetic blockade. It can often be begun on arrival at the replantation center. General anesthesia is sometimes required as a supplement or in children. It is important to avoid any anesthetic that causes postanesthetic shaking, as this may disrupt the anastomoses. Hence, an anesthesiologist familiar with these needs is crucial.

In amputations distal to the wrist, primary repair of essential structures should be attempted. Secondary reconstructive procedures suffer from poorer results. Therefore, a planned sequence of repair is necessary for efficient replantation. Several have been suggested.[141, 144, 148, 149, 152, 153, 156, 157] and Table 20–6 shows our modifications and lists some articles relating to the specific techniques involved.

While a detailed description of the techniques involved in this sequence is beyond our discussion, certain principles deserve emphasis. Atraumatic repair of normal vessels is essential and means that all obviously damaged vessel walls must be resected (Fig. 20–49). Second, tension must be avoided. This is accomplished by bone shortening (up to 1.0 cm), vein grafting, or both. Bone immobilization should precede any repair, as it can be done quickly and it provides a stable scaffold for subsequent repair. Most groups agree that

TABLE 20–6 Sequence of Microvascular Repair

Debridement, both stump and part
Localization and tagging of all essential structures
Bone shortening
Bone stabilization
Extensor tendon repair
Arterial repair*
Venous repair*
Flexor tendon repair
Nerve repair
Loose skin closure

*See text for explanation.

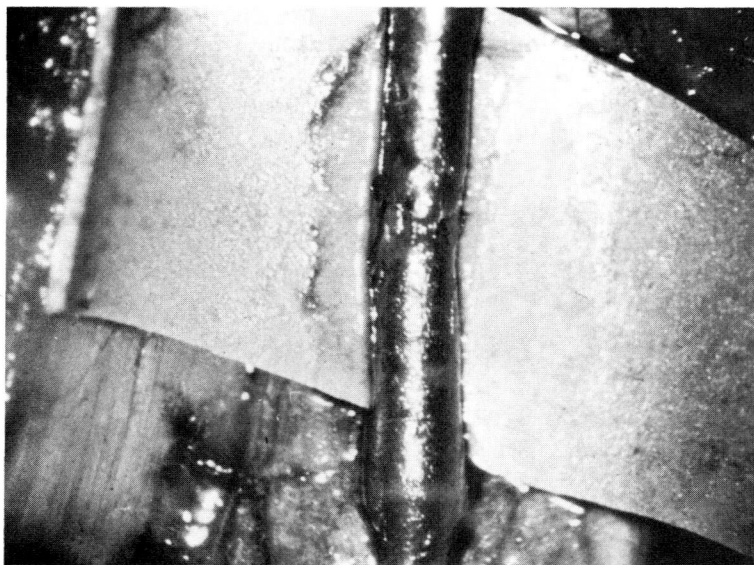

Figure 20–49 Microvascular anastomosis.

as many veins as possible should be repaired, with a minimum of two per artery, but there is conflict concerning the sequence of artery and vein repairs. We favor arterial repair first for the following reasons: (1) Presence of an intact capillary bed with good backflow run-off can be established. A good anastomosis without such flow suggests damage distally in the amputation. (2) Oxygenation and perfusion are reestablished sooner. (3) Venous bleeding makes vein identification much easier. A drawback to utilizing such a sequence is the need for an intermittent tourniquet to prevent excessive blood loss and to allow visualization of the venous repair. Skin defects, especially those with exposed vital structures, should be covered, usually with split-thickness grafts. The extensor tendon is always repaired, as it supplements bony stabilization. Secondary flexor tendon repair is indicated in some amputations, depending on the level of injury.

Postoperative Management

Once restored, circulation may be as quickly lost in the postoperative period as it was with the initial injury. Meticulous attention must be paid to all details, from surgical dressings to the patient's personal habits. A noncircumferential compression dressing reinforced with a well-padded dorsal splint is applied, taking care that the fingertips are exposed. This is essential for the hourly monitoring of circulation as well as for early passive mobilization of the digits. Initially, the extremity is elevated to control the inevitable edema. Subsequent position changes are mediated by vascular sufficiency, with arterial problems requiring more dependency. Methods of monitoring vascular sufficiency include clinical evaluation of skin color, temperature, and capillary refill as well as the more sophisticated Doppler flow meters, pulse volume recorders, and skin temperature electrodes. All have limitations, but a combination of clinical evaluation and skin temperature electrodes has proved to be most practical. Successful replants and normal digits have an average temperature of 32° to 34° C. A recording of less than 30° C is a sure indication of impending anastomotic disaster. The Doppler flow meter is reserved to identify specific vessel failure. A warm ambient room temperature should be maintained.

Bleeding is common in the initial postoperative period and, when dried, may embarass circulation and promote infection. Thus, we believe that dressings should be changed if they are bloody or if the replant looks doubtful. This brings up the problem of vasospasm. The repaired vessels are hypersensitive to any stimulus, and the induced vasospasm can lead to thrombosis. Peripheral or regional sympathetic blockade can moderate this reactivity. The patient should avoid smoking and xanthine stimulants, such as coffee, tea, and soda, which may precipitate vasospasm.

No area of microvascular protocol is more controversial than the use of anticoagulation, and each group approaches the problem with the assuredness of a religion. The controversy has close ties to the debate about the value of anticoagulants in preventing the vascular complications of hip surgery. Anticoagulants include aspirin, Persantin, low molecular weight dextran, heparin given either as a bolus or as a continuous intravenous drip, Coumadin, and urokinase. Review of the literature yields over 20 different protocols.[141, 144, 148, 149, 153, 156, 157] While thrombosis probably underlies most failure, excessive anticoagulation can lead to marked blood loss, tamponade and increased vasospasm of the anastomosis, and systemic complications. The use of nerve blocks increases their morbidity. While as empirical as other protocols, our regimen is: (1) aspirin, 10 gm q 12 hours for its antiplatelet properties; and (2) low molecular weight dextran in a dose of 5 mg per kg begun in the operating room and continued on a slow infusion basis q 12 hours for 4 days. We do not routinely use heparin, but reserve it for an intravenous bolus in the troubled replant or in levels sufficient to raise the partial thromboplastin time to twice normal in cases of distal replants. We also give Thorazine, 25 mg q 8 hours for its tranquilizing and vasodilating properties. Antibiotics are continued for a period of 10 days.

COMPLICATIONS

Early

Vascular Failure. Kleinert[147] has defined a "critical period," emphasizing that failure occurs early, two thirds within the first five days. The relative importance of arterial or venous thrombosis as the cause of failure is still debated. When performed early, Doppler studies are useful with the former type. Any reexploration and revision surgery must be done early to be successful.

The salvage rate averages one third at most centers.

Bleeding. In anticoagulated patients, excessive bleeding can occur. This may cause local anastomotic problems, and its subsequent cessation increases the risk of thromboses.

Infection. Despite the prolonged procedures, adequate microscopic debridement and antibiotics have made this a relative rarity.

Late

Once survival has been achieved, late complications are related to the functional result. Despite the goal of initial primary repair, nearly half of all replants will require secondary surgery. Every tissue plane has its complications: bone, joint, tendon, vessels, and nerve. About 2 per cent of bony nonunion occurs, but malunion with rotational deformity is more common. Joint stiffness is universal and may require capsulectomy or arthrodesis. Flexor tendons stick and require tendolysis or two-stage grafting. All patients experience some cold intolerance, which in a few is disabling. Urbaniak[157] was able to correlate this intolerance with pulse pressure and digital flow, suggesting the need to repair both digital arteries if possible. The degree of sensory recovery of the amputated digit is usually reasonable, and several studies have shown that the majority of replants achieve two-point discrimination under 20 mm.

Unsalvageable Amputations

When replantation is not feasible, the level of the amputation and the finger involved are important. An attempt should always be made to save length, but this is especially critical in the thumb. Index amputations distal to the PIP joint should be covered, but those proximal to it are best treated by primary or secondary index metacarpal ray resection. As was pointed out in the section on isolated index finger replantation, the excessively short or stiff index finger will be bypassed and become more of a cosmetic and functional liability. The same holds true for the small finger, though some controversy exists as to the degree of power grip sacrificed in the fifth ray resection. The long and ring fingers are central to grasp, and an effort should be made to preserve length distal to the PIP joint. Loss of a central digit proximal to the PIP joint may be treated by ray amputation and adjacent finger transposition. Otherwise, coins and small objects may slip from the central defect in the hand.

As mentioned earlier, wound closure may often best be obtained by bone shortening and coverage with local tissue. Some technical points deserve emphasis. If the amputation occurs through a joint, the cartilage and bulbous condylar flares of the proximal bone should be removed. Digital nerves should be pulled distally, cut sharply, and allowed to retract proximally. The practice of suturing the flexor to the extensor tendon over the end of the amputation should be avoided, as this seriously impairs the motion of the adjacent uninjured fingers which share the origins of the extensor and flexor muscles. Lastly, if the amputation occurs through the middle phalanx, the flexor

profundus may retract into the palm and limit proximal interphalangeal flexion by its action on the lumbrical-extensor mechanism. This can be avoided by suturing the profundus to the flexor sheath or by cutting the lumbrical muscle.

RING AVULSION INJURIES

Ring avulsing injuries are devascularizing single digital injuries in which microsurgery may be an option for treatment. Wedding bands are the major culprits, leading to the remark that "a wedding ring can stop your circulation." The mechanism of injury involves catching the ring on an immovable object while the body weight suddenly pulls on the trapped finger. The violence of the force degloves the finger.

Thompson[156] defined four types of injury (Fig. 20–50). Class 1 injuries are straightforward. The treatment of class 2 and class 3 injuries had been frustrating until recent

RING INJURIES

I Crush   II Crush plus
                  one neurovascular bundle

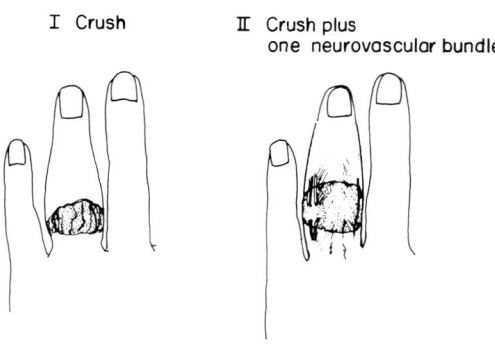

III Crush plus   IV Crush plus
two neurovascular bundles   two neurovascular bundles
                              plus fractures

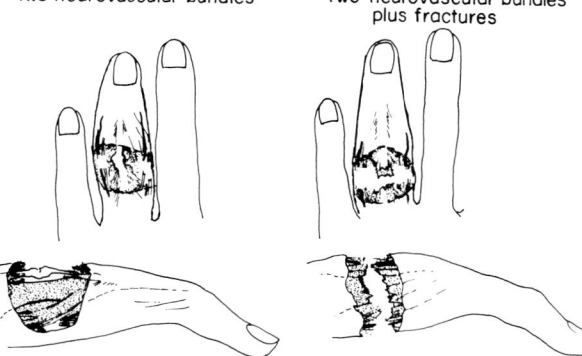

Figure 20–50   Types of ring avulsion injuries.

reports suggesting that all type 2 and one half of type 3 injuries can be salvaged by microsurgical techniques.[153] Despite recent surgical advances, some patients request amputation if the treatment results in a stiff, unesthetic finger.[139] Dorsal vein repair is a key to a successful surgical effort. Class 4 injuries are best handled by ray resection amputation.

REFERENCES

General

1. Boyes, J. H.: Bunnell's Surgery of the Hand. Philadelphia, J. B. Lippincott, 1970.
2. Bureau of Research and Statistics, Harrisburg, Pa., 1970.
3. Eaton, R. G.: Joint Injuries of the Hand. Springfield, C C Thomas, 1971.
4. Flatt, A. E.: The Care of Minor Hand Injuries. St. Louis, C. V. Mosby, 1972.
5. Flynn, J. E.: Hand Surgery. Baltimore, Williams & Wilkins, 1976.
6. Green, D. P., and Rowland, S. A.: Fractures and dislocations in the hand. In: Rockwood, C. A., and Green, D. P. (eds.): Fractures. Philadelphia, J. B. Lippincott, 1975.
7. Milford, L.: The hand. In: Crenshaw, A. H. (ed.): Campbell's Operative Orthopaedics. St. Louis, C. V. Mosby, 1971.
8. Watson-Jones, R.: Fractures and Other Bone and Joint Injuries. Baltimore, Williams & Wilkins, 1940.
9. Weckesser, E. C.: Treatment of Hand Injuries. Chicago, Year Book Medical Publishers, 1974.
10. Workmen's Compensation Board. State of New York, Research and Statistics Bulletin, No. 23, 1968.
11. Zancolli, E.: Structural and Dynamic Bases of Hand Surgery. Philadelphia, J. B. Lippincott, 1968.
12. Backhouse, K. M.: Mechanical factors influencing normal and rheumatoid MP joints. Ann. Rheum. Dis. (Suppl.), 28:15, 1969.

Anatomy and Biomechanics

13. Chao, E., Opgrande, J., and Axmear, F.: Three-dimensional force analysis of finger joints in selected isometric functions. Biomechanics, 9:387, 1976.
14. Cooney, W. P., and Chao, E. Y.: Biomechanical analysis of static forces in the thumb during hand function. J. Bone Joint Surg., 59A:27, 1977.
15. Flatt, A. E., and Fischer, B.: Restraints of the MP joint: A force analysis. Surg. Forum, 19:459, 1967.
16. Hakstian, R., and Tubiana, R.: Ulnar deviation of the fingers. J. Bone Joint Surg., 49A:298, 1967.
17. Kaplan, E. B.: Functional and Surgical Anatomy of the Hand. Philadelphia, J. B. Lippincott, 1953.
18. Kuczynski, K.: The proximal interphalangeal joint. J. Bone Joint Surg., 50B:656, 1968.
19. Kuczynski, K.: Less known aspects of PIP joints of the human hand. Hand, 17:31, 1972.
20. Littler, J. W., Cramer, L. M., and Smith, J. W.: Symposium on Reconstructive Hand Surgery. St. Louis, C. V. Mosby, 1944.
21. Vaughan-Jackson, O. J.: Tendon rupture in the rheumatoid hand. J. Bone Joint Surg., 41B:629, 1959.
22. Wood-Jones, F.: The Principles of Anatomy as Seen in the Hand. Baltimore, Williams & Wilkins, 1942.

Extensor Tendon

23. Dolphin, J. A.: Extensor tenotomy for chronic boutonnière deformity of the finger. J. Bone Joint Surg., 47A:161, 1965.
24. Elliott, R. A.: Injuries to the extensor mechanism of the hand. Orthop. Clin. North Am., 1:335, 1970.
25. Fowler, S. B.: Extensor apparatus of the digits. J. Bone Joint Surg., 31B:477, 1949.
26. Goldner, J. L.: Deformities of the hand incidental to pathological changes of the extensor and intrinsic muscle mechanism. J. Bone Joint Surg., 35A:115, 1953.
27. Landsmeer, J. M. F.: Anatomy of the dorsal aponeurosis of the human fingers and its functional significance. Anat. Rec., 104:31, 1969.
28. Littler, J. W.: Finger extensor mechanism. Surg. Clin. North Am., 47:415, 1967.
29. Littler, J. W., and Eaton, R. G.: Redistribution of forces on correction of boutonnière deformity. J. Bone Joint Surg., 49A:1267, 1967.
30. Matev, I.: Transposition of the lateral slips of the aponeurosis in treatment of long-standing boutonnière deformity. Br. J. Plast. Surg., 17:281, 1964.
31. Milford, L. W., Jr.: Retaining Ligaments of the Digits of the Hand. Philadelphia, W. B. Saunders, 1968.
32. Smith, R. J.: Balance and kinetics of the finger under normal and pathologic conditions. Clin. Orthop., 104:92, 1974.
33. Souter, W. A.: Boutonnière deformity. Clin. Orthop., 104:116, 1974.
34. Stark, H., Boyes, J., and Wilson, J.: Mallet finger. J. Bone Joint Surg., 44A:1061, 1962.
35. Tubiana, R.: Repair of the extensor apparatus of the fingers. Surg. Clin. North Am., 48:1022, 1968.
36. Tubiana, R., and Valentin, P.: Anatomy of the extensor apparatus and the physiology of finger extension. Surg. Clin. North Am., 44:897, 1964.
37. Weeks, P. M.: Chronic boutonnière deformity: Method of repair. Plast. Reconstr. Surg., 40:248, 1968.

Flexor Tendon

38. Burton, R. I., and Eaton, R. G.: Common hand injuries in the athlete. Orthop. Clin. North Am., 4:809, 1973.
39. Carroll, R. E., and Match, R. M.: Avulsion of the flexor profundus tendon insertion. J. Trauma, 10:1109, 1970.

40. Folmar, R. C, Nelson, C. L., and Phalen, G. S.: Ruptures of flexor tendons in the hands of non-rheumatoid patients. J. Bone Joint Surg., *54A*:579, 1972.
41. Green, W. L., and Niebauer, J. J.: Results of primary and secondary repairs in "no man's land." J. Bone Joint Surg., *56A*:1216, 1974.
42. Ketchum, L. D., Martin, N., and Kappel, D.: Factors affecting tendon gap and tendon strength at the site of tendon repair. Plast. Reconstr. Surg., *59*:182, 1977.
43. Lister, G. D., Kleinert, H. E., Kutz, J. E., and Atasoy, E.: Primary flexor tendon repair followed by immediate controlled mobilization. J. Hand Surg., *2*:441, 1977.
44. Schneider, L. H., Hunter, J. M., Norris, T. R., and Nadeau, P.: Delayed flexor tendon repair in "no man's land." J. Hand Surg., *2*:452, 1977.
45. Verdan, C. E.: Half a century of flexor tendon surgery. J. Bone Joint Surg., *54A*:472, 1972.
46. Wenger, D. R.: Avulsion of profundus tendon insertion in football players. Arch. Surg., *106*: 145, 1973.

Collateral Ligaments Exclusive of Thumb

47. Agee, J. M.: Unstable fracture/dislocations of the PIP joints. J. Hand Surg., *3*:386, 1972.
48. Hunt, J. C., Watts, H. B., and Glasgow, J. D.: Dorsal dislocation of the MCP joint of the index finger with reference to open dislocations. J. Bone Joint Surg., *49A*:1572, 1967.
49. Kaplan, E. B.: Dorsal dislocation of the metacarpophalangeal joint of the index finger. J. Bone Joint Surg., *41A*:1081, 1959.
50. McCue, F. C., Honner, R., Johnson, M. C., and Gieck, J. H.: Athletic injuries of the PIP joint requiring surgical treatment. J. Bone Joint Surg., *52A*:937, 1970.
51. McElfresh, E. C., Dobyns, J. H., and O'Brien, E. T.: Management of fracture/dislocations of the PIP joint by extension block splinting. J. Bone Joint Surg., *54A*:1105, 1972.
52. Meyers, M. H.: Dislocations, diagnosis, management, and complications. Surg. Clin. North Am., *48*:1391, 1968.
53. Moberg, E., and Stener, B.: Injuries to the ligaments of the thumb and fingers. Diagnosis, treatment, prognosis. Acta Chir. Scand., *106*: 166, 1954.
54. Murphy, A. F., and Stark, H. H.: Closed dislocation of the MCP joint of the index finger. J. Bone Joint Surg., *49A*:1579, 1967.
55. Pohl, A. L.: Irreducible dislocation of a distal interphalangeal joint. Br. J. Plast. Surg., *29*: 227, 1976.
56. Robertson, R. C., Calley, J. J., and Farris, A. M.: Treatment of fracture/dislocation of the interphalangeal joints of the hand. Am. J. Surg., *50*:563, 1938.
57. Spinner, M., and Choi, B. Y.: Anterior dislocation of PIP joint. J. Bone Joint Surg., *52A*: 1329, 1970.
58. Wiley, A. M.: Instability of the PIP joint following dislocation and fracture/dislocation. Hand, *2*:185, 1970.
59. Wilson, J. N., and Rowland, S. A.: Fracture/dislocation of the PIP joint of the finger. J. Bone Joint Surg., *48A*:493, 1966.

Collateral Ligament of Thumb

60. Bailey, R. A. J.: Some closed injuries of the MCP joint of the thumb. J. Bone Joint Surg., *45B*:428, 1963.
61. Bowers, W. H., and Hurst, L. C.: Gamekeeper's thumb: evaluation by arthrography and stress roentgenography. J. Bone Joint Surg., *59A*:519, 1977.
62. Campbell, C. S.: Gamekeeper's thumb. J. Bone Joint Surg., *37B*:148, 1955.
63. Coonrad, R. W., and Goldner, J. L.: Pathologic findings and treatment in soft tissue injury of the thumb metacarpophalangeal joint. J. Bone Joint Surg., *50A*:439, 1968.
64. Eggers, G. W.: Chronic dislocation of the base of the metacarpal of the thumb. J. Bone Joint Surg., *27*:500, 1945.
65. Neviaser, R. J., Wilson, J. N., and Lievano, A.: Rupture of the ulnar collateral ligament of the thumb (gamekeeper's thumb). J. Bone Joint Surg., *53A*:1357, 1971.
66. Slocum, D. B.: Stabilization of the articulation of the greater multangular and the first metacarpal. J. Bone Joint Surg., *25A*:626, 1943.
67. Smith, R.: Post traumatic instability of the metacarpophalangeal joint of the thumb. J. Bone Joint Surg., *59*:14, 1977.
68. Stener, B.: Displacement of ruptured ulnar collateral ligament of MCP joint of the thumb. J. Bone Joint Surg., *44B*:869, 1962.
69. Tsuge, K., and Shoichi, W.: Locking metacarpophalangeal joint of the thumb. Hand, *6*:255, 1974.

Hand Fractures — General

70. Boland, F. K.: Morsus humanus. J.A.M.A., *116*: 127, 1941.
71. Brown, P. W.: Management of phalangeal and metacarpal fractures. Surg. Clin. North Am., *53*:1393, 1973.
72. Chuinard, R. G., and D'Ambrosia, R. D.: Human bite infections of the hand. J. Bone Joint Surg., *59A*:416, 1977.
73. Goldstein, E. J. C., Miller, T. A., Citron, D. M., and Finegold, S. M.: Infections following clenched fist injury. J. Hand Surg., *3*:455, 1978.
74. James, J. I. P., and Wright, T. A.: Fractures of metacarpals and proximal and middle phalanges of one finger. J. Bone Joint Surg., *48B*:181, 1966.
75. Killbourne, B. C.: Management of complicated hand fractures. Surg. Clin. North Am., *48*:201, 1968.
76. Mann, R. J., Hoffeld, T. A., and Farmer, C. B.: Human bites of the hand: twenty years of experience. J. Hand Surg., *2*:97, 1977.
77. Moberg, E.: Fractures and ligamentous injuries of the thumb and fingers. Surg. Clin. North Am., *40*:297, 1960.
78. Ruedi, T. P., Burri, C., and Pfeiffer, K. M.: Stable internal fixation of fractures of the hand. J. Trauma, *11*:381, 1971.
79. Shields, C., Patzakis, M. J., and Harvey, J. P.: Hand infections secondary to human bites. J. Trauma, *15*:235, 1975.
80. Stark, H. H.: Troublesome fractures and dislocations of the hand. AAOS Instructional Course Lectures, *19*:130, 1970.

81. Swanson, A. B.: Fractures involving the digits of the hand. Orthop. Clin. North Am., *1*:261, 1970.
82. Vom Saal, H. H.: Intramedullary fixation in fractures of the hand and fingers. J. Bone Joint Surg., 35A:5, 1953.
83. Wright, T. A.: Early mobilization in fractures of metacarpals and phalanges. Can. J. Surg., *11*: 491, 1968.

Fractures — Finger Phalanges Including Finger Tip Injuries

84. Atasoy, E., Kutz, J. E., Kleinert, H. E., and Kasdan, M. L.: Reconstruction of the amputated finger tip with a triangular volar flap. J. Bone Joint Surg., 52A:921, 1970.
85. Beasley, R. W.: Reconstruction of amputated fingertips. Plast. Reconstr. Surg., 44:349, 1969.
86. Bloomenstein, R. B.: Individualized treatment of fingertip amputations. Orthop. Rev., 7:27, 1978.
87. Coonrad, R. W., and Pohlman, M. H.: Impacted fractures in the proximal portion of the proximal phalanx. J. Bone Joint Surg., 51A:1291, 1969.
88. Cronin, T. C.: Cross finger flap. Am. Surg., *17:* 419, 1951.
89. Elsahy, N. I.: Replantation of a completely amputated distal segment of thumb. Plast. Reconstr. Surg., 59:579, 1977.
90. Flatt, A. E.: The thenar flap. J. Bone Joint Surg., *39B*:80, 1957.
91. Green, D. P., and Anderson, J. R.: Closed reduction and percutaneous pin fixation of fractured phalanges. J. Bone Joint Surg., 55A: 1651, 1973.
92. Kleinert, H. E., Putcha, S. M., Ashbell, T. S., and Kutz, J. E.: Deformed fingernail. J. Trauma, 7:177, 1967.
93. Kutler, W.: Method for fingertip amputations. J.A.M.A., *133*:29, 1947.
94. Keim, H. A., and Grantham, S. A.: Volar-flap advancement for thumb and fingertip injuries. Clin. Orthop., 66:109, 1969.
95. Lee, M. L. H.: Intraarticular and periarticular fractures of the phalanges. J. Bone Joint Surg., *45B*:103, 1963.
96. Mansoor, I. A.: Fractures of the proximal phalanx of the fingers. J. Bone Joint Surg., 51A: 196, 1969.
97. Newmeyer, W. L., and Kilgore, E. S.: Fingertip injuries. J. Trauma, *14*:58, 1974.
98. Pratt, D. R.: Fingertip injury. *In*: Cramer, L., and Chase, R. (eds.), Symposium on the Hand. Vol. 3. St. Louis, C. V. Mosby, 1971.

Fractures and Dislocations — Finger Metacarpals

99. Berkman, E. F., and Miles, G. H.: Internal fixation of metacarpal fractures exclusive of the thumb. J. Bone Joint Surg., 25:816, 1943.
100. Bora, F. W., Jr., and Didizian, N.: The treatment of the intraarticular fracture of the base of the small finger metacarpal. J. Bone Joint Surg., 56A:1459, 1974.
101. Eichenholtz, S. N., and Rizzo, P. C.: Fracture of the neck of the fifth metacarpal. Is overtreatment justified? J.A.M.A., *178*:425, 1961.
102. Harwin, S. F., Fox, J. M., and Sedlin, E. O.: Volar dislocation of bases of second and third

metacarpals. J. Bone Joint Surg., *57A*:849, 1975.
103. Hazelett, J. W.: Carpometacarpal dislocation other than the thumb. Can. J. Surg., *11*:315, 1968.
104. Hsu, J. O., and Curtis, R. M.: Carpometacarpal dislocation on the ulnar side of the hand. J. Bone Joint Surg., 52A:927, 1970.
105. Hunter, J. M., and Cowen, N. J.: Fifth metacarpal fractures in a compensation clinic population. J. Bone Joint Surg., 52A:1159, 1970.
106. Jahss, S. A.: Fractures of the metacarpals. A new method of reduction and immobilization. J. Bone Joint Surg., 20:178, 1938.
107. Lamb, D. W., Abernethy, P. A., and Raine, D. A.: Unstable fractures of the metacarpals. Hand, 5:43, 1973.
108. Miller, W. R.: Fractures of the metacarpals. Am. J. Orthop., 7:105, 1965.
109. Shorbe, H. B.: Carpometacarpal dislocations. J. Bone Joint Surg., 20:454, 1938.
110. Waugh, R. L., and Yancey, A. G.: Carpometacarpal dislocations. J. Bone Joint Surg., *30A*:397, 1948.

Fractures — Thumb Metacarpal

111. Bennett, E. J.: Fracture of the metacarpal bone of the thumb. Br. Med. J., *12*:2, 1886. Trans. R. Acad. Med. Ireland, *15*:309; Dublin J. Med. Sci., *73*:1882.
112. Gedda, K. O.: Studies on Bennett's fracture: Anatomy, roentgenology, and therapy. Acta Chir. Scand. (Suppl.), *193*:1, 1954.
113. Gedda, K. O., and Moberg, E.: Open reduction and osteosynthesis of Bennett's fracture in the carpometacarpal joint of the thumb. Acta Orthop. Scand., 22:249, 1953.
114. Green, D. P., and O'Brien, E. T.: Fractures of thumb metacarpal. South. Med. J., 65:807, 1972.
115. Griffiths, J. C.: Fractures of the base of the first metacarpal bone. J. Bone Joint Surg., *46B*:712, 1964.
116. Pollen, A. B.: Conservative treatment of Bennett's fracture. J. Bone Joint Surg., *50B*:91, 1968.
117. Rolando, S.: Fracture de la base du premier metacarpien: et principalement sus une varieté non encore dicite. Presse Med., *33*: 303, 1910.
118. Wiggins, H. E., Bundens, W. D., Jr., and Parks, B. J.: Method of treatment of fracture-dislocations of the first metacarpal bone. J. Bone Joint Surg., 36A:810, 1954.

Fractures — Children

119. Blount, W. P.: Fractures in Children. Baltimore, Williams & Wilkins, 1955.
120. Bora, F. W., Jr., Nissenbaum, M., and Ignatius, P. F.: The treatment of epiphyseal fractures in the hand. Orthop. Dig., *4*:11, 1976.
121. Bright, R. W., Burstein, A. H., and Elmore, S. M.: Epiphyseal plate cartilage — an experimental analysis of failure modes. J. Bone Joint Surg., 56A:856, 1974.
122. Brighton, C. T., Cronkey, J. E., and Osterman, A. L.: *In vitro* epiphyseal plate growths in various constant electrical fields. J. Bone Joint Surg., 58A:971, 1976.

123. Brighton, C. T., Chung, S. M. K., and Batterman, S. C.: Shear strength of human femoral capital epiphyseal plate. J. Bone Joint Surg., 58A:94, 1976.
124. Hanlon, C. R., and Estes, W. L.: Fractures in childhood—a statistical analysis. Am. J. Surg., 87:312, 1954.
125. Leonard, M. H., and Dubravcik, P.: Management of fractured fingers in the child. Clin. Orthop. Rel. Res., 73:160, 1970.
126. Salter, R. B., and Harris, R. W.: Epiphysal plate injuries. J. Bone Joint Surg., 45A:587, 1963.

Complications of Hand Fractures

127. Clinkscales, G. S.: Complications in management of fractures in hand injuries. South. Med. J., 63:704, 1970.
128. Curtis, R. M.: Capsulectomy of the interphalangeal joints. J. Bone Joint Surg., 36A:1219, 1954.
129. Dellon, A. L., and Curtis, R. M.: Program for Sensory Reeducation. Baltimore, Johns Hopkins Hospital, 1975.
130. Harrison, D. H.: The stiff interphalangeal joint. Hand, 9:102, 1977.
131. Peacock, E. E., Jr.: Some biochemical and biophysical aspects of joint stiffness. Ann. Surg., 164:1, 1966.
132. Pieron, A. P.: Correction of rotational malunion of a phalanx by metacarpal osteotomy. J. Bone Joint Surg., 54B:512, 1972.
133. Sprague, B. L.: PIP joint contractures and their treatment. J. Trauma, 16:259, 1976.
134. Swanson, A. F.: Flexible implant arthroplasty for arthritic finger joints. J. Bone Joint Surg., 54A:435, 1972.
135. Weckesser, E. C.: Rotational osteotomy of the metacarpal for overlapping fingers. J. Bone Joint Surg., 47A:751, 1965.
136. Wynn Parry, C. B.: Management of the stiff joint. Hand, 3:69, 1971.
137. Wynn Parry, C. B.: Rehabilitation of the Hand. 3rd ed. London, Butterworth, 1973.

Replantation

138. Berger, A., Millesi, H., et al.: Replantation and revascularization of amputated parts of extremities. Clin. Orthop., 133:212, 1978.
139. Buncke, H. J., Chater, N. L., and Szabo, Z.: Manual of Microvascular Surgery. San Francisco, Ralph Davies Microsurgical Unit, 1975.
140. Carroll, R. E.: Ring injuries in the hand. Clin. Orthop., 104:175, 1974.

141. Chien, C. W., Ch'en, Y. C., and Pao, Y. S.: Small vessel anastomosis in reattachment of complete traumatic amputation. Chinese Med., 85: 79, 1972.
142. Daniel, R., and Terzis, J.: Reconstructive Microsurgery. Boston, Little, Brown, 1977.
143. Gelberman, R. H., Urbaniak, J. R., et al.: Digital Sensibility Following Replantation. Paper presented at meeting of American Society for Surgery of the Hand, Dallas, 1978.
144. Hayhurst, J. W., O'Brien, B. McC., et al.: Experimental digital replantation after prolonged cooling. Hand, 6:134, 1974.
145. Ikuta, Y.: Microvascular Surgery. Hiroshima, Lewis Press Co., 1975.
146. Jacobson, J. H., and Suarez, E. L.: Microsurgery in anastomosis of small vessels. Surg. Forum, 11:243, 1960.
147. Kleinert, H. E., Serafin, D., and Daniel, R. K.: The place of microsurgery in hand surgery. Orthop. Clin. North Am., 4:929, 1973.
148. Komatsu, S., and Tamai, S.: Successful replantation of a completely cut off thumb. Plast. Reconstr. Surg., 42:574, 1968.
149. Lucas, G. L. (ed.): Microvascular Surgery and Limb Replantation. Symposium. Clin. Orthop., 133:June 1975.
150. MacLeod, A. M., and O'Brien, B. McC., et al.: Digital replantation. Clin. Orthop., 133:26, 1978.
151. Malt, R. A., and McKhaun, C. F.: Replantation of severed arms. J.A.M.A., 189:716, 1964.
152. Microvascular Symposium. Orthop. Clin. North Am., 8(2), April 1977.
153. O'Brien, B. McC.: Microvascular Reconstructive Surgery. New York, Livingstone and Churchill, 1977.
154. Steichen, J. B., and Russell, R. C.: Revascularization of Ring Injuries by Microvascular Techniques. Paper presented at meeting of American Society for Surgery of the Hand, Dallas, 1978.
155. Tamai, S., et al.: Microvascular anastomosis and its applications on replantation of amputated digits and hands. Clin. Orthop., 133:106, 1978.
156. Thompson, L. K., Posch, J. L., and Lie, K. K.: Ring injuries. Plast. Reconstr. Surg., 42:148, 1968.
157. Urbaniak, J. R., Hayes, M. G., and Bright, D.: Management of bone in digital replantation. Clin. Orthop., 133:184, 1978.

ZACHARY B. FRIEDENBERG, M.D.

Fractures of ————————————— 21
the Pelvis

Pelvic injuries can best be understood if we think of three bones forming a bony ring that has a dual function — transmitting weight from the spinal axis to the lower extremities, and protecting and supporting the organs within the ring. The pelvic girdle is admirably constructed to serve these functions, and when the ring is fractured or displaced, it is because it has been subjected to very severe stresses. Fractures that break the continuity of the ring with or without displacement of the hemipelvis often occur in pedestrians who are struck by speeding autos, in those who suffer crushing injuries, or in individuals struck by heavy weights. The magnitude of the fracturing force is so great that it usually causes serious injuries to other areas of the body in addition to local trauma to the viscera and neurovascular structures contained within the pelvis.

The surgeon caring for such victims must be alert and skilled in the use of resuscitative measures and must possess the diagnostic acumen to assess cranial, thoracic, abdominal, and vascular injuries as well as the skeletal problem. One must not focus on the pelvic fracture until a methodical and thorough evaluation of the total patient has been done. Fractures of the pelvis are the third most common cause of fatal injury from accidents involving motor vehicles; cranial and chest injuries cause more motor vehicle deaths than pelvic injuries. In this chapter, it is emphasized that the treatment of the pelvic skeletal trauma is subsidiary to the treatment of the patient. Injuries to the acetabulum are excluded, as they are discussed elsewhere.

ANATOMY OF THE PELVIS

The pelvic ring is formed by the paired hip bones (innominate bones) separated by the sacrum posteriorly and uniting anteriorly. Each hip bone is flat and fan-shaped and further subdivided into three parts; the flattened ilium articulates with the sacrum posteriorly and reaches the hip joint anteriorly; the ischium forms the inferior portion of the acetabulum and is directed downward and backward to form the lower border of the obturator foramen; the pubis extends forward from the acetabulum to articulate with its paired member anteriorly and has two rami that form the superior and medial bones around the obturator foramen (Fig. 21–1).

The sacrum is wedged between the paired ilii, its broad transverse axis strengthened by the fused alae so that it can resist compressive forces.

The rami of the pubis are thin and drawn out, surrounding the obturator foramen, and this area is vulnerable to direct or transmitted forces applied frontally or laterally.

The sacroiliac articulation is an amphiarthrodial type of joint with a thin covering of articular cartilage that is discontinuous; the surfaces may be united with each other by fibrocartilage in some areas, while in others they are separated by a space containing synovial fluid. These joints permit little motion in adults.

The anterior sacroiliac ligament is sparse, but the interosseous and posterior sacroiliac ligaments are strong and act to resist intrapelvic pressure (Fig. 21–2). The strong posterior sacroiliac ligaments cannot be

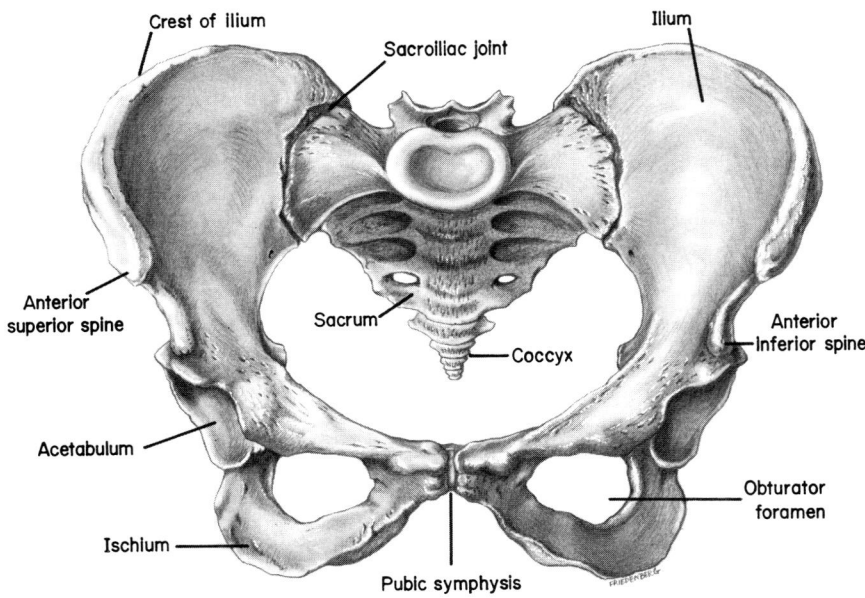

Figure 21-1   The pelvis.

effective unless the ring is intact in front and the well-developed anterior interpubic ligaments keep the symphysis tightly closed, also resisting internal pelvic pressure. The superior and inferior interpubic ligaments are much thinner. The pubic symphysis is also an amphiarthrodial joint.

The hip bone develops from three primary ossification centers, the ilium, ischium, and pubis (Fig. 21-3). These three nuclei converge at the acetabulum and until puberty remain separated from each other

by a Y-shaped cartilage, the triradiate cartilage. Final fusion of the three components occurs about the twentieth year. An apophysis develops along the crest of the ilium early in puberty and fuses between the twentieth and twenty-fifth years.

Apophyses also appear, shortly after puberty, along the spine and tuberosity of the ischium and at the anterior inferior spine of the ilium. All these unite between the seventeenth and twentieth years. A late-appearing apophysis at the margin of the pubis

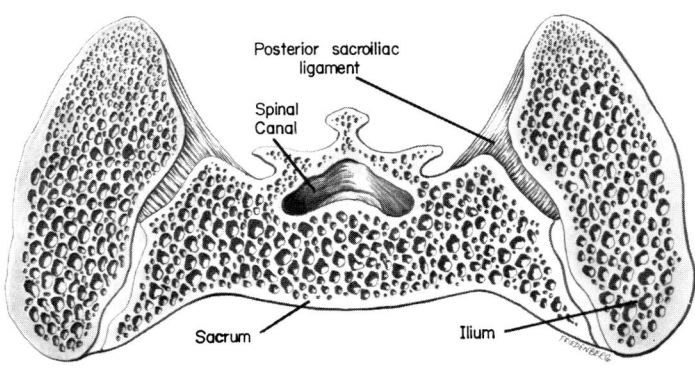

Figure 21-2   The pelvis is constructed to resist internal pressures. The strong posterior sacroiliac ligaments prevent lateral movement of the ilii. The sacrum cannot be displaced backward, as it is firmly gripped by the ilium on each side.

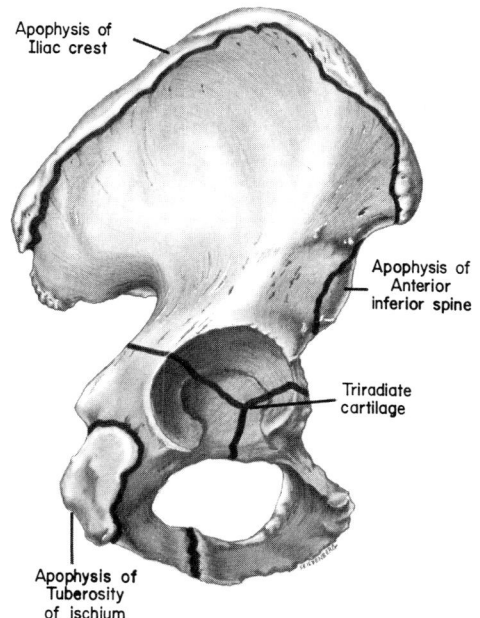

adjacent to the symphysis is seen between the eighteenth and twentieth years and fuses after the twentieth year.

The urethra, bladder, uterus, and rectum are protected within the pelvic ring. On the inner wall of the pelvis the iliac arteries and veins divide, and the numerous branches of the internal iliac vessels are subject to laceration when the pelvis is fractured (Fig. 21–4). Also present on the inner wall of the ilium is the femoral nerve with components from the second, third, and fourth lumbar roots. Branches from the fourth and fifth lumbar nerves form a plexus with the first, second, and third sacral nerves emerging from the sacral foramina, the lumbosacral plexus, which courses along the inner pelvic wall. With the displacement of the pelvic ring, nerve damage can occur at several levels. Traction transmitted to the roots from these nerve structures can cause avulsion of the nerve roots. The lumbosacral plexus and the peripheral nerves themselves may also be damaged. The sympathetic trunk lies on each side of the anterior concave surface of the sacrum, reaching to the coccyx.

Figure 21–3 There are three primary ossification centers of the pelvis; the ilium, ischium, and pubis, which meet in the acetabulum to form the triradiate cartilage. The secondary ossification centers are also shown.

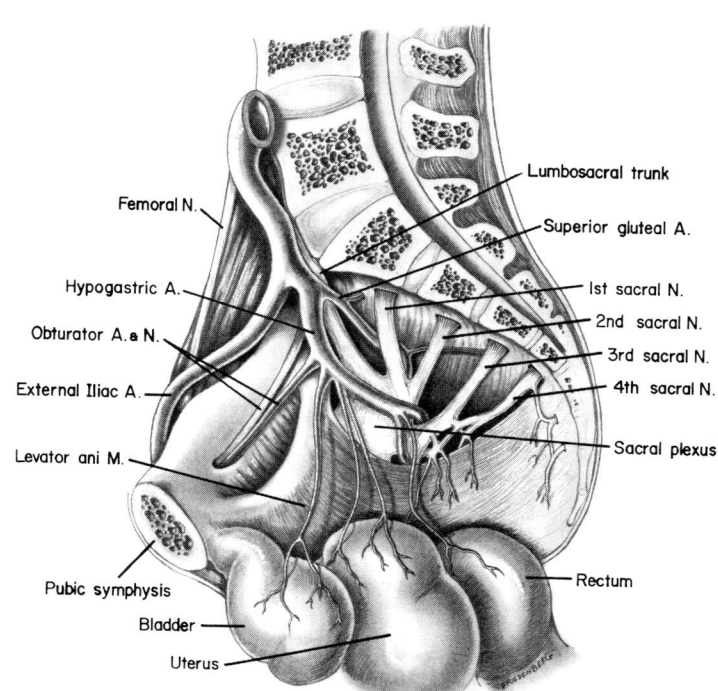

Figure 21–4 The arteries and nerves fixed to the inner wall of the pelvis are thus frequently injured in fractures.

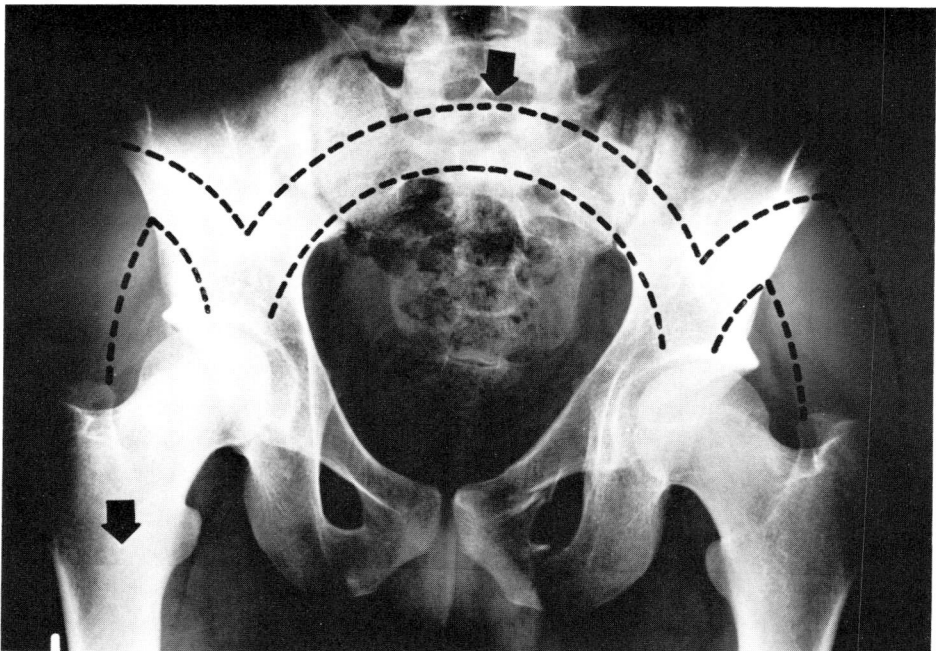

Figure 21–5   The mechanical arches transmit weight from the trunk to the lower extremities. A central primary arch is flanked by two secondary arches, of which the abductor muscles are components. (After G. F. Domisse: Diametric fractures of the pelvis. J. Bone Joint Surg., *42B*:432–443, 1960.)

BIOMECHANICS OF THE PELVIS

The pelvic girdle has a supportive and protective function. It protects the contained viscera and is the medium by which the trunk weight is carried to the lower extremities. The posterior pelvis (posterior to the acetabula) is involved in weight transmission. Patients with congenital aplasia of the forepelvis or those with disease or resection of the forepelvis are mechanically capable of walking. The primary function of the forepelvis is protection.

Domisse has demonstrated the presence of two mechanical arches in the pelvis that correspond to the trabecular pattern of the bone. There is a central primary arch whose apex corresponds to the upper border of the sacrum and which descends on each inner pelvic border to the acetabula (Fig. 21–5). Secondary or lateral arches flank the primary arch, one on each side. The apex of each of these arches is the anterior superior spine, and the medial base is the acetabulum, the lateral base being the greater trochanter. The walls of each of these arches

are the lateral pelvis and the abductor muscles. The apex of the central arch bearing the trunk weight thrusts the wedge-shaped sacrum downward and deeper between the two iliac bones. Posteriorly directed components of this force are resisted by the sacral wedge, which is wider anteriorly. Anterior displacement of the sacrum is resisted by the strong posterior sacroiliac and interosseous ligaments.[5]

The pelvis is constructed to resist internal pressures by virtue of its strong posterior sacroiliac and anterior interpubic ligaments (Fig. 21–6). The sacroiliac joint and the symphysis are so stable that a force *directly* applied to the ring will primarily cause a fracture rather than a dislocation. Once the integrity of the ring has been broken, a continuing force or a rotary component of the original force can spring the joints. It has been shown that the interpubic ligament plays a vital role in linking the two halves of the pelvis and in preventing the sacroiliac joints from opening backward.[5] The interpubic ligament is the clasp holding the two covers of the book closed. When

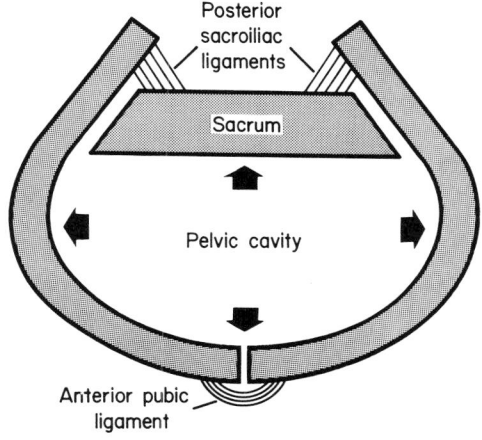

Figure 21–6 A schematic representation of the pelvis shows how internal pressure is strongly resisted by the anterior interpubic ligaments and the posterior sacroiliac ligaments. The blunt, wedge-shaped sacrum cannot be displaced backward because of the ilium.

this anterior tie is disrupted, the weak anterior sacroiliac joints are unable to resist the forces acting to open the pelvis.

Fractures due to *direct* violence may be caused by side-to-side compression, anteroposterior compression, or compression transmitted from below through the ischial tuberosities, as in a fall in the sitting position.

Fractures caused by *indirect* violence usually occur when an axial force is applied to the femur when the knee is struck and the transmitted force is applied to the pelvis. The hip must be in a mildly flexed position

and without any abduction or adduction present. The impact is transmitted to the shelf of the acetabulum, with rupture of the interpubic ligaments or a fracture of the forepelvis followed by rupture of the weak anterior sacroiliac ligaments and opening of the sacroiliac joint (Fig. 21–7). If the hip is sharply flexed and adducted, this force will result in a posterior dislocation of the hip; if the hip was in abduction, a central protrusion of the head into the pelvis will result.

CLASSIFICATION OF FRACTURES OF THE PELVIS

This classification is based primarily on treatment and secondarily on pathomechanics.

Avulsion fractures	Avulsion of anterior superior spine of ilium
	Avulsion of anterior inferior spine of ilium
	Avulsion of tuberosity of ischium
Isolated fractures without separation of the pelvic ring (stable)	Fractures of pubic rami
	Fractures of wing of ilium
	Fractures of sacrum
	Fractures of coccyx

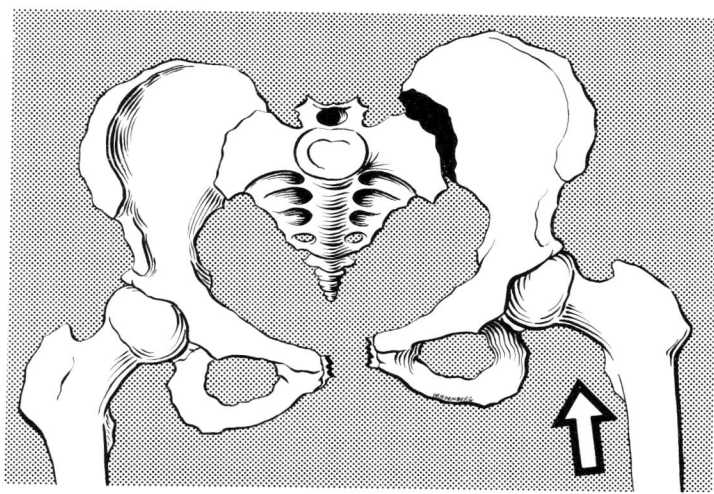

Figure 21–7 An axial force transmitted through the femur displaces the hemipelvis upward, disrupting the pubic symphysis and the sacroiliac joint.

Fractures with loss of continuity of pelvic ring (unstable)

 Fractures of both pubic rami bilaterally (double break in forepelvis)

 Fractures of pubic rami and separation of symphysis

Diametric fractures (unstable)

 Fractures of pubic rami or separation of symphysis with sacroiliac dislocation

 Fractures of pubic rami or separation of symphysis with fracture of ilium

 Overlapped hemipelvis with fracture of pubic rami and fracture of ilium or sacroiliac dislocation

Acetabular fractures (see Chapter 22)

MANAGEMENT OF THE PATIENT WITH A PELVIC FRACTURE

The treatment of a patient with a pelvic fracture taxes the skill of the most competent surgeon. Not only is there a problem with life-threatening pelvic complications, but most patients with pelvic fractures have concomitant injuries to other areas of the body.

Associated Injuries

In a series of 173 patients with pelvic fractures reported by Trunkey and associates, 35 per cent of the injuries were to pedestrians hit by motor vehicles; 25 per cent were to occupants of motor vehicles; 30 per cent occurred in falls, and 10 per cent were to motorcyclists. These 173 patients received 200 injuries outside of the pelvic area, including 36 femoral fractures, 23 spinal fractures, and 24 open fractures. Nine per cent of the patients died.[20]

In another series of 220 pelvic fractures reported by Reynolds and co-workers, 40 per cent were accompanied by skeletal injuries outside the pelvic area. A ruptured bladder or urethra occurred in 8 per cent; the mortality rate in this series was 18 per cent.[16] In a study of blunt trauma to the bladder, it was found that 72 per cent of all such injuries to the bladder were in association with pelvic fractures.[2] Other injuries frequently reported with pelvic fractures are head injuries, crushed chest with hemopneumothorax, liver lacerations, ruptured spleen, massive pelvic or retroperitoneal hemorrhage, perforation of the rectum, rupture of the diaphragm, paralysis due to root or plexus injury, ruptured lumbar disk, uterine injuries in pregnancy, and others.

Immediate Care of the Severely Injured Patient with a Pelvic Fracture

The airway is cleared if necessary. Bleeding and edema in the oropharynx or a flail chest require intubation or tracheostomy. Positive-pressure ventilation may be necessary; open wounds of the chest are closed, and tension pneumothorax is relieved with a large-bore needle.

Intravenous fluids are started with a catheter in a large vein, and a central venous pressure line is also necessary.

A thorough examination is now done with the patient completely undressed. The examiner should proceed in an orderly routine, searching for cranial injuries, spinal injuries, ventilatory malfunction, abdominal injuries, and extremity damage, working down to the feet. The patient is then turned, the back is examined, and a rectal examination is done for blood and to determine rectal tone. The patient is catheterized, and the amount of urine and the presence of blood are noted. A clear return of urine does not necessarily mean that there has been no bladder or urethral injury.

The condition of the patient is monitored regularly; any change in the state of consciousness or neurological changes are noted, and the central venous pressure, urine volume (if the urinary tract is intact), and blood gases are followed. Fractures are splinted. The patient can now be sent to the radiology department for the necessary films.

Urethral and Bladder Injuries

A retrograde cystourethrogram is done. The catheter is advanced to the base of the urethra, and dye is instilled into the urethra before the catheter is passed into the bladder. When laceration of the urethra is present, no attempt should be made to pass the catheter further into the bladder; the patient will require a suprapubic cystostomy. If the urethra is intact, the catheter is introduced into the bladder, 150 ml of water-soluble dye is instilled by gravity technique, the catheter is clamped, and anteroposterior and lateral films are made. In the absence of any overt extravasation, an additional 100 ml of dye is injected to distend the bladder, and additional films are made. The dye is then removed from the bladder and another set of films is made to determine whether an extravasation was hidden behind the bladder shadow.[2]

Bladder injuries may be classified as contusions or as extraperitoneal, intraperitoneal, or combined ruptures. The extravasation is perivesical with extraperitoneal rupture, and in communication with the peritoneal cavity with intraperitoneal rupture. In the combined bladder injury the dye is found around the bladder and in the peritoneal cavity. Operation on the urinary tract can be delayed one or two hours or until the patient's condition is stabilized and can be done in conjunction with other necessary operative procedures.

The bladder may be injured directly by a puncture from a sharp pubic fracture fragment or indirectly by avulsion of the ligaments and the wall when the ring is displaced. Bladder contusions occur frequently with fractures of the pubic rami and ischium. Diametric fracture-dislocations resulted in an equal number of contusions and intra- and extraperitoneal extravasations.[3]

Hemorrhage in Pelvic Fractures

Bleeding surrounding the fracture site is extensive and inevitable, as most of the pelvis is a flat cancellous bone richly supplied with vessels. The bleeding into the pelvic cavity is rarely less than 500 ml and may reach 3000 ml or more.[7] Local massive bleeding has long been recognized as one of the most serious complications of a pelvic fracture, but not until recently has a satisfactory method of controlling it been available. Massive and continuous bleeding is almost always from a lacerated artery and less frequently a result of a venous laceration. It has been estimated that 60 per cent of deaths from pelvic injuries are the result of massive extraperitoneal hemorrhage.[17]

The anatomical proximity of the many branches of the internal iliac artery and vein to the inner wall of the pelvis makes them vulnerable to injury after fracture (see Fig. 21–14). Surgical exploration of the pelvis in a bleeding patient, often one with multiple injuries, in an effort to locate and ligate the torn vessel has had only limited success. Incising the retroperitoneal area already filled with blood and clot and locating the bleeding vessel is difficult, and the manipulation of the tissues and release of the tamponade increases the bleeding. Attempts to control the hemorrhage by ligating the main feeder vessel, the hypogastric artery, have also had a very meager rate of success. The extensive collateral circulation about the pelvis, which is so vital after interruption of the iliac artery, negates the effect of ligation of a major vessel in this area.

Ring and Margolies and their associates have employed angiography to pinpoint the site of bleeding in the pelvis. Most severe hemorrhage after pelvic fracture is arterial. An intraarterial catheter introduced via the femoral or left axillary artery is advanced to the internal iliac artery or just distal to the origin of this vessel. Bleeding vessels are identified by angiography, and the bleeding is controlled with selective embolization using autologous clotted blood deposited proximal to the bleeding vessel or into the internal iliac artery itself. Failure to find an arterial bleeding point or continued bleeding after arterial embolization calls for an examination of the venous system. The precise bleeding site in the vein can be identified by injecting dye into a catheter placed in the femoral vein and advanced to the internal iliac vein, but a clot embolus cannot be injected because of the flow toward the inferior vena cava. A balloon tip may, however, be used to occlude the internal iliac vein.[12, 17]

Neurological Injuries

Nerve lesions with pelvic fractures are often overlooked, as the surgeon's attention is concentrated on the more immediate problems. The necessity of an orderly, thorough, fully recorded examination must again be emphasized. In a series of 633 patients with pelvic fractures, Patterson and Morton found an incidence of 3.5 per cent of neurological complications.[13] The level of the lesion is difficult to place, and there is no specific pattern of neurological impairment or particular nerve structure that is predominantly injured. Neurological complications are seen with the more severe fractures, usually are unilateral and confined to the side of the pelvis that is displaced. About 10 per cent of the neurological complications cause disturbances of bowel and bladder function.

The level of the lesion varies in each case. Displaced pelvic fractures could easily cause a lumbosacral plexus injury, as the plexus rests on the inner side of the wing of the ilium. Root avulsions just distal to the foramen have been reported by Harris and others. In such cases, they found, myelography showed dural diverticula or scarring (Fig. 21–8). They noted that the prognosis for recovery in patients with tears of the dural sleeve was good in contrast to that associated with the same myelographic findings in the cervical spine. As the lumbar roots are more slack than the roots in the cervical column, a dural tear in this area should not be interpreted as a complete tear of the root and the damage need not be irreversible.[8]

Cases of disk rupture have been reported following pelvic fracture, and myelography should be considered to help in the interpretation of nerve damage. Full recovery after nerve lesions due to root or plexus traction or peripheral nerve pressure is infrequent, although some degree of recovery can be expected.

Impotence is a common postfracture complaint. King noted that 43 per cent of patients with pelvic fractures complicated by urethral injury complained of impotence.[11] It would appear that this complaint is related to damage to the penile blood supply or injury to the nervi erigentes rather than to an injury to the autonomic nervous system.

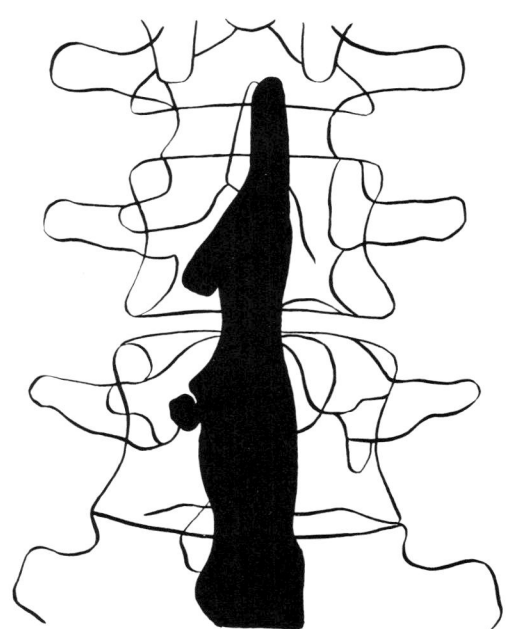

Figure 21–8 Drawing of a myelogram showing dural diverticula of the fourth and fifth lumbar roots resulting from root avulsions following a pelvic fracture.

Pregnancy and Pelvic Fractures

Obstetrical problems arising from a pelvic fracture can threaten an existing pregnancy as well as impair future parturition. Any fracture of the forepelvis or separation of the pelvis will frequently cause an abortion. When such a fracture occurs late in pregnancy it is unwise to attempt a reduction of the fracture until a spontaneous delivery or a cesarian section is done. In pregnancy after a deforming fracture of the pelvis, osteotomies or pelvic realignment are contraindicated in view of the fact that cesarian section has a mortality rate of less than 0.2 per cent when performed electively.

AVULSION FRACTURES

A sudden uncontrolled contraction of any muscle attached to the pelvis may avulse a fragment of bone from the pelvis. Most commonly this injury occurs in an adolescent between puberty and 25 years of age when the developing apophyses have not yet firmly united to the pelvis.

Damage to adjacent structures is rare in this type of injury.

Avulsion of the Anterior Superior Spine

The anterior portion of the iliac crest apophysis can be detached by the pull of the sartorius muscle (Fig. 21–9). This injury usually results from a strenuous effort, as in sprinting or jumping. The individual is forced out of further play be immediate and severe pain localized to the anterior superior spine and the anterior thigh. Flexion and extension of the hip or knee is painful, and swelling followed by ecchymosis develops around the site of the avulsion.

Radiographs show the poorly outlined apophysis separated from the pelvic crest. With minimal separation no radiographic change may be visible, but the diagnosis is not difficult to make on a clinical basis. Comparison with the opposite anterior superior spine may show an asymmetry in the appearance of this structure, and oblique views of the pelvis may show the separation more clearly. Wide displacement of this apophysis is unusual.

Treatment is simply to avoid weight bearing for three weeks with supportive therapy for relief of pain. Fibrous union between the displaced fragment and the pelvis occurs without any functional loss.

Avulsion of the Anterior Inferior Spine

A sudden uncontrolled pull of the rectus femoris muscle can detach the apophysis of the anterior inferior spine (see Fig. 21–9). The adolescent athlete develops sudden groin pain after kicking a football, running, or jumping. Tenderness is localized to the anterior inferior spine, and both active and passive flexion and extension of the hip and knee are painful.

Radiographs show a fragment of bone inferior to the anterior inferior spine. Displacement is usually limited by the reflected head of the rectus femoris, which is anchored to the hip capsule. Under these circumstances the only therapy necessary is to avoid weight bearing for three weeks. If the reflected head is torn, more displacement will occur, permitting the rectus to shorten and thus losing some of its strength.

When the downward displacement is great and the avulsed fragment lies distal to the hip joint, one may be justified in pulling the rectus muscle and the attached bone fragment upward and suturing it to the inferior spine. A single hip spica for four weeks insures that the repair will not disrupt.

Avulsion of the Ischial Tuberosity

This apophysis is avulsed when the adolescent athlete suddenly accelerates when

Figure 21–9 The pelvic apophyses that are most often avulsed. The anterior portion of the iliac crest is detached by the pull of the sartorius muscle, the anterior inferior spine by the rectus femoris, and the tuberosity of the ischium by the hamstrings.

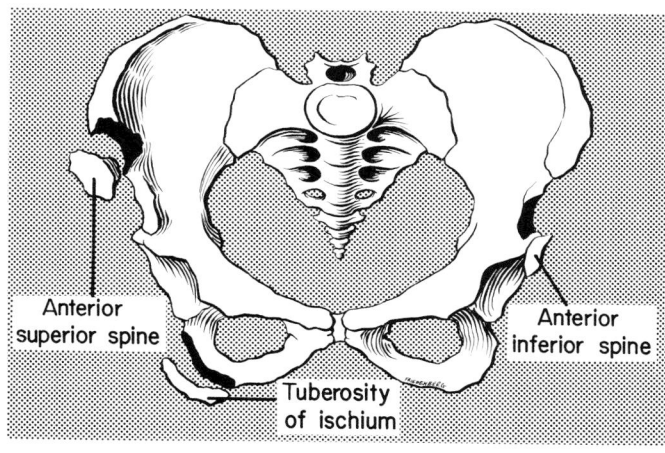

sprinting (see Fig. 21–9). The patient pulls up suddenly and falls to the ground with severe pain in one buttock that radiates into the hamstring muscles. Tenderness is clearly localized to the ischial tuberosity, and attempts to raise the straight leg are very painful. Later, swelling of the buttock and upper thigh with ecchymosis is seen.

Radiographs show the avulsed tuberosity, and varying degrees of separation may be encountered. Avulsions in this area are frequently widely separated.

Those minimally displaced are best treated by avoiding weight bearing for three to four weeks. A tuberosity that is widely separated should be repaired to avoid shortening and loss of strength of the hamstring muscles. It has been shown that those athletes with a wide separation that was not repaired suffered permanent impairment of running ability. Power in the hamstrings one year after injury was reduced 22 per cent.[18] To repair the avulsion, the hamstring with the apophysis is drawn upward to restore its original length, and the apophysis is sutured to the tuberosity. The restoration of length becomes very difficult if more than two weeks has elapsed. A spica cast with the knee flexed and the hip extended is necessary to prevent disruption of the repair.

In any of the avulsions just discussed, the occasional patient will continue to complain of pain at the injury site long afterward, and late excision of the apophysis may be justified. The development of osteochondroma at the site of apophyseal avulsions has also been described.

ISOLATED FRACTURES WITHOUT SEPARATION OF THE PELVIC RING

In this type of injury the break is confined to one part of the ring, and no significant displacement or deformity of the pelvis is possible. Dunn and Morris term this type of injury a stable fracture of the ring. In their series of 115 pelvic fractures, 77 were of this type.[6]

Fractures of the Pubic Rami

Fractures of the pubic rami were most common in this group. One, two, or three

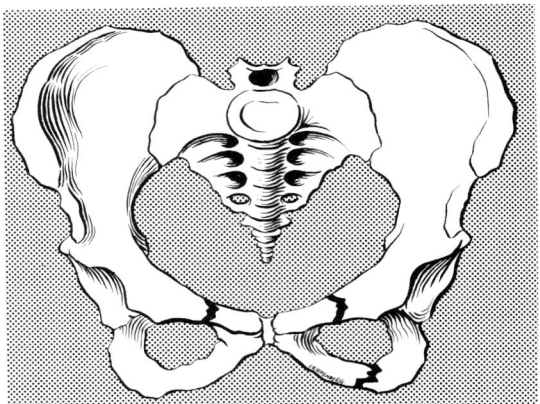

Figure 21–10 Three rami have been fractured, but the ring still retains its stability.

rami may be fractured and the ring will still retain its integrity, but when both rami on each side of the pubic symphysis are fractured, displacement of the forepelvis will result, and this gap in the ring leaves it unstable (Fig. 21–10).

The stable forepelvis fracture results from a blow on the anterior pelvis, and despite the fact that the ring does not yield, it is often associated with serious injury to the contained viscera and severe hemorrhage as well as life-threatening trauma to other areas of the body (Fig. 21–11). Even in those patients with moderate, self-limited retroperitoneal bleeding, ileus occurs frequently, and the use of intravenous fluids and a nasogastric tube is advisable until bowel sounds return.

Unilateral fracture of a single or both pubic rami commonly occurs in elderly patients after a fall. It mimics a hip fracture (Fig. 21–12). Careful examination will readily show that gentle movements of the hip are painless. Abduction and external rotation that stretch the hip adductors will cause pain in the pubic area, and palpation will show focal tenderness over the fracture site.

As the pelvic ring is intact in this type of fracture, no specific therapy is necessary other than recumbency until the pain diminishes. It is unwise to permit the patient to remain immobile in bed until the last vestige of pain has gone, however, as no harm will result from early weight bearing, and prolonged immobility combined with local swelling and the possibility of damage

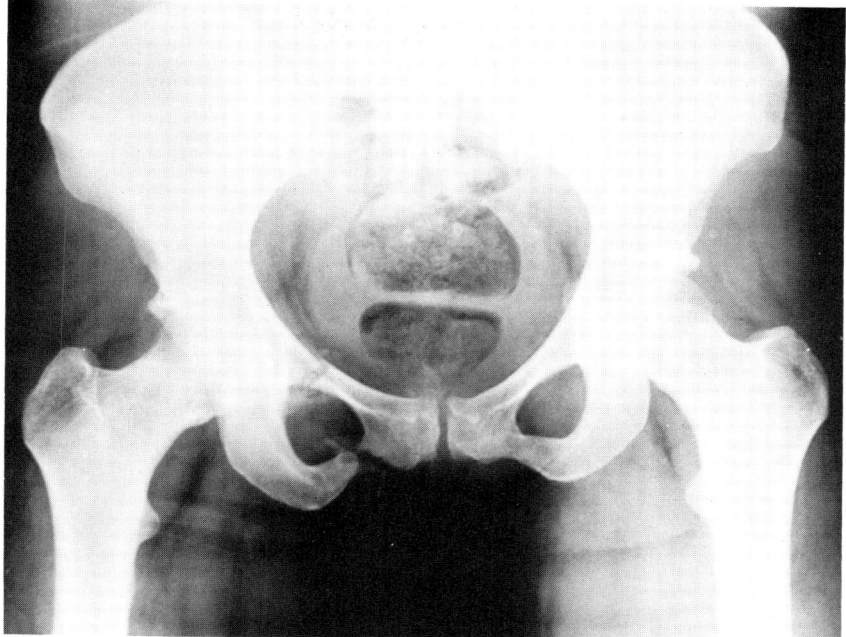

Figure 21-11 Fracture of both pubic rami on the right. Visceral damage is frequent with this type of fracture, but the fracture itself requires no specific therapy.

Figure 21-12 Fracture of both pubic rami from a fall in an 82-year-old white woman who is markedly osteoporotic. Clinically the fracture can be mistaken for a hip fracture.

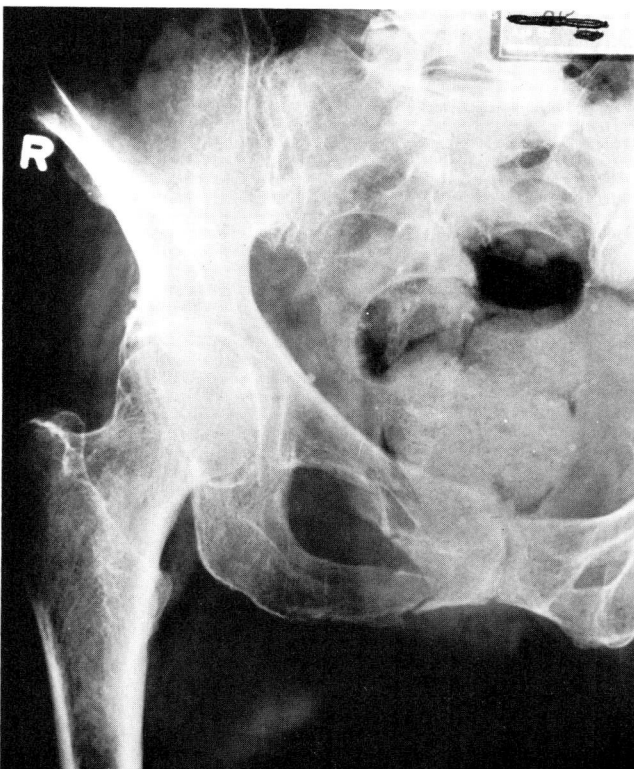

to the pelvic veins may result in thrombosis or embolism. Leg exercises, elastic stockings, and elevation of the bed should be initiated on admission of the patient. When local bleeding is thought to have ceased, the use of anticoagulants should be considered.

Stress fractures of the pubis or ischium may be seen in individuals who have sharply increased their physical activities. Repeated stress due to muscular activity propagates a fine linear crack that spreads across the bone. The patient complains of difficulty in walking due to pain localized to the forepelvis, usually at the ischiopubic junction. Radiographs show a fine crack with a widespread callus reaction. Bed rest or avoidance of weight bearing on the involved side for several weeks permits healing to occur.

Fractures of the Wing of the Ilium

Fractures of the wing of the ilium are usually the result of a fall or a heavy blow directly over this bone (Fig. 21–13). The integrity of the ring remains intact, but severe retroperitoneal hemorrhage and visceral damage are common, and the patient with this condition should be carefully observed and monitored. Tenderness, swelling, and deformity of the ilium are found, and ecchymosis develops later. The patient's activities should be restricted until the pain diminishes. Separation is rarely severe and reduction is usually not indicated (Fig. 21–14).

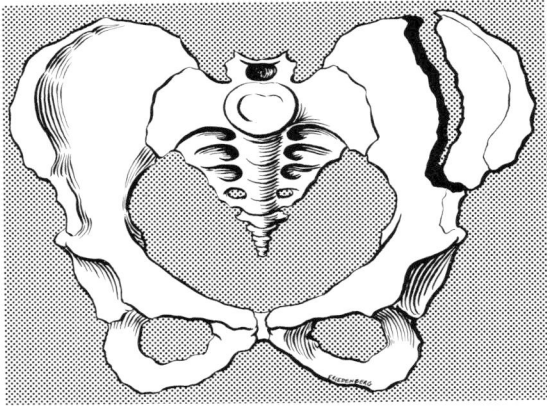

Figure 21–13 Fracture of the wing of the ilium, slightly displaced, the result of a direct blow.

Fractures of the Sacrum

This fracture is the result of a fall in the sitting position or a direct blow to the sacrum (Fig. 21–15). The distal fragment usually angulates forward and is impacted. On examination, pain is well localized to the fracture site; a rectal examination will pinpoint the tenderness at the fracture site, but no abnormal movement can be detected because of the bone impaction. Radiographs are difficult to interpret because of the impaction, but a lateral view will frequently show an angular deviation inconsistent with the normal anterior concavity of the sacrum. Laminography will also more clearly bring out the features of the fracture. No specific therapy is necessary, but the pain may persist for several weeks.

Marked displacement of a sacral fracture is uncommon. Those that have been described are fractures in which the distal segment is angulated forward and may be associated with sacral root impairment and paralysis of the bladder. In these cases, early surgery to free the roots by a wide laminectomy and foraminotomies should be considered.

Fractures of the Coccyx

This fracture follows a fall in the sitting position. The coccyx is composed of four segments, and the fracture may occur as a fracture-dislocation of the sacrococcygeal joint or through any of the segments. Anterior or anterolateral displacement is common. Sitting is very painful, and lying supine may also be painful. Sudden movements in turning and walking may be painful, as the gluteus maximus and the sacrospinous and sacrotuberous ligaments insert on the sides of the coccyx. Tenderness is present over the coccyx; a rectal examination will reveal marked tenderness at the fracture site, and movement at the fracture site can often be appreciated.

Fractures or dislocations are clearly shown on radiographs. The pain may persist for many weeks, and the patient gets most relief from sitting on his posterior thighs, avoiding chair contact with the coccygeal area. The use of an inflatable ring for sitting is helpful. Residual deformity

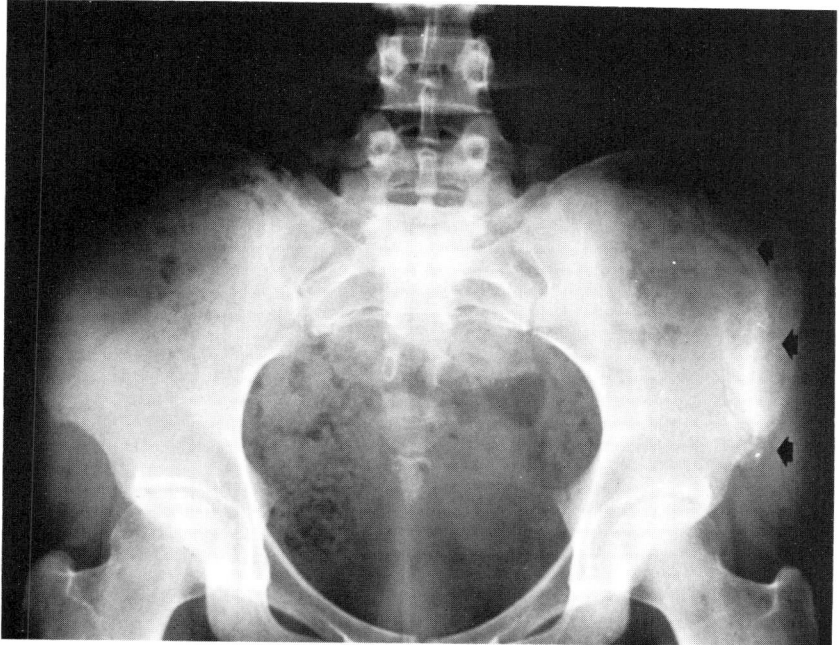

Figure 21–14 An undisplaced fracture of the iliac wing. Hemorrhage and visceral damage may accompany this fracture.

does not cause disability and does not complicate subsequent parturition.

Infrequently, the coccyx remains chronically painful after a fracture. Such patients may get good results from coccygectomy. Coccygectomy for coccygeal pain without a specific antecedent fracture, however, rarely gives relief and has been justly criticized. In many of these patients with long-standing coccygeal pain, the problem is located elsewhere in the spine and is referred to the coccyx.

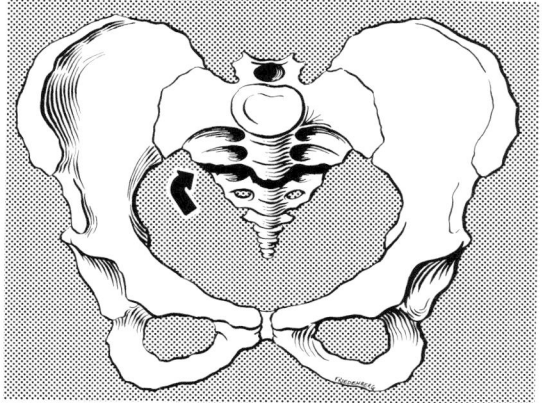

Figure 21–15 Fracture through the sacrum.

FRACTURES WITH LOSS OF CONTINUITY OF PELVIC RING (UNSTABLE)

Double Breaks in the Forepelvis — Bilateral Fractures of Both Pubic Rami

This injury is usually the result of a direct anterior blow or lateral compression of the pelvis (Figs. 21–16 and 21–17). It is an unstable fracture and has been termed a "straddle fracture" by Pennal and Sutherland because of the frequent history of a fall with the impact against the forepelvis.[15] This fracture may involve both pubic rami on each side of the intact symphysis or both pubic rami on one side and a separation at the symphysis. In either type, a segment of the forepelvis loses continuity with the ring. Displacement of the fractured segment is usually not great because of the many muscle attachments to the fractured segment.

Peltier regards this fracture as the most dangerous of all pelvic fractures because of the frequency of associated injuries to the abdominal viscera and severe local hemorrhage. Such fractures constituted 20 per cent of the 186 pelvic fractures in his

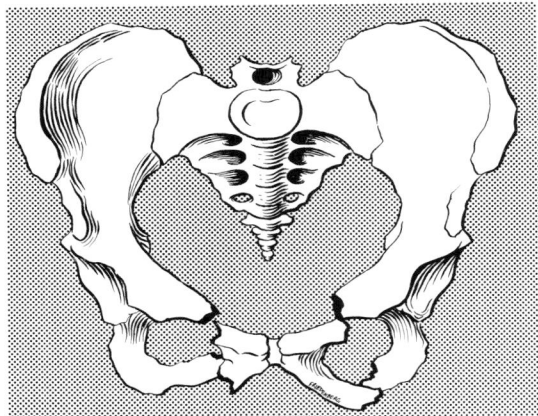

Figure 21–16 Double breaks in the forepelvis. The ring is unstable. This type of fracture is frequently associated with hemorrhage or visceral injury.

series, and 19 per cent of the patients in this group died as a result of complications from associated injuries.[14] Patients with this injury should be observed carefully, as described earlier in this chapter.

The treatment of this fracture or fracture-dislocation is bed rest with the patient in a semisitting position with the thighs flexed and adducted to relax the abdominal and hip adductor muscles that are attached to the fractured fragment. Bed rest should be maintained until the early stage of union can be seen on radiographs. Nonunion is rare, and displacement or failure of union does not interfere with weight bearing. Open reduction is not indicated.

DIAMETRIC FRACTURES

In a diametric fracture two opposite areas of the ring, one anteriorly and one posteriorly on the same side of the pelvis, are broken so that the hemipelvis is free to separate. In such a fracture or fracture-dislocation, the anterior break may be through the separated symphysis or both pubic rami. The posterior break may be through the wing of the ilium, at the sacroiliac joint, or through the sacrum. A fracture of the superior and inferior pubic rami with sacroiliac dislocation is the most common variant.* In a series of fractures with pelvic displacement reported by

_____

*This is called a Malgaigne fracture after the nineteenth century French surgeon.

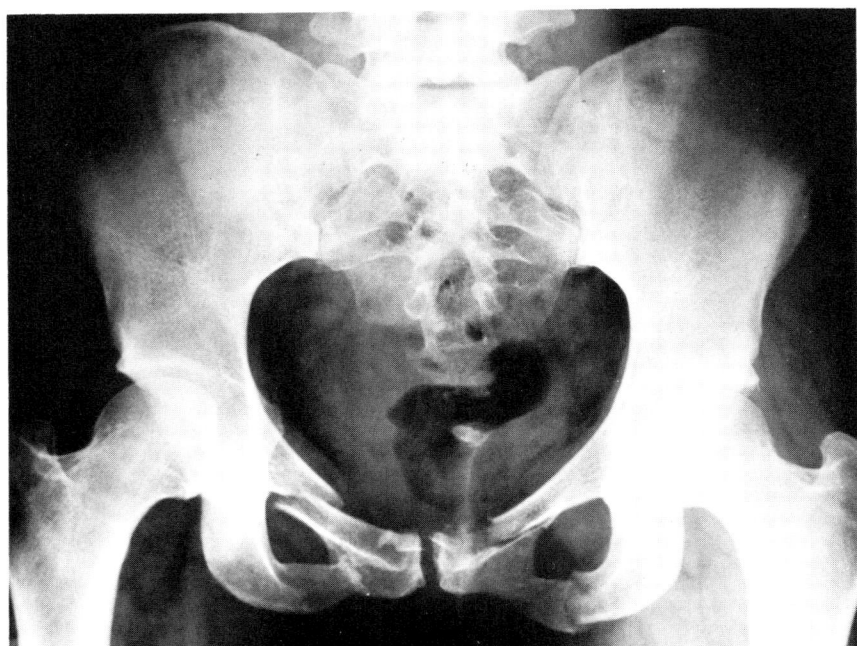

Figure 21–17   A direct blow to the anterior pelvis caused these fractures of both pubic rami on both sides.

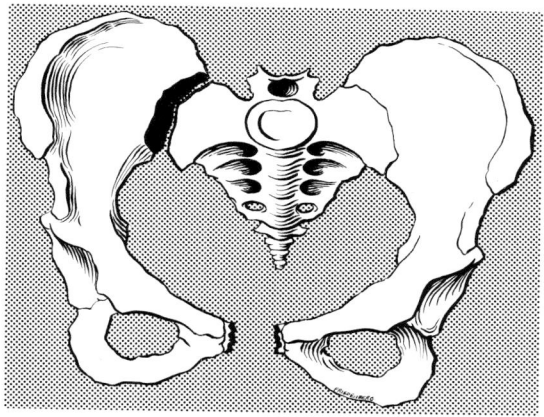

Figure 21-18 A diametric fracture, the right hemipelvis being displaced upward. The anterior injury is a wide separation of the symphysis. The posterior, a sacroiliac dislocation.

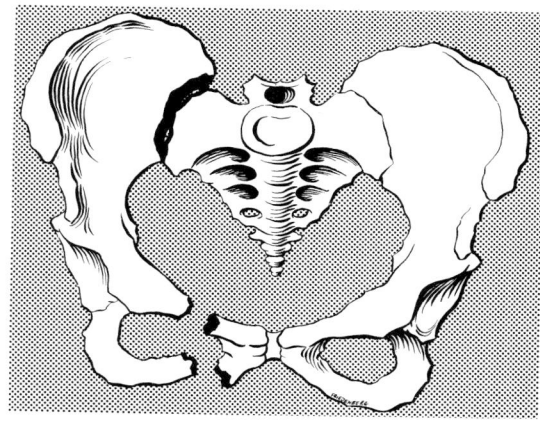

Figure 21-20 A diametric fracture; the anterior separation is a fracture of both pubic rami and the posterior is a sacroiliac dislocation.

Holdsworth, 27 of 42 such injuries showed sacroiliac dislocation associated with a pubic fracture.[9]

Displacement of the hemipelvis is usually upward, with a rotatory component in the sagittal plane opening outward like an open book, the hinge being the posterior fracture or fracture-dislocation. Less often the hemipelvis is displaced inward and overlaps the opposite hemipelvis (Figs. 21-18, 21-19, and 21-20).

A diametric fracture may result from an indirect force transmitted through the femur that is held in a flexed position

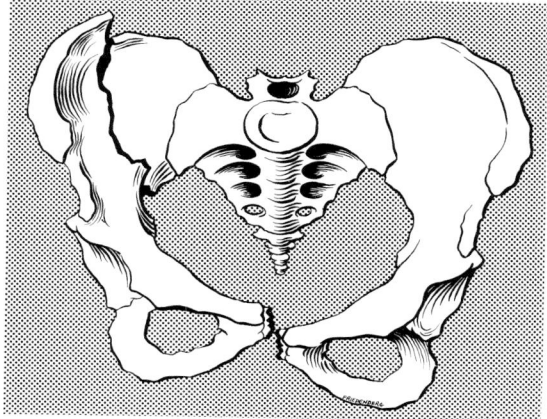

Figure 21-19 A diametric fracture: the anterior separation at the symphysis, the posterior separation a fracture through the ilium.

midway between abduction and adduction. The impact of the femoral head displaces the hemipelvis upward and outward and causes a diastasis anteriorly. This injury may also result from an anterolateral rotatory force or direct lateral compression (Figs. 21-21 and 21-22). In the latter case, the pelvis overlaps and its transverse diameter is narrowed. Overlapping of the pelvis due to lateral compression is an infrequent injury; fracture of the pubic rami without pelvic displacement is most common following lateral compression.

Because visceral injuries and retroperitoneal bleeding are common in diametric fractures, the patient should be fully investigated and carefully observed.

When the hemipelvis is displaced upward and rotated outward, the limb on that side will also be in external rotation. The anterior defect can often be palpated and is sometimes a gap large enough to put a fist through. Movement of the limb is transmitted to the displaced hemipelvis and is painful. Assymmetry of the pelvis may be noted, and tenderness is present both anteriorly and posteriorly. Radiographic examination clearly shows the pelvic separation anteriorly, but the sacroiliac dislocation is not easily seen, as the hemipelvis that is rotated in the sagittal plane is not well shown on the usual radiographic views. Good quality radiographs are required.

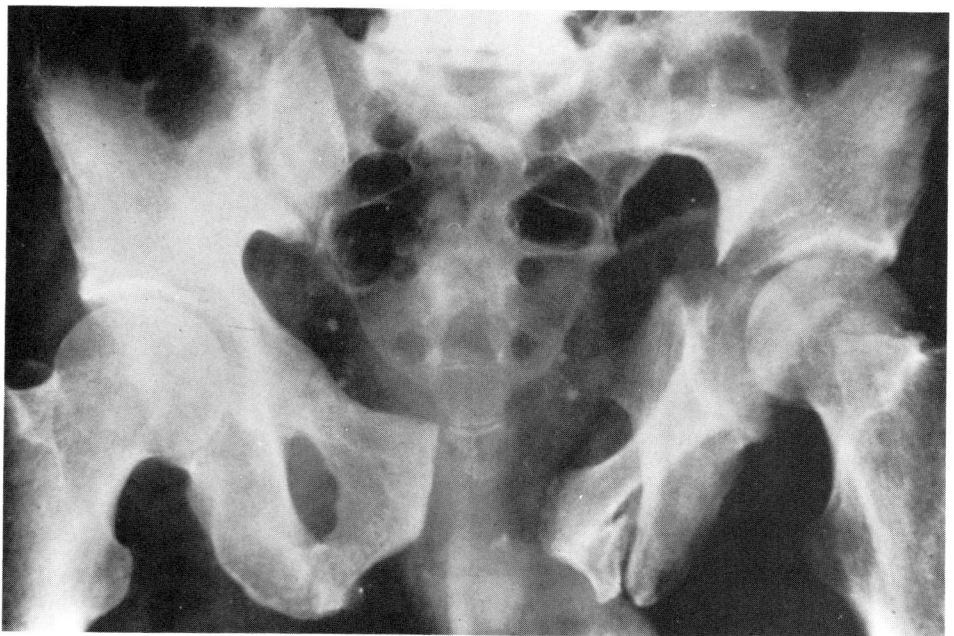

Figure 21–21 A diametric fracture with wide disruption of the symphysis and a dislocation of the sacroiliac joint. The left hemipelvis is displaced upward and externally rotated.

Two methods of treatment for the spread-open pelvis have been used. The sling method was first described by Astley Cooper and also recommended by Bohler.[1, 4] Watson-Jones has advocated the method of lateral recumbency followed by plaster immobilization (Fig. 21–23.)[21]

Watson-Jones recommends that the anesthetized patient be placed in lateral recumbency on his uninjured side, an assis-

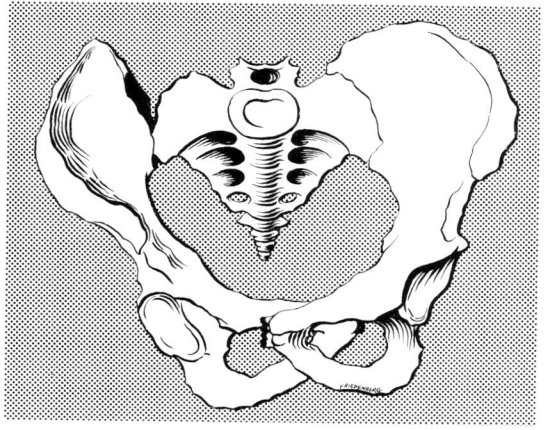

Figure 21–22 Overlapped pelvis.

tant holding one leg over the other. The dislocation is often reduced as soon as the patient is placed in lateral recumbency; if it is not, the surgeon manipulates the pelvis, pushing downward and forward. Radiographs are taken to check the reduction, and the patient is placed in a bilateral short leg hip spica for three months. During anesthesia the bladder and urethra can be repaired if necessary.[21]

The author has found the lateral recumbency and plaster method of Watson-Jones difficult in practice and contraindicated in the seriously injured patient with multiple fractures, visceral, or bleeding complications. The sling method is simple, requires no anesthesia or plaster, and permits continued observation of the abdomen.

A canvas sling extending from the trochanter to just above the iliac crests is passed under the patient's pelvis as a hammock and suspended by weights so that the buttocks just clear the bed. Stiffening rods keep the sling from folding. The sling itself will not close the opened pelvis, however, until it is relieved of the weight of the externally rotated and extended lower limb. A Steinmann pin inserted in

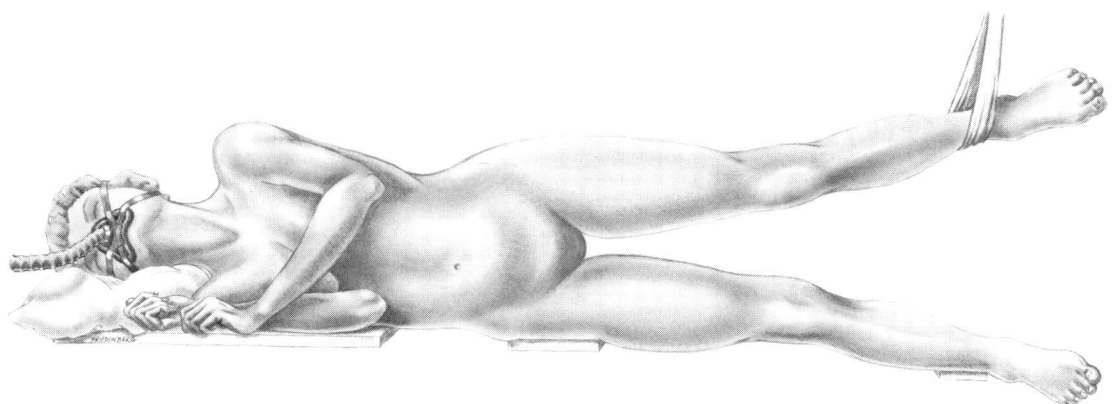

Figure 21–23   The Watson-Jones method of pelvic reduction employing lateral recumbency.

the tibia just distal to the tibial tubercle and attached to weights is used to flex the knee and hip about 30 degrees and maintain neutral rotation. Traction on the pin acts to reduce the upward displacement of the hemipelvis (Fig. 21–24).

Closure of the separated halves of the pelvis is usually well accomplished by this method of sling traction. Therapy can be discontinued after four weeks, and the patient is maintained in a canvas sacroiliac support for an additional four weeks. Fre-

quently, the traction cannot overcome the upward displacement of the hemipelvis when the sacroiliac joint is dislocated. Fractures of the ilium offer no problem in this respect. When the sacroiliac joint remains incompletely reduced, few symptoms develop on weight bearing if full weight bearing is delayed 8 to 10 weeks to permit firm scar tissue and bone to form across the sacroiliac joint. A canvas sacroiliac support should be worn for several months. Delayed weight bearing also per-

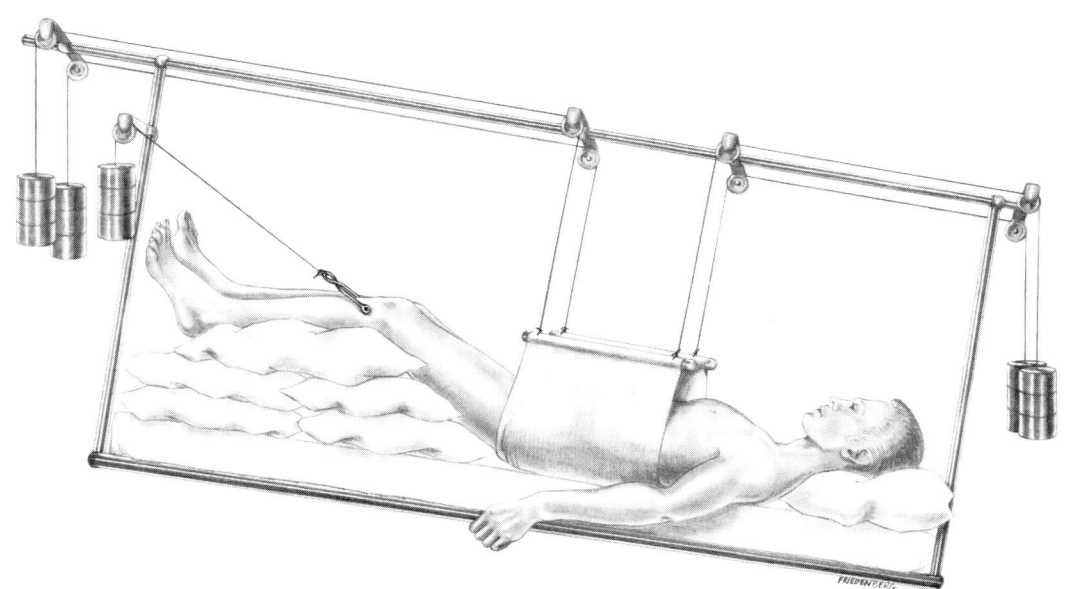

Figure 21–24   Reduction of the displaced pelvis by pelvic sling and traction.

mits firm soft-tissue healing of symphyseal separations and allows pubic fractures to heal. Nonunion is infrequent.

A few patients will continue to complain of sacroiliac pain on weight bearing that is only partially relieved by a pelvic support. Two anteroposterior films of the pelvis, one taken with the weight on one leg and a second with the weight on the other leg, will demonstrate abnormal movement between the two halves of the pelvis. In such a patient with an unstable pelvis, sacroiliac fusion is indicated.

Diametric Fractures with Fracture of the Ilium

Diametric fractures in which the posterior injury is a fracture of the ilium have a better prognosis. The pelvic sling–traction therapy reduces the fracture and may be replaced with a pelvic support after four weeks. The fracture is usually healed at eight weeks, and weight bearing can then be permitted. There is no problem involving anatomical reduction of a joint and no subsequent instability.

Overlapped Hemipelves

This type of a diametric fracture results from a crushing force applied laterally to the pelvis. Visceral injury is common. The pelvic cavity is reduced, and if the posterior injury is a sacroiliac dislocation, the displacement is inward. If the posterior injury is an iliac fracture there is overriding. This type of injury is made worse by a sling, but can be reduced by the turnbuckle method of Jahss (Fig. 21–25) Cylinder casts, well-padded with felt over the adductor area of the thighs and the lateral part of the legs, are applied to both lower extremities, with one turnbuckle connecting the midthigh areas and a second turnbuckle connecting the cylinders at the midleg level. The proximal turnbuckle is gradually opened, the lower turnbuckle closed. A distracting force is applied to the pelvis via the capsule of the hip joints. Reduction is done under x-ray control over a 24 hour period. The cylinders and turnbuckles maintain position for four weeks or may be replaced during this period by a bilateral spica extending to the knees.[10]

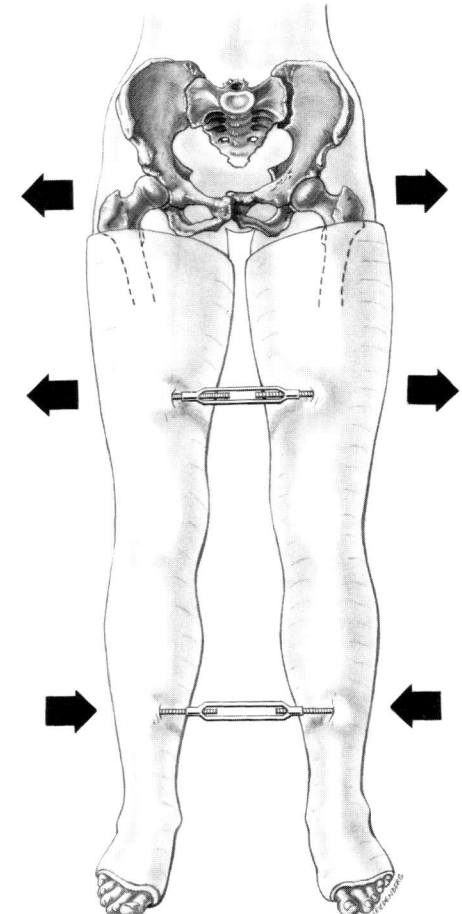

Figure 21–25   The method of Jahss to reduce an overlapped pelvis.

When there is marked overlapping, this method may prove inadequate and an open reduction may be indicated if the patient's condition permits. Through an anterior retroperitoneal incision, the pelvic halves are levered back into place and held in a bilateral spica to the knees.[19]

REFERENCES

1. Bohler, L.: The Treatment of Fractures. 4th Ed. Bristol, John Wright & Sons, 1935.
2. Brosman, S. A., and Fay, R.: Diagnosis and management of bladder trauma. J. Trauma, 13:8: 687–694, 1973.
3. Cass, A. S., and Ireland, G. W.: Bladder trauma associated with pelvic fractures in severely injured patients. J. Trauma, 13:3:205–212, 1973.

4. Cooper, A.: A Treatise on Fractures and Dislocation of Joints. London, J. & A. Churchill, Ltd., 1842.

5. Domisse, G. F.: Diametric fractures of pelvis. J. Bone Joint Surg., *42B*:432–443, 1960.

6. Dunn, A. W., and Morris, H. D.: Fractures and dislocations of the pelvis. J. Bone Joint Surg., *50A*:1639–1648, 1968.

7. Froman, C., and Stein, A.: Complicated crushing injuries of the pelvis. J. Bone Joint Surg., *49B*: 24–32, 1967.

8. Harris, W. R., Rathbun, J. B., Wortzman, G., et al.: Avulsion of lumbar roots complicating fracture of pelvis. J. Bone Joint Surg., *55A*:1436–1442, 1973.

9. Holdsworth, F. H.: Dislocation and fracture-dislocation of the pelvis. J. Bone Joint Surg., *30B*:461–466, 1948.

10. Jahss, S. A.: Injuries involving the ilium; a new treatment. J. Bone Joint Surg., *17*:338–346, 1935.

11. King, J.: Impotence after pelvic fracture. J. Bone Joint Surg., *57A*:1107–1110, 1975.

12. Margolies, M. N., Ring, E. J., Waltman, A. C., et al.: Arteriography in the management of hemorrhage from pelvic fractures. N. Engl. J. Med., *287*:7:317–321, 1972.

13. Patterson, F. P., and Morton, K. S.: Neurological complications of fractures and dislocations of the pelvis. J. Trauma, *12*:12:1013–1016, 1973.

14. Peltier, L. F.: Complications associated with fractures of the pelvis. J. Bone Joint Surg., *47A*: 1060–1072, 1965.

15. Pennal, G. F., and Sutherland, G.: Fractures of pelvis. Motion Picture from American Academy of Orthopaedic Surgery Library, 1961.

16. Reynolds, B. M., Balsano, N. A., and Reynolds, F. X.: Pelvic fractures. J. Trauma, *13*:11:1011–1014, 1973.

17. Ring, E. J., Waltman, A. C., Athanasoulis, C., et al.: Angiography in pelvic trauma. Surg. Gynecol. Obstet., *139*:375–380, 1974.

18. Schlonsky, J., and Olix, M. L.: Avulsion fractures of the ischial epiphysis. J. Bone Joint Surg., *54A*:641–644, 1972.

19. Shanmugasundaram, T. K.: Unusual dislocation of symphysis pubis with locking. J. Bone Joint Surg., *52A*:1669–1671, 1970.

20. Trunkey, D. D., Chapman, M. W., Lim, R. C., Jr., et al.: Management of pelvic fractures in blunt trauma injury. J. Trauma, *14*:11:912–923, 1974.

21. Watson-Jones, R.: Fractures and Joint Injuries. Edinburgh, E. & S. Livingstone, 3rd Ed. 1943.

R. BRUCE HEPPENSTALL, M.D.

22 Fractures and Dislocations of the Hip

Part I — FRACTURES OF THE HIP

The diagnosis and management of fractures of the hip continue to present an important challenge to physicians who treat patients who have suffered trauma. In the past several decades, however, new concepts have evolved in regard to the mechanism of production of this injury, and there are also new ideas about the immediate management of the patient with a fractured hip.

Fracture of the hip is primarily an injury of the aged. It is being seen with increasing frequency because improved medical care has increased the number of elderly persons in the general population, and it is now more important than ever that physicians and the general public recognize the fractured hip, for early diagnosis and treatment are essential to improving survival rates. The trend in recent years has been, through early open reduction and internal fixation, to mobilize these patients as quickly as possible and so to avoid the disastrous complications of prolonged immobilization of these old people. This goal has been accomplished by innovative surgical procedures to obtain stability at the fracture site and improved technical design and quality of metallic devices for internal fixation.

Although the patients are in a high-risk category owing to their advancing age and concomitant medical problems, several studies have revealed a definite decrease in the morbidity and the mortality rate following aggressive surgical treatment. Results to date certainly justify the concept of early treatment and energetic physical therapy to return these patients to an active role in society.

Ambrose Paré (1510-1590) must be given credit as the first physician to diagnose a fracture of the hip and distinguish it from a dislocated hip. His treatment included splints and compresses with bed rest. It was Astley Cooper (1768–1841) who first categorized femoral neck fractures of the hip. He felt that the prognosis was poor with intracapsular fractures, owing to a loss of blood supply, but was better with other types of hip fractures. Von Langenbeck (1850) was the first to utilize a metal device in the treatment of a femoral neck fracture.

In 1902 Whitman introduced the concept of closed manipulation followed by the application of a hip spica. He noted an improved prognosis for union.[213] The most important advance in recent times in the treatment of these injuries came in 1931

630

when Smith-Petersen reported a series of patients treated with a triflange nail.[182] With this development, a new era opened for the internal fixation of hip fractures, and during the following decade both the quality and the type of material utilized underwent improvement.

A further advance was the addition of a side plate to the nail to increase stability. In 1941 Jewett introduced a single nail and plate combination.[112a] Since that time several nail-plate combinations have been reported.

In 1958 Deyerle perfected a side plate that also acted as a template, allowing sliding of multiple pins.[57] The sliding nail concept was further expanded with the introduction of the Pugh nail and the compression hip screw, devices that have enlarged our concept of the treatment of fractures, as they allow compression at the fracture site without protrusion of the nail through the femoral head.[159]

ANATOMY OF THE HIP

The hip joint is a synovial joint of the ball and socket type. It is inherently the most stable joint of this type in the body. This is in part owing to the anatomical configuration of the globular femoral head within the acetabular cavity and the surrounding powerful musculature.

Muscles and Ligaments. The iliopsoas is the main flexor of the hip joint. It is aided in this function by the rectus femoris, sartorius, pectineus, and adductor longus. Extension is provided by the gluteus maximus, the long hamstrings, and the ischial part of the adductor magnus. Hip abduction is provided by the gluteus medius and gluteus minimus together with the tensor fasciae latae. These muscles help to prevent the contralateral pelvic sagging known as "Trendelenburg's sign." Important diagnostically, this sign is produced by having the patient elevate one hip and noting the position of the opposite hip as it holds the entire weight of the body. If the abductor mechanism is paralyzed, the pelvis on the side of the elevated leg will drop because contralateral power of the abductor musculature to balance and control it is lacking. Adduction is provided by the adductors

magnus, longus, and brevis, the pectineus, and the gracilus. External rotation is provided by the gluteus maximus, quadratus femoris, obturator externus, obturator internus, and gemelli. Internal rotation is produced by the tensor fasciae latae and the anterior fibers of the gluteus minimus. The external rotators are significantly more powerful than the internal rotators.

The capsule reaches anteriorly to the intertrochanteric line, but posteriorly the lateral half of the neck is extracapsular. The capsule is reinforced anteriorly by the sturdy iliofemoral ligament of Bigelow. With the hip in 10 degrees of flexion, 10 degrees of abduction, and 10 degrees of external rotation, the capsule is totally slack and maximal joint capacity is present.

Blood Supply. The blood supply to the upper end of the femur is derived from both femoral circumflex arteries, the superior gluteal (probably not the inferior gluteal), the obturator, and the first perforating branch of the profunda. The intertrochanteric area is well supplied by these vessels. The femoral head and neck, however, receive their main blood supply from vessels that lie in the subcapsular area along the femoral neck, where they are exposed to variations in intra-articular pressure that may completely obliterate circulation to this area. The epiphyseal arteries supply most of the blood. Two to six in number, these vessels arise from the vascular ring at the base and run along the superior lateral aspect of the neck. Vasculature in the ligamentum teres is either completely absent or is only adequate to supply a small area surrounding the ligamentous insertion. The inferior lateral quadrant of the femoral head is supplied by two or three metaphyseal arteries.

These specific differences in vascular supply are responsible for the marked differences in healing and avascular necrosis in femoral neck fractures and intertrochanteric fractures; the latter have an excellent blood supply. It is for this reason that several authors have advised aspiration of the hip joint as soon as the diagnosis of a femoral neck fracture is established. The hope is that reducing the increased pressure within the capsular area will relieve the tension on the vessels under the capsule. It has also been suggested that the capsule should be opened during internal fixation to allow a reduction in pressure.

Bone Structure. Structurally, the femoral head is not a perfect sphere; it is slightly compressed in an anterior-posterior direction. The neck of the femur also is not uniform throughout its length. Approximately cylindrical at its junction with the femoral head it becomes increasingly elliptical distally, toward the intertrochanteric area. The cortical shell also changes, being very thin toward the junction with the femoral head and thickest as the femoral shaft is approached. Therefore, the cortical bone is strongest in the inferior portion of the neck.

The internal trabecular system of the femoral head was originally described by Ward.[208a] The orientation of the trabecular structure is produced by the stresses on the femoral head and femoral neck. Three main systems have been described in recent times: a lateral system extending from the lesser trochanteric area and radiating into the trochanteric area along the intertrochanteric line, a medial system originating from the inferior portion of the neck and radiating into the superior portion of the head, and an arcuate system originating from the lateral aspect of the proximal femur and radiating upward to the superior neck and downward into the inferior portion of the femoral head (Fig. 22–1).

Harty's description of the calcar femorale has helped to clarify some previous misconceptions. In the older orthopedic literature the inferior cortex of the femoral neck was often incorrectly designated the calcar. Harty has demonstrated that the calcar femorale is a laminated vertical plate of condensed bone extending laterally from the medial cortex toward the gluteal tubercle. Proximally it blends with the posterior cortex of the neck and distally, beyond the lesser trochanteric area, it fuses with the posterior medial shaft (Fig. 22–2). The significance of the calcar is that it represents a condensed portion of the bone that counteracts the posterior inferior compressive forces of the external rotators.[101] The placement of internal fixation devices in this area has been recommended because of the increased support offered by the thickened bone.

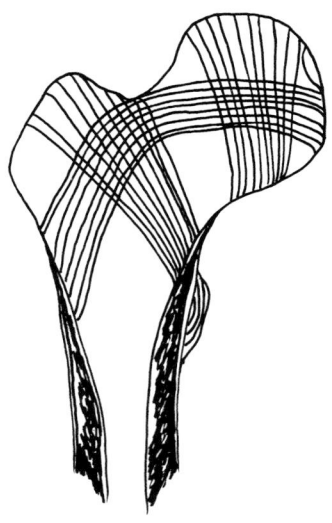

Figure 22–1 Internal trabecular system of the femoral head. Three main systems — a lateral, a medial, and an arcuate — are present.

BIOMECHANICS OF HIP FUNCTION

Rydell has contributed significantly to our understanding of the forces acting on the hip joint, which in the erect position are much greater than the superimposed body weight. This effect is produced by muscular action, particularly the abductor pull, and other dynamic forces acting directly on the joint. By inserting a prosthetic device into the hip joint and, by means of strain gauges, determining the forces acting directly on the femoral head, Rydell has demonstrated that standing on one leg creates a force on the hip joint of approximately two and a half times the body weight. During the swing phase in gait, the force acting on the joint is greater than that predicted by experimental design. The explanation for this interesting finding is that, during the stance phase, the body rolls over the femoral head and the abductors do not have to work as hard as in one-leg support. A definite force peak occurs late in the swing phase when the leg is decelerating, however, and another peak occurs shortly after the stance phase when the leg is accelerating. The dynamic effects of running produce forces up to four and a half to five times body weight. Descending stairs produces the same magnitude of force

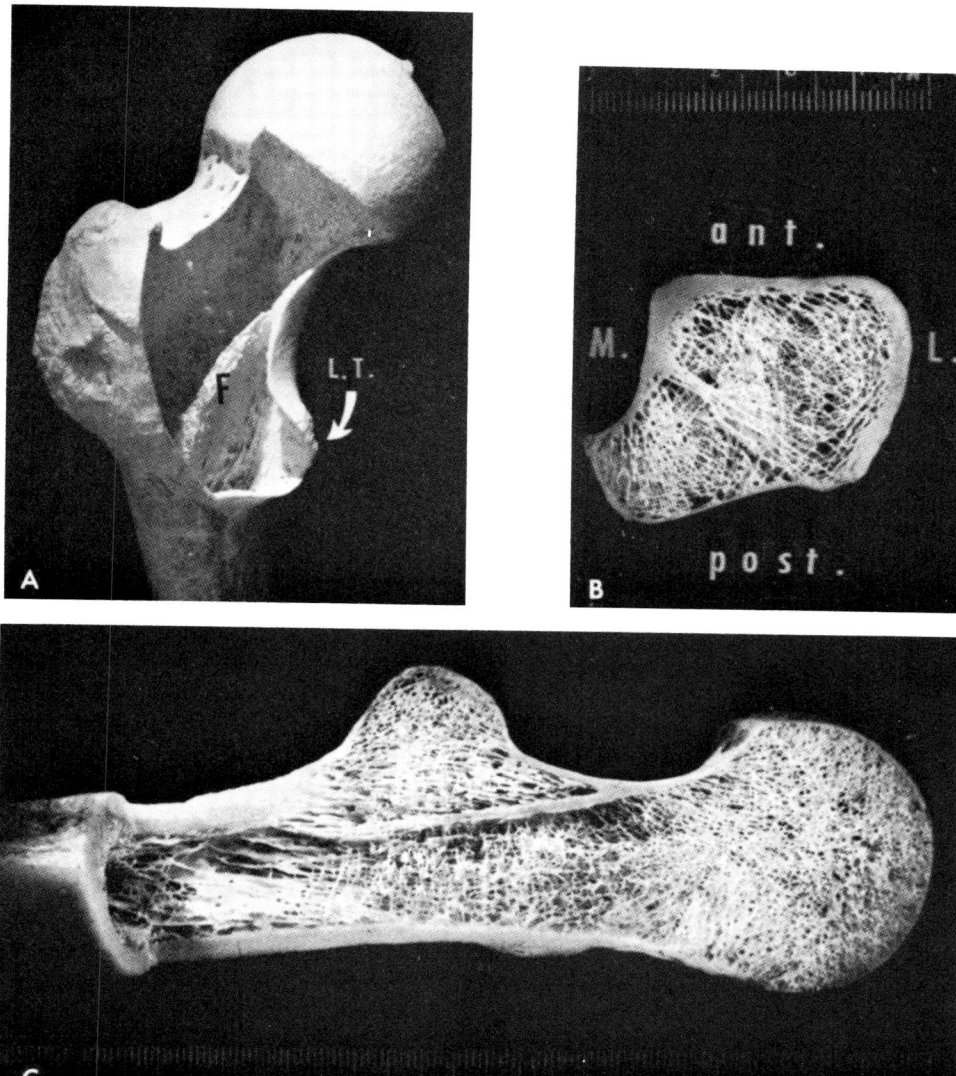

Figure 22–2   *A.* With the lesser trochanter removed, the calcar femorale is evident. *B.* Transverse section at the level of the lesser trochanter shows the calcar extending into the cancellous bone from the medial portion of the cortex. *C.* Lateral view of the lower portion of the neck of the right femur. The calcar and thin-walled intertrochanteric crest are evident. (Courtesy of M. Harty and *Journal of Bone and Joint Surgery*. The calcar femorale and the femoral neck, J.B.J.S., 39A:625–630, 1957.)

on the hip or slightly less than level walking; ascending stairs increases the load to approximately three times body weight.

If a cane is used in the opposite hand during one-leg support, the force acting on the hip joint is reduced to slightly more than body weight. The reduction of the force magnitude occurs because a cane in the opposite hand reduces the abductor force required to retain the hip joint in normal alignment. If the cane is used on the same side, the reduction of force is not as great. The force acting on the hip joint is reduced to approximately one third of body weight when the pressure of the ground is zero (when the weight of the leg is completely balanced by the muscles of the leg). When the leg is completely free of the floor, the force is approximately half of body weight.[167, 168]

A common procedure is to keep patients in bed in an attempt to unload the pressure on the hip joint. With a patient supine in bed, however, flexion of the leg with a straight knee will increase the forces acting on the opposite hip to approximately half of body weight. Abduction of the hip joint increases the force to approximately that of body weight. If traction is applied to the lower extremity with the knee and hip in the slightly flexed position, the force acting on the femoral head will be significantly decreased. This means that the traction counterbalances the muscle pull and unloads the hip joint. It is extremely important to bear these figures in mind during the management of a patient with a fractured hip, because they have a direct bearing on when that patient should be ambulatory and what type of assistive device should be utilized.

INTRACAPSULAR FRACTURES

It is very useful to divide fractures of the proximal femur into intracapsular and extracapsular. This distinction is important not only with respect to their anatomical location but also because fractures in each category differ as to age group affected, incidence, mechanism of injury, treatment, mortality rate, morbidity, and healing potential.

The age of patients with intracapsular fractures is in the middle to late sixties, which is definitely younger than patients with extracapsular fractures. Women appear to have a definite predisposition to intracapsular fractures rather than extracapsular fractures, the former being approximately twice as common as the latter in the female, whereas in the male they occur with equal frequency. The overall incidence of fractured hip is at least twice as great in females as in males.

An interesting unexplained finding is the infrequency of intracapsular fractures among Negroes. This is evident in all large series involving a significant number of Negroes. Another interesting observation is that intracapsular fractures are rare in patients with osteoarthritis of the hip.

MECHANISM OF INJURY

There is a distinct difference between mechanisms of injury in intracapsular and extracapsular fractures. Patients presenting with intracapsular fractures frequently give a history of an indirect injury. At least two basic causes, which may interact are thought to produce this type of injury. The majority of patients with femoral fractures show evidence of generalized osteoporosis or osteomalacia, and several studies have demonstrated a decrease in bone density in patients with intracapsular fractures. Decrease in bone density coupled with a decrease in the trabecular pattern within the femoral neck would certainly predispose to a fracture.

A second explanation may be that these hips are frequently the site of cyclic intermittent loading, which, in the presence of the osteoporosis, may produce microfractures.

Freeman and co-workers were able to demonstrate the presence of trabecular fractures in autopsy material and in femoral heads removed at the time of insertion of prosthetic devices. They noted multiple trabecular fractures at the junction of the femoral head and femoral neck. Predilection for this particular site was readily explicable, since in this area the load-bearing structure undergoes a sharp change in cross section, and this phenomenon is known to cause stress concentration. As age increased the bone density decreased, and the number of trabecular fractures sharply increased when the bone density was less than 0.5 gm per cubic centimeter. It was the feeling of these investigators that an occasional trabecular fracture in the femoral head and neck was a physiological event. When the fatigue fractures increased to more than 10, however, and the bone density was less than 0.5 gm per cubic centimeter, it appeared that the combination of these two factors predisposed the femoral neck to gross fracture.[85]

It has also been suggested that this fracture may be caused by a fall in which the femoral neck is levered over the rim of the posterior acetabulum. It is possible that this mechanism of injury is a cause of the fracture, but it is more likely that this type of

injury superimposed on osteoporotic trabecular fractures produces the majority of
femoral neck fractures.

CLASSIFICATION OF INTRACAPSULAR FRACTURES

Anatomically, these fractures may be categorized according to their levels as: (1)
subcapital—a fracture occurring at the base
of the head or high portion of the neck; (2)
transcervical—a fracture occurring in the
midportion of the neck; and (3) basicervical—a fracture occurring at the base or the
lower portion of the neck.

True subcapital fractures involving the
base of the head but no significant portion of
the femoral neck are not common. Transcervical fractures through the mid and
upper portion of the neck are the most
common. Basicervical fractures occur, but
not nearly as frequently as transcervical
fractures. (In most publications these fractures are "lumped" together and designated
as subcapital.)

This division of femoral neck fractures on
the basis of anatomical location is rather
arbitrary, since all these fractures carry the
risk of loss of the blood supply, producing
both avascular necrosis and nonunion. Although this classification is found in the
orthopedic literature and is still in frequent
use in many hospitals, I do not feel that it is
particularly useful. Far more helpful guidelines have been outlined by Pauwels and by
Garden.

Pauwels Classification. Pauwels divided
intracapsular fractures into three groups on
the basis of obliquity of the fracture: type
1—35 degrees or less from the horizontal;
type 2—between 35 and 60 degrees; type
3—between 60 and 90 degrees. It was his
feeling that the more horizontally placed
fractures have a better prognosis than the
more vertical ones. He also felt that type 1
fractures may heal without internal fixation,
but type 2 and type 3 fractures require
internal stabilization. The percentage of
healing was smaller with the more vertical
fractures.[154]

The major problem with this type of
classification is that it does not take into
account the amount of posterior comminution of the femoral neck. It was adequately
demonstrated by Scheck that posterior
comminution of the femoral neck plays a
very important role in both stability and the
likelihood of healing. His feeling was that
the femoral neck failed in the superior
aspect in tension and in the posterior
inferior aspect in compression.[174] It has
been subsequently stated and it is the
author's feeling that the amount of posterior
femoral neck comminution plays a significant role in the fate of healing. For this
reason, I feel that Pauwel's classification is
incomplete.

Garden Classification. Garden has devised a classification of intracapsular fractures based on the anatomical relationship
of the proximal to the distal fragment rather
than on the apparent location or obliquity of
the fracture line. Type 1, an incomplete
fracture is present with minimal or no
displacement. Type 2, a complete fracture is
present but with minimal or no displacement. Type 3, displacement is present, but
the posterior retinaculum is intact and it has
tethered the proximal fragment, rotating it
to a varus position in relation to the
acetabulum. Type 4, displacement is
present and the retinaculum is disrupted,
which allows the proximal fragment to
remain in normal relationship with the
acetabulum.[88] It has been found in follow-
up studies that the incidence of avascular
necrosis increases with type 3 and type
4, culminating in a rate of more than 50
per cent with type 4.[89] I feel that Pauwels's
classification is important, as it demonstrates that the more vertical a fracture, the
greater the shearing stress and the greater
the instability, with subsequent decrease in
healing rate. On the other hand, the Garden
classification is useful because it demonstrates that the amount of displacement also
is very important for evaluating the amount
of posterior femoral neck comminution; on
this depends the stability of the fracture and
the ultimate result in healing.

PHYSICAL EXAMINATION

Patients presenting with this type of
injury are very apprehensive about motion
of the lower extremity. They are generally
unable to bear weight because of the pain in
the hip. They tend to be more comfortable

with the hip slightly flexed and in external rotation. Characteristically, a patient with a femoral neck fracture has a shortened leg, abduction of the hip, and an external rotation deformity. The external rotation deformity is usually of the magnitude of 30 to 40 degrees, further external rotation being prevented by an intact capsule. This is in contrast to an extracapsular fracture, in which there may be marked external rotation deformity. The patient is generally unable to move the lower extremity without significant pain. A hematoma resulting from the fall may or may not be palpable.

Impacted femoral neck fractures present with different physical findings. The patients will note moderate discomfort in the hip, but are generally able to bear weight. The typical external rotation deformity may not be present if the fracture is impacted in neutral rotation. In fact, the opposite may occur; the extremity may be held in internal rotation because the fracture is impacted with the distal fragment in internal rotation. Generally the examiner is able to move the hip with a moderate amount of pain; the excruciating pain that accompanies an unimpacted fracture is not present, however. It may be difficult to determine any degree of shortening of the limb with an impacted fracture.

Roentgenographic Examination

It can be safely stated that the most important step in the management of a patient with a fracture of the femoral neck is to obtain adequate roentgenographic examination. This includes a true anteroposterior view and a lateral view of the involved hip. The lateral is the most important (Fig. 22–3). This enables the attending physician to determine the extent of posterior femoral neck comminution. It can either be a frog-leg view or a true lateral view. It is preferable to obtain a true lateral view with the cone of the roentgenographic machine under the uninvolved limb, the patient on his back, and the cone directed at the groin of the involved hip. The cone should be at an angle of approximately 30 degrees to the shaft of the femur and directed at a point midway between the greater trochanter and the crest of the ileum on the affected side.

The cassette is then placed with one edge pressed tightly into the flank above the iliac crest and its plane parallel to the fractured femoral neck and perpendicular to the cone. This gives an excellent roentgenograph of the fractured hip and it also is more comfortable for the patient. The frog-leg lateral involves manipulating a hip that is already painful.

It is still common practice in many areas to designate a femoral fracture by its anatomical location in the femoral neck—*subcapital* when it occurs at the junction of the femoral head and femoral neck; *transcervical*, the most common, when it involves the proximal and middle portions of the femoral neck; and *basicervical* when it occurs in the base or lower portion of the neck. More useful classifications, however, are those of Pauwels, defining the obliquity of the fracture (type 1—35 degrees or less from the horizontal; type 2—between 35 and 60 degrees; type 3—between 60 and 90 degrees), and Garden, defining the relationship of the proximal to the distal fragment (type 1—an incomplete fracture with minimal or no displacement; type 2—a complete fracture with minimal or no displacement; type 3—displacement present, but the intact posterior retinaculum tethers the proximal fragment, rotating it to a varus position in relation to the acetabulum; type 4—displacement present, but the disrupted retinaculum allows the proximal fragment and acetabulum to remain in normal relationship). Neither aspect can be ignored. The more vertical a fracture, the greater the shearing stress and the greater the instability, with consequent decrease in healing rate. Equally important, the more displacement and the more posterior femoral neck comminution, the less stable the fracture and the more uncertain the prognosis.

Treatment

Impacted Fractures

Several studies have appeared in the literature dealing with the operative versus nonoperative treatment of impacted femoral neck fractures. Close scrutiny of the results of nonoperative treatment reveals that a

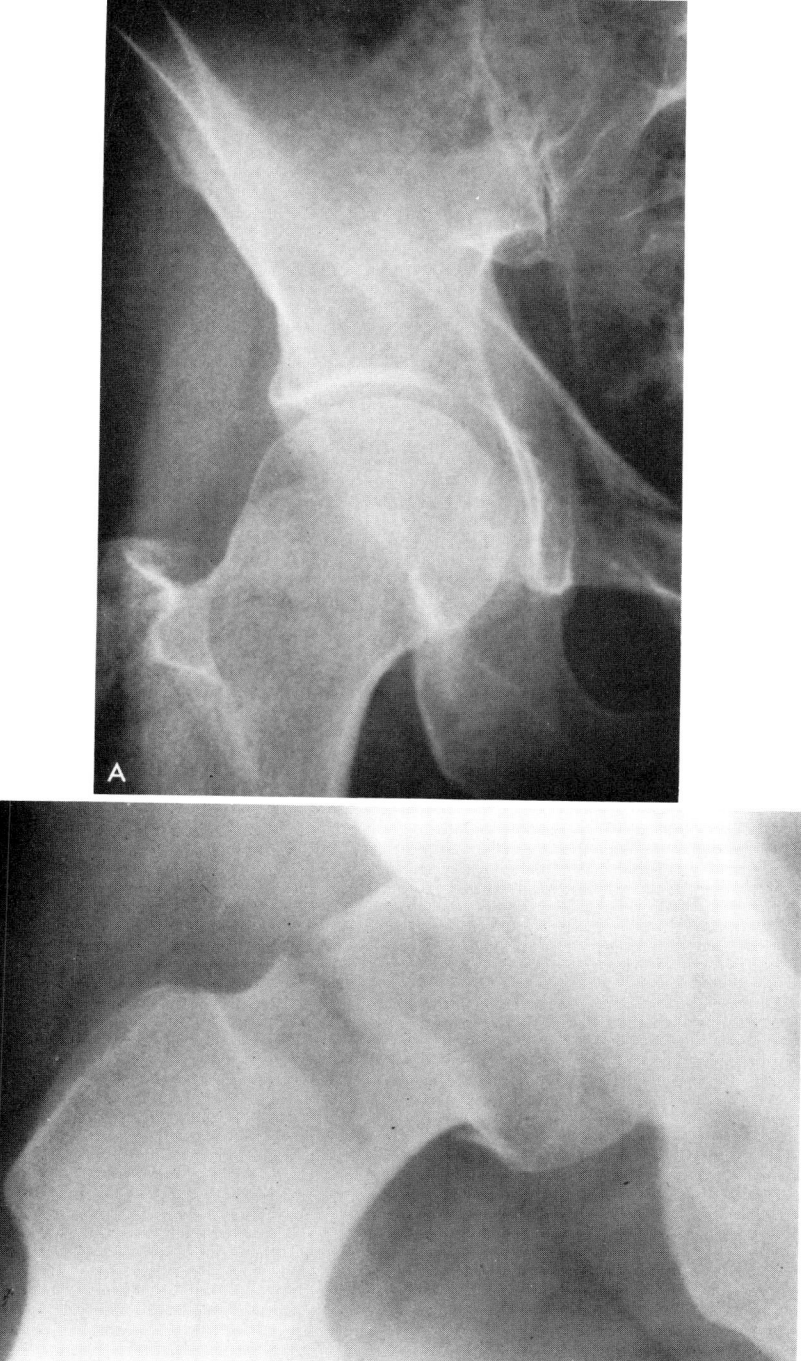

Figure 22–3 *A.* Anteroposterior view of the right hip suggests a subcapital fracture. *B.* Lateral view of the hip demonstrates a definite subcapital fracture.

definite percentage of these fractures "fall apart." This percentage may be small in the truly impacted fractures, but since 100 per cent of them will heal with internal fixation, as opposed to 80 to 90 per cent of those treated by nonoperative methods, internal fixation with multiple pins appears justified. I feel that with improved methods and the use of the image intensifier, the risk of percutaneous pinning is extremely small, and as soon as internal fixation has been accomplished, these patients can be ambulatory and can progress rapidly to full weight bearing.

The majority of impacted fractures are in a slightly valgus position. It is true that there is greater incidence of avascular necrosis of the femoral head with a valgus position. This is due to the displacement of the trabeculae and embarrassment of the blood supply in this position. It is, however, the most stable position, and I do not feel it justified to disimpact the fracture in an attempt to improve the alignment of the femoral head on the femoral neck to lessen the risk of avascular necrosis. The fracture should be pinned in the valgus position with multiple pins that do not displace the fragments (Fig. 22–4). Even if avascular necrosis does develop in the future, the great majority of patients are asymptomatic and do not require further treatment.

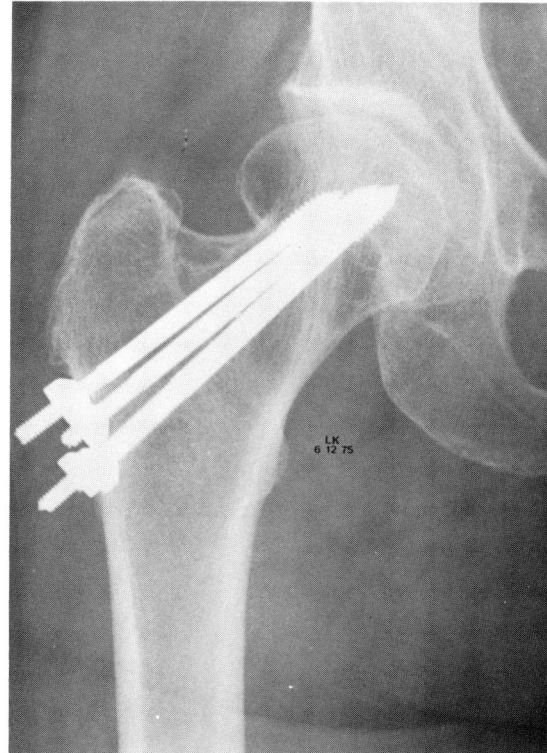

Figure 22–4 An impacted subcapital fracture pinned in stable valgus position without displacement of the impacted fracture.

Displaced Fractures

A fracture of this type should be considered a relative surgical emergency. Most authors feel that any delay in treatment increases the incidence of avascular necrosis. There are very few medical contraindications to early operative intervention, particularly if a spinal anesthetic is used.

Initially, after the patient is admitted to the hospital, a sandbag is placed alongside the lateral aspect of the proximal femur. This prevents excessive external rotation, and patients are generally comfortable in this position; if they are not, gentle Buck's skin traction can be used. Routine blood chemistry determinations are performed. The patient is then taken to the operating room as soon as possible—usually within 12 to 24 hours. Excessive delay for a complete

work-up is not justified. It is best to perform internal fixation early for two reasons. (1) The fracture can be reduced, and further disruption of the blood supply may be prevented. (2) Early mobilization can follow internal fixation, and secondary medical problems can be prevented. One to two units of cross-matched blood should be available, although a blood transfusion is rarely necessary. The surgical preparation of the hip is performed in the operating room under anesthesia. There is no real advantage in attempting to "prep" a painful, immobile hip on the ward prior to surgery. It is extremely important to obtain adequate roentgenographic control prior to the operative procedure, and for this, image intensification has been a major breakthrough. Scout films in both the anteroposterior and lateral planes are obtained in the operating room prior to any preparation and draping. It is important not to

accept anything less than a perfect preoperative reduction of the fracture. There is,
I feel, only one exception to this rule; if an
adequate reduction cannot be obtained
following at least three attempts at closed
reduction, an open reduction and internal
fixation under direct vision are indicated.
This is, however, the exception rather than
the rule. Several methods are available for
manipulative reduction. The author has
found the Leadbetter and Deyerle techniques to be applicable to this type of fracture.

Leadbetter Maneuver. The Leadbetter
technique is performed on the fracture
table. An assistant fixes the pelvis, and
under moderate traction, with the knee
flexed, the hip is slowly flexed to 90 degrees
to relax the capsule and surrounding musculature. The slightly adducted thigh is
then lifted directly upward, which corrects
the posterior displacement and shortening.
The hip is then gently internally rotated 45
degrees to engage the fracture fragments.
The maneuver is completed by circum-
ducting the hip into abduction and extension. Following this type of reduction, the
operator should take the patient's heel in
the open palm of his hand. If a successful
reduction has been obtained, the position of
the hip in abduction with slight internal
rotation can be maintained by supporting
the heel in the palm of the hand. If it cannot,
x-rays will probably reveal inadequate reduction. This becomes important if regular
x-rays are all that are available. Then, if the
open palm test does not demonstrate reduction, a repeat manipulation should be
performed.[126] With an image intensifier,
however, rapid roentgenographic assessment of the reduction is possible.

Deyerle Maneuver. Another useful manipulation is that of Deyerle. The patient is
placed on the fracture table, and a strong
downward pull is exerted on the lower
extremity with the foot in slight external
rotation. This is a direct attempt to pull the
distal fragment below the level of the head
fragment. The foot is placed in internal
rotation until the femoral neck is parallel
with the floor on the lateral x-ray. In the
anteroposterior view the lesser trochanter
will be barely visible. One of the operator's
hands holds the medial side of the knee and
his other hand is placed over the greater

trochanter laterally to apply pressure
against the greater trochanter. This maneuver levers the neck underneath the head
into a slight valgus deformity. The operator
then places both hands just anterior to the
greater trochanter and pushes directly
backward toward the floor. This places the
head in an anatomical or slightly over-
reduced position in a lateral plane. X-rays
are now obtained. The neck must be parallel with the floor in the lateral projection. If
it is not, then the foot should be internally
or externally rotated sufficiently to accomplish this goal.[58] An acceptable anatomical position is extremely important. A varus
position of the femoral head on the femoral
neck is definitely not acceptable and will
doom the procedure to failure (Fig. 22–5). A
slightly valgus or neutral position is preferable. Careful assessment of the reduction on
the lateral view is essential. In this view the
center of the head should be within the

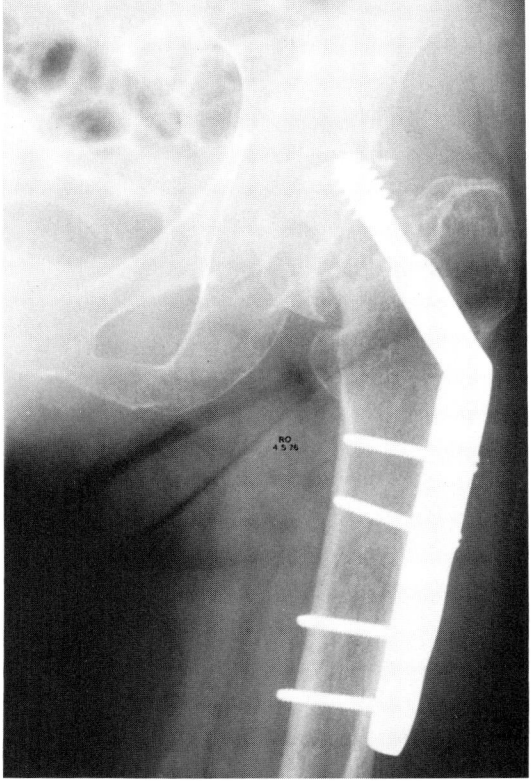

Figure 22–5 A subcapital fracture pinned in a varus
position. The result was a further varus deformity, with
the screw cutting out of the femoral head.

center of the neck; anterior or posterior tilting is not acceptable—is definitely incorrect—but is frequently overlooked when the operator places too much emphasis on the anteroposterior view. I feel that a large portion of the success or failure of internal fixation in this type of fracture depends on adequate reduction verified in both anteroposterior and lateral views. It is well to remember here the words of Nicoll, "No device will hold a badly reduced fracture, and no fracture, however well reduced, will be held by a badly placed nail."[151]

Once the reduction has been adequately accomplished, the operator can proceed with the type of internal fixation that he prefers.

Internal Fixation

Several devices are available for internal fixation for this particular fracture. While it is not the purpose of this text to evaluate the various types of fixation devices, the author prefers the multiple pin technique with modified Hagie pins, the Deyerle multiple pins, and the sliding nail or compression screw devices.

Deyerle Multiple Pin Technique. The Deyerle technique is extremely demanding and, unless the operator pays strict attention to detail, will not produce satisfactory results. If the device is used exactly as Deyerle recommends, however, excellent results can be obtained. The patient is placed on a fracture table and the reduction is performed as just outlined. A lateral incision is made directly over the greater trochanter. A ¼ inch drill hole is made 1½ inches below the flare of the greater trochanter. It is important that this drill hole be through the middle of the shaft. A ⁹/₁₆ inch guide pin 5 inches long, is inserted up the shaft of the neck, parallel with the floor, by using a double-thickness jig. The pin extends across the fracture site in the femoral neck. A set of x-rays is then made in the anteroposterior and lateral planes. These determine which particular hole in the jig to place over the guide pin in order to place the maximum number of pins in the femoral head. The only holes that should not be used for this purpose are the anterior or posterior three or the impacting hole. All the holes are then drilled through the jig

and across the lateral cortex with a ⁹/₁₆ inch drill bit. The three inferior holes along the calcar are drilled only as far as the fracture site. Copious amounts of saline should be utilized to cool the drill bit throughout the drilling. The pin length is calculated so that all the pins are placed approximately ¾ inch from an x-ray shadow of the head seen in the anteroposterior view before impaction. The guide pin is used as a gauge for calculating the length of the pins. A separate 5 inch pin is used to estimate the exact length of the pin that is to replace the guide pin. The length of the rest of the pins is related to this length. The operator must keep in mind that allowance must be made for the thickness of the plate and the jig. The plate is ½ inch in thickness and the jig is 1 inch. The standard size differential of the pins in the various rows is as follows: the proximal row is ½ inch shorter than the next four with the bottom five being ½ inch longer than the middle four.

Following drilling of all holes to the fracture site, the jig is removed. An identical plate is screwed in the same hole that held the jig, and at the same time the plate to be retained is placed over the same guide pin as the jig. The screw is not tightened until another pin has been inserted across the plate to lock it in the most congruous position in relation to the underlying holes that were previously drilled through the jig. Once a minimum of nine pins ⁹/₁₆ inch in diameter have been inserted, the traction apparatus ratchet can be released one or two notches. The impacting punch is then inserted in the impacting hole, and several blows are placed against the plate. The operator will be aware of the appropriate impaction, as the femur will move inward as the fracture impacts. This allows the pins to extrude ¼ to ½ inch in femoral neck fractures. The ⁹/₁₆ inch pins are then advanced further into the head by tightening them gently by hand. Drilling across the fracture site is not necessary, as the pins are self-tapping. *The sine qua non in the use of this device is to maintain the head in a reduced position while impacting the neck up into the head with heavy blows on the impacting plate. This is an essential part of the technique.*

A final set of x-rays is then obtained. It will be noted that the pins come within

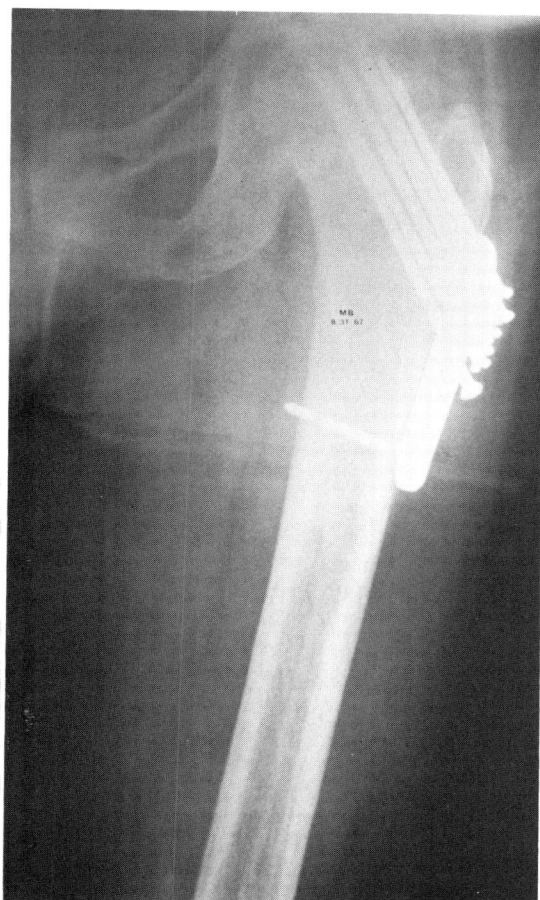

Figure 22-6 A subcapital fracture pinned by the Deyerle technique. In this particular case the pins are slightly more superior than preferred, but the length is appropriate.

¼ inch of the top of the head of the femur (Fig. 22-6). If a broken pin is found at follow-up, this is direct evidence that fixation was inadequate and there has been motion at the fracture site.[58] Again I must stress that this is an excellent technique, but attention must be paid to small details or the results will not be good.

Hagie Pin Technique. Another very useful technique is the insertion of multiple modified large Hagie pins. These pins have a large screw head that has cutting edges on both the proximal and distal portions of the screw for ease of insertion and later removal. The midportion of the screw is smooth, allowing a lag effect. The proximal portion of the pin is threaded to allow compression by a corresponding bolt.

The patient is placed on the fracture table, and the reduction is performed as described previously. A standard lateral incision is made directly over the greater trochanter. At a point approximately 1½ to 2 inches distal to the tip of the greater trochanter a pin is inserted up the femoral neck into the femoral head. The lateral portion of the cortex is the only portion that requires prior drilling, and as a guide to the insertion, the operator's finger can be placed along the inferior border of the neck. Following insertion of the pin, anteroposterior and lateral x-rays are obtained. I do not feel that it is necessary to open the capsule routinely to perform open reduction. This is required only if the attempted closed reduction is not successful. For adequate fixation against a rotational force, I prefer to insert at least four and preferably five or six pins, if at all possible (Fig. 22-7). They should be separated, with an equal distribution in the superior and inferior portions of the neck. Anteroposterior and lateral views are again obtained following insertion of the final pin. It is at this point that any final adjustment of the remaining pins is performed. The bolts are then applied to the threaded proximal portion of the pin and are tightened in an attempt to compress the femoral head on the femoral neck. This is an important point of the procedure, and since the pins do produce a lag effect, definite compression can be obtained. Further settling of the femoral head on the femoral neck may accompany ambulation, but because these pins are smooth in the midportion they will "back out," allowing additional settling and compression at the fracture site. This particular technique of insertion of multiple modified large Hagie pins is preferred by the author for treating high femoral neck fractures. The multiple pins provide better fixation in osteoporotic femoral heads than does the single sliding nail or the compression screw.

Compression Screw Technique. The compression hip screw and the sliding nail concept of Pugh are useful in the treatment of low femoral neck fractures. The most appropriate position for the compression hip screw is directly in the center of the femoral head just above the calcar. With this type of insertion a three-point fixation is

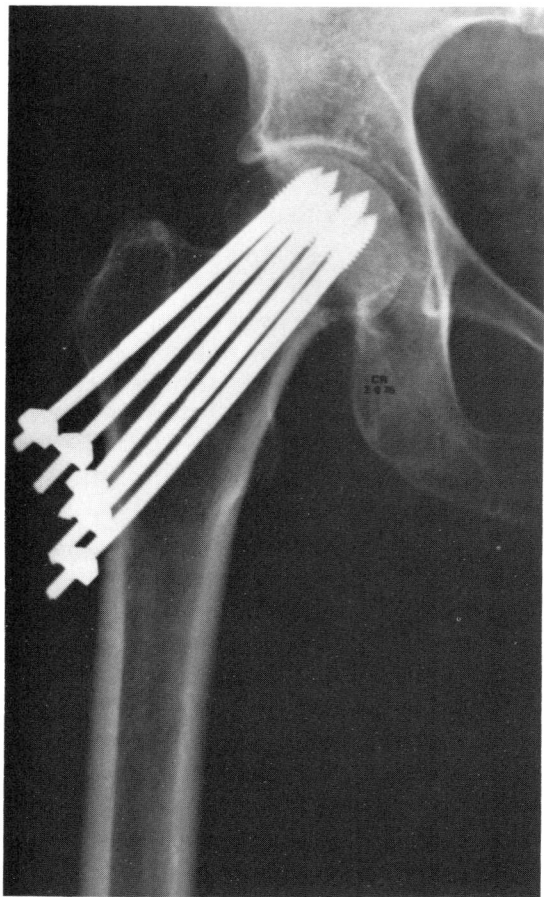

Figure 22-7 A subcapital fracture treated with multiple modified Hagie pins. Note that the pins extend to the subchondral bone.

accomplished. Following adequate reduction on the fracture table, a standard lateral incision is made directly over the greater trochanter. The incision is carried distal to the trochanter for approximately 5 to 6 inches. This is to permit insertion of the side plate. The ideal nail angle is usually approximately 140 degrees to place the screw just above the calcar and in the central portion of the femoral head. A guide pin is then inserted approximately 1½ to 2 inches below the tip of the greater trochanter and driven up into the femoral neck and femoral head. A second guide pin is placed just distal and slightly posterior to the first. Roentgenograms in anteroposterior and lateral planes are then made. The two guide pins are used initially because one

pin invariably is in better position than the other. This saves time in the operative procedure, as the pin with the best position can be left in place and the other pin removed. It is important to remember that the best position for the guide pin and eventually the compression screw is directly in the midportion of the femoral neck and femoral head in the lateral view. If you are to err slightly, it is better to err with the pin in the posterior portion rather than the anterior portion of the head because if the pin cuts out, it usually tends to cut out anteriorly (Fig. 22–8).

If this device is to be used in treating subcapital fractures, the two initial guide pins should be placed through the femoral neck and femoral head and into the acetabulum. These pins are necessary to stabilize the femoral head and prevent rotation during the reaming procedure and the insertion of the compression screw. As stated previously, however, I feel that the multiple pin technique is the best for treatment of high femoral neck fractures.

The guide pin is then advanced to the subchondral portion of the femoral head, and its length within the femoral neck and femoral head is determined. The appropriate compression screw is selected by subtracting ½ inch from the length of the guide pin within the femoral neck and head, and is then put aside to be used following appropriate reaming. The initial reamer is selected, its depth stop is set to the desired length and locked into position, and reaming is carried out over the guide pin until the depth stop is reached. The second, or cortical, reamer is then selected to cut the hole in the proximal portion for the barrel of the side plate. The guide pin is removed, and a cutter is inserted through the prereamed hole up into the femoral neck and head to precut the cancellous bone for insertion of the compression screw. I feel that the cutter should not be advanced up to the subchondral bone but to approximately 1 inch short of it. This is so that when the compression screw is inserted a tight fit will result. If there is excessive torque when the compression screw is advanced toward the subchondral bone, however, the cutter should be reinserted and advanced farther. This is particularly important, as excessive torque during insertion of the screw may

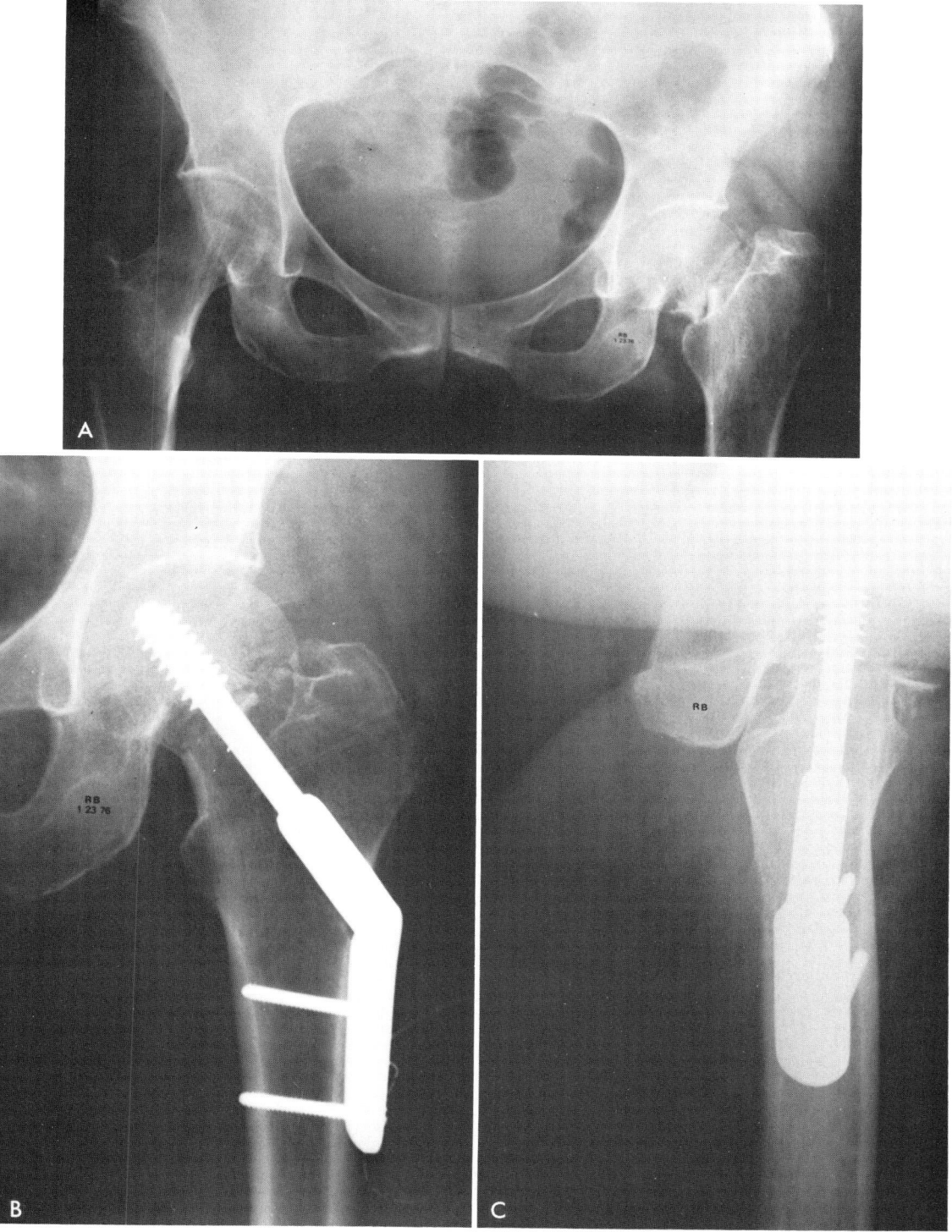

Figure 22–8 *A. A moderately displaced subcapital fracture of the left hip. B. Closed reduction and insertion of a hip compression screw device, anteroposterior view. C. A lateral view demonstrating the position of the compression screw in the femoral head. It is in a slightly posterior position.*

displace the reduced fracture. It is for this reason, too, that guide pins were inserted earlier through the femoral head into the acetabulum to control rotation. The compression screw is inserted with a special wrench that has two grooves on the barrel, the first indicating that the screw is entering the head, and the second, the groove closest to the operator, indicating that the tip of the screw has reached the desired position in the femoral head. It is at this point that the shank of the screw is short by 1/2 inch (i.e., the tip of the shank is located 1/2 inch inward from the lateral cortex). The barrel of the side plate will reach farther than this and will allow the screw to "back out." The compression screw is then turned until the slot in the screw is pointing cephalad, its

correct final position, so that the tongue inside the barrel slides into place and will allow the side plate to be parallel to the shaft of the femur. The appropriately angled side plate is then chosen (135, 140, 145, or 150 degrees). It is frequently difficult to engage the slot of the screw in the tongue of the barrel in the correct position for the screw. I have found that a useful technique is to rotate the screw so that the slot in the screw is facing slightly posteriorly. The barrel can then be easily slipped over the slot without any retractors or muscular attachments pressing against the side plate and preventing the insertion. The entire side plate and screw are then rotated downward back into a position parallel with the shaft of the femur. For high femoral

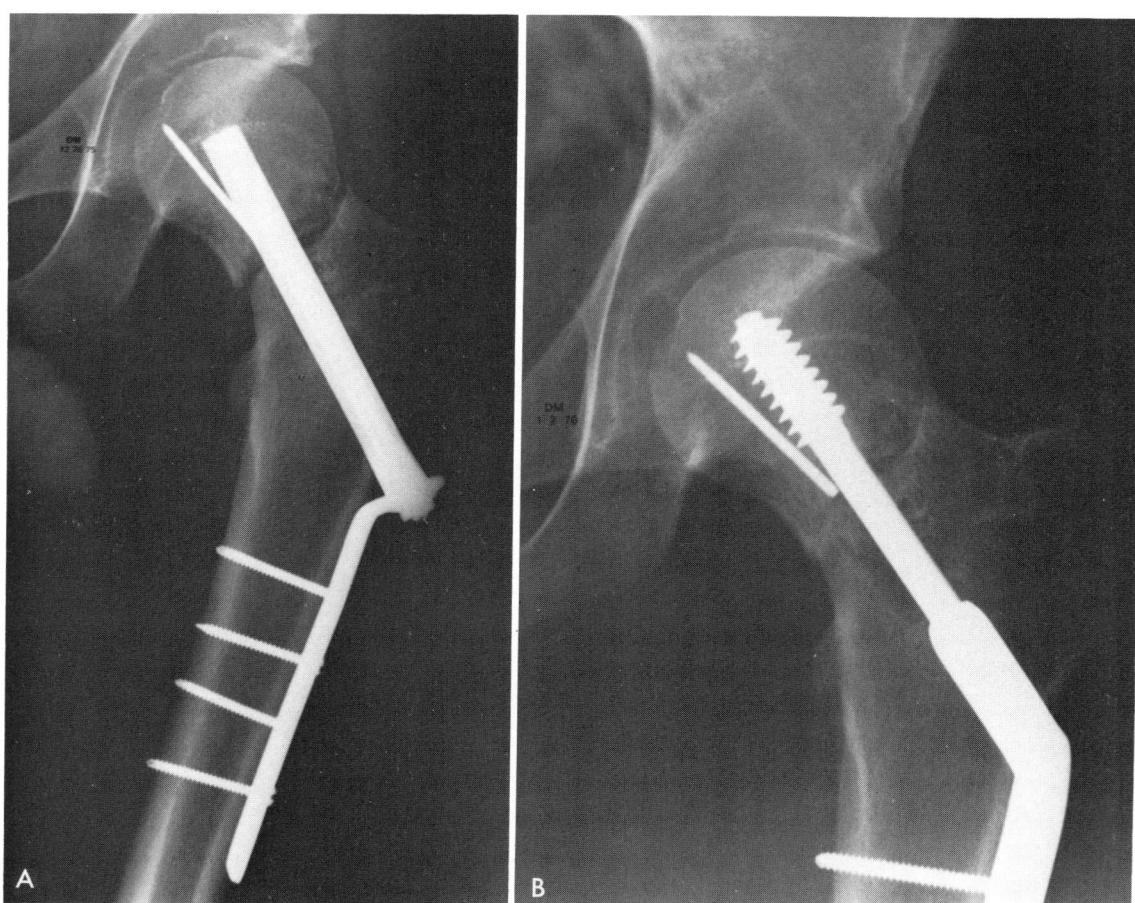

Figure 22–9   A. Subcapital fracture originally treated with a Smith-Petersen nail. Distraction is evident. A guide pin was broken during the procedure and is present. The patient was a 30-year-old man. *B.* The previous device was removed and a compression screw device was inserted, active compression was applied, and a bone graft was added. This went on to uneventful healing.

neck fractures a two-hole side plate is sufficient; a four-hole side plate is selected for treatment of low femoral neck fractures (Fig. 22–9). The side plate is then fixed to the lateral aspect of the femoral shaft with screws. At this point, any traction on the lower extremity must be removed by an assistant. The impacting screw is then inserted into the compression screw and tightened to obtain compression at the fracture site. This forces the nail to slide distally through the barrel of the side plate, allowing impaction of the fracture site.

Two additional methods that appear to have merit are mentioned for completeness' sake. These are the triangular pinning described by Smyth and co-workers, and the cross-screw technique of Garden.[87, 183] These techniques are used frequently in Europe, but seldom in the United States. From a biomechanical standpoint they appear to be sound, but the author has had no experience with them.

POSTOPERATIVE MANAGEMENT

The most important aspect of postoperative treatment is to prevent medical complications in the elderly. It must be kept in mind that the rationale for operating on these patients is to obtain adequate reduction and internal fixation so that they can be active postoperatively to prevent medical complications. Every effort should be exerted to that end. Postoperatively, the patients are kept in bed for 24 to 48 hours until they are comfortable. Balanced suspension with an overhead frame and trapeze does allow the patient to move more easily in bed and utilize the bedpan. Many, however, are comfortable lying free in bed without any suspension or traction. Active pulmonary toilet is initiated immediately after operation to prevent pulmonary complications.

The physical therapy department is consulted for range of motion and strengthening exercises for all major joints and the extremities. It is also important for the therapists to become familiar with the patient as soon as possible, as they play a large role in mobilizing these patients. They can begin transfers to a chair within 24 to 48 hours, depending on the patient's comfort and medical condition. By the third day the patient can usually ambulate with a walker. He is instructed to place a maximum of 20 to 30 lb of weight on the affected lower extremity during ambulation. Patients with high femoral neck fractures are usually not allowed full weight bearing until the fracture heals, but those with low femoral neck fractures can progress to weight bearing rapidly if internal fixation is adequate. Physical and occupational therapy departments provide advice on how to manage with normal activities of daily living. The average length of hospital stay is at least two weeks. By the time of discharge the patient will have managed a walker satisfactorily or will have been advanced to the use of crutches. Roentgenograms are obtained prior to discharge.

The patient is seen in follow-up in one month, when new roentgenograms are taken. These fractures are generally slow to heal, as they rely solely on endosteal callus for healing. The periosteum of the femoral neck does not contain a cambium layer and is unable to form external callus. It must also be remembered that this is an intracapsular fracture; if it is not properly reduced, the fracture site will be bathed with synovial fluid, which may delay repair.

PROGNOSTIC FACTORS

Several interesting findings have emerged from a recent British Medical Research Council study of more than 1500 patients with this type of fracture.[16] The preoperative physical state of the patient is closely related to postoperative mortality; one in five inactive patients died within the first month. A delay in the operative procedure for up to three days did not have any definite effect on the mortality rate. Preoperative hemoglobin levels did not appear to have any influence on morbidity or mortality rates, but preoperative blood urea nitrogen values of 80 mg per 100 ml or more were linked to five times as many deaths as those of less than 40 mg per 100 ml. A mortality rate of 7.4 per cent within the first month postoperatively was found in the female group compared to 13.3 per cent in the male group. Age had a direct influence on the healing of displaced fractures. These fractures healed twice as frequently in patients under 65 as they did in patients over 84 years of age. A surprising finding was that no delay in fracture healing occurred with a delay of internal fixation for up to one week. This is not the impression of most investigators. The fractures more frequently tended to heal when there was a delay before full weight bearing. As expected, the adequacy of reduction was most important to fracture healing: the better the reduction the better the healing. Finally, a central position within the femoral head for the fixation device produced the greatest number of healed fractures.

COMPLICATIONS

Avascular Necrosis

In the majority of studies reported to date avascular necrosis remains the most common complication in the treatment of femoral neck fractures. There is no doubt that at the time of a complete fracture of the femoral neck, with displacement and an increase in intracapsular pressure, a significant portion of the blood supply to the femoral head is disrupted. Most investigators feel that the vessels within the superior retinaculum are the most important to survival of the femoral head. Because of this, patients with these fractures should be operated on as soon as possible. This will prevent further displacement of the fracture fragments and possible further disruption of the already diminished blood supply. Soto-Hall and co-workers found that an increase in the intracapsular pressure caused a definite increase in the incidence of avascular necrosis. They were able to measure the increase in the intra-articular pressure produced by an intracapsular fracture. It was their feeling that the hip joint should be aspirated or that the capsule should be opened to reduce this increased pressure.[185, 186]

Most investigators feel that the blood supply in the ligamentum teres is minimal and may be compromised by an extreme valgus position of the femoral head. This position is associated with an increase in avascular necrosis, the true incidence of which has varied in reported studies. The

least is seen in patients with impacted femoral neck fractures. Overall, however, the range has been reported as from 15 to 40 per cent.

Various authors have attempted to determine the blood supply to the femoral head at the time of the operative procedure, mainly by direct measurement of the oxygen tension within the femoral head or of pressures within the femoral head. These techniques, however, have not been refined sufficiently to allow an accurate determination of the blood supply to the femoral head. Other investigators have attempted to measure the rate of transport of various radioactive elements preoperatively as an index of the blood supply of the femoral head. These studies also have not been of significant benefit.

One must be careful in evaluating reports of the incidence of late segmental collapse, as this complication may occur up to and beyond three years postoperatively. A recent study revealed a 24 per cent incidence at the end of three years in females, compared to 15 per cent in males. Most commonly, it occurs within two years postoperatively. There is no doubt that there is a definitely greater incidence of this complication in Garden's stage 3 and stage 4 femoral neck fractures. The heavier the patient, the more likely is late segmental collapse. As mentioned previously, the valgus position is considered to be more stable for a femoral neck fracture than the varus, but late segmental collapse definitely occurs more frequently with this position. It must be borne in mind, however, that many patients with a small segmental collapse are able to manage with only mild discomfort. Just because he develops late segmental collapse, the patient does not necessarily require a secondary reconstructive procedure.

In an attempt to avoid this complication Judet and co-workers, and Meyers and co-workers devised a muscle pedicle transfer of the quadratus femoris muscle with an underlying portion of the posterior cortex of the greater trochanter, to improve the blood supply and also to help to stabilize these fractures.[115, 142]

If the patient does become symptomatic as avascular necrosis develops, then secondary reconstructive procedures will have to be performed. It has been adequately demonstrated in follow-up that unless the avascular necrosis is recognized before a significant anatomical deformity is present, bone grafting procedures are doomed to failure. The author's feeling is that most symptomatic patients with this complication require conversion to femoral head prosthesis or to a total hip replacement.

Nonunion

Nonunion has been a second problem in the management of patients with fractures of the femoral neck. The incidence has been variously reported as from 10 to 44 per cent. Here again the adequacy of reduction appears to play a major role in the outcome (Fig. 22–10). All series demonstrate a greater incidence of nonunion in patients whose fractures have not been perfectly reduced. It must be kept in mind that this is an intra-articular fracture, and unless it is perfectly reduced and compressed, the fracture site will be bathed with synovial fluid. This appears to be a significant factor in producing nonunion of an intra-articular fracture.

A varus position of the femoral head following open reduction and internal fixation certainly predisposes the patient to nonunion more than does a valgus position or a perfect reduction.

Deyerle feels that adequate reduction, fixation with multiple pins, and impaction at the fracture site result in a significant reduction in the incidence of nonunion.[57, 58]

The proponents of the sliding nail or compression screw devices feel that compressing the femoral head and neck and allowing for some resorption of the fracture site without protrusion of the fixation device also decrease the incidence of nonunion. It has been adequately documented that fractures heal under compression and fail under tension (Fig. 22–10). Thus it appears reasonable that compression with a sliding fixation device aids healing and the prevention of nonunion.

Roentgenographically, nonunion may present as a sclerotic border at the fracture margins, but it may also be seen as resorption at the fracture margin site. In any event, a distinct fracture line remains after a reasonable period of time has passed. This

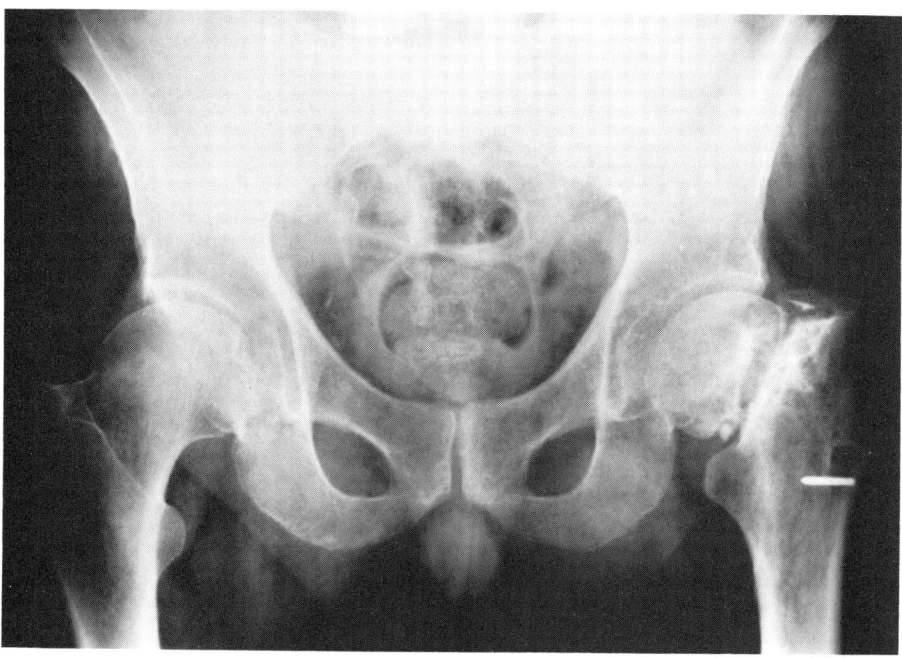

Figure 22–10 Nonunion of subcapital fracture that was pinned in a varus position. The metal device was removed, but the patient continued to complain of pain. Prosthetic revision was required.

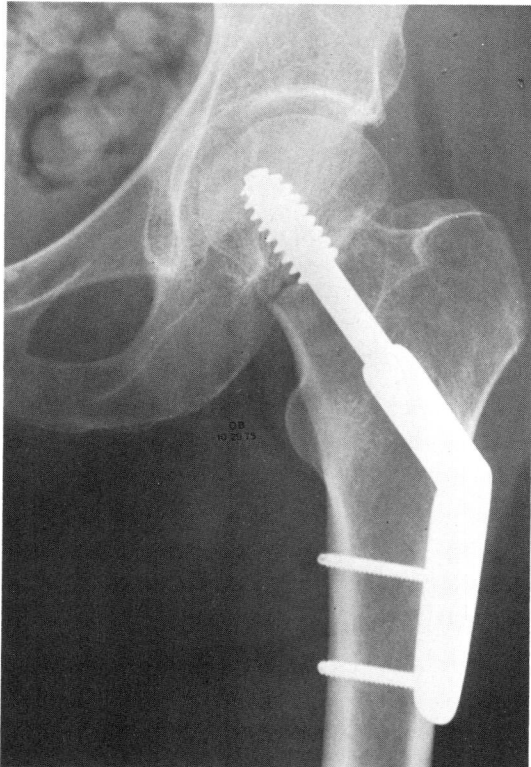

Figure 22–11 A subcapital fracture treated with a compression screw, the threads of which span the fracture. This went on to a nonunion requiring revision. It must be kept in mind that the compression screw must be advanced far enough so the threads do not span the fracture site.

particular fracture should heal normally in from three to six months.

Judet and co-workers, and Meyers and co-workers have treated patients with this problem by muscle pedicle bone grafting and report a significant healing rate with this procedure.[115, 142] This is particularly applicable to the young patient with an established nonunion but with a viable femoral head. Every attempt should be made to preserve the femoral head, as function is never as good with a prosthetic replacement. An alternative method of treating nonunion is to replace the fixation device with a sliding nail and add a bone graft. Femoral head prosthetic replacement is indicated only in the aged and infirm whose life expectancy is short.

Infection

A deep infection is a disaster—and one that is not always evident early in the treatment. The patients may present with moderate discomfort in the hip but without accompanying roentgenographic evidence of infection. They may or may not demonstrate a mild febrile course. A clue in the management of these patients is usually a mild to moderate elevation in the sedimentation rate. Two to three months may pass before roentgenograms reveal evidence suggestive of an infection. An area of radiolucency will frequently develop around the fixation device, which is evidence of motion or infection. There may be demineralization of the subchondral bone in both the femoral head and the acetabular roof. The joint space may gradually diminish.

Treatment of a frank deep infection is difficult. If there is evidence of loss of viability of the femoral head, then the fixation device and the femoral head should be removed and the patient left with a Girdlestone arthroplasty. If the femoral head appears viable, an attempt should be made to preserve this bone stock. Operative decompression with the insertion of an ingress-egress irrigation system and massive intravenous administration of antibiotics is probably the treatment of choice as an initial attempt to preserve the hip joint. If laboratory examination and clinical course give no evidence of improvement, then the metal fixation device must be removed and all dead tissue thoroughly debrided. Fortunately, the incidence of wound infection reported in the majority of series is very low.

INDICATIONS FOR PROSTHETIC REPLACEMENT

Initial prosthetic replacement does have a place in the treatment of femoral neck fractures. In the majority of patients with this problem, however, every effort should be made to perform an open reduction and internal fixation. It is the author's feeling that this should be the initial attempt. There are a very few indications for initial prosthetic replacement. These include the age and feebleness of the debilitated patient, parkinsonism, spastic hemiplegia, the occasional pathological fracture with gross destruction, and the unreduceable comminuted femoral neck fracture.

If the patient is relatively young and has a life expectancy of more than 10 years, I do not feel that supplementary methyl methacrylate is indicated. If, on the other hand, the patient is elderly and his life expectancy is limited, then I feel that supplemental cement fixation aids in the treatment. The problem with methacrylate fixation is that, on follow-up, a significant number of patients will demonstrate a central migration of the prosthesis due to the additional fixation and stresses placed upon the hip.

On the other hand, one of the problems with failure of prosthetic replacement is the complication of loosening. Any motion of the prosthesis, as evidenced radiographically by a halo formation around the prosthetic stem, produces pain. The addition of methyl methacrylate will certainly decrease the likelihood of loosening. Therefore, I feel that if the patient's life expectancy is less than 10 years, then the prosthesis should be cemented in place. A smooth nonfenestrated stem of the Thompson type should be utilized with cement fixation, not a fenestrated stem of the Austin-Moore type. The rationale is that, if the prosthesis must be removed, it is extremely difficult to remove one that is cemented through the fenestrated portion of the stem. It also must be borne in mind that if an infection develops, removal of the cemented prosthesis is more difficult than that of a prosthesis that was inserted without cement.

The majority of patients with a femoral neck fracture do not have significant osteoarthritis of the hip. In the occasional patient who does show evidence of moderate to severe osteoarthritis and has a hip fracture, it would be reasonable to consider a primary total hip replacement. Finally, prosthetic replacement is indicated for the patient in whom internal fixation has failed. This may have resulted from protrusion of the device through the femoral head into the acetabulum, fatigue failure of the fixation device, late development of avascular necrosis with a healed fracture, or unacceptable loss of position of the fracture fragments. If the acetabulum appears to be in satisfactory condition roentgenographically, a femoral head prosthesis may be considered. If there is evidence of deterioration or destruction of the acetabular component, however, I would feel that total hip replacement is the procedure of choice.

In summary, every attempt should be made to perform an open reduction and internal fixation for femoral neck fractures, except when specific contraindications are present. The most recent trend has been to salvage the hip rather than insert a prosthetic replacement, even for displaced fractures.

FEMORAL HEAD FRACTURES

Fractures of the femoral head are not frequent and are usually seen in association with dislocation of the hip. Since the hip is usually dislocated in a posterior direction, associated fractures of the femoral head most commonly occur in the inferior aspect of the head. In an anterior dislocation, the fracture may be in the superior aspect of the head. If the fragment is large and solitary, open reduction and internal fixation should be performed, the best device being a cancellous compression screw that is counter sunk below the articular surface. Removal of the fragment is the procedure of choice if the fragment is not of significant size. Severely comminuted fractures are treated with primary prosthetic or total hip replacement.

EXTRACAPSULAR FRACTURES

The intertrochanteric fracture is the most common and the classic extracapsular fracture. These fractures occur in an older age group than the intracapsular fractures, the average age of patients being 75 years. Many of these people are very inactive prior to their injury. The majority of these fractures are not simple but are comminuted, and the injury is usually more extensive than with an intracapsular fracture. It is a common fracture in the osteoporotic female (women are affected twice as often as men), and several new fixation devices have been developed in an attempt to combat this problem. A more thorough understanding of the biomechanical forces acting on the hip joint has led to improvement in surgical technique for internal fixation. As with the treatment of intracapsular fractures, the main goal is to provide satisfactory fixation in order to mobilize these patients quickly and prevent secondary medical complications. Because these fractures have a better blood supply than intracapsular fractures, they will heal with conservative treatment including bed rest and traction for approximately 12 to 14 weeks. In this age group, however, such treatment is, in the author's opinion, contraindicated because medical complications are more prevalent than with an operative approach.

The anatomy and function of the hip joint were outlined at the beginning of this chapter. As noted then, the intertrochanteric fracture has a better blood supply than the intracapsular fracture. This plays a very significant role in the better healing rate and the infrequency of nonunion with this type of fracture. Characteristically located along the trochanteric line between the greater and lesser trochanters outside the capsule, these are designated as extracapsular fractures. They are not all simple fractures, and many are significantly comminuted.

MECHANISM OF INJURY

The forces that produce this fracture usually differ from those involved in an intracapsular fracture; there is more direct trauma, and the usual history is that the patient stumbled and fell, striking her hip directly. Muscular forces are active and do contribute, but it is usually the direct trauma that accounts for a major portion of the injury. The trochanteric area has a sturdier architectural design than the femoral neck; the cortical bone is thicker, and the degree of osteoporosis is generally less.

It is not uncommon for a patient to have had a syncopal attack, to have fallen and fractured her hip, and then to present with evidence of a mild cerebral vascular accident. The majority, however, will have slipped or tripped, falling directly on the affected extremity.

CLASSIFICATION OF EXTRACAPSULAR FRACTURES

Several classifications have been proposed for extracapsular fractures. In an attempt to simplify a complex problem, Evans originally classified these as stable and unstable fractures.[73a] Although very general, this is basic; it is important to recognize the fractures that are unstable, as their treatment is quite different.

Boyd Classification

Boyd and Anderson attempted to differentiate four types of trochanteric fractures. Type 1 was a linear fracture through the trochanteric region; type 2, a comminuted fracture through the same region; type 3, a trochanteric fracture with an associated subtrochanteric element; and type 4, an oblique fracture of the proximal portion of the shaft of the femur involving the subtrochanteric region (Fig. 22–12).[24] This system is useful because it helps to classify the amount and location of comminution.

Anatomical Classification

I prefer the following basic classification: (1) intertrochanteric, (2) pertrochanteric, and (3) subtrochanteric. This is a simple anatomical division, but it is useful, as the prognosis differs with each different type.

Intertrochanteric Fractures. A simple intertrochanteric fracture lies along the trochanteric line without involving the trochanters per se. This type of fracture is not particularly common and it is relatively easy to manage.

Pertrochanteric Fractures. This is a fracture that extends proximally into the greater trochanter. Both trochanters may be involved, and comminution is generally present. This is by far the most common extracapsular fracture. It is difficult to treat because of the accompanying comminution. The unstable four-part fracture fits into this category. It presents with a head and neck fragment, a lesser trochanteric fragment; a

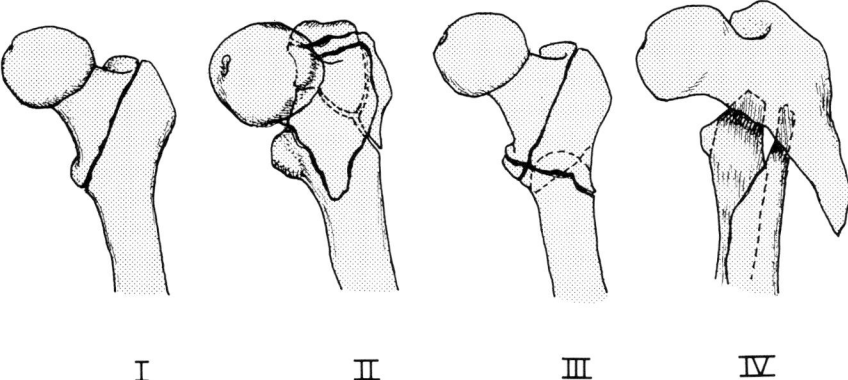

I   II   III   IV

Figure 22-12   Boyd classification of trochanteric fractures. Type 1 is a linear fracture through the trochanteric region; type 2, a comminuted fracture through the same region; type 3, a trochanteric fracture with an associated subtrochanteric element; and type 4, an oblique fracture of the proximal portion of the shaft of the femur involving the subtrochanteric region. (Courtesy of H. Boyd and L. D. Anderson and *Surgery, Gynecology and Obstetrics.* Management of unstable trochanteric fractures, S.G.O., *112*:633–638, 1961.)

greater trochanteric fragment, and the shaft of the femur as a remaining component.

Subtrochanteric Fractures.   A satisfactory working classification of subtrochanteric fractures has been difficult to obtain because there is no precise anatomical definition of the subtrochanteric area. Boyd and Griffin attempted to include these fractures within their overall classification of trochanteric fractures, of which types 1 and 2 were essentially intertrochanteric fractures. Type 3 included a definite subtrochanteric variety, and type 4 consisted of comminuted fractures that extended through the trochanteric area and distally into the subtrochanteric area farther down the shaft.[26]

Fielding and Magliato defined the subtrochanteric area as an area 3 inches in length extending from the proximal border of the lesser trochanter to an area 2 inches distal to the trochanter. They then classified subtrochanteric fractures on the basis of three anatomical locations: type 1 fractures occurring at the level of the lesser trochanter, type 2 fractures occurring in an area 1 to 2 inches below the upper border of the lesser trochanter, and type 3 fractures occurring in an area 2 or 3 inches distal to the upper border of the lesser trochanter (Fig. 22–13). Transverse fractures were relatively easy to classify in this way. The oblique, spiral, and comminuted fractures were then classified according to the level of the major portion of the fracture or the area where the stress of the fracture was concentrated. With this modification, most subtrochanteric fractures could be properly classified. The majority of fractures will fall into the type 1 classification, a decreasing number into type 2, and even fewer into type 3. The incidence of

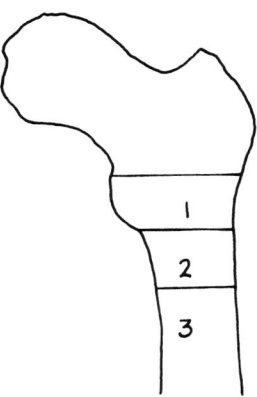

Figure 22-13   Classification of subtrochanteric fractures. Type 1 occurs at the level of the lesser trochanter; type 2, 1 to 2 inches below the upper border of the lesser trochanter; and type 3, 2 to 3 inches distal to the upper border of the lesser trochanter. (Courtesy of J. W. Fielding and H. J. Magliato, and *Surgery, Gynecology and Obstetrics.* Subtrochanteric fractures, S.G.O., *122*:155, 1966.)

union is seen to be the opposite, however, i.e., type 3 fractures are less likely to unite than type 1 and type 2. It must also be kept in mind that medial comminution and a decrease in the medial buttress are usually present in type 3 that are not in type 1 and type 2. This fact along with the great

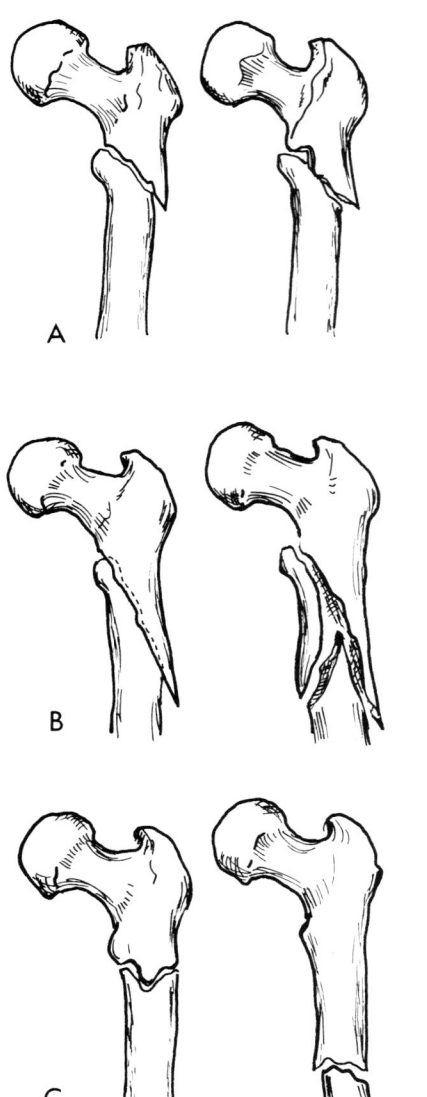

Figure 22–14   Zickel classification of subtrochanteric fractures. *A.* Type 1, short oblique fracture with or without comminution. *B.* Type 2, long oblique fracture with or without comminution. *C.* Type 3, high or low transverse fracture. (Courtesy Zickel, R. E.: J. Bone Joint Surg., 58A:866–872, 1976.)

stresses in the area probably accounts for the decrease in union at this level.[78]

Recently, Zickel has reclassified this type of fracture on the basis of its length and contour, taking into consideration not only the level but also the obliquity and comminution. This is a more functional classification and is probably the one of choice at present. Type 1 is a short oblique fracture with or without comminution. Type 2 is a long oblique fracture with or without comminution. Type 3 is a high or a low transverse fracture (Fig. 22–14).[219]

PHYSICAL EXAMINATION

Extracapsular fractures present in a slightly older age group than intracapsular fractures. Frequently these patients have secondary medical problems that directly complicate treatment and affect the morbidity and mortality rates. Therefore, a thorough medical examination is necessary initially. Evidence of mild heart failure with swelling of the lower extremities is extremely common in this group. Arterial sclerotic vascular disease is likely to be present, and in many patients the pedal pulses are absent. There may be secondary skin changes due to the decreased vasculature. Generalized muscular wasting of the lower extremities due to advanced age is usually evident.

The involved limb is shortened and in external rotation, as with an intracapsular fracture, but the amount of external rotation is generally greater. If the lesser trochanter is intact, the iliopsoas muscle contributes to the external rotation deformity by exerting force on the distal fragment. The capsule of the hip is not involved, and there is no definite structure that limits external rotation. Reflex muscle spasm is present; these patients resist any attempt to put the limb into the neutral position. There may be definite evidence of a hematoma or ecchymosis due to the trauma itself or to the extracapsular extravasation of blood.

It is important to evaluate all the extremities thoroughly in patients with this type of fracture, as many have suffered direct trauma to other parts of the body. Occasionally one will present with a classic Colles' fracture on the same side as the involved hip, this produced by an attempt to break the fall with the outstretched arm.

All these patients urgently require a thorough neurological examination. As mentioned previously, they may have had a syncopal attack that has indirectly caused the fracture. It may well be that a mild cerebral vascular accident caused the fall, and unless a proper neurological examination is performed initially, the exact diagnosis will be missed. Not uncommonly, patients in this age group become extremely confused immediately postoperatively — with or without a neurological deficit. On many occasions the confusion or the neurological deficit or both are blamed on the anesthesia required for the operative procedure when, in fact, the initial event was precipitated by mild cerebral ischemia or a frank cerebral vascular accident.

ROENTGENOGRAPHIC EXAMINATION

As with intracapsular fractures, it is extremely important to obtain adequate roentgenographic views to determine the amount of comminution present, for its extent will directly affect the stability at the fracture site. Moore, Cram, and Dimon and Hughston have recently stressed the importance of comminution of the medial and posteromedial femoral cortex and its subsequent relationship to collapse and varus deformity at the fracture site.[53a, 61] The lateral roentgenogram is the tool for determining the amount of comminution present. If the patient is obese, the lateral roentgenograms obtained may be inadequate. It is a *definite error* to accept such roentgenograms, as they may make it impossible to determine the stability of the fracture preoperatively and the result may be that an incorrect operative procedure is performed. The general roentgenographic appearance is that of a hip in varus position because of the extracapsular fracture.

TREATMENT

These fractures will generally heal with conservative therapy because of the abundant blood supply. Since these patients are generally older than those with intracap-

sular fractures, however, it is even more important to obtain adequate fixation of the fracture in order to initiate early ambulation to prevent secondary medical complications. Therefore, operative treatment becomes the "conservative" approach in dealing with them. With this in mind, the object is to determine the amount of stability at the fracture site and then decide which particular surgical technique will provide the most stability.

Several new devices for the treatment of these fractures have been described in the orthopedic literature in recent years. It is not the purpose of this text to comment on each particular one. Rather, it is well to remember the old proverb, "There is more than one way to skin a cat."

The two most important advances in the management of these fractures in the past two decades have been the development of a sliding compression screw device and the biomechanical concept of a medial displacement osteotomy as proposed by Dimon and Hughston. Both have had a profound effect on the results obtained in treatment of patients with this particular injury.

Intertrochanteric Fractures

As stated earlier, this is not seen frequently. It presents as a simple fracture along the intertrochanteric line without major involvement of the trochanters per se. It may be in relatively anatomical position when first seen. The usual pattern is for the hip to be in a mild varus position owing to the deforming muscular forces. The patient is placed on the fracture table in the operating room, slight traction is applied, and scout roentgenograms are obtained. If the position is anatomically acceptable, the operator can then proceed with internal fixation. A mild to moderate varus deformity can be corrected by further longitudinal traction with slight abduction. If this is still not sufficient to accomplish adequate reduction, mild external rotation can be added, but care must be taken not to pin the hip in excessive external rotation.

I prefer the sliding compression screw with the accompanying side plate for treating these fractures. Although the technique of insertion is essentially the same as

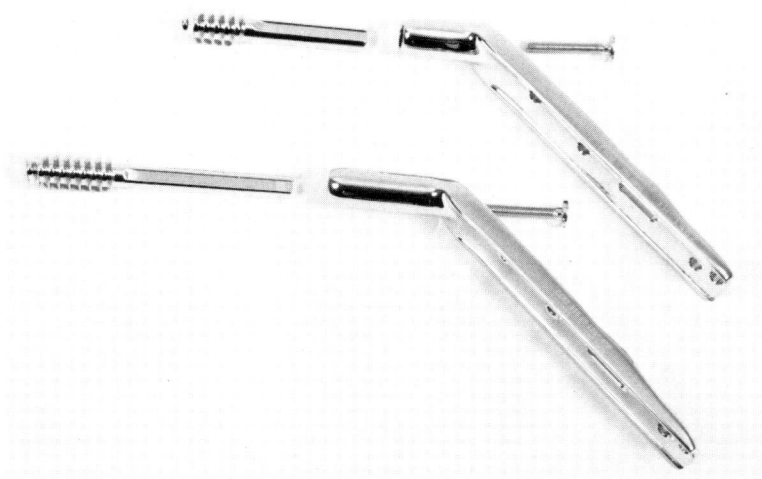

Figure 22–15 The two types of compression screws and accompanying barrels. The top screw is of a short thread design with a short barrel on the side plate. The bottom screw is of a long thread design with a regular barrel side plate.

already outlined in the treatment of femoral neck fractures, there are a few technical considerations. The compression screw comes in two designs, one with a short thread length, and the other with a longer thread length (Fig. 22–15). The long thread length is chosen for this fracture because it provides sturdier fixation. Similarly, the barrel of the side plate comes in two different lengths, one short and one long. The long-barreled side plate is satisfactory for these fractures. It must be remembered that there must be an adequate amount of space between the most distal aspect of the threaded portion of the screw and the barrel of the side plate to allow for impaction at the fracture site and permit the nail to "back out" (Fig. 22–16). If this space is not provided, the screw cannot back out as settling occurs at the fracture site, and the screw will protrude through the femoral head. As in the treatment of intracapsular fractures, the screw should be advanced to the subchondral area. It is important not to advance it through the femoral head, as this will not only damage the articular surface but will also result in loss of fixation. The final point to remember is that you have only "one shot" with this device. If the screw is inadvertently introduced into the incorrect portion of the femoral head and is

then removed and reinserted in a different area, the amount of fixation is significantly decreased. The guide pin must be properly used to avoid this complication. A four-hole side plate is preferable for this fracture.

The Jewett device has been used for the treatment of this type of fracture (Fig. 22–17). This, however, is a single solid unit and it does not allow for settling at the fracture site. We have all seen examples of the Jewett nail protruding through the femoral head as the fracture settles. Although not as pronounced with this particular fracture as it is with unstable fractures, this problem has caused many surgeons to abandon the device.

Pertrochanteric Fractures

This is the most common type of extracapsular fracture seen in clinical practice. The fracture line extends into the greater trochanter and may involve both trochanters and there may be attending comminution. The lesser trochanter may be avulsed by the iliopsoas tendon with a significant portion of the medial cortex. Similarly there may be a large fragment posteriorly that interferes with stability. It is of the utmost importance

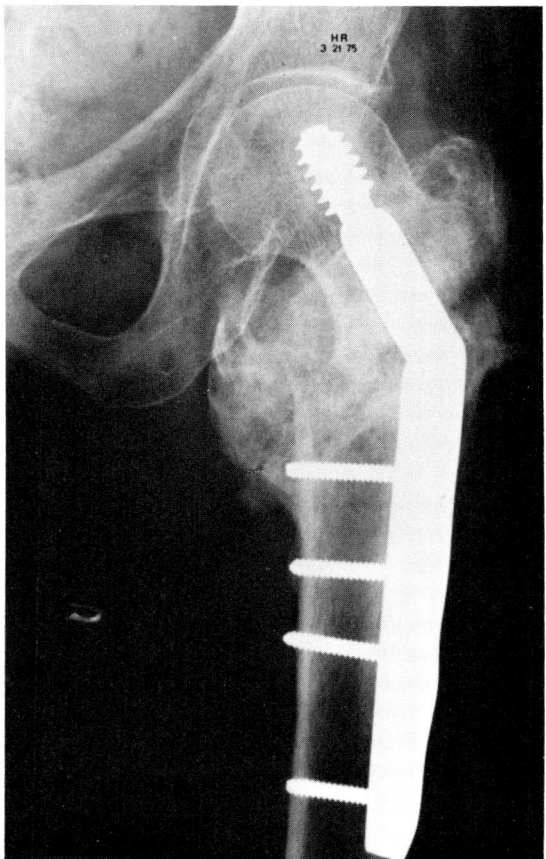

Figure 22–16 An extracapsular fracture treated with compression screw device. Note that significant collapse of the fracture along with the medial displacement has occurred and the compression screw has collapsed into the barrel. This collapse and 'backing out' of the screw allowed settling at the fracture site. Had the screw been unable to collapse into the barrel, it would have protruded through the femoral head as the fracture settled.

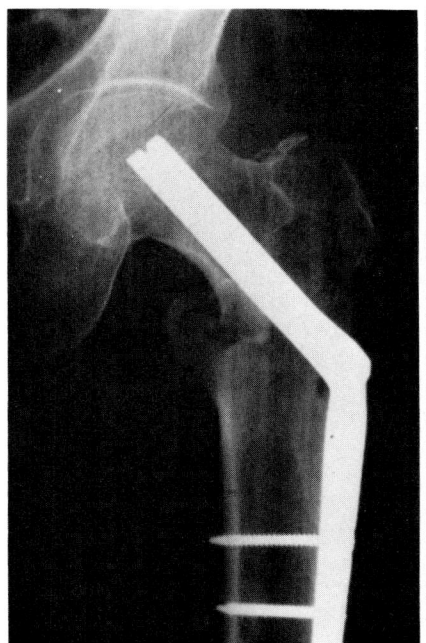
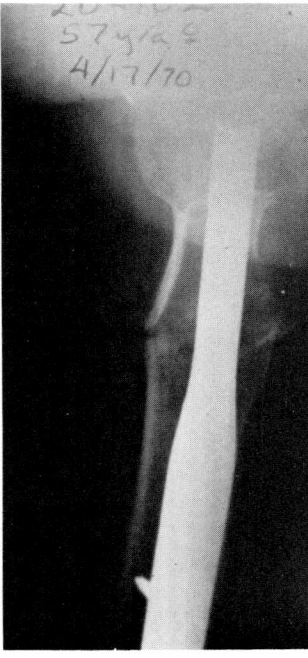

Figure 22–17 Extracapsular fracture treated with a Jewett one-unit device. It does not allow for settling at the fracture site. If this does occur the nail may penetrate the femoral head.

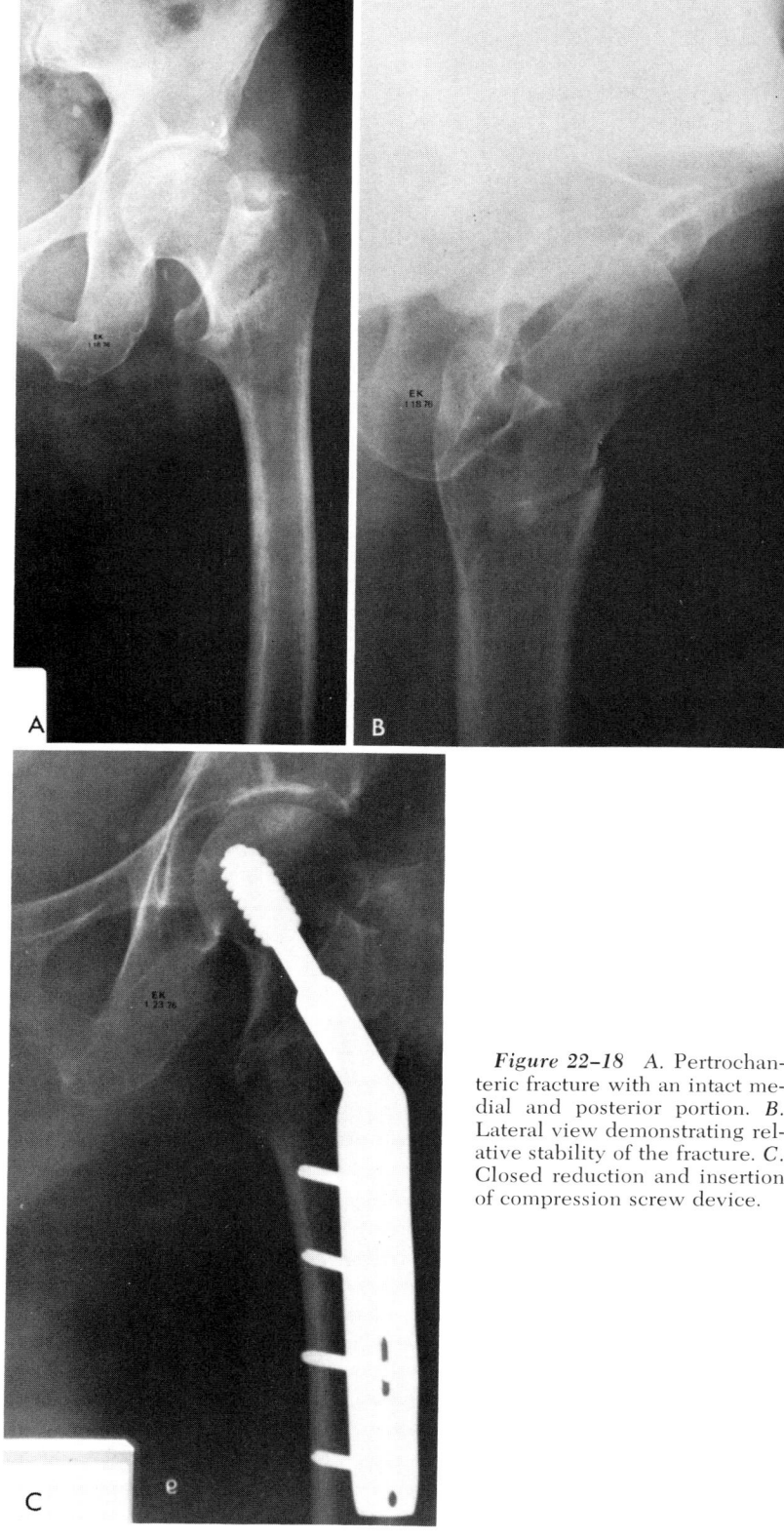

Figure 22–18 *A.* Pertrochanteric fracture with an intact medial and posterior portion. *B.* Lateral view demonstrating relative stability of the fracture. *C.* Closed reduction and insertion of compression screw device.

to determine whether these fractures are stable or unstable; they should be considered unstable if there is significant comminution on the medial or posterior aspects.

If the fracture appears to be stable, with intact medial and posterior portions, a standard reduction can be performed and the sliding compression screw device can be inserted as outlined previously (Fig. 22–18).

This is not the case with an unstable fracture. An anatomical reduction and internal fixation in the presence of instability may well lead to disaster. The four-part fracture consisting of a head and neck fragment, a lesser trochanteric fragment, a greater trochanteric fragment, and the remaining shaft of the femur is an excellent example of an unstable extracapsular fracture. The final determination of stability may have to be made during the operative procedure. It is important to expose the anterior and posterior portions of the proximal femur to determine whether there is a defect medially or posteriorly. Occasionally a fracture will appear stable on routine roentgenograms, but at the operative procedure, a defect will be noted along the medial cortex of the proximal femur. It is for this reason that I cannot stress firmly enough that all fractures of this type should be thoroughly evaluated at the time of operation. If a large medial fragment remains unappreciated and an anatomical reduction is performed, there will be no buttress effect at the fracture site, and the fixation device will take all the stress and may eventually end with fatigue failure.

Compression Screw and Medial Displacement Osteotomy. It is true that the sliding compression screw does allow for some "give and take" at the fracture site. I have seen cases in which an unstable intertrochanteric fracture with a medial osseous defect was anatomically reduced with the sliding compression screw and the distal fragment gradually became displaced medially during the healing process. Other internal fixation devices do not allow for this type of settling and will usually protrude through the femoral head, cut out of the femoral head, or break because of fatigue failure.

I feel the best treatment for the unstable

fracture is a medial displacement osteotomy, as described by Dimon and Hughston, combined with the sliding compression screw (Fig. 22–19).[61] This combination of procedures, in which the inferior portion of the femoral neck is inserted into the shaft of the femur with compression of the cortical bone of the femoral neck against the cortical aspect of the medial portion of the shaft of the femur, is excellent from a biomechanical standpoint.

Sarmiento Method. Another good method for providing stability with an unstable fracture without a medial displacement osteotomy has been advocated by Sarmiento and Williams. In this technique an oblique osteotomy of the proximal femur is performed. The head and neck fragment is then opposed to the shaft, producing medial cortical apposition and allowing for impaction (Fig. 22–20). This technique does permit use of a fixed-angle nail. Sarmiento advocates a 135 degree I beam nail for this procedure.[173]

Holt Method. Holt has produced an extremely strong fixed nail that is attached to the shaft of the femur with bolts. He felt that with such a beefed-up nail the tendency for the device to fail should be decreased.[108] This is not the problem, however. Biomechanical testing has shown the Holt nail to be extremely strong, but the strength of the nail is less crucial than the adequacy of reduction so that the nail does not take all the force directly. If the reduction is not stable, no matter how strong the nail is, it may not fail but it may easily "cut out" of the femoral neck and head fragment. We are reminded of the excellent advice of Nicoll, "no device will hold a badly reduced fracture, and no fracture, however well reduced, will be held by a badly placed nail."[151]

Harrington and Johnston Method. Harrington and Johnston have recently reported a new technique for managing the unstable intertrochanteric fracture by utilizing a medial displacement osteotomy with a sliding compression screw device. This is a slight modification of the technique of Dimon and Hughston. In dealing with a large population of alcoholics who were completely unreliable, they realized that they had to devise a technique that would allow full weight-bearing postopera-

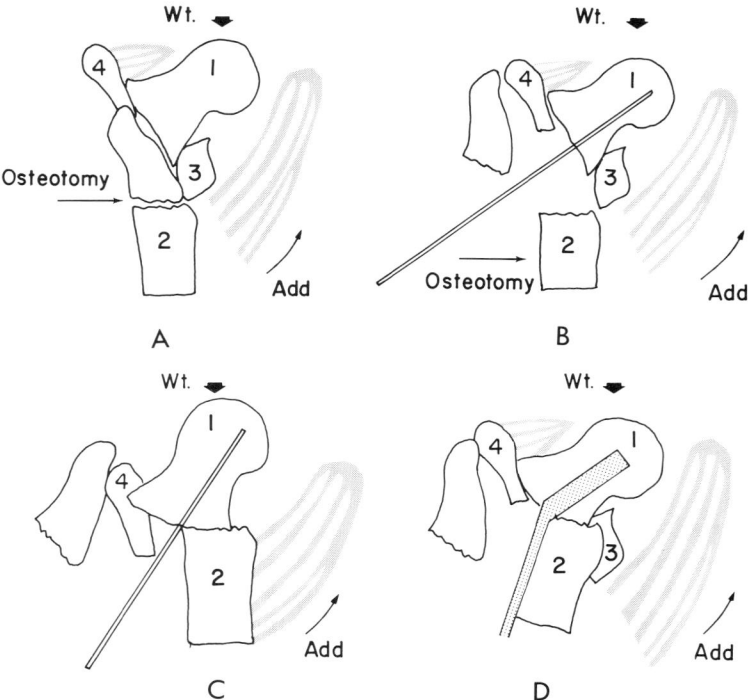

Figure 22–19 Medial displacement fixation. *A.* Osteotomy of spike on shaft fragment (when present). *B.* Placement of guide wire. *C.* Shaft displaced over the spike of the head and neck segment. *D.* Impaction of fracture and fixation with nail. (Courtesy of J. Dimon, III, and J. C. Hughston and *Journal of Bone and Joint Surgery.* Unstable intertrochanteric fractures of the hip, J.B.J.S., *49-A:*440–450, 1967.)

tively.They perform the operative procedure with the patient in a lateral decubitus position with the affected thigh draped free because they feel that this makes it easier to impact the fracture fragments without difficulty. The only danger with this position is that a permanent fixed rotation deformity of the lower extremity may result. This may be compensated for by fixing the side plate to the shaft with the shaft internally rotated approximately 15 to 20 degrees (Fig. 22–21).[98] I feel that this is an excellent technique for the treatment of the unstable fracture. Its only drawback, a minor one, is that the patient may ultimately have slight shortening of the involved extremity—a small price to pay for healing of a typical unstable four-part fracture.

I prefer to have the patient in the supine position. This adds traction to accomplish the medial displacement without requiring an assistant to pull on the lower extremity.

It also allows for ease of roentgenographic control, particularly if an image intensifier is available. Following appropriate anesthesia (most of these patients are elderly, and spinal anesthesia is preferred), the patient is placed on the fracture table and the roentgenographic device is positioned to obtain adequate anteroposterior and lateral views. A lateral incision is made directly over the greater trochanter. The trochanteric fragment is identified, and the proximal femur is stripped of its muscular attachments for approximately 4 inches to allow for insertion of the side plate. An osteotomy of the lateral spike is then performed on the distal fragment at a level at or slightly above the level of the intact cortex on the medial side. The fragment of the greater trochanter and the lateral cortex are retracted in a cephalad direction, allowing direct inspection of the neck portion of the head and neck fragment. Two guide

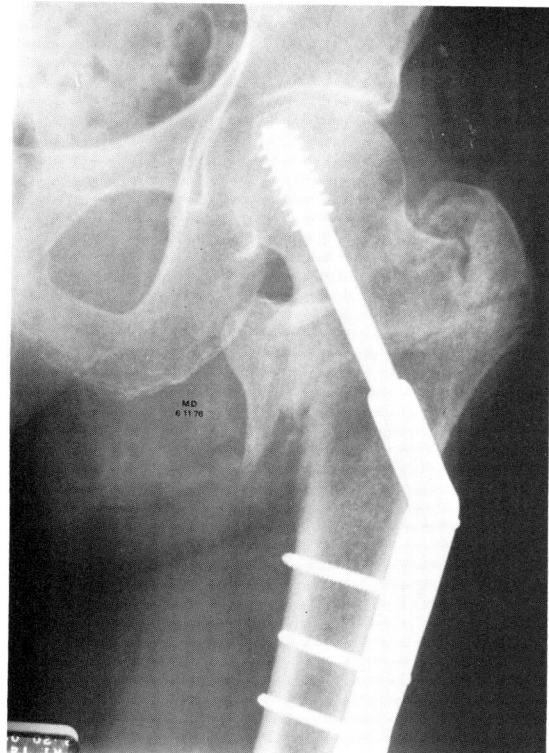

Figure 22–20 An extracapsular fracture treated by an oblique osteotomy of the proximal shaft of the femur with a valgus reduction of the head and neck fragment and insertion of the compression screw and side plate. The oblique fracture has been converted to a more acceptable horizontal fracture giving added stability.

side plate. This is an extremely important point in the procedure. Without this notch, the barrel will not lie correctly, and the femoral head will be forced into a varus position. The femoral neck is then impacted into the femoral shaft, and a side plate is selected. A 135 degree short-barrel side plate is usually required (the long-barrel one is not used for this particular technique, as it does not allow the compression screw to "back out"). A four-hole plate is satisfactory. It is then fixed to the lateral aspect of the femoral shaft. The impaction screw is then inserted into the compression screw and tightened sufficiently to compress the medial portion of the femoral neck tightly

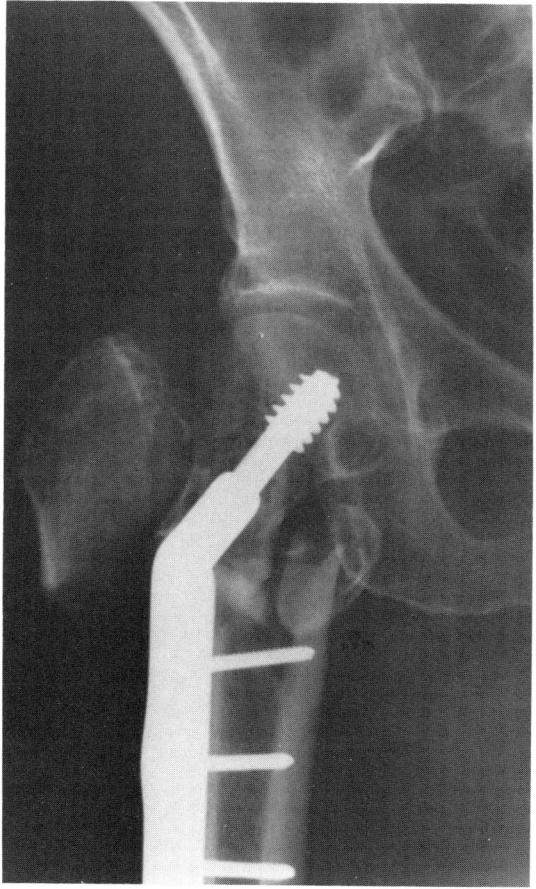

Figure 22–21 An unstable four-part extracapsular fracture. Osteotomy of the greater trochanteric fragment has been performed. The shaft has been displaced medially, and the inferior spike of the neck has been driven down the shaft. The compression screw and a short-barrelled side plate were then applied. The patient went on to uneventful healing.

wires are then inserted into the femoral neck and head; roentgenograms reveal which is in the best position.

The central portion of the femoral head is the best location for the compression screw, the length of which is determined by the length of the guide wire within the femoral head and neck up to the subchondral area—5 to 6 cm on an average. The compression screw comes in two thread lengths; in this particular fracture the short length is appropriate. At this point the traction should be completely released from the lower extremity to enable the operator to impact the femoral neck fragment into the shaft of the femur so that the inferior portion of the neck abuts against the medial portion of the femoral shaft. Prior to impaction a notch is created in the lateral aspect of the distal fragment to accept the barrel of the

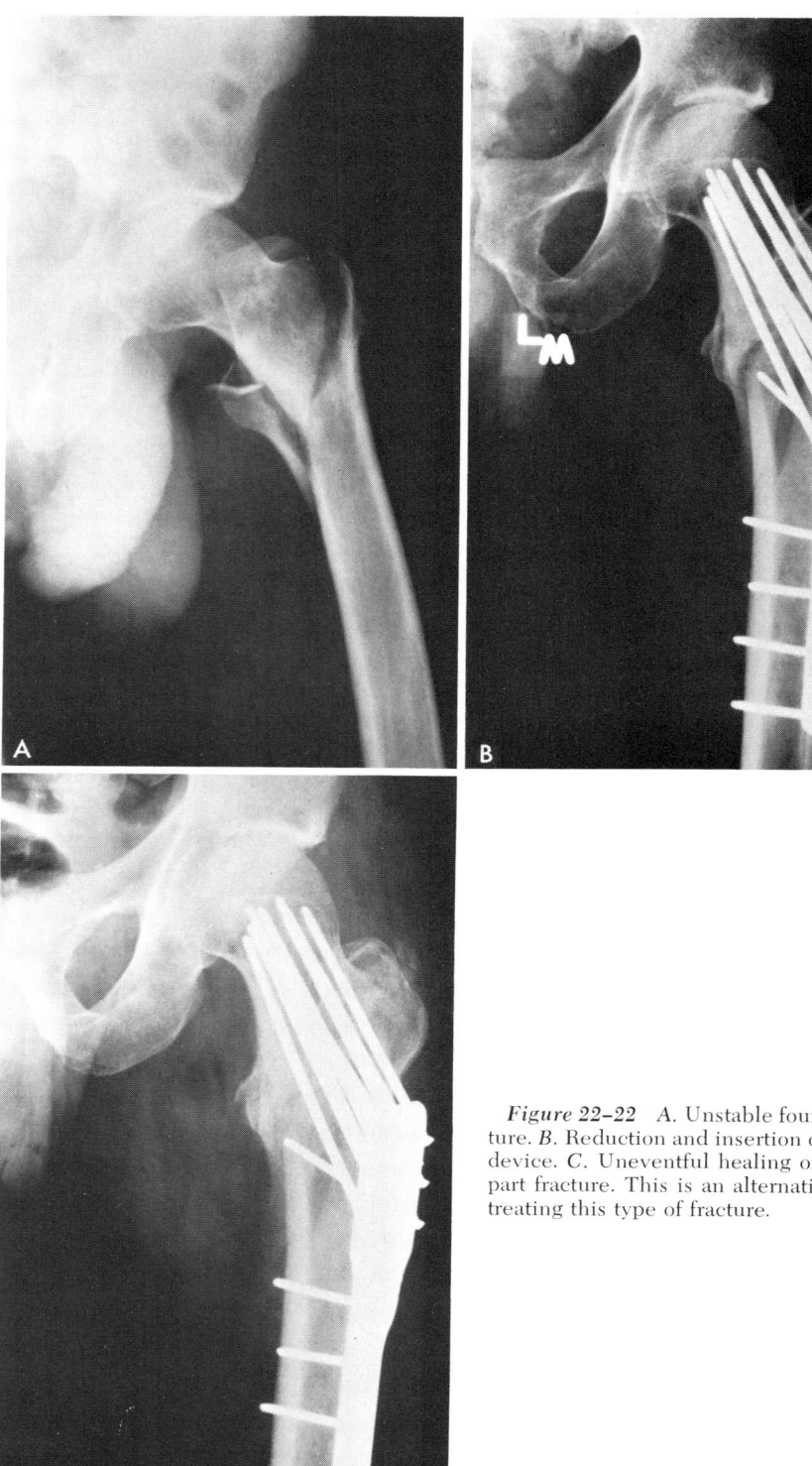

Figure 22–22   A. Unstable four-part fracture. B. Reduction and insertion of Deyerle device. C. Uneventful healing of the four-part fracture. This is an alternative way of treating this type of fracture.

against the medial cortex of the distal femoral shaft. This medial buttress effect supplies additional support against the deforming forces normally present in the hip so that the compression screw does not bear the full brunt. This is an excellent concept, and I feel the procedure is the treatment of choice for this type of unstable four-part fracture.

Isolated Fractures of the Trochanters

Isolated fractures of the greater or lesser trochanter are usually due to avulsion injuries. The following rule of thumb is useful: displacements of more than 1 cm for the greater trochanter or 2 cm for the lesser trochanter should be treated by open reduction and internal fixation with a compression screw. The only exception to this rule is in the very elderly patient in whom operative fixation is rarely necessary. These fractures are usually seen in the young. They may be managed by four to five days of bed rest followed by gradual ambulation with crutches. A total of three to four weeks of protective weight bearing with crutches is, on the average, all that is necessary (Fig. 22–23).

If operative reduction is performed, the patient is usually kept in bed until comfortable and then allowed to be ambulatory without weight bearing for a total of three to four weeks. At the end of this time he can advance to partial weight bearing for approximately three weeks. By then, full weight bearing without support is usually possible.

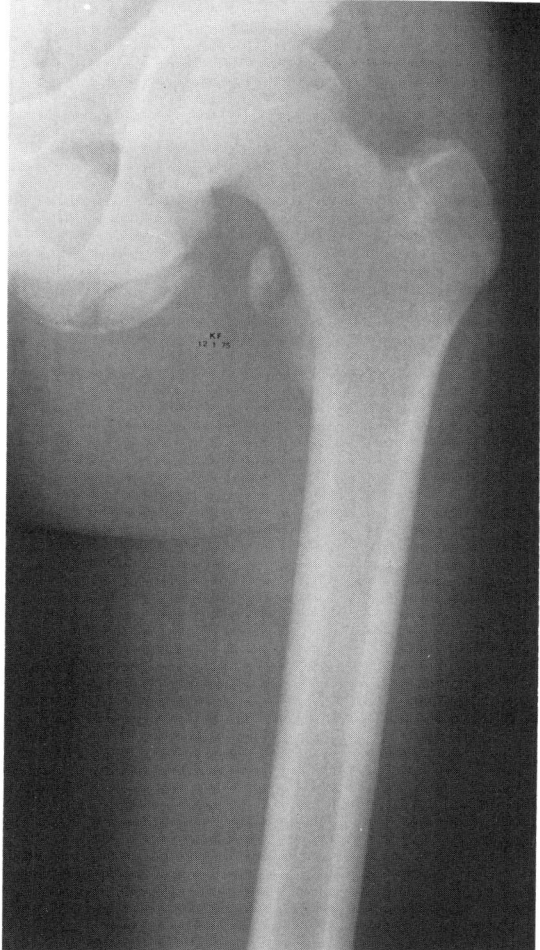

Figure 22-23 Avulsion fracture of the lesser trochanter in a teen-age patient. Treated conservatively with five days of bed rest. Recovery was uneventful.

Subtrochanteric Fractures

These fractures are notoriously difficult to classify and treat properly. The major problem in the management of patients with subtrochanteric fractures is the magnitude of the stresses normally generated in this particular area. Koch determined that the forces acting in this area produce a compression stress medially and a tensile stress laterally, and calculated those present in the medial subtrochanteric area, finding them to exceed 1200 psi (pounds per square inch) at a level 1 to 3 inches distal to the lesser trochanter. He calculated the tensile stresses laterally to be approximately 20 per cent less in magnitude.[121a] On the other hand, it must be remembered that fractures occurring at a level 1 to 3 inches distal to the lesser trochanter occur in an area of cortical bone rather than one of cancellous bone, as in pertrochanteric fractures. Thus, the body attempts to increase the amount of osseous stock present to combat the enormous stresses produced in this area.

These fractures characteristically are due in the young to severe direct trauma and in the elderly to a combination of osteoporosis and direct trauma.

The main goal in treatment is to obtain sufficient stability with internal fixation to allow early mobilization and subsequent healing. Occasionally, in the presence of severe comminution of the medial aspect or a medical condition contraindicating surgery, these fractures are treated with traction. The problem with this program is the very high incidence of malunion and nonunion. It must also be borne in mind, particularly with the elderly, that the conservative approach requires bed rest in traction for a period ranging from two to four months. This prolonged bed rest and the concommitant secondary medical complications must be weighed against the chance of producing sufficient stability to allow early mobilization.

Since union is seriously affected by both the level and the amount of medial comminution, the treatment is not uniform for all subtrochanteric fractures. The four types of internal fixation devices that have been employed in an attempt to obtain stability are a heavy Jewett device with a long side plate, a sliding compression screw with a long side plate, a compression blade plate, and a Küntscher nail or a Zickel nail. It may be easily appreciated that there is no single universal device at present for treating all subtrochanteric fractures.

The anatomical deformity that is present depends on the level of the fracture and the accompanying muscular forces. The operator must remember that in a properly reduced fracture the medial portion is subject to compression forces while the lateral aspect is subject to tensile forces. Therefore, the extramedullary devices are placed along the lateral aspect of the proximal shaft of the femur to act as a tension band. This principally requires a satisfactory medial buttress to be successful. Intramedullary devices, on the other hand, attempt to compensate for these compressive and tensile forces by producing resistance to them within the medullary portion of the bone. In the following discussion of treatment methods, Zickel's classification, taking into account the level, the obliquity, and the comminution, is used: type 1, a short oblique fracture with or without comminution; type 2, a long oblique fracture with or without comminution; and type 3, a high or low transverse fracture.

Type 1 fractures can be anatomically reduced and treated with a sliding compression screw and a long side plate or a compression blade plate. Either of these techniques will produce satisfactory internal fixation, and union occurs in more than 90 per cent of cases. If there is comminution present, I prefer to treat this with a sliding compression screw with a long side plate, which will allow for medial displacement at the fracture site during healing.

The presence of a long oblique fracture with or without comminution along the medial aspect, type 2, presents a much more difficult treatment problem (Fig. 22–24). If there is a segmental fragment along the medial aspect, then every attempt should be made to transfix this fragment to the proximal and distal major fragments. This can be accomplished with cancellous compression screws. Another method is to fix this fragment with a Parham band, and circlage wires can also be used to bring the medial fragments together. I, however, do not prefer this type of treatment. Once the medial buttress has been reestablished, a compression blade plate or an intramedullary device can be inserted. I feel that in the presence of comminution at this level a supplementary bone graft should be added in all cases. This is because, in the presence of severe comminution, the internal fixation device must withstand all the stresses in the area, which will inevitably lead to fatigue fracture of the stressed device. In this situation the operator and the patient are in a race against time. With a supplementary bone graft added, the fracture will heal more rapidly, and once healing is established the stress on the fixation device will be decreased. If, on the other hand, the bone graft is not added and healing is delayed, the likelihood of failure due to stress fatigue is increased significantly. A further aid to obtaining increased stability, in addition to the internal device and the bone graft, is to select a large plate with at least six holes to be placed along the anterior aspect of the shaft of the proximal femur spanning the fracture area. It cannot be emphasized enough that every attempt should be made to gain all possible stability in this area because of the high concentration of stresses normally present.

Type 3 fractures are more stable than

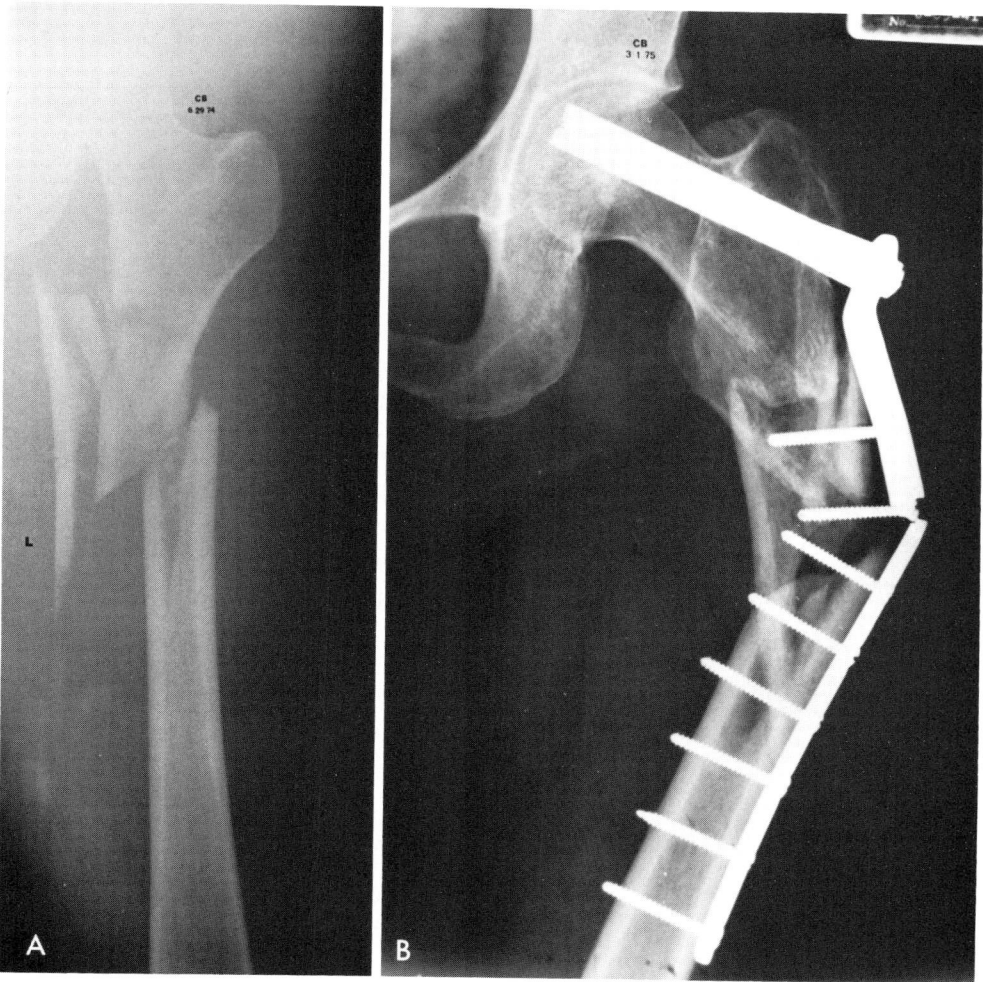

Figure 22-24 A. Type 2 fracture with a large medial butterfly fragment. This is the type that can be treated with a Zickel nail and circlage wires. B. A deliberate attempt to form a medial buttress was not made, and the thin long side plate did not provide enough stability. This was the wrong type of device for this particular fracture.

types 1 and 2 because of their horizontal nature. In the high fracture I prefer the Zickel nail, as the femoral canal is wide in this location and an intramedullary rod alone may not provide enough stability. The Zickel nail, by virtue of the combined fixation of the nail in the femoral neck and the rod down the shaft, will provide the necessary stability (Fig. 22-25). In the low type 3 transverse fracture an intramedullary rod such as the Sampson, the Hansen-Street, or the Küntscher may be utilized, or a Zickel nail may also be considered (Fig. 22-26). Bone grafting is not necessary with this type of fracture.

Overall in treating type 2 and type 3 fractures, I have found the Zickel nail or the compression blade plate to be most helpful in obtaining stability in this difficult location. The Zickel device consists of an intramedullary rod with a tunnel drilled into the rod through its proximal portion. A triflanged nail is inserted through the tunnel and locked in place with a set screw at the upper end of the rod. This combination of intramedullary rod and proximal transfixing nail supports both the proximal and distal fragments.

The patient is placed on a regular operating table in the lateral decubitus position.

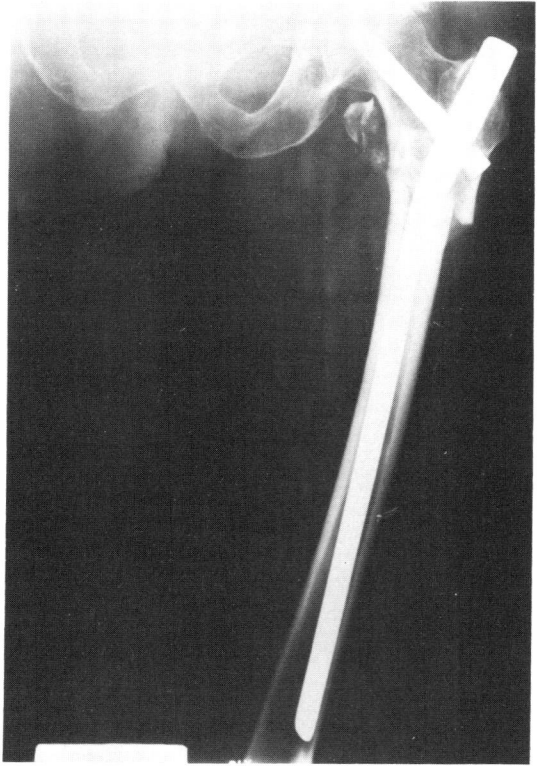

Figure 22–25 A type 2 fracture treated appropriately with a Zickel nail. Healing was uneventful.

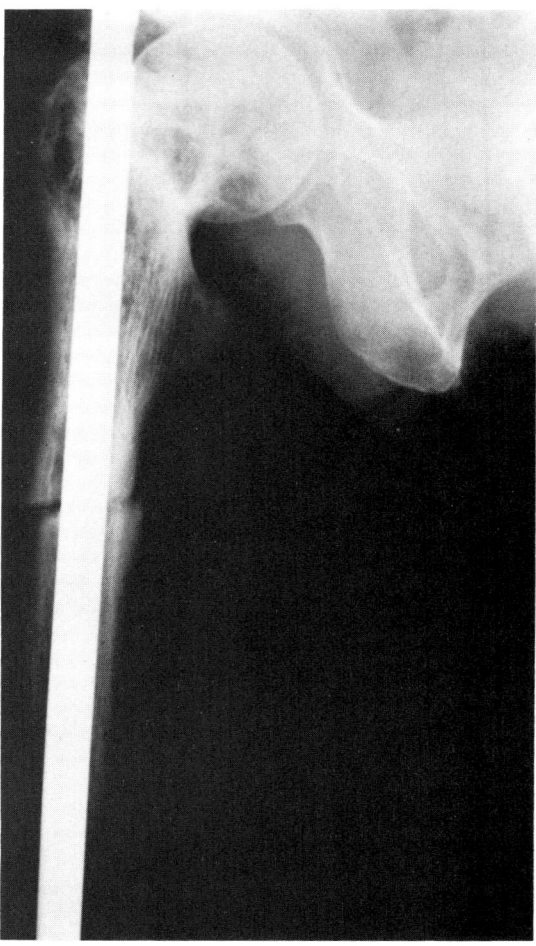

Figure 22–26 A low type 3 fracture treated with a Küntscher rod. Healing was uneventful.

A standard lateral incision is used to expose the area of the greater trochanter and the proximal femur. The fracture is identified and anatomically reduced as well as possible. The amount of medial comminution is then determined; if it is acceptable, then the proximal and distal fragments are reamed to accommodate the intramedullary rod. The rod is then inserted through the trochanter and driven in to the appropriate depth. A special device supplied to locate the hole in the proximal portion of the nail indicates the exact location on the lateral cortex of the proximal femur for insertion of the triflanged nail. After being inserted through the hole in the intramedullary rod up into the femoral neck and head, the nail is locked into position with a set screw in the proximal end of the intramedullary rod. This prevents motion of the triflanged nail within the intramedullary rod. Satisfactory stability is usually obtained with this device.

If there is excessive medial comminution and a medial buttress cannot be created, a Zickel nail or a sliding compression screw and side plate with an added bone graft and an anterior six-hole plate is recommended for this difficult fracture.

POSTOPERATIVE MANAGEMENT

The entire principle underlying the operative treatment of patients with extracapsular fractures is that satisfactory internal fixation will allow early ambulation, avoiding secondary medical complications. The entire postoperative course is directly influenced by the amount of stability obtained at the time of internal fixation. The two major questions involved in the postoperative rehabilitation of these patients are: (1) When is it safe for these patients to be transferred from bed to chair? (2) At what time can these patients be ambulatory with supportive devices and when can they begin weight bearing? The answers to these questions are directly determined by the amount of stability obtained during the operative procedure.

Intertrochanteric Fractures

Patients with intertrochanteric fractures are usually treated without suspension postoperatively. They can be transferred from bed to chair within 24 to 48 hours, and can then progress to early ambulation with a walker. Touchdown gait with the walker is initiated next. The majority of patients are capable of this stage of rehabilitation by the second to third day. Those with nondisplaced fractures treated with a sliding compression screw device can then progress rapidly to full weight bearing. These patients are usually discharged 10 to 14 days postoperatively, depending on their progress at physical therapy. Some of them are able to manage crutch walking prior to their discharge. If there is any hesitancy in obtaining balance, however, these patients should continue using a walker until they are seen in routine follow-up at one month with new x-rays.

Pertrochanteric Fractures

The postoperative management of patients with pertrochanteric fractures also depends on the amount of stability obtained. If there was an element of comminution present and a sliding compression screw device has been inserted, these patients can progress rapidly to active ambulation like those in the foregoing group. In the presence of comminution, however, it is best to keep them at partial weight bearing for six weeks; generally, they are able to tolerate 50 per cent weight bearing on the involved limb without difficulty. If a significant amount of comminution is present along the posterior or medial aspect and a medial displacement osteotomy has not been performed, then these

patients should not progress to full weight bearing until there is radiological evidence of beginning osseous union across the fracture site. Some of them will show evidence of medial displacement of the distal fragment if the sliding compression screw has been utilized. In other words, this type of device allows the patient to perform his own medial displacement osteotomy with settling at the fracture site. In the presence of a true unstable four-part fracture, the amount of weight bearing is definitely influenced by the operative technique. If a medial displacement technique along with the sliding compression screw has been employed, as in the technique of Harrington and Johnston, then there will be additional support along the medial aspect to compensate for the comminution, and early active weight bearing can be initiated. Progression to active weight bearing with this type of fracture, however, depends on the amount of stability and the buttressing effect obtained along the medial aspect. If this has not been adequate and firm impaction is not present, then these patients should be kept at partial weight bearing for a period of six to eight weeks.

Subtrochanteric Fractures

For patients with type 1 subtrochanteric fractures treated with a sliding compression screw, ambulation and early weight bearing are initiated within the first week. These patients usually have little difficulty in achieving full weight bearing status within two to three weeks. Those with type 3 transverse fractures are started with early active ambulation and full weight bearing within two to three weeks. On the other hand, oblique and comminuted fractures of types 2 and 3 may require additional protection. If the operator is of the opinion that adequate stability was obtained at the operative procedure, then these patients are allowed partial weight bearing within one week; if internal fixation has been accomplished but significant stability along the medial aspect is lacking, then they are not. If they are elderly, they are managed as bed to chair patients with physical therapy to maintain motion of all major joints. If a patient is young and unreliable about weight bearing, then consideration should be given to the application of a one and a half hip spica.

COMPLICATIONS

Nonunion

The rate of nonunion of intertrochanteric and pertrochanteric fractures is very low owing to the presence of an excellent blood supply and adequate cancellous bone. This is not the case with subtrochanteric fractures. On Fielding and Maglioto's classification, type 1 has a less than 10 per cent nonunion rate, while types 2 and 3 have rates varying from 34 to 57 per cent.[78] This is mainly because the bone at the type 2 and type 3 levels is cortical and that at the type 1 level is cancellous.

If the internal fixation appears adequate, nonunion is treated with a bone grafting procedure. The internal fixation device is not altered if it is providing adequate fixation, but if it does not appear to be, it is replaced by a similar device or a new device is chosen as outlined previously and a supplementary bone graft is added.

Infection

Infection is another dreaded complication in the operative management of hip fractures. The main requisite is to identify the offending organism. Appropriate intravenous antibiotics are then initiated. The internal fixation device is not removed if the fracture has not healed; every attempt should be made to maintain the internal fixation device until healing does occur. This can usually be accomplished by thorough debridement and insertion of an ingress-egress irrigation system. The irrigation system accompanied by intravenous administration of appropriate antibiotics will bring the infection under control in a significant number of cases. If the infection cannot be brought under control with these measures, then the internal fixation device must be removed. Reconstructive arthroplasty is not performed until all evidence of infection has been eliminated and a satisfactory time interval has passed.

The only satisfactory way to avoid infection is by using meticulous surgical technique and prophylactic antibiotics. There is in the literature ample evidence of the usefulness of intravenous prophylactic antibiotics in the management of patients with hip fractures. The confusion in the past has been over when to initiate the antibiotic therapy. Recent evidence has definitely demonstrated that if prophylactic antibiotics are to be utilized they must be started preoperatively and carried through the operative procedure and into the early postoperative interval. The prime time for antibiotic coverage is during the operative procedure, and it is important to obtain an adequate therapeutic blood level prior to making the skin incision. Most authors in this field feel that the antibiotic therapy can be discontinued within 24 to 48 hours postoperatively. I have been satisfied with the results of intravenous cephazolin (Ancef) or cephalothin (Keflin).

Part II HIP DISLOCATIONS, FRACTURE-DISLOCATIONS, AND ACETABULAR FRACTURES

This type of injury results from direct trauma. The force required to produce it is major, and for this reason patients frequently present with multiple injuries. There is no specific age group, as both the young and the elderly are subject to such trauma. Most series indicate a male predominance, and auto accidents are, by far, the most common cause. All series indicate an increased incidence with high-speed vehicular accidents. Although it has been adequately demonstrated that the use of seat belts decreases this type of trauma, many drivers refuse to wear them, and automobiles now do not demand their use while in motion. For this reason, these injuries will continue to be seen in the future.

Depending on the degree and direction of the force, the hip may be dislocated anteriorly or posteriorly, or a central fracture-dislocation may involve the acetabulum.

In the initial evaluation of these patients a thorough physical examination is indicated, as many of them have injuries to other systems. Occasionally the hip injury will be overlooked if an obvious life-threatening problem exists. To prevent this, in many medical centers throughout the country, a roentgenogram of the pelvis is obtained for all patients who have sustained severe trauma. Acetabular injury may present along with an associated fracture of the ipsilateral femur, and attention being focused on the obvious fracture of the femur, the dislocated hip may not be detected. This error may be avoided by adhering to the old dictum that a roentgenogram should visualize the proximal and distal joints involved in all diaphysial fractures—an excellent rule and very applicable to this type of trauma. A simple clinical maneuver can differentiate a fractured femur from a dislocated hip. With a dislocated hip, motion of the lower extremity at the hip will be severely restricted because of associated pain and muscular spasm. This is not the case with a fractured femur; the examiner can produce motion at the fracture site. The danger in this differentiation is that a dislocated hip may be missed in the presence of a fractured femur. Taking standard roentgenograms of the hip and knee whenever there is a femoral shaft fracture will prevent this.

The dislocated hip should be reduced *as soon as possible.* The first 24 to 48 hours following injury is a golden period. If at all possible the hip should be relocated within the first 24 hours; if reduction must be delayed because of other severe medical complications, it is definitely more difficult after 48 to 72 hours. Similarly, future hip function is decreased with a delay in reduction.

ANTERIOR DISLOCATIONS

Anterior dislocations constitute approximately 10 per cent of all dislocations of the hip. This type of injury is caused by direct trauma, the first of two common mechanisms being an automobile accident in which the patient's knee is driven against the dashboard with the thigh in a position of abduction. The impact will usually cause the knee to rotate into further abduction and external rotation, which leads to an anterior dislocation. The second mechanism is a direct blow on the posterior aspect of the abducted and externally rotated thigh, as caused by a fall from a height.

CLASSIFICATION

A useful working classification of anterior dislocations is (1) obturator, (2) iliac, and (3) pubic.

PHYSICAL EXAMINATION

The typical deformity of an anterior dislocation is flexion, abduction, and external rotation of the involved lower extremity (Fig. 22–27). The flexion is not as marked with an iliac or pubic dislocation as with an obturator dislocation. If the patient is not obese, the femoral head may be palpated in the groin in a pubic dislocation or in the vicinity of the anterior iliac spine in an iliac dislocation. There may not be any shortening of the leg, particularly in an obturator dislocation. Assessment of shortening is difficult because of the flexed attitude of the hip and knee. If the injury has been caused by striking the dashboard, examination of the knee will frequently demonstrate evidence of direct trauma to the anterior aspect of the knee—a visible laceration or abrasion. The knee should be thoroughly examined to rule out an associated injury. If the mechanism was a fall in which the posterior aspect of the thigh or buttock area was

ANTERIOR   **POSTERIOR**

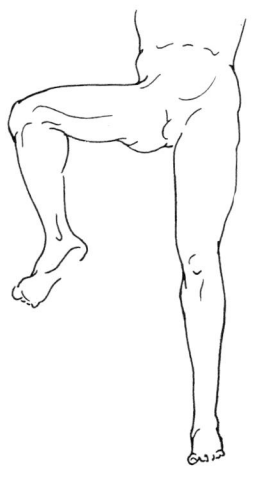
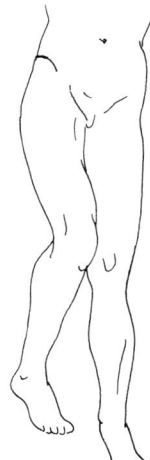

Figure 22–27   The attitude of the lower extremity in anterior and posterior dislocation.

injured, a hematoma or abrasion may be visible. The neurovascular status of the lower extremity should be evaluated carefully.

ROENTGENOGRAPHIC EXAMINATION

Standard anteroposterior and lateral roentgenograms of the hip will reveal the anterior dislocation of the hip and the position of the femoral head. Once the head escapes through the capsule of the joint, it may migrate either upward or downward. If it migrates downward, it may be seen in the obturator foramen. If there has been further progression and the Y ligament of Bigelow has been partly torn, the femoral head may be seen projecting into the perineum. On the other hand, it may not project downward and may be seen along the body of the pubis.

TREATMENT

As stated earlier, this injury should be reduced as soon as possible. The reduction should be performed under a spinal or general anesthetic if the patient's general condition will allow such anesthesia. If there are severe associated chest or head injuries, reduction may have to be attempted without anesthesia.

Allis Method of Reduction. The Allis method of reduction, which requires the operator and an assistant, is preferred by the author. The patient is placed on the operating table in the supine position, his thigh in mild abduction and flexion, and the operator applies traction in the line of the femur. The assistant applies pressure in an outward direction over the inner surface and upper third of the thigh and groin. The operator then completes the reduction by adducting and internally rotating the extremity (Fig. 22–28). If the initial reduction is not satisfactory it can be repeated one time, but forceful repeated attempts at closed reduction are not indicated. If, at the end of a second trial of the procedure, the hip remains dislocated, then the patient should be prepared for an open reduction. A failed reduction usually implies that a defect is present in the anterior portion of the capsule and that reduction attempts close the defect, producing a buttonhole effect. If repeated forceful attempts are

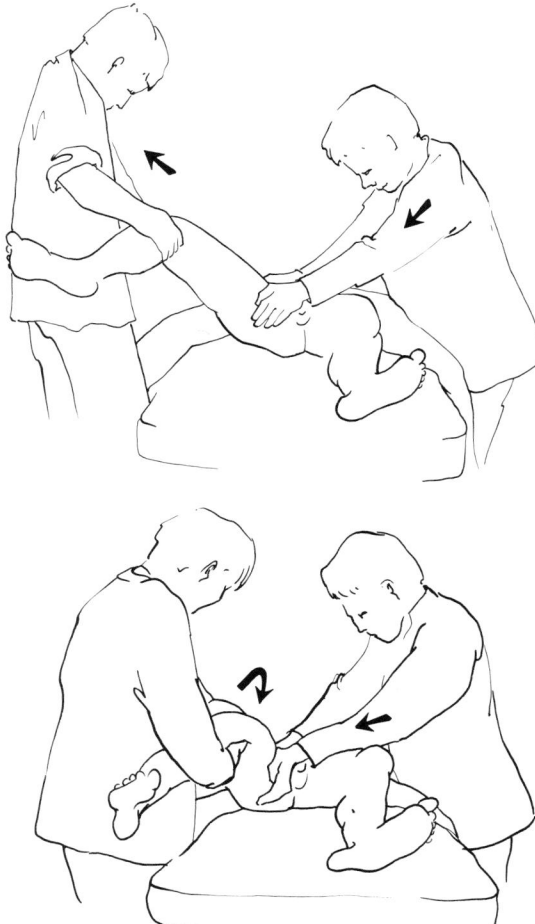

Figure 22–28 Allis method of reducing anterior dislocation of the hip.

continued, further damage to the femoral head and associated soft-tissue structures may occur.

Once the hip has been reduced it is usually stable. The recurrence rate following an anterior dislocation is extremely low. If redislocation does occur, an anterior repair of the capsular defect is indicated.

Aftercare. The aftercare following reduction is relatively simple. The patients are kept in bed, the affected hip and knee in a neutral position with Bucks traction. They appear to be more comfortable with this traction apparatus. Muscle setting progress-

ing to active motion and light resistance exercises is instituted immediately. A rule of thumb is not to allow the patient to ambulate until hip motion approximates normal and the hip appears to be free of signs of joint irritation. Soft-tissue healing should be accomplished prior to protected weight bearing. The time interval required to obtain this goal varies between patients. Protective weight bearing should be continued from 10 to 12 weeks. Salicylate therapy is initiated following reduction in an attempt to protect the injured cartilage, starting with .06 gm orally four times a day. It is felt that this also offers some protection against phlebitis.

POSTERIOR DISLOCATIONS

Posterior dislocations of the hip are far more frequent than anterior dislocations. The exact incidence varies from series to series but approximates a rate of 85 to 90 per cent of all hip dislocations.

The vast majority of these injuries are caused by automobile accidents in which the patient's knee strikes the dashboard directly. The mechanism of injury is a force transmitted through the flexed knee and down the slightly adducted and internally rotated femur to the hip joint. Since the most common cause of injury is an automobile accident, these patients, like those with anterior dislocations, must have thorough physical examinations. It is not uncommon for other major systems to be involved. As with anterior dislocations, it is extremely important to reduce a posterior dislocation as soon as possible, and the follow-up results are similar in that the earlier the reduction the better the prognosis. Reduction should be carried out within 24 hours of injury if at all possible.

CLASSIFICATION

Posterior dislocations may be classified (after Thompson and Epstein) into five types: (1) those with or without a minor fracture; (2) those with a large single fracture of the posterior acetabular rim; (3) those with a comminuted fracture of the rim of the acetabulum, with or without a major fragment; (4) those with a fracture of the acetabular rim and floor; and (5) those with a fracture of the femoral head.[198]

PHYSICAL EXAMINATION

With a posterior dislocation of the hip, the typical deformity is a shortened, adducted, and internally rotated extremity. This is partially due to the intact iliofemoral ligament. A careful physical examination must be performed to rule out an ipsilateral fracture of the femur. Like an anterior dislocation, a posterior dislocation is a relatively fixed deformity, while if the femur is fractured the lower extremity can usually be manipulated. This is an important diagnostic clinical sign. Since a significant number of sciatic nerve injuries follow dislocations of the hip, a careful neurological examination of the lower extremity is indicated to rule this out. The nerve injury can be due to direct contusion, partial laceration, or a traction-type injury. If there is any neurological deficit, this should be classified as an emergency and the reduction should be performed as soon as possible. An injured nerve here, as in other parts of the body, does not tolerate direct pressure or traction for any period of time. Therefore, immediate reduction to relieve the pressure on the nerve is mandatory.

ROENTGENOGRAPHIC EXAMINATION

Standard anteroposterior and lateral roentgenograms will reveal posterior dislocation. In order to assess the status of the acetabulum the three-quarter internal and external oblique views of Judet are obtained by rolling the patient 45 degrees to the left and then 45 degrees to the right. The obturator oblique view is obtained when the patient is rolled away from the injured side, the iliac-wing view when the patient is rolled toward the injured hip. The former demonstrates the entire anterior column along with the posterior lip of the acetabulum and the obturator foramen. The latter demonstrates the entire posterior margin of the innominate bone, the anterior lip of the acetabulum, and the entire iliac wing and crest.

The standard anteroposterior and lateral roentgenograms will demonstrate the femoral head behind and above the acetabulum (Fig. 22–29).

TREATMENT

Type 1 Dislocations

The three common types of maneuver employed to reduce a dislocated hip are the Allis, the Bigelow, and the Stimson.

Allis Method of Reduction. In the Allis method of reduction, the head of the femur is mobilized into place by direct traction on the flexed thigh (Fig. 22–30). The patient is given a spinal or general anesthetic and is then placed supine on his back with the pelvis immobilized by an assistant pressing downward on the anterior superior iliac spines. The operator then flexes the hip and knee to a right angle while maintaining the lower extremity in slight adduction and internal rotation. The flexed extremity is then lifted upward, drawing the head of the femur over the rim of the acetabulum and through the rent in the capsule, which allows it to slip back into proper position. The extremity is then gently lowered. If the operator encounters increased resistance in lifting the thigh, the adduction and internal rotation are increased to relax the capsule and disengage the head from the pelvis. By adduction and gentle rotation, the femoral head can usually be freed from its confines and the reduction completed.

Bigelow Method of Reduction. Bigelow's method of reduction relaxes the Y ligament of Bigelow by flexion of the hip and then utilizes the ligament as a fulcrum to lever the head into the acetabulum. This method is not for routine use, as it may rupture the Y ligament or damage the sciatic nerve or soft tissues posterior to the hip joint.

Stimson Method of Reduction. Stimson's method is excellent and should be employed more frequently than at present. As in other Stimson methods, the concept is to use the weight of the extremity to aid in the reduction (Fig. 22–31). This does not always require general anesthesia. It can frequently be performed with intravenous morphine or diazepam (Valium). The pa-

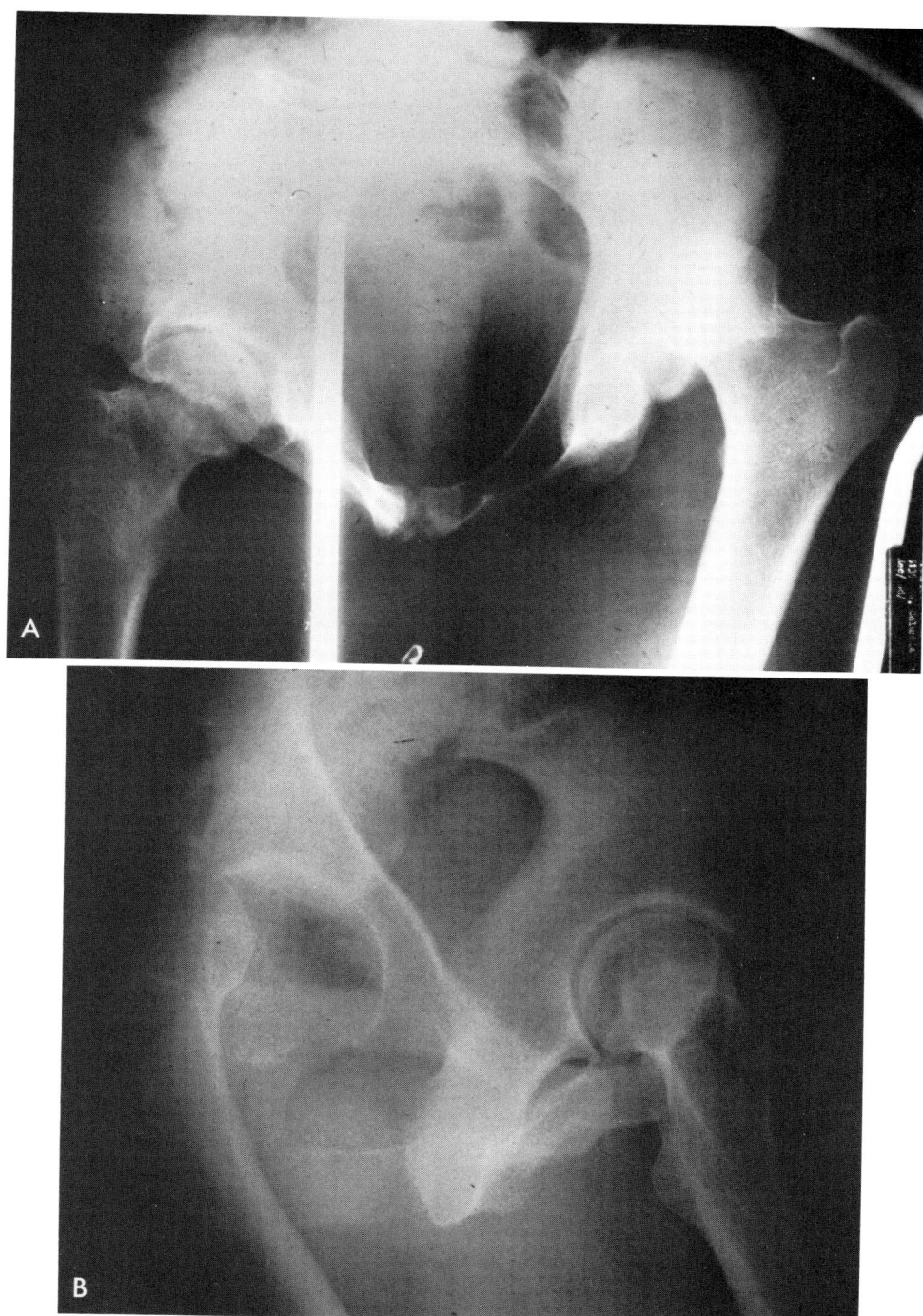

Figure 22-29 *A.* Anteroposterior view demonstrating posterior dislocation of hip. *B.* Oblique view demonstrating posterior dislocation of hip.

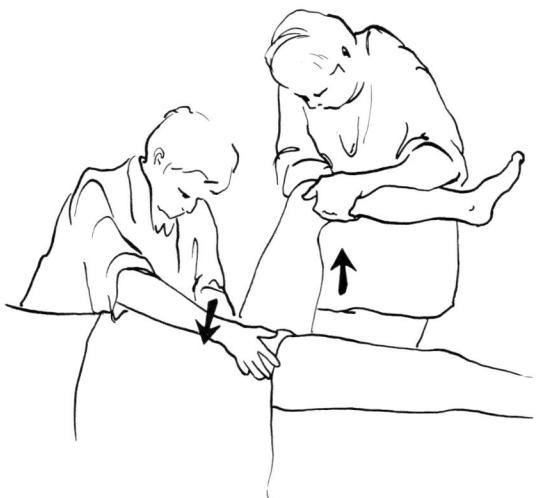

Figure 22–30 Allis method of reducing posterior dislocation of the hip.

tient is placed face down on a table with his lower extremities hanging over the edge. An assistant balances the uninvolved leg in slight flexion at the hip and knee, while the operator grasps the ankle of the involved limb with one hand and flexes the knee to a right angle. The hip is now at 90 degrees of flexion with the weight of the extremity directly downward. This weight provides the required traction. Once the muscles surrounding the hip relax, the hip will be relocated without difficulty. If it is not, the operator can apply gentle pressure on the posterior aspect of the calf to increase the downward force enough to pull the hip back into position. This is an excellent maneuver; it requires little effort on the part of the

operator or the patient, and an added advantage is that anesthesia is not always required. Once it is relocated, all that is necessary is to prevent adduction and flexion of the involved hip—by an abduction pillow between the knees or by gentle Buck's traction in slight abduction. Physical therapy is then initiated as in anterior dislocations. Once the soft-tissue structures have had a chance to heal and the patient demonstrates painless motion of the hip, he can be ambulatory with crutches. Protective weight bearing is then carried on for a total of 10 to 12 weeks.

Type 2 Through Type 5 Dislocations

The treatment of these particular injuries has been very controversial in the past. The recent studies by Epstein, d'Aubigne, and Judet as well as the Scandinavian series have, however, demonstrated the advantages of primary open reduction. These authors feel that the articular cartilage has initially received severe trauma and that joint debris from associated fractures may be present within the joint, predisposing it to future degenerative arthritis. The open reduction method allows for reconstitution of the primary architecture of the hip joint. It is important that large fragments be anatomically reduced and held in place by internal fixation devices (Fig. 22–32).[8, 71–73, 116]

The posterior surgical approach as outlined by Epstein allows excellent exposure of the posterior aspect of the hip. The patient is given a general anesthetic and

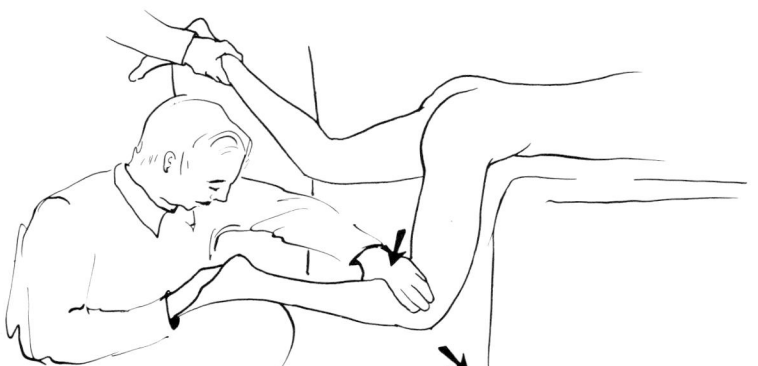

Figure 22–31 Stimson method of reduction for posterior dislocation of the hip. This is the preferred method.

then placed in prone position. The incision extends from the posterior superior iliac spine outward and downward to the region of the greater trochanter. If further exposure is necessary the incision may be extended laterally through the aponeurosis of the gluteus maximus and the tensor fascia lata. In the gluteus maximus muscle it is deepened by blunt rather than by sharp dissection, decreasing the amount of bleeding. Areolar and fatty tissues are removed from the peritrochanteric bursa. At this point the most important step is to identify the sciatic nerve and retract it out of harm's way. Once this has been done, the short rotator muscles can be incised from their attachment to the trochanteric fossa. The hip joint can then be adequately visualized. If further exposure is required the gluteus medius may be removed from its attachment to the greater trochanter. The posterior approach has several advantages. It allows excellent exposure of the hip joint, the operator can easily visualize the acetabulum to locate loose fragments and to transfix the fractured acetabular rim if necessary, and it does not interfere with the anterior blood supply.

The end result of all types of internal fixation devices is to provide secure anatomical reduction. Cancellous bone screws appear to be extremely useful for large posterior fragments, and various European authors have advised the use of a small plate with multiple screws.

Roentgenograms are obtained immediately after reduction to document the status of the reduction and demonstrate the presence or absence of loose fragments within the joint.

The treatment of subsequent avascular necrosis or traumatic arthritis is generally the same as that for primary avascular necrosis or degenerative arthritis. The majority of the patients who develop these complications will require total hip replacement in the future. It is the author's feeling that there is no place for primary total hip replacement; this can always be performed later as an elective secondary procedure if required.

The treatment of sciatic nerve injuries follows the principles outlined in Chapter 34.

Old Dislocations

Dislocations that have been "missed" are not frequent, but they do occur. A general rule of thumb is that up to six weeks following the original injury an attempt at reduction by conservative measures including traction and manipulation may be

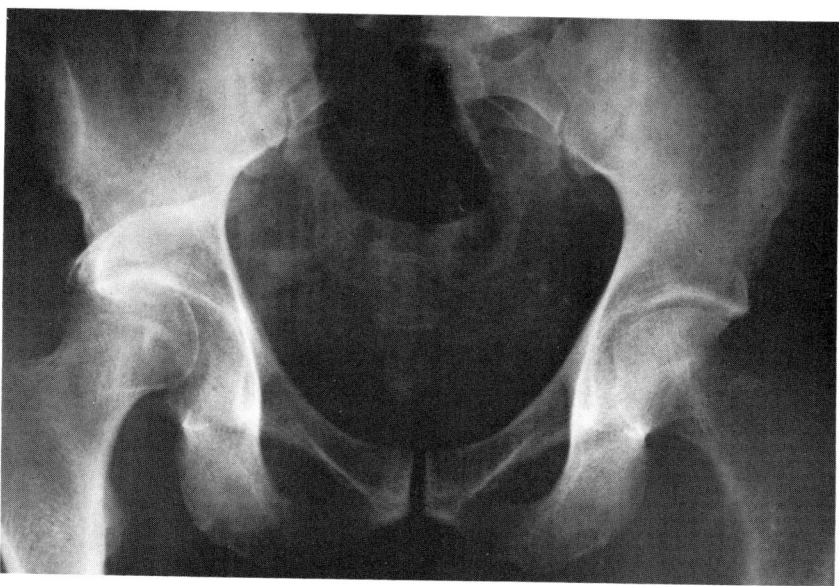

Figure 22–32   Posterior dislocation of the hip associated with a large posterior fragment. An extremely unstable injury, it required operative fixation of the posterior fragment with large cancellous bone screws.

successful. If the dislocation has been present for longer than six weeks, or in an elderly patient for a shorter time, skeletal traction should be employed in an attempt to pull the head of the femur down to the vicinity of the hip joint prior to any attempt at reduction. It is true that the femoral head in a dislocation that has been unreduced for more than six weeks runs a very high risk of avascular necrosis and degenerative arthritis. Even so, however, the treatment of choice is to perform a reduction in an attempt to salvage the hip. Closed reduction following skeletal traction may not be successful, and the patient may require an open reduction, which is still the procedure of choice following a failed closed reduction for an old dislocated hip. Obviously, there must be a point at which reduction would be futile. If the dislocation has been unreduced for several months, an arthroplasty will probably be indicated. The initial step in performing an arthroplasty, however, would be to bring the head down to the level of the acetabulum by preoperative skeletal traction or by muscular sectioning procedures.

Occasionally, a patient will present with an ipsilateral fracture of the femur as well as a dislocated hip. There are two generally accepted procedures for treating this injury. In the first, a heavy screw is inserted through the lateral trochanter into the femoral neck. This allows control of the femoral head for manipulative purposes. Once the femoral head has been reduced, the femoral shaft fracture can be treated as described in Chapter 23. I feel, however, that the procedure of choice is an open reduction and internal fixation of the femoral shaft fracture followed by a closed reduction of the dislocated hip. If the fracture is in the midportion of the femur, a Küntscher nail may be employed for the internal fixation.

COMPLICATIONS

The two most feared complications of posterior dislocations of the hip are sciatic nerve injury and avascular necrosis of the femoral head. As stated previously, the sciatic nerve can be damaged by direct contusion, by partial laceration, or by a traction injury. Since nerve tissue does not respond well to continued pressure, immediate reduction of the dislocation is required to prevent further nerve injury.

The second major complication is avascular necrosis of the femoral head. This occurs in from 20 to 30 per cent of cases, according to various reports. The only significant finding consistent with all reports is that the earlier the reduction is performed, the better the result. If the hip is reduced within 24 hours there is a high percentage of good results; if there is a delay in reduction, that percentage decreases significantly. In this light, dislocated hips should be considered a surgical emergency.

CENTRAL FRACTURE-DISLOCATIONS AND ACETABULAR FRACTURES

It is fair to state that the treatment of these fractures remains controversial. Several reports have appeared recently justifying either an open reduction and internal fixation approach or a closed reduction with prolonged skeletal traction. Because these injuries are frequently associated with other multiple-system injuries, the definitive treatment of the fracture-dislocation of the hip may have to be delayed. The consensus in the United States appears to be that the majority of these fractures may be treated conservatively by closed reduction and prolonged skeletal traction — in contrast to the surgical approach advocated by Judet and Letournel in Europe. The latter authors have, however, helped to clarify the exact anatomical distortion produced by these severe injuries.

This type of fracture is seen in all age groups. The average age of the patients is in the early forties. There is a slightly higher rate of incidence in males.

MECHANISMS OF INJURY

Automobile accidents continue to account for the majority of these injuries. A direct lateral blow to the trochanteric area may produce a central fracture-dislocation of the hip by driving the femoral head horizontally directly through the inner wall and into the pelvis. Typically, this type of injury occurs when a pedestrian is struck along the trochanteric area by the bumper or fender of an oncoming car; when a person falls from a height, landing on the trochanteric area; or when a passenger or driver in an automobile accident, is in the seated position, and is thrust forward so that a direct longitudinal force is driven along the femur as the knee strikes the dashboard. If the lower extremity is in slight internal rotation when this happens, the femoral head may be driven directly posteriorly, causing a posterior acetabular fracture. If the limb is in slight external rotation and abduction, the femoral head may be driven upward and inward, producing a bursting or shattering type of fracture that may involve all areas of the acetabulum, including the inner wall, the superior dome, and the posterior wall. Although the femoral head may appear to be resting centrally in the pelvis with a bursting-type fracture, it is often actually found to be in a posterior and upward location.

CLASSIFICATION

Several classifications have been proposed to clarify the type of injury, the treatment, and the prognosis. A good working classification must also take into account the exact anatomical location of the fracture within the acetabulum as this definitely affects the form of treatment chosen for these patients. A simple one is: type 1—fractures of the inner wall (pubic division) with and without intrapelvic protrusion of the femoral head; type 2—fractures of the posterior wall (ischial division) with and without posterior dislocation of the femoral head; type 3—fractures of the superior dome (iliac division) with and without displacement of the femoral head; and type 4—bursting or shattering fractures, which involve disruption of all portions of the acetabulum, including the pubic, iliac, and ischial segments. This system is not entirely academic; it has a direct application in that treatment of these injuries as based on the anatomical location of the fracture. Other classifications have been advocated, but this is the easiest to apply clinically.

Type 1 — Inner Wall Fractures. This type

of fracture occurs when the femoral head is driven through the thin central portion of the acetabulum. The femoral head may then rest within the pelvis, producing a intrapelvic protrusion or creating a fracture of the central portion of the acetabulum while remaining located in its normal position. The most important feature of this fracture is that the superior dome of the acetabulum is not altered. This has a direct bearing on the prognosis, as the direct weight-bearing surface is not affected, and the results are good if the femoral head is relocated under the superior dome.

Type 2 — Posterior Wall Fractures. Like type 1 fractures, these injuries do not involve the superior weight-bearing surface of the acetabulum. The posterior portion of the acetabulum provides stability for the femoral head. As mentioned previously in regard to posterior dislocations of the hip associated with fracture of the posterior acetabulum, the sciatic nerve may be injured. If the fracture is not reduced quickly avascular necrosis of the femoral head may result.

Type 3 — Superior Dome Fractures. This type of fracture carries a poor prognosis, as it involves the weight-bearing superior dome of the acetabulum. It is for this reason that a more aggressive approach to treatment is undertaken in an attempt to recreate a superior dome that will withstand weight bearing.

Type 4 — Bursting or Shattering Fractures. This type of injury carries the worst prognosis. This is due to the gross disruption of the acetabulum that is produced. Like type 3 injuries, these require a more aggressive approach to treatment in an attempt to reconstruct a weight-bearing surface and inner wall of the acetabulum that will conform to the shape of the femoral head in order to prevent future arthritis.

PHYSICAL EXAMINATION

These patients have sustained significant trauma and frequently present with symptoms and signs of hypovolemic shock. It is not unusual for them to have lost several units of blood into the hip and pelvic area, and it is therefore important to examine them for signs of imminent shock.

Physical examination of the involved hip will usually reveal local evidence of injury with a central fracture-dislocation of the hip. A large hematoma may well be present along the lateral aspect of the proximal femur. There may also be evidence of a skin abrasion caused by direct lateral trauma. Any attempt to move the hip joint proper will elicit severe pain. The attitude of the lower extremity depends upon the particular type of acetabular fracture; if intrapelvic protrusion is present, shortening will be evident, while in a posterior fracture-dislocation of the hip, the lower limb is usually both grossly shortened and in internal rotation.

A careful neurovascular assessment of the involved extremity should be performed. The vasculature of the limb is usually intact, but a neurological deficit may be present, particularly with a posterior fracture-dislocation of the hip in which there is direct pressure on the sciatic nerve by the femoral head. As mentioned previously, it is important to record any neurological deficit with this type of injury, as this may have a direct bearing on the type of treatment selected for this particular patient.

It is also important to examine the abdomen for bowel sounds, as reflex ileus may be present with severe intrapelvic protrusion.

ROENTGENOGRAPHIC EXAMINATION

It is extremely important to obtain adequate roentgenographic evaluation of all patients with acetabular fractures. Judet, Judet, and Letournel have described the four views that they feel are most appropriate for assessing these injuries: (1) an anteroposterior view of the pelvis in order to identify any fractures of the opposite side (Fig. 22–33); (2) an anteroposterior view of the involved hip; (3) the obturator oblique view, which is obtained by having the patient supine but rolled 45 degrees away from the injured hip (Fig. 22–34); and (4) the iliac wing view, which is obtained by having the patient supine but rolled 45 degrees toward the affected hip.[116]

In the anteroposterior view of the pelvis the anterior lip, the posterior lip, and the roof of the acetabulum can be assessed. The ilioischial line formed by the posterior portion of the quadrilateral surface of the ischium behind the inner portion of the

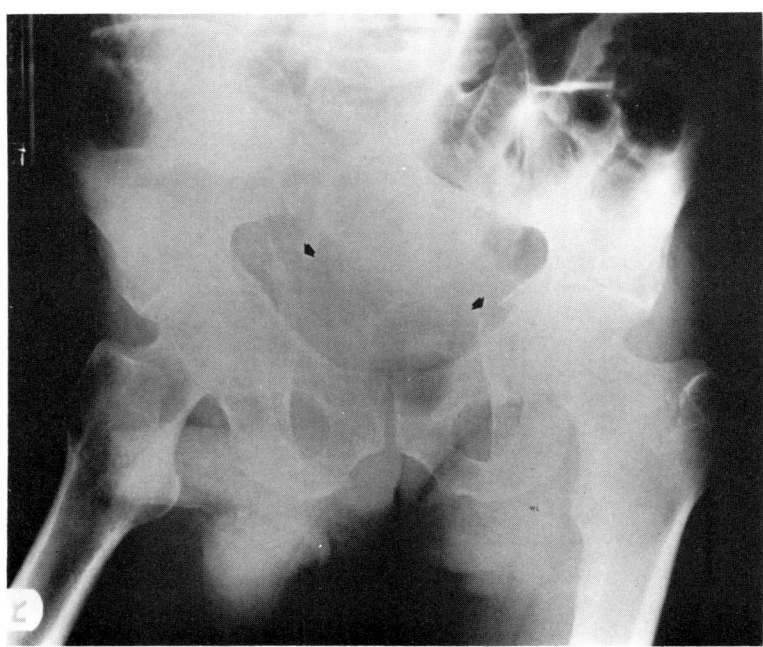

Figure 22–33 Anteroposterior view demonstrating bilateral central fracture-dislocations of the pelvis (arrows).

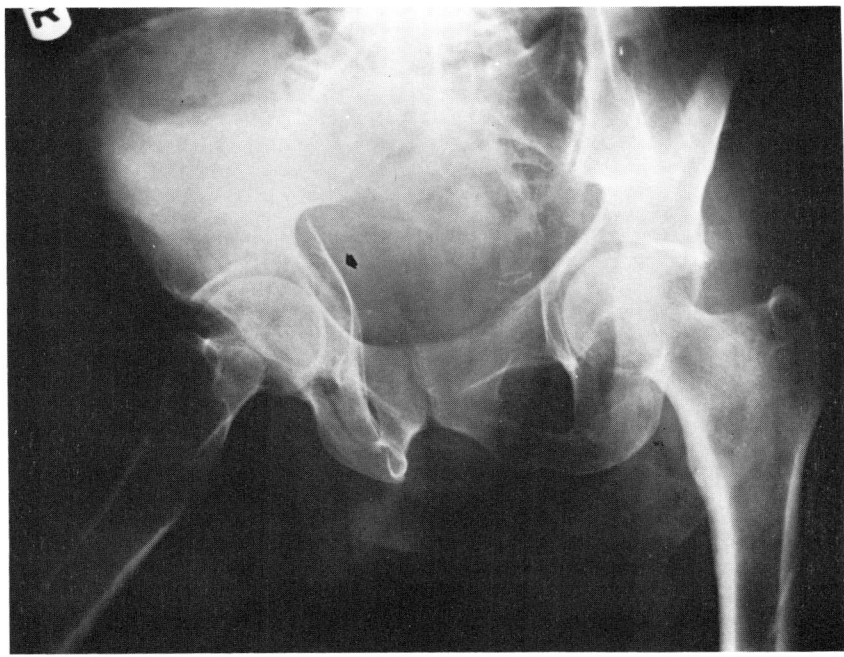

Figure 22–34 Obturator view demonstrating intact posterior wall on the left and visualizing the central fracture-dislocation on the right (arrow).

socket and the iliopectineal line that corresponds for its largest portion to the anatomical superior channel may be properly evaluated. The obturator oblique view is obtained to assess the anterior column, the posterior lip of the acetabulum and obturator foramen, and the wing of the ilium. The iliac wing view is used to assess the posterior margin of the innominate bone, the anterior lip of the acetabulum, and the entire iliac wing and crest.

These views allow the attending physician to determine the extent of the injury and to decide which particular type of fracture is present. The oblique views have been particularly valuable in determining the amount of comminution present and the degree of involvement of both the anterior and posterior columns.

TREATMENT

General Management

As stated previously, many patients with this particular type of injury present with signs and symptoms of hypovolemic shock due to blood loss. It is important to secure sufficient blood for hemoglobin studies and also to start transfusion of an adequate amount of cross-matched blood. It is generally a good rule of thumb to obtain at least two units of cross-matched blood for patients presenting with these fractures.

Specimens for routine laboratory studies are obtained, and the patients are placed in temporary Buck's traction in order to make them comfortable so that appropriate roentgenograms can be taken and also to attempt to stabilize the pelvic fragments and thereby decrease the amount of hemorrhage. Eight pounds of skin traction is usually adequate for comfort, and the patients can then be transported to the radiology department. It is important that a member of the medical staff accompany the patient to the radiology department, as hypovolemic shock may develop during the time interval required to obtain adequate roentgenograms. Once the roentgenograms have been obtained, an appropriate course of treatment can be selected and initiated.

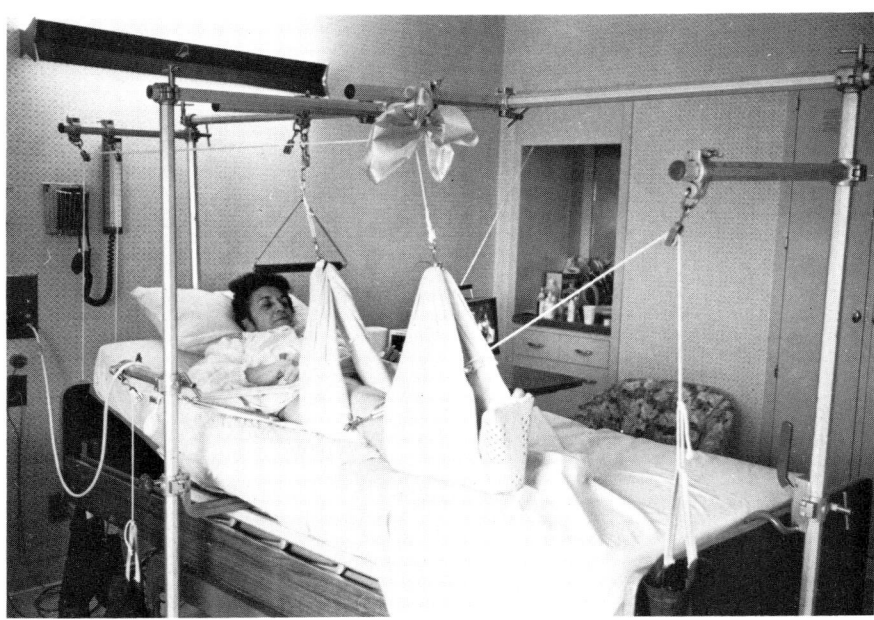

Figure 22–35 A patient with a central fracture-dislocation of the hip was removed from her Thomas splint and Pearson knee attachment at four weeks and maintained in skeletal traction with slings to suspend the lower extremity. Lateral traction is provided through a large sling around the proximal femur.

Type 1 – Inner Wall Fractures

These fractures can generally be managed by closed reduction. A sling is placed around the medial aspect of the proximal thigh and pulled in a lateral direction. This will tend to pull the femoral head out of the pelvis back into normal alignment under the superior dome. If the femoral head is not within the pelvis, a Kirschner wire may be inserted through the tibial tubercle for skeletal traction. The leg is then placed in balanced skeletal suspension with a Thomas splint and a Pearson knee attachment. The pull on the Kirschner wire is in direct line with the normal position of the leg in relation to the body. A large sling around the medial aspect of the proximal femur may be used for continuous lateral traction if there is any tendency toward central displacement of the femoral head (Fig. 22–35). If this is not adequate, a trochanteric screw may be inserted for direct lateral traction (Fig. 22–36).

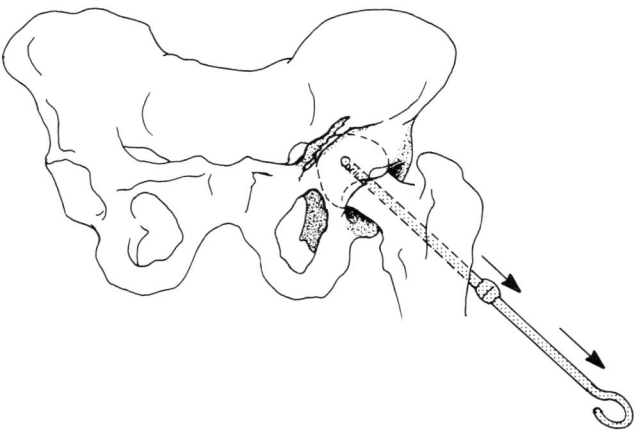

Figure 22–36 A large trochanteric screw may be inserted up the femoral neck into the femoral head for direct lateral skeletal traction.

In general it is appropriate to begin with approximately 15 to 20 lb of skeletal traction through the tibial wire and 8 to 10 lb of lateral traction. This can always be altered as indicated by appropriate roentgenograms. Several other devices have been advocated for lateral traction. A heavy Kirschner wire may be placed through the trochanter in an anterior-posterior direction and a traction bow attached for direct lateral traction. Lipscomb has advocated placing two pins in the proximal lateral portion of the femur with one pointing cephalad and the other more caudad, producing a scissoring effect that prevents them from pulling out.[127a] All the aforementioned methods of obtaining lateral traction are satisfactory and should be employed if there is evidence of central migration of the femoral head.[199]

Patients are usually maintained in skeletal traction for a minimum of six weeks. At that time the traction apparatus may be removed and the patient started on hip motion in bed. These patients are gradually allowed to ambulate without weight bearing initially and then to progress to partial weight bearing after four weeks. They are not allowed full weight bearing until at least three months postinjury. Open reduction and internal fixation are infrequently necessary with this type of fracture, as the major superior weight-bearing portion of the acetabulum is not directly affected. The prognosis following treatment is excellent.

Type 2—Posterior Wall Fractures

As has been mentioned previously, the posterior portion of the acetabulum plays an important role in the stability of the hip. This portion of the acetabulum is generally fairly thick compared to the thinner inner wall. It is vitally important to treat a posterior fracture-dislocation as an emergency, as immediate reduction will definitely decrease the likelihood of avascular necrosis of the femoral head. The longer the femoral head remains dislocated, the more likely is avascular necrosis. These patients are given a general anesthetic, and the dislocation is gently reduced. Following reduction, the stability of the hip is evaluated. If there is a tendency toward redislo-

cation, with a small fragmented portion of a posterior lip present, the patient should be placed in balanced skeletal suspension. If a large posterior acetabular fragment is present and the hip is not stable, it is reasonable to proceed with an open reduction and internal fixation with multiple screws. Care must also be taken to remove any free osseous fragments from within the acetabulum at the time of the open reduction. This type of treatment has been discussed earlier in this chapter.

Type 3—Superior Dome Fractures

These fractures are difficult to manage, as the fracture itself involves the major weight-bearing surface of the acetabulum. It is for this reason that an adequate reduction must be performed to establish a congruent superior dome. Occasionally this can be done by balanced longitudinal skeletal traction combined with lateral skeletal traction. If, however, there is any tendency toward a step-off deformity in the superior dome area, then open reduction and internal fixation should be performed. This type of surgical approach, according to previous follow-up studies, produces good to excellent results, provided that the superior dome congruency has been reestablished. Judet, Judet, and Letournel have advocated early open reduction and internal fixation with large cancellous bone screws or a curved compression plate.[116] There has been a trend, recently, toward early open reduction and adequate internal fixation for this type of fracture. Judet's results would certainly support this approach.

It is also important to remember that if closed reduction is attempted with these fractures it should be performed early, as the best chance of success exists within the first 72 hours. Following that interval the likelihood of obtaining an adequate closed reduction decreases. As I stated previously, however, many patients with this type of fracture also have other injuries, and a proper reduction may have to be delayed in order to treat the more life-threatening wounds. In this situation it is best to treat the life-threatening conditions, and once these are stable, proceed with an open reduction and internal fixation. The ilioinguinal approach of Judet, as described in his original article, is preferred for the open treatment of this fracture.[116]

The postoperative management depends upon the security of the internal fixation. If this is adequate, the patient may be managed with Buck's skin traction for two to three weeks with gentle motion of the hip initiated early postoperatively. On the other hand, if the attending surgeon does not feel the internal fixation to be adequate, then the patient should be placed in skeletal traction for four to six weeks and should start early general range of motion exercises while in traction. He is then allowed to be ambulatory without weight bearing for an additional three weeks, before progressing to partial weight bearing. It is best to keep these patients from full weight bearing for 10 to 12 weeks postoperatively.

Type 4 – Bursting or Shattering Fractures

This type of fracture carries the poorest prognosis. It is a severe injury and involves disruption of all three major components of the acetabulum. As with management of

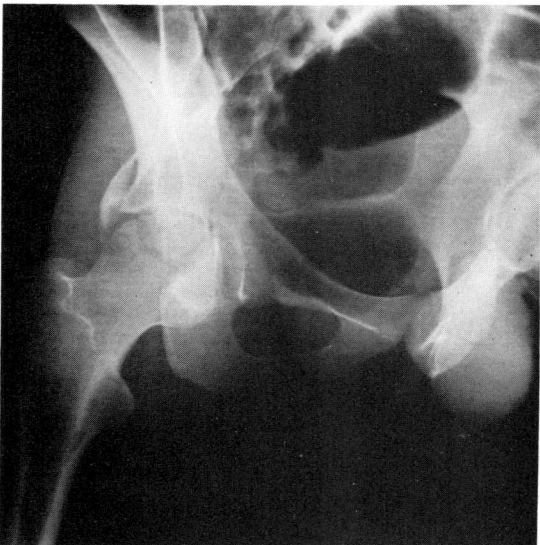

Figure 22–37 A bursting fracture following lateral traction to reduce the femoral head from within the pelvis back into a normal relationship. The central fracture as well as a large posterior lip segment is evident. This was unstable and required open reduction and internal fixation.

type 3 fractures, it is extremely important to attempt to reconstitute the superior dome and inner wall of the acetabulum (Fig. 22–37). If this goal is not obtained, severe degenerative arthritis of the hip is frequently the end result at an early date.

These patients are taken to the operating room, a general anesthetic is administered, a closed manipulation of the central fracture-dislocation of the hip is performed, and a skeletal wire is inserted through the tibial tubercle for skeletal traction. A lateral trochanteric screw is usually inserted at this time for direct lateral skeletal traction. Appropriate roentgenograms are then obtained in the operating room following the reduction. The amount of traction on the tibial pin and the lateral femoral screw will have to be altered, depending on follow-up roentgenographic examination. It is generally best to begin with 20 to 25 lb of traction through the tibial wire and 10 to 12 lb of traction through the lateral trochanteric screw.

Some authors recommend open reduction and internal fixation for these severe injuries. This aggressive operative approach has been advocated by Judet, Judet, and Letournel.[116] Many of these fractures are severely comminuted, however, and it is extremely difficult to obtain adequate fixation at the time of the open reduction. On the other hand, the reduction obtained with a closed method will not be satisfactory if several large portions of the acetabulum remain within the pelvis. In this particular circumstance it is appropriate to attempt by open reduction and internal fixation to replace the displaced acetabular fragments in proper alignment. This may require both an anterior and a posterior approach. If there is gross disruption and it is difficult to obtain a medial buttressing effect, then I feel it is advantageous to perform a bone graft utilizing a piece of iliac crest bone at that time in case total hip replacement is required at a later date. This will allow a thick medial buttress to form. If it is not done and the medial acetabular fragments are allowed to remain within the pelvis, a very thin inner pelvic wall with central protrusion is the final result—a situation that makes it very difficult later to perform a total hip replacement without predisposing the patient to further central migration of the acetabular component of the total hip. If a previous bone grafting procedure has been performed to build up the inner wall, the total hip replacement can usually be performed at a later date without excessive technical difficulty.

If closed reduction is selected and performed, then prolonged skeletal traction of at least 10 to 12 weeks should be carried out. I feel there is no doubt that the longer the traction is maintained the less the likelihood that the femoral head will migrate centrally once the traction is released. It is also beneficial to keep these patients from weight bearing for an additional four to eight weeks following removal of the skeletal traction. If the traction is removed too soon, and if weight bearing is instituted too early, the femoral head will have a tendency toward central protrusion, which certainly predisposes the hip to early severe arthritis requiring total replacement.

PROGNOSIS

The prognosis and management of patients with fractures of the acetabulum, like those with injuries of other weight-bearing joints, to a large extent depend upon the adequacy of the reduction and the final congruency of the joint. There can be no doubt that the severe forces required to produce these injuries definitely affect the articular cartilage of the femoral head and the acetabulum. If an adequate reduction is obtained, however, the results are good in at least 80 per cent of cases. If there is a step-off deformity of the articular surfaces, the results are significantly less satisfactory. The final stability following treatment is also important to the final outcome. When there is a tendency toward instability of the fracture fragments the incidence of osteoarthritis increases. In posterior dislocation of the femoral head associated with fractures of the acetabulum, the incidence of avascular necrosis of the femoral head increases with increasing delay in reduction. This type of fracture-dislocation should be considered a surgical emergency, and the femoral head should be relocated as quickly as possible. This is the only way that the dreaded complication of avascular

necrosis of the femoral head can be avoided. I might also point out that avascular necrosis of the femoral head may not manifest itself for as long as one to two years postinjury. If it does develop then, the results are definitely worse.

COMPLICATIONS

Arthritis

Severe degenerative arthritis of the hip is a recognized complication of these fractures (Fig. 22–38). Although this does affect the overall results, these patients may later be treated with total hip replacements if the arthritis is severe. As I stated previously, one of the problems in the follow-up management of patients with central protrusion of the femoral head is a very thin medial wall associated with a central protrusion, which makes it very difficult to perform a total hip replacement. When this problem exists, primary bone grafting to obtain a thick medial buttress should be considered prior to total hip replacement. If it is not done, there is a strong possibility that future central migration of the entire total hip replacement may occur.

Thrombophlebitis

Thrombophlebitis of the pelvic and leg veins is a recognized complication of these fractures. All patients should be treated with anticoagulant medication, because their prolonged bed rest does have a tendency to invite this complication. We must also not lose sight of the fact that the significant soft-tissue disruption along the inner wall of the pelvis associated with these fractures may or may not affect the iliac veins, which are in close proximity. Heparin has been demonstrated to delay fracture healing, but it is probably best to start off with heparin initially and then gradually switch to warfarin (Coumadin). There is significant controversy at the present time as to exactly what form of anticoagulative measure is appropriate, but there is a widespread feeling that some measure should be taken against this problem.

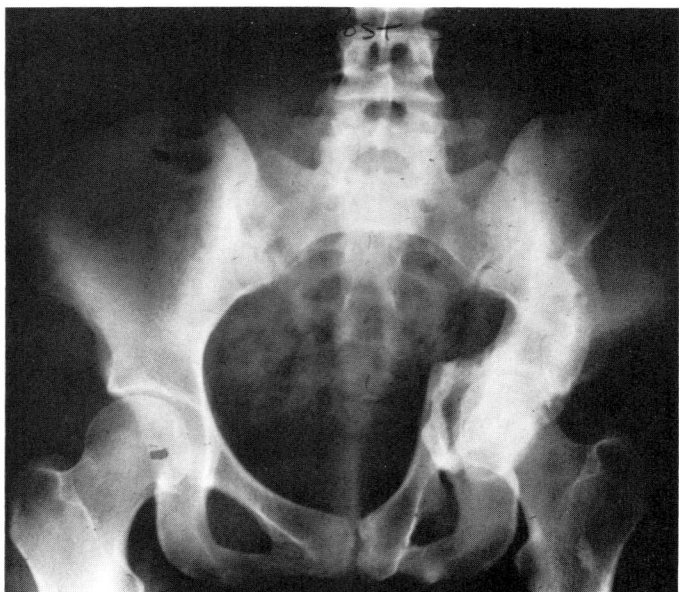

Figure 22–38 Painful degenerative arthritis of the hip following a central fracture-dislocation that ultimately required total hip replacement.

Myositis Ossificans

Myositis ossificans is a reported complication of these fractures. The exact incidence has been variously reported as 34 per cent in cases treated with open reduction and less than 10 per cent in cases treated by closed reduction.

Infection

If open reduction of these fractures has been performed, the possibility of infection always exists. The rate has been variously reported to be less than 10 per cent. This problem may be decreased by the preoperative and intraoperative use of prophylactic antibiotics. As in other areas, it is extremely important to obtain a high blood level of the antibiotic prior to performing the operative procedure. Antibiotic irrigation solutions can also be employed to reduce this possibility.

Fat Embolism

Fat embolism is also a recognized complication, particularly in association with other long bone fractures. The treatment of this complication is outlined in Chapter 36.

Nerve Injury

Sciatic nerve injuries may be associated with posterior acetabular fractures and dislocation of the hip. The majority of these involve the peroneal distribution of the nerve and do eventually recover. This may, however, take a period of two to three months for spontaneous recovery. On the other hand, traumatic transection and delayed repair of the sciatic nerve are not followed by good results. The most important aspect in the treatment of these injuries is to relieve the pressure on the sciatic nerve caused by the posterior dislocation of the hip. Nerve tissue does not tolerate constant pressure.

REFERENCES

1. Aggarwall, N. D., and Singh, H.: Unreduced anterior dislocation of the hip. J. Bone Joint Surg., 49B:288–292, 1967.
2. Ambrose, G. B., Garcia, A., and Neer, C. S.: Displaced intracapsular fracture of the neck of the femur. J. Trauma, 3:361–369, 1963.
3. Anderson, L. D., Hansa, W. R., and Waring, T. L.: Femoral head prosthesis. J. Bone Joint Surg., 46A:1049–1065, 1964.
4. Arden, G. P.: Radioactive isotopes in fractures of the neck of the femur. J. Bone Joint Surg., 42B:21–27, 1960.

5. Armstrong, J. R.: Traumatic dislocation of the hip joint. J. Bone Joint Surg., *30B*:429–445, 1948.

6. Arnoldi, C. C., and Linderholm, H.: Fractures of the femoral neck. I. Vascular disturbance in different types of fractures, assessed by measurement of the intraosseous pressures. Clin. Orthop., *84*:116–127, 1972.

7. Arnold, W. D., Lyden, J. P., Minkoff, J.: Treatment of intracapsular fractures of the femoral neck. J. Bone Joint Surg., *56A*:254–262, 1974.

8. d'Aubigne, R. M.: Management of acetabular fractures in multiple trauma. J. Trauma, 8:333–349, 1968.

9. Aufranc, O. E., Jones, W. N., and Harris, W. H.: Complicated fracture dislocation of the acetabulum. J.A.M.A., *182*:858–861, 1962.

10. Backman, S.: The proximal end of the femur. Acta Radiol., *146*[Suppl.]:1–166, 1957.

11. Badgley, C. E.: Fractures of the hip joint; some causes for failure and suggestions for success. AAOS Instructional Course Lectures, *17*:106, 1960.

12. Banks, H. H.: Factors influencing the result in fractures of the femoral neck. J. Bone Joint Surg., *44A*:931–964, 1962.

13. Banks, H. H.: The healing of intra-articular fractures. Clin. Orthop., *40*:17–29, 1965.

14. Banks, S. W.: Aseptic necrosis of the femoral head following traumatic dislocation of the hip. J. Bone Joint Surg., 23:753–781, 1941.

15. Barnes, R.: Fracture of the neck of the femur. J. Bone Joint Surg., *49B*:607–617, 1967.

16. Barnes, R., Brown, J. T., Garden, R. S., and Nicoll, E. A.: Subcapital fractures of the femur. A prospective review. J. Bone Joint Surg., *58B*:2–24, 1976.

17. Barr, J. S.: Experiences with a sliding nail in femoral neck fractures. Clin. Orthop., *92*:63–68, 1973.

18. Barry, T. J., Potter, G. D., and Stinchfield, F. E.: Roentgenographic assessment of periacetabular bone. J. Bone Joint Surg., *51A*:533–538, 1969.

19. Basset, F. M.: Normal vascular anatomy of the head of the femur. J. Bone Joint Surg., *51A*:1139–1153, 1969.

20. Bentley, G.: Impacted fractures of the neck and femur. J. Bone Joint Surg., *50B*:551–561, 1968.

21. Bohr, H., and Larsen, E. H.: On necrosis of the femoral head after fracture of the neck of the femur. J. Bone Joint Surg., *47B*:330–338, 1965.

22. Bonfiglio, M., and Bardenstein, M. B.: Treatment by bone grafting of aseptic necrosis of the femoral head and non-union of the femoral neck. J. Bone Joint Surg., *40A*:1329–1346, 1958.

23. Bonfiglio, M., and Voke, E. M.: Aseptic necrosis of the femoral head and non-union of the femoral neck. J. Bone Joint Surg., *50A*:48–66, 1968.

24. Boyd, H., and Anderson, L. D.: Management of unstable trochanteric fractures. Surg. Gynecol. Obstet., *112*:633–638, 1961.

25. Boyd, H. B., and Calandruccio, R. A.: Further observations on the use of radioactive phosphorus (P³²) to determine the viability of the head of the femur. J. Bone Joint Surg., *45A*:445–460, 1963.

26. Boyd, H. B., and Griffin, L. L.: Classification and treatment of trochanteric fractures. Arch. Surg., 58:853–866, 1949.

27. Boyd, H. B., and Salvatore, J. E.: Acute fracture of the femoral neck: Internal fixation or prosthesis? J. Bone Joint Surg., *46A*:1066–1068, 1964.

28. Boyd, H. B., Zilversmit, D. B., and Calandruccio, R. A.: The use of radioactive phosphorus (P³²) to determine the viability of the head of the femur. J. Bone Joint Surg., *37A*:260–269, 1955.

29. Boyd, K. S., Burke, J. F., and Colton, T.: A double-blind clinical trial of prophylactic antibiotics in hip fractures. J. Bone Joint Surg., *55A*:1251–1258, 1973.

30. Brav, E. A.: Traumatic dislocation of the hip joint. J. Bone Joint Surg., *44A*:1115–1134, 1962.

31. Brodetti, A.: An experimental study on the use of nails and bolt screws in the fixation of fractures of the femoral neck. Acta Orthop. Scand., *31*:247–271, 1961.

32. Brookes, M., and Wardle, E. N.: Muscle action and the shape of the femur. J. Bone Joint Surg., *44B*:398–411, 1962.

33. Brown, J. T., and Abrami, G.: Transcervical femoral fracture. J. Bone Joint Surg., *46B*:648–663, 1964.

34. Bruckman, R. A., Marek, F. M., and Schien, A. J.: Treatment of displaced intracapsular fractures of the neck of the femur, with the sliding nail. Clin. Orthop., *81*:185, 1971.

35. Burwell, H. N.: Replacement of the femoral head by a prosthesis in subcapital fractures. Br. J. Surg., *54*:741–749, 1967.

36. Cassebaum, W. M., and Nugent, T.: Predictability of bony union in displaced intracapsular fractures of the hip. J. Trauma, 3:421–424, 1963.

37. Catto, M.: Histological study of avascular necrosis of femoral head after transcervical fracture. J. Bone Joint. Surg., *47B*:749–776, 1965.

38. Catto, M.: The histological appearances of late segmental collapse of the femoral head after transcervical fracture. J. Bone Joint Surg., *47B*:777–791, 1965.

39. Chandler, S. B., and Kreuscher, P. H.: The blood supply of the ligamentum teres. J. Bone Joint Surg., *14*:834–846, 1932.

40. Charnley, J.: Treatment of fractures of neck of femur by compression. J. Bone Joint Surg., *38B*:772, 1956.

41. Charnley, J., Blockey, N. S., and Purser, D. W.: The treatment of displaced fractures of the neck of the femur by compression. A preliminary report. J. Bone Joint Surg., *39B*:45–65, 1957.

42. Chrisman, O. S., and Snook, G. A.: Studies of the protective effect of aspirin against degeneration of human articular cartilage. Clin. Orthop., 56:77–82, 1968.

43. Claffey, T. J.: Avascular necrosis of the femoral head. J. Bone Joint Surg., *42B*:802–809, 1960.

44. Clawson, D. K.: Trochanteric fractures treated by the sliding screw plate fixation method. J. Trauma, 4:737–752, 1964.

45. Clawson, D. K.: Intracapsular fractures of the femur treated by the sliding screw plate fixation method. J. Trauma, 4:753–756, 1964.
46. Clawson, D. K., Davis, F. J., and Hansen, S. T., Jr.: Treatment of chronic osteomyelitis with emphasis on closed suction-irrigation technic. Clin. Orthop., 96:88–97, 1973.
47. Cleveland, M., and Fielding, J. W.: A continuing end result study of intracapsular fractures of the neck of the femur. J. Bone Joint Surg., 36A:1020–1030, 1954.
48. Cleveland, M., Bosworth, D. M., Thompson, F. G., Wilson, H. J., and Ishizuka, T.: A ten-year analysis of intertrochanteric fractures of the femur. J. Bone Joint Surg., 41A:1399–1408, 1959.
49. Coleman, S., and Compere, C.: Femoral neck fractures. Pathogenesis of avascular necrosis, nonunion, and late degenerative changes. J. Bone Joint Surg., 39A:1419, 1957.
50. Compere, E. L., and Wallace, G.: Etiology of aseptic necrosis of the head of the femur after transcervical fracture. J. Bone Joint Surg., 24:831–841, 1942.
51. Conolly, W. B., and Hedberg, E. A.: Observations on fractures of the pelvis. J. Trauma, 9:104–111, 1969.
52. Conrad, J. J., and Tanin, A. H.: Experiences with the use of a Massie nail. Clin. Orthop., 81:186, 1971.
53. Cotton, F. J., and Morrison, G. N.: Hip fractures. Valgus position. Accidental or engineered. J. Bone Joint Surg., 20:461–468, 1938.
53a. Cram, R. H.: The unstable intertrochanteric fracture. Surg. Gynecol. Obstet., 101:15–19, 1955.
54. Crawford, H. B.: Experience with the non-operative treatment of impacted fractures of the neck of the femur. J. Bone Joint Surg., 47A:830–831, 1965.
55. Dehne, E.: The weight-bearing principle in treatment of lower-extremity fractures, 1885–1972. J. Trauma, 12:539–540, 1972.
56. Dehne, E., and Immerman, E. W.: Dislocation of the hip combined with fracture of the shaft of the femur on the same side. J. Bone Joint Surg., 33A:731–745, 1951.
57. Deyerle, W. M.: Absolute fixation with contact compression in hip fractures. Clin. Orthop., 13:279–297, 1959.
58. Deyerle, W. M.: Multiple pin peripheral fixation in the fractures of the neck of the femur: Immediate weight-bearing. Clin. Orthop., 39:135–156, 1965.
59. Dickson, J. A.: The high geometric osteotomy with rotation and bone graft for ununited fractures of the neck of the femur. J. Bone Joint Surg., 29:1005–1018, 1947.
60. Dimon, J. H.: The unstable intertrochanteric fracture. Clin. Orthop., 92:100–107, 1973.
61. Dimon, J. H., and Hughston, J. C.: Unstable intertrochanteric fractures of the hip. J. Bone Joint Surg., 49A:440–450, 1967.
62. Dingley, A. F., and Denham, R. H.: Pubic dislocation of the hip. J. Bone Joint Surg., 46A:865–867, 1964.
63. DiStefano, V. J., Nixon, J. E., and Klien, K. S.:

64. Stable fixation of the difficult subtrochanteric fractures. J. Trauma, 12:1066–1070, 1972.
65. Eaton, G. O.: Internal fixation in displaced intracapsular fractures of the femoral neck. J. Bone Joint Surg., 38A:23–32, 1956.
65. Ecker, M. L., Joyce, J. J., and Kohl, E. J.: The treatment of trochanteric fractures using a compression screw. J. Bone Joint Surg., 57A:23–27, 1975.
66. Eggers, G. W., Shindler, T. O., and Pomerat, C. M.: The influence of contact-compression factor on osteogenesis in surgical fractures. J. Bone Joint Surg., 31A:693–716, 1949.
67. Eichenholtz, S. N., and Stark, R. M.: Central acetabular fractures. J. Bone Joint Surg., 46A:695–714, 1964.
68. Elliot, R. B.: Central fractures of the acetabulum. Clin. Orthop., 7:189–202, 1966.
69. Ellis, J.: Central dislocation of the femur. J. Bone Joint Surg., 47B:595, 1965.
70. Emmett, J.: Measurements of the acetabulum. Clin. Orthop., 53:171, 1967.
71. Epstein, H. C.: Posterior fracture dislocations of the hip. J. Bone Joint Surg., 43A:1079–1098, 1961.
72. Epstein, H. C.: Traumatic dislocations of the hip. Clin. Orthop., 92:116–142, 1973.
73. Epstein, H. C.: Posterior fracture-dislocations of the hip: long-term follow-up. J. Bone Joint Surg., 56A:1103–1127, 1974.
73a. Evans, E. M.: The treatment of trochanteric fractures of the femur. J. Bone Joint Surg., 31B:190–203, 1949.
74. Evarts, C. M., and Feil, E. J.: Prevention of the thromboembolic disease after elective surgery of the hip. J. Bone Joint Surg., 53A:1271–1280, 1971.
75. Eyre-Brook, A. L., and Pridie, K. H.: Intracapsular fractures of the neck of the femur. Final results of 75 consecutive cases treated by the closed method of pinning. Br. J. Surg., 29:115–138, 1941.
76. Farkas, A., Wilson, M. S., and Hayner, J. C.: An anatomical study of the mechanics, pathology, and healing of fractures of the femoral neck. J. Bone Joint Surg., 30A:53, 1948.
77. Fielding, J. W.: Subtrochanteric fractures. Clin. Orthop., 92:86, 1973.
78. Fielding, J. W., and Magliato, H. J.: Subtrochanteric fractures. Surg. Gynecol. Obstet., 122:155, 1966.
79. Fielding, J. W.: Wilson, S. A., and Ratzan, S.: A continuing end-result study of displaced intracapsular fractures of the neck of the femur treated with the Pugh nail. J. Bone Joint Surg., 56A:1464–1472, 1974.
80. Fielding, J. W., Wilson, H. J., and Zickel, R. E.: A continuing end-result study of intra-capsular fracture of the neck of the femur. J. Bone Joint Surg., 44A:965, 1962.
81. Fina, C. P., and Kelly, P. J.: Dislocations of the hip with fractures of the proximal femur. J. Trauma, 10:77, 1970.
82. Frangakis, E. K.: Intracapsular fractures of the neck of the femur. J. Bone Joint Surg., 48B:17, 1966.

83. Frankel, V. H.: Mechanical fixation of unstable fractures about the proximal end of the femur. Bull. Hosp. Joint Dis., 24:1, 1963.
84. Frankel, V. H., and Burstein, A. H.: Orthopaedic Biomechanics. Philadelphia, Lea & Febiger, 1970.
85. Freeman, M., Todd, R. C., and Pirie, C. J.: The role of fatigue in the pathogenesis of senile femoral neck fractures. J. Bone Joint Surg., 56B:698–702, 1974.
86. Gallie, W. E.: Avascular necrosis involving articular surfaces. J. Bone Joint Surg., 38A:732–737, 1956.
87. Garden, R. S.: Low-angle fixation in fractures of the femoral neck. J. Bone Joint Surg., 43B:647–663, 1961.
88. Garden, R. S.: Stability and union in subcapital fractures of the femur. J. Bone Joint Surg., 46B:630–647, 1964.
89. Garden, R. S.: Malreduction and avascular necrosis in subcapital fractures of the femur. J. Bone Joint Surg., 53B:183–197, 1971.
90. Goodfellow, J. W., and Bullough, P.: The interpretation of the radiological joint space. J. Bone Joint Surg., 50B:877, 1968.
91. Goodman, A. H., and Sherman, M. S.: Postirradiation fractures of the femoral neck. J. Bone Joint Surg., 45A:723–730, 1963.
92. Gossling, H. R., and Hardy, J. H.: Fractures of the femoral neck: A comparative study of methods of treatment in 400 consecutive cases. J. Trauma, 9:423–429, 1969.
93. Gothlin, G., and Hindmarsh, J.: Studies of hip joint by means of lateral acetabular roentgenograms. J. Bone Joint Surg., 38A:1218–1230, 1956.
94. Graham, J.: Early or delayed weight-bearing after internal fixation of transcervical fracture of the femur. J. Bone Joint Surg., 50B:562–569, 1968.
95. Green, J. T., and Gay, F. H.: High femoral neck fractures treated by multiple nail fixation. Clin. Orthop., 11:177–184, 1958.
96. Greenwald, A. S., and Haynes, D. W.: Weight-bearing areas in the human hip joint. J. Bone Joint Surg., 54B:157–163, 1972.
97. Harmon, P. H., Baker, D. R., and Reno, J. H.: Experiments on the holding powers of various types of metallic internal fixation for transcervical fractures of the femur. Am. J. Surg., 76:515–524, 1948.
98. Harrington, K. D., and Johnston, J. O.: The management of comminuted unstable intertrochanteric fractures. J. Bone Joint Surg., 55A:1367–1376, 1973.
99. Harris, W. H.: A new lateral approach to the hip joint. J. Bone Joint Surg., 49A:891–898, 1967.
100. Harty, M.: Blood supply to the femoral head. Br. Med. J., 2:1236, 1953.
101. Harty, M.: The calcar femorale and the femoral neck. J. Bone Joint Surg., 39A:625–630, 1957.
102. Harty, M.: Some aspects of the surgical anatomy of the hip joint. J. Bone Joint Surg., 48A:197–202, 1966.
103. Harty, M., and Joyce, J. J.: Surgical approaches to the hip and femur. J. Bone Joint Surg., 45A:175–190, 1963.
104. Helal, B., and Akevis, X.: Unrecognized disloca-

105. tion of the hip in fractures of the femoral shaft. J. Bone Joint Surg., 49B:293–300, 1967.
105. Hewson, J. S.: Treatment of intracapsular fracture of the hip with primary pedicle bone graft from greater trochanter. Clin. Orthop., 76:100–110, 1971.
106. Hinchey, J. J., and Day, P. L.: Primary prosthetic replacement in fresh femoral neck fractures. J. Bone Joint Surg., 46A:223–240, 1964.
107. Hirsch, C., and Frankel, V. H.: Analysis of forces producing fractures of the proximal end of the femur. J. Bone Joint Surg., 42B:633–640, 1960.
108. Holt, E. P.: Hip fractures in the trochanteric region. Treatment with strong nail and early weight bearing. J. Bone Joint Surg., 45A:681–705, 1963.
109. Howe, W. W., Lacey, T., II, and Schwartz, R. P.: A study of the gross anatomy of the arteries supplying the proximal portion of the femur and the acetabulum. J. Bone Joint Surg., 32A:856–866, 1950.
110. Hudson, O. C.: Complications of acetabular fractures following posterior dislocation of the hip. Am. J. Surg., 93:131–132, 1957.
111. Hunter, G. A.: Posterior dislocation and fracture dislocation of the hip. J. Bone Joint Surg., 51B:38–44, 1969.
112. Jeffrey, C. C.: Spontaneous fractures of the femoral neck. J. Bone Joint Surg., 44B:543–549, 1962.
112a. Jewett, E. L.: One piece angle nail for trochanteric fractures. J. Bone Joint Surg., 23:803–810, 1941.
113. Johnson, J. T., and Crothers, O.: Nail versus prosthesis for femoral-neck fractures. J. Bone Joint Surg., 57A:686–692, 1975.
114. Johnston, R. C., and Smidt, G. L.: Measurement of hip-joint motion during walking. J. Bone Joint Surg., 51A:1083–1094, 1969.
115. Judet, J., Judet, R., Lagrange, J., and Dunover, J.: A study of the arterial vascularization of the femoral neck in the adult. J. Bone Joint Surg., 37A:663–680, 1955.
116. Judet, R., Judet, J., and Letournel, E.: Fractures of the acetabulum: Classification and surgical approaches for open reduction. J. Bone Joint Surg., 46A:1615–1646, 1964.
117. Kaufer, H., Matthews, L. S., and Sonstegard, D.: Stable fixation of intertrochanteric fractures. J. Bone Joint Surg., 56A:899–907, 1974.
118. Kimbrough, E. E.: Concomitant unilateral hip and femoral-shaft fractures—a too frequently unrecognized syndrome. J. Bone Joint Surg., 43A:443–449, 1961.
119. Kleiman, S. G., Stevens, J., Kolb, L., and Pankovich, A.: Late sciatic nerve palsy following posterior dislocation of the hip. J. Bone Joint Surg., 53A:781–782, 1971.
120. Klenerman, L., and Marcuson, R. W.: Intracapsular fractures of the neck of the femur. J. Bone Joint Surg., 52B:514–517, 1970.
121. Knight, R. A., and Smith, H.: Operative management of central acetabular fractures. J. Bone Joint Surg., 39A:1430–1431, 1957.
121a. Koch, J. C.: The Laws of bone architecture. J. Anat., 21:177, 1917.
122. Kranendonk, D. H., Jurist, J. M., and Ha, G. L.:

Femoral trabecular patterns and bone mineral content. J. Bone Joint Surg., *54A*:1472–1478, 1972.

123. Laing, P. G., and Ferguson, A. B., Jr.: Radio-sodium clearance rates as indicators of femoral head vascularity. J. Bone Joint Surg., *41A*: 1409–1422, 1959.

124. Larson, C.: Fracture dislocation of the hip. Clin. Orthop., 92:147–154, 1973.

125. Leadbetter, G. W.: A treatment for fracture of the neck of the femur. J. Bone Joint Surg., *15*:931–940, 1933.

126. Leadbetter, G. W.: Closed reduction of fractures of the neck of the femur. J. Bone Joint Surg., *20*:108–113, 1938.

127. Linton, P.: Types of displacement in fractures of the femoral neck. J. Bone Joint Surg., *31B*:184–189, 1949.

127a. Lipscomb, P. R.: Fracture-dislocation of the hip. *In*: I. C. L., The American Academy of Orthopaedic Surgeons. Vol. 18, pp. 102–109. St. Louis, C. V. Mosby, 1961.

128. Lorenzo, F. A.: Molybdenum steel lag screw in internal fixation of fractured neck of femur. Surg. Gynecol. Obstet., 73:98–104, 1941.

129. Lowell, J. D., and Aufranc, O. E.: Anterior approach to the hip joint. Clin. Orthop., *61*:193–198, 1968.

130. Lunceford, E. M.: Use of the Moore self-locking Vitallium prosthesis in acute fractures of the femoral neck. J. Bone Joint Surg., *47A*:832–841, 1965.

131. Lyddon, D. W., Jr., and Hartman, J. T.: Traumatic dislocation of the hip with ipsilateral femoral fractures. J. Bone Joint Surg., *53A*:1012–1016, 1971.

132. McElvenny, R. T.: The roentgenographic interpretation of what constitutes adequate reduction of the femur neck. Surg. Gynecol. Obstet., *80*:97–106, 1945.

133. McElvenny, R. T.: The immediate treatment of intracapsular hip fractures. Clin. Orthop., *10*: 289–325, 1957.

134. McKibbin, W. B.: An ambulatory method of treatment for intertrochanteric fractures of the femur. Surg. Gynecol. Obstet., 76:343–346, 1943.

135. McMullen, H. L.: Acetabular fractures. J. Bone Joint Surg., *53B*:556, 1971.

136. Massie, W. K.: Functional fixation of femoral neck fractures; telescoping nail technique. Clin. Orthop., *12*:230–255, 1958.

137. Massie, W. K.: Extracapsular fractures of the hip treated by impaction, using a sliding nail plate fixation. Clin. Orthop., *22*:180–202, 1962.

138. Massie, W. K.: Fractures of the hip. J. Bone Joint Surg., *46A*:658–690, 1964.

139. Massie, W. K.: Treatment of femoral neck fractures emphasizing long term follow-up observations on aseptic necrosis. Clin. Orthop., 92:16–62, 1973.

140. May, J. M. B., and Chacha, P. B.: Displacements of trochanteric fractures and their influence on reduction. J. Bone Joint Surg., *50B*:318–323, 1968.

141. Merchant, A. C.: Hip abductor muscle force. J. Bone Joint Surg., *47A*:462–476, 1965.

142. Meyers, M. H., Harvey, J. P., and Moore, T. M.: The muscle pedicle bone graft in the treatment of displaced fractures of the femoral neck: Indications, operative technique and results. Orthop. Clin. North Am., 5:779–792, 1974.

143. Moore, A. T.: Fractures of the hip joint (intracapsular); a new method of skeletal fixation. J. S. C. Med. Assoc., 30:199–205, 1934.

144. Moore, A. T.: The self-locking metal hip prosthesis. J. Bone Joint Surg., *39A*:811–827, 1957.

145. Mulholland, R. C., and Gunn, D. R.: Sliding screw-plate fixation of intertrochanteric femoral fractures. J. Trauma, *12*:581–591, 1972.

146. Müller, M. E., Allgöwer, M., and Willenegger, H.: Manual of Internal Fixation. New York, Springer-Verlag, 1970.

147. Murray, R. C., and Frew, J. F. M.: Trochanteric fractures of the femur. J. Bone Joint Surg., *31B*:204–219, 1949.

148. Naiman, P. T., Schien, A. J., and Siffert, R. S.: Medial displacement fixation for severely comminuted intertrochanteric fractures. Clin. Orthop., 62:151–155, 1969.

149. Nicoll, E. A.: Traumatic dislocation of the hip. J. Bone Joint Surg., *34B*:503–505, 1952.

150. Nicoll, E. A.: Acetabular fractures and dislocation of the hip. J. Bone Joint Surg., *35B*:147, 1953.

151. Nicoll, E. A.: The unsolved fracture. J. Bone Joint Surg., *45B*:239–241, 1963.

152. Niemann, K. M. W., and Mankin, H. J.: Fractures about the hip in an institutionalized patient population. J. Bone Joint Surg., *50A*:1327–1340, 1968.

153. Paus, B.: Traumatic dislocation of the hip. Acta Orthop. Scand., *21*:99–112, 1951.

154. Pauwels, F.: Der Schenkenholsbruck, ein mechanisches Problem. Grundlagen des Heilungsvorganges. Prognose und kausale Therapie. Stuttgart, Beilageheft zur Zeitschrift fur Orthopaedische Chirurgie, Ferdinand Enke, 1935.

155. Pearson, J. R., and Hargadon, E. J.: Fractures of the pelvis involving floor of acetabulum. J. Bone Joint Surg., *44B*:550–561, 1962.

156. Persson, B. M.: Trochanteric side traction for acetabular fractures—a pinholding device. Acta Orthop. Scand., 36:219–220, 1965.

157. Phemister, D. B.: Repair of bone in aseptic necrosis. J. Bone Joint Surg., *12*:769–787, 1954.

158. Pigeott, M.: A method of forecasting capital avascular necrosis after fracture of the neck of the femur. J. Bone Joint Surg., *47B*:375, 1965.

159. Pugh, W. L.: A self-adjusting nail-plate for fractures about the hip joint. J. Bone Joint Surg., *37A*:1085–1093, 1955.

160. Ray, R. D., Sankaran, B., and Fetrow, K. O.: Delayed union and non-union of fractures. J. Bone Joint Surg., *46A*:627–643, 1964.

161. Ray, R. D., Degge, J., Gloyd, P., and Mooney, G.: Bone regeneration, an experimental study of bone-grafting materials. J. Bone Joint Surg., *34A*:638–647, 1952.

162. Reich, R. S.: The selection of patients with hip fractures for prosthetic or other types of hip reconstruction (high osteotomy or bone graft or both). J. Bone Joint Surg., *48A*:203–210, 1966.

163. Riska, E. B.: Prosthetic replacement in the treatment of subcapital fractures of the femur. Acta Orthop. Scand., 42:281–290, 1971.

164. Roberts, A., Rooney, T., Loupe, J., Roberts, F., and Wickstrom, V.: A comparison of the functional results of anatomic and medial displacement valgus nailing of intertrochanteric fractures of the femur. J. Trauma, 12:341–346, 1972.

165. Rowe, C. R.: The management of fractures in elderly patients is different. J. Bone Joint Surg., 47A:1043–1059, 1965.

166. Rowe, C. R., and Lowell, J. D.: Prognosis of fractures of acetabulum. J. Bone Joint Surg., 43A:30–59, 1961.

167. Rydell, N.: Forces acting on the femoral head prothesis. Acta Orthop. Scand., 88[Suppl.]:7–132, 1966.

168. Rydell, N.: Biomechanics of the hip joint. Clin. Orthop., 92:6, 1973.

169. Salzman, E. W., Harris, W. H., and DeSanctis, R. W.: Anticoagulation for prevention of thromboembolism following fractures of the hip. N. Engl. J. Med., 275:122–130, 1966.

170. Sarmiento, A.: Avoidance of complications of internal fixation of intertrochanteric fractures. Clin. Orthop., 53:47–59, 1967.

171. Sarmiento, A.: Unstable intertrochanteric fractures of the femur. Clin. Orthop., 92:77–85, 1973.

172. Sarmiento, A., and Laird, C. A.: Posterior fracture dislocation of the femoral head. Clin. Orthop., 92:143–146, 1973.

173. Sarmiento, A., and Williams, E. M.: The unstable intertrochanteric fracture: Treatment with a valgus osteotomy and I-beam nail-plate. J. Bone Joint Surg., 52A:1309–1318, 1970.

174. Scheck, M.: Management of fractures of the femoral neck. J. Bone Joint Surg., 47A:819–829, 1965.

175. Seddon, H.: Surgical Disorders of the Peripheral Nerves. Baltimore, Williams & Wilkins, 1972.

176. Senn, N.: The treatment of fractures of the neck of the femur by immediate reductions and permanent fixation. J.A.M.A., 13:150, 1889.

177. Sevitt, S.: Avascular necrosis and revascularization of the femoral head after intracapsular fractures. J. Bone Joint Surg., 46B:270–296, 1964.

178. Sherman, M., and Phemister, D. B.: The pathology of ununited fractures of the neck of the femur. J. Bone Joint Surg., 29:19–40, 1947.

179. Smith, F. B.: Effects of rotary and valgus malpositions on blood supply to the femoral head. J. Bone Joint Surg., 41A:800–815, 1959.

180. Smith, L. D.: Role of muscle contraction or intrinsic forces in the causation of fractures of the femoral neck. J. Bone Joint Surg., 35A:367–383, 1953.

181. Smith-Petersen, M. N.: Treatment of fractures of the neck of the femur by internal fixation. Surg. Gynecol. Obstet., 64:287–295, 1937.

182. Smith-Petersen, M. N., Cave, E. F., and Van Gorder, W.: Intracapsular fracture of the neck of the femur. Arch. Surg., 23:715–759, 1931.

183. Smyth, E. H. J., Ellis, J. S., Manifold, M. C., and Dewey, P. R.: Triangle pinning for fracture of the femoral neck. J. Bone Joint Surg., 46B:664–673, 1964.

184. Solonen, K. A.: Prophylactic anticoagulation therapy in the treatment of lower limb fractures. Acta Orthop. Scand., 33:329–341, 1963.

185. Soto-Hall, R., Johnson, L. H., and Johnson, R.: Alterations in the intra-articular pressures in transcervical fractures. J. Bone Joint Surg., 46A:662, 1963.

186. Soto-Hall, R., Johnson, L. H., and Johnson, R. A.: Variations in the intra-articular pressure of the hip joint in injury and disease. J. Bone Joint Surg., 46A:509–516, 1964.

187. Speed, J. S.: Central fractures of the neck of the femur. J.A.M.A., 104:2059–2063, 1935.

188. Stevens, D. B.: Postoperative orthopaedic infections—a study of etiological mechanisms. J. Bone Joint Surg., 46A:96–102, 1964.

189. Stevens, J., Freeman, P. A., Nordin, B. E. C., and Barnett, E.: The incidence of osteoporosis in patients with femoral neck fracture. J. Bone Joint Surg., 44B:520–524, 1962.

190. Stevens, J. S., Fardin, F. R., and Freeark, R. J.: Lower extremity thrombophlebitis in patients with femoral neck fractures: A venographic investigation and a review of the early and late significance of the findings. J. Trauma, 8:527–534, 1968.

191. Stewart, M. J., and McCarroll, H. R.: Fracture dislocation of the hip: A follow up and comparative study. J. Bone Joint Surg., 52B:773–774, 1970.

192. Stewart, M. J., and Milford, L. W.: Fracture-dislocation of the hip. J. Bone Joint Surg., 36A:315–342, 1954.

193. Stimson, B. B.: Manual of Fractures and Dislocations. Philadelphia, Lea & Febiger, 1939.

194. Stimson, L. A.: A Treatise on Fractures. Philadelphia, H. C. Lea's Son & Co., 1883.

195. Sullivan, R. C., Bickel, W. H., and Lipscomb, P. R.: Recurrent dislocation of the hip. J. Bone Joint Surg., 37A:1266–1270, 1955.

196. Taylor, G. W., Neufeld, A. J., and Nickel, V. L.: Complications and failures in the operative treatment of intertrochanteric fractures of the femur. J. Bone Joint Surg., 37A:306–316, 1955.

197. Thompson, F. R.: Indications and contraindications for the early use of an intramedullary hip prosthesis. Clin. Orthop., 6:9–16, 1955.

198. Thompson, V. P., and Epstein, H. C.: Traumatic dislocation of the hip. J. Bone Joint Surg., 33A:746–778, 1951.

199. Tipton, W., D'Ambrosia, A. R., and Ryle, G.: Nonoperative management of central fracture-dislocations of the hip. J. Bone Joint Surg., 57A:888–893, 1975.

200. Tobin, W. J.: An atlas of the comparative anatomy of the upper end of the femur. Clin. Orthop., 56:83–103, 1968.

201. Todd, R. C., Freeman, M. A. R., and Pirie, C. J.: Isolated trabecular fatigue fractures in the femoral head. J. Bone Joint Surg., 54B:723–728, 1972.

202. Tovee, E. B., and Gendron, E.: The use of radioactive phosphorus in the determination of

the viability of the femoral head in dogs after subcapital fractures. J. Bone Joint Surg., 36A: 185, 1954.

203. Trueta, J.: Appraisal of the vascular factor in the healing of fractures of the femoral neck. J. Bone Joint Surg., 39B:3–5, 1957.

204. Trueta, J.: The normal vascular anatomy of the human femoral head during growth. J. Bone Joint Surg., 39B:358–394, 1957.

205. Trueta, J., and Harrison, M. H. M.: The normal vascular anatomy of the femoral head in adult man. J. Bone Joint Surg., 35B:442–461, 1953.

206. Tucker, F. R.: Arterial supply to the femoral head and its clinical importance. J. Bone Joint Surg., 31B:82–93, 1949.

207. Urist, M. R.: Fracture-dislocation of the hip joint. J. Bone Joint Surg., 30A:699–727, 1948.

208. Urist, M. R.: Fractures of the acetabulum. Ann. Surg., 127:1150–1164, 1948.

208a. Ward, F. O.: Human Anatomy. London, Renshaw, 1838.

209. Watson, H. K., Campbell, R. D., and Preston, A. W.: Classification, treatment and complications of the adult subtrochanteric fracture. J. Trauma, 4:457–480, 1964.

210. Watson, M.: Microfractures in the head of the femur. J. Bone Joint Surg., 57A:696–698, 1975.

211. Weissman, S. L., and Salama, R.: Trochanteric fractures of the femur: Treatment with a strong nail and early weight-bearing. Clin. Orthop., 67:143–150, 1969.

212. Wertheimer, L. G., and Lopez, S. de L. F.: Arterial supply of the femoral head. J. Bone Joint Surg., 53A:545–556, 1971.

213. Whitman, R.: A new method of treatment for fractures of the neck of the femur. Am. J. Surg., 36:746, 1902.

214. Whitman, R.: The abduction method as the exponent of a treatment for all forms of fractures at the hip in accord with surgical principle. Am. J. Surg., 21:335–344, 1933.

215. Whittaker, R., Abeshaus, M. M., Scholl, M. W., and Chung, S. M. K.: Fifteen years' experience with metallic endoprosthetic replacement of the femoral head for femoral neck fractures. J. Trauma, 12:799–806, 1972.

216. Wilson, H. J., Fielding, W., and Zickel, R. C.: Pugh nail fixation of displaced intracapsular fractures of the femoral neck. J. Bone Joint Surg., 46A:1373, 1964.

217. Wiltberger, B. R., Mitchell, C. L., and Medrick, D. W.: Fracture of the femoral shaft complicated by hip dislocation. A method of treatment. J. Bone Joint Surg., 30A:225–228, 1948.

218. Zickel, R. E.: A new fixation device for subtrochanteric fractures of the femur. A preliminary report. Clin. Orthop., 54:115–123, 1957.

219. Zickel, R. E.: An intramedullary fixation device for the proximal femur. Nine years' experience. J. Bone Joint Surg., 58A:866–872, 1976.

R. BRUCE HEPPENSTALL, M.D.

Fractures of the ————————————— 23
Femur

Fractures of the shaft of the femur are regularly encountered in everyday orthopedic practice. The recent trend has been toward early ambulatory treatment of patients with these fractures, a goal achieved by early operative internal fixation or the use of skeletal traction followed by the application of a cast brace. The concept of early ambulation in the treatment of femoral fractures is not entirely new. In the mid-eighteenth century, Dr. Smith of Philadelphia became concerned over the significant morbidity and high death rate among patients treated with splinting devices. He developed a fracture brace that was designed to allow early mobilization of patients with fractured femora and noted a significant decrease in the morbidity and mortality. He also was able to achieve union in all cases reported.[70] His method was not considered standard therapy at that time, and the concept was not widely accepted. It was, however, a very important milestone, as cast bracing is one of the most exciting developments in the treatment of femoral fractures today. Obviously, Dr. Smith was a physician ahead of his time.

In 1940, Küntscher reported the results of intramedullary rod fixation of fractured femora. This too was an important milestone, as it "opened the door" to the concept of stable internal fixation and early ambulation in the treatment of these fractures. Since that time many new internal fixation devices and operative methods have been developed to implement that concept. This has led to a definite decrease in morbidity, hospital stay, and recovery time.

SURGICAL ANATOMY

Muscles. The femur is surrounded by heavy muscles that are in turn encased in a tough sheath of dense fibrous tissue, the fascia lata. This strong supporting tissue is attached to Poupart's ligament anteriorly and extends to the gluteal region posteriorly. Distally, it is continuous with the deep fascia of the leg. The iliotibial band is a thick portion along the lateral surface that receives the insertion of the tensor fasciae latae. Thick bands of fibrous tissue project inward from the fascia lata; the most important are the internal and external intermuscular septa. These divide the thigh into anterior and posterior muscular compartments. The internal intermuscular septum forms the floor of Hunter's canal in its deeper portion. The femoral vessels and nerves pass through this canal. The flexor group of muscles includes the biceps femoris, the semimembranosus, and the semitendinosis—collectively known as the hamstrings. The extensor group is composed of the four parts of the quadriceps muscle. Abduction of the thigh is accomplished by the gluteus medius through its insertion into the greater trochanter. Adduction is produced by the musculature that arises from the ischiopubic ramus and extends down to the adductor tubercle.

Bone Structure. The shaft of the femur is roughly cylindrical in cross section throughout most of its extent. The linea aspera, an elevated ridge extending along the posterior border of the shaft, serves as the attachment for the musculature. The bone is not entirely straight, but is bowed in a forward and outward direction. This anterolateral bowing is important and must be preserved when fractures are treated or the biomechanical stresses at the hip and knee will be altered. The thickness of the cortex decreases both proximally and distally. This is associated with a definite increase in the proportion of cancellous bone in the supracondylar area. It is this distal area that may be predisposed to fracture in the elderly because of an alteration in the rate of bone turnover. The level of the fracture has a profound influence on the type of rotational deformity present. In fractures of the proximal femoral shaft the gluteus muscles tend to produce an abduction deformity, while the iliopsoas tends to create a flexion and external rotation type of deformity. Midshaft fractures may be associated with a varus deformity owing to the adductor musculature. Distal femoral fractures may be associated with a flexion deformity of the femoral condyles caused by the gastrocnemius musculature.

Blood Supply. The blood supply to the femur has been extensively studied by Rhinelander and Laing.[46, 62] Like that of other tubular bones, the basic blood supply comes from the metaphyseal, periosteal, and endosteal vessels. The periosteal component is associated with the multiple muscular attachments along the shaft, each nutrient artery perforating the linea aspera to gain access to the midportion of the shaft. These arteries originate from the proliferating branches of the profunda femoris artery which lie posterior to the femur. The main femoral artery continues distally to the junction of the middle and distal thirds of the thigh, where it turns backward, approaches the femur, and passes through the insertion of the adductor magnus muscle to reach the popliteal space. It is in this location that the artery may be exposed to injury during a fracture of the distal third of the femur. The sciatic nerve runs posteriorly beneath the hamstrings and may occasionally be injured in severe fractures of the femur.

Rhinelander has made several outstanding contributions to our understanding of the microvasculature. He has found that the majority of the cortical diaphyseal bone is supplied by the nutrient vessel system. The outer one third to one quarter of the cortex is supplied by the periosteal vessels. He demonstrated that the intramedullary vasculature was greatly altered during insertion of intramedullary fixation devices. With destruction of the endosteal circulation, the periosteal blood supply increases and may support most of the diaphysis. Similarly, if the periosteum is "stripped," the endosteal blood supply will expand to cover this function. Rhinelander found that circlage wires did not produce severe embarrassment of the blood supply, but that Parham bands may create necrosis by altering the periosteal blood supply, and he was able to demonstrate that the best type of intramedullary device is of a "fluted" design that will allow control of rotation but at the same time allow new endosteal vessels to form between the flutes. This device is available today as the Sampson nail.[62]

MECHANISMS OF INJURY

A fracture in this area is associated with severe trauma. Most commonly, it is caused by a vehicular accident or a fall from a height, and frequently, it is associated with multiple system injuries. The typical patient is a child or a young adult with a history of direct violence. Males predominate in most series. This fracture is infrequently seen in the elderly, as they are more likely to sustain a fracture of the proximal or distal femoral areas. With advancing age and decreased bone turnover, both the osseous mass and the cortical thickness are decreased, particularly in the supracondylar area, accounting for the predilection for fracture in this location in the elderly.

Occasionally a fracture of the shaft of the femur will be associated with a dislocation of the hip. It is important to bear this in mind during the initial evaluation of a patient with a femoral fracture.

CLASSIFICATION OF FEMORAL FRACTURES

A useful working classification for fractures of the femoral shaft divides them into two large groups, open and closed. Each group can then be further subdivided into transverse, oblique, spiral, and comminuted types.

The open type may be created by injury from the fracture fragments or by external trauma causing soft tissue loss that exposes the fracture site. This division is not only academic, but important clinically, as the amount of contamination is increased in the external trauma type with secondary soft tissue loss, and the amount of necrotic tissue is also increased. Open fractures created by injury from within the extremity are also contaminated, but to a lesser degree.

The various patterns of fracture may occur in both the open and closed injuries. It is extremely important to evaluate the amount of comminution accurately. This has a direct bearing on the final result, particularly when open reduction and internal fixation are employed. It is not uncommon, for example, for the surgeon to misinterpret the roentgenograms of a "butterfly" fracture in which the fracture line is not complete and be lulled into a false sense of security, feeling that he can accomplish rigid internal fixation. When the fracture site is exposed, however, the true nature of the butterfly fragment becomes evident. Careful study of the roentgenograms prior to proceeding with an open reduction is mandatory.

PHYSICAL EXAMINATION

The diagnosis of a fracture of the femoral shaft is usually fairly straightforward. Patients present with a hematoma and gross enlargement of the thigh, compared to the normal extremity. There is tenderness at the fracture site, and the characteristic deformity is anterior and lateral angulation. The patient may show evidence of impending shock. Loss of two to three units of blood at the fracture site and into the soft tissues is not unusual with this type of injury. Since there are frequently associated injuries to other systems, a patient in frank shock is not uncommon.

As with other fractures, it is important to examine the proximal and distal joints carefully. Occasionally the femoral shaft fracture will be accompanied by a dislocated hip. The knee may also have sustained severe ligamentous injury, depending on the type of accident. The neurovascular status of the injured extremity should be recorded. Sciatic nerve injury is not frequent, but has been seen in association with femoral shaft fractures. A major vascular injury may also be present. The femoral artery may be injured in the vicinity of the adductor hiatus. Careful examination of the popliteal and pedal pulses is important. If either is absent, then the surgeon must be aware that a vascular injury may be present. Careful assessment of the capillary return to the foot will aid in determining whether the blood supply to the distal extremity is adequate. If there is any doubt, a femoral arteriogram or consultation with a vascular surgeon is in order.

ROENTGENOGRAPHIC EXAMINATION

It is important to obtain adequate roentgenograms to evaluate this injury. As stated earlier, a dislocated hip can occasionally be associated with a fracture of the femur. Therefore, it is mandatory to have anteroposterior and lateral views of the femur that also visualize the hip and knee joints. If these cannot be obtained on one large cassette, then a separate x-ray of the hip and knee should be obtained. As mentioned previously, it is important to determine the amount of comminution present. If there is a suggestion of a butterfly fragment, then oblique views of the femur may be indicated.

Since this injury is caused by direct major trauma, it is a good rule to obtain an anteroposterior roentgenogram of the pelvis. This will help to reveal whether a pelvic fracture is present or whether there is an associated dislocation of the hip.

TREATMENT OF FEMORAL FRACTURES

Traction

Traction is a necessary and important part in the treatment of all femoral shaft fractures. Skin traction is useful in transporting patients with this type of injury.

Skin Traction

Thomas Splint with Skin Traction. A common method is to utilize a combination

692 FRACTURES OF THE FEMUR

of a Thomas splint and skin traction. The injured extremity is placed in the Thomas splint and the skin traction is applied through adhesive strips and then pulled down to and fastened to the distal end of the splint. Counter traction is obtained through the ring of the Thomas splint, in the groin, and the actual traction is obtained by fastening the skin traction to the distal end of the splint. This is a satisfactory way to transport patients from the scene of an accident to the hospital. It also provides a means of temporary immobilization in the emergency room in order to facilitate proper roentgenograms. It is not useful in the definitive treatment of these fractures, as it maintains the lower extremity in full extension and it is difficult, in this position, to control the deforming muscular forces.

Russell Traction. A variation in skin traction was developed by Russell in an attempt to produce a traction force in line with the femoral shaft, with the knee in the position of flexion (Fig. 23–1). This is a much more comfortable position than Buck's-type traction. Russell traction is occasionally useful in older children. It is set up with one traction rope. The calf of the injured extremity is elevated on a couple of

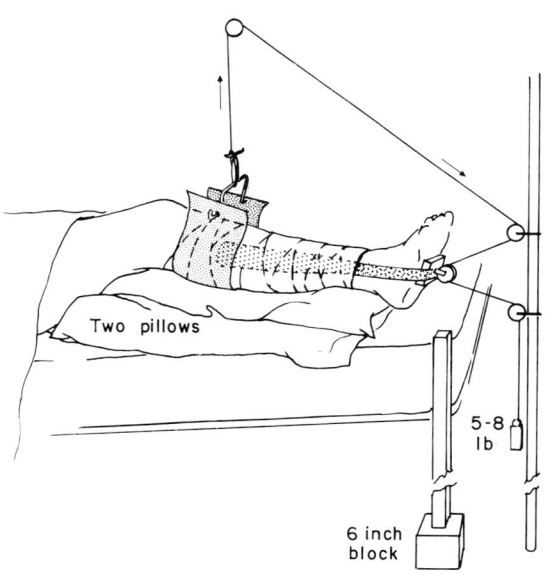

Figure 23–1 Russell traction. A single rope provides the required traction. Upward traction is provided by the overhead pulley, and distal traction is provided through the three-pulley system at the foot of the bed.

pillows, and a padded sling is placed under the knee with an overhead pulley slightly distal to the knee. Buck's traction apparatus is then applied to the tibial area. The single traction rope is adjusted so that it pulls in an upward and slightly distal direction and then downward to a three-pulley system, providing distal traction through the tibial skin traction. A weight of approximately 8 lb is applied to the traction rope. In order to add mechanical advantage, the lower end of the bed is usually elevated approximately 6 inches. Split Russell traction with the use of a skeletal traction wire has a greater clinical application.

Skeletal Traction. An integral part of all treatment programs for fractured femora, skeletal traction is useful in the early management to produce overdistraction at the fracture site if internal fixation is the treatment of choice. It is also useful in the initial management prior to the application of cast braces. The three common methods of obtaining skeletal traction for this injury are split Russell traction through a skeletal wire, suspension traction, and 90–90–90 traction.

Split Russell Traction. Split Russell traction may be obtained by the insertion of a Kirschner wire through the tibial tubercle. The extremity is placed in a Thomas splint with a Pearson knee attachment. Vertical traction is then applied through a traction bow attached to the Kirschner wire, and horizontal traction is obtained through straps attached to the traction bow (Fig. 23-2).

Suspension Traction. Suspension traction is obtained with the use of a Kirschner wire pulling in the line of direction of the femur with the extremity suspended in a Thomas splint with a Pearson knee attachment (Fig. 23–3). In this way knee motion can be instituted early while skeletal traction in line with the femur is still maintained with the wire through the tibial tubercle. Skeletal traction through the supracondylar area is seldom if ever indicated with this type of traction.

90–90–90 Traction. This is an extremely useful method for treating the patient with an open contaminated fracture with soft-tissue loss along the posterior aspect of the thigh and buttock areas. It allows for ease of soft-tissue wound care and is comfortable

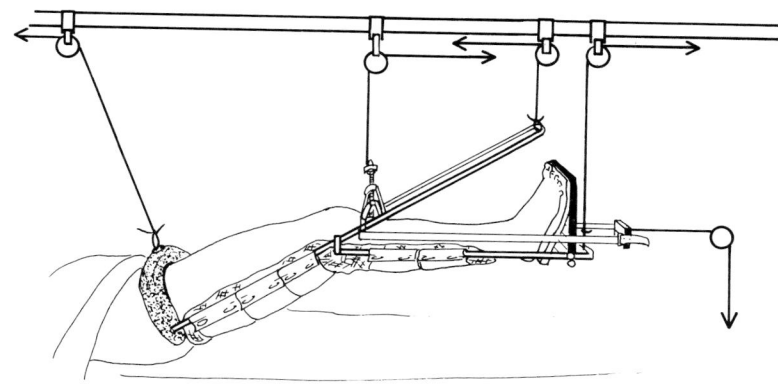

Figure 23–2 Split Russell traction. A Kirschner wire is inserted into the tibial tubercle, and the extremity is placed in a Thomas splint with a Pearson knee attachment. Vertical traction is provided by the overhead pulley; horizontal traction is provided through the straps attached to the traction bow.

for the patient. It is also useful in the older, heavier child. In this method a Kirschner wire is inserted in the supracondylar area. The below-the-knee portion of the lower extremity is suspended in a horizontal position by means of a plaster cast and slings. The traction is applied through the supracondylar area and the extremity is positioned so that the knee, hip, and ankle are in 90 degrees of flexion (Fig. 23–4). In this position the distal fragment is well controlled by the traction wire and suspended lower leg. One of the disadvantages of this technique, however, is the use of a supracondylar wire, which may predispose to stiffening of the knee. This type of traction must be observed carefully in the young pediatric group, as avascular changes

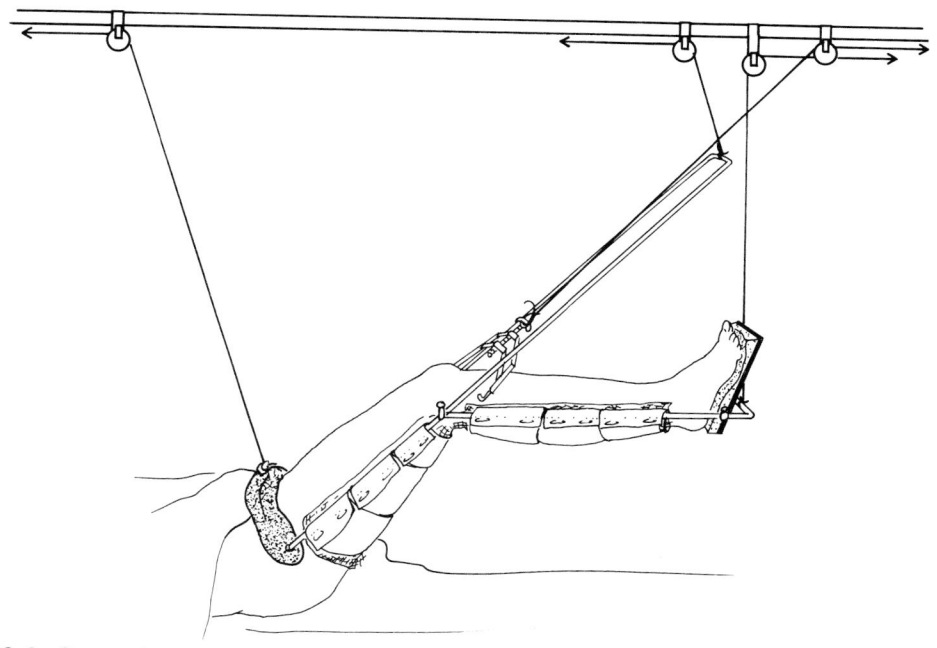

Figure 23–3 Suspension traction. A Kirschner wire is inserted into the tibial tubercle area, and traction is provided in the line of direction of the femur. The extremity is suspended in a Thomas splint and Pearson knee attachment.

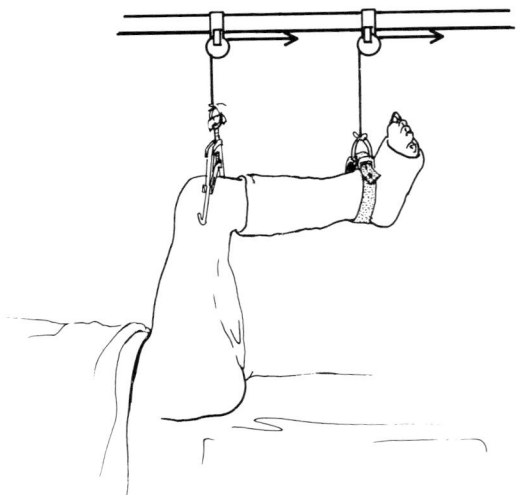

Figure 23–4 90–90–90 traction. An excellent method for treating the patient with an open fracture and soft-tissue loss along the posterior aspect of the thigh. A Kirschner wire is inserted into the supracondylar area. The extremity is then positioned with 90 degrees of flexion at the hip and 90 degrees of flexion at the knee, with the ankle maintained at 90 degrees. The tibial area is supported in the horizontal plane by a short leg cast, and the leg is suspended by an overhead pulley. This method must be used with caution in the young pediatric age group.

may be produced in the suspended extremity.

Internal Fixation

Intramedullary Fixation. Intramedullary nail fixation has a definite place in the treatment of femoral shaft fractures. The method was initially popularized by Küntscher, who in 1940, reported the results of utilizing his rod for intramedullary fixation.[44a] The initial rod was a V-shaped device; this was subsequently changed to the cloverleaf design. He obtained the advantages of internal fixation with the use of a limited incision. A small incision was made at the greater trochanter, and a guide wire was inserted, under roentgenographic control, through the medial portion of the greater trochanter down the femoral shaft. Küntscher then reamed over the guide wire to enlarge the intramedullary canal and inserted a stainless steel V-rod over the guide wire, down the femoral shaft and across the fracture site (Fig. 23–5). His aim

was to obtain rigid internal fixation by extensive reaming of the medullary canal and the insertion of a tight-fitting rod. The concept of a limited incision did not gain widespread acceptance in North America initially, owing to the difficulty of inserting the rod across the fracture site with two-plane x-ray. The development of the image intensifier has, however, enhanced the technical ability of most surgeons to perform this internal fixation through a limited incision, and several recent studies have indicated the excellent results that can be obtained with this technique. The infection rate is definitely diminished compared

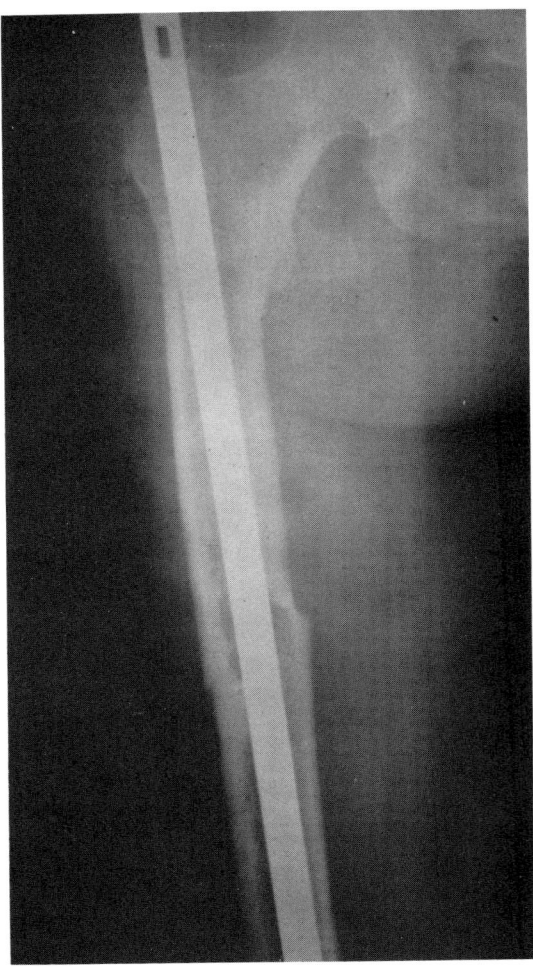

Figure 23–5 "Closed" insertion of a Küntscher rod in a fractured femur. In this case the rod could have been a larger size to provide a tighter fit. The rod extends just above the tip of the trochanter and down to the level of the upper border of the patella.

to that of formal open reduction. Nevertheless, open reduction is still employed in several centers today. Not all centers or peripheral hospitals have image intensifiers at their disposal. Therefore, open reduction and internal fixation with intramedullary rods will continue to have a place in the treatment of femoral shaft fractures.

Prior to open or closed reduction and internal fixation with an intramedullary device, the patient is maintained in skeletal traction while a definite attempt is made to overdistract the fracture fragments. The rationale behind this method is that purposeful distraction of the fracture fragments will stretch the soft tissues surrounding the fracture site and make it relatively easy to accomplish reduction and internal fixation. If overdistraction has not been accomplished, it is frequently difficult to reduce the fracture, owing to overlap of the fragments with contraction of the soft tissues. The patient is initially placed in 20 lb of skeletal traction. Following an appropriate time interval, a roentgenogram is obtained. If there is not satisfactory evidence of reduction, an additional 10 lb is added and follow-up roentgenograms are obtained. Ten pounds is again added until there is satisfactory evidence of reduction with distraction of the fracture fragments.

The timing of the reduction and internal fixation has been controversial in the past. In the majority of reported series, a wait of between 7 and 10 days prior to internal fixation has been preferred. There appears to be a definite increase in the union rate and a decrease in the infection rate in patients treated in this manner. Many of these patients have sustained significant trauma and have injuries to other systems. Frequently, under these conditions, blood replacement is necessary. In a study on oxygen transport to standardized wounds in a series of control patients, elective operative patients, and multiple trauma patients, the author found that the multiple trauma patients had a definite decrease in the oxygen supply to the standard soft-tissue wound (Fig. 23–6). This was correlated with the cardiac output and the inherent red blood cell function. In spite of an increase in cardiac output, the trauma patients still demonstrated a decrease in oxygen supply. This deficit was present for approximately five to six days after injury.[37] It has been conclusively demonstrated that hypoxia delays wound repair and increases susceptibility to infection in soft tissue. If one extrapolates these findings to the patient with a fractured femur and associated injuries, it becomes obvious that wound healing may be delayed and the patient may be more susceptible to infection in the early period than after a delay of seven to ten days. These studies fit well with the clinical experience that delayed open reduction and internal fixation has a better prognosis than immediate open reduction and internal fixation. This may not apply to the closed reduction and limited incision of Küntscher in which the fracture site is not open and no large wound is present. It is for these reasons, that I prefer a delay of seven days prior to open reduction and internal fixation if this treatment program is selected.

Figure 23–6 Oxygen tension measurements in standardized wounds in a control group of patients and a group of patients sustaining multiple trauma. Note that there is a significant decrease in the local wound oxygen tension in the patients with multiple trauma compared to the control group. It has been adequately demonstrated that hypoxia in soft tissue wounds increases the incidence of infection and delays repair. This finding may explain why it is better to wait seven days before open reduction to avoid wound healing complications. (Courtesy of R. B. Heppenstall, F. N. Littooy, R. Fuchs, et al. and *Surgery*. Gas tensions in healing tissues of traumatized patients, Surgery, 75:874–880, 1974.)

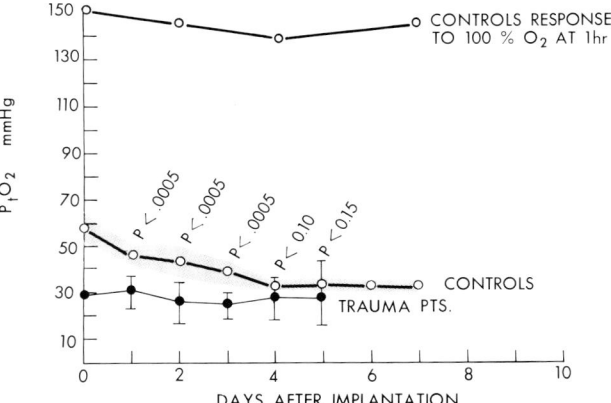

Open Reduction and Intramedullary Rod Fixation. A spinal or general anesthetic is administered and the patient is placed in a lateral decubitus position with the affected extremity up. The fracture site is exposed by a standard posterolateral incision. The intermuscular septum is identified and followed to bone. The soft-tissue structures are reflected anteriorly. The fracture site is identified, the fracture fragments are mobilized, and the distal fragment is delivered from the wound. The medullary canal is reamed in a standard fashion. The proximal fragment is then delivered from the wound and appropriately reamed. Next, guide wire is passed retrograde up the femoral shaft to exit at the base of the superior portion of the neck. An incision is then placed proximal to the trochanter where the guide wire is palpable. A reamer is inserted over the guide wire to drill a hole at the junction of the neck and the trochanter. Once this hole is drilled, the medullary rod is passed over the guide pin with the eye of the rod facing posteromedially and the rod is driven into the trochanteric region of the femur. Strength testing of the cloverleaf rod by Soto-Hall and McCloy revealed that the cloverleaf was weakest with the open side facing the compression side.[72] It is for this reason that the rod is driven into the femur in this fashion. Once the rod has been inserted to the fracture site, the fracture is reduced and the rod is driven across the site (Fig. 23–7). It is imperative that the intramedullary fixation device have a tight grip within the intramedullary canal. This requires adequate reaming of the medullary canal and the insertion of a proper-sized device. The rod is inserted with the eye facing posteromedially and extends distally to the level of the proximal edge of the patella. Not more than 1 inch of the rod should be palpable proximal to the trochanter.

Three other devices are at present available for intramedullary fixation. The Schneider rod is a four-flanged rod with its own cutting broaches. This provides satisfactory resistance to tortion (Fig. 23–8). Hanson and Street devised a diamond-shaped rod for which a specially designed cutting broach is used. Finally, a heavy-duty fluted rod has been developed and is known as the Sampson rod. The advantages

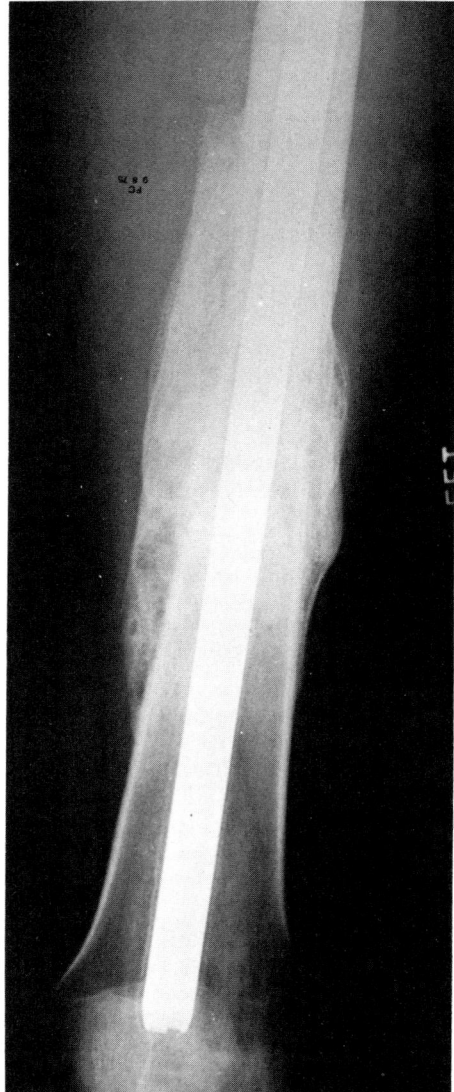

Figure 23–7 A fracture of the lower midportion of the femur treated with a snug-fitting Küntscher rod. This fracture was comminuted, and a bone graft was applied at the time. Extensive bone formation is evident, extending both proximally and distally from the fracture site.

of this rod, as outlined by Rhinelander, are that it provides rotational stability by virtue of the flutes and also allows ingrowth of a new endosteal blood supply between the flutes.[62] This rod has a sound scientific design and appears to be becoming more popular. It is probably important, however, to become familiar with one type of rod and employ it when internal fixation is indicated.

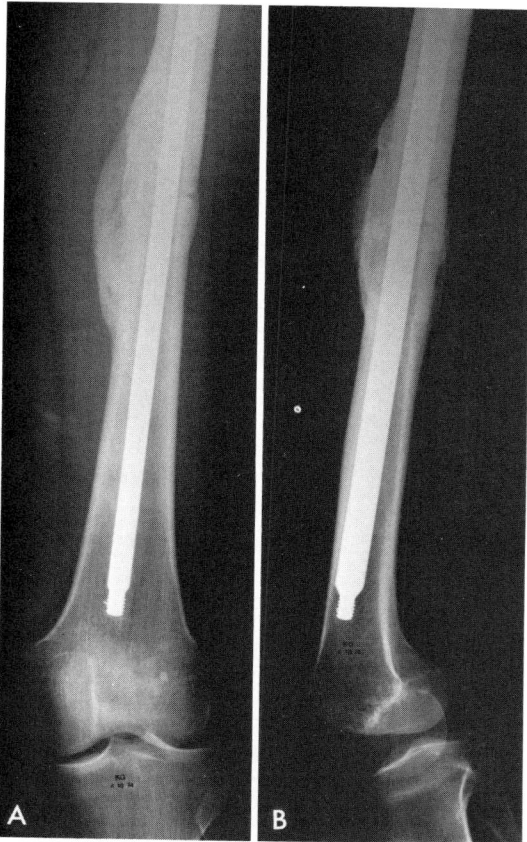

Figure 23-8 A. Anteroposterior view of a transverse fracture of the midshaft of the femur treated with an intramedullary rod. Note the excess bone formation on the medial side of the femur, which is the compression side. B. Lateral roentgenogram of the same fracture revealing evidence of healing. Note the snug fit of the rod.

Closed Nailing. Several centers have reported excellent results with closed nailing of femoral shaft fractures. This technique is similar to that originally outlined by Küntscher in that it involves a limited incision proximal to the greater trochanter for the insertion of an intramedullary fixation device through the proximal shaft, across the fracture site, and into the distal shaft. The fracture site is *not* exposed in this technique, which has several advantages. It does not disturb the fracture site proper and therefore does not involve stripping of the periosteal attachments to gain exposure for insertion of the intramedullary device. No large wound is produced, and the possibility of infection is greatly diminished. The

disadvantage is that it requires the use of an image intensifier (Fig. 23-9). It can be performed with two-plane regular roentgenograms, but this is much more difficult. The procedure may be performed with the patient in the prone position on the extension fracture table with the thigh flexed at 80 degrees and 20 to 30 degrees of adduction. Traction is maintained through a distal femoral or proximal tibial pin. The procedure may also be performed with the patient supine on a regular fracture table, also with traction applied through a distal pin. An incision 5 to 8 cm in length is made along the central axis of the femur, extending cephalad from the tip of the greater trochanter. The tip of the greater trochanter is identified, and an awl is inserted inside it and is directed toward the midportion of the knee joint. A guide wire is then placed down the shaft of the proximal femur, a reamer is placed over the guide wire in the intramedullary canal, and the proximal portion of the femur is reamed to appropriate size. The fracture is reduced, and the

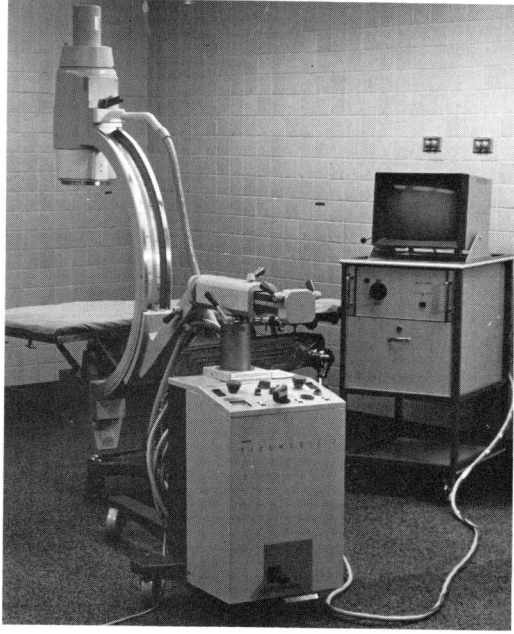

Figure 23-9 One of the commercially available image intensifiers in the operating room. The large C arm may be maneuvered with ease to produce an anteroposterior or lateral projection. The memory bank is seen in the far right-hand corner. This allows the image to be held on the screen until the next picture is taken.

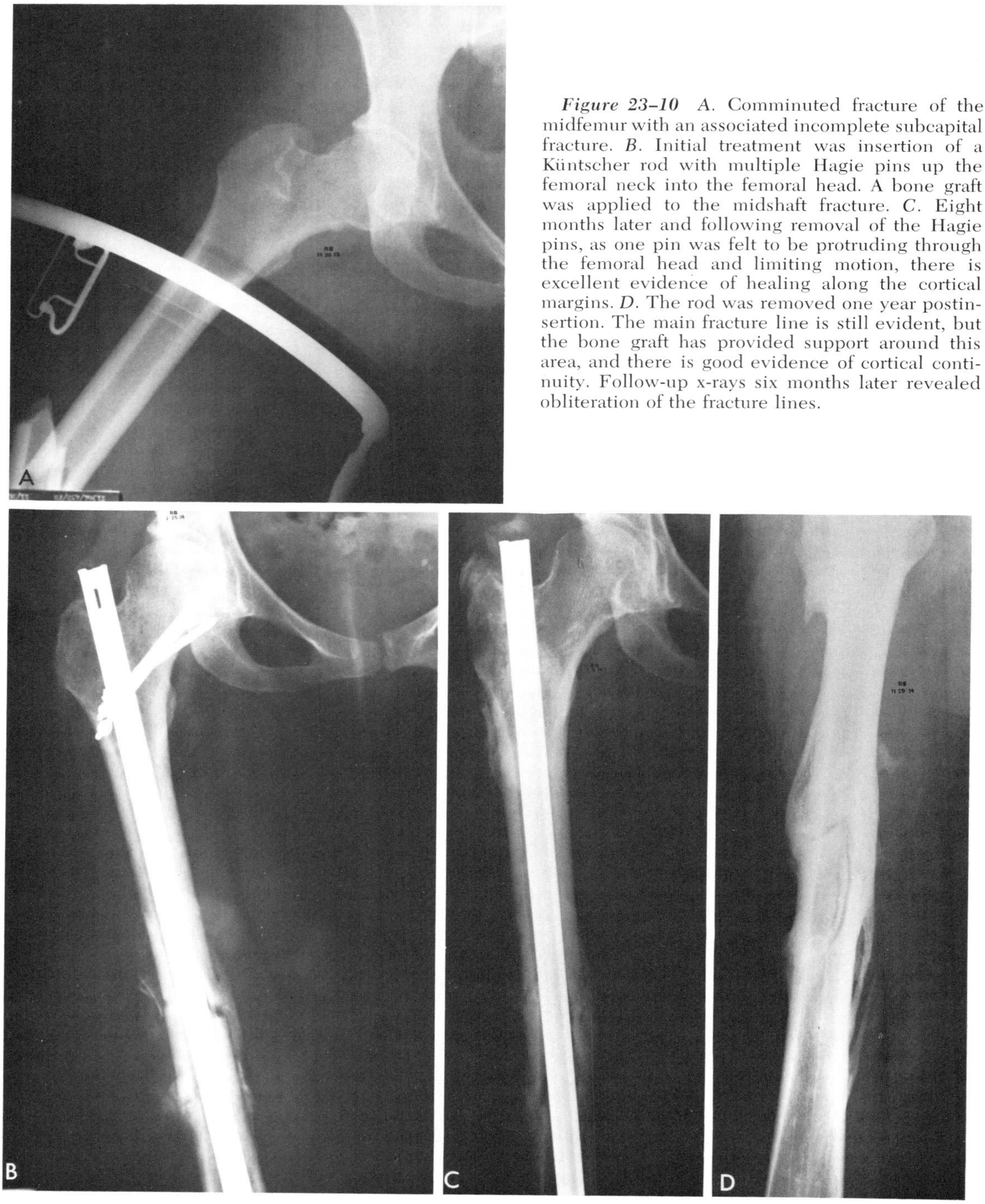

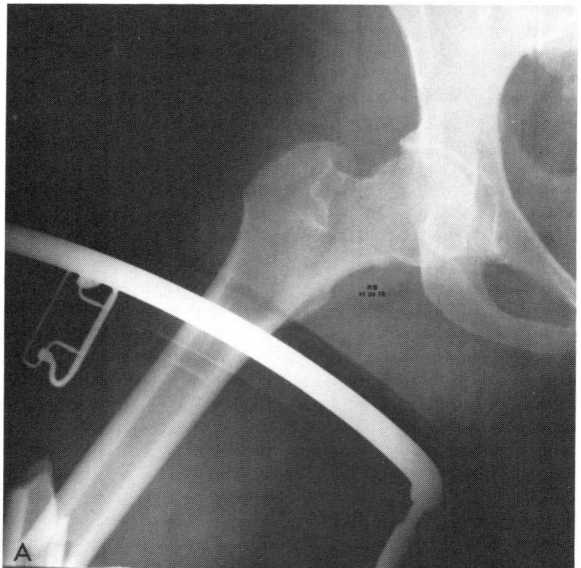

Figure 23–10 A. Comminuted fracture of the midfemur with an associated incomplete subcapital fracture. B. Initial treatment was insertion of a Küntscher rod with multiple Hagie pins up the femoral neck into the femoral head. A bone graft was applied to the midshaft fracture. C. Eight months later and following removal of the Hagie pins, as one pin was felt to be protruding through the femoral head and limiting motion, there is excellent evidence of healing along the cortical margins. D. The rod was removed one year postinsertion. The main fracture line is still evident, but the bone graft has provided support around this area, and there is good evidence of cortical continuity. Follow-up x-rays six months later revealed obliteration of the fracture lines.

reaming is continued across the fracture site. Flexible reamers are a definite advantage for this. The nail is then driven across the fracture site and into the distal shaft of the femur.

The entire operative procedure can be

performed fairly rapidly with the use of the image intensifier. It does require an assistant to mobilize the distal fragment through the traction apparatus and manipulate it into the proper position so that the guide wire and Küntscher rod can be placed across the fracture site. It has, however, definite advantages in the very limited incision and the fact that the fracture site is not exposed.

All of the foregoing methods allow adequate internal fixation and early mobilization. There is no doubt that muscular contractions across the fracture site aid in fracture healing. Active muscular contractions augment the blood supply to the area and also generate an electrical potential across the fracture site. Both of these are felt to be important in the healing process, as outlined in Chapter 2.

Intramedullary fixation with the use of crossed Rush rods is not discussed here, as it does not provide satisfactory fixation and has lost its popularity in the treatment of femoral fractures.

Bone Grafting. What place, if any, does bone grafting play in the treatment of fractured femora? This question is still very controversial in regard to open reduction and internal fixation. It is the author's feeling that if internal fixation is selected for treatment and comminution is present at the fracture site, this is a primary indication for bone grafting. This is particularly true in the presence of a butterfly fragment. It is true that the majority of cells do not survive following a bone grafting procedure. They do, however, provide the appropriate scaffolding for new osseous "creeping substitution." We have all seen evidence of healing due to the bone graft around a butterfly fragment while the fracture line remained evident and only gradually diminished with passing of time (Fig. 23–10). This finding suggests that if the bone graft had not been added at the time of the operative procedure, the fracture might well have progressed to nonunion.

Compression Plates. Compression plating has a limited application for treating femoral fractures. First, if a single plate is to be positioned along the lateral aspect of the femur, there must be no comminution of the medial portion of the femur. The plate acts as a tension band, and if comminution is present along the medial portion there will be no resistance to further compression. Second, a single compression plate is not sufficient to leave the patient out of plaster. If a single compression plate is applied to the lateral aspect of the femur for a fracture,

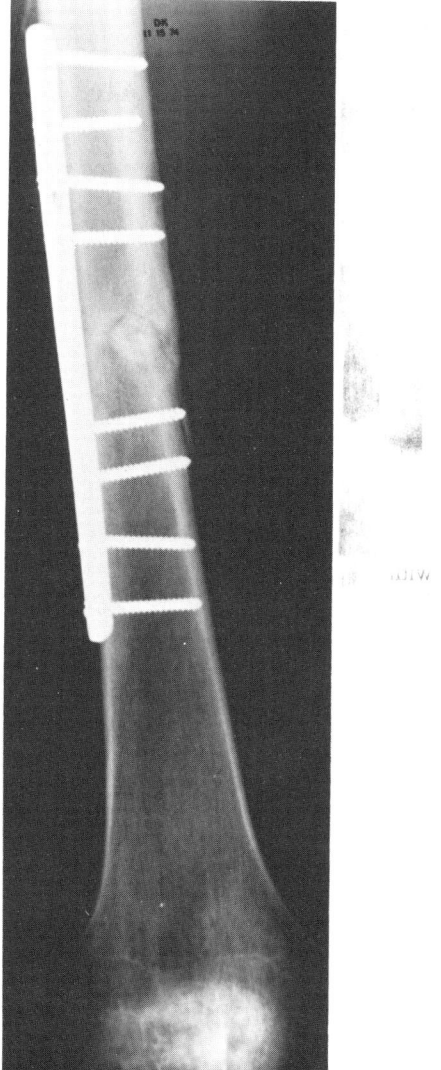

Figure 23–11 A transverse fracture of the midportion of the femur treated with a single compression plate along the lateral aspect of the femur. It is important that at least four screws be inserted proximal and distal to the fracture site. This mode of fixation requires application of a cast brace or a hip spica. A single plate does not provide enough support without plaster.

supplementary external support in the form of a cast or cast brace should be supplied (Fig. 23–11). To obtain firm fixation while avoiding the use of supplementary external devices, dual compression plating is necessary. In the past, 90–90 plating of the femur was advocated. This does supply adequate

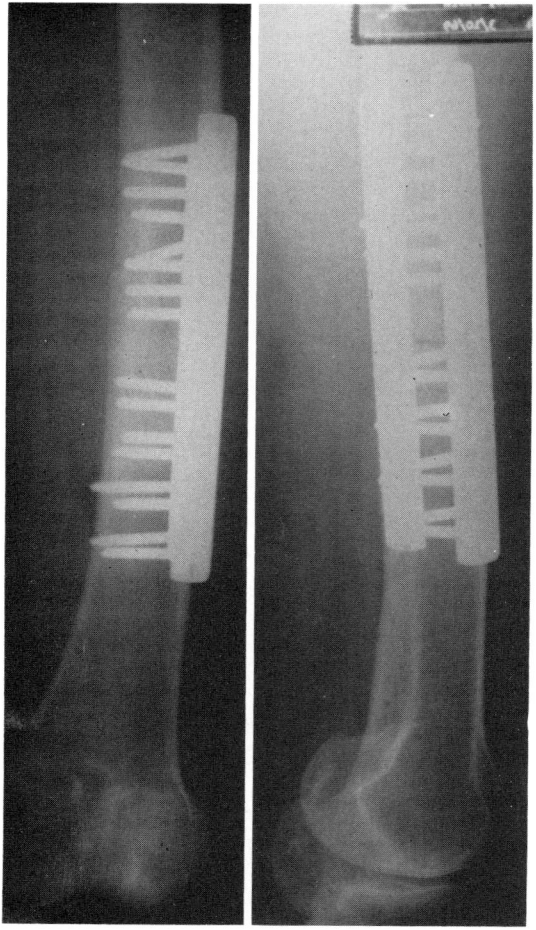

Figure 23–12 Midshaft femoral fracture treated with dual 90–90 plates. Additional external support is not required with this type of fixation.

fixation without the use of a cast (Fig. 23–12). The plates must eventually be removed, however, and when they are, they must be removed one plate at a time with two to three months intervening. If both plates are removed at once, the bone will be severely weakened through the screw holes, as the cortex is not accustomed to resisting normal forces because a major portion of the load has been taken by the compression plates. It has been adequately demonstrated that disuse osteoporosis exists underneath heavy compression plates. For these reasons, one plate must be removed at a time and support must be given in the form of crutches or a cane

during the four to six week interval required for the bone to adapt to the new forces.

One of the relative indications for use of the compression plate may be the presence of concomitant intracapsular fractures. Internal fixation in the form of multiple pins may be used in the treatment of the intracapsular fracture. A compression plate could then be applied to the femoral shaft fracture. The alternative to this method is to treat the femoral fracture with an intramedullary rod and then treat the intracapsular fracture with multiple pins positioned around the rod. This is technically very difficult but can be accomplished. If the femoral shaft fracture is below the isthmus, however, the indications for the intramedullary rod may not be present. This would be an indication for a compression plate.

Nonoperative Approach – The Cast Brace

This title is a bit of a misnomer, as the conservative management of these fractures requires the insertion of a skeletal traction pin. Nonoperative treatment at the fracture site proper is, however, implied. Three methods exist for this approach.

The first method is to maintain the patient in skeletal pin traction until the fracture has healed. A second is to maintain the skeletal traction until there is enough stability at the fracture site to discontinue its use and apply a hip spica. I feel that the indication for this method has decreased in modern orthopedic care. The third method is to apply a cast brace. This has all but eliminated the other forms of therapy. The incidence of secondary medical complications with the first and second treatment programs is significant when compared to that with the cast brace treatment program. In addition, it is felt that fracture healing is stimulated by active mobilization with the use of a cast brace.

Compressive forces are applied across the fracture site with this treatment. The total contact by the thigh component of the cast brace provides a hydraulic effect as the thigh, compressed within the rigid confines of the cast brace, becomes a semi-rigid fluid-filled tube with the fluid constantly maintained under pressure. The compressed soft tissue then tends to provide an even distribution of forces across the fracture site. Connolly and co-workers have demonstrated excellent results with treatment of femoral fractures in this manner but have also demonstrated that motion across the fracture site does occur.[21, 22] Motion at the fracture site does not seem to matter as long as it occurs with a compressive contractile force produced by active muscle contraction with ambulation. The quadrilateral socket at the proximal portion of the cast brace is not meant to function as an ischial weight-bearing device, but rather to control rotation at the fracture site and also to provide a rigid support, maintaining the hydraulic effect. This technique is particularly applicable to fractures in the middle and the distal half of the femoral shaft. Recently, it has also been utilized for fractures of the proximal shaft, but in this case the cast requires a hinge at its proximal end connecting it to a pelvic band. For the usual fractures in the mid and distal portion of the femur the pelvic band and hinge in the hip area are not required. Several studies including those of Connolly and co-workers, Mooney and co-workers, and Burkhalter have demonstrated the beneficial effect on fracture healing of the use of a cast brace.[12, 21–23, 51, 52]

Timing of Application of Brace. When this technique was being developed, the cast brace was applied at approximately the same time that a hip spica would be applied (six to eight weeks). As more experience was gained, however, it became obvious that such a delay was not justified. For the novice it is probably best to wait five to seven weeks before applying the cast brace. At the end of this time the fracture site is "sticky" and there is less discomfort associated with the application of the brace, but once experience has been gained with using this technique, the brace may be applied as early as one to two weeks following injury. Initially, a proximal tibial pin is inserted for skeletal traction in bed with the use of a Thomas splint and Pearson knee attachment. Once the swelling about the fracture site subsides and the pain diminishes, then that is the time to apply the cast brace. The procedure usually requires some type of supplemental analgesia and a muscle relaxant. Occasionally, a patient will have significant discomfort and

light anesthesia may have to be administered. I feel that the sooner the brace can be applied and ambulation started, the better the treatment. There is no question that return of the patient to a functional ambulatory state has a positive stimulatory effect on the fracture healing process. This effect is outlined in Chapter 2.

Application of Cast Brace. This technique will produce good results only if strict attention is paid to details. As stated earlier, the cast brace functions on a hydrodynamic principle. This requires that the thigh portion fit very snugly; the hydraulic effect will not be produced by a loosely applied brace. Some provision must also be made to prevent the cast from slipping down. This is done by including both the thigh and the lower leg, the two portions of plaster then being connected with a polycentric metal joint at the knee to allow free motion of the knee joint (Fig. 23–13).

The cast brace is applied with the patient lying supine in bed. A Spandex sock is drawn over the proximal thigh area. This is the same type of sock that is worn over an

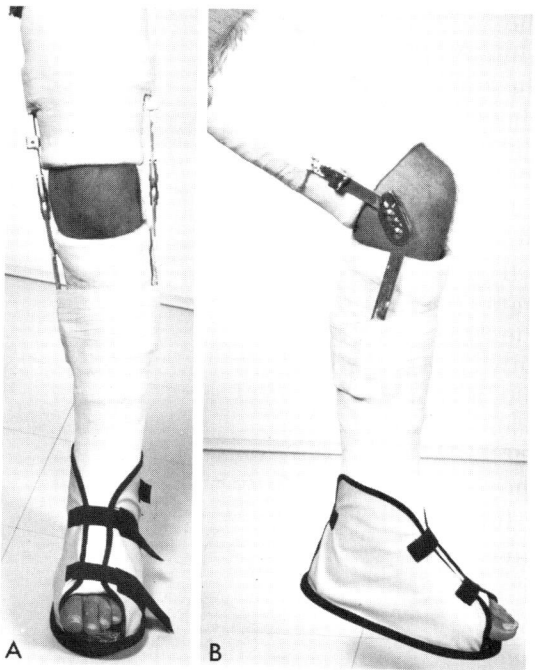

Figure 23–13 A. Anterior view of a properly applied cast brace. B. Lateral view of the same patient. Note the position of the polycentric hinge allowing flexion of the knee.

amputation stump under a prosthesis, and it provides an excellent interface between the skin and plaster. It is important that there not be a lot of bulky material in this area or a snug-fitting cast will be impossible. A small amount of Webril may be added to the very proximal portion of the thigh to fit under the adjustable plastic quadrilateral socket. A quadrilateral socket is not entirely necessary for the application of the cast brace, but it does help in controlling rotation. Elastic plaster is then wrapped circumferentially around the proximal thigh. If the socket is available, it is incorporated; if it is not, then the elastic plaster may be molded firmly to form an ischial seat and fit snugly into the Scarpa triangle area and over the greater trochanter. The plaster is then extended down the entire leg, incorporating the knee, tibia, ankle, and foot. The foot is held at 90 degrees to the tibia. Once the plaster has set, sufficient plaster must be removed at the knee to allow at least 90 degrees of flexion and full extension. Metal polycentric hinges are then applied. Various jigs are available to align the hinges to allow ease of motion at the knee. The metal joint should be positioned at the level of the adductor tubercle, which is normally located at the midpatellar region. They should also be placed approximately $1/2$ inch posterior to the midportion of the leg to reproduce a physiologically normal anatomical axis at the joint. If the attending surgeon is worried about the amount of comminution and the stability at the fracture site, then the proximal tibial pin can remain in place, allowing intermittent skeletal traction when the patient is supine in bed. The pin may also be left in when the foot and ankle are not included in plaster. The pin then suspends the plaster portion of the cast and prevents any distal slippage. With the foot and ankle included in plaster, however, this is not usually a problem, and in the majority of cases the pin may be removed at the time the cast brace is applied.

Routine roentgenograms are obtained following application of the cast brace. If there has been a shift of alignment, appropriate wedging of the thigh portion of the cast is necessary to correct the malalignment. Mooney has adequately demonstrated that an opening wedge type of correction produces the fewest skin problems.[51] This is performed at the level of the fracture site with the open part of the wedge corresponding to the varus portion of the fracture. In other words, if there is significant lateral bowing, a medial opening wedge is performed; if there is significant medial bowing, then a lateral opening wedge is performed. The patient may then ambulate as soon as he is comfortable in the cast brace.

Initially minimal partial weight bearing is encouraged. Full weight bearing should follow as tolerated. It is extremely important to explain to these patients the necessity for full weight bearing to stimulate the fracture healing process. Some pistoning does occur at the fracture site with active ambulation and weight bearing, but most studies have revealed that no large amount of shortening is produced with this type of treatment. In comparison with the results of anatomical reduction and internal fixation, there is slightly more shortening with the cast brace technique. We must bear in mind, however, that the cast brace is generally reserved for the more comminuted and displaced fractures, and therefore many series reflect this bias when the two methods are compared.

The patient is discharged from hospital when comfortable. This is usually two to three weeks following application of the brace. While he is still in hospital, appropriate wedging to obtain the best alignment possible must be performed. Several cast wedging or manipulation procedures may be required, and if performed during the early phase of fracture healing, are probably not detrimental to fracture repair. I must stress the early phase, as manipulation performed three to four weeks following application of the brace probably does interfere with the fracture healing process. The brace is usually left in place for 12 to 14 weeks. At the end of this time the majority of fractures have healed. Mooney has stressed the importance of taking into account the state of function of the limb at this time rather than relying solely on the roentgenographic evaluation.[51] The patient who is nontender at the fracture site and who shows no evidence of motion and has no pain associated with full weight bearing can usually be left out of plaster, but the majority of surgeons are a little skeptical about leaving patients out of plaster before there is definite evidence of obliteration of the fracture site roentgenographically. The point to be made is that the fracture may be healed even though the fracture site is still faintly visible. If there is some doubt about the status of the fracture roentgenographically, the safest course is to return the patient to a cast brace for an additional three to four weeks.

This type of early ambulatory treatment restores the patient to active social life and significantly decreases the cost of hospitalization. These advantages—the early discharge from the hospital and the significant financial saving to the patient, compared to previous traditional skeletal traction methods—make this type of treatment extremely appealing in orthopedics today.

Operative Versus Nonoperative Treatment

As already pointed out, it is extremely difficult to improve on the excellent results obtained with the cast bracing technique. Any type of operative procedure, however, also carries operative and postoperative complications. The major complication with internal fixation for femoral fractures is infection. In most series reported to date there is a definite incidence of infection associated with this treatment program. On the other hand, fractures in the proximal half of the femur are difficult to treat with a cast brace and a pelvic band with a hinge at the hip. In this area, also, they are subjected to significant pressures, as previously outlined in the treatment of subtrochanteric fractures. The author has found the Zickel apparatus as well as the other types of intramedullary rods to be helpful for treating fractures in the proximal half of the femur (Fig. 23–14). If comminution is present, then in addition to the intramedullary rod, circlage wires may be applied in order to approximate butterfly or loose fragments.

There is a place for operative treatment in fractures of the shaft of the femur associated with ipsilateral hip fractures. An intramedullary rod may be inserted with multiple pins around the rod into the femoral neck and femoral head to stabilize the hip fracture. An alternative method is to treat

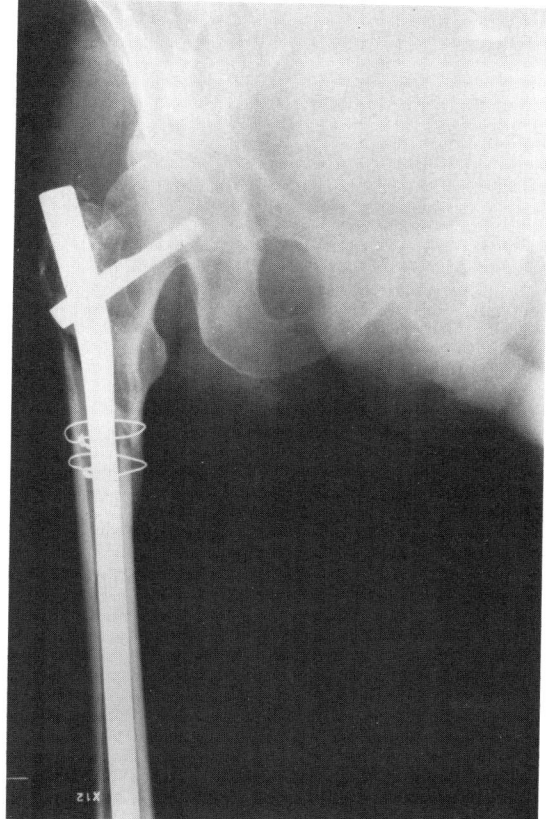

Figure 23–14 A proximal femoral fracture treated with a Zickel nail.

the femoral shaft fracture with two compression plates and then treat the hip fracture with multiple pins.

The "closed" treatment, in which an intramedullary device is inserted as originally outlined by Küntscher, has been received with enthusiasm in the United States in recent years. This has been brought about by the development and use of the image intensifier, which has greatly simplified management of patients with this technique. The very limited incision required in the proximal trochanteric area to insert the rod without exposure of the fracture is a definitely appealing feature because it avoids the dreaded complication of infection. This method also provides for stable internal fixation with an intramedullary rod and allows early active ambulation and early return to function. Therefore, its use will probably increase in many centers around the country.

As I have stated previously, it is very difficult to improve on the excellent results of using a cast brace for treating femoral fractures in the midshaft and distal half of the femur. This method will continue to be very popular, and its use is certainly increasing in all centers. Suffice it to say, the majority of femoral shaft fractures can and should be managed with this technique.

COMPLICATIONS IN FEMORAL FRACTURES

Malunion

This type of complication is relatively common in femoral shaft fractures. There is a great deal of muscular force involved in the femoral shaft area, and a tendency toward migration definitely exists. It is seen most in association with conservative methods, including skeletal traction and plaster immobilization; operative methods usually obtain satisfactory position at the fracture site, and the incidence of malunion is not quite as significant. We must keep in mind that there is a normal anterolateral bow to the femur and this is not malunion. This is normal. In addition to this normal state, an anterior bow of 15 degrees is certainly acceptable. This does not apply to lateral bowing, as this will affect alignment and stresses at the knee (Fig. 23–15).

Once significant malunion has developed, it is no easy task to correct the deformity. This is usually best accomplished by an open osteotomy at the site of the malunion, appropriate correction, and the application of either a compression plate or an intramedullary device to provide rigid internal fixation. The amount of correction required should be calculated preoperatively from the roentgenogram, and the wedge of bone should be predetermined. In this way, good correction may be obtained.

Knee function must be maintained. This

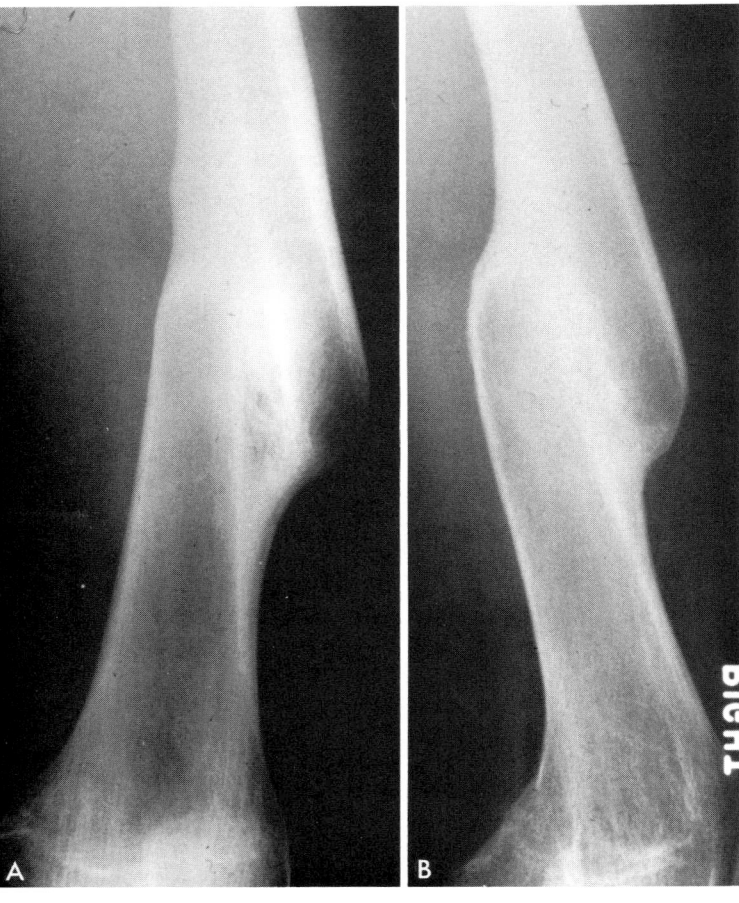

Figure 23–15 A. Anteroposterior view of malunion of a midfemoral fracture. The fracture healed, but the patient required an osteotomy and compression plate fixation for realignment to decrease the abnormal stress on the knee due to the malalignment. B. The position in the lateral view is acceptable.

will deteriorate rapidly if significant malunion is present in the femoral shaft because of the additional abnormal stresses placed on the knee.

Nonunion

Nonunion must be treated by some type of operative intervention or it will not heal. Most nonunions in the middle and distal portion of the femur may be treated with compression plates and bone grafting procedures. The alternative is an intramedullary rod with a bone graft procedure. It is usually not sufficient to utilize only the bone at the fracture site by turning back slivers of bone from both the proximal and distal shaft areas. I prefer to obtain a good supply of cancellous bone from the ipsilateral iliac crest for insertion at the fracture site following the internal fixation procedure. If a fibrous union is already present, this does not have to be "taken down." All that is necessary, if there is acceptable alignment, is to decorticate the bone around the shaft in both the proximal and distal fragments and apply a good portion of cancellous bone graft in this area.

If a pseudoarthrosis is present, with a definite false joint, then this must be removed as in other areas of the body prior to internal fixation.

The nonunion rate varies. In most series, with present techniques, it approximates 1 to 5 per cent.

Delayed Union

Femoral fractures should demonstrate a decrease in pain and some stability at the fracture site by three to four months. If this has not occurred by four months, the observer must entertain the possibility of a delayed union. This does not mean that all fractures that do not demonstrate some stability and significant pain relief by four months will definitely go on to nonunion. One should simply be wary of this complication at this particular time.

Operative intervention is not indicated by four months, but the patient with a cast brace should be actively encouraged to bear full weight if at all possible. The rationale of weight bearing and its stimulatory effect on the fracture repair process must be thoroughly explained to the patient if cooperation is to be expected.

Infection

This complication is seen with internal fixation of femoral fractures and also with the treatment of open fractures in this area. All series reported on internal fixation for these fractures reveal a definite incidence of infection, which varies with the various case reports.

The patient usually has an intramedullary rod or a compression plate. It has been adequately demonstrated that if stability is present at the fracture site and is being provided by the internal fixation, then this should *not* be removed in an attempt to control the infection. Removing the internal fixation device in the presence of infection may well produce a disaster; not only is an infection present but there is also gross instability at the fracture site as well. It is more sound physiologically to leave the internal fixation in place and perform a debridement with insertion of an irrigation system. The device may then be removed following evidence of stability at the fracture site.

This is not to say that the internal fixation device should never be removed in order to gain control of infection. If extreme, life-threatening sepsis is present and all attempts at debridement and irrigation have failed to control it, then the internal fixation device must be removed and a thorough debridement performed. This is not the usual set of circumstances, however. Most patients are febrile, but extreme sepsis is rare with this problem. Occasionally if there is no evidence of good fixation provided by the internal device, it may be removed and replaced with a more appropriate one. For example, if an intramedullary rod is present that is too small to give stability at the fracture site, then it should be replaced with a more acceptable larger rod.

Antibiotics should be administered in appropriate amounts on the basis of operative cultures. The majority of investigators recommend a six week course of parenteral antibiotics in hospital followed by three to six months of oral antibiotics for this particular problem.

The other circumstances in which infection may be a complication is an open fracture that may not have been treated with internal fixation. This type of problem can be avoided by thorough debridement and irrigation at the time of the injury. If there is any doubt about the degree of contamination present, then it is sound to leave the wound open and perform a secondary closure at a later date when there is evidence that good granulation tissue is present. The secret to control of this type of problem is thorough debridement with or without an irrigation system and appropriate antibiotics.

It is not wise to attempt internal fixation in an open fracture. It is true that in Europe primary debridement of open fractures followed by immediate internal fixation has met with significant success. In general, this has not been the experience in North America. A far more physiological approach is to perform a debridement with or without a secondary closure and follow it at a later date by internal fixation if necessary when there is no longer any evidence of infection. A sobering fact in this regard is the high rate of infection reported with primary internal fixation in the presence of open fractures in the various series from North America. This has varied from 5 to 14 per cent. Needless to say, these are significant figures; they should be a deterrent to primary internal fixation of open fractures.

REFERENCES

1. Allen, W. C., Piotrowski, G., Burstein, A. H., and Frankel, V. H.: Biomechanical principles of intramedullary fixation. Clin. Orthop., 60:13–20, 1968.
2. Allgower, M., Ehrsam, R., Ganz, R., Matter, P., and Perren, S. M.: Clinical experience with a new compression plate "DCP." Acta Orthop. Scand., 36(Suppl.):277–279, 1969.
3. Anderson, R.: An ambulatory method of treating fractures of the shaft of the femur. Surg. Gynecol. Obstet., 62:865, 1936.
4. Anderson, R. L.: Conservative treatment of fractures of the femur. J. Bone Joint Surg., 49A:1371–1375, 1967.
5. Bohler, J.: Results in medullary nailing of ninety-five fresh fractures of the femur. J. Bone Joint Surg., 33A:670–678, 1951.
6. Bohler, J.: Percutaneous internal fixation utilizing the x-ray image amplifier. J. Trauma, 5:150–155, 1965.
7. Bohler, J.: Closed intramedullary nailing of the femur. Clin. Orthop., 60:51–67, 1968.

8. Boyd, H. B., Anderson, L. D., and Johnson, D. S.: Changing concepts in the treatment of non-union. Clin. Orthop., 43:37–54, 1966.
9. Brav, E. A.: Further evaluation of the use of intramedullary nailing in the treatment of gun-shot fractures of the extremities. J. Bone Joint Surg., 39A:513–520, 1957.
10. Brav, E. A.: The use of intramedullary nailing for nonunion of the femur. Clin. Orthop., 60:69–75, 1968.
11. Brooks, D. B., Burstein, A. H., and Frankel, V. H.: The bio-mechanics of torsional fractures. The stress concentration effect of a drill hole. J. Bone Joint Surg., 52A:507–514, 1970.
12. Burkhalter, W. E.: Experience with brace-cast for femoral fractures. Cast-bracing of fractures. A report of a workshop sponsored by the Committee on Prosthetics Research and Development, Division of Engineering, National Research Council, Washington, D.C., 1971.
13. Burstein, A. H., Currey, J., Frankel, V. H., Heiple, K. G., Lunseth, P., and Vessely, J. C.: Bone strength—the effect of screw holes. J. Bone Joint Surg., 54A:1143–1156, 1972.
14. Burwell, H. N.: Internal fixation in the treatment of fractures of the femoral shaft. Injury, 2:235, 1971.
15. Carr, C. R., and Wingo, C. H.: Fractures of the femoral diaphysis. A retrospective study of the results and costs of treatment by intramedullary nailing and by traction and a spica cast. J. Bone Joint Surg., 55A:690–700, 1973.
16. Castle, M. E., and Orinion, E. A.: Prophylactic anticoagulation in fractures. J. Bone Joint Surg., 52A:521–528, 1970.
17. Charnley, J.: Knee movement following fractures of the femoral shaft. J. Bone Joint Surg., 29:679–686, 1947.
18. Charnley, J.: The Closed Treatment of Common Fractures. 3rd Ed. Baltimore, Williams & Wilkins Co., 1961.
19. Charnley, J., and Guindy, A.: Delayed operation in the open reduction of fractures of the long bones. J. Bone Joint Surg., 43B:664–671, 1961.
20. Clawson, D. K., Smith, R. F., and Hansen, S. T.: Closed intramedullary nailing of the femur. J. Bone Joint Surg., 53A:681–692, 1971.
21. Connolly, J. F., and King, P.: Closed reduction and early cast-brace ambulation in the treatment of femoral fractures. Part I. An in vivo quantitative analysis of immobilization in skeletal traction and a cast-brace. J. Bone Joint Surg., 55A:1559–1580, 1973.
22. Connolly, J. F., Dehne, E., Lafollette, B.: Closed reduction and early cast-brace ambulation in the treatment of femoral fractures. Part II. Results in one hundred and forty-three fractures. J. Bone Joint Surg., 55A:1581–1599, 1973.
23. Connolly, J. F., Whittaker, D., and Williams, E.: Femoral and tibial fractures combined with injuries to the femoral or popliteal artery: A review of the literature and analysis of 14 cases. J. Bone Joint Surg., 53A:56–58, 1971.
24. Danckwardt-Lilliestrom, G.: Reaming of medullary cavity and its effect on diaphysial bone: Fluorochromic, microangiographic and histologic study on the rabbit tibia and dog femur. Acta Orthop. Scand., 50, (Suppl.):128, 1969.

25. DeLorme, T. L., West, F. E., and Schriber, W. J.: Influence of progressive-resistance exercises on knee function following femoral fractures. J. Bone Joint Surg., 32A:910–924, 1950.

26. Dencker, H.: Shaft fractures of the femur: A comparative study of the results of various methods of treatment in 1,003 cases. Acta Chir. Scand., 130:173–184, 1965.

27. Doporto, J. M., and Rafique, M.: Vascular insufficiency complicating trauma to the lower limb. J. Bone Joint Surg., 51B:680–685, 1969.

28. Drombrowski, E. T., and Dunn, A. W.: Treatment of osteomyelitis by debridement and closed wound irrigation suction. Clin. Orthop., 43:215–231, 1965.

29. Evans, F. G., Pedersen, H. E., and Lissner, H. R.: The role of tensile stress in the mechanism of femoral fractures. J. Bone Joint Surg., 33A:485–501, 1951.

30. Fisk, G. R.: The fractured femoral shaft—new approach to the problem. Lancet, 1:659, 1944.

31. Funk, F. J., Wells, R. E., and Street, D. M.: Supplementary fixation of femoral fractures. Clin. Orthop., 60:41–49, 1968.

32. Funsten, R. V., and Lee, R. W.: Healing time in fractures of the shafts of the tibia and femur. J. Bone Joint Surg., 27:395–400, 1945.

33. Gant, G. C., Shaftan, G. W., and Herbsman, H.: Experience with the ASIF compression plate in the management of femoral shaft fractures. J. Trauma, 10:458–471, 1970.

34. Grundy, M.: Fractures of the femur in Paget's disease of bone—their etiology and treatment. J. Bone Joint Surg., 52B:252–262, 1970.

35. Hampton, O. P.: Delayed internal fixation of compound battle fractures in the Mediterranean theatre of operations. Ann. Surg., 123:1–24, 1946.

36. Hartmann, E. R., and Brav, E. A.: The problem of refracture in fractures of the femoral shaft. J. Bone Joint Surg., 36A:1071–1079, 1954.

37. Heppenstall, R. B., Littooy, F. N., Fuchs, R., et al.: Gas tensions in healing tissues of traumatized patients. Surgery, 75:874–880, 1974.

38. Herndon, J. H., Tolo, V. T., Lanoue, A. M., and Deffer, P. A.: Management of fractured femora in acute amputees. J. Bone Joint Surg., 55A:1600–1613, 1973.

39. Hirsch, C., Cavandias, A., and Nachemson, A.: An attempt to explain fracture types. Experimental studies on rabbit bones. Acta Orthop. Scand., 24:8–29, 1955.

40. Howland, W. S., Jr., and Ritchey, S. J.: Gunshot fractures in civilian practice. An evaluation of the results of limited surgical treatment. J. Bone Joint Surg., 53A:47–55, 1971.

41. Hubbard, M. J. S.: The treatment of femoral shaft fractures in the elderly. J. Bone Joint Surg., 56B:96–101, 1974.

42. Inman, V. T.: Functional aspects of the abductor muscles of the hip. J. Bone Joint Surg., 29:607–614, 1947.

43. Kaufer, H.: Nonoperative ambulatory treatment for fracture of the shaft of the femur. Clin. Orthop., 87:192–199, 1972.

44. Kennedy, R. H.: Traction-suspension treatment in fractures—certain commonly-neglected factors. J. Bone Joint Surg., 15:320–326, 1933.

45. Küntscher, G.: The intramedullary nailing of fractures. Clin. Orthop., 60:5–12, 1968.

46. Laing, P. G.: The blood supply of the femoral shaft: Anatomical study. J. Bone Joint Surg., 35B:462–466, 1953.

47. Lam, S. J.: The place of delayed internal fixation in the treatment of fractures of the long bones. J. Bone Joint Surg., 46B:393–397, 1964.

48. Lyddon, D. W., Jr., and Hartman, J. T.: Traumatic dislocation of the hip with ipsilateral femoral fracture. A case report. J. Bone Joint Surg., 53A:1012–1016, 1971.

49. MacAusland, W. R., Jr., and Eaton, R. G.: The management of sepsis following intramedullary fixation for fractures of the femur. J. Bone Joint Surg., 45A:1643–1650, 1963.

50. McNeur, J. C.: The management of open skeletal trauma with particular reference to internal fixation. J. Bone Joint Surg., 52B:54–60, 1970.

51. Mooney, V.: Cast bracing. Clin. Orthop., 102:159–166, 1974.

52. Mooney, V., Nickel, V. L., Harvey, J. P., and Snelson, R.: Cast-brace treatment for fractures of the distal part of the femur. J. Bone Joint Surg., 52A:1563–1578, 1970.

53. Müller, M. E., Allgower, M., and Willenegger, H.: Technique of Internal Fixation of Fractures. New York, Springer-Verlag, 1965.

54. Neer, C. S., II, Grantham, S. A., and Shelton, M.: Supracondylar fracture of the adult femur. A study of 110 cases. J. Bone Joint Surg., 49A:591–613, 1967.

55. Nichols, P. J. R.: Rehabilitation after fractures of the shaft of the femur. J. Bone Joint Surg., 45B:96–102, 1963.

56. Nicoll, E. A.: Quadricepsplasty. J. Bone Joint Surg., 45B:483–490, 1963.

57. Olerud, S., and Danckwardt-Lilliestrom, G.: Fracture healing in compression osteosynthesis in the dog. J. Bone Joint Surg., 50B:844–851, 1968.

58. Parham, F. W.: Circular constriction in the treatment of fractures of the long bones. Surg. Gynecol. Obstet., 23:541–544, 1916.

59. Pedersen, H. E., and Serra, J. B.: Injury to the collateral ligaments of the knee associated with femoral shaft fractures. Clin. Orthop., 60:119–121, 1968.

60. Perren, S. M., Huggler, A., Russenberger, M., Allgower, M., Mathys, R., Schenk, R., Willenegger, H., and Müller, M. E.: The reaction of cortical bone to compression. Acta Orthop. Scand., 36(Suppl.):125, 1969.

61. Rascher, J. J., Nahigian, S. H., Macys, J. R., and Brown, J. E.: Closed nailing of femoral-shaft fractures. J. Bone Joint Surg., 54A:534–544, 1972.

62. Rhinelander, F. W.: Effects of medullary nailing on the normal blood supply of diaphyseal cortex. AAOS Instructional Course Lecture, Vol. 22, pp. 161–187. St. Louis, Mosby, 1973.

63. Rokkanen, P., Slates, P., and Vankka, E.: Closed or open intramedullary nailing of femoral shaft fractures? A comparison of conservatively

treated cases. J. Bone Joint Surg., *51B*:313–323, 1969.

64. Sage, F. P.: The second decade of experience with the Küntscher medullary nail in the femur. Clin. Orthop., *60*:77–85, 1968.

65. Schatzker, J., and Barrington, T. W.: Fractures of the femoral neck associated with fractures of the same femoral shaft. Can. J. Surg., *11*:297, 1968.

66. Schneider, H. W.: Use of the four-flanged self-cutting intramedullary nail for fixation of femoral fractures. Clin. Orthop., *60*:29–39, 1968.

67. Scott, R. D., Turner, R. H., Leitzes, S. M., Aufranc, O. E.: Femoral fractures in conjunction with total hip replacement. J. Bone Joint Surg., *57A*:494–501, 1975.

68. Scudese, V. A.: Femoral shaft fractures, percutaneous multiple pin fixation, thigh cylinder plaster cast and early weight bearing. Clin. Orthop., *77*:164–178, 1971.

69. Seimon, L. P.: Refracture of the shaft of the femur. J. Bone Joint Surg., *46B*:32–39, 1964.

70. Smith, H.: On the treatment of ununited fractures by means of artificial limbs which combine the principle of pressure and motion at the seat of fracture and lead to the formation of an ensheathing callus. Am. J. Med. Sci., *29*:102–119, 1855.

71. Smith, J. E. M.: The results of early and delayed internal fixation of fractures of the shaft of the femur. J. Bone Joint Surg., *46B*:28–31, 1964.

72. Soto-Hall, R., and McCloy, N. P.: Cause and treatment of angulation of femoral intramedullary nails. Clin. Orthop., *2*:66, 1953.

73. Steinmann, F. R.: Eine neue Extensionsmethode in der Frakturenbehandlung. Zentralbl. Chir., *34*:938–942, 1907.

74. Street, D. M.: One hundred fractures of the femur treated by means of the diamond-shaped medullary nail. J. Bone Joint Surg., *33A*:659–669, 1951.

75. Stryker, W. S., Russell, M. E., and West, H. D.: Comparison of the results of operative and non-operative treatment of diaphyseal fractures of the femur at the Naval hospital, San Diego, over a five-year period. J. Bone Joint Surg., *52A*:815, 1970.

76. Taylor, L. W.: Principles of treatment of fractures and non-union of the shaft of the femur. J. Bone Joint Surg., *45A*:191–198, 1963.

77. Weil, G. S., Kuehner, H. G., and Henry, J. P.: The treatment of 278 consecutive fractures of the femur. Surg. Gynecol. Obstet., *62*:435–441, 1936.

78. Wickstrom, J., and Corban, M. S.: Intramedullary fixation for fractures of the femoral shaft. J. Trauma, *7*:551, 1967.

79. Wickstrom, J., Corban, M. S., and Vise, G. T., Jr.: Complications following intramedullary fixation of 324 fractured femurs. Clin. Orthop., *60*:103–113, 1968.

80. Wilson, J. N.: The management of infection after Küntscher nailing of the femur. J. Bone Joint Surg., *48B*:112–116, 1966.

JAMES E. NIXON, M.D.

and

VINCENT J. DISTEFANO, M.D.

Injuries of the Knee _____ 24

INTRODUCTION

The knee is frequently involved in athletic injuries and industrial accidents. Unlike the hip, which is stabilized by a ball-and-socket articulation, the knee is dependent on surrounding ligamentous structures for stability. Consequently, serious knee injuries are commonly encountered.

This chapter deals primarily with osseous injuries about the knee and includes a brief section on sprain fractures. Acute ligamentous and meniscal injuries are not within the scope of the discussion. The content is divided into five subjects: (1) fractures of the distal femur; (2) fractures of the proximal tibia; (3) fractures of the patella; (4) sprain fractures; and (5) dislocations of the knee.

FRACTURES OF THE DISTAL FEMUR

SUPRACONDYLAR FRACTURES

The fracture area is above the condyle, extending to the junction of the femoral tubular shaft or diaphysis. The distal femoral fragment is vulnerable to the action of those muscles that are directly attached as well as to the contracting forces working distal to the uncontrolled knee joint.[1] The contracting thigh muscles tend to cause fracture overriding, shortening, and exter-

nal rotation of the proximal shaft fragment. The distal fragment may be flexed by the gastrocnemius and the angulation reinforced by the quadriceps and hamstrings. The assumption of gross flexion is not seen in clinical practice and is as much a product of anterior overriding as of gastrocnemius pull.[2] The femoral condylar muscle attachments introduce rotational elements into the condyle. With fracture penetrance into the joint (condylar separation), the displacement problem becomes more severe.[3]

Historical Aspects

Splinting is a traditional method of fracture treatment. Early treatment of femoral fractures was not dictated by anatomical location but rather was influenced by splint preference, methods of attachment, time of application, complementary physical therapy, and similar penumbral elements. Historically, the results with splint treatment were poor, and the fixed splint gave way to combined splinting and traction.[4] Because the results were unsatisfactory from the standpoint of shortening, patient acceptance, and position commitment, relative splinting and dynamic skin traction were employed.[5] An extension of skin (Russell traction) allowed manipulation and angular modification.[6] Direct application to the bone of contramuscular forces, or corrective traction, was introduced in 1907 and 1909 by Steinmann and Kirschner.[7, 8] In time the method became popular and fracture care improved, as this chronic invasive technique proved to have few problems.

In World War II, the high incidence of supracondylar femoral fractures and the frustrating problem of control of the distal fragment resulted in a modification of skeletal traction. Skeletal reduction was accomplished with vertical traction on the distal femoral fragment combined with double pin application to the proximal tibia and distal femur.[9] Open reduction of single condylar fractures was an obvious early treatment because of the generally poor results with traction.[10] When fixation devices improved one area of femoral fracture care—the hip—they were introduced in other areas,[11, 12] and internal fixation, used in cases of nonunion, was logically extended to fresh fractures.

Classification

Since it can be used as a basis for therapeutic guidelines and for establishing a prognosis, the system developed by Neer, Grantham, and Shelton is the most satisfactory one for classifying supracondylar fractures of the femur (Fig. 24–1).[2] These injuries are categorized as follows:

Type 1: Impacted with minimal displacement

Type 2:
  A: Medial displacement of the condyles
  B: Lateral displacement of the condyles
Type 3: Comminuted fractures of the distal shaft

Type 1 fractures accounted for about 30 per cent of all supracondylar fractures in this series.[2] Almost 90 per cent of the patients were women, 50 per cent of whom were over 65 years of age. Intercondylar T-fractures were present in fifteen patients, but only one required reduction.

Type 2A fractures occurred in another 30 per cent of the patients; 60 per cent in this group were women, and 40 per cent were over 65 years of age. In contrast to the absence of associated injuries in type 1 fractures, almost 40 per cent of type 2A fractures were accompanied by multiple injuries. Multiple injuries were also common in patients with type 2B fractures. Of the twelve patients with concomitant fractures, six had comminuted tibial shaft fractures in the same extremity, and one had bilateral supracondylar fractures. About 75 per cent of these patients were men, and only 18 per cent were over 65 years of age. The type B fracture was found in about 20 per cent of these patients.

Type 3 fractures (Fig. 24–2), which com-

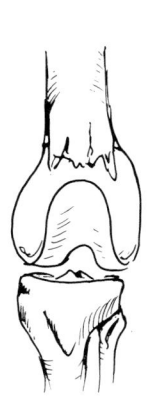 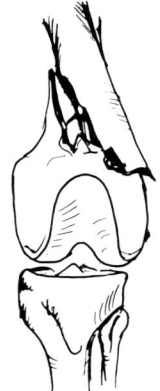 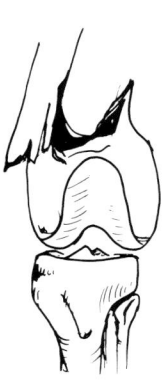 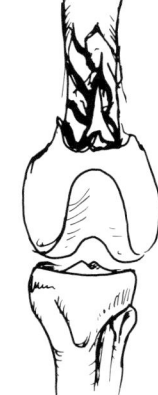

| Impacted Minimal Displacement | Medial Displacement Of Condyles | Lateral Displacement Of Condyles | Mixed Supracondylar And Shaft |

Figure 24–1   Classification after Neer. (Courtesy of the *Journal of Bone and Joint Surgery.* J. Bone Joint Surg., 49A:595, 1967.

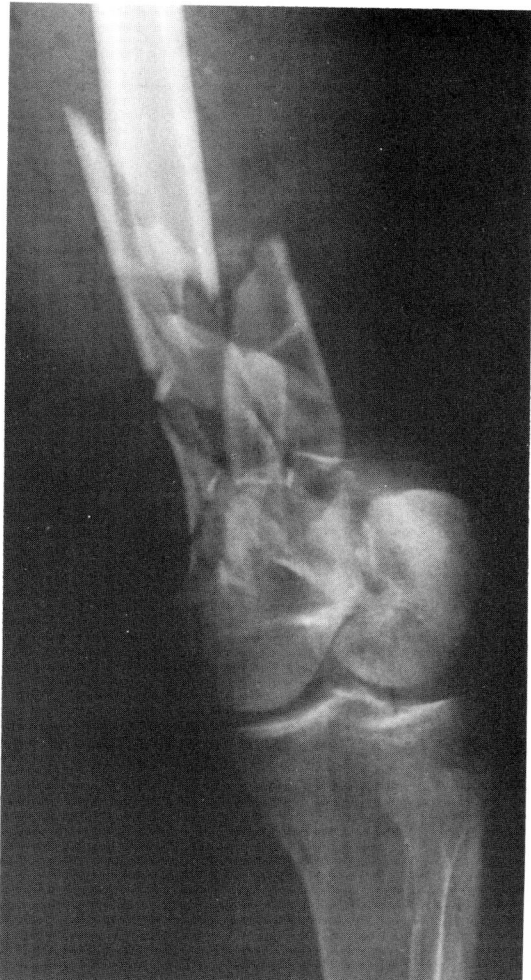

Figure 24-2 Comminuted supracondylar-condylar and undisplaced lateral plateau fracture. The patient had a bilateral supracondylar fracture.

prised about 20 per cent of the fractures in this series, occurred in equal numbers in men and women. Only 14 per cent of the patients were over 65 years old, and the majority had multiple injuries, including fractures of the ipsilateral tibial shaft (six cases), ankle (five cases), patella (four cases), and hip (two cases).

Mechanisms of Injury

The type of trauma that produces most supracondylar fractures of the femur is related to the type of population. In hospi-

tals located near interstate highways, the majority of patients are victims of high-velocity vehicular accidents; in geriatric communities, falls in the home are the most common mechanism. Falls or jumps from heights, such as scaffolds, roofs, and fire escapes, are frequent causes in urban centers.[3]

In the series of Neer, Grantham, and Shelton, the majority of patients with minimally displaced type 1 fractures were injured by falling on a flexed knee at home. These patients had osteoporosis as a result of age, arthritis, vascular disease, paralysis, or a previous fracture at another level in the same extremity.

More violent force exerted on the anterolateral aspect of a flexed knee resulted in a fracture with medial displacement of the condyles (type 2A). These fractures were often produced by the impact of an automobile dashboard or a fall from a height, but a fairly large percentage of patients had osteoporosis and less severe trauma.

Most patients with type 2B fractures (lateral displacement of the femoral condyles) had been struck on the lateral aspect of an extended leg by an automobile. In a smaller number of cases, this type of injury also resulted from a hard blow to the medial side of the flexed knee. With the exception of some type 2A fractures in which the femoral shaft was driven through the lateral part of the extensor expansion, damage to the extensor apparatus was rare in type 1 and 2 fractures.

Comminuted fractures (type 3) resulted from the exertion of extreme force on the anterior aspect of the flexed knee or, in two cases, crush injuries. In contrast to type 1 and 2, type 3 injuries were often accompanied by severe damage to the quadriceps tendon (Fig. 24–3) and concomitant fractures of other bones in the same extremity. Neurovascular complications, malunion, and nonunion were also more common with this injury than with types 1 and 2.[2]

Clinical Findings

In most cases, the traumatic episode is followed immediately by inability to bear weight, deformity in the supracondylar area, and malalignment of the extremity.

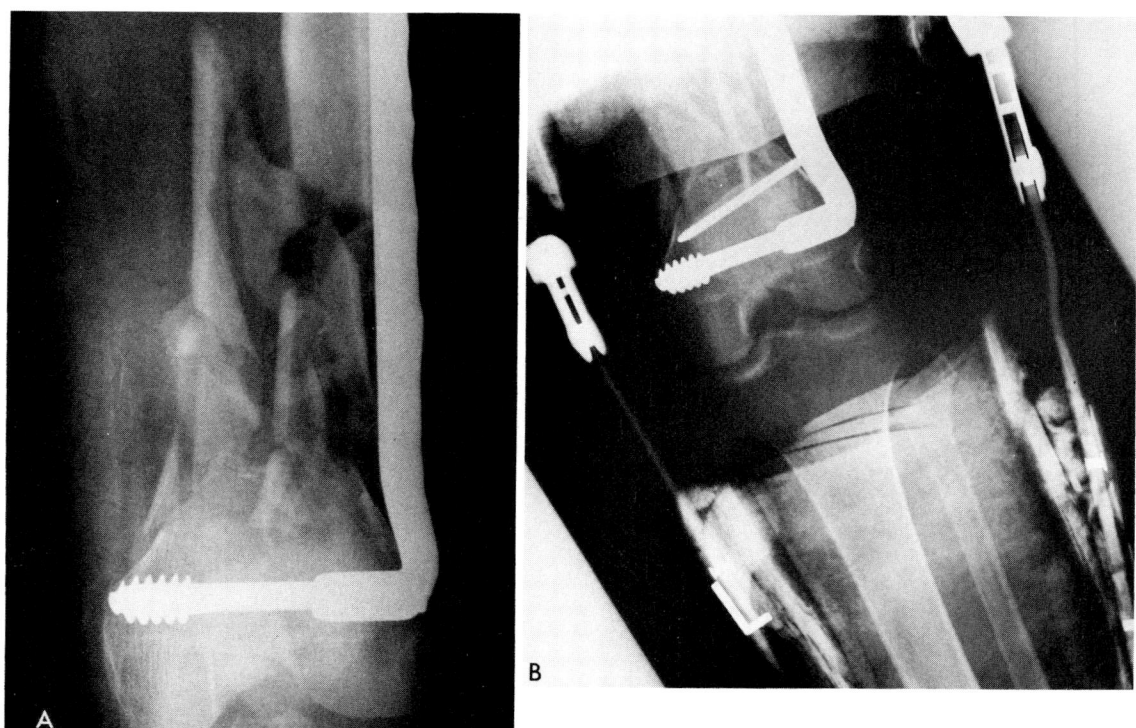

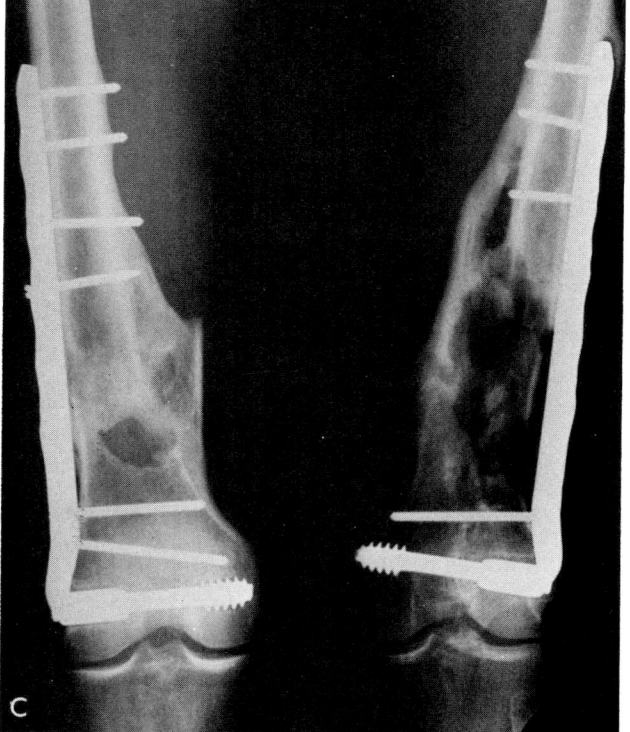

Figure 24-3 *A.* Reduction after resolution of soft tissue trauma for complicated trauma of left knee. *B.* Cast brace after six weeks. *C.* Restriction of knee motion to 60 degrees despite use of a cast brace. Additional bone grafting and quadricepsplasty were required.

Foreshortening of the extremity, preternatural motion, swelling, and crepitus may also be noted. However, none of these findings may be evident in impacted or nondisplaced type 1 fractures, which are most common in elderly women.

Neurovascular Complications. One of the misconceptions about supracondylar fractures of the femur is that they are frequently accompanied by vascular injuries. Actually, vascular injuries are relatively rare with fractures in this area. In the series of Neer, Grantham, and Shelton, only 1 of 110 patients developed a vascular complication; this was a patient with a comminuted supracondylar fracture. In this case the sharp end of the femoral shaft severed the popliteal artery under the arch of the adductor magnus where the artery is bound closely to the femur. This type of vascular injury occurs more often when the fracture site is higher up on the femoral shaft, at the level of the arch of the adductor magnus.[2]

In spite of their low incidence in supracondylar fractures, the possibility of vascular complications should always be borne in mind because of their life-threatening nature. Any unusual tense swelling in the popliteal area, constant pain, absence of pulse, loss of color, and coldness of the skin in the affected limb suggest that vessels at or adjacent to the fracture site have ruptured. Because vascular occlusion may occur either immediately after trauma or hours to days later, the vascular status of the affected extremity should be evaluated repeatedly.

Vascular injury calls for prompt and decisive action by orthopedic and vascular surgeons. The site of the injury can be visualized by arteriography, but this procedure is not mandatory. A medial approach is employed, the fracture is firmly fixed, the pes anserinus is taken down, a compartment release is performed, and the vessel is repaired by grafting or excision and reanastomosis. Failure to treat vascular injuries promptly results in disaster.[15, 16] The reader is referred to Chapter 33 for further information on vascular injuries and fractures.

Nerve injuries, which are generally of the fracture type and resolve within three months, are usually managed by watchful waiting. Early assessment with electromyography and nerve conduction studies may be useful in establishing a prognosis.

Roentgenographic Findings

In general, most supracondylar fractures of the femur are clearly visualized on standard anteroposterior and lateral films. However, additional views should be taken to fix the fracture planes and to aid preoperative planning for patients with displaced and comminuted fractures that are to be treated by open reduction and internal fixation. It is particularly important to delineate fractures that penetrate into the knee joint, because the articular surface must be anatomically restored to obtain optimal results. Because patients who have supracondylar fractures may have concomitant injuries, it is a good policy to x-ray the entire femoral shaft and hip joint so that other fractures and dislocations can be diagnosed and treated.

Treatment

General Principles. Unless treatment permits early active motion of the knee, patients with supracondylar fractures tend to lose some knee motion, particularly flexion. In addition to allowing active motion, any treatment method should accomplish rapid, solid bone healing, so that the patient can ambulate without support in approximately three months. If the treatment falls short of these goals, it must be reassessed. Age, agility, obesity, and social considerations determine methods of treatment as much as the roentgen pattern does. Therefore, therapeutic guidelines should not be inflexible.

In 1956, White and Russin proposed that supracondylar fractures "should be regarded in the same category as intertrochanteric fractures in which internal fixation is the standard method of treatment."[11a] This dictum ran counter to accepted methods of conservative care, which had long been fostered by the "Liverpool tradition" of great orthopedists, beginning with Hugh Owen Thomas through Robert Jones to Watson-Jones. The conservative approach agrees with data in the literature claiming that the results of surgical intervention were not the equal of those of conservative treatment.

A review of the literature suggests the following: (1) Not all fractures in this area are problems. Approximately 30 per cent respond to simple treatment with prompt healing. (2) A remarkably long period elapses before an adequate number of cases is available for analysis. (3) There are currently too few recorded cases to identify those fractures that are best treated surgically. Time not only affords a number of cases but also shadows the results with the subtle intrusion of change in technique as well as advancements in surgery. Time also introduces the elements of social force that tend to condition the acceptability of care.

Casting. Following aspiration of the knee, if necessary, most impacted, minimally displaced supracondylar fractures, including stable Y- and T-fractures, are best treated with a well-molded, long leg cylinder cast. Although neurovascular complications are rare, particularly with simple type 1 supracondylar fractures, the patient should be hospitalized so that the status of the fractured limb can be closely monitored. Again, it should be emphasized that vascular complications do not always occur immediately after injury: In some cases a blood clot forms several days later, and unless prompt action is taken the outcome can be catastrophic. Simple type 1 supracondylar fractures in osteoporotic females usually require about one week of hospitalization. With the initial cylinder cast, the patient is instructed to use a touch-down gait or to bear weight to tolerance.

After collagen has consolidated around the fracture, usually within two to three weeks, hinges are applied to convert the cast to a cast brace. This promotes bone healing by permitting early weight bearing and active knee motion. It also prevents adhesions and contractures from developing in the soft tissues surrounding the knee.

If the patient is obese, casting alone does not usually provide adequate immobilization, because the plaster can never be applied tightly enough. It is therefore advisable to apply a full-length compression dressing before casting. In extremely obese patients, light traction assures stability prior to the application of plaster.

Traction. Skeletal traction applied to the proximal tibia has been the traditional method for the treatment of unstable or malaligned supracondylar fractures. However, because of its many disadvantages we prefer to reserve traction for unstable fractures, in which open reduction and internal fixation are contraindicated. Contraindications include open fractures in which the wound is grossly contaminated or is accompanied by soft tissue loss.

Because the patient's general condition must be stable enough for him to withstand surgery, traction may be the best treatment, at least initially, for victims of severe trauma who have sustained other injuries. Elderly patients may not be suitable candidates for surgery either, but their medical condition should be carefully assessed before a treatment program is selected. Not infrequently, the age of the patient is based upon the physician's, not the patient's, perception.

It is easiest to apply traction when the patient is still in the emergency room, first moving the bed there and carefully transferring the patient to it. Customarily, the fractured extremity is supported in a Thomas splint and a Pearson attachment.[17, 18] The knee should be flexed to only about 20 degrees.[2] A pin is inserted in the proximal tibia and a weight of 10 to 20 lb is applied in a horizontal direction.

In the series of Neer and co-workers[2] the most common sequela of traction was a varus internal rotation of the distal fragment, which is believed to be increased by the unopposed lateral pull of the adductor magnus. To prevent this deformity, the distal fragment should be rotated externally, not held in the neutral position, since the hip joint and femoral shaft fall into external rotation. It is recommended that the pin be inserted somewhat more posteriorly in the medial aspect of the tibia so that it emerges more anteriorly near the crest of the tibia on the lateral aspect (Fig. 24–4).

Standard anteroposterior and lateral views of the fractured femur should be obtained while the patient is in traction. This is difficult because of the angle between the knee joint and the thigh and because of the external rotation of the fractured extremity. It has been demonstrated experimentally that angulation of the x-ray tube to either side of the true

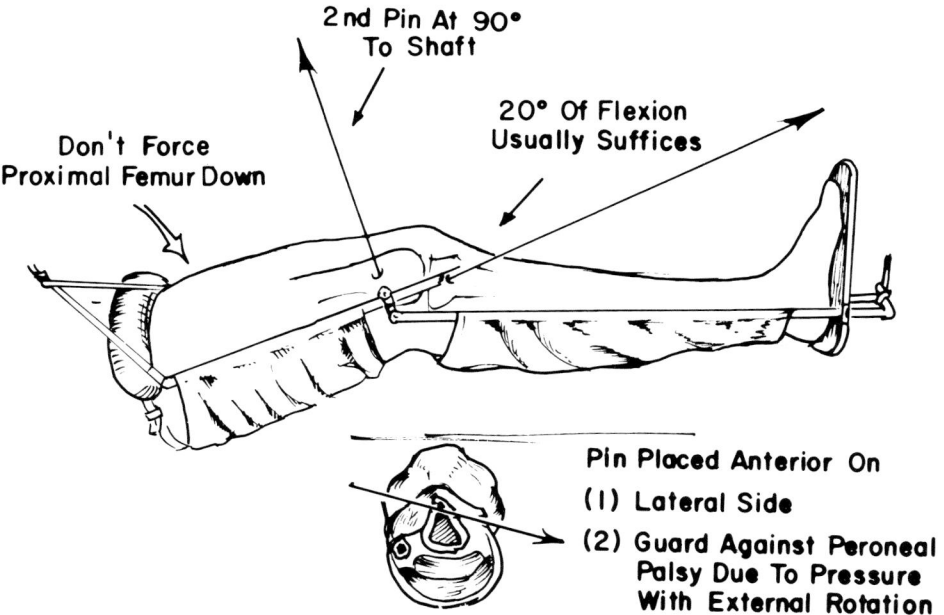

Figure 24–4 Skeletal traction techniques.

anteroposterior or lateral projection produces distortion, causing the fracture to appear highly displaced when it is actually reduced.[2] If the patient can be anesthetized, it is better to reduce the fracture under x-ray control at the time traction is applied rather than to rely on multiple series of portable, and at times inadequate, films to check the results of traction manipulation.

If the fracture cannot be reduced or if reduction cannot be maintained by traction, a second pin may be placed in the distal femoral fragment (Fig. 24–5). The pin is inserted directly into the bone, starting on the medial aspect to avoid injuring the femoral blood vessels. The pin is run parallel to the knee joint, using the upper triangular apex of the adductor tubercle as a landmark. This places the pin just above the axis of rotation of the knee, above the synovial reflections of the joint, and below the distal flare of the suprapatellar pouch. Vertical traction is placed on the femoral pin in a direction that forms an angle of about 90 degrees with the long axis of the femur.[9] In our experience, placing the pin in this site usually does not bring it too close to the supracondylar fracture. When we have used this two-pin method no vascular complications have occurred, as they occa-

sionally do if the pin is placed in the distal femoral shaft; moreover, none of our patients developed an infection in the fracture site or knee joint.[16]

The two-pin method is particularly useful when the distal fragment is displaced posteriorly. This relatively rare fracture is probably caused by the impact of the injury or by pressure from an overriding shaft that has been displaced anteriorly. In treating this injury, it is important not to flex the knee too far, since excessive flexion often results in even greater posterior displacement of the distal fragment (see Fig. 24–4).[2]

To prevent fixation of the quadriceps and to promote bone healing, the patient is encouraged to move the knee while in traction. If traction is to be maintained until bone healing is adequate for mobilization, the patient must be hospitalized for eight to twelve weeks. A hip spica applied after three to six weeks, when the bone begins to unite, is an alternative to the expense and disability of prolonged traction in the hospital.

Traction, however, may be the only method that can be used initially for patients with obviously contaminated open fractures, wounds with soft tissue loss, and severe trauma with multiple injuries. In

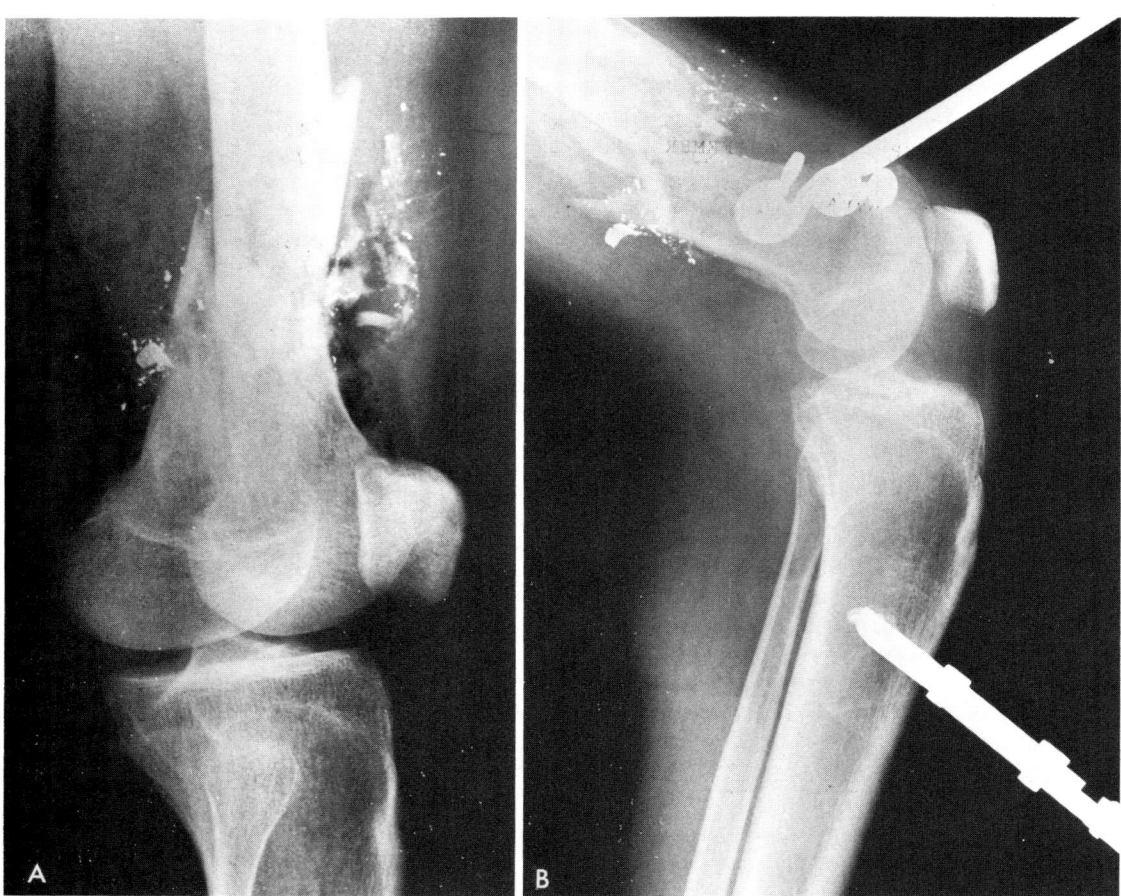

Figure 24–5 A.   Open comminuted fracture in the supracondylar area. Traction was instituted after debridement of the entrance. *B.*   The position was lost and a second pin was inserted. (1) Insertion was too late, (2) traction should be placed at 90 degrees to the femoral shaft; (3) the knee is in too much flexion.

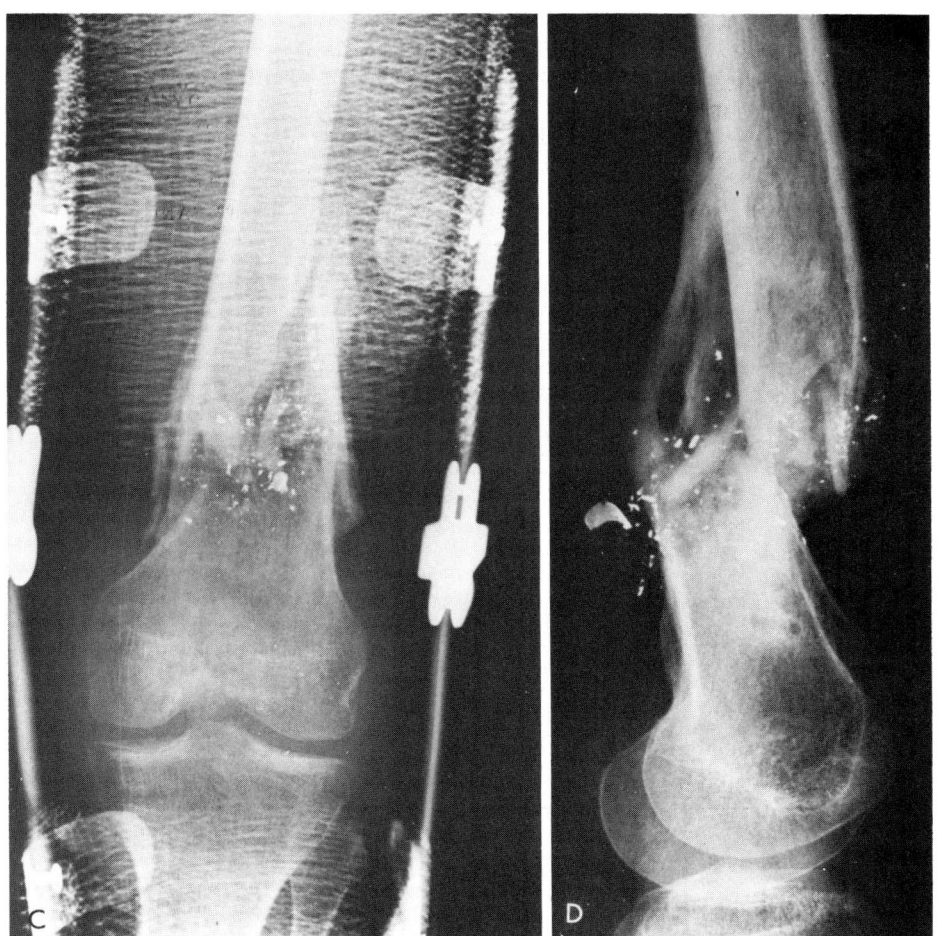

Figure 24–5 Continued.   C. Ambulation in cast brace. D, Healing at six months with persistent posterior angulation.

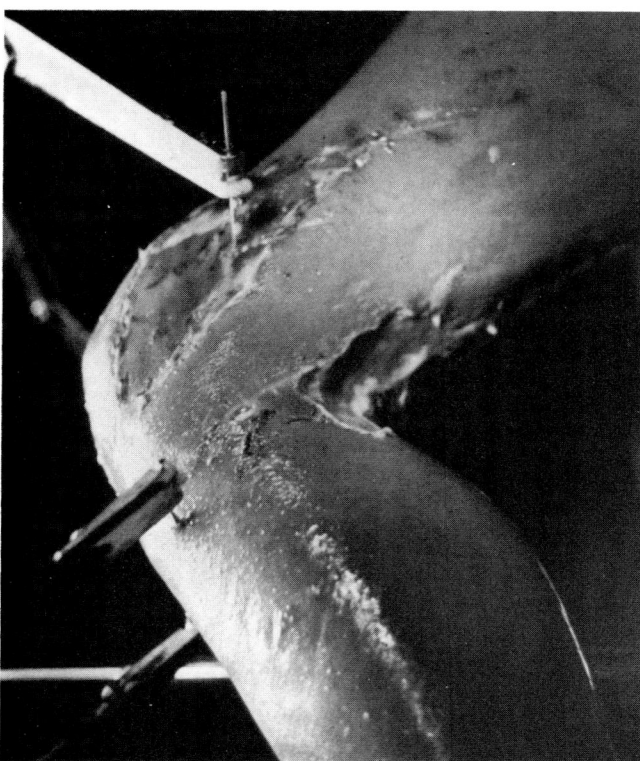

Figure 24-6 Combined relaxation incision and skin graft to close wound. At one week the wounds are "closed."

these cases it is advisable to debride the wound and allow it to close by either primary or secondary intention. Whenever possible, an aggressive approach should be taken to wound closure: This may include tissue advancement, relaxing incisions, and skin grafting (Fig. 24–6).

The average lengths of hospitalization for conservatively treated supracondylar fractures of the distal femur are as follows:

Type 1: 8 days
Type 2: 60 days with traction
Type 3: 42 to 60 days in traction; discharged in plaster

The simple undisplaced supracondylar fracture in the osteoporotic female may involve a hospital stay of approximately one week. Open reduction necessitates three weeks of hospital care, whereas uncomplicated extended-traction treatment requires hospitalization for two months. The cost of conservative treatment may compel evaluation of alternative methods and force more creative means of care.

Cast Bracing. The cast brace is one of these innovative means of care. After initial traction, it allows ambulatory treatment of the fractured distal femur once the patient's fracture is stable (out of traction), clinically firm, and no longer painful.[20-22] The device provides external support during the maturation of fracture callus. It improves union over the use of the plaster spica and permits continued muscle and joint function while protecting the fracture from destructive forces. The cast brace is a total-contact device. With ambulation, a painless but bothersome effusion may develop in distal fractures. Intermittent elevation or an elastic knee support will combat the knee effusion. Successful utilization of the cast brace depends in part on the availability of appropriate technical help.

The cast brace is the second part in the primary phase of traction reduction and fracture stabilization. It should not be limited to traction cases, because it is also useful in those fractures stabilized by internal fixation (Fig. 24–7).

Open Reduction and Internal Fixation. Unless surgery is contraindicated,

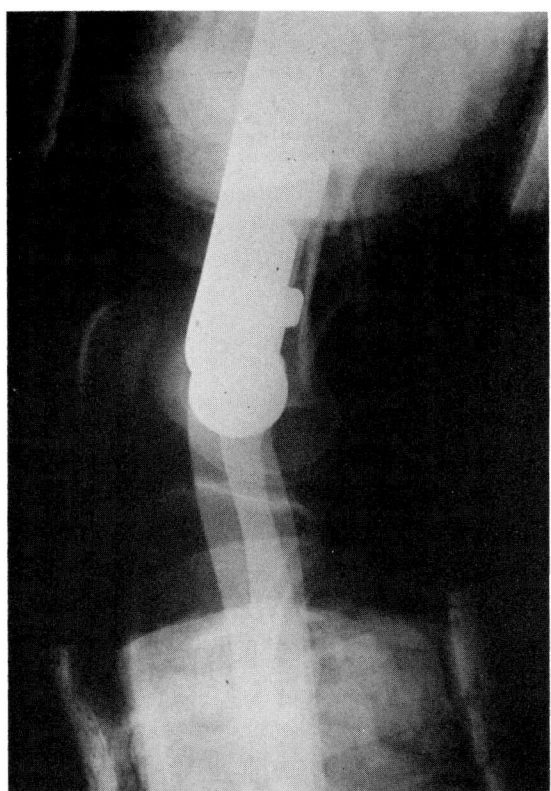

Figure 24–7   Cast brace augmenting internal fixation.

good results can be obtained by immediate open reduction and internal fixation of displaced and comminuted supracondylar fractures. Surgery makes it possible to obtain anatomical reduction of the fracture, and the fixation device acts as an internal splint for the bone until it heals (Fig. 24–8). This "splint" allows the patient to ambulate, permits early knee motion, and shortens the length of hospitalization.

The distal contours of the femur combined with distortions produced by trauma make replacement of a fixation device difficult. When selecting such a device, the surgeon should bear in mind that it must provide maximum strength and firm fixation (Fig. 24–9). Fixation devices that have been employed for supracondylar fractures of the femur include conventional and split pins, intramedullary rods, and blade plates and their variants.

The difficulty with conventional and split pins is their failure to penetrate and grasp the bone in the short-broad distal fragment

of the femur. If the fracture is comminuted and unstable, this problem is intensified. Pins may be satisfactory for transverse fractures, which are inherently more stable.

If an intramedullary device, such as Rush pins, is inserted from above the fracture site, the curved distal ends of the pins must pass each other in the isthmus of the femur and are difficult to place accurately in the broad distal fragment. Image intensification is essential for the placement of such devices. Unfortunately, distal insertion of the intramedullary pins further weakens the fragile cortical bone that overlies mushy cancellous bone in the distal fragment. Finally, intramedullary pins generally do not afford firm or continued stability with motion. This necessitates postoperative traction or casting until the bone heals, defeating the purpose of internal fixation.

We have not yet evaluated the recently introduced Zickel device.[23] This method awaits a significant trial before taking its place in the treatment of femoral fractures.

Blade plates, such as the Elliot,[24] the AO,[25] and the Richards right-angle screw plate, are currently widely used. The AO plate bender enables one to contour the plate close to the bone and to correct blade error, but placement in the distal fragment can be difficult (Fig. 24–10). If they are improperly inserted, fixed blade plates may produce varus or valgus angulation. Attempts to reinsert these devices or to correct their length or angle result in an unstable mushy hole in the distal fragment. Rigid adherence to technical detail is the only way to prevent these complications.

The Richards supracondylar compression plate system is equipped with a guide pin to orient placement in the distal fragment (Fig. 24–11). In addition, a compression screw provides firm fixation for bicondylar fractures (Fig. 24–12). The Richards device has a twofold disadvantage: It is difficult to adjust to the contours of the femur, particularly if placed low in the condyle, and the distal fragment may rotate unless two-point fixation can be obtained.

When surgery must be delayed to permit wound closure, open reduction and internal fixation should probably be combined with insertion of a cancellous bone graft. Bone grafting should definitely be performed on patients undergoing open reduction of a

Text continued on page 729.

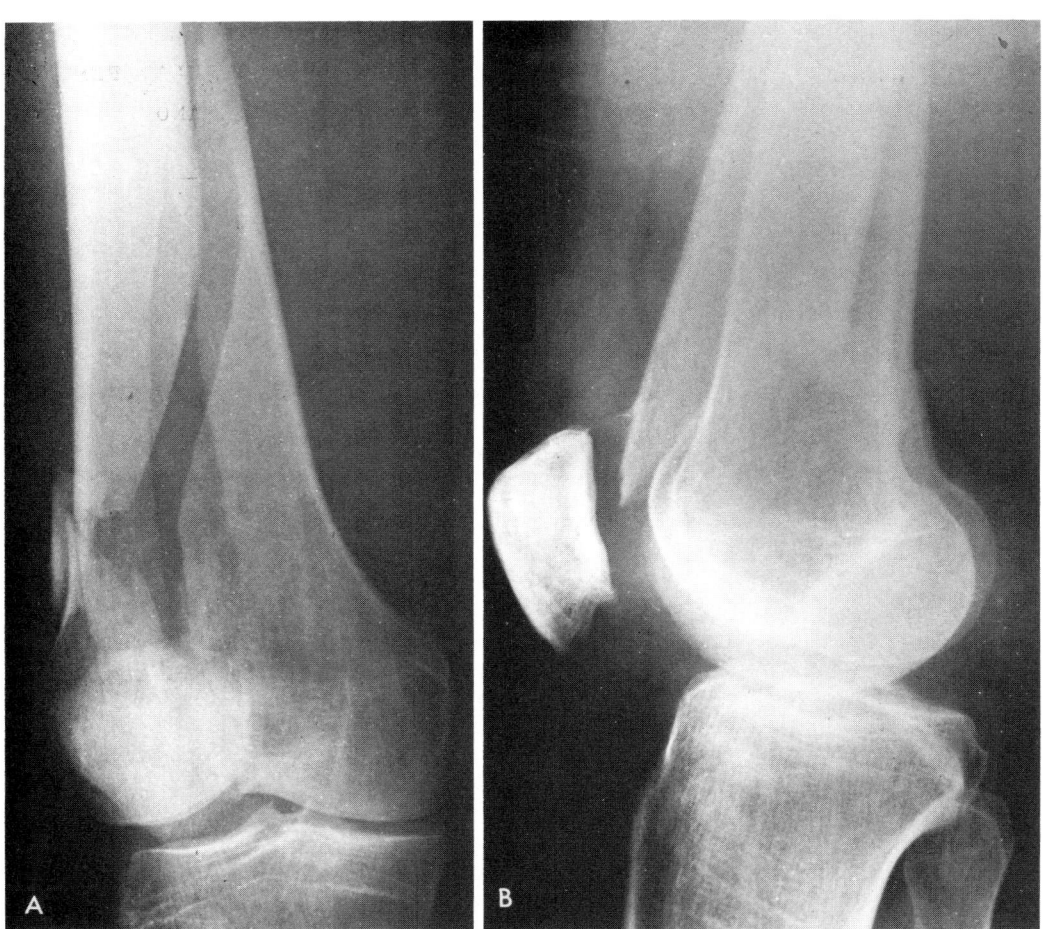

Figure 24–8   *A* and *B.*   Supracondylar-lateral condyle fracture with spiral shaft fracture in osteoporotic bone. Anteroposterior and lateral views.

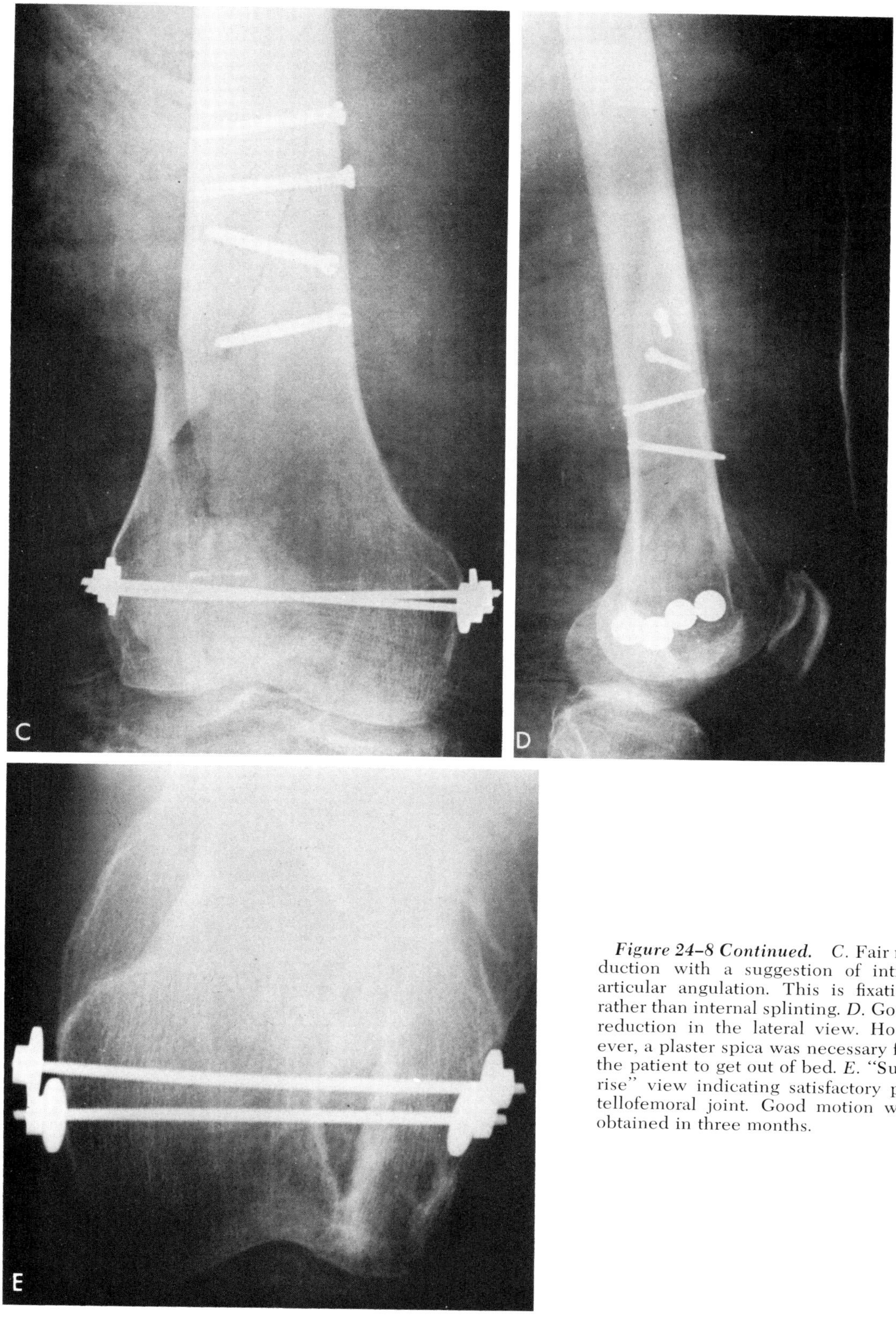

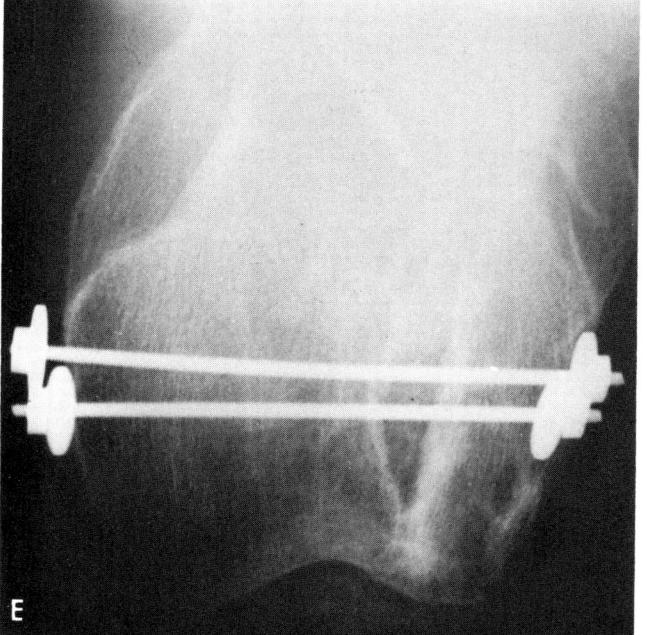

Figure 24–8 Continued. C. Fair reduction with a suggestion of intra-articular angulation. This is fixation rather than internal splinting. *D.* Good reduction in the lateral view. However, a plaster spica was necessary for the patient to get out of bed. *E.* "Sunrise" view indicating satisfactory patellofemoral joint. Good motion was obtained in three months.

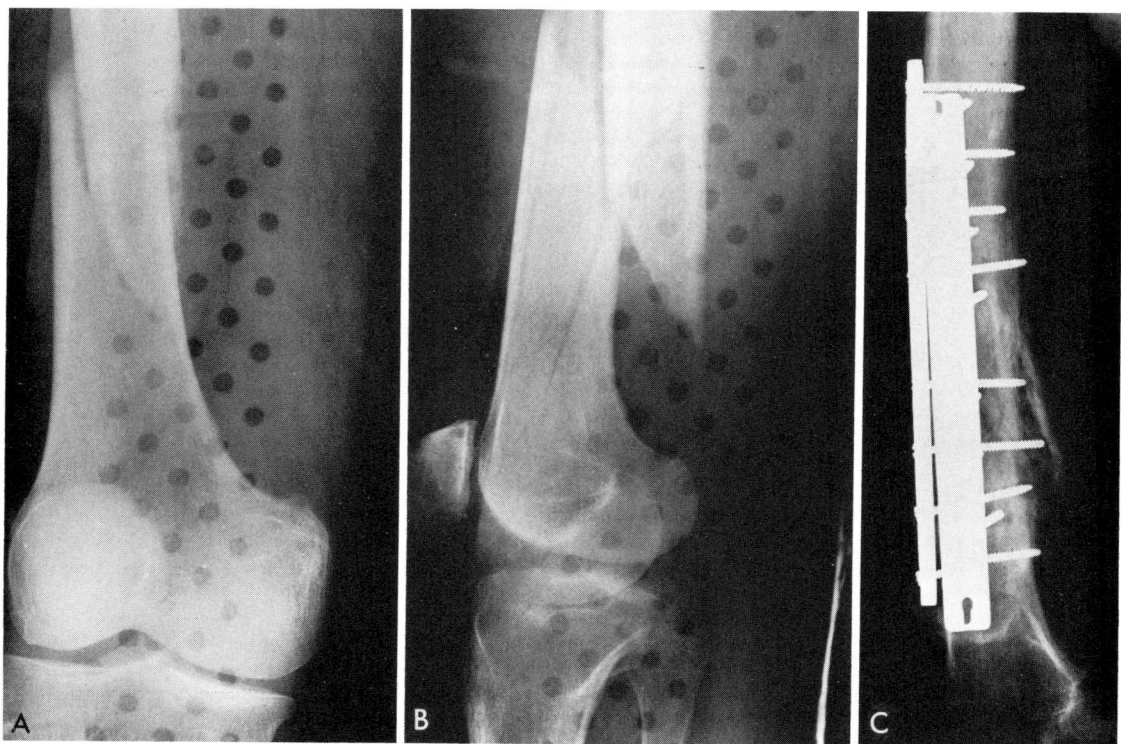

Figure 24–9   *A* and *B*. Anteroposterior and lateral views of a distal femoral fracture fragmenting into the supra-condylar region. *C*. Lateral view shows satisfactory healing at eight weeks.

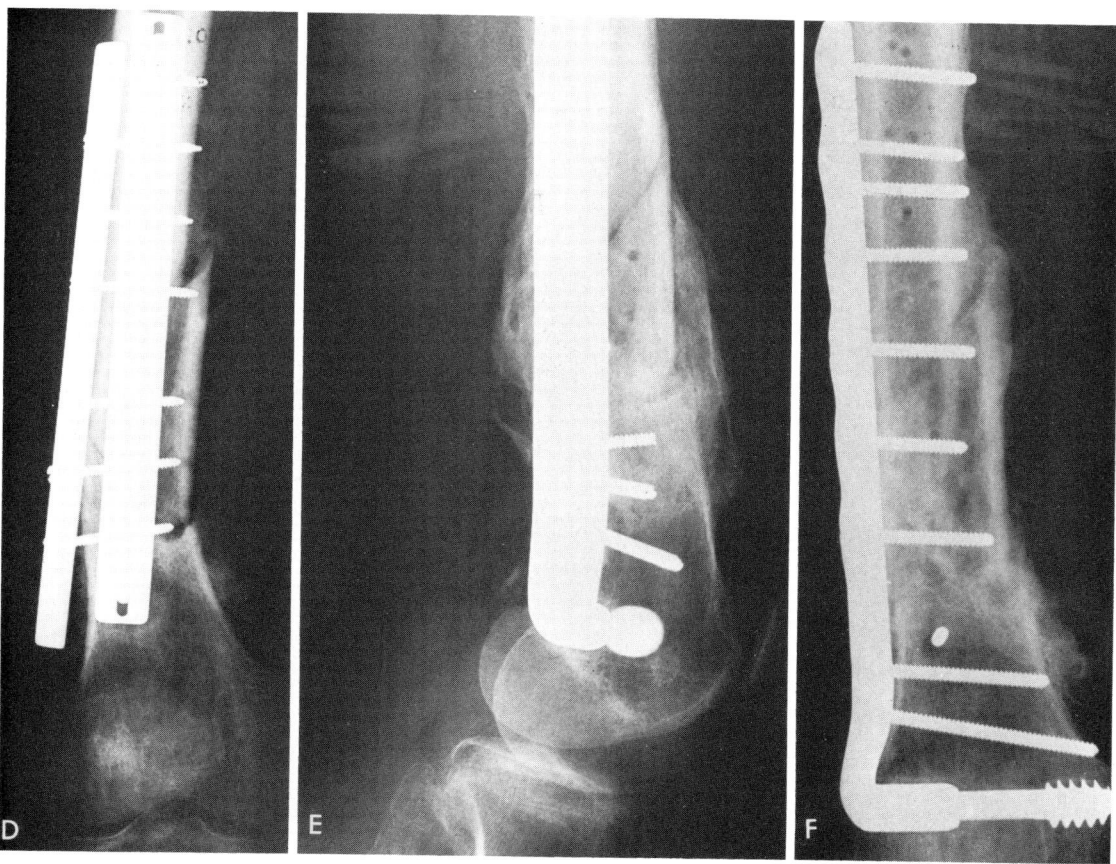

Figure 24–9 Continued. D. Anteroposterior view demonstrates poor choice of fixation with fracture penetration into the cancellous supracondylar area. *E* and *F*. Satisfactory healing after application of an appropriate device.

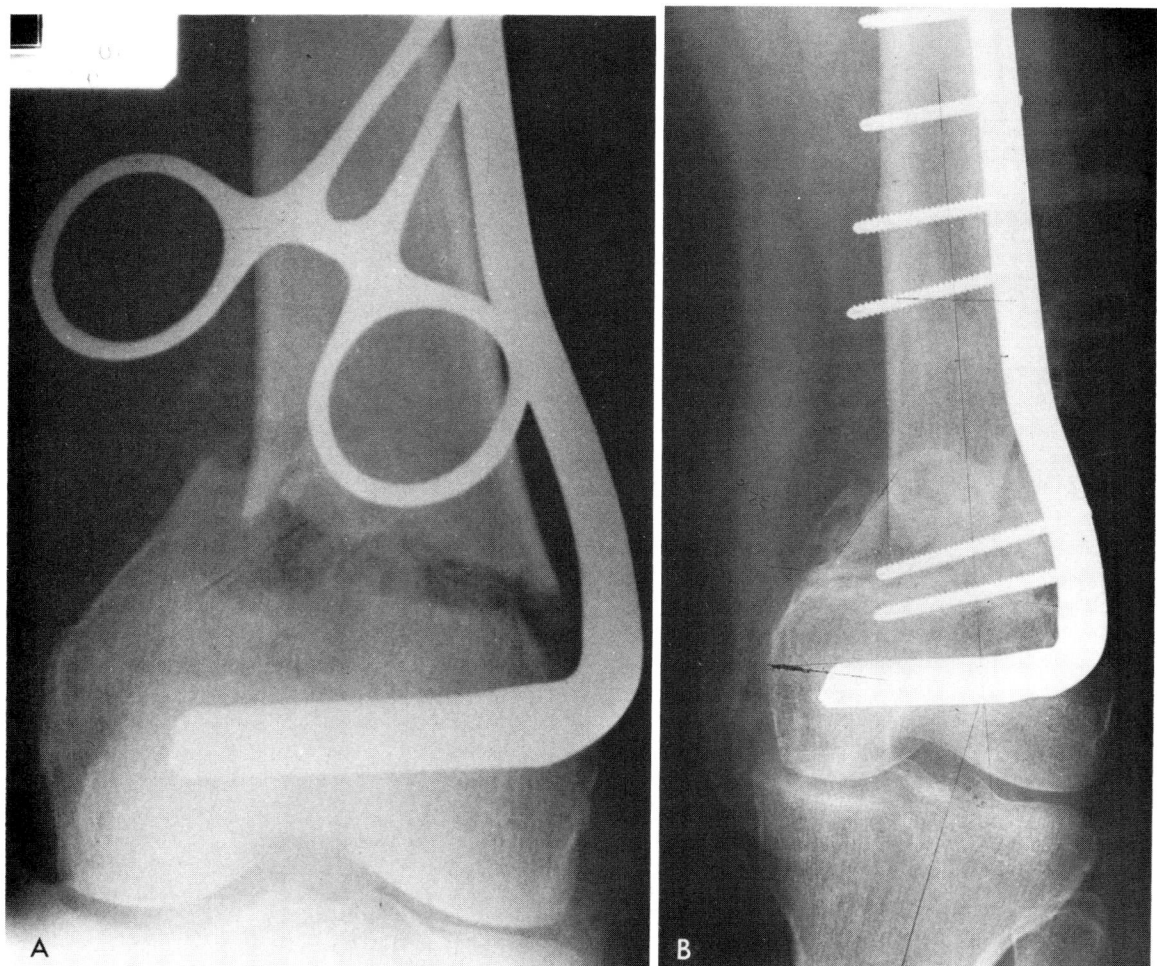

Figure 24–10   *A.* Insertion of fixed blade plate at surgery. *B.* Postoperative view shows slight settling.

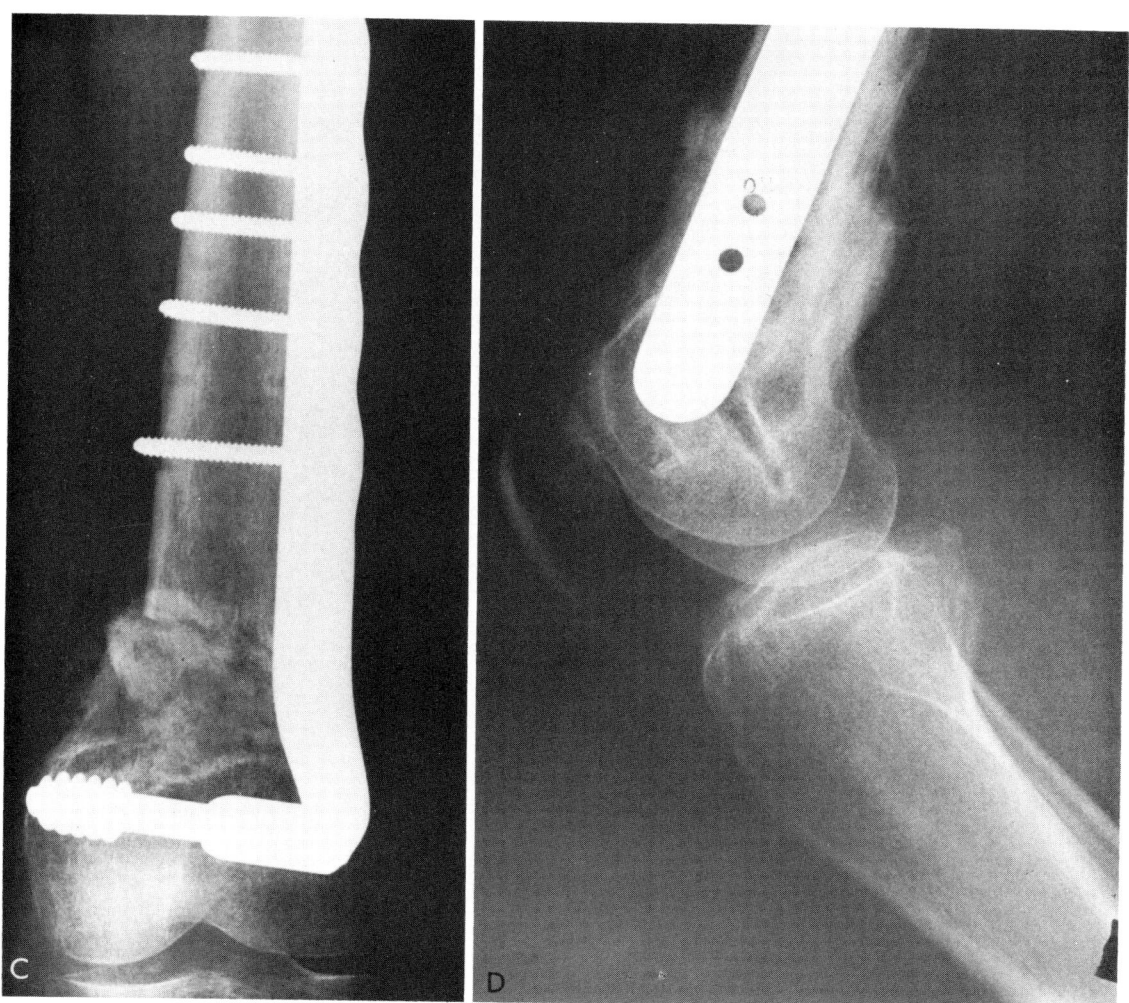

Figure 24–10 Continued.   C and D. Corrected osteotomy with new device and bone grafting.

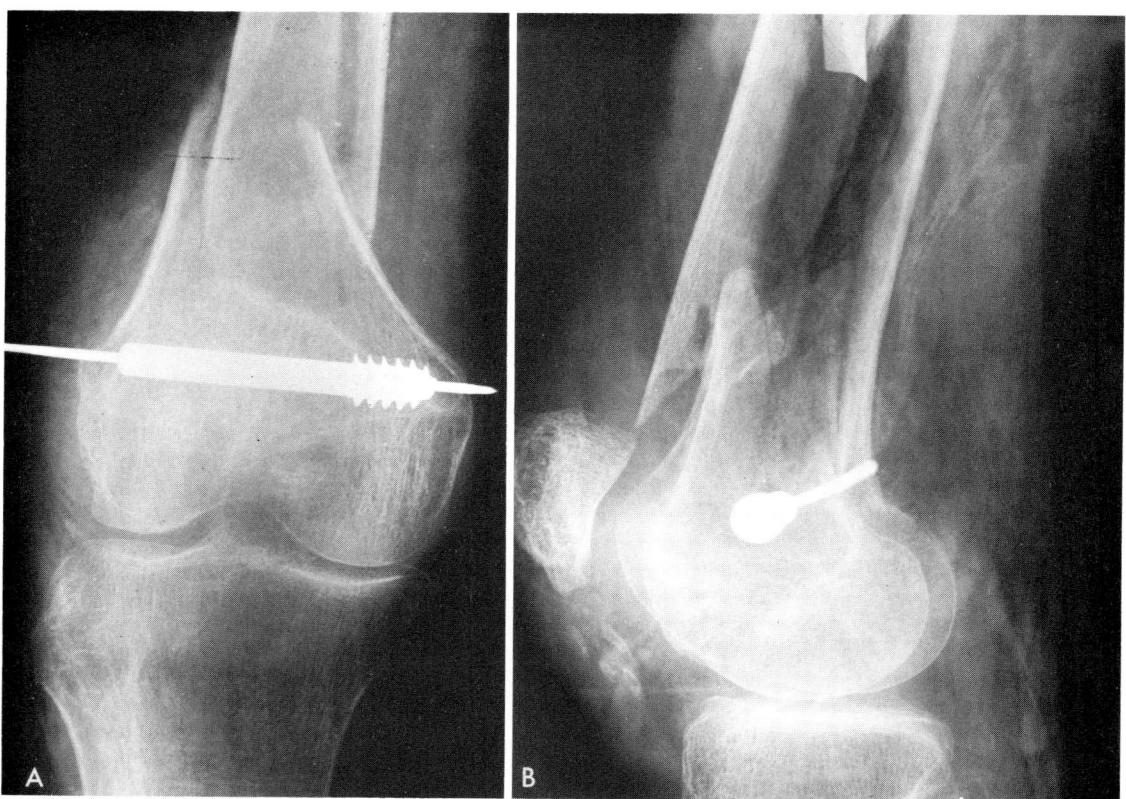

Figure 24–11   A and B. Anteroposterior and lateral views. A guide pin allows good positioning.

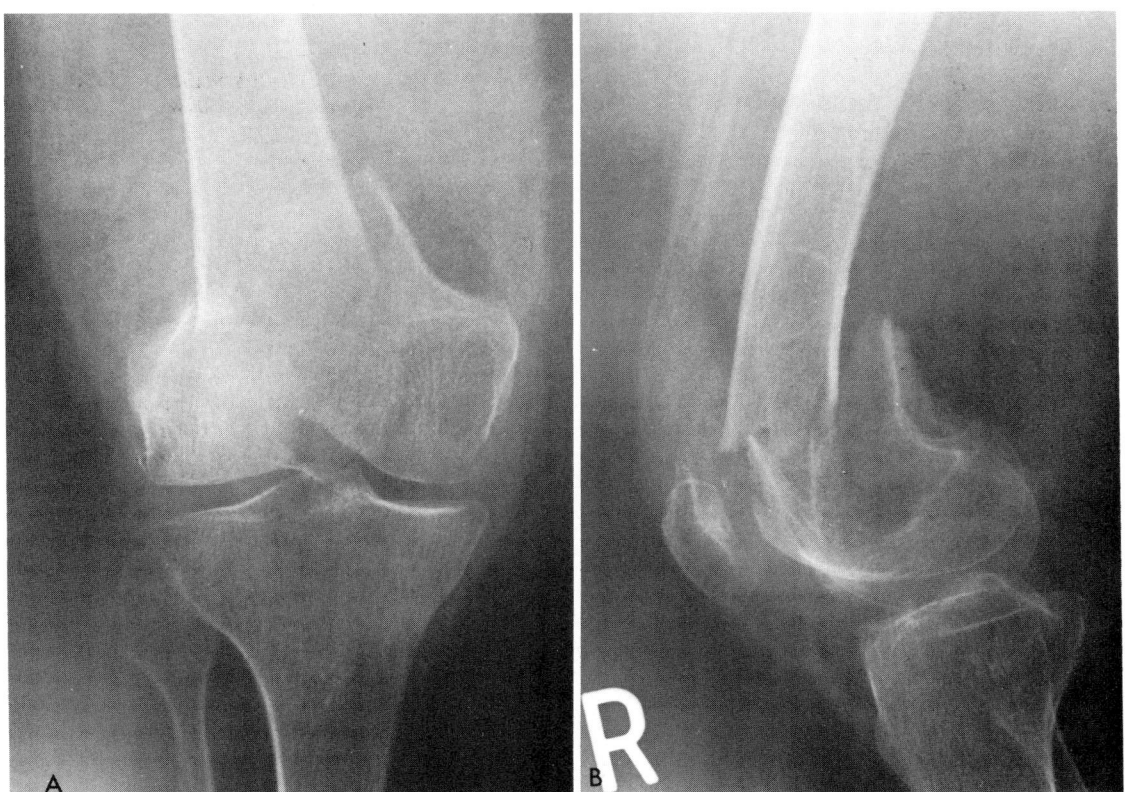

Figure 24–12 *A* and *B*. Anteroposterior and lateral views of supra- and intracondylar fracture in an aged osteo-porotic female with residual effects of polio.

Illustration continued on the following page

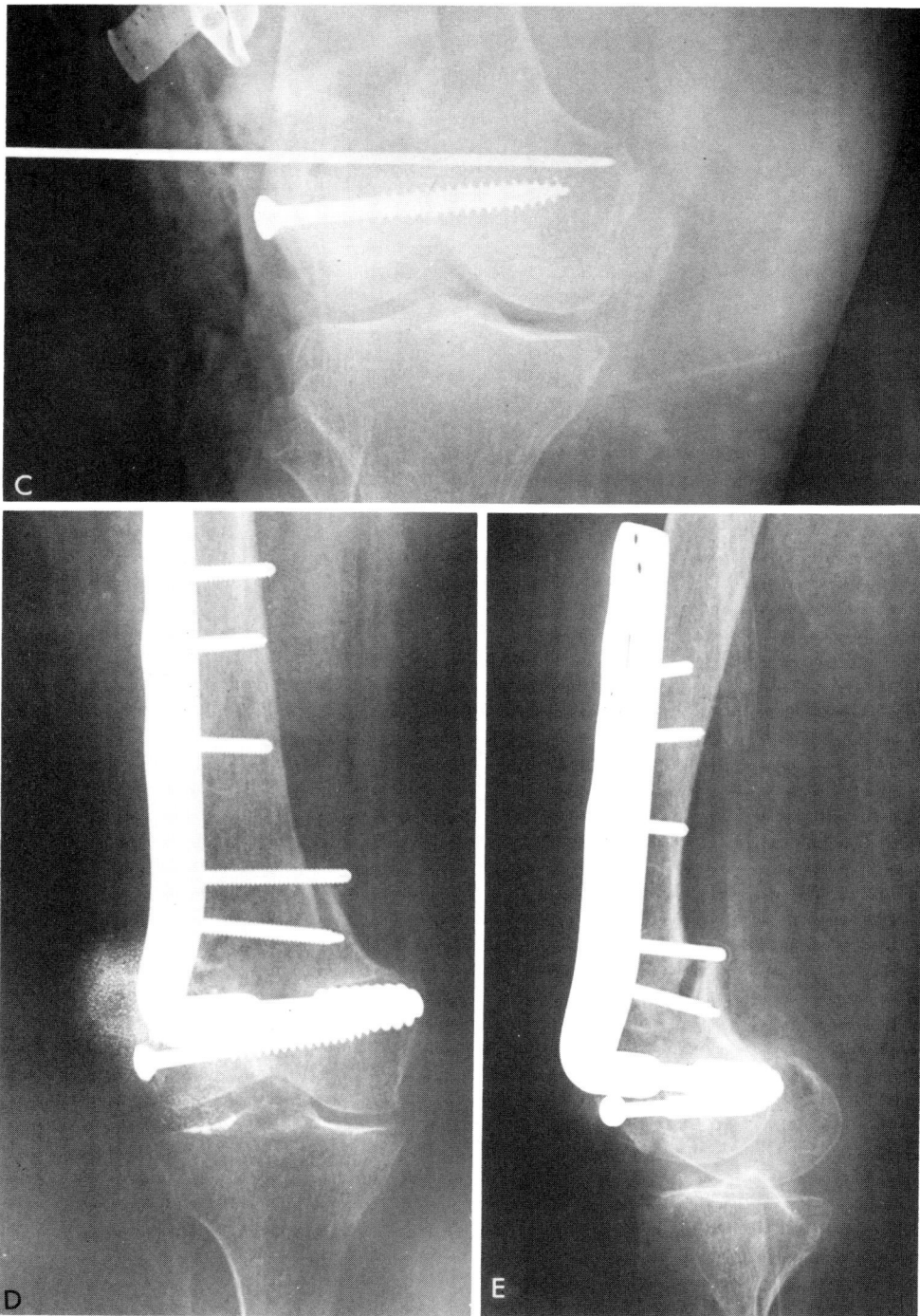

Figure 24–12 Continued. *C.* Intraarticular reduction and fixation with a lag screw. A guide pin is in position. *D* and *E.* Anteroposterior and lateral views of internal fixation. This osteoporotic patient treated with cast bracing at one week was removed from plaster at eight weeks and went on to full knee motion.

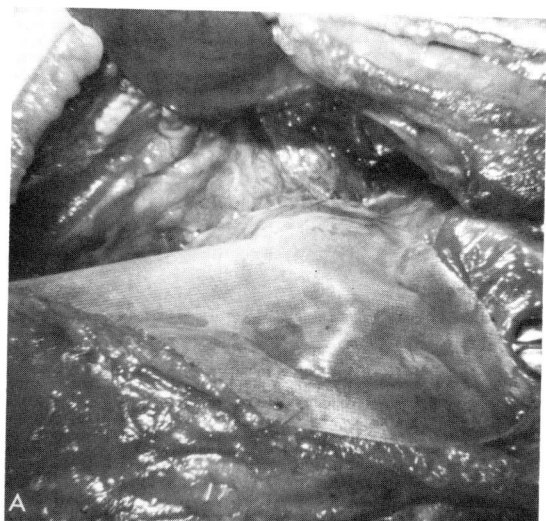

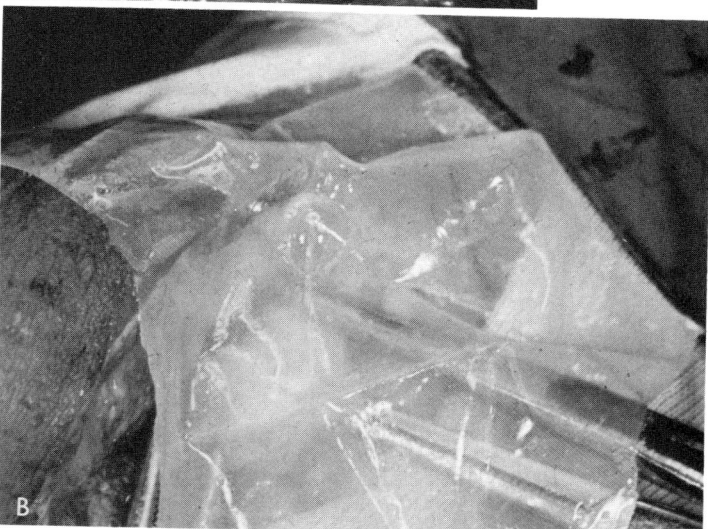

Figure 24–13 A. Silicone membrane tacked onto suprapatellar pouch. A screw was placed in the distal condylar fracture. B. Silicone membrane upon removal, with 100 degrees of knee motion.

comminuted fracture that involves or extends into the distal shaft of the femur. Surgical treatment of a patient with osteoporotic bone might include methyl methacylate reinforcement to improve fixation of the tip of the device in the cancellous bone.

If the quadriceps has become scarred, as it does in cases of delayed surgery and in delayed union or nonunion, it can be repaired by the insertion of dural substitute, a silicone membrane.

Since bone grows from bone, its separation from portions of the surrounding soft tissue does not materially interfere with healing. With early or late need to separate

the suprapatellar space from bone, an interposed membrane of silicone (Fig. 24–13) is inserted in the shape of the synovial pouch over and about the distal shaft of the femur, surrounding the condyles above and below the collateral ligamentous structures.

POSTOPERATIVE CARE. Firm, full-length compression dressings and resting splints are required for the *wound* until the early phase of soft tissue healing occurs (seven to ten days). Once this initial healing is completed, internal fixation may be augmented with a walking cast or cast brace. The purpose of internal fixation is to restore anatomical relationships above the knee joint and to make the patient, not

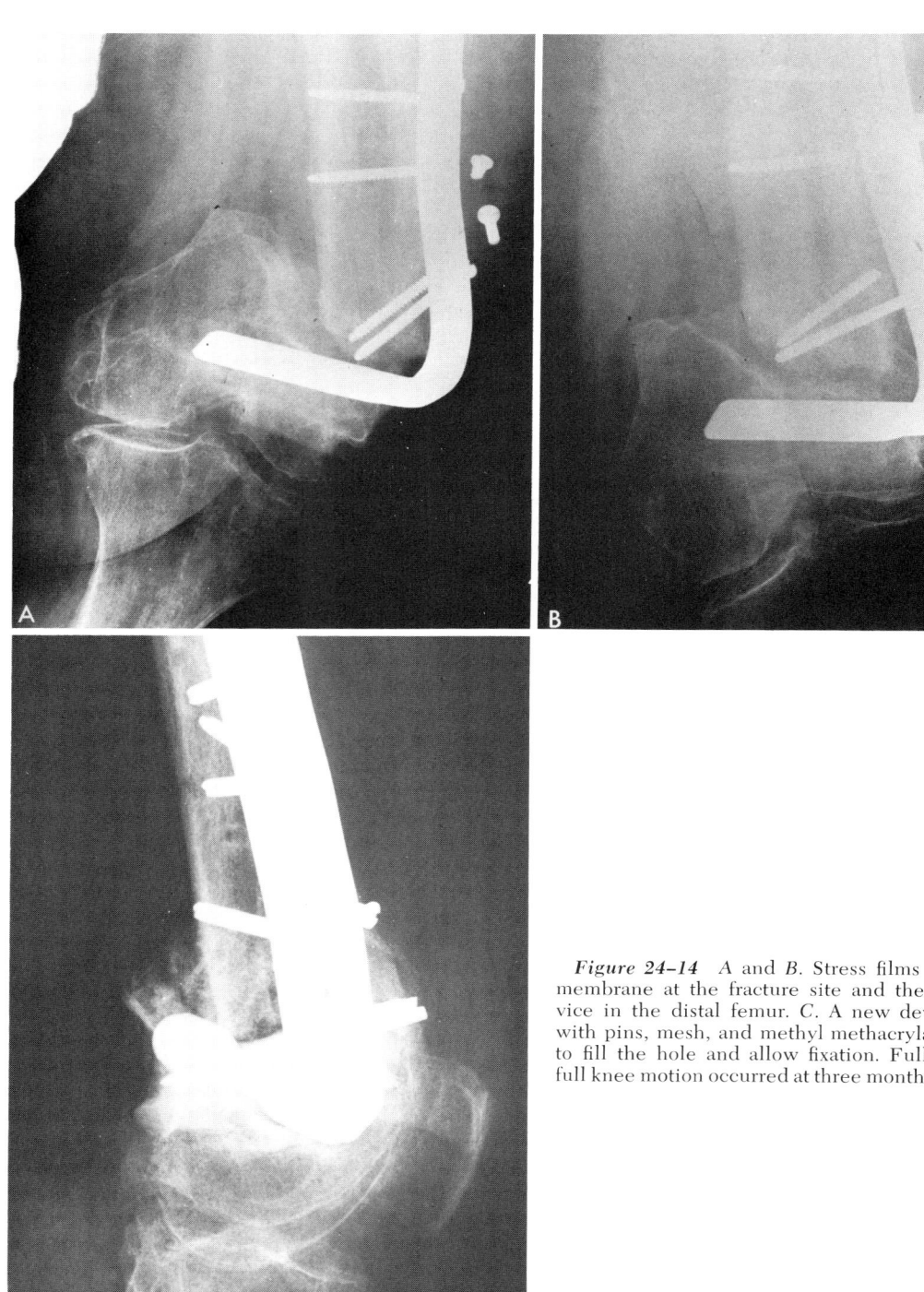

Figure 24–14 A and B. Stress films demonstrate membrane at the fracture site and the fixation device in the distal femur. C. A new device secured with pins, mesh, and methyl methacrylate was used to fill the hole and allow fixation. Full union with full knee motion occurred at three months.

necessarily the limb, ambulatory. Weight bearing should be delayed until there is good radiological evidence of healing. In contrast to patients treated with traction, who require six to eight weeks of hospitalization, those treated with open reduction and internal fixation are usually discharged after 21 days.

POSTOPERATIVE COMPLICATIONS. It should be pointed out that internal fixation does not rule out the development of nonunion. If the fracture fragments have not united within three months, prompt surgery and bone grafting should be considered. They may be combined with interposition of silicone membrane to reconstruct the soft tissues around the knee (Fig. 24–14). Unfortunately, surgery for the correction of postoperative complications is even more difficult than that for the original fracture.

INTRAARTICULAR FRACTURES

A fracture of the supracondylar area of the femur combined with a condylar fracture poses a challenging and complex therapeutic problem. The end result depends upon (1) the initial damage to the joint, and (2) the surgeon's success in restoring the anatomical congruity of the femoral condyle and glide surface for the patella. These injuries, commonly called Y- or T-fractures, occur in a variety of patterns, but the simple classification system based on anatomy is the most useful (Fig. 24–15).[2]

Clinical Findings

In addition to the signs and symptoms of supracondylar fractures, swelling and deformity of the knee joint develop, and motion or translocation of the patella may be obstructed. Movement of the tibia may elicit marked, harsh crepitus.

Roentgenographic Findings

Unless intraarticular fractures are impacted, multiple views are needed to define the displacement of the condylar fracture fragments.

Treatment

In treating intraarticular fractures, the goal is to reestablish anatomical relationships within the knee joint. Traditionally, these fractures are treated with traction if the fragments can be aligned. Although anatomical reduction can be achieved by traction, the late restriction of knee motion that often follows conservative treatment

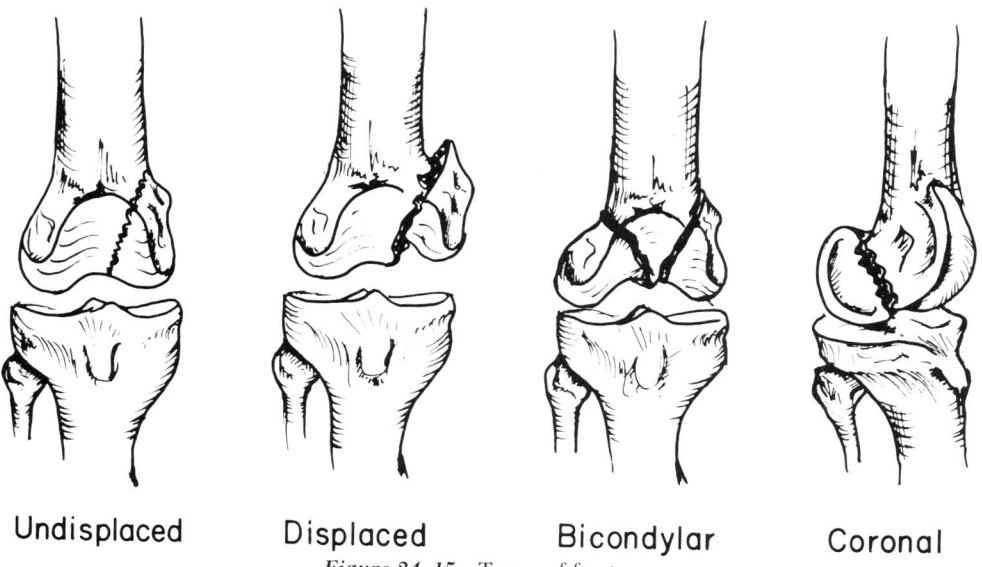

Undisplaced   Displaced   Bicondylar   Coronal

Figure 24–15 Types of fractures.

suggests that open reduction gives better results in young, healthy patients who have good bone stock. Surgical reduction is mandatory if the condylar fragments cannot be aligned by traction (Fig. 24–16).

At the time of surgery an open reduction may also be performed on the supracondylar fracture, or surgery may be limited to transfixation of the condylar fragment, with the supracondylar fracture treated by traction. The latter approach is definitely useful for open fractures in which the extensive surgery required for fixation of the supracondylar element is contraindicated.

Accurate anatomical reduction is essential, but it may not be easy to attain. Compression screws and the more stable bladeplate combinations now available have made it possible to improve stability throughout the fracture area. If the distal intercondylar fragments are stable, early motion is allowed. When the supracondylar fracture has also been stabilized with internal fixation, early active mobility of the knee joint can be achieved.

CONDYLAR FRACTURES

Isolated fractures of the femoral condyle are rare and occur more frequently in the lateral condyle. The mechanism producing this fracture is a combination of hyperabduction and adduction with axial loading. Malposition of the condylar fragment produces a deformity that is likely to result in nonunion.

Depending upon the mechanism of injury, the plane of the fracture may be either sagittal or coronal. In coronal fractures, the posterior portion of the condyle is generally split away. In some cases, the injury may be a combination of sagittal and coronal fractures. The rarest type of condylar fracture is that involving both the lateral and the medial condyles.

A patient with a condylar fracture cannot walk and develops a hemarthrosis of the knee immediately after the injury. Crepitus may be noted, and with a segmental loss an obvious varus deformity is seen.

Standard anteroposterior and lateral

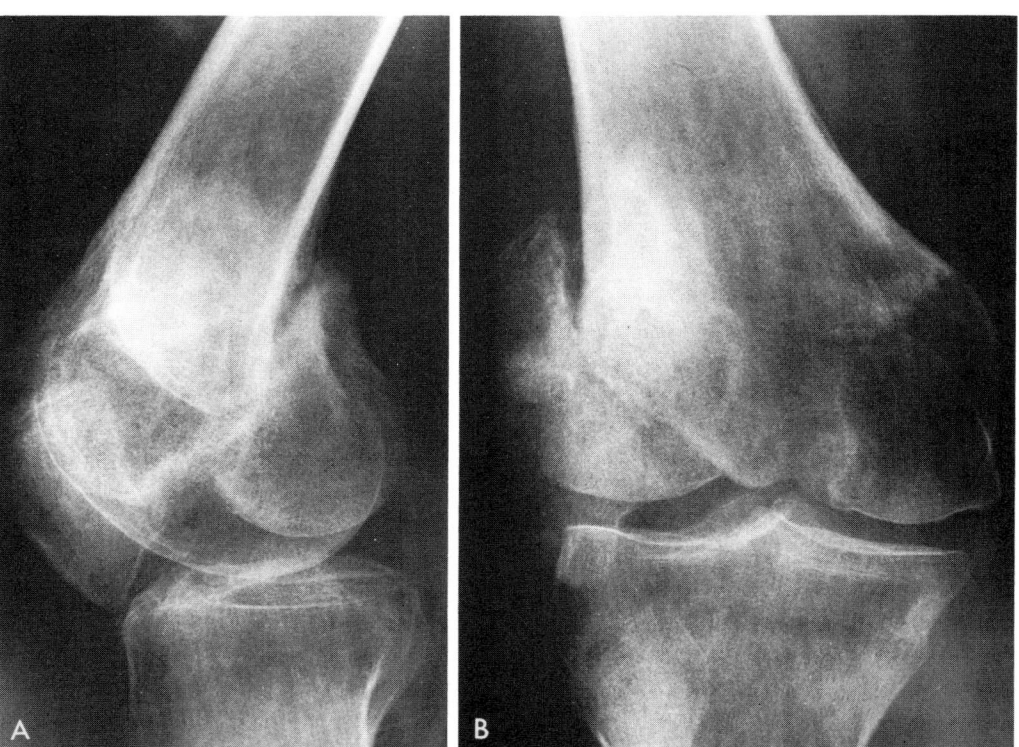

Figure 24–16   *A.* Lateral view of nonunion of a condylar fracture. Note position of the patella. *B.* Oblique view. Note angulation. There is a double fragment and displacement of the patella laterally and distally into the gap.

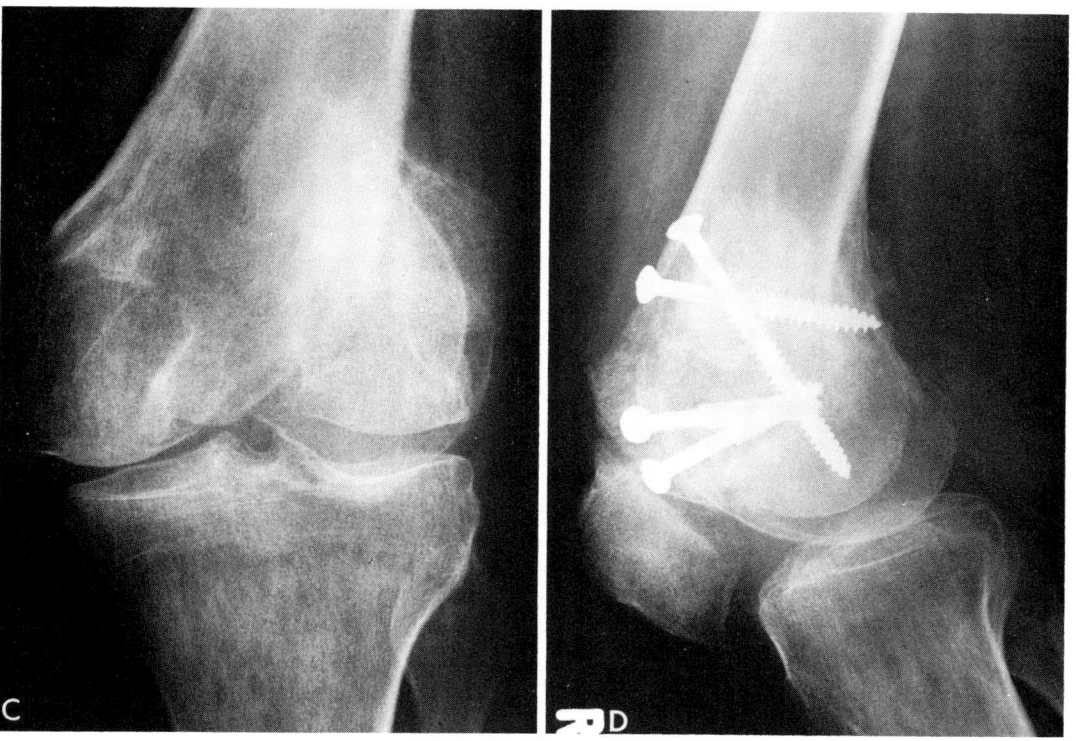

Figure 24–16 Continued. C. Anteroposterior view shows angulation and displacement of the patella. *D.* Lateral view. Open reduction and internal fixation. Note the position of the patella. The patellar tendon is fixed distally, but the patella is centralized.

Illustration continued on the following page

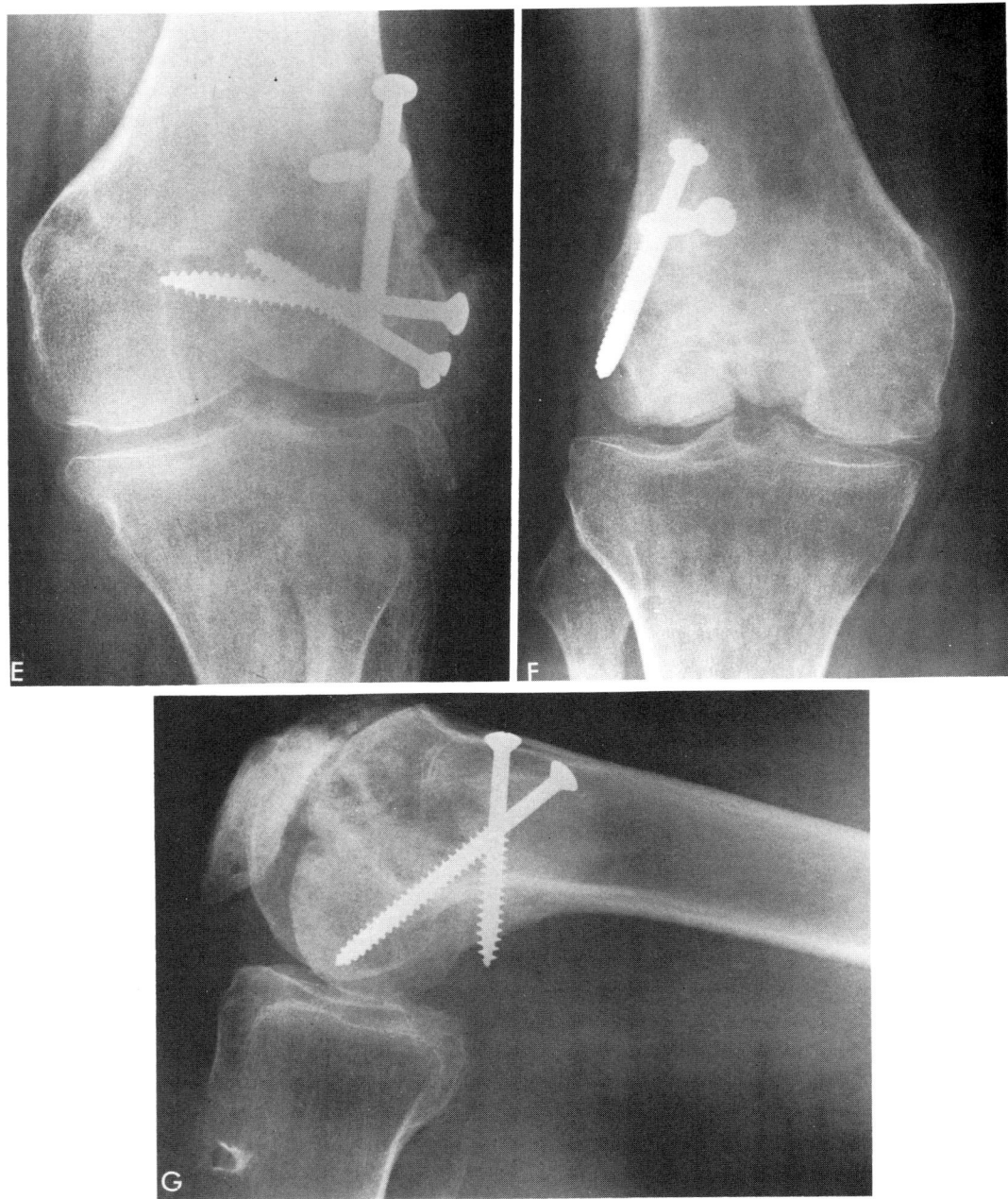

Figure 24–16 Continued. *E.* Overriding of patella on oblique view. *F.* Anteroposterior view shows smooth union. Quadriceps plate and patellar tendon lengthening are achieved. The patella is centralized and relatively upright. *G.* Lateral view. Dry crepitus of the joint is seen. Note degree of flexion and relative satisfactory position of the patella.

films usually show the fracture. However, additional views are necessary to fix the fracture planes and to allow preoperative planning.

When a condylar fracture is undisplaced or minimally displaced, it might be thought that cast treatment would suffice. However, as with unstable, nonimpacted interarticular fractures, the congruity of the joint surface is disrupted. Unless congruity is restored by anatomical reduction, disabling degenerative changes will develop. Thus, open reduction with internal fixation is the only dependable treatment. Cast bracing and traction are unsuitable methods for treating condylar fractures because of the high risk of delayed union and nonunion. Fixation with appropriate bolts or cancellous screws permits early knee motion, but the patient should not be allowed to bear weight on the affected extremity until union is established. Bicondylar fractures are best fixed with the Richards supracondylar compression plate.

FRACTURES OF THE PROXIMAL TIBIA

SURGICAL ANATOMY

The transverse diameter of the articular surface of the femoral condyle is less anterior than it is posterior. In the flexed knee the wider portion articulates; in extension the narrower, wedged-shaped anterior surface opposes the tibia. The femur is internally rotated on the tibia in the last few degrees of extension. The narrow anterior part of the lateral femoral condyle exposes a portion of the upper articular surface of the lateral tibial plateau with this rotation. Klin[27] states that the surface of the lateral tibial condyle extends about 0.5 cm beyond the femoral condyle.

The upper surface of the lateral tibial plateau is uniformly convex when seen from the lateral side. It is a saddle-shaped facet, convex in the sagittal plane and concave in the coronal plane.[28]

The knee joint is the largest joint in the body. It consists of two condyloid joints (femoral and tibial) with an arthroidal joint (patellofemoral) in between. The knee is stabilized by intra- and extraarticular liga-

ments and by muscular attachment.[29] Its weakness, from the standpoint of vulnerability to fracture, is the expanded cancellous condyles supported by the relatively narrow tibial shaft. The upper tibial flares provide a relatively flat articular surface to support the femoral condyles. Attachment to the flares is manifest by bony prominences for tendon and ligament attachments. In addition to its medial and anterior flares, the tibia projects backward beyond its supporting column and is deficient anteriorly above the tibial tubercle. Although the intercondylar eminences of the proximal tibia are nonarticular, the spine projections medially and laterally are not. The interarticular eminences provide attachment for the menisci and ligaments and abut the adjacent intercondylar "nonarticular" bone.

According to Bohler,[30] with roentgenographic confirmation by Moore, and Harvey,[31] the tibial plateaus slope posteroinferiorly 10 to 15 degrees from the horizontal, such that the angle between the longitudinal axis of the tibia and the plane of the plateaus is approximately 80 degrees.

MECHANISM OF INJURY

Experimental studies have shown that forced abduction and compression are important in the production of fractures of the lateral tibial plateau.[32] Forced abduction may cause the external margin of the lateral femoral condyle to press against the lateral tibial plateau. The leverage of the femur acts on the plateau against the resistng force of the tensed medial collateral and anterior cruciate ligaments. Should the load on the lever exceed the tensile strength of the tissues, the lesion may be a fracture, resulting from pressure between the condyles, a rupture, caused by tension in the ligaments, or concomitant fracture and rupture. Since the medial collateral ligament becomes less taut and abduction forces are dissipated, injuries are less likely to occur when the knee is moderately flexed. In experimental studies, gross soft tissue injuries were infrequent, occurring in only 2 of 44 cases in which valgus stress, axial loading, or both were applied.[32] Stress fractures, which are more likely to develop in the medial tibial plateau, may also occur.[33, 34]

Since vehicular accidents are responsible for most tibial plateau fractures, these injuries have been called fender fractures.[35, 36] In other series, falls as well as sudden, direct application of force to the knee have been reported to be the primary cause.[31, 38] Because falls force the femoral condyles against the tibial plateau with varus and valgus stress and heavy axial loading, they too can produce these injuries. Pure forces exerted across the joint may rupture the ligaments, and pure axial loading may result in bicondylar fractures. Certainly the location and extent of depression of a compression fracture depends upon both the angle of the knee at the time of injury and the duration of the forces that are exerted.

CLASSIFICATION

Fractures are classified to guide the surgeon in (1) establishing a diagnosis; (2) choosing the optimal method of treatment; (3) evaluating the course of healing; and (4) establishing a prognosis. The classification system developed by Mason Hohl[44] is a useful guide to treatment of fractures of the tibial condyles (Fig. 24–17 and Table 24–1). He groups these fractures as follows:

1. Undisplaced—those with 0 to 4 mm of depression or widening
2. Displaced—those with 5 mm or more of depression
    a. local articular
    b. split depressed
    c. split
    d. centrally depressed
    e. comminuted bilateral

The simple and descriptive system of Courvoisier also meets a clinical need.[46] Both Hohl and Courvoisier found approximately the same distribution of fracture types. Hohl[44] found that about 25 per cent of fractures of the tibial condyles were undisplaced; the remaining 75 per cent, which were displaced, included 25 per cent with central depressions and 25 per cent with split depressions. Centrally depressed and comminuted bilateral fractures each accounted for about 10 per cent of the total, split fractures constituting the rest.

There are other classification systems based on the mechanism of injury.[45] How-

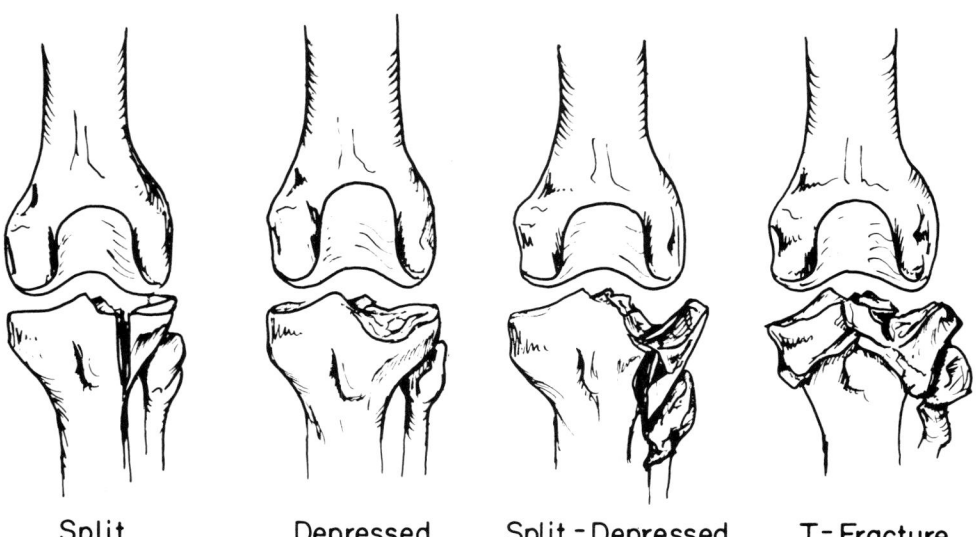

Split   **Depressed**   **Split - Depressed**   **T - Fracture**

Figure 24–17 Classification of proximal tibia fractures. (Courtesy of M. Hohl and The *Journal of Bone and Joint Surgery*. J. Bone Joint Surg., *38A*:1001–1017, 1956.)

ever, since the mechanisms are complex, rarely being either direct or indirect, the value of these systems is more limited.

CLINICAL FINDINGS

Injuries of the knee joint produce tenderness and hemarthrosis. Preternatural motion may be expected because of the fracture. Although most patients with fractures of the tibial plateau have rather evident pain and disability, these symptoms may be absent in alcoholics. Suspicion of collateral ligament rupture should be aroused by tenderness along the course of these ligaments, and subluxation of the femur on the tibia may be noted if the medial collateral and anterior cruciate ligaments are torn.

TABLE 24–1 Classification and Treatment of Fractures of the Tibial Condyle*

Type	Incidence (per cent)	Extent of Depression	Roentgenographic Studies	Treatment	Time until Healing
Undisplaced	24	0–4 mm of depression or widening	Stress films Laminography	Aspiration Soft cast or cylinder cast Knee motion— 4 weeks	4–12 weeks non–weight bearing
Displaced Local depression	26	+5–10 mm	Stress films Laminography	Surgery— dependent on age, demands of daily living Grafting, internal fixation Cast brace— 2nd to 8th week	12 weeks non– weight bearing
Split depression	26		Stress films	Surgery— grafting Bolts— supporting plate Cast brace— 2nd to 8th week	12 weeks non– weight bearing
Total depression	11		Stress films O.R.	Surgery—internal fixation, supportive fixation Cast brace 2nd to 8th week	12 weeks
Split 1. 2.	3	Depressed 1. 0–4 mm 2. +5 mm below tibial plateau	Stress films Laminography	1. Soft cast 8–10 weeks 2. Surgery— internal fixation	12 weeks 12 weeks
Comminuted	10		Stress films O.R.	Surgery— supportive fixation, grafting Cast brace	12+ weeks non–weight bearing

*After Hohl, M.: Tibial condylar fractures. J. Bone Joint Surg., 49A:1455–1467, 1967.

ROENTGENOGRAPHIC FINDINGS

Although standard anteroposterior and lateral films visualize most tibial plateau fractures, occasional fractures are best demonstrated on oblique views. Laminographs are most useful in assessing central depressions. The tibial plateau view, a 15 degree caudal anteroposterior view, is needed to accurately measure the extent of articular depression (Fig. 24–18).[31] Unless a full set of x-rays is obtained, an occasional fracture will go undiagnosed.

Initial films may give clues to both ligamentous instability and ligamentous avulsion. Retrospective examination of x-rays of minimally displaced fractures that healed with varus or valgus deformities may disclose a ligamentous rupture.

Stress roentgenograms offer the best and most accurate means of assessing ligamentous injuries. These films should be obtained after the induction of anesthesia in operative cases and should be seriously considered in nonoperative cases in which there is distinct tenderness and hypersensitivity and failure of the anterior cruciate end-point. The structures should be evalu-

ated in both flexion and full extension. If the tibial plateau is depressed and the ligaments are intact, gentle abduction stress applied to the extended knee should not open the joint space more than 1 mm. Experimental studies do not suggest that the extent of joint space opening is a reflection of cruciate ligament stability.[35, 47] In stress testing, it is essential to compare the extent of joint space opening in the normal and the injured knee because of individual variation in the laxity of the medial collateral ligament. The medial collateral ligament is more likely to be ruptured in split fractures of the lateral condyle, while the anterior cruciate is more often injured in medial condylar and bicondylar fractures.[48]

TREATMENT

General Principles

Surgeons experienced in fracture therapy emphasize that the most important element of treatment is not so much the details of the method but the principles on which the method is based. It is also important to understand that treatment principles do not remain static but change with time. The surgeon must choose that method or combination of methods best suited to the clinical situation, basing the choice on the reasonable demands of the patient as well as medical condition, age, and physical capabilities and on his own professional experience and the facilities available to him.

In no other aspect of orthopedic care does Bruce Gill's aphorism so aptly apply as in the treatment of fractures: "Study principles rather than methods. A mind that grasps principles will devise its own method." Progressive refinements in fracture care over the past 200 years have resulted from advances in the field of experimental osteogenesis; the development of new surgical materials and equipment, radiological techniques, and antibiotics; and improvements in medical care and anesthesia support.

The treatment of all types of intraarticular fractures aims at restoration of normal joint function and prevention of late,

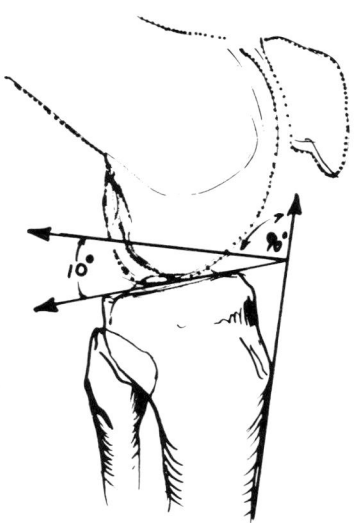

Angles

Figure 24–18 Knee angle.

posttraumatic osteoarthritis. Permanent or progressive disability in the knee is caused by (1) instability, (2) angular deformity, (3) restricted motion, and (4) pain resulting from traumatic arthritis.

Many surgeons claim that the best way to prevent late disability is stable anatomical restoration of the joint surface and stable internal fixation to allow early motion.[39-41] However, there is some doubt as to the absolute validity of this claim. Several long-term follow-up studies have demonstrated that good functional results can be obtained with nonoperative treatment even if anatomical and roentgenographic results are imperfect.[28, 37, 42]

When deciding between conservative and operative treatment, the surgeon should bear the following facts in mind.

1. Restricted motion results from pericapsular scarring, intraarticular adhesions, and myostatic contractures, all of which develop with prolonged immobilization of the knee. Since union usually follows active knee motion, prolonged immobilization is rarely indicated.

2. Muscle weakness is a corollary of immobilization, disuse, and pain. Insistence on early active use and muscle reeducation eliminates weakness.

3. Initial instability implies that the knee joint is functionally impaired. If this instability remains uncorrected, results will be less than optimal.

4. Residual malalignment results in therapeutic failure. There is a close association between angular deformity and osteoarthritis of the knee joint.[41]

5. Incapacitating pain is generally associated with roentgenographically evident osteoarthritis; pain and roentgenographic changes correlate closely with instability and angulation. This is particularly true of varus angulation.

If the patient can be treated so as to prevent angular deformity and to allow early motion without surgery, this is the method of choice. If, however, surgical treatment cannot assure anatomical correction and stabilization sufficient to allow early motion, it is unjustified. In cases in which the patient would otherwise be doomed to malalignment, instability, and prolonged immobilization, surgery should be performed.

If the purpose of surgical fixation is to reproduce exact joint anatomy and to assume stability with early motion, and the method is not to augment fixed cast treatment but to dispense with it or shorten the time of application, then the operative approach is valid. Otherwise, surgical fixation is intrusive and inappropriate.

Although they are useful, these guidelines are an oversimplification of the choices open to the surgeon. Other factors must be considered, including minimizing the danger of further deterioration in the patient's condition, especially in those who have undergone severe trauma, those who are elderly, and those who are poor surgical risks. Local conditions may also preclude surgery, necessitating an alternative to open anatomical restoration.

The surgeon's attitude also determines the choice of treatment. The more conservatively minded will reserve surgery for cases in which nonoperative care would result in unequivocal failure, while the surgically inclined will tend to choose open procedures. However, unsuccessful, long-continued conservative treatment of tibial plateau fractures may jeopardize the success of surgery when it is finally undertaken or may rule it out entirely. By the same token, it is equally disastrous to adopt the attitude, "A chance to cut is a chance to cure." Surgery *always* reveals problems more complex than those evident on x-rays and should not be undertaken with an untrained team or limited resources or as an emergency procedure.

Conservative Treatment

If there are no injuries of the supporting ligamentous structures, conservative treatment is indicated for undisplaced (0 to 4 mm depression) fractures of the tibial condyles. Patients with simple or minimally displaced impacted fractures are first aspirated to relieve the pressure and pain caused by hemarthrosis. They are then placed in a well-molded cylinder or, with appropriate instruction, in a Jones compression dressing for two to four weeks. Because loss of the patient to clinical and roentgenographic follow-up after casting invites changes that may be irremedial, these patients should be seen weekly with early x-ray control. This is particularly important for fractures that penetrate into circumferential cortical bone, resulting in loss of the buttress for the undepressed cancellous bone.

With these minor fractures, patients should soon be released from the plaster cylinder, which may then be used as a bivalved "brace." To rehabilitate the muscles and restore motion, the patient is encouraged to actively move the knee.

After four to eight weeks, there should be sufficient consolidation to allow partial weight bearing, but full weight bearing should be postponed until eight to twelve weeks postinjury.

In the elderly patient with a minor compression fracture and a stable knee, short-term immobilization for pain, followed by supported ambulation, is the method of choice.

Traction is useful for treating patients with contaminated wounds and those with doubtful skin viability or skin loss. Wound closure can be accomplished by one of several methods: debridement and closure, secondary intention, or a vigorous plastic approach involving flap procedures, relaxing incisions, or skin grafting. Traction is applied until the wound closes. When the fracture is "sticky," after approximately three to six weeks, the patient may be converted to a cast brace. Muscle exercises should be started early and the patient maintained on a non–weight-bearing status for 12 weeks.

Surgical Treatment

Stable, minimally displaced fractures that respond well to conservative treatment account for about 25 per cent of all tibial plateau fractures. Another 50 per cent of these fractures can be managed by relatively limited surgery.

In a recent series, approximately 25 per cent of the patients who underwent surgery for tibial plateau fractures also had ligamentous and capsular injuries, some of which were extensive. Tears of the medial collateral ligament were the most common type of soft tissue injury, occurring primarily in fractures of the lateral condyle. Tears of the anterior cruciate ligament and mul-

tiligament injuries were also common. In about 12 per cent of these cases, tears of the anterior cruciate were found in conjunction with fractures of the lateral condyle.[48]

In minimally displaced fractures accompanied by ligament injuries, early reconstruction and repair of soft tissue damage is essential for good results. Provided that all concomitant ligamentous injuries are diagnosed and repaired early, the prognosis is good. However, the surgeon's fear of producing additional "scar" all too often results in inadequate exposure of the joint, leading to incomplete identification of all of the injuries and to inadequate repair. The approach chosen as well as the extent of exposure should be dictated by the results of preoperative examination and surgical exploration.

Because it is extensive enough to afford access to the tibial shaft and plateau and the knee joint and to permit repair of the ligamentous elements, we prefer to use either a "lazy S" incision (Fig. 24–19)[56] or the utility incision of Hughston.[57] We make the proximal arm of the "S" just behind the adductor tubercle or laterally along the course of the biceps tendon, then swing anteriorly and almost horizontal at the joint line, and finally proceed distally and down-

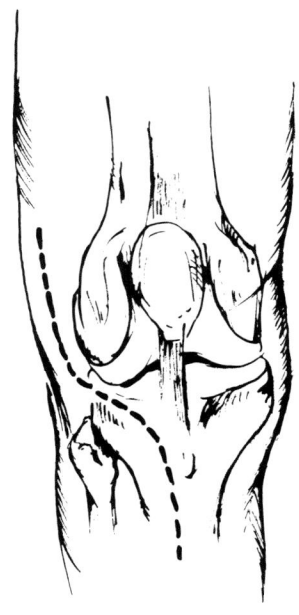

Lazy-S

Figure 24-19   "Lazy S" incision.

ward along the tibial tubercle and crest of the tibia. The skin must be incised to the level of the deep fascia, and all vessels in the suprafascial areolar tissue must be protected. If the soft tissue injuries are so extensive that two incisions must be made, the "S" is shifted somewhat posteriorly to enlarge the anterior bridge of tissue.

In addition to conventional medial and lateral exposures for such routine procedures as osteotomy or ligamentous reconstruction, the tibial tubercle may be osteotomized and the knee joint opened anteriorly.[51] Since it involves flap or vascular problems or both, we are reluctant to use the "Y" or champagne-cup incision.

A variety of internal fixation devices have been employed in tibial plateau fractures. Closed reduction and traction methods have been augmented by percutaneous introduction of wires or pins under roentgenographic control.[58] Percutaneous bolting of minimally displaced fractures also has its advocates. When this method is used, sur-

gery is preceded by application of traction for a few days.[59]

After pure split or separation fractures are surgically reduced, bolts or cancellous screws can be employed to provide nontilt transverse fixation of the bone. However, if the cortical bone is defective a supporting plate is necessary.

More extensive exposure is required for the use of cerclage or wire containment. When the joint is exposed sufficiently for visual reduction of the fragments, multiple wires may be inserted for multiplane stability.[60, 61] Any bolt or pin alone or in combination may also be used with exposure of this type.

Many depressed fractures (depression of 5 mm or more) require bone grafting as well as internal fixation (Fig. 24–20). Simple open reduction creates a subarticular cavity, and remarkably large quantities of bone are required to fill these cavities. If surgery is being contemplated for this type of fracture, the patient's condition must be sufficiently

Text continued on page 745.

Figure 24–20 Maturing cancellous bone graft, seen best in the lateral view. The residual "hole" to be filled is quite large, with cortical bone above and cancellous bone below. This patient has full range of motion, and experiences minor aches with prolonged sitting.

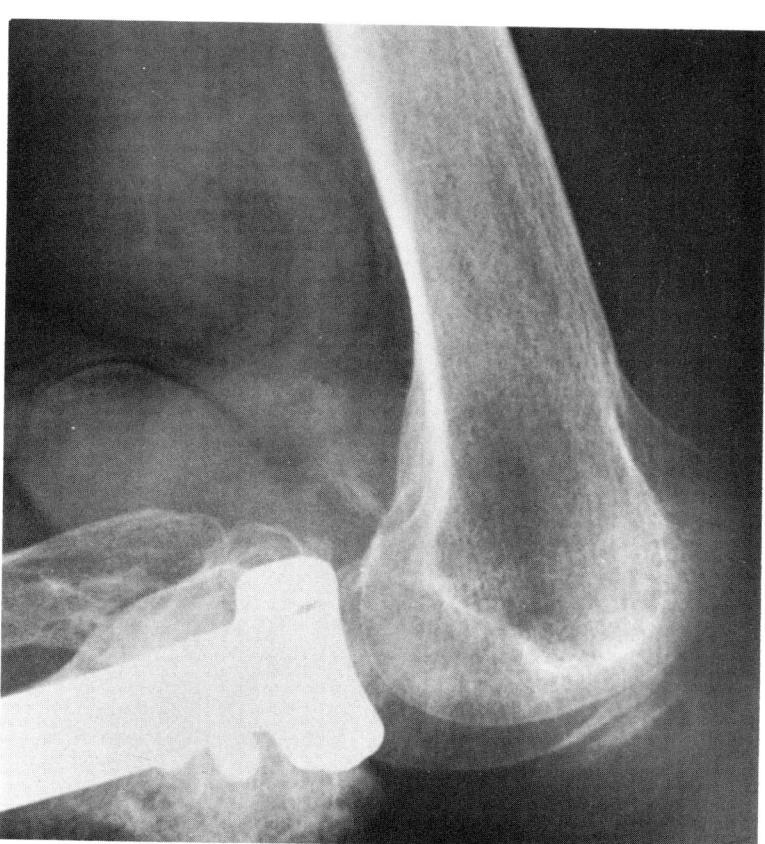

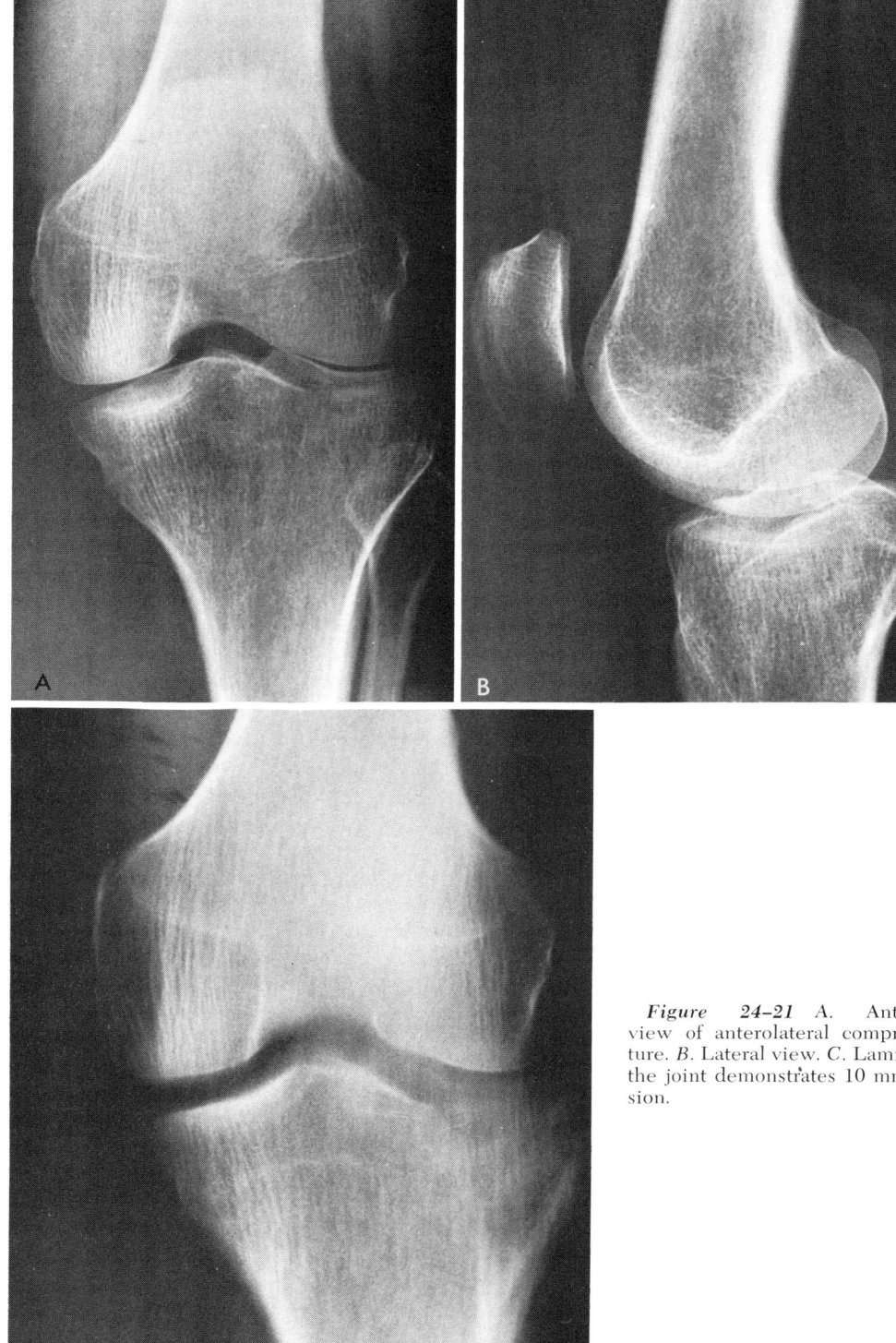

Figure 24–21 A. Anteroposterior view of anterolateral compression fracture. *B*. Lateral view. *C*. Laminography of the joint demonstrates 10 mm of depression.

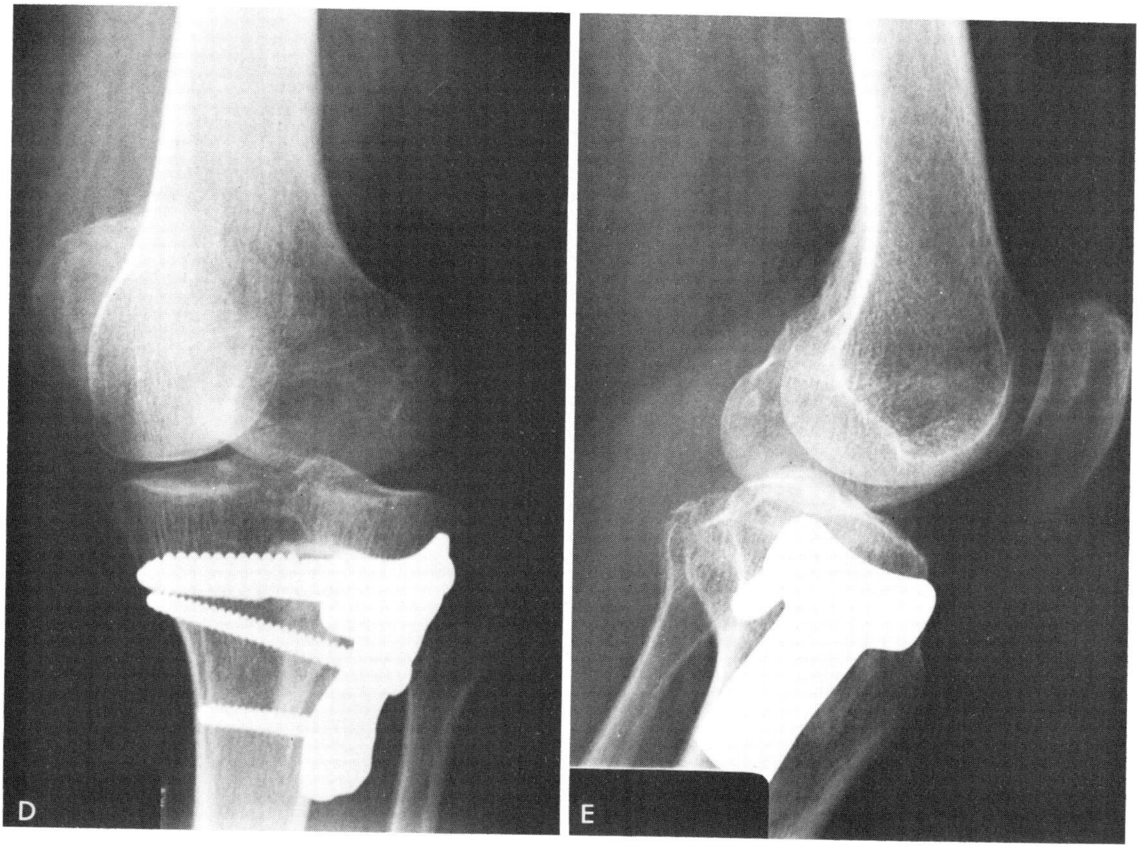

Depressed-Split

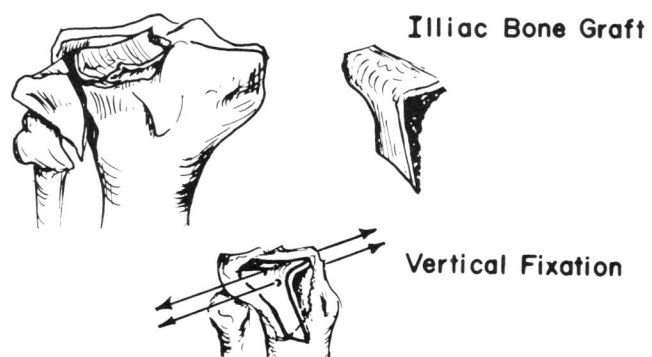

Illiac Bone Graft

Vertical Fixation

Surface Depression

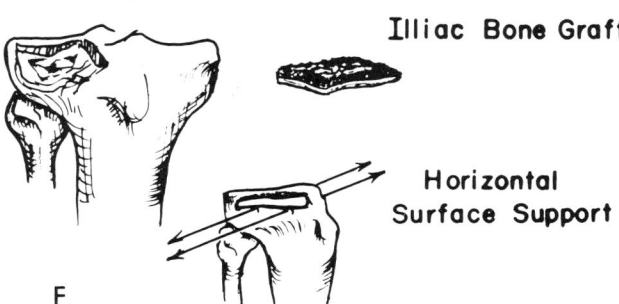

Illiac Bone Graft

Horizontal Surface Support

F

Figure 24–21 Continued. D and E. Oblique view demonstrates maturing vertical cortical graft extending from front to back. It is fixed by a screw and acts as a prop to the joint surface. F. Grafting.

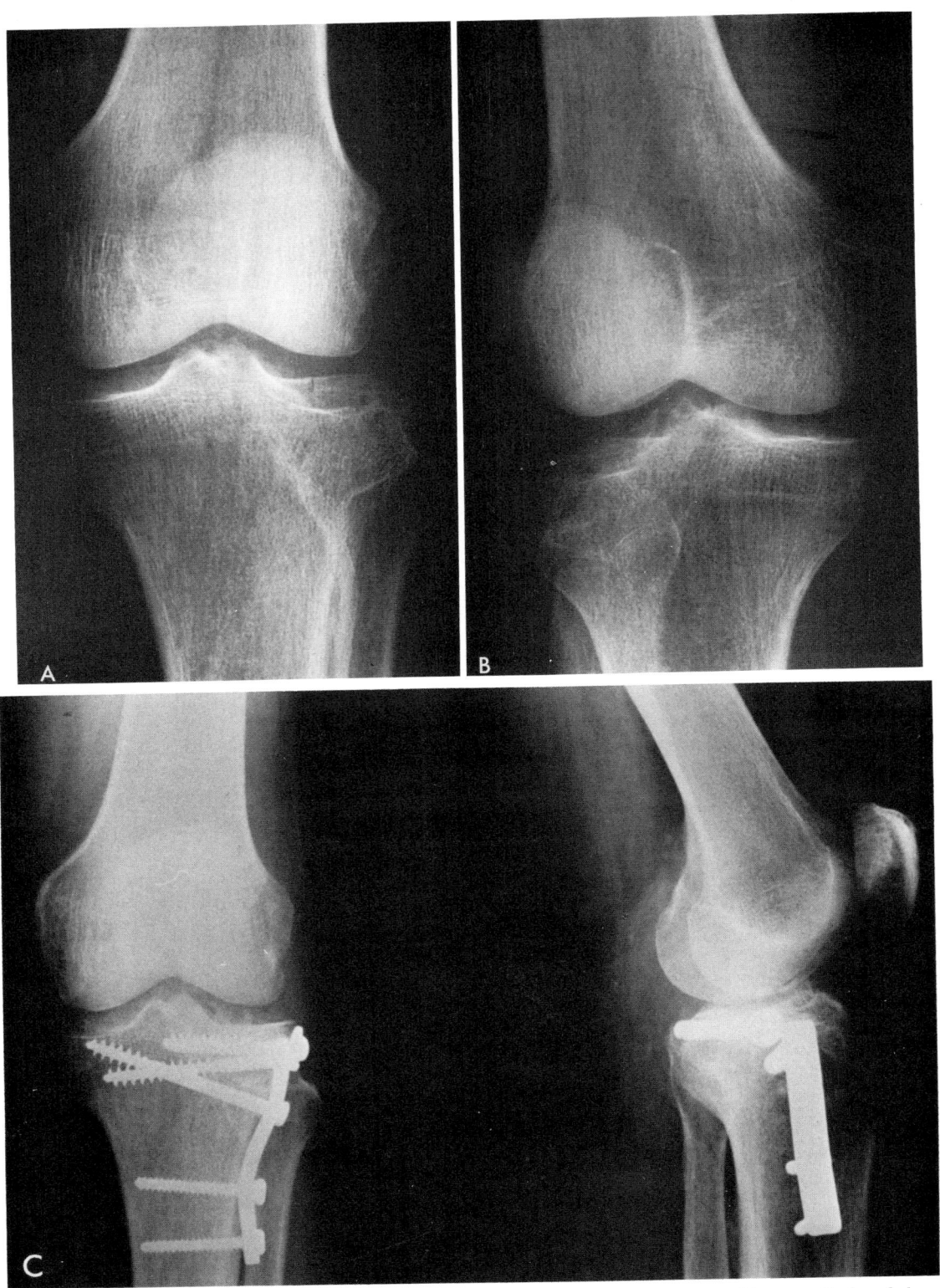

Figure 24–22   A and B. Fragmented rim with primary central depression. C. Horizontal bone graft placed above the screws. Screws give posterolateral compression as well as medial compression and support the graft above.

stable to permit the removal of bone from the iliac crest for grafting. Because cancellous bone used alone tends to collapse upon firm compaction, particularly in elderly osteoportic patients with deficiencies of both the bone supply and the bed, it is desirable to use a combination of cortical and cancellous bone. Autogenous bone may be augmented with bank bone, and in very rare cases methyl methacrylate may have to be used.

If the lateral cortex is stable and can act as a buttress for the elevated fragments and supporting cortical and cancellous bone grafts, any device that has a broad compression surface that will provide firm contralateral fixation is sufficient. Wire loops,[53] bolts and washers,[54] Knowles pins,[28] and plates and bolts[55] have been employed as internal fixation devices.

If necessary, the anterior tibial condyle can be readily opened to permit exposure and packing of the cavity. To provide maximum stability, screws or bolts, placed horizontally along the top of the cavity beneath the weight-bearing areas of the tibia, can be used to support cortical bone. This surface is then propped up with morcellized bone from the iliac crest, which is pounded into the cavity to fill the interstices. The more distal, and generally better, cortical fragment should be fixed first lest it angle with proximal compression. Comminuted and unstable depressed fractures are best treated by bolting both surfaces of the shaft together.

In mixed fractures (separation and depression) the separated fragment is opened like the cover of a book: this is followed by elevation of the joint surface and packing (Fig. 24–21). Cortical bone can be placed either vertically or horizontally if it is supported from below. The fracture is then fixed as for a simple separation. If stability cannot be assured, a supporting plate may be required (Fig. 24–22).

Although the operative approach is the same, serious problems may be encountered in the surgical treatment of Y- or T-fractures. In the proximal plateaus the problem is approached by attempting to create a single fracture and then joining the fragments to their mates on the opposite side. This may be accomplished by tempo-

rary pinning or definitive screwing of the anatomically reduced fragments. The following principles should be considered in determining the level of fixation: (a) provision of support for depressed areas, (b) compression of the vertical fracture, and (c) assurance of cortical support from below by plates. If both proximal cortices are defective, two plates, joined by bolts, must be employed (Fig. 24–23). There is no reason for this, however, unless the surgeon intends to reestablish anatomical conditions that will permit early, if guarded, motion.

While these guidelines suffice for 75 per cent of tibial plateau fractures, the remaining 25 per cent of grossly comminuted and bicondylar fractures require multifaceted treatment, including surgery. It may be necessary to use the whole spectrum of therapeutic measures: traction, followed by surgery, and finally, application of a cast brace. In this way, treatment can be designed for each individual case (Figs. 24–24 and 24–25). Delayed surgery may be considered if the skin wound is extensive enough to create problems with primary healing and to increase the risk of infection. In these cases the major problem is wound healing, and immediate treatment, consisting of distal traction, bulky compressive dressings, and splint immobilization, assures stability of the wound until the patient's condition improves sufficiently to permit surgery. Fortunately, fractures of this type are uncommon.

FRACTURES OF THE PATELLA

INCIDENCE

Fractures of the patella constitute approximately 1 per cent of all skeletal injuries. Traffic accidents may account for as much as 25 per cent of these fractures, which are found predominantly in younger adults.[74, 75] The mean age is approximately 40 years, males tending to be slightly younger and females older. Approximately 65 per cent of these injuries occur in males. Neither side is affected more often than the other, and bilateral fractures are uncommon.[74]

Text continued on page 751.

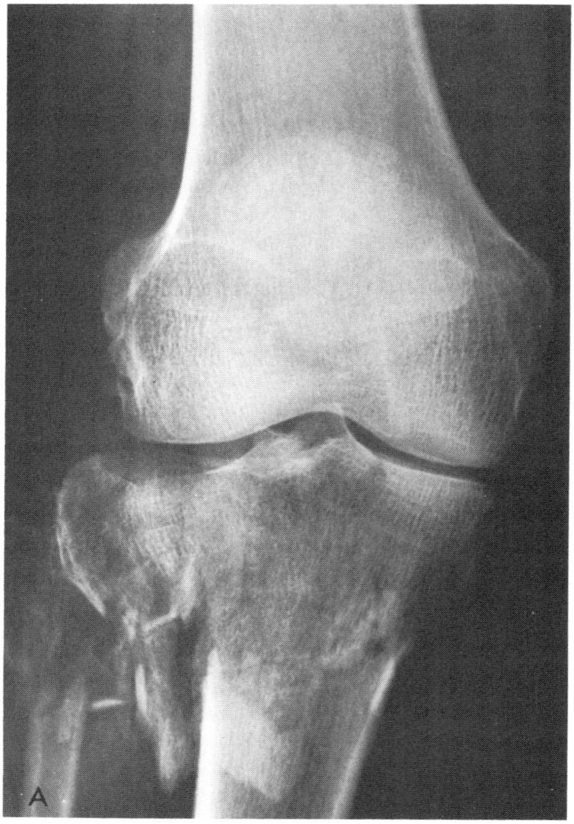

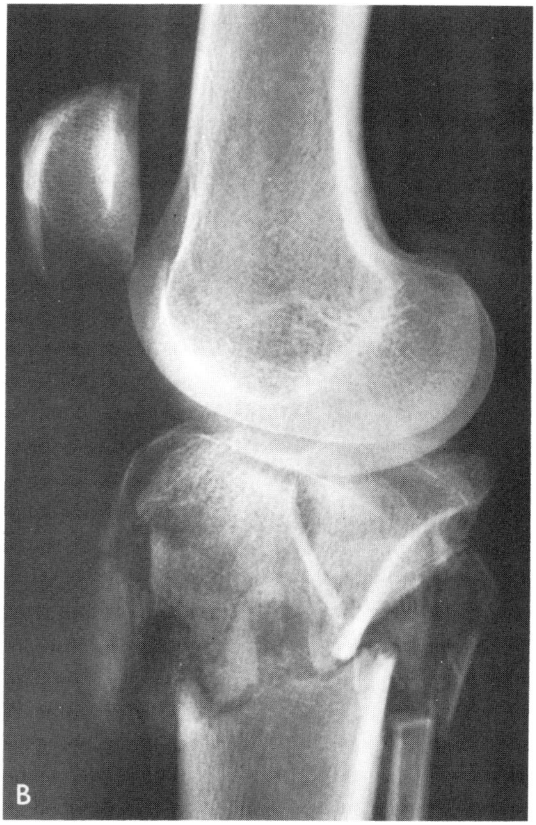

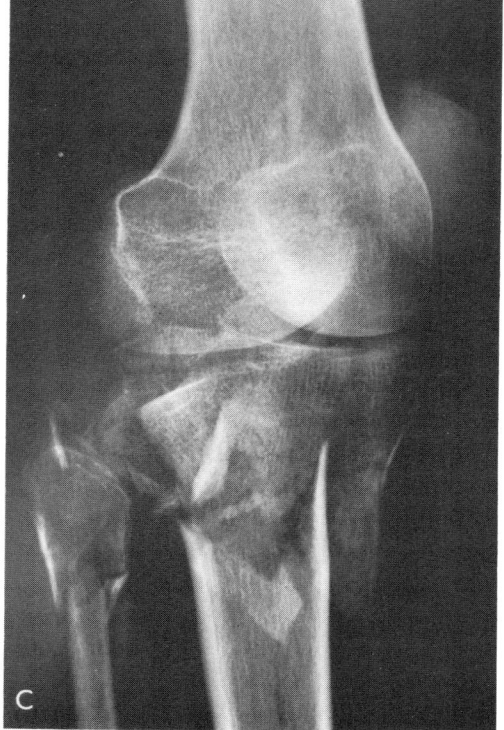

Figure 24–23   A. Anteroposterior view of the knee. B. Lateral view. C. Comminuted fracture of the plateau.

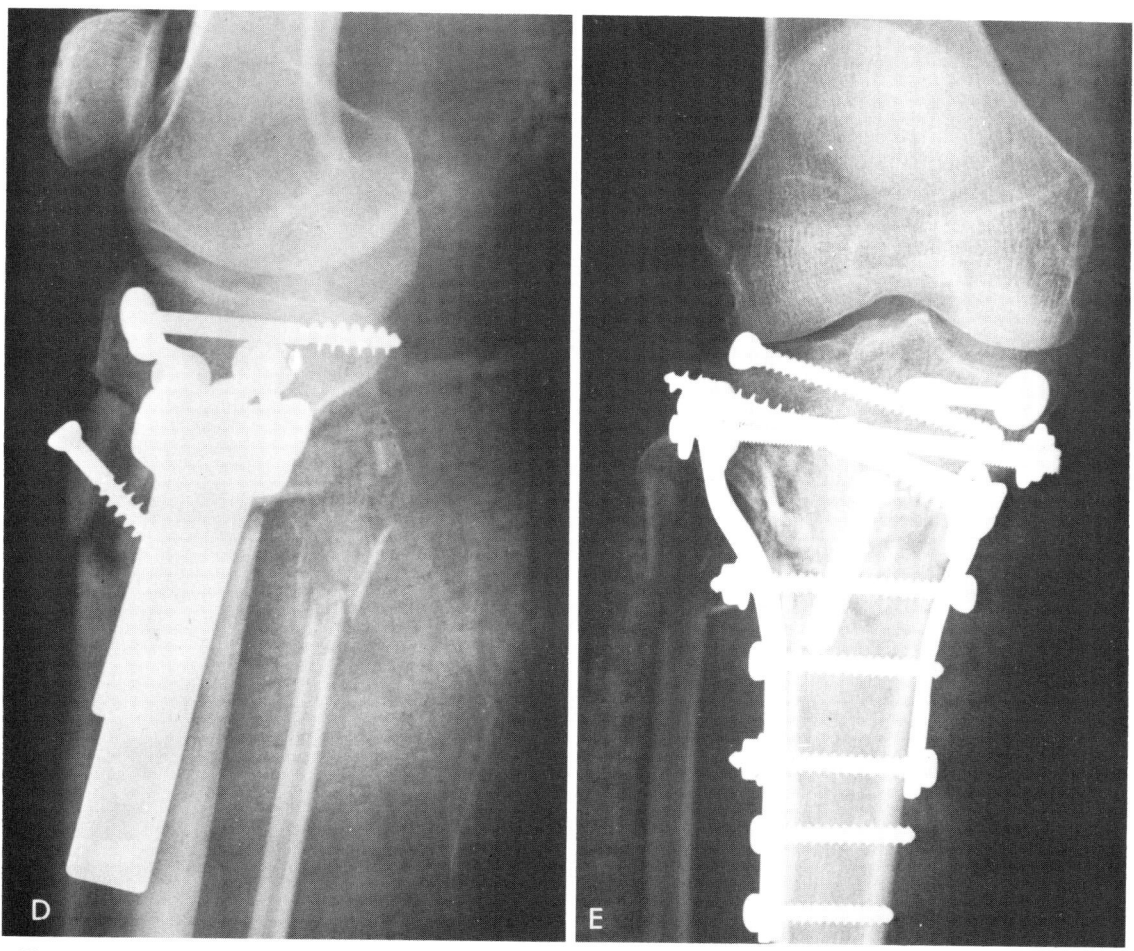

Figure 24–23 Continued. D and E. Stabilizing internal fixation through the plateau maintains integrity, with support from the shaft below.

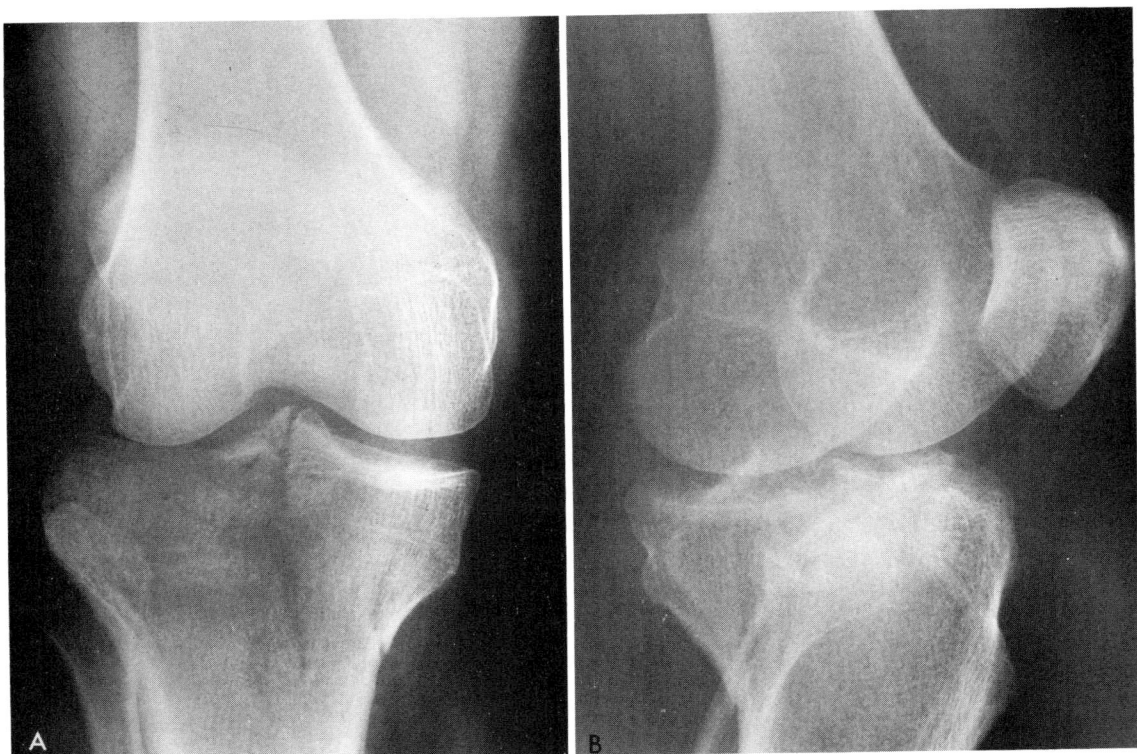

Figure 24-24 *A* to *D*. This is a poor bolt technique because of the comminution and failure of support from below. Poor results can be expected.

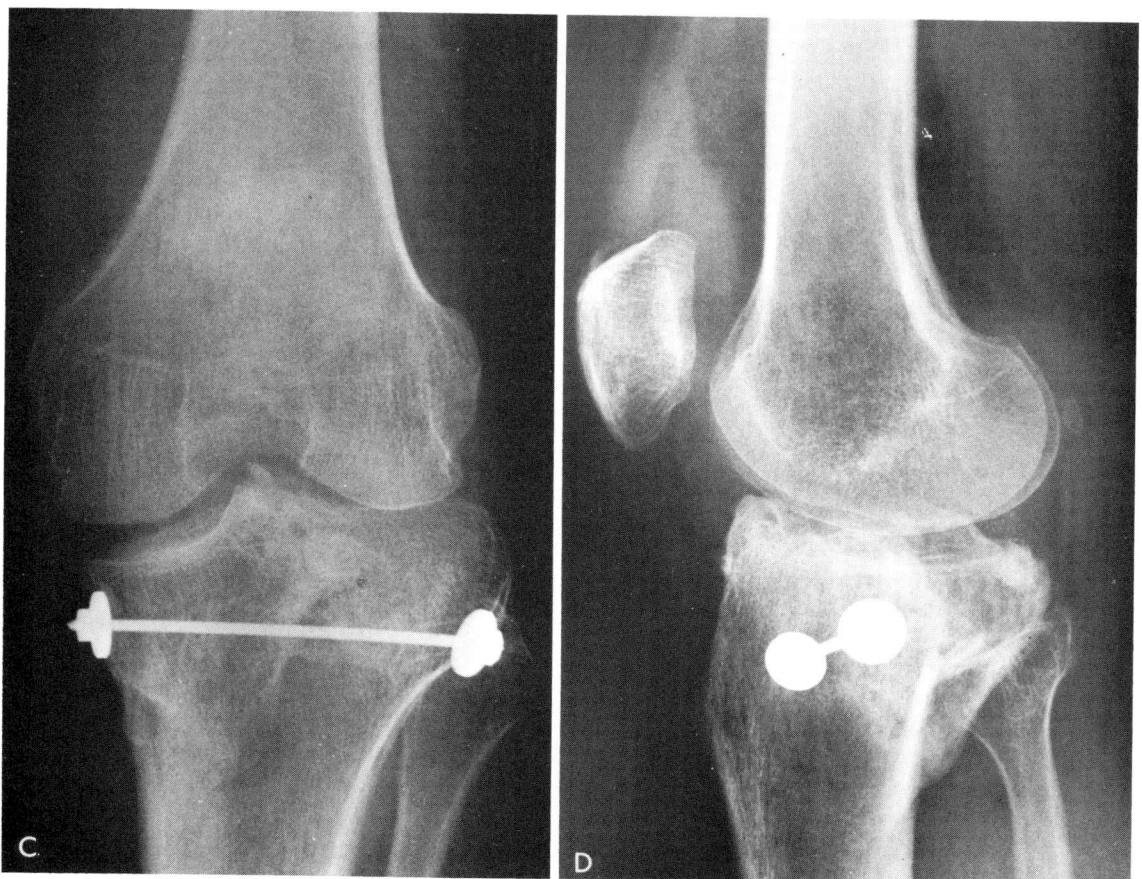

Figure 24–24 Continued.

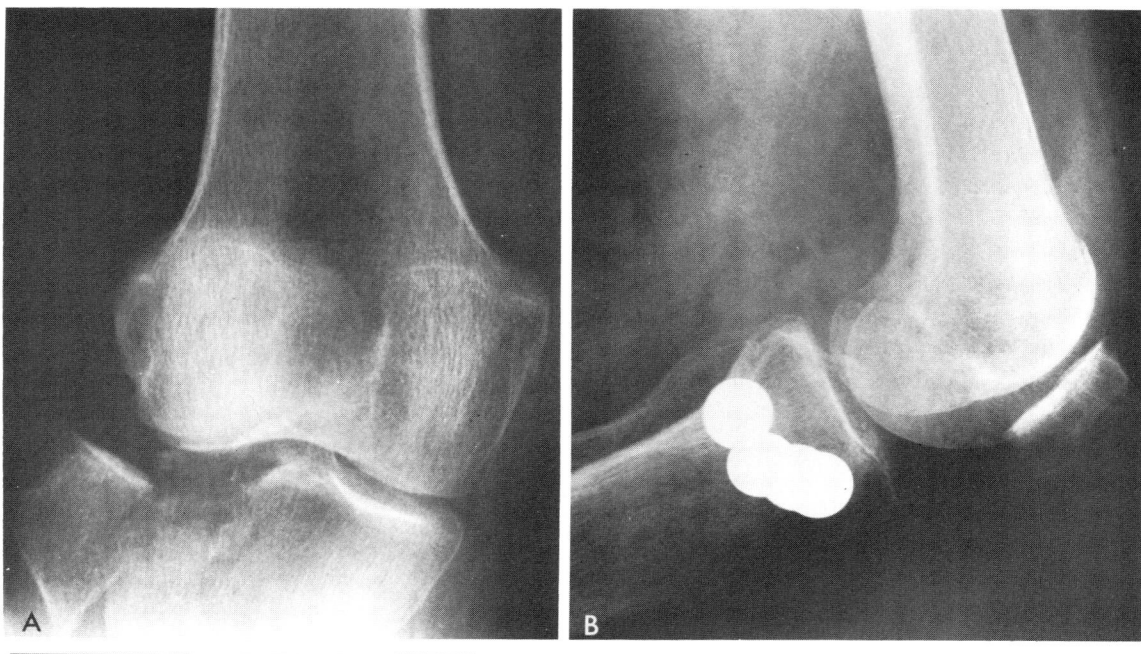

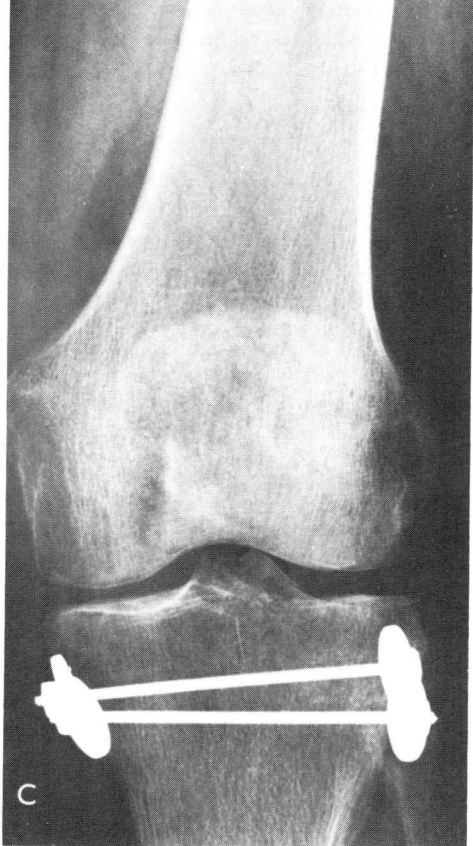

Figure 24–25 A to C. Bolts may give excellent fixation if the contralateral side is good. This patient underwent repair of the medial collateral ligament.

SURGICAL ANATOMY

The inferior part of the patella, a triangular-shaped bone with rounded edges, has a relatively flat surface on its anterior aspect. The apex is joined to the tibial tuberosity by the patellar ligament. The superior third of the anterior surface, which is convex, is covered with fibers from the quadriceps tendon that extend into the superficial layers of the patellar ligament. The cartilaginous articulating surface, facing the femur, is divided into a small medial and a larger lateral portion by a verticle ridge. A narrow strip runs along the medial margin of this surface, with the remainder divided into two lower, two middle, and two upper facets by the vertical ridge.[63, 64] Wiberg[65] found that the posterior surface of the patella may assume three different forms (Fig. 24–26): type 1 having a central ridge, type 2 a more medial ridge and a smaller medial facet, and type 3 an even more medial displacement of the ridge and a medial facet that slopes steeply forward and medially. In types 2 and 3, the trochlea is also situated more medially than in type 1.

The contact surface between the patella and the distal femur varies with different positions of the knee joint. In the extended

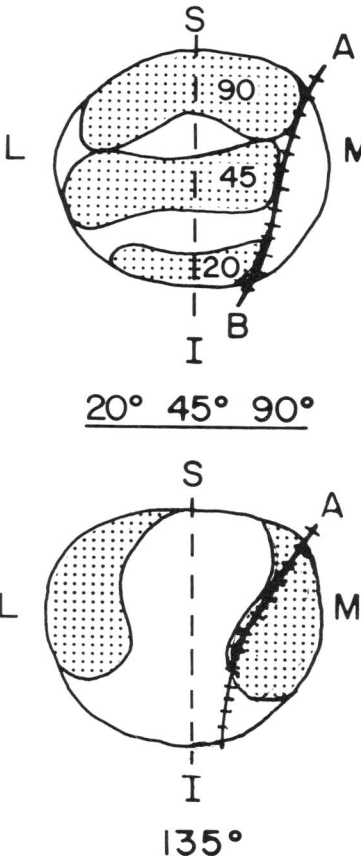

Figure 24–27   Contact surface of the patella with degrees of flexion (after Goodfellow).

position, only the lower facets articulate, while increasing flexion brings progressively larger areas into contact with the femur. At maximal flexion, the patella nestles between the femoral condyles with slight lateral displacement. It is then that the upper facets articulate with the articular surface of the distal femur (Fig. 24–27).

The vascular supply consists of a patellar rete composed of the superior, medial, and inferior geniculate arteries. The rete penetrates the lower pole and central bone of the anterior patellar surface; the upper pole is supplied by the central penetrating artery. Marginal penetration is minimal.[66, 67]

The patella is incorporated into the tendon system of the quadriceps muscle, which consists of the rectus femoris, vastus intermedius, vastus lateralis, and vastus medialis. There is a clinical difference between the vastus medialis longus and the

Types Of Patellar Contours

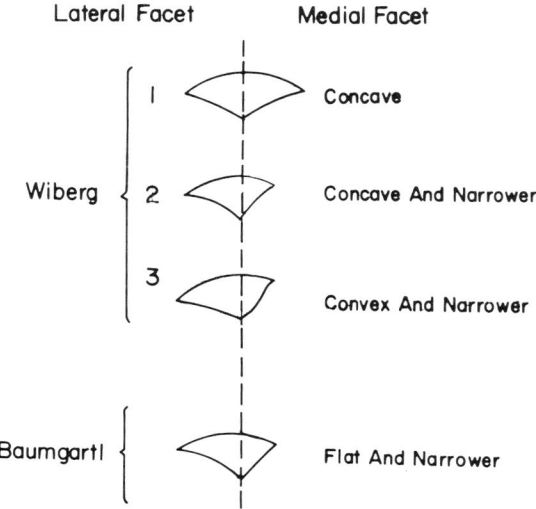

Figure 24–26   Shapes of the posterior surface of the patella. (Courtesy of G. Wiberg and *Acta Orthopaedica Scandinavica*. Acta Orthop. Scand., *12*:319–410, 1941.)

vastus medialis: The former is longitudinally directed, and the latter is more transverse.[68] The strong quadriceps tendon inserting into the proximal base of the patella includes all four components of the quadriceps, the most anterior being the rectus femoris and the most posterior the vastus intermedius. Some superficial tendinous fibers from the rectus femoris continue across the anterior surface of the patella and insert directly into the patellar tendon, whereas the deeper, stronger fibers insert into the anterior base of the patella and the proximal third of its anterior surface. The vastus medialis and vastus lateralis continue along the medial and lateral aspects of the patella, inserting directly into the tibia. These fibers together with deep transverse fibers originating in the femoral epicondyles form the patellar retinacula. The lateral expansions of the quadriceps apparatus together with the iliotibial band serve as an auxiliary extensor of the knee joint. Provided that the patellar retinacula are preserved, patients with injuries of the extensor apparatus can walk and lift the leg from a supine position, even if the patella is fractured and the infrapatellar tendon ruptured.

MECHANISMS OF INJURY AND TYPES OF FRACTURES

The question arises as to whether a fracture of the patella is caused by direct or indirect violence or by a combination of both. In the past, most authors[70-72] divided fractures of the patella into two main types on the basis of the traumatic mechanism. In general, transverse fractures were believed to result from indirect trauma, whereas comminuted fractures were attributed to direct injury. However, it is now recognized that other factors, such as the degree of knee flexion at the time of trauma, are important in determining the type of fracture produced.[64] At 30 degrees of flexion the patella is tilted, and transverse support is narrowed. Pressure exerted against the femur by the tensile forces of the quadriceps and patellar ligaments increases progressively

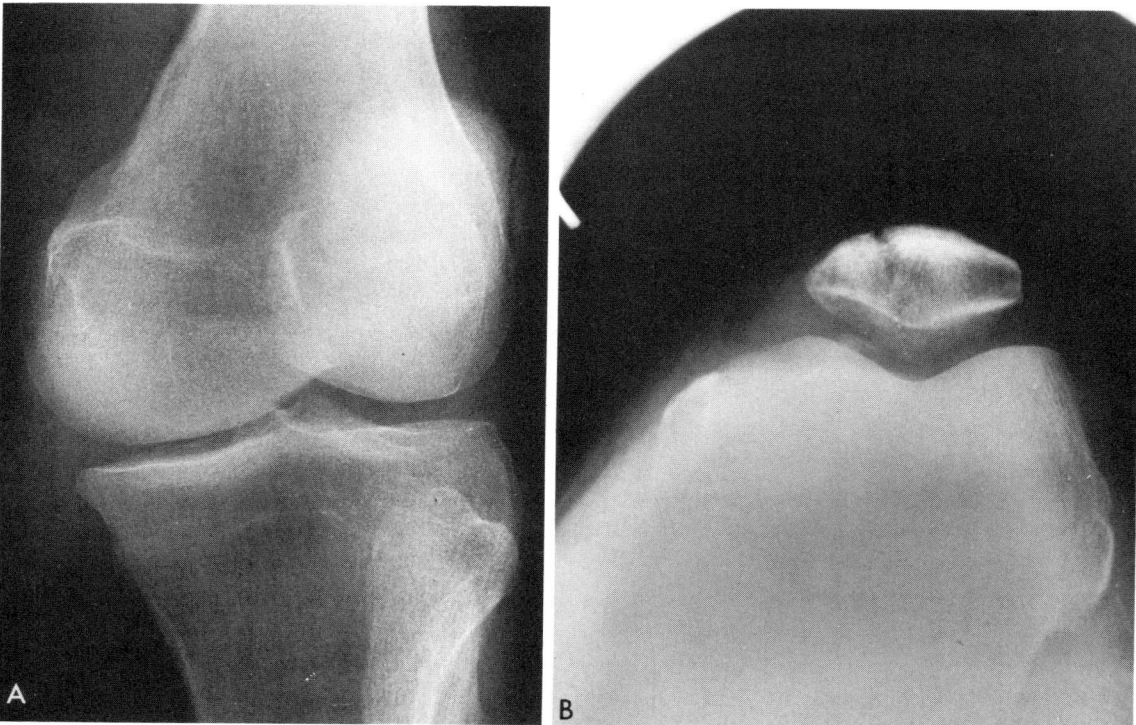

Figure 24-28   A and B. Longitudinal fracture requires oblique views or the "sunrise" view in order to be seen with certainty.

with increasing flexion.[69] More recently it has been recognized that a number of different types of fracture may result from the same mode of injury.[63, 74, 75]

In 1910 transverse patellar fractures were reported to be the most common type, occurring in approximately 70 per cent of patients.[73] However, most recent studies indicate that transverse fractures occur most often in older patients, in whom transverse and comminuted fractures are about equally common.[74] In Bostrom's series,[75] transverse fractures accounted for only 25 per cent of the total, while comminuted fractures constituted 16 per cent and longitudinal fractures 28 per cent. These figures suggest that longitudinal fractures are not as uncommon as previously reported (Fig. 24–28).[76] Since direct trauma is considered to be the most frequent cause of longitudinal fractures of the patella,[77] this indicates that direct injuries, such as dashboard injuries, account for an increasing percentage of patellar fractures.

The typical "indirect" fracture is transverse, with some comminution of the nonarticular surface. When the accelerated limb, controlled by the musculotendinous unit, is stopped suddenly, patellar fractures generally result from the effect of indirect forces. Chondromalacia may momentarily impede the joint surfaces from gliding when the individual stumbles or partially falls or when the extremity is suddenly obstructed in the performance of a purposeful, powerful action (Fig. 24–29). In our experience, the superolateral pole of the patella may actually be ruptured by uncontrolled muscular contraction during athletic activity. This type of trauma may produce a fracture with a pattern resembling the one seen in most patients with bipartite patella (Fig. 24–30). After the fracture occurs, collapse of the knee against muscle tension probably accounts for tearing of the quadriceps expansion and fragment separation.

Although fractures resulting from direct trauma are typically stellate or comminuted, incomplete or displaced fractures may also be produced by the same mechanism. A combination of trauma, muscle contraction, and joint collapse results in surface comminution and fragment separation. It should be noted that comminuted fractures are not invariably accompanied by rupture of the quadriceps expansion, even though the patella may be severely crushed (Fig. 24–31).

The literature suggests that osteochondral fractures of the patella are rare.[74] First reported by Kroner in 1905,[78] such fractures have been reported only sporadically since then.[79-82] Widespread participation in competitive athletics by both sexes may lead to an increased incidence of these fractures, however (Fig. 24–32).[83, 84] Since osteochondral fractures invariably occur on the medial aspect of the patella, lateral hypermobility of the patella is considered a prerequisite for their production. While these fractures are not easily detected on conventional x-rays and are difficult to identify,[86] joint aspiration, clinical signs referable to the medial margin, arthrography, and arthroscopic evaluation should enable earlier and more accurate diagnosis.[87]

CLINICAL FINDINGS

The diagnosis of a fresh patellar fracture usually involves no difficulties. If the fragments are widely separated a defect may be palpated. The joint is distended by a hemarthrosis which, when aspirated, yields a frankly bloody fluid with large floating fat globules. Owing to hemorrhagic translation into the soft tissues, wide separation of the fragments may limit distention of the knee. A typical finding is the patient's inability to lift the leg with the knee extended. However, in fractures in which the quadriceps mechanism is intact, the diagnosis may be more difficult. These include longitudinal and marginal fractures as well as fractures of the distal nonarticular pole. The physician should request a rigorous roentgenographic evaluation[88] or, if necessary, perform an arthroscopic examination when patellar trauma is associated with a bloody aspirate containing large amounts of fat.

ROENTGENOGRAPHIC FINDINGS

In the comminuted or transversely split patella in which the fragments are separated, plain films are diagnostic. However, a roentgenographic study is incomplete un-

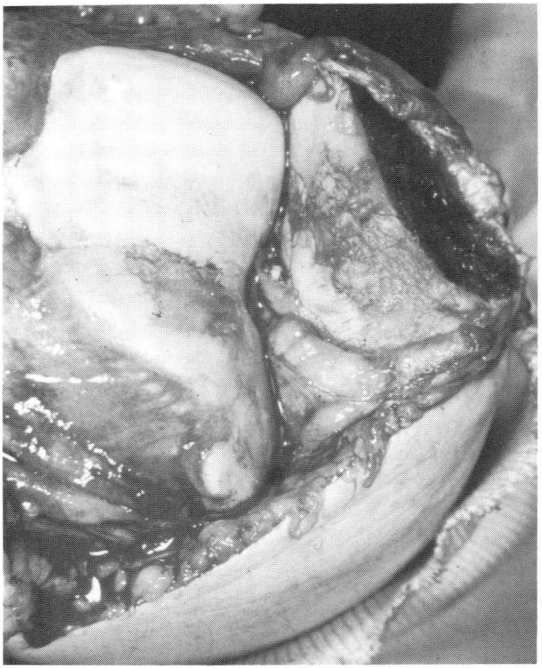

Figure 24-29 Leaping ballet dancer whose foot struck choreographic tape fixed to the floor, "snapping" the patella.

less it includes oblique views, and the axial or "sunrise" view is necessary to rule out or define longitudinal and marginal fractures. If there is doubt as to the integrity of the lateral expansion of the quadriceps, a flexion view may be helpful in determining whether conservative or surgical care is needed. Since vertical marginal fractures may not produce specific clinical signs, x-rays are required. Most fractures of this type are located laterally, at the junction between the middle and the lateral third of the patella (Fig. 24-33).[89] It should be noted that the typical site of this fracture differs from the location of the accessory ossification center in bipartite patella. In the latter condition, which is a normal variant, a line similar to that seen in fractures runs obliquely over the superolateral margin of the patella. In addition, bipartite patella is not infrequently bilateral and symmetrical.[89]

CONSERVATIVE TREATMENT

In fractures in which the fragments are minimally separated and the extensor

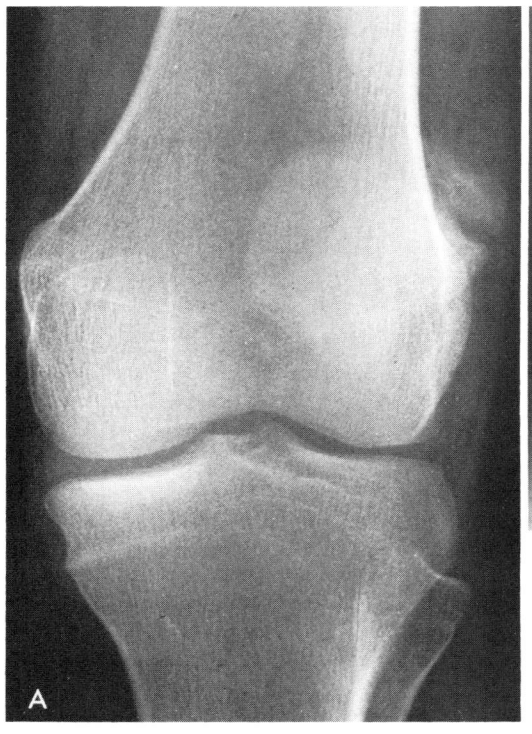

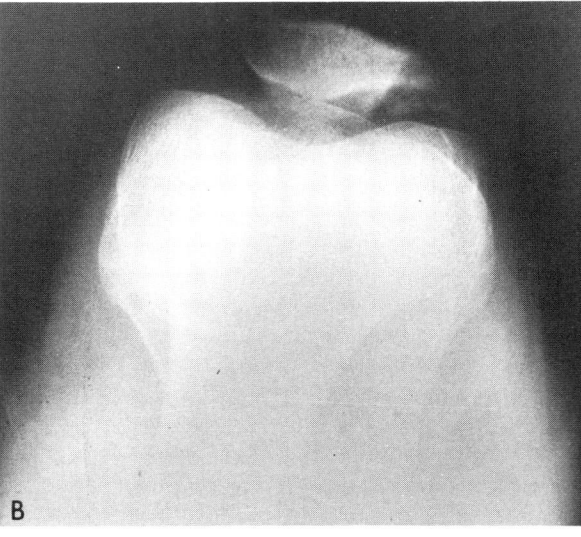

Figure 24-30 A and B. Sustained sudden pain with quick dismount from a horse. The pain, which became chronic, was consistent with fracture.

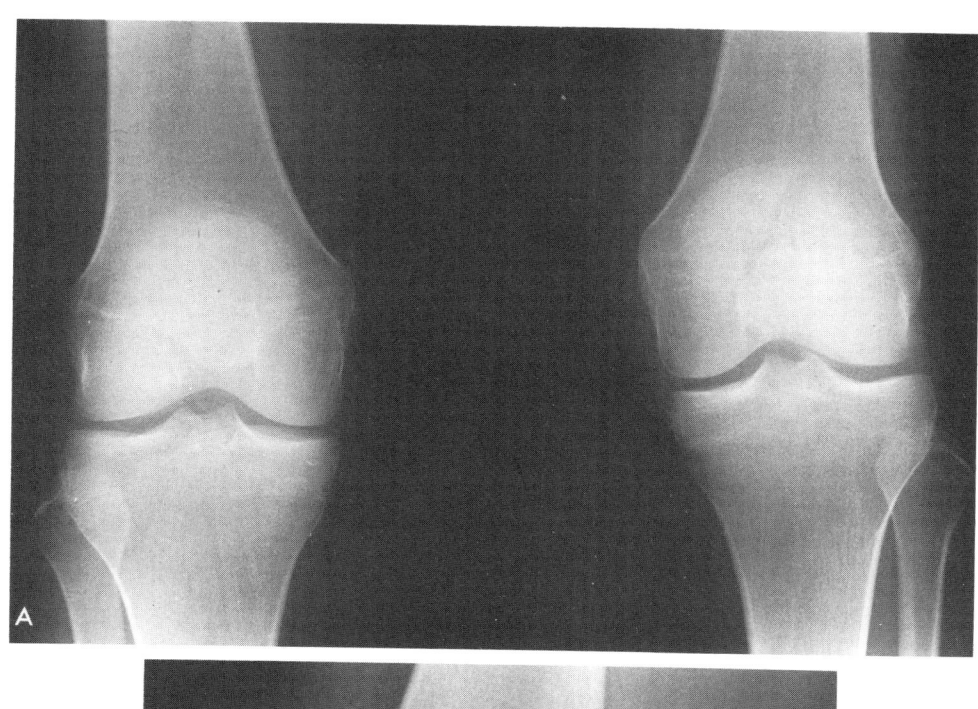

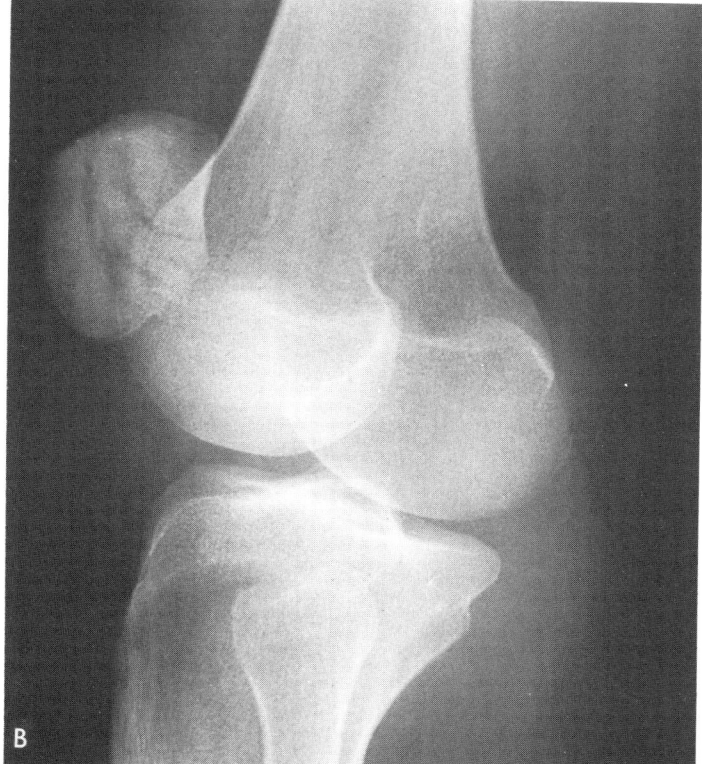

Figure 24-31 A. Bilateral impaction on automobile dashboard resulted in a single patellar fracture. *B.* Oblique views demonstrate undisplaced but multiple fractures. One might expect chondral changes with this degree of crushing and comminution.

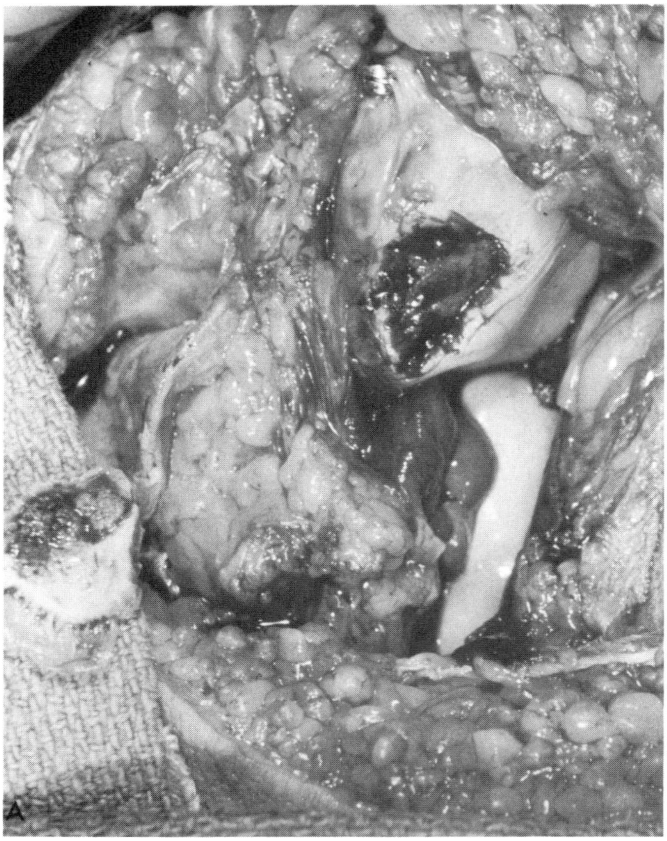

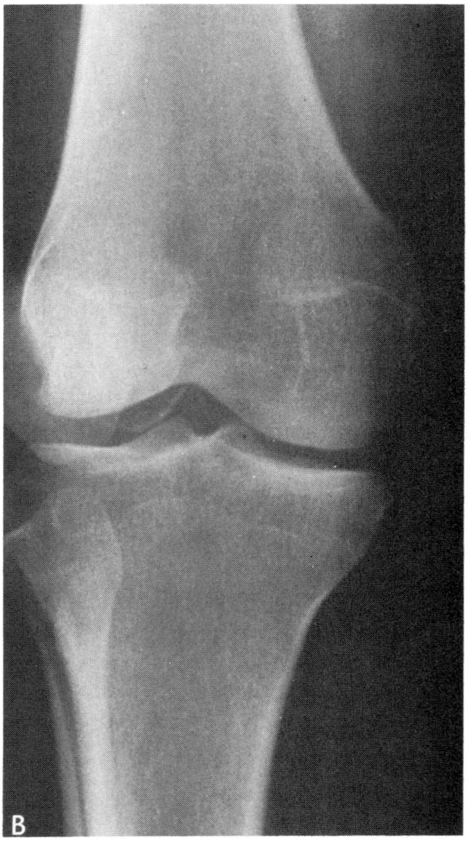

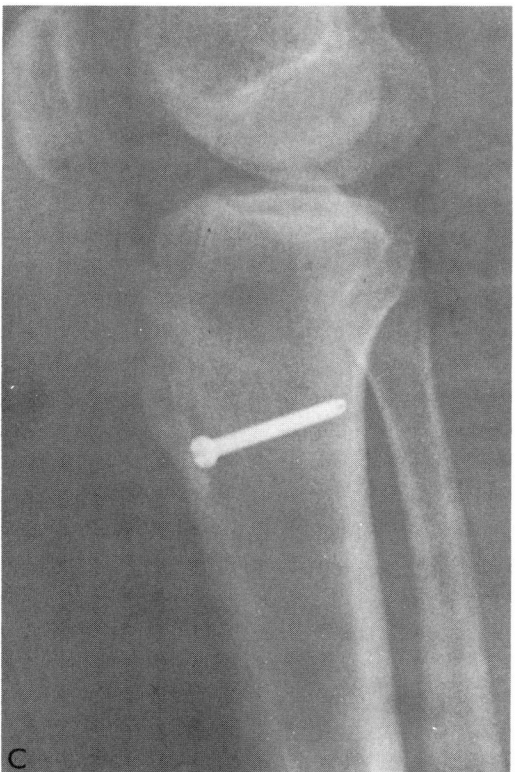

Figure 24-32 *A.* Osteochondral fracture. *B.* The oblique view is the only profile that demonstrates the osteochondral fracture. This fracture fragment was quite large. *C.* Postoperative view of corrective surgery following removal of the fragment.

756

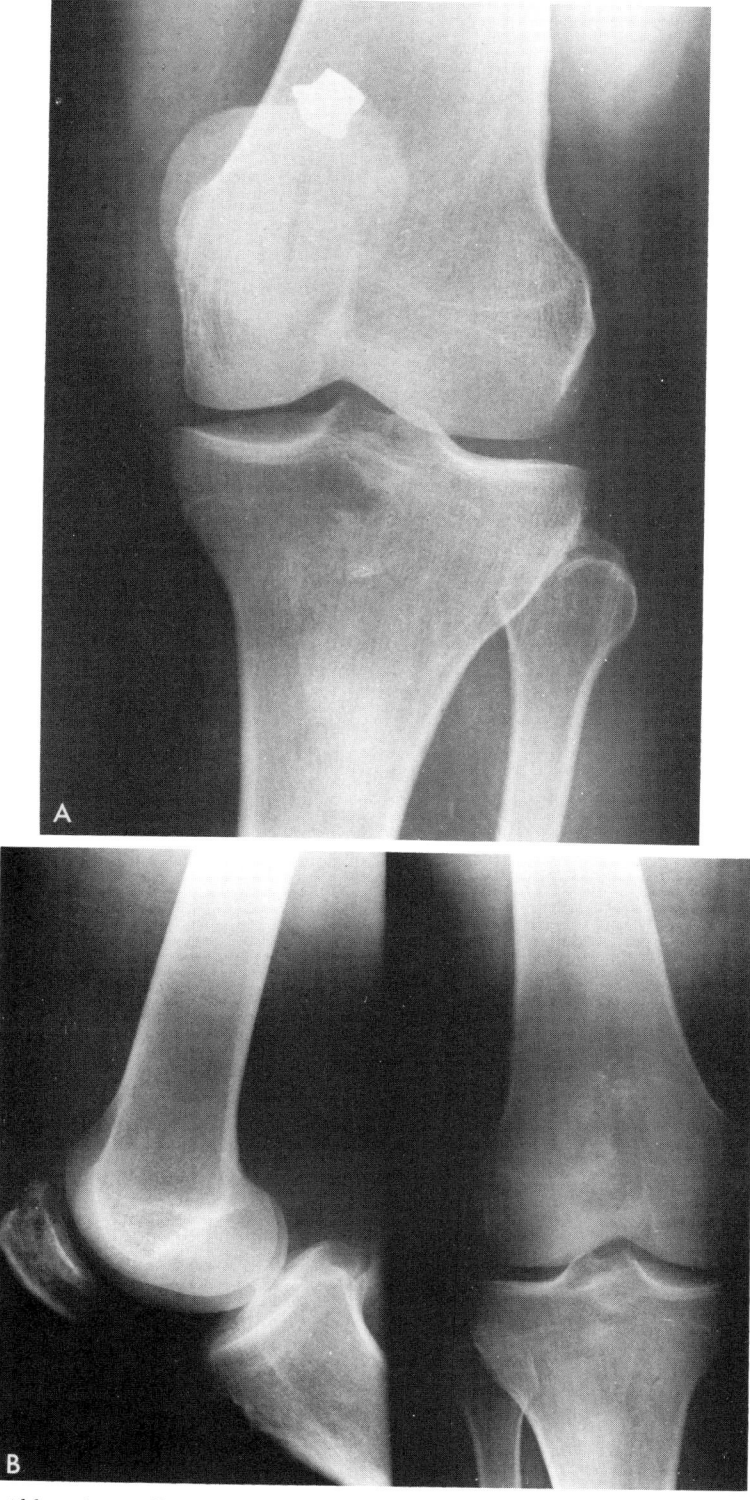

Figure 24–33 *A.* Although not all vertical fractures are on the lateral side, some are obvious on the lateral x-ray. *B.* Vertical shadow in the patella persists despite clinical healing.

mechanism is intact, nonoperative treatment gives excellent results.[63, 64] Aspiration of the hemarthrosis resolves the acute pain. This is followed by application of a compression bandage and splints and, two to three days later, by a well-molded plaster cylinder, applied with the knee held in a few degrees of flexion, from the ankle to the groin. Tromboning of the cast is prevented by molding the plaster firmly about the condyles and incorporating a cast brace hinge at the ankle. The patient is maintained in the cylinder for four to six weeks and is encouraged to place full weight on the affected side. When the plaster is removed, a progressive and intensive pro-

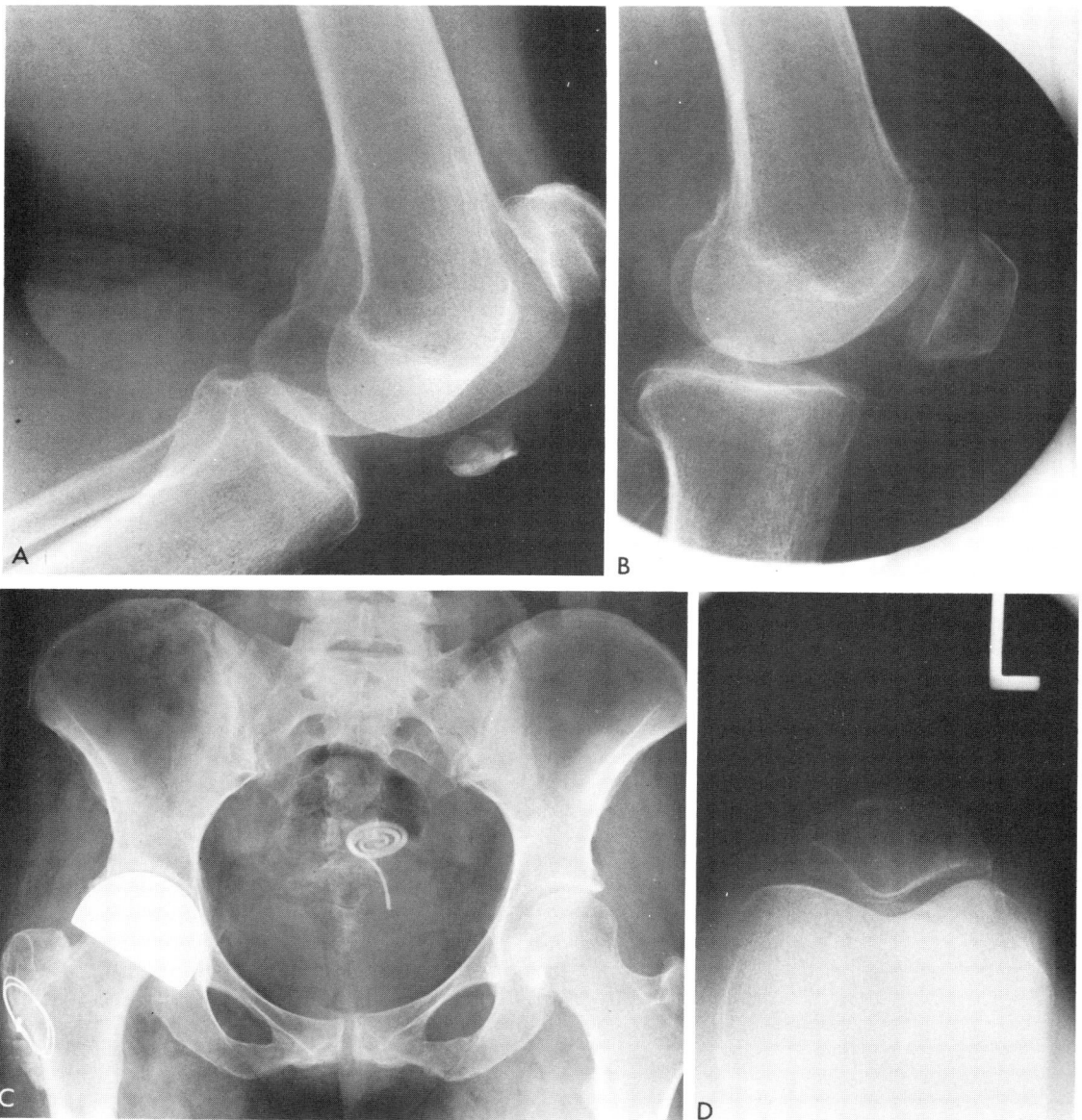

Figure 24–34   A. Flexion view demonstrates wide separation of the fragment. B. The lower pole is excised. C. Concern with this patient's minor fracture is increased because of an excellent cup arthroplasty present for seven years. Not infrequently, multiple fracture problems evolve as a consequence of one another. D. Repair of the quadriceps expansion and multilayer suturing of the bone and the patellar tendon allows beginning motion at three weeks upon removal of a walking cylinder.

gram of exercises for the knee extensors and flexors is instituted.

Early release from splints or plaster and institution of joint motion should be augmented by medical observation until sound union is realized. Age and infirmity together with posttraumatic weakness, pain, and restricted joint motion may interact to reproduce the injury (Fig. 24–34).

OPERATIVE TREATMENT

Historical Aspects

Until the 1850's, all patellar fractures were treated with compression bandages, splints, and elevation of the extremity. Percutaneous clamps, aimed at holding the fragments together, were applied.[91]

Cameron of Glasgow performed the first open operation on a patellar fracture in 1877.[92] In 1892, Berger first employed cerclage, encircling the patella with a metal wire. Partial patellectomy was introduced by Thompson in 1935,[94] and total patellectomy was popularized by the writings of Blodgett and Fairchild[95] and Brooke[96] in the mid-1930's.

In 1909, Heineck laid down the criteria that surgical procedures must meet.[97]

1. The fracture must be reduced.
2. The fragments must be maintained in initimate opposition until union has been effected.
3. The continuity of the soft tissues must be reestablished.
4. The function of the knee joint must be restored.

Operative treatment is indicated when extensor function is completely or partially lost. Three surgical methods have been advocated:

1. Restoration of normal anatomy with union of the patella.
2. Repair of the quadriceps apparatus with retention of the major fragment.
3. Total excision of the patella.

The extent of damage to the lateral expansion of the quadriceps must be assessed and anatomical restoration achieved. Restoration of normal anatomy has also

been recommended for transverse fractures with large fragments, in which the integrity of the articular surface can readily be established.

For transverse fractures, cerclage as well as wire inserted through lontitudinally drilled holes is commonly used and is recommended by Anderson.[98] Bohler has recommended transverse drill holes.[71] The AO group introduced the anterior insertion of one or two wires through drill holes or through the insertion of the quadriceps and patellar tendon.[99] Tightening of these "tension bands" overreduces the fracture, but when the knee is flexed or the quadriceps contracted the pressure of the femoral condyles against the patella compresses the bony fragments together. The use of these tension bands is not restricted to simple transverse fractures. They may also be used in comminuted fractures if combined with two Kirschner wires to give lateral stability; occasionally, partial patellectomy is recommended with this technique. The advantage of this method over conventional circumferential cerclage of the patella is that the fragments do not come apart on the anterior surface. Although we have had no experience with this method; the institution of early motion that is possible with the use of tension bands is appealing. In other methods of wire fixation a plaster cast is applied after the repair. Full weight bearing with crutch support is begun by the second week, and the plaster is removed after four to six weeks.

Because the superior pole of the patella is supplied only by the central penetrating artery, any procedures that involve freeing soft tissue or denuding the bone may compromise the vasculature. Consequently, the wisdom of retaining small superior fragments is questionable because of the possibility of postoperative avascular necrosis. Partial patellectomy with repair of the quadriceps is recommended in fractures with one large and one small fragment, those with one large and a smaller comminuted segment, and those in which a large fragment can be salvaged.[63, 64, 98] To prevent tilting of the fragments, an overlapping repair of the aponeurosis is done after a broad surface of the underlying bone has been denuded (Fig. 24–35).[100] Most authors recommend removal of the lower pole.[63, 64, 94, 98]

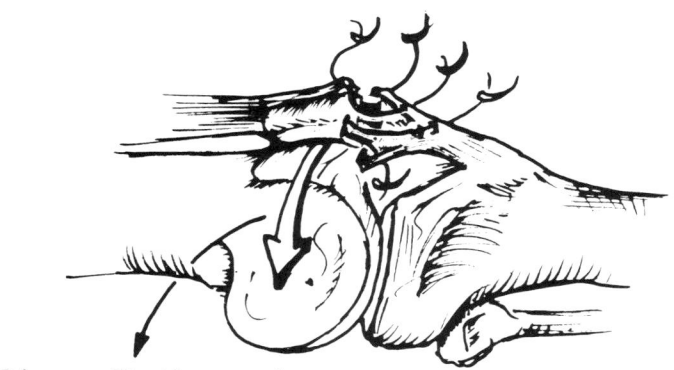

Close Retinaculum

Nestle The Bone Within The Tendon To Prevent Tilting

Figure 24-35   Proper repair of tendon to prevent tilting of fragment.

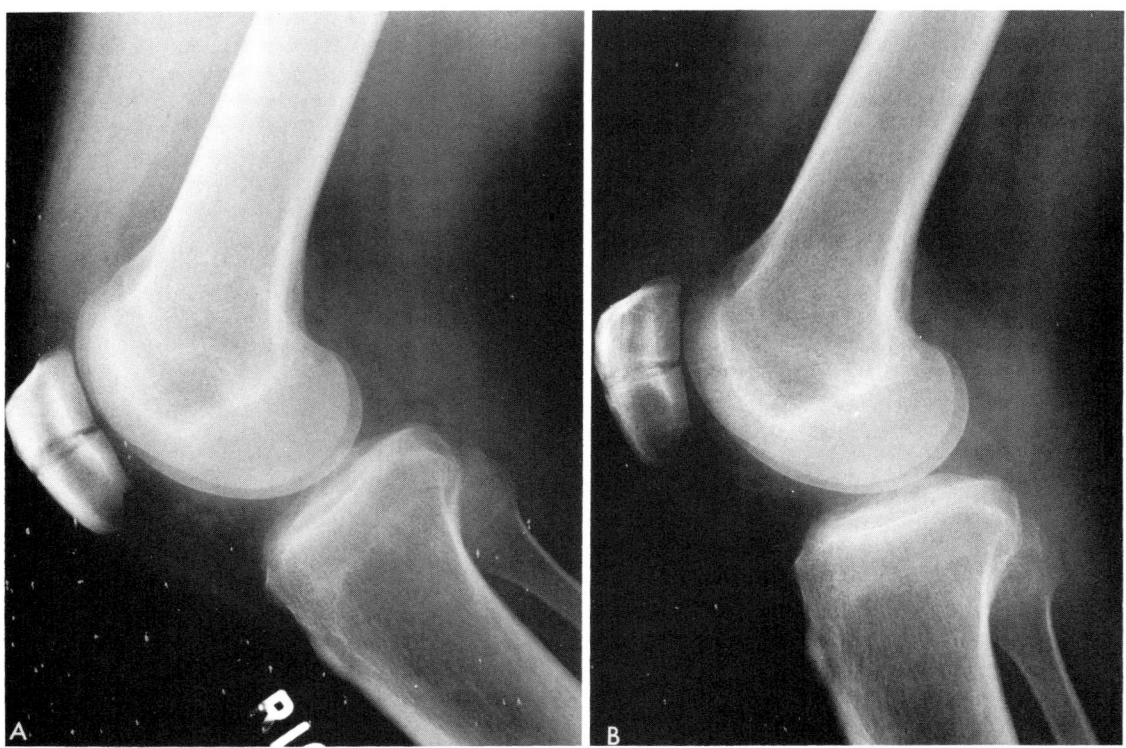

Figure 24-36   *A.* Undisplaced fracture. Quadriceps expansion is maintained. *B.* Removal from plaster at six weeks. The fracture progressed to uneventful healing.

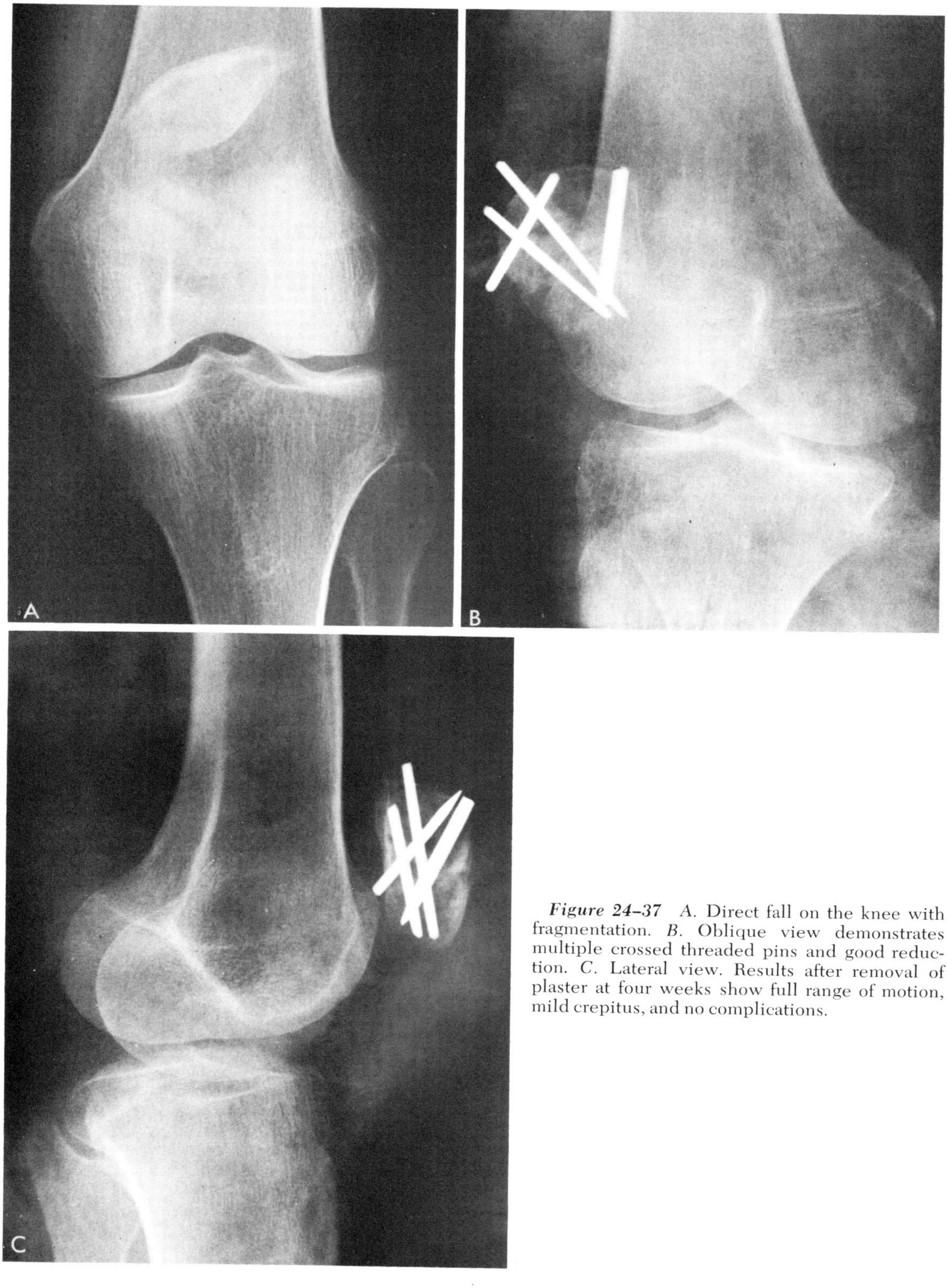

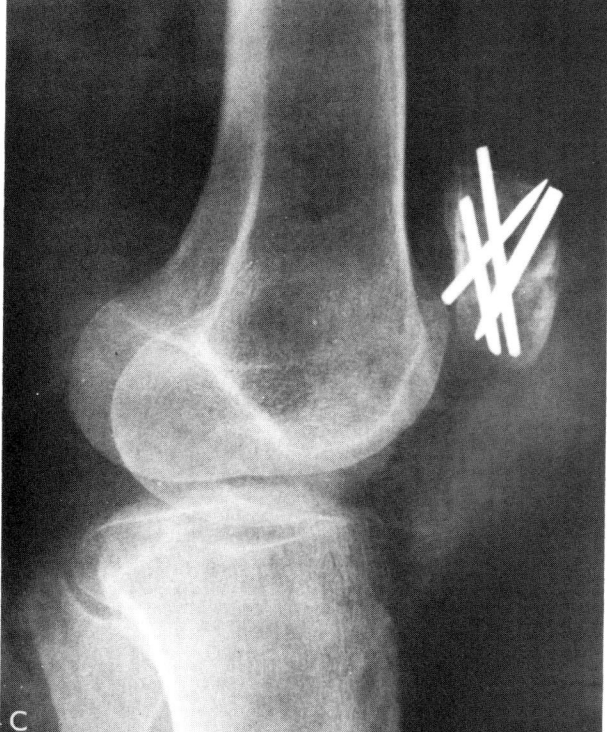

Figure 24-37 A. Direct fall on the knee with fragmentation. B. Oblique view demonstrates multiple crossed threaded pins and good reduction. C. Lateral view. Results after removal of plaster at four weeks show full range of motion, mild crepitus, and no complications.

In comminuted fractures with no large fragments, total excision of the patella is recommended.[63, 64] The gap is closed by suturing the quadriceps tendon to the patellar ligament, with an attempt to avoid laxity in the repair. Plastic methods have also been described.[101]

Recommended Approach

The treatment of patellar fractures and the results depend upon the severity of the initial trauma. When extension is preserved, the fragments separated by less than 3 mm, and the offset less than 2 mm, good to excellent results can be expected from nonoperative treatment (Fig. 24–36).

Since the literature does not suggest one clearly superior method of osteosynthesis, the choice of operative technique is probably of less consequence than the mode of injury. The method selected should assure anatomical restoration and continued stability of the fragments in addition to early removal from plaster, preferably after four weeks, with early institution of active motion. Anatomical and firm repair of the quadriceps expansion should permit early mobilization and should condition the release from plaster, rather than roentgenographic signs of union. If firm fixation is provided and anatomical repair of the quadriceps established, the only reason to restrict early weight bearing is immediate postoperative inflammation. Crutches should be used to aid ambulation, not to substitute for it.

To fix transverse fractures and fractures in which the articular surface is well maintained, we have for many years used threaded, crossed Kirschner wires and Steinmann pins with satisfactory results (Fig. 24–37). When partial excision of the patella is necessary, multiple drill holes are bored and the tendon fixed to the retained fragment by nestling the bone into the tendon in a layered fashion. If this is not possible, as is sometimes the case in badly comminuted fractures, all of the fragments should be discarded. The attendant loss of quadriceps function, which may cause difficulty in descending stairs, slopes, and ramps, is definitely preferable to the results of delayed patellectomy. These can include chronic quadriceps wasting, chronic synovitis, and eventual osteoarthritis. Patellectomy performed immediately permits proper repair of the quadriceps mechanism and affords more rapid rehabilitation of supporting muscle and return of function, particularly in younger patients.

SPRAIN FRACTURES

Sprain fractures are a special kind of ligament-bone injury that is most often seen in adolescents and young children. These fractures are caused by ligament stress, which results in the avulsion of a fragment or fragments of bone at the site of ligamentous insertion. Displacement of the avulsed fragments represents a third-degree ligamentous injury that is reflected in joint instability. The true significance of these injuries is sometimes lost in the general diagnosis of "chip fracture."

CRUCIATE LIGAMENTS

Sprain fractures involving the cruciate ligaments occur at their rather extensive tibial insertions, and the avulsed fragments have measured up to 24 by 11 mm.[102] Mechanical interference with joint motion, ligamentous laxity, and acute hemarthrosis are the clinical manifestations of displaced fractures, but one should remain alert to the possibility of concomitant internal derangement of the capsuloligamentous complexes and of the menisci. Open reduction is the treatment of choice for displaced fractures. At the time of surgery the anterior horn of either meniscus may be found interposed between the fragments and in such instances should be retracted, but not excised, to allow fracture reduction (Figs. 24–38 and 24–39).

MISCELLANEOUS AVULSION FRACTURES

Avulsion fractures occur about the skeletally mature knee at the site of tendon or ligament insertion and are significant to the extent that they influence knee stability.

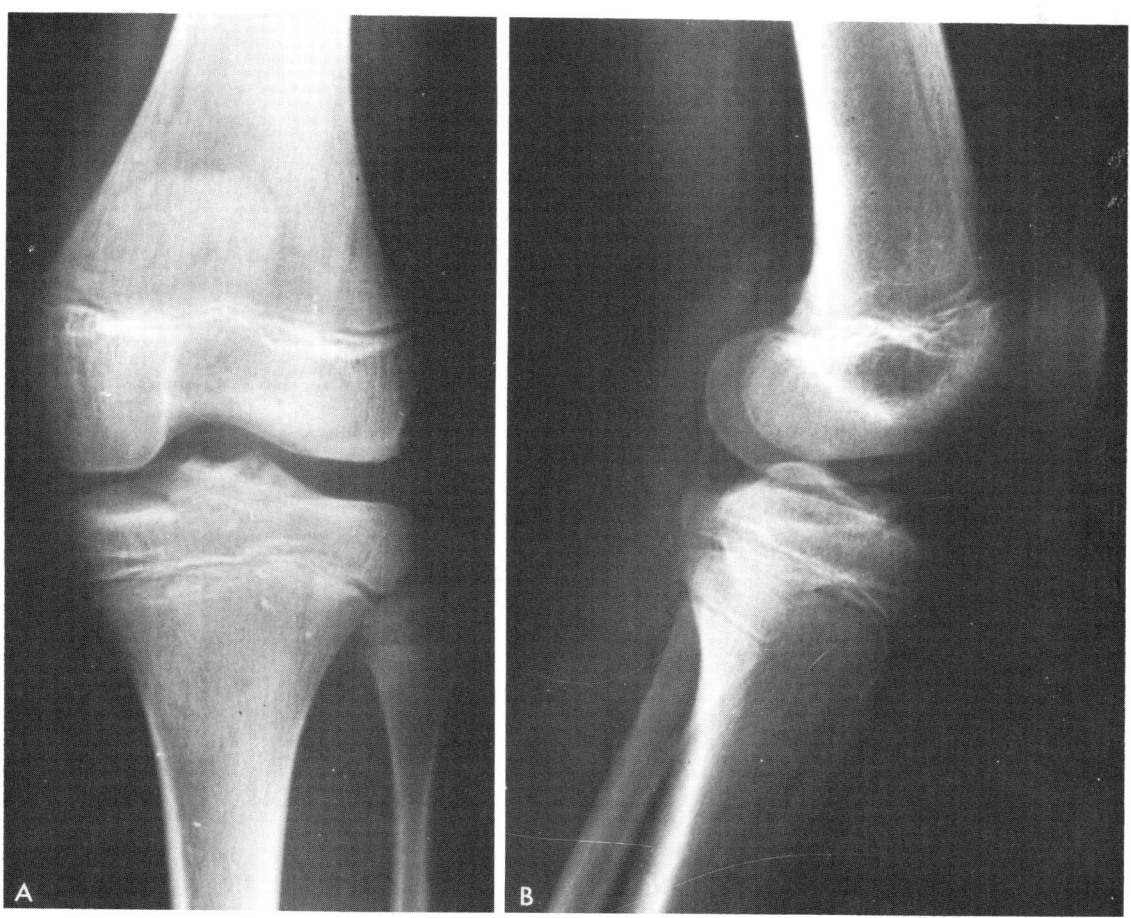

Figure 24–38 Sprain fracture of anterior tibial spine involving the tibial attachment of the anterior cruciate ligament as seen in the anteroposterior (A) and lateral (B) projections.

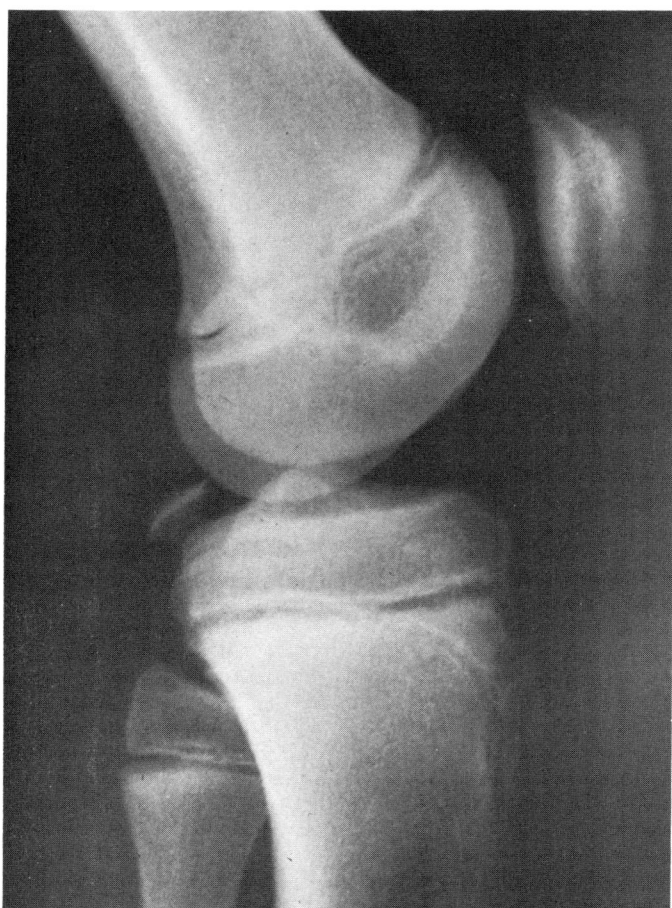

Figure 24–39   Sprain fracture involving the tibial attachment of the posterior cruciate ligament. It was treated by primary open reduction and internal fixation through a posterior approach.

Avulsion Fracture of the Fibular Head

These fractures (Fig. 24–40) may involve the insertions of the conjoined tendon of the biceps femoris muscle and the fibular collateral ligament. As a consequence of varus stress there may be associated injury to the lateral structures of the knee, including the arcuate ligament complex, anterior cruciate ligament, lateral capsular ligament, iliotibial band, posterior cruciate ligament, and popliteus tendon as well as the gastrocnemius muscle and menisci. The injury produces posterolateral or combined anterolateral-posterolateral rotary instability of the knee. It is essential that the function of the common peroneal nerve be fully assessed and documented at the time of initial evaluation and surgery and its status carefully monitored during the early postoperative period. Preoperative varus stress films should be obtained with great caution to avoid added injury to the nerve. Primary soft tissue repair and fracture reduction are required to restore optimal stability, but residual neural deficit following injury to the peroneal nerve is not uncommon.[103]

Avulsion Fractures of the Tubercle of Gerdy

These fractures involve the tibial insertion of the iliotibial band and usually result in varus instability. There may be concomitant damage to any of the lateral structures of the knee; these injuries are best treated by prompt open reduction and fixation and soft tissue repair.

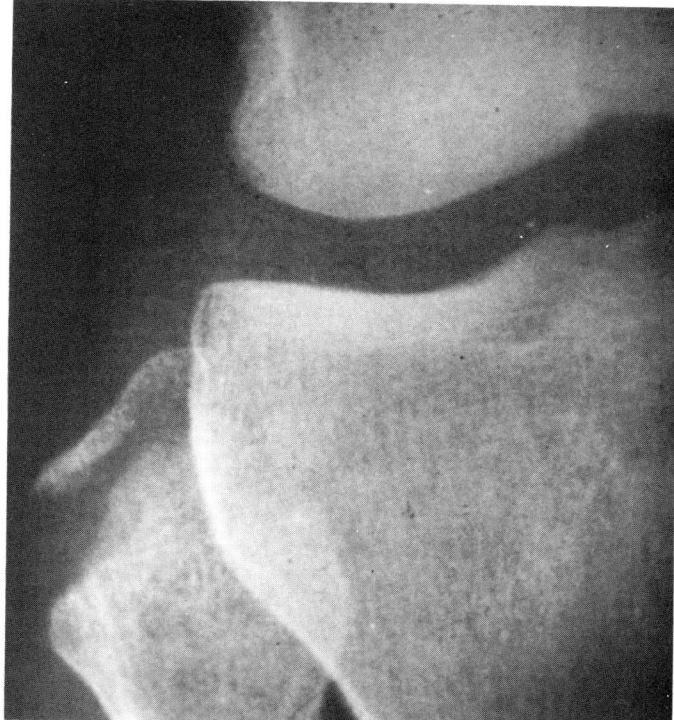

Figure 24–40 Avulsion fracture of the fibular head involving the conjoined tendon and fibular collateral ligament. It was treated by primary reduction.

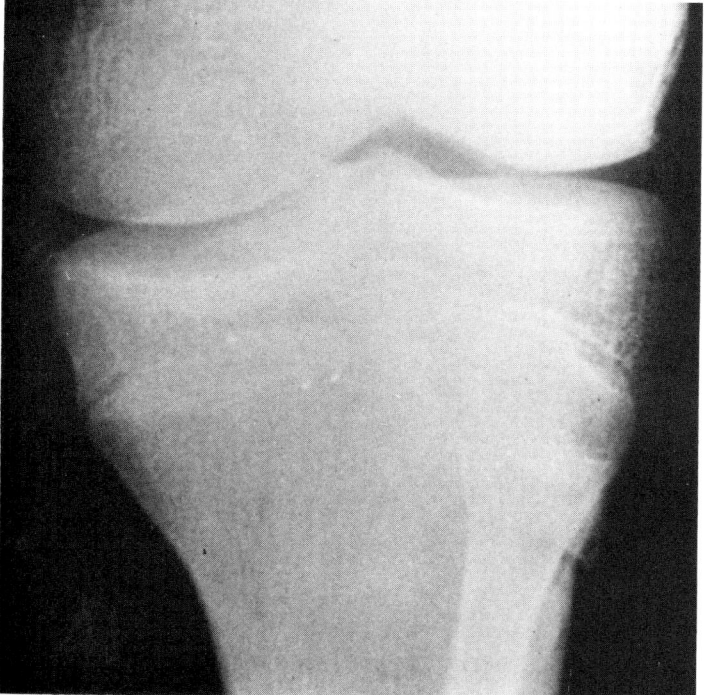

Figure 24–41 Sprain fracture. Medial capsular ligament is seen on the oblique view but is not visualized on the standard posteroanterior view.

Sprain Fracture of the Medial Capsular Ligament

A torsional valgus injury to the knee may result in disruption of the meniscotibial component of the medial capsular ligament, with avulsion of the distal end from the tibia.[104] The peripheral meniscal attachment is usually intact in such cases, but failure to relocate the avulsed fragment may result in a hypermobile meniscus, rendering it vulnerable to injury and producing joint dysfunction. Radiographically, the lesion appears as a small osseous fragment medially adjacent to the joint margin. Since the lesion may be obscured by the tibia on the standard anteroposterior view, an oblique view is usually necessary to disclose it. The importance of a complete roentgenographic examination of the injured knee cannot be overemphasized (Fig. 24–41).

FRACTURE VARIANTS INVOLVING THE PATELLA AND DISTAL KNEE EXTENSOR MECHANISM

Tibial Tubercle

These fractures, caused by avulsion of the quadriceps mechanism, are uncommon, and for the most part are seen before closure of the proximal tibial epiphysis in the 12- to 16-year age group.[105] The fracture variants have been classified by Watson-Jones[106] and by Hand and co-workers.[107] Basically, they fall into two categories: those that involve the tibial tubercle as a separate ossification center, and those that extend cephalad into the proximal tibial epiphysis. The latter are in effect Salter 3 fractures. If the tibial tubercle is completely cartilaginous, x-rays may at first be misleading. However, the diagnosis can be established by a history of sudden, well-localized pain associated with vigorous quadriceps contraction with the foot fixed and subsequent inability to support full weight on the extremity. These findings are coupled with the physical signs of hemarthrosis, local swelling, and tenderness and radiographic evidence of patella alta on the lateral view with the knee flexed 30 degrees.

Treatment consists of accurate reduction of displaced fractures. Growth disturbances, such as leg length inequality and genu

recurvatum due to epiphyseal injury, are theoretically possible but seldom observed.

Partite Patella

Persistence of separate patellar ossification centers may cause difficulty in evaluating the knee following trauma. Bipartite and tripartite anomalies are most common, but multiple divisions are possible. Although these are usually asymptomatic developmental variants, they can on occasion give rise to disability (Fig. 24–42). The symptoms may be gradual in onset, as seen in athletes, or may develop suddenly after direct trauma. Symptoms include localized pain and pressure and, less often, painful catching and swelling. Symptoms are believed to be caused by abnormal mobility at the synchondrosis between the osseous fragments. The most common physical findings are localized tenderness and a bony prominence over the superolateral aspect of the patella with effusion and occasional palpable creptitation during active motion. In Weaver's series of 21 cases of symptomatic bipartite patella, 10 were unilateral.[108] The lesion may involve the distal patellar pole, the lateral margin, or the superolateral pole,[109] the latter being by far the most common. Acute fracture can be excluded radiographically, as the opposing edges of the partite patella are smooth and rounded. Clinically, acute hemarthrosis is absent. Persistent symptoms, unresponsive to a nonoperative regimen of initial rest followed by quadriceps rehabilitation, are best treated by excision of the accessory fragment or fragments and reattachment of the vastus lateralis tendon to the parent patella.

Peripheral Fractures of the Patella

Fractures of the patella involving only small portions of the periphery, i.e., the superior and inferior poles and the medial and lateral margins, represent strain or sprain injuries at the attachment of tendon or capsule-retinaculum complexes and result from indirect violence.

Fractures of the lateral margin of the patella may be produced by direct force, since the bone is thinner and more vulner-

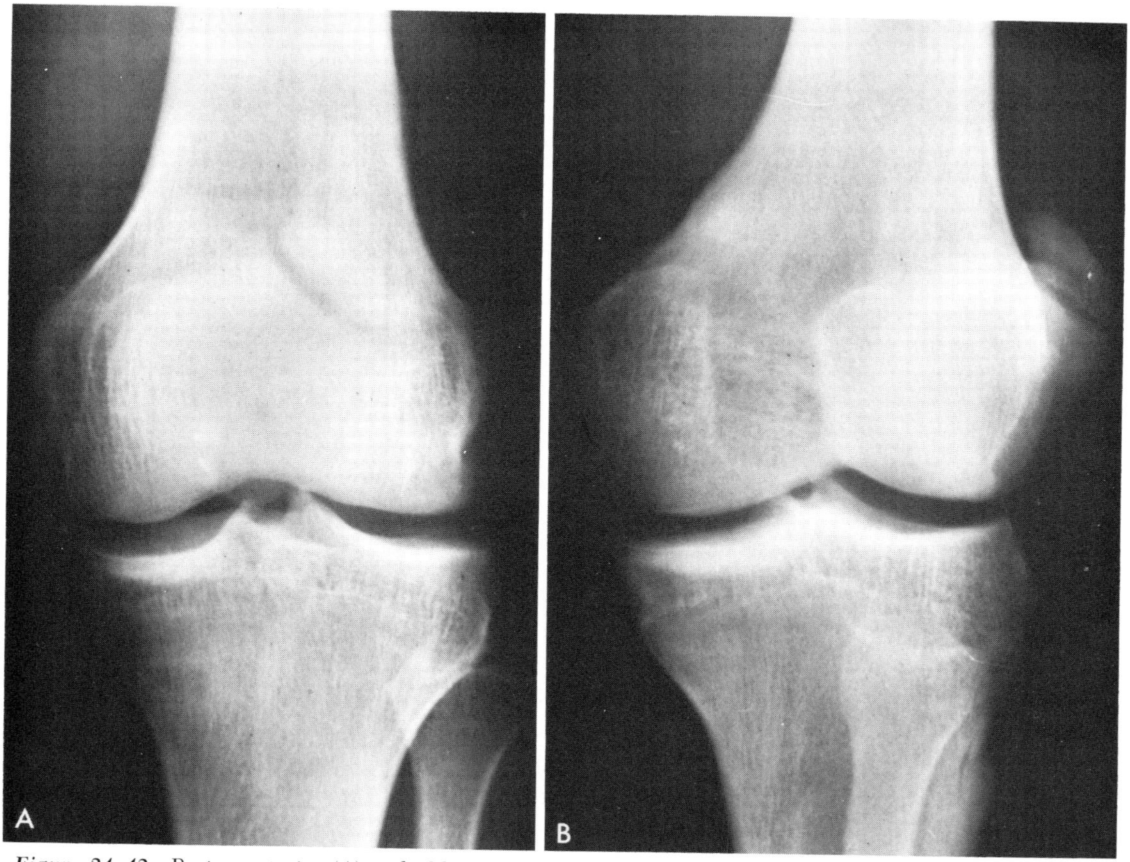

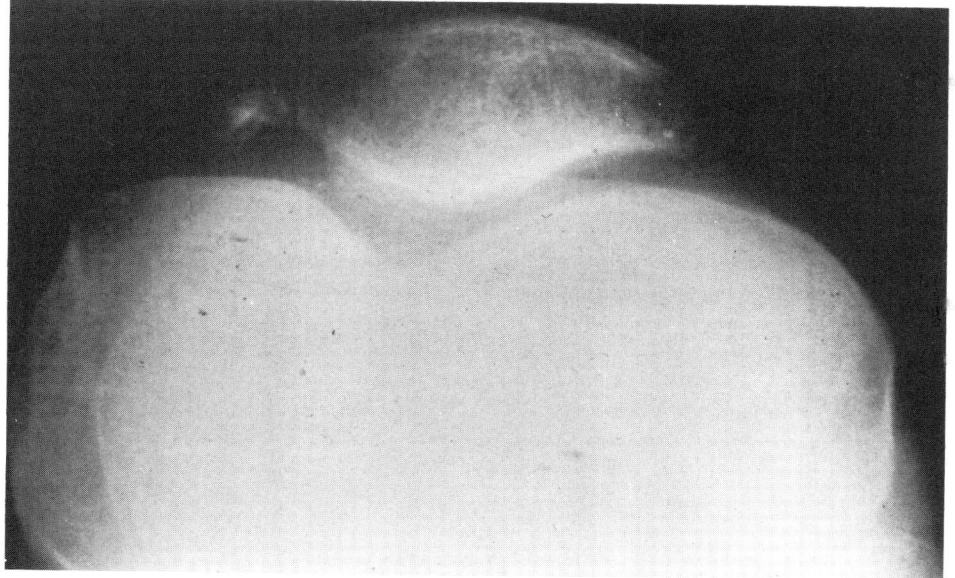

Figure 24–42 Posteroanterior (A) and oblique (B) projections of a bipartite patella in a professional athlete, rendered symptomatic by a direct blow to the anterior aspect of the knee. Treated nonsurgically.

Figure 24–43 Skyline view of the patella in a patient with chronic lateral dislocation, revealing heterotopic bone formation contiguous with the medial aspect of the patella.

767

able in this area, particularly with the knee acutely flexed.[110] Standard anteroposterior and oblique x-rays of the knees may not disclose the fracture, but a skyline view of the patellofemoral joint is usually diagnostic (Fig. 24–43). Treatment consists of excision of the osseous fragment and repair of the lateral retinaculum and capsule. An intraoperative search should be made for an accompanying chondral injury to the articular surface of the patella with loose body formation.

Avulsion fractures of the medial margin of the patella with the medial retinaculum may occur as the patella is forcefully dislocated laterally. Coleman reported that this osteochondral fracture of the medial aspect of the patella had a propensity to form a loose body within the knee joint and claimed the lesion was diagnostic of recurrent patellar dislocation.[111] The lesion representative of lateral dislocation of the patella may also take the form of single or multiple bony ossicles in the same location; these form as a consequence of hematomatous ossification at the site of tearing of the medial retinaculum from the periosteum as the patella dislocates laterally. Such lesions require time to develop and are not seen on skyline films taken shortly after the original injury.[112] An osteochondral fracture associated with acute lateral dislocation supports opinion favoring primary surgical repair for patellar dislocations. The lesion should be excised at the time of surgery. Continued knee disability with locking may develop following dislocations of the patella treated nonoperatively. This results from radiographically invisible chondral loose bodies shorn from the undersurface of the patella or articular surface of the lateral femoral condyle at the time of injury.

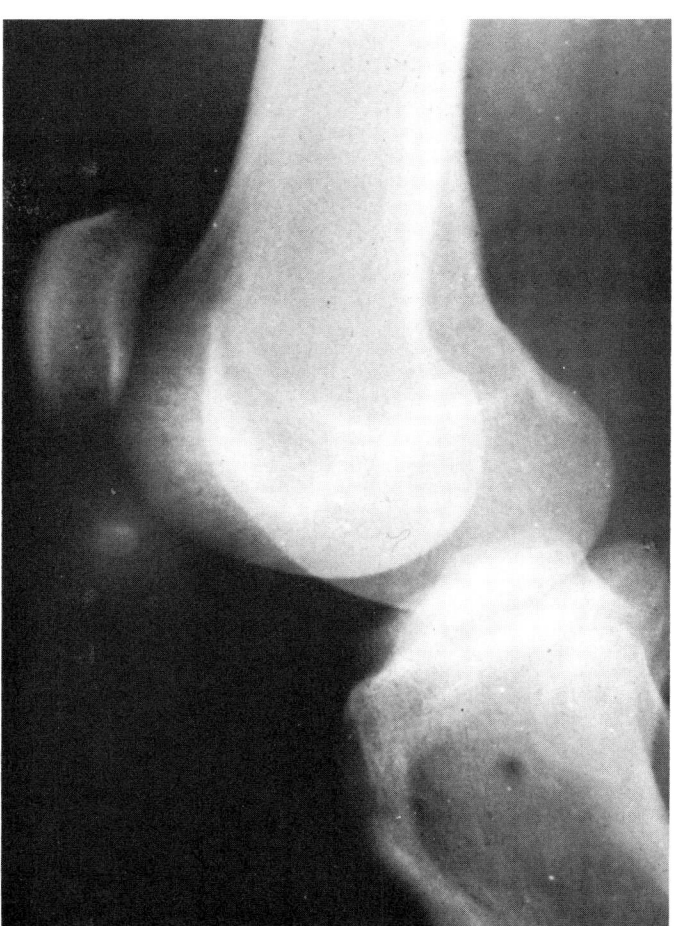

Figure 24–44   Complete rupture of the infrapatellar tendon. A small ossicle marks the normal station of the patella.

Avulsion fractures of the superior and inferior poles of the patella are significant to the extent that they compromise function of the quadriceps and patellar tendons, respectively.

As a result of violent quadriceps contraction with the knee fixed or actively flexing, the quadriceps insertion onto the superior pole of the patella may pull loose, with a shell of cortical bone visible on the lateral x-ray. The clinical picture of incomplete avulsions is one of localized pain aggravated by active quadriceps contraction and passive stretch. As swelling subsides, a defect may be palpable immediately supradjacent to the patella, particularly during active contraction of the quadriceps. Partial injuries with good quadriceps function may be treated nonoperatively, but complete avulsion of the quadriceps mechanism with extensor loss requires reattachment of the quadriceps aponeurosis to the patella.

A similar injury may occur at the inferior pole of the patella from avulsion of the patellar tendon with an accompanying fragment of bone. In some cases there will be a long-standing history of patellar tendinitis, the so-called jumper's knee. A lateral x-ray shows the avulsed fragment at the normal station of the inferior pole and patella alta of the parent patella (Fig. 24–44). Surgical repair is necessary to restore normal function to the extensor mechanism. A retention wire passed through the patella and tibial tubercle may be used to maintain the proper positon of the patella against the pull of the quadriceps muscle and protect the repair site during the early stages of healing.

DISLOCATIONS OF THE KNEE

Dislocations of the knee, as reported in the literature, are a rare injury. Kennedy, reviewing the records of 700,000 compensation injuries for the period from 1955 to 1957, was able to trace just two cases.[113] Hoover found only 14 cases admitted over 48 years to the Mayo Clinic.[114] Clinical diagnosis of knee dislocations is not difficult. Roentgenograms, taken to confirm the clinical impression and to exclude associated fractures, demonstrate the dislocation, but the severely injured knee may be anatomically oriented by muscular contrac-

ture when first seen. It may well be that dislocation is more common than the literature attests, the specific diagnosis being reserved for those unreduced dislocations noted clinically in the emergency room.

SURGICAL ANATOMY

It seems likely that complete dislocation cannot occur if either of the cruciate ligaments is intact. According to Palmar, the posterior cruciate ligament prevents excessive internal rotation of the tibia on the femur, and the anterior cruciate ligament prevents abnormal external rotation of the tibia on the femur.[115] Hughston believes that the anterior cruciate prevents hyperextension of the knee and that the posterior cruciate is the basic stabilizer of the knee.[116]

The medial collateral ligament is the largest ligament in the region of the knee. Since some portions of the medial collateral ligament are taut during the entire range of knee motion., it helps to stabilize the knee against both anteroposterior and mediolateral displacement.[117] The lateral collateral ligament serves primarily as a stabilizer of the knee on its lateral aspect during the first 20 or 30 degrees of flexion. The posterior capsule, reinforced by the oblique popliteal and popliteal ligaments, stabilizes the knee posteromedially and medially. When the medial collateral ligament is completely ruptured it is reasonable to expect a tear in the posterior capsule (Fig. 24–45). The importance of the posterior capsule has been emphasized by O'Donoghue and Kennedy.[118, 119]

The severity of injury in knee dislocations is ultimately related to the damage sustained by the contents of the popliteal space. Injury to the popliteal artery is related to the peculiar anatomy of the region. The popliteal artery originates at the tendinous hiatus of the adductor magnum muscle, by which it is firmly anchored to the femoral shaft. Within the popliteal space it gives off five arterial branches: paired superior and inferior genicular and unpaired middle genicular arteries. The arteries arise immediately above and below the knee joint. The popliteal artery passes distally below the heads of the gastrocnemius mus-

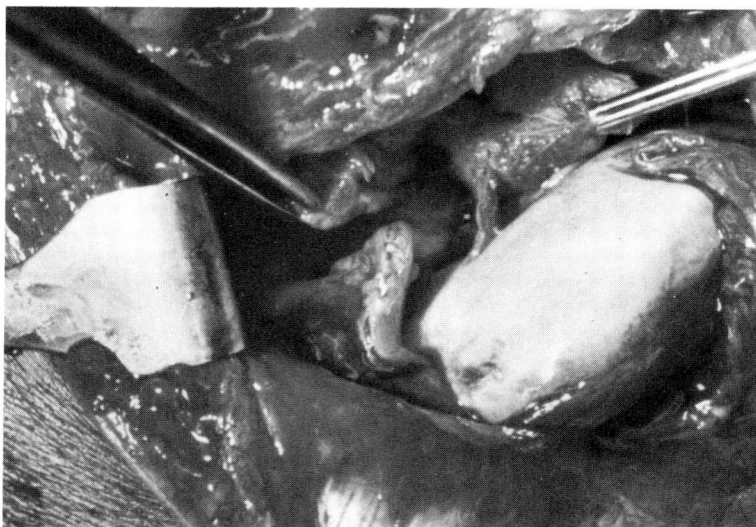

Figure 24–45 Ligamentous injury. Ruptured anterior and posterior cruciate ligaments, involving menisci joint capsule as well as medial joint.

cle and then beneath the tendinous arch of the soleus muscle, by which it is held firmly against the underlying bone. At this point the artery ends by division into posterior and anterior tibial arteries. The latter passes immediately through the interosseous membrane. Moored at either end, the popliteal artery passes like a bowstring across the popliteal space. Arterial rupture tends to occur at the point of emergence of a major branch. Skeletal dislocation causes stretching of the popliteal artery. The nerves in the popliteal space are not anatomically fixed and therefore are less likely to be distinguished. Injury to the nerve, if it occurs, is usually traction in continuity, which is not irreparable.

MECHANISM OF INJURY

Complete dislocation of the knee is caused by severe direct or indirect violence. The type of dislocation depends upon the direction and location of the force. Fractures are frequently accompanied by dislocation. Attempts have been made to use stress machines and cadaver knees to delineate the mechanics of injury.[113] It was demonstrated that anterior dislocation could result from hyperextension of the knee, since the popliteal artery ruptured at 50 degrees of hyperextension. A posterior dislocation was more difficult to produce, however.[113]

A review of the histories of patients with dislocations identifies vehicular injuries (motorcycles, automobiles, and tractors) as a major contributor in approximately 50 per cent of cases. Entrapment of the extremity, falls, and sports injuries are other causes.

CLASSIFICATION

Dislocations are described in terms of tibial displacement with respect to other structures about the knee. Using this terminology, there are five main types of dislocation: anterior, posterior, lateral, medial, and rotary.[113, 120] It is the concensus of more recent reviewers that this terminology avoids confusion.[121, 122]

TREATMENT

All authors advocate immediate reduction of the knee dislocation. In most instances the reduction is accomplished quite easily by gentle but sustained traction. Following reduction, a careful evaluation of the circulatory status of the extremity must be carried out. The initial view of the extremity cannot be used to indicate the probability of rupture of the popliteal vessels. This is because the overwhelming force producing the dislocation and the immediate deformity are invariably much greater than was realized at the time of examination, when the joint "evidence" has been reduced to at least a relative alignment.[123]

The presence of warm skin over the dorsum of the foot and toes is not evidence of an intact blood supply, since it may be found in the presence of complete arterial occlusion.[124] The presence of full dorsalis pedis and posteror tibial pulses following reduction does not invariably mean that there has been no injury to the popliteal vessels. Contusion of the arteries or severe injury to the intimal and medial layers without the loss of continuity is a common consequence of fracture injury, and thrombosis formation may ensue within a few hours to several days.[125, 126]

The period during which an extremity deprived of its major source of blood remains ischemic strongly influences the chances for survival upon restoration of circulation. Progress in the field of early definitive surgery was disappointing in World War II.[127] Gangrene has been reported to occur in 70 per cent of patients with ligation of the femoral and popliteal arteries.[128]

The time lag between occlusion and restoration of circulation is critical. Experimental studies[129] suggest that the maximum allowable delay is from six to eight hours if permanent ischemic lesions are to be averted.

The methods of arterial repair depend upon local conditions. The importance of adequate debridement of the damaged artery has been stressed.[130] Delay in effective restoration of circulation is frequently the result of faulty diagnosis. The signs of distal arterial insufficiency are: diminished or absent pulsation below the knee; ischemic pain distal to the injury; numbness; parasthenia or complete absence of cutaneous sensation; pallor; coolness; paralysis; and absence of pulsation on oscillometry. Concomitant peripheral edema may confuse the issue. The need for a definitive diagnosis is greatest when it is most difficult—in the case with multiple injuries. In these and all other cases, arteriography offers significant advantages.[131]

Although attitudes toward ligamentous injury to the knee have changed over time, a

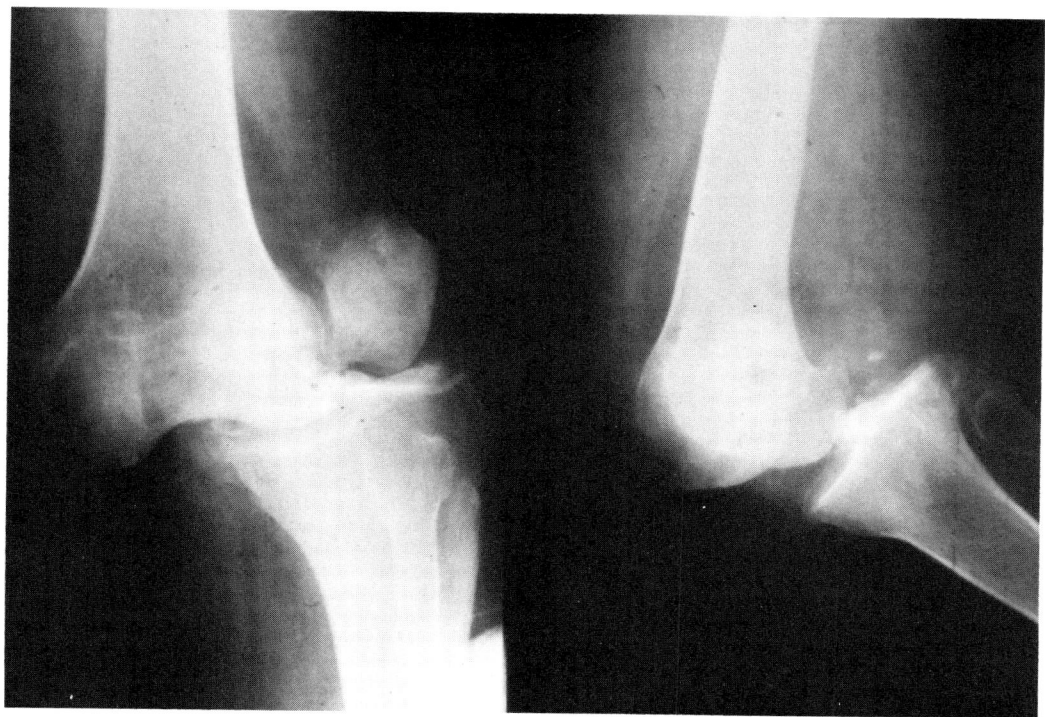

Figure 24-46 Posterior dislocation.

recent paper suggests that the results of conservative care are acceptable in uncomplicated cases.[132] In general, immobilization for long periods tends to reduce movement. In contradistinction to the reports of conservative care, a closely followed series, gathered over a short time, led to the conclusions that prompt closed reduction, early repair of all damaged ligaments, and careful evaluation and monitoring of the peripheral circulation, with vascular repair when necessary, achieve optimal results.

Posterolateral dislocations differ from other types of dislocations in several respects (Fig. 24–46). This injury is primarily a rotary dislocation without significant displacement. It is accompanied by buttonholing of the medial femoral condyle through the medial capsule and invagination of the tibial collateral ligaments within the joint.[133] Clinical findings are constant. The extremity lies in 30 to 40 degrees of medial rotation and some flexion. The medial femoral condyle is prominent and easily palpated under the skin. Immediately distal to the bulging femoral condyle the skin is puckered and drawn into a transverse groove. The groove becomes more pronounced when attempts are made to reduce the dislocation. There is generally no evidence of injury to nerves or vessels. In this injury, a sudden force produces abduction and medial rotation of the tibia on the femur when the knee is flexed. The literature suggests that these medial dislocations are rare, anterior dislocations being most common. The most usual neurological lesion is peroneal palsy.

Recommended Treatment

It is our position that the recommendation of Meyers and Harvey[134] be carried out, in light of the excellent results with repair of ruptured ligaments of the knee and the realization that reconstruction is a poor substitute for immediate repair. The medial approach described by O'Donoghue[135] allows repair of the anterior cruciate and medial collateral ligaments. A smaller lateral incision is needed to suture the anterior cruciate lesion and to allow exploration of the lateral arcuate ligament. Repair of all torn ligaments is accomplished as soon as it

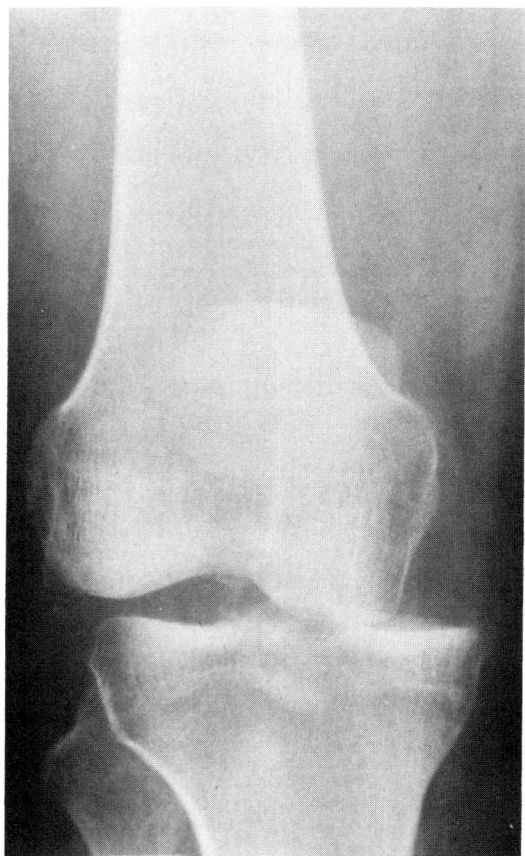

Figure 24–47 Lateral dislocation of the knee partially reduced in the emergency room.

is certain that the popliteal vessels have not been damaged.

If there are doubts after arteriography, the vessels should be explored. To assure stability during repair a transfixing intercondylar pin may be used in the nonarticular space of the joint. The extremity is placed in plaster for six weeks. Progressive motion is gained with supportive weight bearing over the next six weeks.

REFERENCES

Distal Femur

1. Pott, P.: Some Few General Remarks on Fractures and Dislocations. 2nd Ed. London, 1773, p. 37.
2. Neer, C. S., Grantham, S. A., and Shelton, M. L.: Supracondylar fractures of the adult femur. J. Bone Joint Surg., *49A*:591–613, 1967.

3. Wade, P. A., and Okinaka, A. J.: The problem of the femur in the aged person. Am. J. Surg., 97:499–512, 1959.
4. Smith, N.: Observations on fractures of the femur with an account of a new splint. *In*: Smith, N. R. (ed.): Medical and Surgical Memoirs. Baltimore, William A. Francis, 1831, p. 139.
5. Buck, G.: An improved method of treating fractures of the thigh. Trans. N. Y. Acad. Med., 2:232–250, 1861.
6. Russell, R. H.: Theory and method in extension of the thigh. Br. Med. J., 2:637–638, 1921.
7. Steinmann, F. R.: Eine neue extension methode in der frakturenbehandlung. Zentralbl. Chir., 34:938–942, 1907.
8. Kirschner, M.: Ueber Nagelextension. Beitr. Klin. Chir., 64:266–279, 1909.
9. Modlin, J.: Double skeletal traction in battle fractures of the lower femur. Bull. U. S. Army Med. Dept., 4:119–120, 1945.
10. Mahorner, H. R., and Bradburn, M.: Fractures of the femur. Report of 308 cases. Surg. Gynecol. Obstet., 56:1066–1079, 1933.
11. Umansky, A. L.: Blade-plate internal fixation for fracture of the distal end of the femur. Bull. Hosp. Joint Dis., 9:18–21, 1948.
11a. White, E. H., and Russin, L. A.: Supracondylar fractures of femur. Am. Surg., 22:801–820, 1956.
12. Aetenberg, A. R., and Shorkey, R. L.: Blade-plate fixation in non-union and in complicated fractures of the supracondylar region of the femur. J. Bone Joint Surg., 31A:312–316, 1949.
13. Scuderi, C., and Ippolito, A.: Non-union of supracondylar fractures of the femur. J. Int. Coll. Surg., 17:1–18, 1952.
14. Klingensmith, W., Oles, P., and Martinez, H.: Arterial injuries associated with dislocation of the knee or fracture of the lower femur. Surg. Gynecol. Obstet., 120:961–964, 1965.
15. Hoover, N. W.: Injuries of the popliteal artery associated with fractures and dislocations. Surg. Clin. North Am., 41:1099–1112, 1961.
16. Bergan, F.: Traumatic initial rupture of the popliteal artery with acute ischemia of the limb in cases with supracondylar fractures of the femur. J. Cardiovasc. Surg., 4:300–302, 1963.
17. Thomas, H. J.: The Treatment of Deformities. Fractures and Disease of Bones in the Lower Extremities. London, H. K. Lewis, 1890.
18. Pearson, M. C., and Drummond, J.: Fractured Femurs: Their Treatment by Caliper Extensions. London, Oxford University Press, 1919.
19. Nicholson, J. T.: Personal communication.
20. Mooney, V., Nickel, V. L., Harvey, J. P., and Snelson, R.: Cast brace treatment for fractures of the distal part of the femur. J. Bone Joint Surg., 52A:1563–1578, 1970.
21. Moll, J. H.: The cast brace walking treatment of open and closed femoral fractures. South. Med. J., 66:345–352, 1973.
22. Connolly, J. F., Dehne, E., and LaFollette, B.: Closed reduction and early cast brace ambulation in the treatment of femoral fractures. J. Bone Joint Surg., 55A:1581–1599, 1973.
23. Zickel, R. E., Fietti, V. G., Lawsing, J. F. III., and Cochran, G. V.: A new intramedullary fixation device for the distal third of the femur. J. Bone Joint Surg., 59B:505, 1977.
24. Elliot, R. B.: Fractures of the femoral condyles. Experiments with a new design femoral condyle blade plate. South. Med. J., 52:80–95, 1959.
25. Muller, M. R., Allgower, M., and Willenegger, H.: Technique of Internal Fixation of Fractures. New York, Springer-Verlag, 1970.
26. Olerud, S.: Operative treatment of supracondylar-condylar fractures of the femur. J. Bone Joint Surg., 54A:1015–1032, 1972.

Proximal Tibia

27. Klin, R.: Usual etiology of "fender fractures." N. Engl. J. Med., 210:480–481, 1934.
28. Roberts, J. M.: Fractures of the condyles of the tibia. An anatomical and clinical end result study of one hundred cases. J. Bone Joint Surg., 50A:1505–1521, 1968.
29. Frazer, J. E.: Frazer's Anatomy of the Human Skeleton. Breathnach, A. S. (ed.): 5th Ed. London, J & A Churchill, Ltd., 1958.
30. Bohler, L.: The Treatment of Fractures. Vol. 3. New York, Grune & Stratton, 1956, pp. 1650–1651.
31. Moore, T. M., and Harvey, J. P.: Roentgenographic measurements of tibial plateau depression due to fracture. J. Bone Joint Surg., 56A:155–160, 1974.
32. Kennedy, J. C., and Bailey, W. H.: Experimental tibial plateau fractures. J. Bone Joint Surg., 50A:1527–1534, 1968.
33. Levitin, J.: March fractures of the articular surface of the tibia and its relation to osteoarthropathy. Radiology, 46:273–275, 1946.
34. Cornell, C. M., and Hardy, R. C.: Plateau fractures of the tibia. Surgery, 28:735–743, 1950.
35. Cotton, F. J., and Berg, R.: "Fender fractures" of the tibia at the knee. N. Engl. J. Med., 201:989–995, 1929.
36. Hohl, M., and Luck, V.: Fractures of the tibial condyle: a clinical and experimental study. J. Bone Joint Surg., 38A:1001–1017, 1956.
37. Apley, A. G.: Fractures of the lateral tibial condyle treated by skeletal traction and early mobilization. J. Bone Joint Surg., 38B:699–708, 1956.
38. Solonen, K. A.: Fractures of the tibial condyles. Acta Orthop. Scand. (Suppl.), 63:7–32, 1963.
39. Slee, G. C.: Fractures of the tibial condyles. J. Bone Joint Surg., 37B:427–437, 1955.
40. Palmer, I.: Compression fractures of the lateral tibial condyle and their treatment. J. Bone Joint Surg., 21:674–680, 1939.
41. Rasmussen, P. S.: Tibial condylar fractures. J. Bone Joint Surg., 55A:1331–1350, 1973.
42. Weisman, S. L., and Herold, Z. H.: Fractures of the tibial plateau. Clin. Orthop. Rel. Res., 33:194–200, 1964.
43. Burrows, H.: Fractures of the lateral condyle of the tibia. Br. J. Bone Joint Surg., 38B:612–613, 1956.
44. Hohl, M.: Tibial condylar fractures. J. Bone Joint Surg., 49A:1455–1467, 1967.
45. Nerviaser, J. S., and Eisenberg, S. H.: Diagnostic and therapeutic obstacles encountered in

tibial plateau fractures. Bull Hosp. Joint Dis., *17*:48–57, 1956.

46. Fractures of the tibial tubercle: a clinical study, treatment based on 129 cases. A. O. Bull., 1973.

47. Martin, A. F.: The pathomechanics of the knee joint. The medial collateral ligament and lateral tibial plateau fractures. J. Bone Joint Surg., *42A*:13–22, 1960.

48. Wilpula, E., and Bakalim, G.: Ligamentous tear concomitant with tibial condylar fracture. Acta Orthop. Scand., *43*:292–300, 1972.

49. Fagerberg, S.: Tomographic analysis of depressed fractures within the knee joint, and injuries of the cruciate ligaments. Acta Orthop. Scand., 27:219–227, 1958.

50. Schioler, G.: Tibial condylar fractures with a particular view to the value of tomography. Acta Orthop. Scand., *42*:462, 1971.

51. Olerud, S.: Osteotomy of the tibial tuberosity in fractures of the tibial condyle. Acta Orthop. Scand., *42*:430–432, 1971.

52. Lee, H. G.: Osteoplastic reconstruction in severe fractures of the tibial condyles. Am. J. Surg., *94*:940–944, 1957.

53. Gottfries, A., Hagert, C. G., and Sörensen, S. E.: T & Y fractures of the tibial condyles. A follow-up study of cases treated by closed reduction and surgical fixation with a wire loop. Injury, 3:56–63, 1971.

54. Barr, J. S.: New technique. Br. Med. J., 2:365, 1938.

55. Rombold, C.: Depressed fractures of the tibial plateau. J. Bone Joint Surg., *42A*:783–797, 1960.

56. DePalma, A. F.: Disease of the Knee. Philadelphia, J. B. Lippincott, 1954.

57. Hughston, J. C., and Eilers, A.: The role of the posterior oblique ligament in repair of acute medial collateral ligamentous tears of the knee. J. Bone Joint Surg., 55A:923–940, 1973.

58. Miler, T. S.: Du traitement des fractures des condyles du fémur et du tibia par embrochange. Lyon Chir., *61*:89–92, 1965.

59. Merle D'Aubigne, R.: Formes anatomiques et traitement des fractures de l'extrémité supérieures du tibia. Rev. Chir. Orthop., *46*: 289–318, 1960.

60. Fryjordet, A.: Operative treatment of tibial condyle fractures. Acta Chir. Scand., *133*:17–24, 1967.

61. Wolf, M. D., and White, E. H.: Depressed fractures of the tibial plateau. Surg. Gynecol. Obstet., *116*:457–462, 1963.

62. Wittebol, P.: Treatment of fractures of the tibial plateau. Arch. Chir. Scand., *20*:253–267, 1968.

Patella

63. Smillie, I. S.: Injuries of the Knee Joint. 4th Ed. Edinburgh, Churchill Livingstone, 1970.

64. DePalma, A. F.: Diseases of the Knee. Philadelphia, J. B. Lippincott, 1954.

65. Wiberg, G.: Roentgenographic and anatomic studies on the femoropatellar joint. Acta Orthop. Scand., *12*:319–410, 1941.

66. Crock, H. V.: The arterial supply and venous drainage of the bones of the human knee joint. Anat. Rec., *144*:199–218, 1962.

67. Scapinelli, R.: Blood supply of the human patella. Its relation to ischaemic necrosis after fracture. J. Bone Joint Surg., *49B*:563–570, 1967.

68. Lieb, I. J., and Perry, J.: Quadriceps function. An anatomical and mechanical study using amputated limbs. J. Bone Joint Surg., *50A*: 1535–1548, 1968.

69. Morrison, J. B.: Functions of the knee joint in various activities. Biomed. Eng., *4*:573–580, 1969.

70. Adams, C. C.: Outline of Fractures. 5th Ed. Edinburgh, E & S Livingstone, 1968.

71. Bohler, L.: Die Technik der Knochenbruchbehandlung. 12th–13th Ed. Vienna, Wilhelm Maudrich Verlag, 1957.

72. Watson-Jones, R.: Fractures and Joint Injuries. 5th Ed. Edinburgh, E & S Livingstone, 1952.

73. Corner, E. M.: Figures about fractures and refractures of the patella. Ann. Surg., *52*:707–709, 1910.

74. Nummi, J.: Fracture of the patella. A clinical study of 707 patellar fractures. Ann. Chir. Gynaecol. (Suppl.), *179*:1–85, 1971.

75. Bostrom, A.: Fractures of the patella. A study of 422 patellar fractures. Acta Orthop. Scand. (Suppl.), 1–80, 1972.

76. Cave, E. F.: Fractures and other Injuries. Chicago, Year Book Publishing Co., 1958.

77. Koppell, N. P., and Thompson, W. H. L.: Patellar fractures and repair of the patellar retinacula. Gen. Pract., *26*:112–115, 1962.

78. Kroner, M.: Ein Fall von Flächenfraktur und luxation der patella. Dtsch. Med. Wochenschr., *31*:996–997, 1905.

79. Stewart, S. F.: Frontal fractures of the patella. Ann. Surg., *81*:536–539, 1925.

80. Milgram, J. E.: Tangential osteochondral fracture of the patella. J. Bone Joint Surg., *25*:271–280, 1943.

81. Millard, D. C., and Lee, T. H.: "The twist" fracture-dislocation of the patella. N. Engl. J. Med., *267*:246–247, 1962.

82. Freiberger, R. H., and Kotzen, L. M.: Fracture of the medial margin of the patella. A finding diagnostic of lateral dislocation. Radiology, 88:902–904, 1967.

83. O'Donoghue, D. H.: Treatment of Injuries to Athletes. 2nd Ed. Philadelphia, W. B. Saunders, 1970.

84. Hughston, J. C.: Recurring dislocation of the patella in young athletes. South. Med. J., *57*: 623–628, 1964.

85. Ahlstrom, J. P.: Osteochondral fracture of the knee joint associated with hypermobility and dislocation of the patella. J. Bone Joint Surg., *47A*:1491–1502, 1965.

86. O'Donoghue, D. H.: Chondral and osteochondral fractures. J. Trauma, 6:469–481, 1966.

87. Ashby, M. E., Shields, C. L., and Karmy, J. R.: Diagnosis of osteochondral fractures in acute traumatic patellar dislocations using air arthrography. J. Trauma, *15*:1032–1033, 1975.

88. Gregg, J. R., Nixon, J. E., and DiStefano, V. D.: Neutral fat globules in traumatized knees. Clin. Orthop. Rel. Res., *132*:219–224, 1978.

89. Lapidus, P. W.: Longitudinal fractures of the patella. J. Bone Joint Surg., *14*:351–379, 1932.

90. Black, J. K., and Conners, J. D.: Vertical fractures of the patella. South. Med. J., *62*:76–77, 1969.

91. Malgaigne, J. F.: Treatise on Fractures. Philadelphia, J. B. Lippincott, 1859.

92. Lister, J.: A new operation for fracture of the patella. Br. Med. J., *2*:850, 1877.

93. Berger, B., and Quenu, B.: Suture de la rotule par un nouveau (cerclage de la rotule). Soc. Chir. Paris, *18*:523–525, 1892.

94. Thompson, J. E. M.: Comminuted fractures of the patella. Treatment of cases presenting one large fragment and several small fragments. J. Bone Joint Surg., *17*:431–434, 1935.

95. Blodgett, W. E., and Fairchild, R. D.: Results of total and partial excisions of the patella for acute fractures. J.A.M.A., *106*:2121–2125, 1936.

96. Brooke, R.: The treatment of fractured patella by excision. A study of morphology and function. Br. J. Surg., *24*:733–747, 1936–1937.

97. Heineck, A. P.: The modern operative treatment of fracture of the patella. Surg. Gynecol. Obstet., *9*:177–248, 1909.

98. Anderson, L. D.: Campell's Operative Orthopaedics. 5th Ed. St. Louis, C. V. Mosby Co., 1971.

99. Muller, E., Allgower, M., and Willenegger, H.: Manual of Internal Fixation Techniques. Berlin, Springer-Verlag, 1969.

100. Duthie, H. L., and Hutchinson, J. R.: The results of partial and total excision of the patella. J. Bone Joint Surg., *40B*:75–81, 1958.

101. Shorbe, H. B., and Dobson, C. H.: Patellectomy. Repair of the extensor mechanism. J. Bone Joint Surg., *40A*:1281–1284, 1958.

Sprain Fracture

102. Zaricznyj, B.: Avulsion fracture of the tibial eminence: treatment by open reduction and pinning. J. Bone Joint Surg., *59A*:1111–1114, 1977.

103. Towne, L. C., Blazina, M. E., Marmor, L., and Lawrence, J. F.: Lateral compartment syndrome of the knee. Clin. Orthop., *76*:160–168, 1971.

104. Price, C. T., and Allen, W. C.: Ligament repair in the knee with preservation of the meniscus. J. Bone Joint Surg., *60A*:61–65, 1978.

105. Levi, J. H., and Coleman, C. R.: Fracture of the tibial tubercle. J. Sports Med., *4*:254–263, 1976.

106. Watson-Jones, R.: Fractures and Joint Injuries. 4th Ed. Vol. 2. Baltimore, Williams & Wilkins, 1955.

107. Hand, W. L., Hand, C. R., and Dunn, A. W.: Avulsion fractures of the tibial tubercle. J. Bone Joint Surg., *53A*:1579–1583, 1971.

108. Weaver, J. K.: Bipartite patella as a cause of disability in the athlete. J. Sports Med., *5*:137–143, 1977.

109. Saupe, H.: Primare Knochenmarkseiterung der Kniescheibe. Dtsch. Z. Chir., *258*:386, 1943.

110. O'Donoghue, D. H.: Treatment of Injuries to Athletes. 3rd Ed. Philadelphia, W. B. Saunders, 1976, p. 644.

111. Coleman, H. M.: Recurrent osteochondral fracture of the patella. J. Bone Joint Surg., *30B*:153, 1948.

112. McDougall, A., and Brown, D. J.: Radiologic sign of recurrent dislocation of the patella. J. Bone Joint Surg., *50B*:841–843, 1968.

Dislocations

113. Kennedy, J. C.: Complete dislocation of the knee joint. J. Bone Joint Surg., *45A*:899–904, 1963.

114. Hoover, N. W.: Injuries of the popliteal artery associated with fracture and dislocations. Surg. Clin. North Am., *41*:1099–1112, 1961.

115. Palmar, I.: On injury to the ligaments of the knee joint. A clinical study. Acta Chir. Scand. (Suppl.), 53, 1938.

116. Hughston, J. C.: The posterior cruciate in knee joint stability. J. Bone Joint Surg., *51A*:1045–1046, 1969.

117. Brantigan, O. C., and Voshell, H. F.: The mechanics of the ligaments and menisci of the knee joint. J. Bone Joint Surg., *23*:44–46, 1941.

118. O'Donoghue, D. H.: Surgical treatment of injuries to the knee. Clin. Orthop., *18*:11–36, 1960.

119. Kennedy, J. C., and Grainger, R. W.: The posterior cruciate ligament. J. Trauma, *7*:367–377, 1967.

120. Reckling, F. W., and Peltier, L. F.: Acute knee dislocations and their complications. J. Trauma, *9*:181–191, 1969.

121. Anderson, R. L.: Dislocation of the knee. Report of four cases. Arch. Surg., *46*:598–603, 1943.

122. Conwell, H. E., and Allredge, R. H.: Complete dislocations of the knee joint. A report of seven cases with end results. Surg. Gynecol. Obstet., *64*:94–101, 1937.

123. Myles, J. W.: Seven cases of traumatic dislocation of the knee. Proc. R. Soc. Med., *60*:279–281, 1967.

124. Morton, J. H., Southgate, W. A., and Deweese, J. A.: Arterial injuries of the extremities. Surg. Gynecol. Obstet., *123*:611–622, 1966.

125. Bassett, F. H., and Silvers, D.: Arterial injuries associated with fracture. Arch. Surg., *92*:13–19, 1966.

126. Klingensmith, W., Oles, P., and Martinez, H.: Arterial injuries associated with dislocations of the knee or fracture of the lower femur. Surg. Gynecol. Obstet., *120*:961–964, 1965.

127. DeBakey, M. E., and Simone, F. A.: Battle injuries of arteries in World War II. Ann. Surg., *123*:534–579, 1946.

128. Rose, E. A., Hess, O. W., and Welch, C. S.: Vascular injuries of the extremities in battle casualties. Ann. Surg., *123*:161–179, 1946.

129. Miller, H. H., and Welch, C. S.: Quantitative studies on the time factor in arterial injuries. Ann. Surg., *130*:428–438, 1949.

130. Jones, E. L., Peters, A. F., and Gasior, R. M.: Early management of battle casualties in Vietnam. Arch. Surg., 97:1–15, 1968.
131. MacClean, L. D.: The diagnosis and treatment of arterial injuries. Can. Med. Assoc., 88:1091–1101, 1963.
132. Taylor, A. R., Hylesburg, G. P., Arden, W., and Rainey, H. A.: Traumatic dislocation of the knee. A report of 43 cases with special reference to conservative care. J. Bone Joint Surg., 54B:96–102, 1972.
133. Quinlan, A. G., and Sharrard, W. J. W.: Posterolateral dislocation of the knee with capsular interposition. J. Bone Joint Surg., 40B:660–663, 1958.
134. Meyers, M. H., and Harvey, J. P.: Traumatic dislocations of the knee joint. J. Bone Joint Surg., 53A:16–29, 1971.
135. O'Donoghue, D. H.: Treatment of Injury to Athletes. 3rd Ed. Philadelphia, W. B. Saunders, 1976.

R. BRUCE HEPPENSTALL, M.D.

Fractures of the _____ 25
Tibia and
Fibula

Tibial fractures are among the injuries seen most frequently in orthopedic practice today. They occur in all age groups and are the result of direct trauma. Previously they were frequently associated with skiing injuries, but with the improvement of skiing equipment their frequency has decreased in recent times.

In the past, it was felt that nonunion occurred frequently in fractures of the distal third of the tibia, and because of this, their treatment remained controversial. The proponents of open reduction and internal fixation claimed a decreased incidence of nonunion, particularly with fractures located in the distal third of the tibia, while advocates of various nonoperative methods also claimed similar improved overall results.

Recently, a new method of nonoperative management has been advocated. This is a treatment program consisting of early closed reduction followed by the application of a short or long leg cast early, active, full weight bearing, as tolerated. It has been employed by Dehne, Brown, Sarmiento, and Nicoll with very impressive results.[17, 30–32, 89, 98–100] The rationale of this particular type of treatment program is that return of the injured limb to early active function circumvents the problems of disuse osteoporosis and muscular atrophy following immobilization and nonweight bearing.

The overall results of this nonoperative early ambulatory program have been so impressive that there has been a definite trend toward nonoperative treatment in the past decade. It is difficult to justify operative methods with all the associated complications of an operative procedure in the face of the excellent results obtained with conservative treatment. This does not mean that operative methods are totally condemned, but rather are relegated to use for very specific indications. Operative methods, including bone grafting, are still the treatment of choice for nonunion of the tibia.

This chapter deals primarily with the management of tibial fractures, as fibular fractures infrequently occur as isolated injuries.

SURGICAL ANATOMY

Bone Structure. The anterior aspect of the shaft of the tibia is subcutaneous through its entire length and is very vulnerable to injury in this location. It is a long tube of heavy bone that abruptly enlarges at each end. The midportion of the shaft consists of thick compact bone, while the ends are largely cancellous in structure with a thin surrounding cortex. There is a marked difference in the shape and size of the bone in the proximal portion compared to the distal third. A cross section of the proximal portion of the tibia is approximately triangular, while the distal third reveals a cross section that is rounded and much smaller in diameter. The majority of fractures occur in

777

the distal third, in the area where the shaft is narrow and has less supporting strength.

The fibula is a very slender column of bone compared to the tibia. It is similar to the tibia in that the shaft is the narrowest portion and there is an expansion at each end. The proximal expanded portion, the head of the fibula, articulates with the lateral portion of the tibia and protects the common peroneal nerve, which travels immediately lateral to and under it. At the distal end the shaft expands to form the lateral malleolus. The interosseous membrane, a firm sheet of connective tissue, fills in the gap between the tibia and fibula. In its proximal portion the membrane has a small opening through which pass the anterior tibial vessels. The membrane serves to prevent separation of the osseous structures with fractures. Since most of the fibers run downward and outward, they tend to distribute indirect forces acting on the tibia and fibula. The membrane is felt to play an active role in preventing overriding of fracture fragments and in evening distribution of forces along the tibia and fibula during early ambulatory treatment of fractures in this area.

Muscles. The musculature of the leg is classically divided into four different groups of muscles, each group being contained in its own separate fascial compartment.

The extensor group of muscles, contained within the anterior compartment situated on the front of the leg, includes the tibialis anterior, the extensor digitorum longus, the extensor hallucis longus, and the peroneus tertius. The anterior tibial artery and the deep peroneal nerve are also contained in the anterior compartment. A very specific syndrome called the anterior tibial compartment syndrome is produced when the tissue pressure increases within the compartment proper, producing ischemic changes in the contained musculature. The increased tissue pressure may be caused by active bleeding inside the compartment from a laceration of the anterior tibial artery or by muscle swelling in response to injury. In either event, the increased pressure results in a decrease in active oxygen supply to the contained muscles and ischemic necrosis.

The abductor group of muscles is located in the lateral compartment. These are the peroneus longus and brevis, which are located lateral to the anterior group of muscles and anterior to the external intermuscular septum. The peroneal muscles are supplied by the superficial peroneal nerve, and the peroneus longus frequently receives additional nerve supply from a branch of the common peroneal or the deep peroneal nerve. The peroneal muscles are the chief everters of the foot and serve a protective function for the fibula because of their location.

The posterior group of muscles is contained within two separate compartments. The calf group proper consists of the soleus, the gastrocnemius, and the plantaris. The deep flexor group, which is situated beneath the calf group and separated from it by an intermuscular septum, consists of the tibialis posterior, the flexor digitorum longus, and the flexor hallucis longus. The posterior tibial artery and its large branch (the peroneal artery) traverse the posterior compartment. The posterior tibial nerve is also contained in this compartment.

Blood Supply. The blood supply to the tibial shaft deserves special emphasis. The shaft is supplied by the nutrient artery (a branch of the posterior tibial artery) and the periosteal vessels. The nutrient artery enters the posterolateral cortex at the level of origin of the soleus muscle, directly below the oblique line of the tibia posteriorly. Once the artery has pierced the cortical bone, it divides into four distinct branches. Three of these ascend proximally, and only one main branch descends distally. Several smaller branches do originate off the main descending branch to supply the endosteal surface. The periosteum receives blood from branches of the anterior tibial artery during its course down the interosseous membrane. The main blood supply involved in fracture healing originates from the intramedullary vasculature, as in other bones. Nelson and co-workers and Rhinelander, in separate studies, adequately demonstrated that the intramedullary vascular supply plays the most important role in the healing of tibial fractures.[88, 95] It is important to realize that the tibia has less potential than other long bones for obtaining an extraosseous blood supply, owing to the paucity of soft tissues in the distal extremity, particularly in the distal third of the tibia. Rhinelander demonstrated that with disruption of the intramedullary vascular supply, the periosteal blood vessels increase in number and size in order to take an active role in new bone formation. He was also able to demonstrate that a fluted intramedullary nail offers large channels for regeneration of the medullary arteries, while the broad surface of a cloverleaf nail keeps the nutrient arterial blood supply suppressed. Olerud and Karlström investigated the blood supply to artificially created segmental fractures of the tibia. They created segmental fractures of the tibia by dual osteotomies with a Gigli saw. Following production of the fracture they applied compression plate fixation and were able to observe excellent revascularization of the intermediate fragment, four fifths of it by medullary arterials.[90] Rhinelander's studies revealed that compression plating was the least disturbing to the blood supply compared to other methods of internal fixation.[95]

MECHANISMS OF INJURY

Fractures of the shaft of the tibia may be caused by direct or indirect violence. Direct injuries result from major trauma such as vehicular accidents or gunshot wounds. Indirect injuries are produced by a fall from a height in which the patient lands on his feet, or by a torsional injury in which the thigh or foot is fixed while the opposite end of the bone is subjected to a twisting force. As stated previously, one of the more frequent types of indirect injury is related to skiing accidents in which the foot becomes fixed in the binding and ski boot while the remainder of the body rotates.

The injuries resulting from direct violence carry poorer prognoses than those resulting from indirect violence. The greater force associated with direct violence generates two distinct problems. First, it produces greater displacement of the fracture fragments as well as more comminution. Second, since the subcutaneous tissue along the anterior aspect of the tibia is sparse, severe soft-tissue loss may compound the problem with an open injury secondary to skin loss. This is a very difficult situation to manage. The prognosis associated with a compound fracture is definitely poorer than that associated with a simple fracture.

High-energy injuries tend to produce transverse fractures with significant comminution. Injuries secondary to indirect violence are more likely to be long oblique or spiral fractures. Again, the tissue destruction is much less with a low-energy spiral fracture than with a high-energy transverse or comminuted fracture.

The majority of fibular fractures are produced by the same mechanism of injury as the tibial fracture. Occasionally, one sees a fracture of the fibula that has been caused by direct trauma to the lateral side of the leg and is unassociated with a fracture of the tibia. This is usually a transverse fracture at the level at which the violence occurred and shows little tendency toward displacement (Fig. 25–1). The remainder of isolated fractures of the fibula are usually associated with ankle injuries due to leverage action and with a tear of the interosseous membrane. This type is known as a Maisonneuve fracture and is discussed further with fractures of the ankle joint.

CLASSIFICATION OF TIBIAL FRACTURES

Several classifications have been proposed to predict the type of treatment required for the prognosis associated with all fractures of the tibia. As for those of the hip, some authors have advocated classifying them as stable and unstable fractures. Fractures of the tibia cannot be compared to intertrochanteric fractures in this way, however, because the majority of those previously classified as unstable can be treated with reduction and early functional weight bearing. The situation is obviously different in the tibia than in the hip. Specific surgical procedures have been advocated to increase stability in the hip, as outlined in Chapter 22. The problems encountered in fractures of the tibia are different, as gross shortening or having the fracture "fall apart," is an unusual occurrance when proper nonoperative treatment methods have been used.

The classification outlined by Ellis is preferred by the author. Ellis found that the

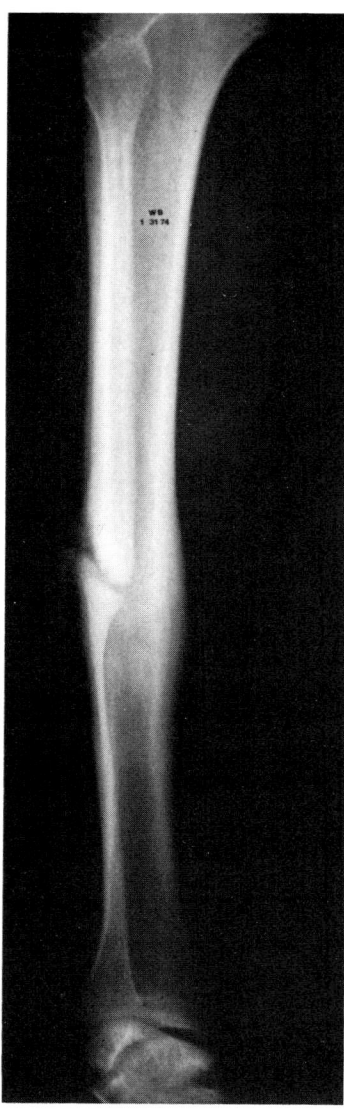

Figure 25–1   Fracture of the midshaft of the fibula due to direct violence. Nonunion developed, an unusual feature.

severity of injury directly influenced the healing time of the fracture. He noted that the severity of the injury was directly influenced by three factors. These included: (1) The presence of displacement. If there was significant displacement associated with the fracture there was an increase in the delay of fracture healing. (2) The presence or absence of severe open wounding. If there was a definite open fracture that was severe, this definitely de-

layed the healing process. (3) The amount of comminution. The fractures associated with more comminution showed a definite delay in the fracture healing process.

Keeping these factors in mind, Ellis then produced a classification based on the degree of severity of the fracture. Minor severity included an undisplaced, unangulated fracture with minor comminution or a minor open wound. Moderate severity comprised a fracture that was completely displaced or angulated with a moderate degree of comminution or a minor open wound. Major severity included complete displacement associated with major comminution or a major open wound. Ellis was able to document the time to healing of the fracture as well as the incidence of delayed union. In the minor severity group he found that bony union occurred at 10 weeks with a delayed union rate of 2 per cent. In the moderate severity group he found that bony healing occurred at 15 weeks with an 11 per cent rate of delayed union. In the major severity group healing took 23 weeks and there was a significantly delayed union rate of 60 per cent.[41-43] This is an extremely useful classification, as it allows one to predict how long the fracture will take to heal as well as the probability of delayed union. A final very important point is that Ellis was unable to demonstrate any difference in the healing time of fractures related to the anatomical location in the tibia.

PHYSICAL EXAMINATION

Patients with fractures of the tibia have significant pain at the fracture site. The pain is present without weight bearing, but it is greatly accentuated with weight bearing. Localization of the site of pain is usually very specific.

Deformity of the shaft is usually present. Motion at the fracture site increases the pain. Hematoma develops early and is easily palpable because the tibia lies closely beneath the skin. It is for this reason that localization of the fracture site is not difficult. A careful assessment of the soft-tissue structures is very important. If the fracture has been caused by direct violence, the overlying soft tissue may appear damaged; a bumper injury, for example, will produce a severe soft-tissue injury, in addition to the fracture. Frequently, however, the full extent of the injury is not evident, and if it is not fully appreciated on initial examination, the proper treatment may not be selected. This possibility must always be kept in mind when, during the course of treatment, an unexplained febrile episode may indicate the presence of soft tissue necrosis with subsequent grossly open fracture in a cast-enclosed extremity. The presence or absence of a puncture wound should be recorded. The treatment and the prognosis are definitely different for an open fracture and for a simple fracture, and frequently the only evidence that the fracture is open may be an easily overlooked small puncture wound. A careful neurological examination of the lower extremities should be performed. Nerve injuries associated with fracture of the tibia are not common, but occasionally a peroneal nerve injury will be seen with a fracture of the proximal fibula. This may be manifest by the inability to dorsiflex the great toe or by a decrease in sensation in the first web space, indicating an injury to the deep peroneal nerve.

Much more important is the assessment of the status of the vascular supply to the lower extremity. Particularly with comminuted fractures of the proximal third of the tibia, the anterior tibial artery may be injured during its course through the interosseous membrane. There may be complete laceration or severe contusion of the artery at this level, which is the type of injury that leads to an anterior compartment syndrome. One must also remember that the distal pulses may be palpable, owing to collateral circulation, in the presence of complete severance of the anterior tibial artery. Therefore, it is mandatory to record both the amount of tenderness and the amount of tension directly over the anterior compartment. The adequacy of distal capillary filling should be assessed in all tibial fractures.

ROENTGENOGRAPHIC EXAMINATION

All patients presenting with a history of an injury followed by pain in the tibial area should have standard roentgenographic examination. Standard anteroposterior and lateral views are all that are generally required in the initial assessment. The views must include not only the entire tibia and fibula but also the knee and ankle joints. The technician must not come down on the area of tenderness, as a fracture of the fibula in the proximal area may be missed. It is also important to obtain views of the knee and ankle, as the amount of angulation at the fracture site can then be properly determined. During the course of treatment, if the amount of healing cannot be fully determined by standard views, then oblique views or tomograms of the area are usually helpful. There are several important points about the fracture that must be documented. The level of fracture, whether in the proximal, middle, or distal third of the tibia, should be recorded. The direction of the fracture should also be recorded; it may be a simple transverse or a spiral or oblique fracture. The presence or absence of comminution must be determined. The amount of angulation present at the fracture site is important. The amount of displacement at the fracture site is an indication of the severity of the injury and must be determined in both the anteroposterior and lateral views. For instance, the displacement may not be appreciated in a routine anteroposterior view while there is a significant amount present in a lateral view. The amount of rotation should be assessed both clinically and roentgenographically. The presence or absence of a concomitant fibular fracture is important, as the amount of displacement of the tibial fragments is less in the presence of an intact fibula and the associated soft-tissue damage is also decreased.

Finally, the presence or absence of foreign material in the soft tissues must be noted.

TREATMENT OF TIBIAL FRACTURES

As stated at the beginning of this chapter, there has been a definite trend toward nonoperative treatment of these fractures. In the 1950s a surgical approach was advocated for many of them. Following the excellent reports of Dehne and Brown and their co-workers, Sarmiento, and Nicoll, however, it is difficult to justify an operative approach today.[17, 30-32, 89, 98-100] The single most important advance in the treatment of tibial fractures is the concept of a closed reduction and cast application followed by early ambulation and rapid return to full weight bearing. There is no doubt that this concept has revolutionized the treatment of fractures of the tibia. Gratitude must be extended to Dehne and Brown and their associates, and to Sarmiento for developing this important concept which has been further extended by Sarmiento. He has advocated the use, initially, of a long leg cast for two weeks, followed by a snug below-knee total-contact cast for an additional two weeks, followed by a below-knee brace with a free ankle. He feels that this is the most expedient way to return the limb to its normal functional state and he has had excellent results with this method.[98-100]

Reduction and Cast Application in Simple Fractures

The initial management of a patient with a simple noncomminuted fracture depends on the presence or absence of: (1) the amount of displacement present at the fracture site, (2) the degree of angulation at the fracture site, and (3) the degree of rotation at the fracture site. The initial amount of displacement at the fracture site determines the severity of the injury: the greater the displacement, the more serious the injury.

It is not entirely necessary to achieve perfect anatomical reduction. It is true that every physician treating this injury attempts to obtain 100 per cent reduction, but, this is not necessary as far as displacement is concerned. A certain amount of leeway is allowable in this instance, a useful working rule being to obtain at least 50 per cent apposition of the fracture fragments.

Angulation, on the other hand, is more specific and must be controlled more carefully. I prefer not to accept more than 5 to 10 degrees either in the anteroposterior or the lateral plane. Greater angulation than this will interfere with normal function. It is important to maintain the knee and ankle joint surfaces parallel to each other to prevent alteration in the weight-bearing stresses applied to both the knee and the

ankle (Fig. 25-2). It is also important to observe the configuration of the normal, uninjured extremity. In a patient with a mild varus deformity in the uninjured leg, it would be an error to accept a 5 to 10 degree valgus angulation at the fracture site in the injured one. In other words, a definite attempt should be made to "match up" the lower extremities.

Rotation must be corrected to a nearly

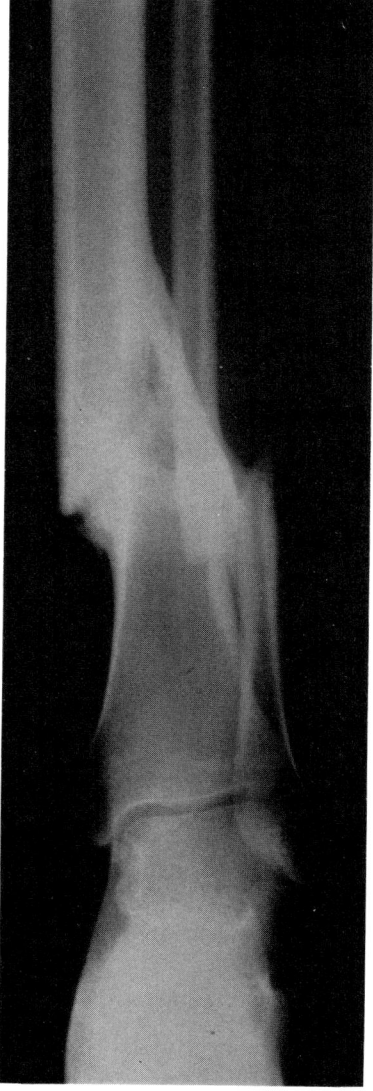

Figure 25-2 Angulation of the fracture site may produce an alteration in weight bearing at the ankle owing to a change in position of the horizontal axis of the ankle joint. Angulation greater than 5 to 10 degrees should not be accepted.

perfect position. There is no room for error in this regard—a patient is extremely unhappy with a lower extremity that is internally or externally rotated in comparison with the uninjured normal one. Clinical evaluation is the best guide here. A mental image of the patient's uninjured limb should always be maintained during the reduction of a fracture of the opposite tibia. Once the reduction is completed and the cast applied, the amount of rotation should be carefully compared with that of the normal uninjured extremity.

The initial reduction is performed by having the patient supine with the involved extremity hanging over the end of the stretcher or table so that the weight of the leg itself provides the correct amount of traction for reduction. This principle is similar to that of the Stimson method for reduction of dislocations of the shoulder and hip. It is also helpful to have the normal lower extremity also over the end of the table so that the operator can compare the position following reduction with it.

Gentle traction may be applied to the involved lower extremity through the ankle and foot. To best achieve this, the operator should be in the seated position on a stool. If the patient is unable to tolerate the attempt at closed reduction because of increased pain, then spinal or general anesthesia will be necessary to provide adequate relaxation to obtain the proper reduction. Once the reduction is obtained, Webril is applied from the toes to the knee. A standard below-knee cast is applied while the operator maintains the reduction. The foot is usually in the neutral position. If it becomes evident that placing the foot in the neutral position causes posterior angulation at the fracture site, however, a slight equinus inclination is acceptable for a period of four to six weeks. Once the plaster has set from the knee to the toes, the cast is extended to the groin. I feel it is best to keep the knee in almost full extension during application of the long leg cast. It is true that 20 to 30 degrees of flexion of the knee is more comfortable for the patient. I feel, however, that almost full extension of the knee provides a better position for direct transmission of weight through the fracture site. Ambulation and weight bearing are then allowed as soon as they can be tolerated. Most patients are able to bear full weight by 7 to 10 days. The rationale for early weight bearing is that tissue edema is decreased and the circulation is increased by having the injured limb back in functional use. Additional factors may be the direct stresses across the fracture site and an alteration of the electrical potential across the fracture site with active weight bearing. Electrical potentials and fracture healing are discussed further in Chapter 3.

It was Dehne, in the United States, who first popularized the early weight bearing principle for the treatment of fractures of the tibia. This concept was further expanded by Sarmiento, who in the laboratory, investigated the exact action of weight bearing on the soft tissues and the effect on fracture healing. It was his contention that this form of treatment acted on a hydrostatic principle; the equal compression of the soft-tissue parts by the snugly applied cast distributed the forces across the fracture site equally and decreased the tendency toward displacement.[98-100]

Follow-up roentgenograms are obtained the day following reduction and at one and three weeks postreduction. Full weight bearing is continued, and at the end of one month the long leg cast is changed to a Sarmiento-type patellar tendon-bearing cast. This is a snug, form-fitting cast with an extension over the patella, and it is carefully molded around the tibial condyles and the patella in an attempt to control rotation. It has been adequately demonstrated that the patellar tendon-bearing cast does not significantly reduce the weight borne on the tibial condyles; its purpose is not to unload the fracture site entirely because compression at the fracture site stimulates healing. The patellar tendon-bearing cast is maintained until there is evidence of healing at the fracture site, both by clinical determination and by roentgenographic corroboration.

An alternative form of therapy is to apply a short leg brace with a free ankle at six to eight weeks following the initial fracture. The advantage of this type of treatment is that motion at the ankle can then be started early. It is the author's feeling, however, that the majority of patients with tibial fractures do not have difficulty in regaining ankle motion.

An additional protective device occasionally applied in the treatment of tibial fractures is the Delbet gaiter. This is applied when it is felt that the fracture is healing satisfactorily but has not yet healed quite sufficiently to allow weight bearing without some support. In simple terms, it is a cylindrical tibial cast with extensions over both malleoli. The extensions allow control of rotation. It is useful in a young, aggressive individual who will stress the healing fracture excessively, as it provides added protection.

Shortening. Shortening does not seem to be a particularly significant problem when a long leg cast is used and is followed by a patellar tendon-bearing cast. Sarmiento has demonstrated that very few patients ultimately have a significant degree of shortening, and loss of position is not frequent.[98–100] If shortening does occur early because of the obliquity of the fracture, the pins and plaster technique may be applied (Fig. 25–3). It is important to prevent distraction at the fracture site.

Cast Wedging. Wedging of casts is an old art and is still useful in modern practice. Although the number of physicians who utilize it has definitely decreased in the past two or three decades, it is a useful technique and should be employed in the management of fractures of the tibia. It is particularly useful if a reduction is difficult to hold and the operator is still faced with significant angulation at the fracture site. Under these conditions, wedging is probably preferable to removal of the cast, a new reduction, and then application of a new cast. There are two differing techniques for wedging the cast. Charnley has advocated wedging the cast at the intersection of the long axis of the two fragments.[23] This is the technique that I prefer. Watson-Jones, on the other hand, wedged the cast directly over the fracture site.[111]

Roentgenograms are obtained in which several metal markers on the cast make it possible to determine the exact fracture site. A closing or an opening wedge may be performed; I prefer the opening wedge, as it does not have the theoretical disadvantage of pinching the skin at the wedge site as the closing wedge may. The long axes of the two fragments are drawn on the cast and the wedge is cut at the intersection. In an open-ing wedge the cast is cut on the concave side, leaving the fulcrum on the convex side. For example, if a varus angulation of the tibia is to be corrected, the apex of the wedge is based on the lateral aspect of the tibia. The plaster is then opened anteriorly, posteriorly, and medially, but left intact on the lateral side, which then acts as a fulcrum. The most distal fragment is angulated into a more neutral position, thus opening the medial side of the cast. The defect in the cast is then held in position by plaster or a small piece of wood, and the entire area is rewrapped in plaster and a new roentgenogram is obtained. The only theoretical disadvantage of an opening wedge is that distraction may occur at the fracture site. I have not found this to be a problem.

Operative Treatment

The majority of fractures of the tibia can be handled very successfully with closed reduction and cast application. There are, however, certain specific instances in which either the procedure is not appropriate or the reduction cannot be maintained. Under these circumstances operative methods are certainly indicated. Several of the techniques with the appropriate indications follow.

Pins and Plaster. The pins and plaster technique is useful in the problem cases in which it is difficult to maintain a satisfactory reduction. Variations of this technique have been described in the past by Stader, Anderson and Hutchins, and Böhler.[4, 12] Two distinct concepts emerged. Stader and Anderson popularized the use of pins above and below the fracture site with an external apparatus to control motion of the pins.[6] Böhler, on the other hand, described a method of treating these fractures by placing pins above and below the fracture site and then incorporating the pins in a plaster cast.[12]

These techniques may be applied to the treatment of tibial fractures in which the reduction is difficult to maintain. The Stader or Anderson method is particularly useful for tibial fractures with associated severe soft-tissue loss; the pins maintain the reduction and can be held by an external apparatus that allows inspection and treatment of the areas devoid of soft tissue. This

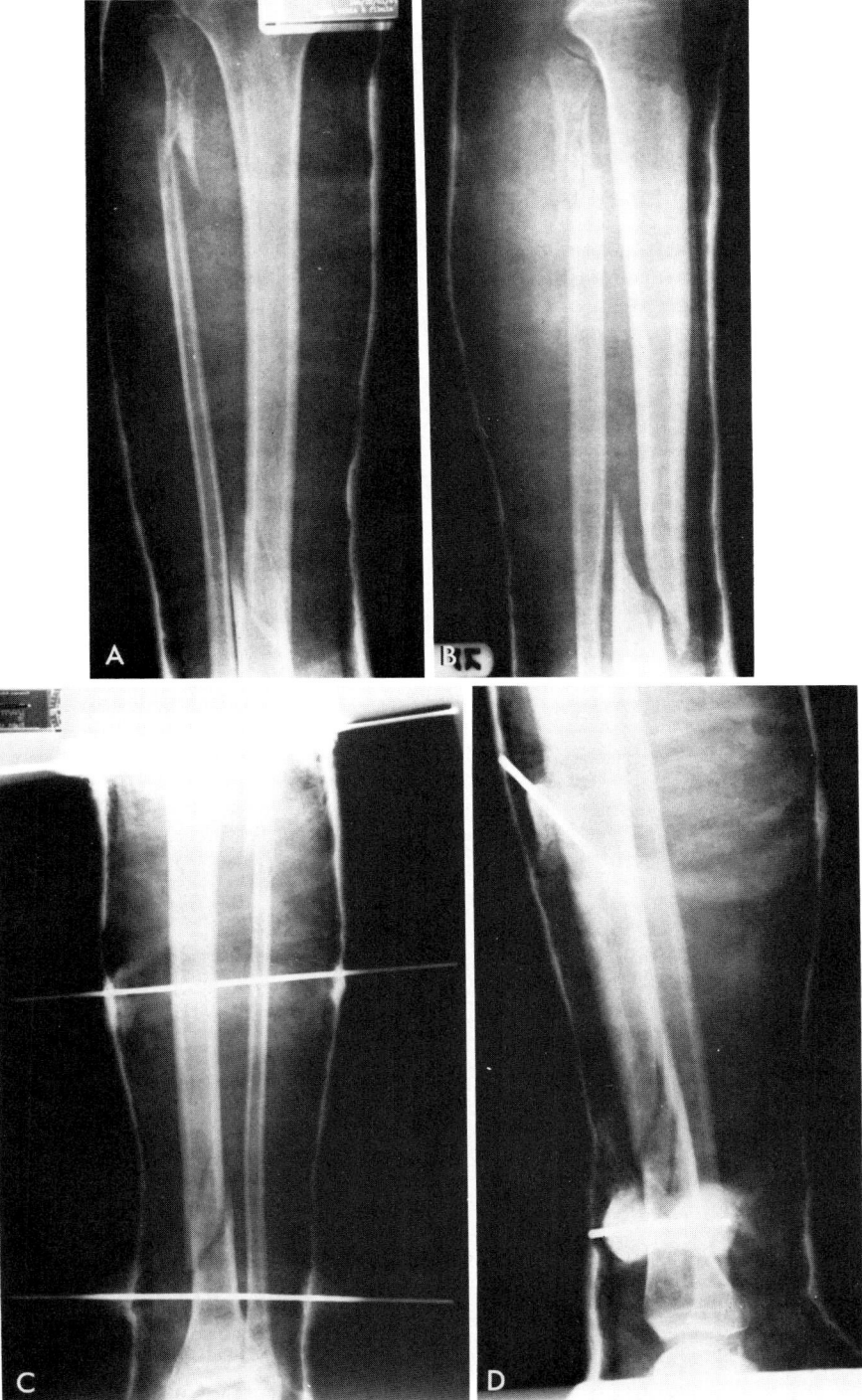

Figure 25–3 A. Anteroposterior view of a long spiral fracture of the distal tibia. *B.* There was loss of length in a cast. *C.* Anteroposterior view following application of pins and plaster to correct the shortening. *D.* Lateral view demonstrating satisfactory position with T pins in place.

does not occur frequently, but when it does it is a very difficult situation to manage and this technique allows appropriate treatment of both problems. Recently a new device, the Hoffman apparatus, has become available and is very useful in treating these injuries.

In the pins and plaster technique, some authors prefer two pins above and one pin below the fracture site (Fig. 25–4). I feel, however, that there is better control of the fragments with two pins above and two pins below the fracture site. The procedure is simple to perform. An appropriate anesthetic is administered, and two nonthreaded Steinmann pins, 3/32 inch in diameter, are drilled across the proximal tibial fragment above the fracture site under sterile conditions. The pins should be separated at least 4 to 5 cm if possible. In a similar fashion, two Steinmann pins are placed through the distal fragment parallel to the proximal pins. The surgeon will then have improved control of the fracture fragments, and these may be reduced satisfac-

torily with appropriate manipulation. There is usually no problem in obtaining sufficient traction to reduce the fracture with the distal pins. A standard below-knee cast is then applied, incorporating the pins. Roentgenograms are obtained to check the position of the fracture fragments. If the reduction is not satisfactory, the cast is removed, a new reduction is performed, a new cast is applied, and repeated roentgenograms are taken. Once satisfactory reduction has been obtained the cast is extended into a long leg cast. There has been little problem with the pins incorporated in plaster. The infection rate is extremely low, but if a pin-tract infection does develop around one of the pins, that pin can always be removed and the reduction maintained with the plaster.

There is controversy at the present time about when these patients should be allowed to bear weight. Since this technique is not employed unless there is difficulty in maintaining reduction or a large displacement of the fracture fragments indicating severe soft tissue injury, I prefer to keep

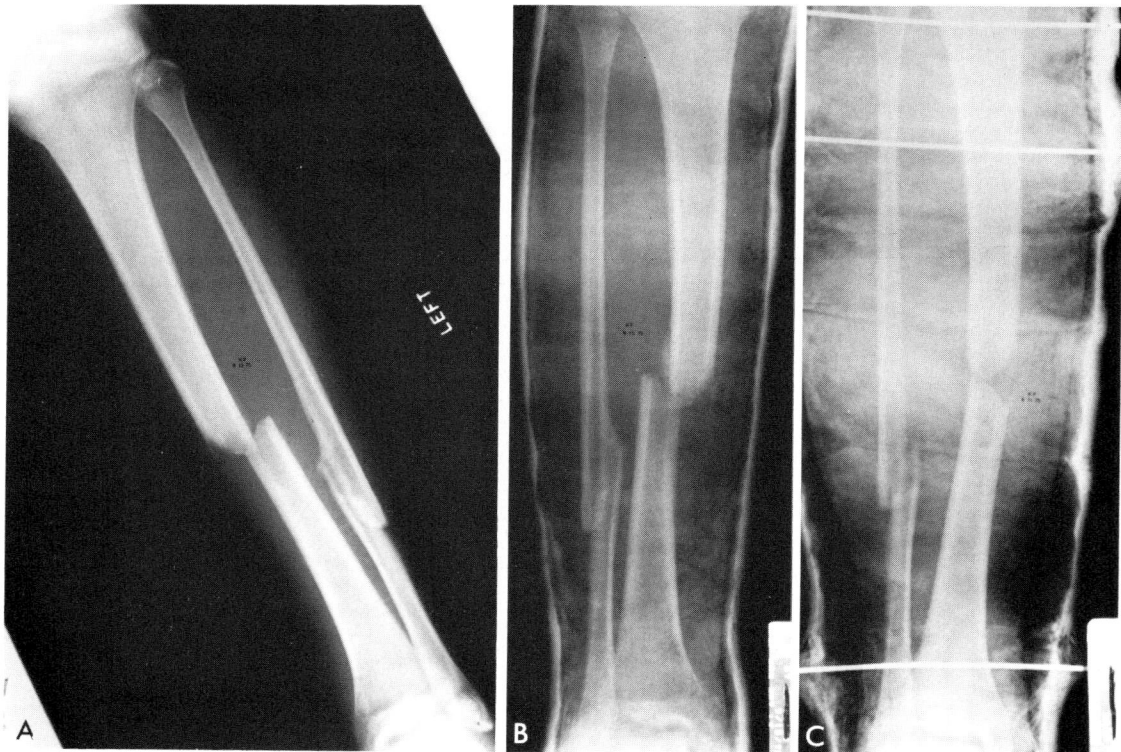

Figure 25–4 *A.* An open fracture with loss of bone stock producing gross shortening and difficulty in maintaining reduction. Note the overlap of the fibula fracture due to the loss of bone at the tibial fracture site. *B.* Position in plaster following two weeks of debridement of the open wound. The position could not be maintained adequately. *C.* Pins and plaster used to control rotation and attempt to regain length. It is important to prevent distraction, or nonunion may result.

these patients from weight bearing for a period of six weeks. At this time the pins are removed and the patient is allowed full active weight bearing in the cast. The long leg cast is maintained for an additional three weeks, when it is changed to a well-molded patellar tendon-bearing cast. The patient then wears this cast until there is roentgenographic evidence of healing.

When a severe soft-tissue loss requires that external apparatus be applied to the pins, the apparatus is maintained until satisfactory treatment of the soft-tissue loss allows the application of a cast incorporating the pins. The external apparatus is then removed.

Pin Traction. This particular technique is useful in cases in which there has been significant trauma to the anterior aspect of the tibia, such as bumper injuries or open fractures, and is also useful in allowing examination to determine whether an anterior compartment syndrome is developing. Direct inspection of the anterior aspect of the tibia is possible as well as the application of dressings or debridement.

A ⅛ inch in diameter Steinmann pin is drilled across the os calcis under sterile conditions and appropriate anesthesia. A traction bow is then attached to the os calcis pin, and appropriate traction is applied. Eight pounds is usually sufficient to maintain reduction. The lower extremity is suspended on a Thomas splint or a Böhler frame. Roentgenograms are obtained following application of the traction, and the amount of traction is adjusted to produce satisfactory reduction. In the meantime, close inspection of the anterior compartment may reveal undue swelling or excessive tenderness indicative of an impending anterior compartment syndrome. If the syndrome does occur, appropriate operative treatment may be started and the extremity may be maintained in the os calcis traction during the operative procedure and postoperatively. To treat severe soft-tissue loss along the anterior aspect of the tibia, Betadine soaks can be applied and intermittent debridement carried out while the fracture fragments are held in appropriate position. Once there is evidence of satisfactory healing of the soft-tissue structures, a cast can be applied incorporating the os calcis pin.

Hoffman External Fixation. The Hoffman device has been very useful for the management of unstable, comminuted, and

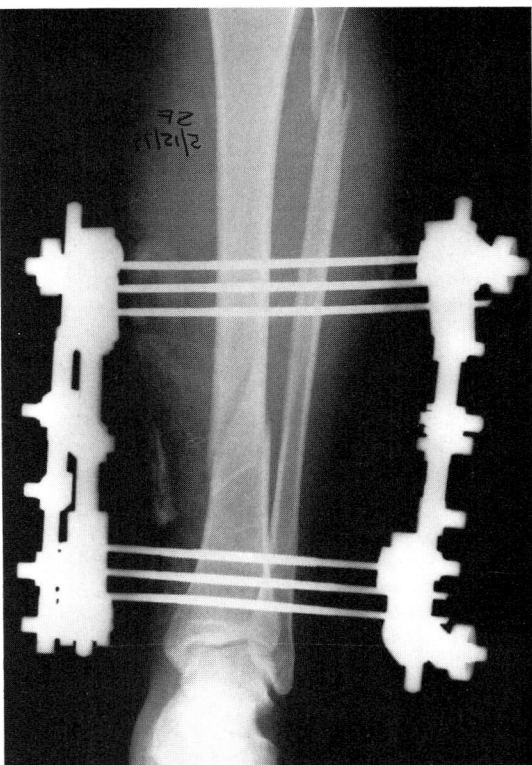

Figure 25–5 An open fracture of the tibia managed with the insertion of a Hoffman device.

open tibial fractures (Fig. 25–5). Its advantages are several: (1) It provides excellent stability at the fracture site through the use of multiple pins and outrigger bars that form a rigid external frame. It is approximately 40 times more stable than pins and plaster fixation. (2) An unstable segmental fragment may be secured with a separate pin attached to a side bar. (3) Active compression at the fracture site may be obtained by compression of the outrigger bars. (4) Segmental defects may be securely immobilized while a bone graft is inserted into the defect. (5) Partial weight bearing is possible with this device in the absence of plaster. (6) It allows full inspection and access to soft tissue defects for skin grafting or appropriate dressing of the wound. (7) Motion of the knee and ankle is encouraged to stimulate healing and prevent contractures.

Routinely, three pins are inserted above and three below the fracture site. The pins are threaded in the midportion and connected by an outrigger system of bars that may be manipulated in all planes. This device should not be employed for routine fractures, as conventional casting and early weight bearing are satisfactory. Therefore, I must stress that it is only used for difficult tibial fractures and is an excellent method under these circumstances.

Intramedullary Fixation. This particular technique has a very limited application in modern treatment of tibial fractures. Lottes has been the principal advocate of intramedullary nailing of the tibia in the United States and has developed his own particular device.[73, 74] Küntscher also popularized this technique in the past in Europe. Its use today is very limited, however, because of the high success rate obtained with the well-applied total-contact cast. The only clinical situation in which this method has proved to be useful is the treatment of segmental fractures in which the reduction has been difficult to maintain (Fig. 25–6). The best results have been obtained with

closed nailing, which usually requires the use of an image intensifier and produces little trauma under these circumstances. If the fracture site has to be openly reduced to obtain intramedullary fixation, however, the remaining blood supply to the segmental fracture is severely diminished, while the total blood supply to the fragment is grossly altered by the insertion of the intramedullary device in any case.

The Lottes procedure is performed with the patient under appropriate anesthesia, usually spinal. A small incision is made in the vicinity of the tibial tubercle. A hole is drilled in this area to accept a Lottes nail, which is then passed in a distal direction down the medullary canal and across the fracture site into the distal fragment. The risk of infection is certainly decreased by this method because the fracture site is not

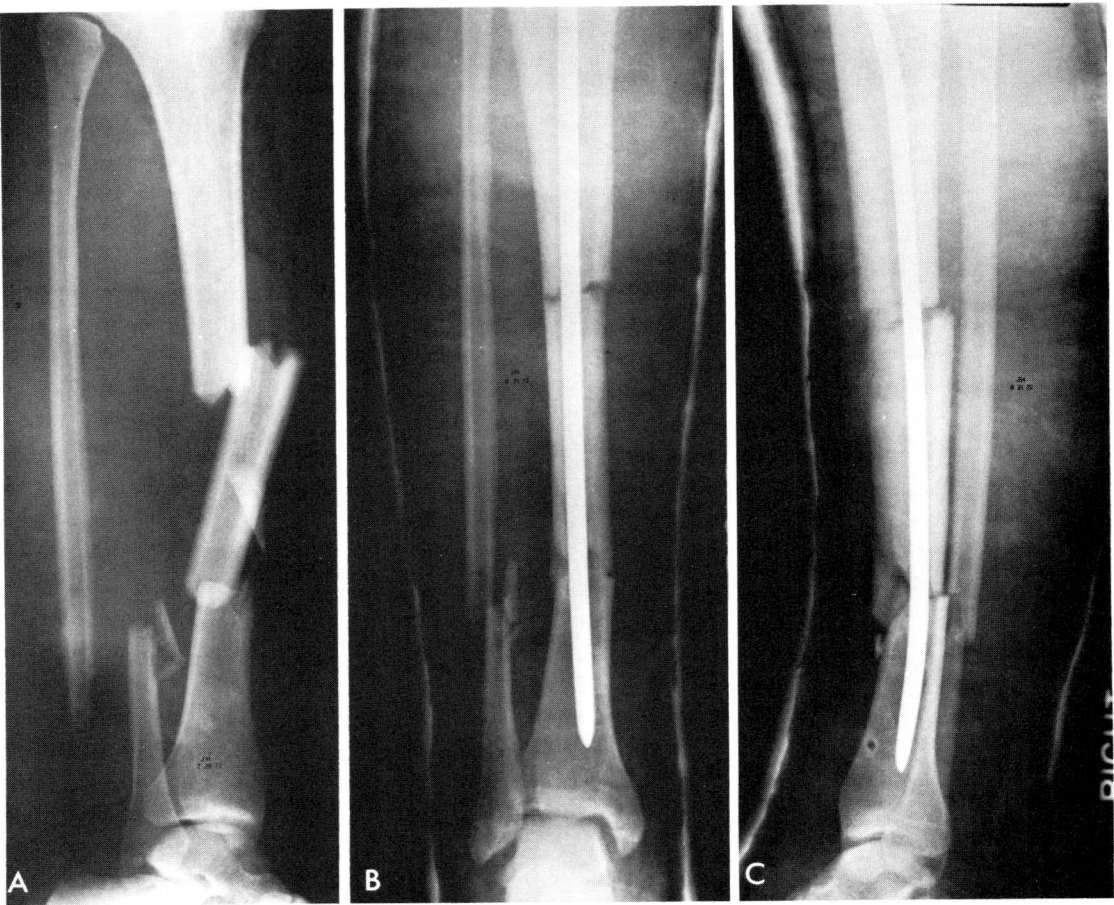

Figure 25–6 A. A grossly displaced segmental fracture of the tibia and associated fibular fracture. Satisfactory reduction was difficult to maintain with closed measures. B. An anteroposterior view of the tibia following closed Lottes nailing of the segmental fracture. C. Lateral view of the segmental fracture with the Lottes nail in place reveals no evidence of significant angulation.

exposed. A major drawback, however, is that this technique does not provide firm fixation. The same concept that applies to the femur also applies to the tibia. The nail does not obtain a tight purchase in the distal fragment, as the tibia tends to flare in its distal third. It is for this reason that most surgeons who use this technique also apply a cast for ambulation. Immediate total weight bearing can then be begun with the cast.

Again, I must stress that intramedullary fixation has very limited application in the overall management of tibial fractures but is useful in unstable segmental fractures.

Open Reduction and Compression Fixation. Like intramedullary fixation, open reduction and internal fixation with compression plates find limited use in the overall management of fractures of the tibia. This technique has received ardent support in Switzerland and France and has been outlined and approved by various European centers. There is no doubt that their statistics are very impressive; the results with this technique, however, compared to those with closed reduction and early ambulation, are certainly not as impressive in the United States (Fig. 25–7). The major problem to be feared with this particular method is infection. It must be remembered that when a closed fracture is treated by open reduction and internal fixation the fracture is converted from a "closed" fracture to an "open" fracture. As with all operative procedures, there is a definite risk of infection. When this technique is used, strict attention must be paid to detail, as outlined by the AO group, if results are to be satisfactory. I feel that the only clinical situations to which it is applicable are the difficult to maintain reduction and the established nonunion treated with the addition of a bone graft. Occasionally, it is difficult to maintain the reduction of a segmental fracture, and compression plating may have to be performed. The technique has been received with enthusiasm in the United States for the treatment of nonunion of the tibia, for which it is combined with a bone graft procedure.

Postoperatively, patients treated with a compression plating technique require plaster support for ambulation. It must also be borne in mind that significant osteoporosis occurs under a rigid compression plate and, once the fracture has healed, the strength of the bone may be appreciably

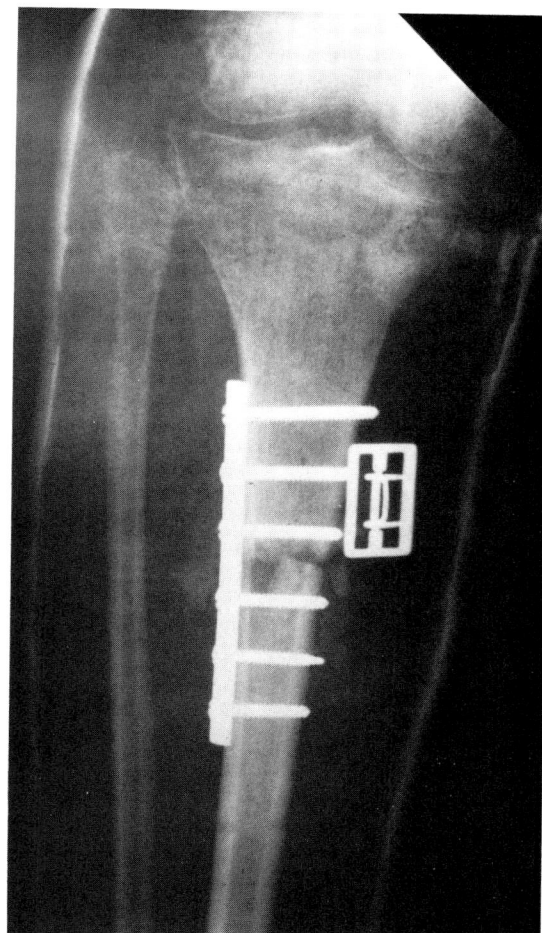

Figure 25–7 A tibial fracture treated with a single compression plate. This technique has been received enthusiastically in European centers but not in North America, except for cases in which it is difficult to maintain a satisfactory reduction by closed measures.

altered. It is for this reason that all compression plates should be removed as soon as the fracture has healed in young people. This applies particularly to ski injuries, as these patients will return to skiing following healing of the fracture, and the osteoporosis under the compression plate may predispose the tibia to another fracture while skiing.

Alternative Methods of Internal Fixation. I include these methods for completeness sake. I do not advocate their use in any tibial fracture.

Parham bands were popular in the past, particularly for treatment of oblique and small segmental fractures. It has since been adequately demonstrated that these bands diminish the blood supply to the surrounding bone. Rhinelander documented the decrease in blood supply caused by these devices and demonstrated that the circlage wire is preferable in the treatment of these fractures, as it does not significantly reduce the blood supply to the bone.[95] This technique, however, does not provide rigid fixation, and for this reason it has not received widespread acceptance.

Compression screws have been advocated for the treatment of oblique, spiral, and segmental fractures. The same criticism applies to this technique as to the circlage wires, it does not provide rigid fixation.

Both these techniques expose the patient to infection and they do not obtain significant fixation. It is for these reasons that they have not been widely accepted in the United States.

Special Problems

Combined Femoral and Tibial Fractures. This combination is not exceedingly rare. It is usually produced by severe trauma such as occurs in a fall down a flight of stairs or a vehicular accident. It presents a special problem in that it is difficult to obtain and hold reduction in both the femoral and tibial areas. If the femoral fracture is at a level satisfactory for intramedullary fixation, I have found it useful to proceed as follows. The patient is given a spinal anesthetic and is then placed on a fracture table. A thigh rest is used to support the femoral fracture, while the knee is flexed to 90 degrees. A $3/32$ inch Steinmann pin is placed through the proximal tibial fragment at the level of the tibial tubercle. The tibial fracture is then reduced and a below-knee cast is applied incorporating the proximal tibial pin. A traction bow is attached to the proximal pin and a traction apparatus is set up to support the thigh. Next, the hip is prepared and draped in the usual manner for blind rodding of the femur. If an image intensifier is available, this procedure can be performed quickly and will provide satisfactory fixation of the femoral fracture. The intramedullary rod is passed down the femoral shaft and across the fracture site into the distal fragment as outlined in Chapter 24. Postoperatively, the patient may ambulate with crutches on the second or third day. I advise active weight bearing to tolerance after the first week. The advantage of this particular method is that it allows early weight bearing and provides early active motion of the knee. The risk of infection following closed rodding of the femur is very small.

The alternative method of treatment is closed reduction of the tibial fracture with a proximal tibial pin incorporated in the below-knee cast followed by traction through the tibial pin for the femoral fracture for approximately two to three weeks. The patient may then be ambulatory with a cast brace for both the femoral and tibial fractures. This form of treatment is also satisfactory, allows relatively early motion of the knee, and does avoid the small risk of infection associated with intramedullary fixation of the femur. It is currently arousing widespread enthusiasm.

Segmental Fractures. These fractures are frequently "bumper" injuries. They are associated with severe trauma. For this reason there is also significant associated injury to the soft tissue in the pretibial area. This must always be borne in mind or devastating results may occur. These fractures may be initially treated with closed reduction and the application of a long leg cast of which the anterior tibial portion has been removed to allow inspection of the soft-tissue structures and assessment of an impending anterior compartment syndrome. Gross disruption of the tissues with a segmental fracture does reduce the incidence of the anterior compartment syndrome by allowing the escape of blood out of the previously closed compartment. If a standard long leg cast is used for these fractures, the patient's temperature must be monitored carefully. Several cases have been reported in which significant soft-tissue slough due to the associated injury occurred under the cast.

If a satisfactory reduction has been obtained the patient may be ambulatory but not start weight bearing, initially. After a period of four weeks he is allowed partial weight bearing progressing gradually to full weight bearing (Fig. 25–8).

As mentioned previously, if there is significant difficulty in obtaining and maintaining reduction of the segmental fracture, consideration may be given to intramedullary fixation or compression plating. I prefer compression plating for small segmental fractures, but if there is a large segmental fracture, the intramedullary technique of Lottes may be indicated.

In the past, the incidence of nonunion

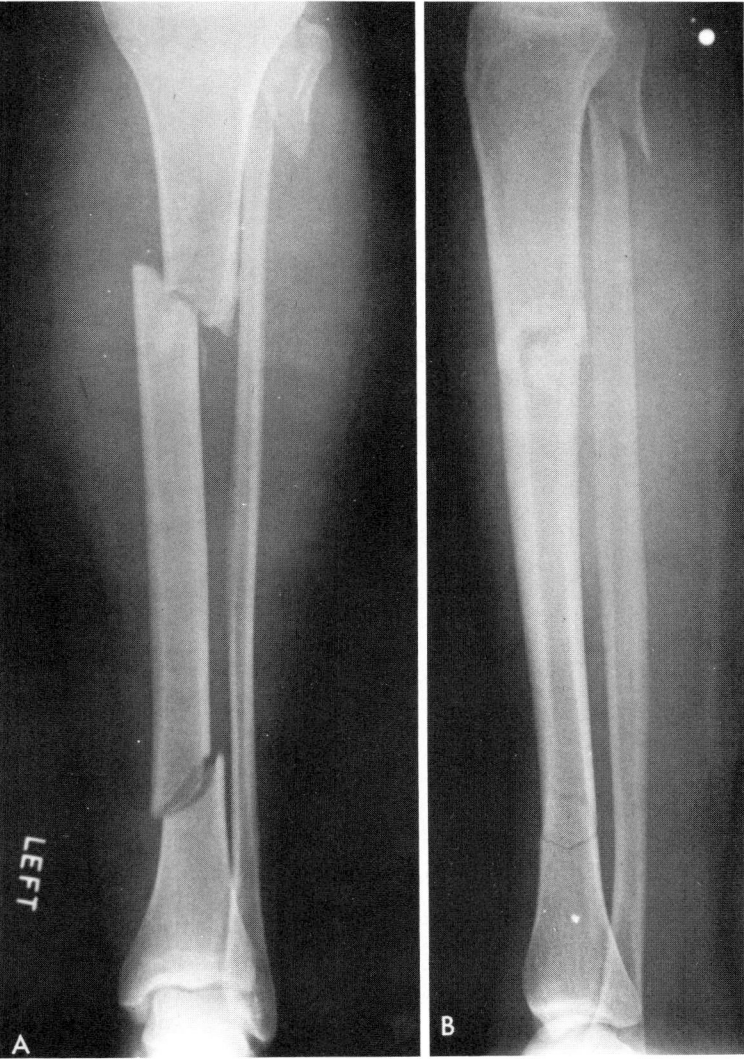

Figure 25–8 *A.* Anteroposterior view of a large segmental tibial fracture. Fortunately there is satisfactory osseous contact with very minimal angulation. *B.* Lateral roentgenogram revealing no evidence of anterior or posterior angulation of the segmental fracture. This healed satisfactorily with a long leg cast and partial weight bearing at five weeks postinjury.

with these fractures ranged from 20 to 60 per cent. In recent years and with a closed reduction, application of a snug-fitting cast, and early weight bearing, however, the incidence of nonunion has decreased to less than 20 per cent.

Soft-Tissue Injuries and Open Fractures. Severe soft-tissue injuries may occur along the anterior aspect of the tibia in association with segmental fracture due to bumper injuries. These can usually be controlled in a long leg cast with its anterior portion removed over the involved area. This is to allow for inspection of the soft-tissue structures and debridement of any necrotic tissue. This same technique can also be adapted for treatment of severe soft-tissue loss along the posterior aspect of the tibia by

removing a large segment of the plaster from the posterior part of the cast (Fig. 25–9).

The treatment of open fractures of the tibia deserves special attention. As with open fractures elsewhere, thorough debridement of the open injury to remove necrotic and contaminated tissue is extremely important if the dreaded complication of gas gangrene is to be avoided. It is not sufficient to remove the superficial portion of the skin wound, as the necrotic and contaminated tissue deep within the wound is the perfect culture medium for bacterial growth. I feel very strongly that these patients should be taken to the operating room, and there, under appropriate anesthesia, a thorough and careful

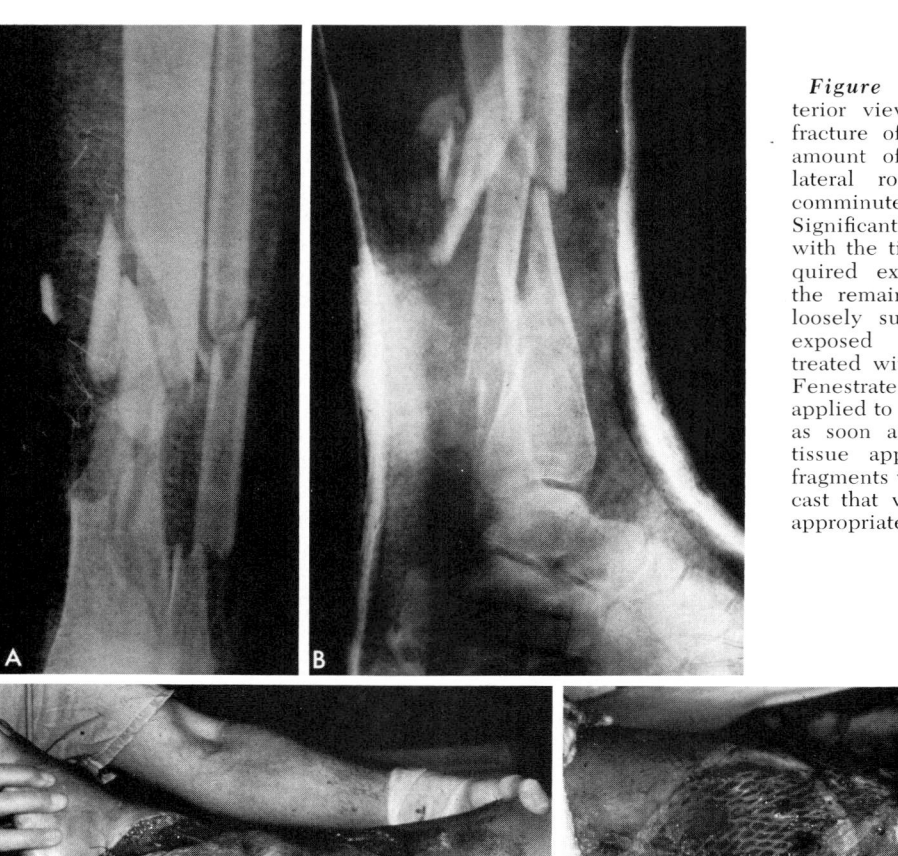

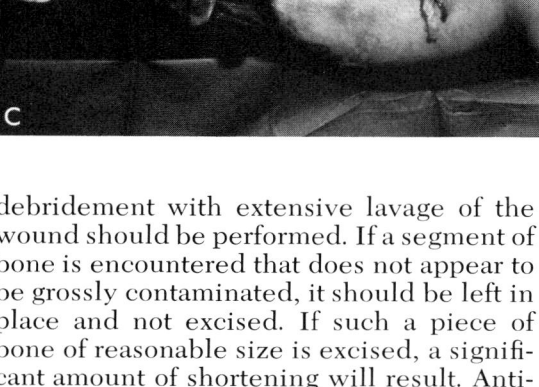

Figure 25–9 *A.* Anteroposterior view of a severe open fracture of the tibia. Note the amount of comminution. *B.* A lateral roentgenogram of the comminuted open fracture. *C.* Significant skin loss associated with the tibial fracture. This required extensive debridement; the remaining viable skin was loosely sutured in place. The exposed muscle areas were treated with Betadine soaks. *D.* Fenestrated skin grafts were then applied to the open muscle areas as soon as healthy granulation tissue appeared. The fracture fragments were controlled with a cast that was windowed in the appropriate areas.

debridement with extensive lavage of the wound should be performed. If a segment of bone is encountered that does not appear to be grossly contaminated, it should be left in place and not excised. If such a piece of bone of reasonable size is excised, a significant amount of shortening will result. Antibiotics may be added to the irrigating solution, but it is felt that the mechanical irrigation is the important factor in removing a large portion of the bacteria that may be present.

The treatment of a large open fracture with significant skin loss is a little more controversial. Several authors feel that it is important to obtain adequate soft-tissue coverage over the exposed fracture surfaces. This is usually accomplished by swinging a skin flap over the defect and using a relaxing incision. Other authors feel that it

is best to treat these injuries with wide debridement followed by the application of Betadine soaks. I favor the latter method of treating these injuries by applying wet Betadine soaks that are changed daily. Once the wound appears "clean," a secondary closure or a skin flap with a relaxing incision may be employed to close the defect. I am against closing the wound initially because a frank infection may occur under the soft-tissue flap. If closure is delayed, the majority of the contaminated tissue will have already been removed. This method appears to offer the soft tissues the best chance for healing. A final method that I have used on several occasions is to apply Betadine soaks to the open wound and follow this with the application of a long leg cast and early ambulation. This treatment has been demonstrated to be very beneficial, as reported in several articles published from the armed services. It returns the limb to active function without paying specific attention to the soft-tissue wound. The dressings are changed, not daily but weekly or every other week. The rationale behind this is that the return of the limb to functional activity improves the blood supply to the soft-tissue structures, and the wounds gradually heal by secondary intention. It is an excellent method of treating these severe injuries and should certainly have a place in the overall treatment of open fractures of the tibia.

The pins and plaster technique is also useful in the management of open injuries associated with significant comminution at the fracture site in which it is difficult to maintain reduction. The wound is thoroughly debrided. The limb is prepared again and redraped, and pins are inserted above and below the fracture site through normal tissue. The wound is then packed open with Betadine soaks and a long leg cast is applied, incorporating the pins. The patient then ambulates as soon as possible, without weight bearing on the involved extremity. A window is placed over the area of skin loss, and the wound is inspected every other day until there is evidence that it is "clean," at which time the window may be replastered. Repeat inspection is carried out in one to two weeks but the cast itself is not changed until four to six weeks, provided it is maintaining proper alignment of the fracture fragments. If there is significant loss of position of the fragments, however, then the cast is removed, a proper reduction is performed, and a new cast is applied, incorporating the pins as before.

A final method for management of these injuries is debridement of the area followed by the insertion of a pin in the os calcis for gentle traction, to be applied on a Böhler frame. This method was popular following World War II. Its popularity has decreased recently however, and it has been largely supplemented by either pins and plaster or debridement followed by the application of wet soaks to the area of soft-tissue loss and a long leg cast.

If there has been significant soft-tissue loss on both the anterior and posterior aspects of the tibia, pins and plaster may be applied and immobilized with an external apparatus similar to the Roger-Anderson device connecting the pins. This allows for proper debridement and adequate care of the soft-tissue wounds while still maintaining the reduction.

Recently, there has been a wave of enthusiasm for the management of large open fractures with skin loss by the following technique. A Hoffman external fixation device is applied for fracture stability. An arteriogram is performed, and if there are at least two patent vessels present in the tibial area a free skin graft is applied to the tibial soft tissue defect with its attendant artery and vein, from the medial thigh or iliac crest area. Microvascular techniques are required to anastomose the artery and vein of the flap to the corresponding vessels in the tibial area. This provides for an active live flap for coverage of the defect. A composite bone and skin graft may be obtained from the iliac crest to provide live bone and soft tissue to fill in the defect. The combined procedure has been performed by the author on several severe open tibial fractures with excellent results. These cases should be referred to medical centers where this expertise is available.

I do not feel that there is any indication for open reduction and internal fixation in an open injury. There is no doubt that the incidence of infection is definitely increased with this treatment, and it is an approach difficult to justify in the face of the excellent results reported with the use of a long leg cast followed by early weight bearing as reported by Brown and Urban.[17]

PROGNOSIS

The prognosis in regard to fractures of the tibia has changed greatly over the past decade. This has been largely attributed to the concept of managing these injuries with early ambulation and early return to active weight bearing. This approach allows a quick return of the injured limb to a functional status. It is felt that the even distribution of the forces acting around the fracture site decreases the amount of edema secondary to the injury and it has also been postulated that the early return to active weight bearing produces compression across the fracture surface that stimulates the healing process. Prior to the advent of this concept patients were treated with a long leg cast and prolonged avoidance of weight bearing. Comparison of older studies with the newer studies reveals a definite difference in the incidence of delayed union and nonunion. A significant reduction in the development of these two complications has been reported in all recent studies of the early weight bearing technique.[17, 30–32, 98–100]

Several factors appear to play a prominent role in the prognosis of these fractures. These have been identified and outlined by Ellis. He was able to demonstrate at follow-up that three factors appear to influence the healing rates with these injuries. First, the amount of displacement has a direct effect on the healing rate. The greater the displacement, the greater the injury and associated soft-tissue disruption. Second, the presence or absence of a compound injury directly influences the healing rate. There was a definite delay in healing associated with open fractures as compared to simple closed injuries. Finally, severe comminution at the fracture site adversely affects the healing rate. Ellis felt that all three factors taken together were an indication of the severity of the injury.[42] An additional factor in determining the healing rate is the presence or absence of distraction at the fracture site. If distraction is present, the incidence of delayed union and nonunion increases. This adverse effect has also been demonstrated with traction per se. These two findings are part of the reason why treatment of these injuries with skeletal traction through an os calcis pin has become less popular in recent times.

There is great controversy at present about when union of these fractures is delayed. I feel that there should be significant evidence of healing both clinically and radiologically by 20 weeks. If at that time such evidence is lacking, I feel it is an indication of delayed healing. Nonunion, however, is a clinical diagnosis and is dependent on the clinical and roentgenographic findings outlined in Chapter 4.

In the past, the level of the fracture was thought to play a significant role in the fracture healing process. I feel, however, that it has been adequately demonstrated in recent studies that the level is not of signal importance in healing of fractures of the tibia. The notion that an increased incidence of delayed union and nonunion is associated with fractures in the distal third of the tibia is longer accurate. This incorrect impression is still given in many older textbooks and is still retained by many practicing physicians. It is true that the distal third of the tibia is a common site for the development of congenital pseudarthrosis, but it is not true that the distal third is associated with a significantly increased incidence of nonunion of fractures of the tibia treated by modern methods.

In a similar manner the pattern of the fracture line has received particular attention. The three common patterns of tibial fractures are transverse, oblique, and spiral. Transverse fractures are usually the result of direct trauma, and for this reason are frequently associated with more direct force and soft-tissue destruction. Oblique and spiral fractures, on the other hand, are associated with indirect injuries associated with a significant amount of torque. These do not have the severe soft-tissue disruption and energy absorption that are associated with displaced transverse fractures. I do not feel that the direction of the fracture line in itself is important as a prognostic indicator, provided there has been no significant displacement.

Segmental fractures appear to have a greater incidence of delayed union than simple fractures. It must be kept in mind that these are, by definition, comminuted fractures and are the result of more significant direct trauma than other types of tibial fractures. The amount of soft-tissue disruption with these injuries certainly must have some bearing on the increased incidence of delayed union. Another most important factor in the healing of this type of fracture has been demonstrated by Rhinelander. He was able to document the fact that the intramedullary vasculature is the most important source of blood in healing tibial fractures. This main blood supply is completely disrupted with a segmental fracture and must be reconstituted across two distinct fracture sites. This by itself could easily account for a delay in healing. It must be kept in mind that, in many of these fractures, this adverse factor is also associated with significant soft-tissue disruption so that both the intramedullary and periosteal blood supplies may well be affected. It is frequently difficult to maintain a proper reduction with this type of injury, and occasionally a compression plate or an intramedullary rod is required. In closed rodding, the periosteal blood supply is not significantly altered. If, however, an open reduction with exposure of the fracture sites for insertion of the intramedullary device is required, then both the intramedullary and periosteal blood supplies are altered. This has a pronounced adverse effect on healing of the fracture. Several of the older studies found a 20 to 60 per cent incidence of nonunion associated with the management of these fractures. More recent studies have demonstrated a greater incidence of nonunion than in simple fractures, but have variously set the rate at 5 to 20 per cent.

As stated previously, distraction at the fracture site is detrimental to healing of tibial fractures. Ellis, in his excellent review, felt that distraction of only 1.5 mm adversely affected fracture healing. This certainly fits in with recent concepts that direct apposition or actual compression at the fracture site enhances the healing process.

The management of the patient with an intact fibula in the presence of a fracture of the tibia has remained controversial to the present time. Several authors have felt that the presence of an intact fibula indirectly indicates a less severe injury. The fibula may then act as an internal strut to aid in maintaining the alignment of the tibial fragments. This concept may be true, but it is also true that an intact fibula may be detrimental to fracture repair by reducing the amount of compression on the tibial fracture site. I feel very strongly that if a patient with an intact fibula demonstrates evidence of a delay in healing, an improved prognosis may be seen with a limited resection of the fibula to allow compression of the tibial fragments. It is for this reason that I always pay special attention to fractures of the tibia associated with an intact fibula and do not hesitate to resect a portion of the fibula if there is no evidence of healing by 20 weeks.

In conclusion, there is an overall improvement in healing of tibial fractures with appropriate reduction and return to active ambulation with early weight bearing, as substantiated by the studies of Ellis, Weissman, Nicoll, Dehne and co-workers, Brown and Urban, and Sarmiento.[17, 30–32, 41–43, 89, 98–100, 112]

Part of the problem in defining the exact incidence is the controversy surrounding the exact time interval after which this complication is present. I feel that delayed union is present if there is no evidence of clinical union by 20 weeks. This does not mean that the fracture will inevitably go on to nonunion; many patients who show no definite evidence of healing at 20 weeks will eventually go on to union. The 20 week time interval is useful in that it cautions the attending surgeon that this fracture "may" go on to nonunion. Not all patients presenting at this time interval should have an operative procedure in an attempt to stimulate healing. If, however, there is evidence of healing of an associated fibular fracture with slight distraction at the tibial fracture site, then I feel it is reasonable to resect a limited portion of the fibula to allow compression at the tibial fracture site (Fig. 25–10). This is a very benign procedure and has resulted in many fractures' progressing to full union. It is important to resect a portion of the fibula rather than to perform a simple fibular osteotomy; removal of the segment of the fibula allows for adequate compression at the fracture site, which is not always the case with a simple osteotomy of the fibula. It also prevents rapid healing of the fibula prior to healing of the tibial fracture.

Again, I must stress that every attempt should be made to have patients bearing full weight on their tibial fractures as soon as possible. If a patient has been kept from weight bearing for the initial 10 to 12 weeks following the fracture, it is most important to encourage him in full weight bearing in the cast. The majority of patients who show evidence of delayed union at 20 weeks and who have not been weight bearing for a significant percentage of that time may progress to uneventful fracture healing following an interval of full weight bearing.

COMPLICATIONS IN TIBIAL FRACTURES

Delayed Union

The exact incidence of delayed union has varied in several published reports.

Nonunion

A diagnosis of nonunion is based on a combination of clinical and roentgenographic examination. A small number of fractures in which union is delayed will progress to nonunion. I feel that this diagnosis should be entertained if there is no

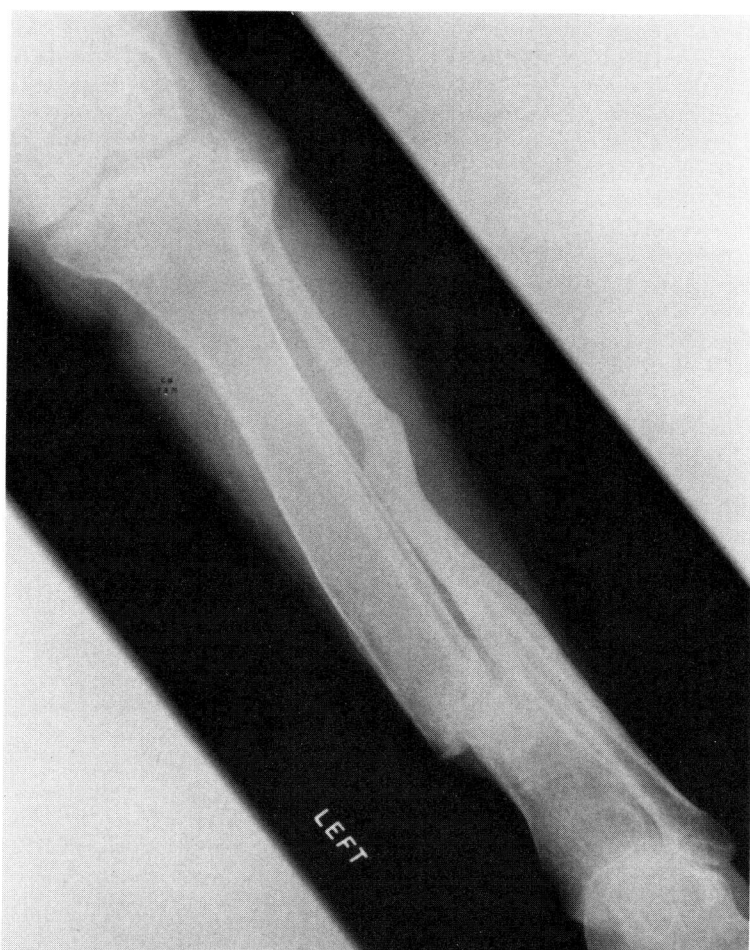

Figure 25–10 A fracture of the tibia and fibula. The fibular fracture healed and produced slight distraction at the tibial fracture site, resulting in eventual nonunion. Note the hypertrophy of the fibula in response to the added stress. Frequently, if a section of the fibula is excised, active compression can occur at the tibial fracture site, stimulating healing.

evidence of healing by 26 weeks. The clinical manifestations include pain and tenderness at the fracture site; there may or may not be active motion at the fracture site with stress. Pain may be present with active weight bearing. The roentgenographic signs of nonunion as outlined previously, include sclerosis or flaring at the fracture site without evidence of actual continuity of bone. As in delayed union, there may be evidence of healing of an associated fibular fracture and slight distraction at the tibial fracture site. At this late date, however, I feel that something more than resection of the fibula is required. Following World War II it was not uncommon to use an anterior approach for the insertion of cancellous bone grafts with or without a direct attempt to take

down the fracture site. More recently, the posterolateral approach of Harmon has become very popular for the treatment of nonunion in this area.[54] This is an excellent approach, as it provides adequate soft-tissue coverage and the problems related to skin slough and delayed healing of the soft-tissue wound by the anterior approach are avoided.

The Harmon posterolateral approach to the tibia may be made with the patient prone or on his side with the affected extremity up. Technically it is easiest with the patient prone, but this requires good anesthesia, as the patient must be intubated. The skin incision is placed along the lateral border of the gastrocnemius on the posterolateral aspect of the extremity. The peroneal musculature is situated anteriorly, and the gastrocnemius, soleus, and flexor hallucis longus muscles are situated posteriorly. The interval between the anterior peroneal muscles and the posterior muscle group is identified. The soleus and flexor hallucis longus muscles are reflected medially, exposing the posterior surface of the fibula, and the tibialis posterior is dissected from its origin on the posterior aspect of the interosseous membrane. The muscles are then stripped subperiosteally from the posterior aspect of the tibia. Care must be taken in the management of the proximal portion of the wound, as the large muscular branches of the peroneal artery lie in close association with the peroneal muscles at this level. The posterior tibial artery and vein and the tibial nerve have been retracted medially in the posterior muscle mass. The operator should not visualize these structures directly, as they are situated between the flexor hallucis longus and tibialis posterior muscles. The posterior aspect of the tibial shaft is almost completely exposed except for its proximal quarter. The nonunion site is identified; if it appears to be relatively stable, the nonunion is not "taken down." It is my feeling that if adequate stability is present a bone graft is all that is required. If, on the other hand, there is gross motion at the nonunion site with minimal stability, then I feel that a compression plate should be applied in addition to a bone graft. If a simple bone grafting procedure is all that is required, which may be the case, the posterior aspect of the tibia proximal and distal to the nonunion site is decorticated. The medial border of the posterior aspect of the fibula is also decorticated above and below the nonunion site. An adequate amount of cancellous bone from the iliac crest is placed along the proximal and distal portions of the tibia, extending over to the decorticated fibula. The reflected muscles are then allowed to retract into proper position. The deep fascia is closed on the lateral aspect of the leg. I prefer to apply a posterior splint in the immediate postoperative period. This will allow for some swelling at the operative site. On the third to fourth postoperative day the patient is placed in the sitting position in bed with the extremities dangling over the edge of the bed. A careful inspection of the wound is made and a snug long leg cast is applied. The patient is then encouraged to begin weight bearing as soon as it can be tolerated. At four to six weeks the long leg cast is converted to a snug patellar tendon-bearing cast. This type of cast is maintained until there is evidence of union. Clinical evidence of union may take five to seven months postoperatively (Fig. 25–11).

I have had no experience with the use of a Lottes nail along with resection of a portion of the fibula in the management of nonunion. Good results have been reported in the hands of surgeons accustomed to this method.

If there is a significant loss of osseous substance at the nonunion site, I feel that the dual onlay bone graft method of Boyd is the treatment of choice.[13] Cancellous bone chips are also placed in the defect between the dual onlay grafts.

The management of infected nonunion is a little more difficult. Recently, Freeland and Mutz have successfully treated 23 patients with infected nonunion of the tibia by a posterior bone grafting procedure. If there is drainage from the anterior aspect of the tibia, local debridement of this area is performed prior to formal bone grafting. At the time of operation the anterior wound is sealed off with an adherent drape. Preoperative, intraoperative, and postoperative antibiotics should be administered for this surgical procedure. The approach is essentially the Harmon posterolateral approach, but if the nonunion is in the proximal portion of the tibia a posteromedial approach is advocated. Compression plates are not recommended. A simple bone grafting procedure, as outlined previously, is performed. The postoperative treatment is similar except that these patients continue to receive large doses of antibiotics. Freeland and Mutz found that the average time for osseous union was five and a half months and it occurred in all patients.[47] This provides an excellent method of treatment for a difficult problem.

Anterior Compartment Syndrome

This syndrome is a very serious complication that may occur in patients with tibial fractures. Increased intracompartmen-

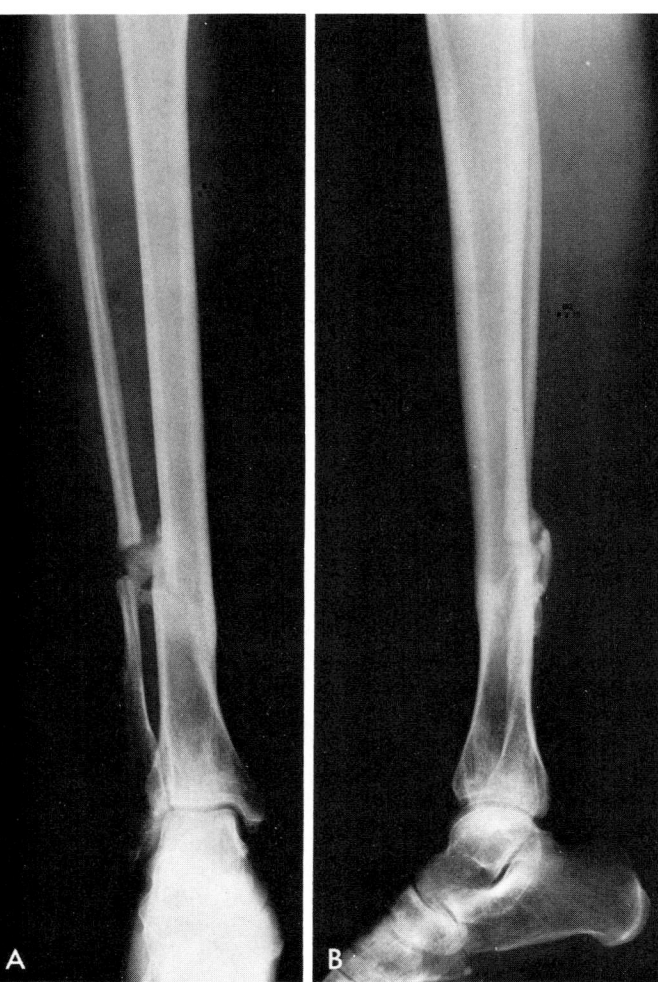

Figure 25–11 A. Anteroposterior view of nonunion of the distal tibia treated by a posterolateral Harmon approach and insertion of bone graft along with sleeve resection of the fibula. Solid union of the tibia is evident five months postoperatively. *B.* Lateral view revealing evidence of solid union at the previous nonunion site.

tal pressure is the underlying pathogenetic factor. This produces a true surgical emergency. The increased pressure within the muscular compartment prevents venous return, which causes edema and further increases the pressure until it is high enough to block arterial inflow in the extremity. If the fibula has also been fractured, the muscle compartment may be violated, allowing blood to escape into the subcutaneous tissues and effecting self-decompression. The onset of the condition may be heralded in by an increase in pain in the extremity along with parasthesiae. The pain may subside with further progression and be replaced by a decrease or lack of sensation in the affected limb. It is important to test the muscular strength of the digits and also to determine whether

passive muscle stretching produces pain. The compartment will feel tense to direct palpation. Peripheral pulses are not a good guide, as collateral flow can maintain the pedal pulses, giving a false sense of security. Careful assessment of the capillary return to the toes is important and may provide an early warning signal (Fig. 25–12).

The compartmental pressures can be measured directly by the method of Whitesides and co-workers or by the wick catheter technique.[113] If the pressures approach 40 to 60 mm Hg or higher, a fasciotomy should be performed, *the sooner the better.* This should include a thorough release of the fascia overlying the compartment. As open release including the skin is preferred. A skin graft can always be

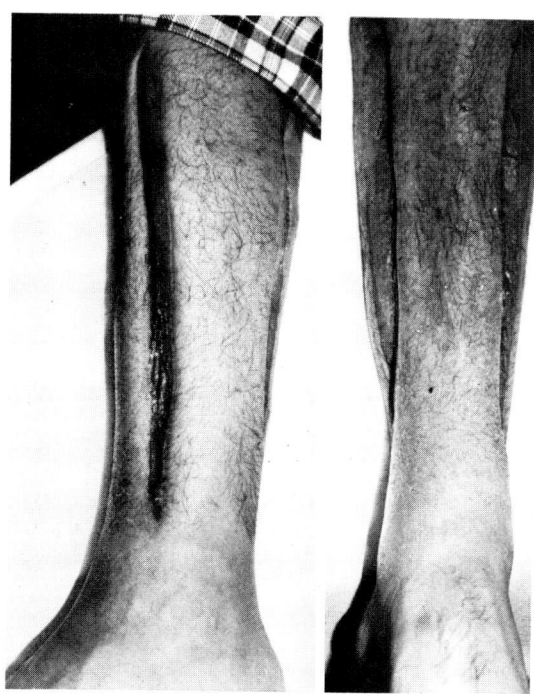

Figure 25–12 The appearance of the lower extremity following an adequate fasciotomy for an anterior compartment syndrome. The patient retained full function.

applied to the skin defect. This will allow the contained muscle to expand, providing an improvement in the circulation. If the fasciotomy is performed prior to 12 hours following the development of the syndrome, the function of the nerve and muscle will be preserved. If more than 12 hours elapse, residual sensory and motor deficits will occur. I cannot stress strongly enough that this is a true surgical emergency and an adequate fascial release must be performed as soon as possible.

The syndrome may also result from a crush injury to the lower extremity without a fracture, by the same mechanism of increased compartmental pressures. It may also be seen when swelling has occurred under a snug cast. If there is any indication of this syndrome developing, the cast must be removed for proper assessment and for pressure readings. The Whiteside technique provides a quick reliable method of measuring the compartmental pressures directly.[113]

REFERENCES

1. Abbot, L. C.: The use of iliac bone in the treatment of ununited fractures. AAOS Instructional Course Lectures, Vol. 2. Ann Arbor, J. W. Edwards, 1944.
2. Adler, J. B., Shaftan, G. W., Rabinowitz, J. G., and Herbsman, H.: Treatment of tibial fractures. J. Trauma, 2:59–75, 1962.
3. Albert, M.: Delayed union in fractures of the tibia and fibula. J. Bone Joint Surg., 26:566–578, 1944.
4. Anderson, L. D., and Hutchins, W. C.: Fractures of the tibia and fibula treated with casts and transfixing pins. South. Med. J., 59:1026–1032, 1966.
5. Anderson, M. K., McDonald, K., and Stephens, J. G.: A study of the effect of open and closed treatment on rate of healing and complications in fractures of the tibial shaft. J. Trauma, 1: 290–297, 1961.
6. Anderson, R.: An automatic method of treatment for fractures of the tibia and fibula. Surg. Gynecol. Obstet., 58:639–646, 1934.
7. d'Aubigne, R. M.: Surgical treatment of nonunion of long bones. J. Bone Joint Surg., 31A: 256–266, 1949.
8. d'Aubigne, R. M.: Infection in the treatment of ununited fractures. Clin. Orthop., 43:77–82, 1965.
9. Bauer, G. C. H., and Edwards, P.: Fracture of the shaft of the tibia. Incidence of complications as a function of age and sex. Acta Orthop. Scand., 36:95–103, 1965–1966.
10. Bergentz, S. E., and Thureborn, E.: Shaft fractures of the lower leg: Open versus closed reduction. Analysis of a twenty-year series. Acta Chir. Scand., 114:235–241, 1957.
11. Blockey, N. J.: The value of rigid fixation in the treatment of fractures of the adult tibial shaft. J. Bone Joint Surg., 38B:518–527, 1956.
12. Böhler, J.: Treatment of non-union of the tibia with closed and semiclosed intramedullary nailing. Clin. Orthop., 43:92–102, 1965.
13. Boyd, H. B.: The treatment of difficult and unusual non-unions. With special reference to the bridging of defects. J. Bone Joint Surg., 25: 535–552, 1943.
14. Boyd, H. B., Anderson, L. D., and Johnston, D. S.: Changing concepts in the treatment of non-union. Clinical Orthopaedics and Related Research, 43:37–54, 1965.
15. Boyd, H. B., Lipinski, S. W., and Wiley, J. H.: Observations of non-union of the shafts of the long bones with a statistical analysis of 842 patients. J. Bone Joint Surg., 43A:159–168, 1961.
16. Boylston, B. F., and Milam, R.: Segmental fractures of the tibia: An analysis of thirty cases. South. Med. J., 50:969–975, 1957.
17. Brown, P. W., and Urban, J. G.: Early weight-bearing treatment of open fractures of the tibia. J. Bone Joint Surg., 51A:59–75, 1969.
18. Burwell, H. N.: Plate fixation of tibial shaft fractures — a survey of 181 injuries. J. Bone Joint Surg., 53B:258–271, 1971.

19. Campbell, W. C.: Transference of the fibula as an adjunct to free bone graft in tibial deficiency. Report of three cases. Am. J. Orthop. Surg., 1:625–631, 1919.
20. Carpenter, E. B.: Management of fractures of the shaft of the tibia and fibula. J. Bone Joint Surg., 48A:1640–1646, 1966.
21. Carpenter, E. B., Dobbie, J. J., and Siewers, C. F.: Fractures of the shaft of the tibia and fibula. Comparative end-results from various types of treatment in a teaching hospital. Arch. Surg., 64:443–456, 1952.
22. Carrell, W. B.: Transplantation of fibula in the same leg. J. Bone Joint Surg., 41A:887–914, 1938.
23. Charnley, J.: The Closed Treatment of Common Fractures. 3rd Ed. Edinburgh, E. & S. Livingstone, 1961.
24. Chrisman, O. D., and Snook, G. A.: The problem of refracture of the tibia. Clin. Orthop., 60:217–219, 1968.
25. Codivilla, A.: On the care of congenital pseudoarthrosis of the tibia by means of periosteal transplantation. Am. J. Orthop. Surg., 4:163–169, 1906.
26. Companacci, M., and Zanoli, S.: Double tibiofibular synotosis for non-union and delayed union of the tibia. J. Bone Joint Surg., 48A:44–56, 1966.
27. Connolly, J. F., Whittaker, D., and Williams, E.: Femoral and tibial fractures combined with injuries to the femoral or popliteal artery. J. Bone Joint Surg., 53A:56–67, 1971.
28. Crellin, R. Q., and Tsapogas, M. J. C.: Traumatic aneurysm of the anterior tibial artery. Report of a case. J. Bone Joint Surg., 45B:142–144, 1963.
29. Davis, A. G.: Fibular substitution for tibial defects. J. Bone Joint Surg., 26:229–237, 1944.
30. Dehne, E.: Treatment of fractures of the tibial shaft. Clin. Orthop., 66:159–173, 1969.
31. Dehne, E., Metz, C. W., Deffer, P. A., and Hall, R. M.: Nonoperative treatment of the fractured tibia by immediate weight bearing. J. Trauma, 1:514–533, 1961.
32. Dehne, E., Deffer, P. A., Hall, R. M., Brown, P. W., and Johnson, E. V.: The natural history of the fractured tibia. Surg. Clin. North Am., 41:1495–1513, 1961.
33. Devas, M. B.: Stress fractures of the tibia in athletes or "shin soreness." J. Bone Joint Surg., 40B:227–239, 1958.
34. Devas, M. B.: Shin splints or stress fractures of the metacarpal bone in horses and shin soreness or stress fractures of the tibia in man. J. Bone Joint Surg., 49B:310–313, 1967.
35. Devas, M. B., and Sweetman, R.: Stress fractures of the fibula—a review of fifty cases in athletes. J. Bone Joint Surg., 38B:818–829, 1956.
36. Dickerson, R. C.: Recent developments in the study and treatment of fractures. Surg. Gynecol. Obstet., 131:537–554, 1970.
37. Dooley, B. J., Menelaus, M. B., and Paterson, D. C.: Congenital pseudarthrosis and bowing of the fibula. J. Bone Joint Surg., 56B:739–743, 1974.
38. Edwards, P.: Fracture of the shaft of the tibia:

39. Edwards, P., Baver, G., and Widmark, P. H.: The time of disability following fracture of the shaft of the tibia. Acta Orthop. Scand., 40:501–506, 1969.
40. Eggers, G. W. N., Shindler, T. O., and Pomerat, C. M.: The influence of the contact-compression factor on osteogenesis in surgical fractures. J. Bone Joint Surg., 31A:693–716, 1949.
41. Ellis, H.: Disabilities after tibial shaft fractures. J. Bone Joint Surg., 40B:190–197, 1958.
42. Ellis, H.: The speed of healing after fracture of the tibial shaft. J. Bone Joint Surg., 40B:42–46, 1958.
43. Ellis, J.: Treatment of fractures of the tibial shaft. J. Bone Joint Surg., 46B:371–372, 1954.
44. Fernandez-Palazzi, F.: Fibular resection in delayed union of tibial fractures. Acta Orthop. Scand., 40:105–118, 1969.
45. Flanagan, J. J., and Burem, H. S.: Reconstruction of defects of the tibia and femur with apposing massive grafts from the affected bone. J. Bone Joint Surg., 29:587–597, 1947.
46. Forbes, D. B.: Subcortical iliac bone grafts in fracture of the tibia. J. Bone Joint Surg., 43B:672–679, 1961.
47. Freeland, A. E., and Mutz, S. B.: Posterior bone-grafting for infected ununited fracture of the tibia. J. Bone Joint Surg., 58A:653–657, 1976.
48. Gustilo, R. B., Simpson, L., Nixon, R., et al.: Analysis of 511 open fractures. Clin. Orthop., 66:148–154, 1969.
49. Gustilo, R. B., Simpson, L., Nixon, R., Ruiz, A., and Indeck, W.: An analysis of 511 open fractures at Hennepin County General Hospital. J. Bone Joint Surg., 50A:830–831, 1968.
50. Hampton, O. P., Jr., and Holt, E. P., Jr.: The present status of intramedullary nailing of fractures of the tibia. Am. J. Surg., 93:597–603, 1957.
51. Hand, F. M.: Crisscross tibiofibular graft for non-union of the tibia. Clin. Orthop., 1:154–160, 1953.
52. Hanson, L. W., and Eppright, R. H.: Posterior bone grafting of the tibia for non-union. A review of twenty-four cases. J. Bone Joint Surg., 48A:27–43, 1966.
53. Harkins, H. N., and Phemister, D. B.: Simplified technique of onlay grafts. For all ununited fractures in acceptable position. J.A.M.A., 109:1501–1506, 1937.
54. Harmon, P. H.: A simplified approach to the posterior tibia for bone grafting and fibular transferral. J. Bone Joint Surg., 27:496–498, 1945.
55. Harvey, F. J., Hodgkinson, A. H. T., and Harvey, P. M.: Intramedullary nailing in the treatment of open fractures of the tibia and fibula. J. Bone Joint Surg., 57A:909–915, 1975.
56. Hedenberg, I., and Pompeius, R.: Shaft fractures of the lower leg. Comparing the early results of open and closed treatment in 120 cases. Acta Chir. Scand., 118:339–348, 1960.
57. Hicks, J. H.: Amputation in fractures of the tibia. J. Bone Joint Surg., 46B:388–392, 1964.

492 consecutive cases in adults. Importance of soft tissue injury. Acta Orthop. Scand., (Suppl. 76), 1965.

58. Hjelmsted, A.: Fractures of the tibial shaft. A study of primary and late results in 105 cases. Acta Chir. Scand., 121:511–516, 1961.

59. Hoaglund, F. T., and States, J. D.: Factors influencing the rate of healing in tibial shaft fractures. Surg. Gynecol. Obstet., 124:71–76, 1967.

60. Holden, C. E. A.: Bone grafts in the treatment of delayed union of tibial shaft fractures. Injury, 4:175–179, 1972.

61. Huntington, T. W.: Case of bone transference. Use of a segment of fibula to supply a defect in the tibia. Ann. Surg., 41:249–251, 1905.

62. Jackson, R. W., and Macnab, I.: Fractures of the shaft of the tibia. A clinical and experimental study. Am. J. Surg., 97:543–557, 1959.

63. Jefferys, C. C.: Spasm of the posterior tibial artery after injury. J. Bone Joint Surg., 45B: 223, 1963.

64. Jones, K. G.: Treatment of infected non-union of the tibia, through the postero-lateral approach. Clin. Orthop., 43:103–109, 1965.

65. Jones, K. G., and Barnett, H.C.: Cancellous-bone grafting for non-union of the tibia through the posterolateral approach. J. Bone Joint Surg., 37A:1250–1260, 1955.

66. Karlström, G., and Olerud, S.: Percutaneous pin fixation of open tibial fractures. Double-frame anchorage using the Vidal-Adrey method. J. Bone Joint Surg., 57A:915–923, 1975.

67. Kratochvil, B. L., and Premer, R. F.: The Delbet split: A report of three cases. Clin. Orthop., 36:151–155, 1964.

68. Lam, S. J.: The place of delayed internal fixation in the treatment of fractures of the long bones. J. Bone Joint Surg., 46B:393–397, 1964.

69. Lamb, R. H.: Posterolateral bone graft for nonunion of the tibia. Clin. Orthop., 64:114–120, 1969.

70. Landoff, G. A.: A comparative study of methods of treatment of diaphyseal fractures of the leg. Acta Orthop. Scand., 18:37–60, 1948.

71. Laurence, M., Freeman, M. A., and Swanson, S. A.: Engineering considerations in the internal fixation of fractures of the tibial shaft. J. Bone Joint Surg., 51B:754–768, 1969.

72. Leach, R. E., Hammond, G., and Stryker, W. S.: Anterior tibial compartment syndrome—acute and chronic. J. Bone Joint Surg., 49A:451–462, 1967.

73. Lottes, J. O.: Intramedullary nailing of the tibia. AAOS Instructional Course Lectures, Vol. 15. Ann Arbor, J. W. Edwards, 1958.

74. Lottes, J. O.: Treatment of delayed or nonunion fractures of the tibia by medullary nail. Clin. Orthop., 43:111–128, 1965.

75. Lucas, K., and Todd, C.: Closed adult tibial shaft fractures. J. Bone Joint Surg., 55B:878, 1973.

76. McCarroll, H. R.: The surgical management of ununited fractures of the tibia. J.A.M.A., 175: 578–583, 1961.

77. McLaughlin, H. L., Gaston, S. R., Neer, C. S., and Craig, F. S.: Open reduction and internal fixation of fractures of the long bones. J. Bone joint Surg., 31A:94–114, 1949.

78. McMaster, P. E., and Hohl, M.: Tibiofibular cross-peg grafting. J. Bone Joint Surg., 47A: 1146–1158, 1965.

79. McMaster, P. E., and Hohl, M.: Tibiofibular cross-peg grafting. Follow-up notes. J. Bone Joint Surg., 57A:720–721, 1975.

80. MacNab, I.: Blood supply of the tibia. J. Bone Joint Surg., 39B:799, 1957.

81. McNeur, J. C.: The management of open skeletal trauma with particular reference to internal fixation. J. Bone Joint Surg., 52B:54–60, 1970.

82. Maisonneuve, M. J. G.: Recherches sur la fracture du perone. Arch. Gen. Med., 7:165–187, 433–473, 1840.

83. Matsen, F. A. Compartmental syndrome. An unified concept. Clin. Orthop., 113:8–14, 1975.

84. Milch, H.: Tibiofibular synostosis for nonunion of the tibia. Surgery, 27:770–779, 1950.

85. Moore, S. T., Storts, R. A., and Spencer, J. D.: Fractures of the tibial shaft in adults: A ten year survey of such fractures. South Med. J., 55:1178–1183, 1962.

86. Moritz, J. R., Saviers, G. B., Earle, A. S., and Ball, J. D.: Spiral fractures of the tibia: long term results of Parham band fixation. J. Trauma, 2:147–161, 1962.

87. Müller, M. E., Allgower, M., and Willenegger, H.: Technique of Internal Fixation of Fractures. New York, Springer-Verlag, 1965.

88. Nelson, G., Kelly, P., Paterson, L., and Janes, J.: Blood supply of the human tibia. J. Bone Joint Surg., 42A:625–635, 1960.

89. Nicoll, E. A.: Fractures of the tibial shaft. A survey of 705 cases. J. Bone Joint Surg., 46B: 373–387, 1964.

90. Olerud, S., and Karlström, G.: Secondary intramedullary nailing of tibial fractures. J. Bone Joint Surg., 54A:1419–1428, 1972.

91. Owen, R., and Tsimboukis, B.: Incidence of ischemic contracture following closed injuries to the calf. J. Bone Joint Surg., 49B:268–275, 1967.

92. Pankovich, A. M.: Maisonneuve fracture of the fibula. J. Bone Joint Surg., 58A:337–342, 1976.

93. Phemister, D. B.: Treatment of ununited fractures by onlay bone grafts without screw or tie fixation and without breaking down of the fibrous union. J. Bone Joint Surg., 29A:946–960, 1947.

94. Ratliff, A. H. C.: Fractures of femur and tibia in same limb. J. Bone Joint Surg., 47B:586, 1965.

95. Rhinelander, F. W.: Tibial blood supply in relation to fracture healing. Clin. Orthop, 105:34–80, 1974.

96. Rorabeck, C. H., and MacNab, I.: Anterior tibial-compartment syndrome complicating fractures of the shaft of the tibia. J. Bone Joint Surg., 58A:549–550, 1976.

97. Sakellarides, H. T., Freeman, P. A., and Grant, B. D.: Delayed union and nonunion of tibial-shaft fractures. A review of 100 cases. J. Bone Joint Surg., 46A:557–569, 1964.

98. Sarmiento, A.: A functional below-the-knee cast for tibial fractures. J. Bone Joint Surg., 49A: 855–875, 1967.

99. Sarmiento, A.: A functional below-the knee brace for tibial fractures. A report on its use in

one hundred and thirty-five cases. J. Bone Joint Surg., 52A:295–311, 1970.

100. Sarmiento, A.: Functional bracing of tibial and femoral shaft fractures. Clin. Orthop., 82:2–13, 1972.

101. Scudese, V. A., Birotte, A., and Gialenella, J.: Tibial shaft fractures: Percutaneous multiple pin fixation, short leg cast and immediate weight bearing. Clin. Orthop., 72:271–282, 1970.

102. Seddon, H. J.: Volkmann's ischaemia in the lower limb. J. Bone Joint Surg., 48B:627–636, 1966.

103. Shaar, C. M., Krenz, F. P., Jr., and Jones, D. T.: Fractures of the tibia and fibula—treatment with the Stader reduction and fixation splint. Surg. Clin. North Am., 23:599–630, 1943.

104. Sheridan, G. W., and Matsen, F. A.: Fasciotomy in the treatment of the acute compartment syndrome. J. Bone Joint Surg., 58A:112–114, 1976.

105. Smith, J. E. M.: Results of early and delayed internal fixation for tibial shaft fractures. J. Bone Joint Surg., 56B:469–477, 1974.

106. Stephens, J. G., and Anderson, M. N.: An analysis of open and closed treatment of fractures of the tibial shaft. Can. J. Surg., 4:65–68, 1960.

107. Tucker, J. T., Watkins, F. P., and Carpenter, E. B.: Conservative treatment of fractures of the shaft of the tibia. J.A.M.A., 178:802–805, 1961.

108. Urist, M. R.: End result observations influencing treatment of fractures of shaft of tibia. J.A.M.A., 159:1088–1093, 1955.

109. Urist, M. R., Mazet, R., Jr., and McLean, F. C.: The pathogenesis and treatment of delayed union and non-union. A survey of eighty-five ununited fractures of the shaft of the tibia and one hundred control cases with similar injuries. J. Bone Joint Surg., 36A:931–967, 1954.

110. Veliskakis, K. P.: Primary internal fixation in open fractures of the tibial shaft. The problem of wound healing. J. Bone Joint Surg., 41B:342–354, 1959.

111. Watson-Jones, R., and Coltart, W. D.: Slow union of fractures. With a study of 804 fractures of the shafts of the tibia and femur. Br. J. Surg., 30:260–276, 1942.

112. Weissman, S. L., Herold, H. Z., and Engelberg, M.: Fractures of the middle two-thirds of the tibial shaft. Results of treatment without internal fixation in 140 consecutive cases. J. Bone Joint Surg., 48A:257–267, 1966.

113. Whitesides, T. E., Haney, T. C., Morimoto, K., and Harada, H.: Tissue pressure measurements as a determinant for the need of fasciotomy. Clin. Orthop., 113:43–51, 1975.

114. Witschi, T. H., and Omer, G. E.: The treatment of open tibial shaft fractures from Vietnam war. J. Trauma, 10:105–111, 1970.

115. Zucman, J., and Maurer, P.: Two-level fractures of the tibia. J. Bone Joint Surg., 51B:686–693, 1969.

R. BRUCE HEPPENSTALL, M.D.

Injuries _____ 26
of the
Ankle

Ankle injuries are encountered daily in both civilian and military practices. They include not only fractures but soft tissue ligamentous injuries as well. The ankle is extremely susceptible to injury owing to the fact that the foot is the only part of the body in contact with the ground surface in the stance and walking phases of gait. An irregular or slippery surface will predispose to ankle injuries. This is compounded by the fact that while the foot is firmly fixed to the ground during walking or running the rest of the body may act as a fulcrum to apply excessive torque at the ankle joint.

Because there appear to be some misconceptions regarding several of the pioneers in the field of ankle injury, the author will attempt to summarize their various contributions. In a monograph on fractures and dislocations published in 1768,[55] Sir Percivall Pott described a fracture of the fibula occurring 2 or 3 inches proximal to the most distal aspect which included a tear of the deltoid ligament with a lateral subluxation of the talus. It was his apparent belief that this was the most common type of ankle fracture. The problem with his concept is that he did not feel there was any damage to the distal tibiofibular syndesmosis. In fact, the fracture he described—one with an intact syndesmosis—probably does not occur. This description should not be used as a term for bimalleolar fractures as it has been in many institutions in the past. However, it will probably continue to be used as a generic term for all fractures of the ankle caused by external rotation forces.

Probably Pott's most significant contribution is that he was the first to place an injured part midway between the extremes of flexion and extension to relax the deforming muscular forces at the fracture site. Previously the definitive treatment had been to place all fractured limbs in full extension. His concept, a radical departure from standard therapy at that time, is still practiced today.

It remained for Dupuytren early in the 1800's to appreciate the importance of the distal syndesmosis in ankle injuries.[27] The fracture bearing his name is a fracture of the fibula that occurs 2 1/2 inches proximal to the most distal aspect of the lateral malleolus, and is thought to be secondary to an outward motion of the foot and ankle in relation to the tibia. Dupuytren believed that the fibular fracture followed a tear of the deltoid ligament or a fracture of the medial malleolus. He observed correctly that in order for a lateral dislocation of the talus to occur as part of the injury there must be a complete rupture of the tibiofibular ligaments.

In 1840 Maisonneuve, a pupil of Dupuytren, was able to produce in a series of cadaver experiments an oblique fracture of the fibula that had not been described previoulsy.[47] He applied external rotatory forces to the foot and then observed the various injuries produced about the ankle. He contended that an external rotation force applied to the ankle could rupture the deltoid ligament. The same force could cause a fracture of the medial malleolus, with a rupture of the tibiofibular ligament in the absence of a fracture of the lateral malleolus. The force would then be transmitted proximally to cause a fracture of the fibula in the proximal third. This injury has come to be known as the Maisonneuve fracture, and its presence calls for a careful assessment of the ankle. If a Maisonneuve fracture is observed clinically and roentgenographically the practitioner must rule out the presence of both a frank diastasis at the ankle joint secondary to a rupture of the tibiofibular ligament and a torn deltoid or fractured medial malleolus. The reader may feel this is overemphatic, but it is not uncommon to see severe ankle injuries that have been "missed," even though the proximal fibular fracture has been observed.

In 1915 Cotton described a fracture of the posterior articular margin of the tibia.[23] In spite of his describing this particular fracture it has become commonplace to refer to a trimalleolar fracture as a Cotton's fracture.

In 1922 Ashhurst and Bromer reported on a very extensive investigation into the mechanism of fractures of the ankle and published a classification which is still used by many practitioners.[1] In 1950 Lauge-Hansen described a further set of cadaver experiments and produced a new working classification which is widely used today.[41]

SURGICAL ANATOMY

The ankle joint is very complex, and a full understanding not only of the osseous structure but also of the major stabilizing ligaments is essential. The ankle joint is made up of three basic osseous structures. (1) The distal aspect of the tibia provides a relatively horizontal surface at its distal articulation as well as at the distal projection of the medial malleolus. (2) The lateral malleolus forms the outer boundary of the ankle joint. Together the fibula and the distal aspect of the tibia are termed the ankle mortise. (3) The talus is surrounded by the ankle mortise and constitutes the remaining portion of the ankle joint proper.

The ankle mortise is wider in its anterior aspect than in its posterior aspect. The anatomical configuration provides for motion of the talus in the ankle mortise, as the talus is also wider in its anterior aspect. This is an extremely important fact to bear in mind in the management of ankle fractures. If the foot is placed in plantar flexion and the fractured malleoli are secured tight against the talus in this position, the ankle mortise will be compromised. The talus will be unable to dorsiflex, since it presents the wide anterior surface during dorsiflexion. Therefore, it is essential to test the ankle motion once internal fixation is secured to insure that dorsiflexion is not restricted by too tight an ankle mortise. This should not occur if anatomical restoration is complete.

The distal end of the tibia provides a relatively horizontal plane for articulation with the talus (Fig. 26-1). This aspect of the articular surface is called the tibial plafond. It has a direct bearing on the stability of the ankle following fractures of the medial malleolus. If the medial malleolar fracture

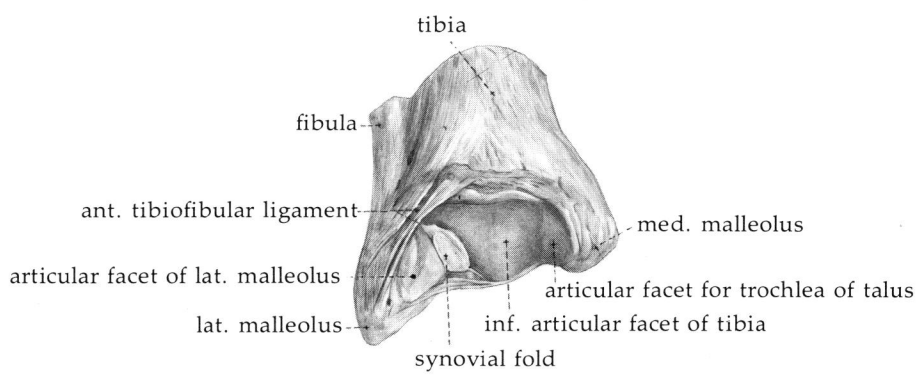

Figure 26-1 Articular surfaces of the tibia and fibula in the right ankle joint. (Courtesy of J. Langman and M. W. Woerdeman and W. B. Saunders Co., Philadelphia, Pa. *Atlas of Medical Anatomy*, 1978.)

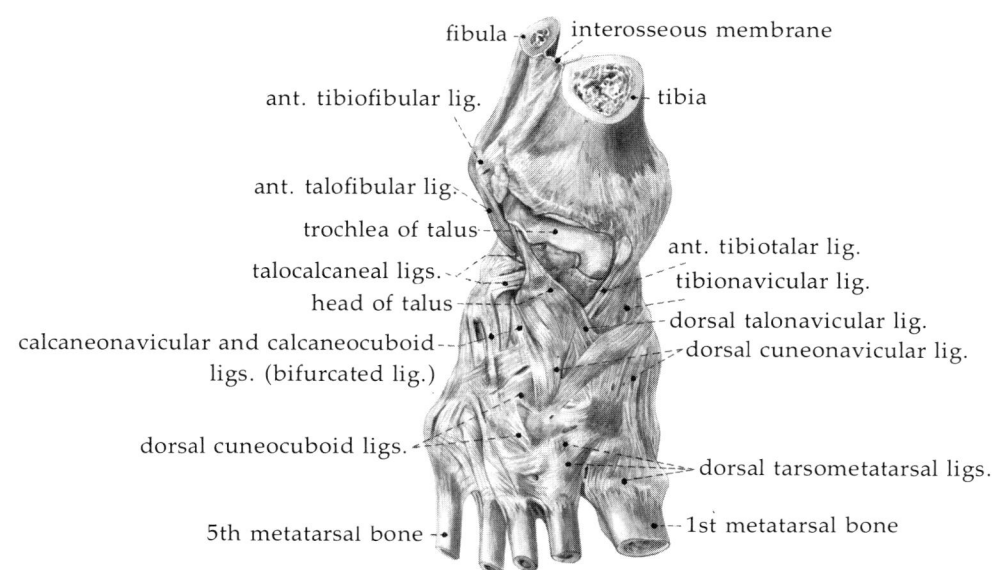

Figure 26-2 Dorsal view of the right ankle. (Courtesy of J. Langman and M. W. Woerdeman and W. B. Saunders Co., Philadelphia, Pa. *Atlas of Medical Anatomy*, 1978.)

occurs at the level of the tibial plafond, or if it extends above the level of the tibial plafond, the ankle joint is considered to be very unstable. However, if the fracture of the medial malleolus is an avulsion injury, with a portion of the medial malleolus remaining intact distal to the tibial plafond, then the talus is considered to be relatively stable within the ankle mortise. Therefore, the tibial plafond has an important bearing on the assessment of whether the ankle injury is stable or unstable, and whether or not it requires internal fixation.

The inner portions of the medial and lateral malleoli are lined with articular cartilage to allow motion of the talus in the ankle mortise. The lateral malleolus tends to be situated in a slightly posterior position in relation to the medial malleolus in a lateral projection, extending approximately 1 cm distal to the medial malleolus.

The talus provides a relatively convexed superior articular surface. It has a wedge-shaped appearance. The anterior aspect is distinctly wider than the posterior to accommodate the similar configuration of the ankle mortise. The superior aspect of the talus is also wider below than above. This wedge shape contributes to stability within the ankle mortise.

The surrounding ligamentous structures furnish significant stability to the ankle joint. These structures include the interosseous ligament, the tibiofibular ligaments, the inferior transverse ligament, and the medial and lateral collateral ligaments (Figs. 26–2 and 26–3).

The interosseous ligament is a distal projection of the interosseous membrane, and the fibers run in an oblique downward direction from the tibia to the fibula. This ligament provides significant strength to the syndesmosis.

The tibiofibular ligament includes anterior and posterior portions. The anterior tibiofibular ligament consists of fibers that project downward between the tibia and fibula along the anterior aspect. The posterior tibiofibular ligament is a similar structure, although not quite as large on the posterior aspect extending between the tibia and fibula. The inferior transverse ligament is located along the posterior portion of the distal tibia and fibula and spans the area between the lateral malleolus and the posterior aspect of the distal tibia. This is a strong ligament, and its proximal fibers tend to merge with the posterior tibiofibular ligament. All these ligaments permit some slight motion at the

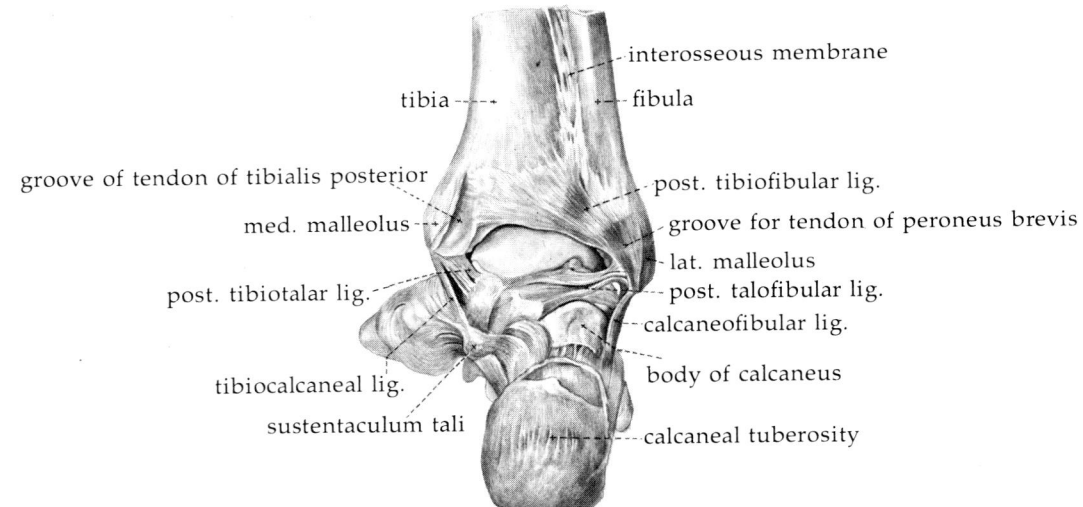

Figure 26-3 Right ankle seen from the back. (Courtesy of J. Langman and M. W. Woerdeman and W. B. Saunders Co., Philadelphia, Pa. *Atlas of Medical Anatomy, 1978.*)

distal tibiofibular syndesmosis. This is a very important concept in fracture management since a patient cannot be allowed to bear weight if an internal fixation device is placed across the distal syndesmosis. A slight amount of motion occurs normally at the syndesmosis. If the patient with a surgical device that spans the distal syndesmosis is allowed to bear weight, the

internal fixation device will probably break. Therefore, all such patients must remain non–weight-bearing until the metallic device is removed.

The medial collateral ligament is also known as the deltoid ligament. It consists of a superficial and a deep portion (Figs. 26–4 and 26–5). The superficial fibers originate from the tip of the medial malleolus and

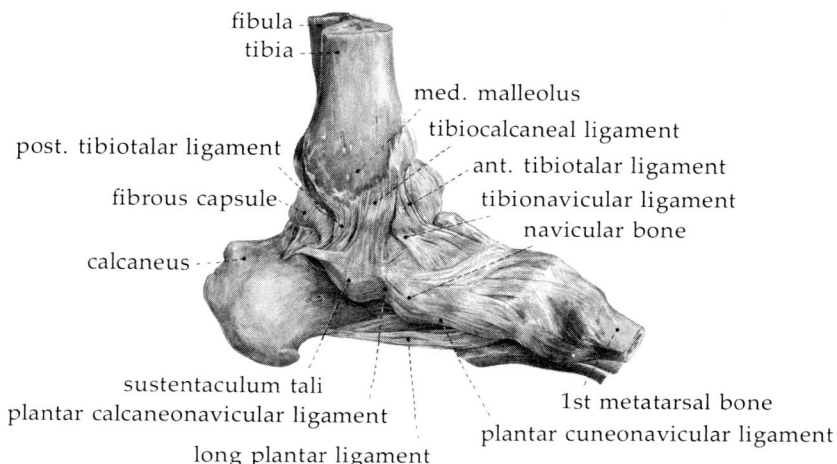

Figure 26-4 Medical view of the ligaments of the ankle. (Courtesy of J. Langman and M. W. Woerdeman and W. B. Saunders Co., Philadelphia, Pa. *Atlas of Medical Anatomy, 1978.*)

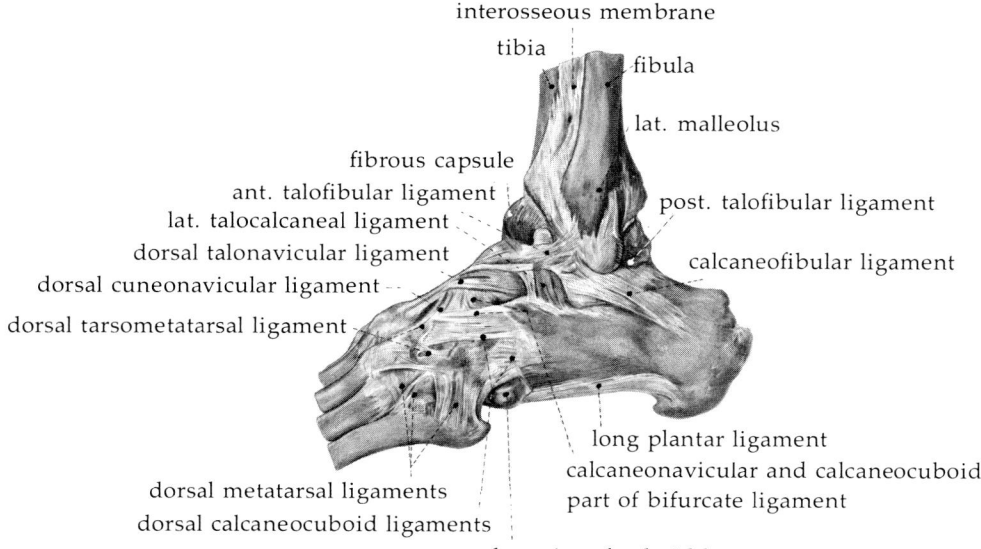

interosseous membrane
tibia
fibula
lat. malleolus
fibrous capsule
ant. talofibular ligament
lat. talocalcaneal ligament
dorsal talonavicular ligament
dorsal cuneonavicular ligament
dorsal tarsometatarsal ligament
post. talofibular ligament
calcaneofibular ligament
long plantar ligament
calcaneonavicular and calcaneocuboid
part of bifurcate ligament
dorsal metatarsal ligaments
dorsal calcaneocuboid ligaments
tuberosity of cuboid bone

Figure 26–5   Lateral view of the ligaments of the ankle. (Courtesy of J. Langman and M. W. Woerdeman and W. B. Saunders Co., Philadelphia, Pa. *Atlas of Medical Anatomy*, 1978.)

insert on the navicular, sustentaculum tali navicular, and the talus proper. The deep portion of the medial collateral ligament extends from the medial malleolus across to the medial aspect of the talus. The two segments of the medial collateral ligament provide a very strong structure which resists external rotation and abduction forces. Each portion of the ligament must be sutured separately in the operative repair of a torn medial collateral ligament.

The lateral collateral ligament is made up of three portions, including the anterior and posterior talofibular ligaments and the calcaneofibular ligament. The anterior talofibular ligament extends from the anterior portion of the lateral malleolus across to the talus, and is situated slightly anterior to the lateral articular facet of the talus. The posterior talofibular ligament extends from the posterior portion of the lateral malleolus across to the posterior aspect of the talus, and is situated slightly lateral to the groove in the talus for the flexor hallucis longus tendon. The calcaneofibular ligament is the middle portion of the lateral collateral ligament, extending distally from the lateral malleolus to the lateral aspect of the calcaneus.

BIOMECHANICS OF THE ANKLE

The ankle is a modified hinge joint, with the primary motions of flexion and extension. The amount of motion at the ankle joint is measured in relation to the foot being maintained at a right angle to the tibia. For example, when the foot is at a right angle to the tibia it is in the neutral position, and measurements are made from this point. Normally, approximately 20 degrees of dorsiflexion (extension) and approximately 50 degrees of plantar flexion are present. This amount of motion is required during the normal gait cycle.

In the stance phase the foot is in approximately the neutral position. However, during the normal push-off phase the tibia tends to rotate forward over the talus. In this position the wide portion of the wedge-shaped talus comes into direct contact with the distal tibial articular surface. At the extreme of dorsiflexion this functions as a mechanical block to further extension. This, in conjunction with strong muscle contraction of the posterior calf group of muscles, provides stability and allows for firm push-off during the gait cycle. A dorsiflexion movement at the ankle joint is accompanied by a slight posterior rotation of the fibula along with proximal motion of the fibula. This compensatory effect results from the anatomical wedge shape of the talus. Thus, there is motion at the distal syndesmosis with normal dorsiflexion of the ankle. This type of motion allows for some widening to occur at the ankle mortise as the broad wedge-shaped portion of the talus articulates with the distal tibia. In plantar flexion the fibula has a slight amount of external rotation and also slight distal migration.

If these motions at the distal syndesmosis are kept in mind, it is not difficult to understand why an internal fixation device should not be inserted across the syndesmosis if weight bearing is to be allowed. The predictable result is that the internal fixation device will break. Therefore, if operative internal fixation for a diastasis is

performed the patient must be kept non–weight-bearing until the device is removed. The standard treatment is to allow a six-week interval, followed by removal of the internal fixation device, and then active full weight bearing in a below-knee cast.

CLASSIFICATION BY MECHANISM OF INJURY

Several working classifications of ankle injuries have appeared in the literature. Basically, they have included one or more of the following: (1) the anatomical deformity present; (2) the principal deforming force applied; and (3) the position of the ankle and foot at the time of injury. The significance of classifying ankle injuries is that treatment is based on attempting to

TABLE 26–1   Ashhurst and Bromer — Classification of Three Hundred Ankle Fractures [*]

A. Fractures by External Rotation
1. First Degree: Lower end of fibula only ("mixed oblique").. 79   (26%)
2. Second Degree: Same, *plus* rupture of internal lateral ligament or fracture of internal malleolus ("low Dupuytren")... 100   (33%)
   (a) Internal lateral ligament, uncomplicated.. 13
       Internal lateral ligament complicated by posterior marginal fragment of tibia........... 13
   (b) Internal malleolus, uncomplicated.. 32
       Internal malleolus complicated by posterior marginal fragment of tibia 42
3. Third Degree: Same, *plus* fracture of whole lower end of tibia, representing the internal malleolus.. 5   (1.7%)
Total Fractures by External Rotation... 184   (61%)

B. Fractures by Abduction (Fibular Flexion)
1. First Degree: Internal malleolus only 20   (6.6%)
2. Second Degree: Same *plus* fracture of fibula (transverse, above or below tibiofibular joint) 41   (13.7%)
   (a) Below inferior tibiofibular joint (no diastasis) ("bimalleolar fracture") 13
   (b) Above inferior tibiofibular joint (with diastasis) ("Pott's fracture," "Dupuytren type") 28
3. Third Degree: Internal malleolus represented by whole lower end of tibia......................... 2   (0.66%)
Total Fractures by Abduction... 63   (21%)

C. Fractures by Adduction (Tibial Flexion)
1. First Degree: External malleolus only, transverse, at or below level of tibial plafond............ 27   (9%)
2. Second Degree: Same, *plus*
   (a) Internal malleolus below level of tibial plafond ("bimalleolar fracture")...................... 3
   (b) Median surface of tibia up and in from joint surface.. 8   (3.6%)
3. Third Degree: Same, *plus* whole lower end of tibia ("supramalleolar fracture by adduction").. 2   (0.66%)
Total Fractures by Adduction... 40   (13.3%)

D. Fractures by Compression in Long Axis of Leg
1. Isolated Marginal Fractures 1
2. Comminution of tibial plafond... 3
3. T or Y-fractures ("V-fractures of Gosselin")... 4
Total Fractures by Compression in Long Axis of Leg... 8   (2.7%)

E. Fractures by Direct Violence (Supramalleolar types).. 5   (1.7%)

[*]*From: Ashhurst, A. P. C., and Bromer, R. S.: Classification and mechanism of fractures of the leg bone involving the ankle. Arch. Surg., 4:51, 1922. Courtesy of *Archives of Surgery*.

reverse the deforming force in order to obtain appropriate reduction. Also, if treatment methods are to be properly evaluated some form of consistent classification must be applied. For this reason a working classification is not just academic but is vital for the proper evaluation, treatment, and follow-up of these injuries. The purely anatomical classification was in vogue during the 19th century, when emphasis was placed on the osseous injury, with no particular importance attached to the associated ligamentous injury.

It remained for Ashhurst and Bromer in 1922 to review and classify 300 cases of ankle injuries on the basis of their mechanism of injury (Table 26–1).[1] They found that external rotation was a significant factor in injury in their series. Their original classification is included in this chapter so that the reader may appreciate this first intelligent attempt at categorization. One major criticism of this type of classification is that it does not take into account a combination of forces. Rather, it is based on the concept of a unidirectional force. Today it is obvious that ankle injuries are produced by a combination of complex forces acting on the ankle joint. This concept has developed as our understanding of the biomechanics of the musculoskeletal system has expanded, particularly over the past two decades.

A much more useful working classification was proposed by Lauge-Hansen,[41] who developed it following an excellent series of cadaver experiments. The reader is referred to this outstanding approach to the problem. Not only did he include the major force involved, but he also took into consideration the position of the foot at the time of injury. As the injuries are subclassified, the first word relates to the position of the foot at the time of injury, and the second word relates to the direction of the deforming force. Since its publication it has become evident that not all injuries can be neatly fitted into this original classification. Therefore, a modified Lauge-Hansen classification was proposed in an effort to include all types of ankle injuries (Table 26–2). This is an excellent working classification, and one that the author has found extremely useful in understanding the mechanism of injury and then formulating the appropriate treatment. Recently, Pankovich has attempted to follow the Lauge-

Hansen terminology to evaluate and group the three different types of fractures of the fibula proximal to the distal tibiofibular syndesmosis.[52] This has been very useful

TABLE 26–2   Modified Lauge-Hansen Classification of Ankle Injuries

Supination-External Rotation
  Rupture of the anterior tibiofibular ligament, or avulsion fracture of one of its bone insertions. Rupture of the interosseous ligament.

  Fracture of the fibula above the syndesmosis.

  Rupture of the posterior tibiofibular ligament, or fracture of the posterior tubercle or margin of the tibia.

  Fracture of the medial malleolus, or rupture of the deltoid ligament.

Supination-Adduction Rotation
  Traction fracture of the lateral malleolus at or below the level of the ankle joint, or rupture of talofibular ligaments.

  Fracture of medial malleolus (tibial plafond vertical fracture).

Pronation-External Rotation
  Fracture of the medial malleolus or rupture of the deltoid ligament.

  Rupture of the anterior tibiofibular ligament, or avulsion fracture of its bone insertion; rupture of the interosseous ligament.

  Fracture of the fibula above the syndesmosis.

  Rupture of the posterior tibiofibular ligament, or fracture of the posterior tibial margin.

Pronation-Abduction
  Rupture of the deltoid ligament or fracture of the medial malleolus.

  Rupture of all ligaments of the syndesmosis, or avulsion fracture of one of the bone insertions.

  Fracture of the fibula proximal to the syndesmosis.

Pronation-Dorsiflexion
  Fracture of the medial malleolus.

  Fracture of the anterior articular margin of tibia.

  Fracture of the distal tibia extending into the articular surface, with a supramalleolar fracture of the fibula.

and will be included in the discussion. Another recent advance has been the recognition by Yablon and co-workers of the key role played by the lateral malleolus in displaced fractures of the ankle.[65]

TREATMENT OF ANKLE INJURIES

In the past, the usual practice was to make an initial attempt at closed reduction of the ankle injury and then to consider operative reduction if this failed. Relatively stable ankle injuries may be treated in this fashion. However, the more unstable injury is definitely disposed to redisplacement in the cast as the swelling subsides. Therefore, if this method is employed, careful follow-up and frequent cast changing, when indicated, are necessary. Kristensen noted that approximately 10 per cent of unstable ankle fractures redisplaced after appropriate closed reduction and satisfactory casting.[38] Braunstein and Wade found that 70 per cent of their cases had evidence of loss of position in the cast following reduction.[6] They found that this usually occurred in the first three days and was repeated at the end of two weeks. Cedell reviewed the results with operative versus nonoperative management of supination-external rotation injuries and found that degenerative arthritis of the ankle occurred twice as frequently in the conservatively treated group as in the operatively treated group.[14, 15]

There has been a more aggressive operative approach in recent times, particularly with unstable injuries. This approach is similar to others described throughout this book which aim at returning the patient to functional activity as quickly as possible, since this appears to have a beneficial effect on fracture healing. The downside risks in the operative approach to unstable injuries involve the possibility of anesthetic complications and the development of infection. These risks must be balanced against the positive aspects, which include anatomical restoration of the injured joint surfaces and adequate internal fixation to allow early motion and early active weight bearing. That is not to state that open reduction will guarantee a good result. It is important to stress the fact that if operative treatment is selected, adequate direct anatomical restoration is necessary, followed by significant internal fixation. The worst of both worlds is to perform an operation and not attain these two goals. Under these circumstances the patient is exposed to the risks of an anesthetic and infection without the advantages of open reduction and internal fixation.

The degree of internal fixation obtained must be individualized and is determined at the time of the operative procedure. The treating physician must then determine when to initiate active motion of the ankle joint and when to allow partial and full weight bearing on the involved extremity. Active motion of the ankle joint is thought to be a significant factor in nutrition of the articular cartilage. Rigid immobilization of the ankle, on the other hand, probably has a detrimental effect on articular cartilage nutrition. If this is coupled with the fact that rigid immobilization produces fibrous scarring around the ankle joint and may in itself limit motion, the benefit of early active motion is not difficult to comprehend. Functional weight bearing and active contraction of the surrounding musculature is thought to be a definite factor in stimulating healing of fractures, as outlined in other sections of this book. The only exception to allowing full active weight bearing following internal fixation is if a fixation device has been placed across the syndesmosis. Under these circumstances, weight bearing will have to be delayed until the device is removed.

Since the ankle is functionally a weight-bearing joint and is subject to significant stresses, the author favors the operative approach for unstable injuries in order to obtain as good an anatomical reduction as possible and to prevent future arthritis. Although many of these injuries could be managed by closed reduction, this approach requires meticulous attention to the casting technique and very close follow-up along with frequent cast changes in order to avoid the dread complication of redisplacement.

As stated previously, a minor modification of the Lauge-Hansen classification provides very useful guidelines to the management of ankle injuries. The first word refers to the position of the foot at the time of injury, and the second to the direction of the injuring force. Pronation and supination refer to the position of the foot attained by rotational movement around the axis of the subtalar joint. Abduction and adduction indicate rotational movements of the talus around its long axis. Internal and external rotation of the talus refer to the movements around the vertical axis of the tibia.

SUPINATION-EXTERNAL ROTATION INJURIES

MECHANISM OF INJURY

This injury occurs with the foot in a position of supination at the time an external rotation deforming force is applied. Four distinct stages have been identified.

As the deforming force is exerted a stage 1 injury occurs, with rupture of the anterior tibiofibular ligament or avulsion fracture of one of its bone insertions. There is also a rupture of the interosseous ligament. Stage 2 is a fracture of the fibula above the syndesmosis. Stage 3 is a rupture of the posterior tibiofibular ligament or fracture of the posterior tubercle of the tibia. Stage 4 is a fracture of the medial malleolus or rupture of the deltoid ligament.

PHYSICAL EXAMINATION

In stage 1 injuries, patients will usually present with pain and swelling along the dorsolateral aspect of the ankle. The tenderness is localized to an area that corresponds to the anterior tibiofibular ligament and the interosseous ligament. There is no tenderness to direct palpation along the posterior aspect of the ankle, indicating that the posterior tibiofibular ligament is intact. There is also no evidence of instability of the ankle joint.

A stage 2 injury presents with swelling along the dorsolateral aspect of the ankle, extending upward in a proximal direction. There is localized tenderness to direct palpation over the torn anterior tibiofibular ligament, and there is also exquisite tenderness to direct palpation over the fracture of the distal fibula. A step-off deformity is usually not present with this particular injury.

Stage 3 presents with quite marked swelling along the entire anterior aspect of the ankle, extending in a proximal direction over the fracture area of the distal fibula. With this type of injury the ligamentous support to the distal syndesmosis is disrupted, accounting for the increased swelling. Frequently a palpable defect or step-off deformity is seen at the level of the fibular fracture as well as marked tenderness to direct palpation along the anterior and posterior portions of the ankle. Attempted weight bearing is extremely painful. The area of ecchymosis may extend for quite a distance proximally owing to the significant soft tissue and osseous disruption.

A stage 4 injury presents all of the typical findings of stage 3 with the added factor that the talus is unstable in the ankle mortise. In other words, a lateral displacement of the talus may occur with an abduction force applied to the ankle. There is gross swelling along the entire aspect of the ankle, with acute tenderness to direct palpation over the deltoid ligament or medial malleolus as well as over the area of the syndesmosis and the portion of the fibula that is fractured.

ROENTGENOGRAPHIC EXAMINATION

All injuries of the ankle require a minimum of three roentgenograms. These include anteroposterior, lateral, and mortise views. The anteroposterior roentgenogram is obtained in a similar fashion to anteroposterior roentgenograms in other areas. This is extremely useful in delineating any fractures of the malleoli and in determining whether or not the ankle mortise is intact (Fig. 26–6).

The lateral roentgenogram is also taken in a standard manner. A specific normal finding with this view is that the fibula is superimposed on the posterior half of the tibia. In other words, its anatomical configuration is slightly posterior in alignment to the tibia. This view is helpful in delineating any fractures of the anterior or posterior margins of the distal tibia. The fibula is superimposed on the tibia and talus, and therefore fractures of this bone are not well visualized in the lateral projection.

The mortise view enables the examiner to evaluate the status of the mortise per se. It is

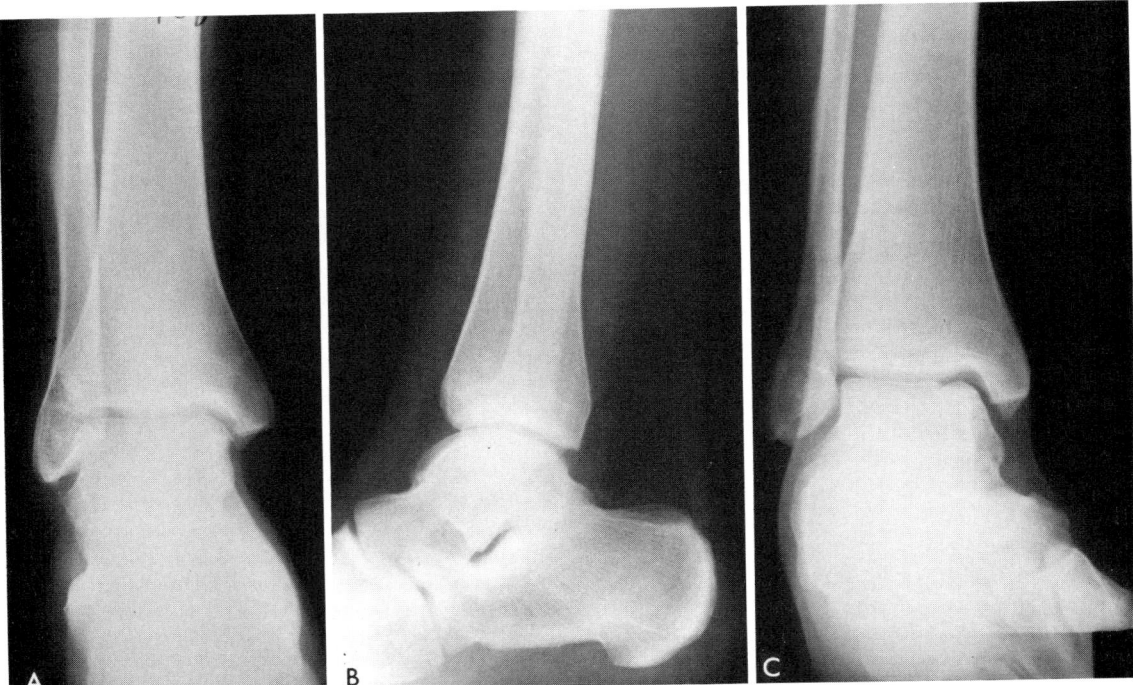

Figure 26–6 A. Routine anteroposterior view of the ankle. Note the area of osteochondritis dessicans of the medial dome of the talus. *B.* Routine lateral view of the ankle. *C.* Mortise view obtained with the foot placed in 20 degrees of internal rotation.

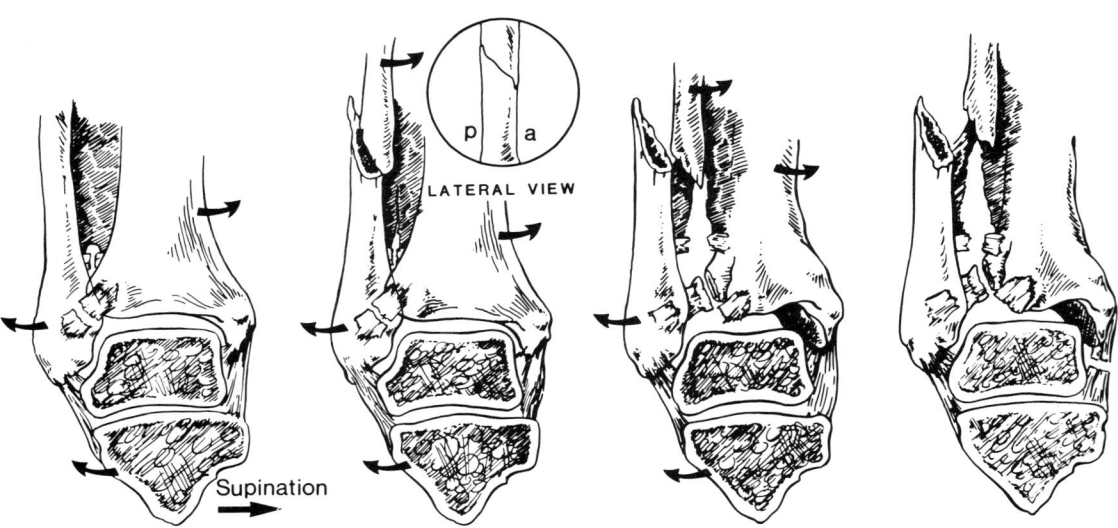

Figure 26–7 Fractures of the fibula proximal to the distal tibial fibular syndesmosis. Mechanism of injury and lesions in various stages of supination-external rotation fractures. (Courtesy of A. M. Pankovich and *Journal of Bone and Joint Surgery.* J. Bone Joint Surg., *60A:221–229, 1978.)*

obtained through an anteroposterior projection with the foot placed in 20 degrees of internal rotation. If a clear space is evident at the syndesmosis in this view, the examiner should suspect a diastasis. A true diastasis is definitely present if the width between the two bones exceeds 3 mm in the mortise view. This view is also useful in detecting any talar dome fractures. Once again, all injuries of the ankle should have these three roentgenographic studies performed for proper evaluation.

Stage 1 injuries fail to reveal any specific roentgenographic signs apart from a soft tissue swelling visible along the dorsolateral aspect of the ankle. Stage 2 demonstrates the fracture of the distal fibula (Fig. 26–7). The fracture line has a specific direction if it occurs proximal to the syndesmosis, as outlined by Pankovich.[52] It is spiral and variably oblique, extending from the anterior edge in a posterosuperior direction. The anterior edge of the fracture is usually located 4 cm or more proximal to the distal end of the fibula. Stage 3 demonstrates the same type of fibular fracture along with evidence of mild separation at the syndesmosis. Stage 4 reveals a definite diastasis, and the talus may be shifted laterally in the ankle mortise.

TREATMENT

Stage 1 Injury

Stage 1 injuries may be treated in a conservative fashion. The posterior tibiofibular ligament complex is still intact. The anterior tibiofibular and interosseous ligaments will heal with conservative management in approximately six weeks. If the patient has significant swelling along the dorsal aspect of the ankle an Ace bandage may be advised, along with crutches for partial weight bearing for two weeks. The alternative is to place the patient in a below-knee weight-bearing cast for comfort. If there is significant tenderness along the anterolateral aspect of the ankle and the patient is unable to place full weight without significant discomfort, a walking cast may be indicated for approximately four weeks.

Stage 2 Injury

A stage 2 injury may be treated with the use of a below-knee cast for eight weeks (Fig. 26–8). Since the deltoid ligament and medial malleolus are intact, this is considered a relatively stable injury. Partial

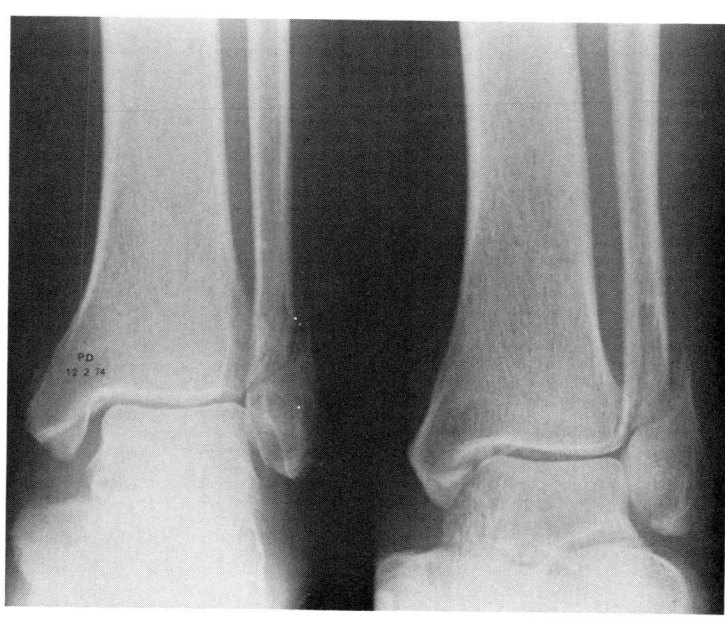

Figure 26–8 A stage 2 supination-external rotation injury. Treated with closed reduction of the fibula fracture and application of a below-knee cast.

weight bearing for two to three weeks is recommended, followed by full weight bearing as tolerated. The usual outcome is uneventful healing of the fibular fracture and fibrous repair of the ligamentous structures.

Stage 3 Injury

Stage 3 injuries may be treated by closed reduction with a snug formfitting long leg cast. In this fracture the ligamentous structures of the syndesmosis are completely disrupted, but the deltoid and lateral ligaments remain intact. If the reduction is satisfactory and can be maintained, patients are placed on non–weight-bearing for four weeks, when the cast is changed to a below-knee weight-bearing cast for an additional four weeks. If the reduction is not complete or if follow-up roentgenograms reveal separation of the syndesmosis, operative intervention is advised. This involves the insertion of a long oblique compression screw from the lateral malleolous at the level of the tibial plafond. The screw is then turned in a slightly proximal direction, spanning the syndesmosis into the adjacent tibia to secure the distal syndesmosis.

A Webb bolt may also be utilized for this purpose. The bolt is inserted in a horizontal plane just above the tibial plafond, spanning the distal fibula, across the syndesmosis, and through the adjacent tibia. The bolt may then be tightened to close the syndesmosis. However, it is extremely important to realize that overcorrection of this defect may result if the bolt is too tight. Therefore, the bolt must be applied with the foot in a neutral or slightly dorsiflexed position so that the broad surface of the talus occupies the ankle mortise. If the device is tightened with the foot in forced plantar flexion, it is conceivable that an overcorrection may occur, blocking dorsiflexion of the ankle by the anatomical configuration of the talus in the tight ankle mortise.

Postoperatively, the patient is maintained on non–weight-bearing for six weeks. At this time the internal fixation device is removed, and full weight bearing in a temporary below-knee cast for two weeks is permitted. The patient is then able to bear weight without support.

Stage 4 Injury

Stage 4 injuries are classified as unstable owing to the fact the deltoid ligament is torn or the medial malleolus is fractured, in addition to other injuries. Under these conditions the talus may be displaced laterally in the ankle mortise. These injuries should be managed with operative repair of the deltoid ligament or internal fixation of the fractured medial malleolus and stabilization of the syndesmosis (Fig. 26–9). In short, both the medial and lateral aspects of the ankle joint are exposed, and the injury is identified. It used to be thought that if the medial aspect of the joint could be stabilized, the lateral aspect of the joint could be molded against the stabilized medial portion with the use of plaster. However, as Yablon and co-workers have demonstrated, particular attention should be paid to the lateral malleolar injury, as the talus tends to follow the lateral malleolar fragment.[65]

These investigators showed that if the deltoid ligament alone was divided no instability of the ankle resulted. Resection of the medial malleolus at the level of the joint line allowed approximately 10 degrees of rotatory displacement of the ankle, but very little valgus instability. If only the fibular collateral ligaments were divided, there was approximately 30 degrees of external rotatory instability and marked talar instability. Finally, resecting the lateral malleolus produced marked rotatory and valgus instability. They also found that when bimalleolar fractures were created in cadavers the talus could be anatomically repositioned only when the lateral malleolus was accurately reduced. It was their opinion that the key to anatomical reduction of bimalleolar fractures was to internally fix the lateral malleolus in anatomical position, as the displacement of the talus followed that of the lateral malleolus. A small 4-holed plate will certainly allow adequate stability of the distal malleolar fracture. The author prefers to treat this injury in the following manner.

The medial aspect of the joint is exposed through a Broomhead[7] or a Colonna and Ralston[20] type of incision. If the deltoid ligament has been torn, a portion of it may be tucked back under the medial malleolus, perhaps explaining why a closed reduction is not always successful in correcting this

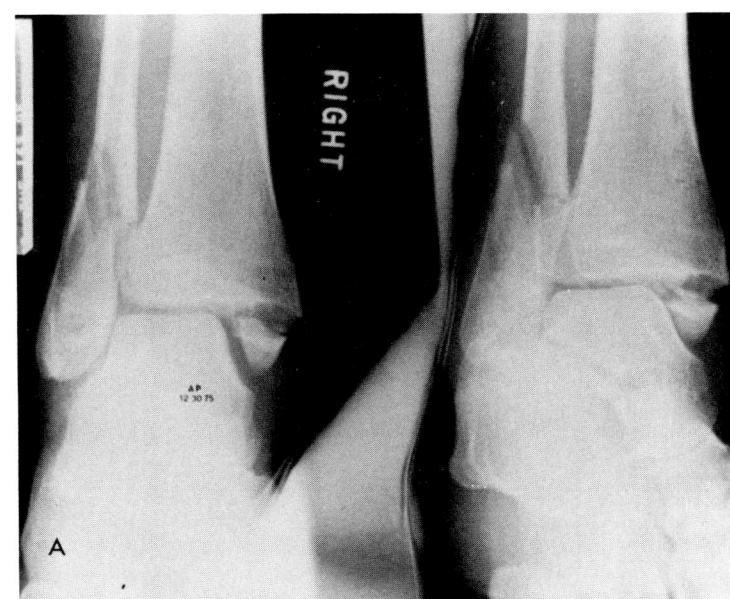

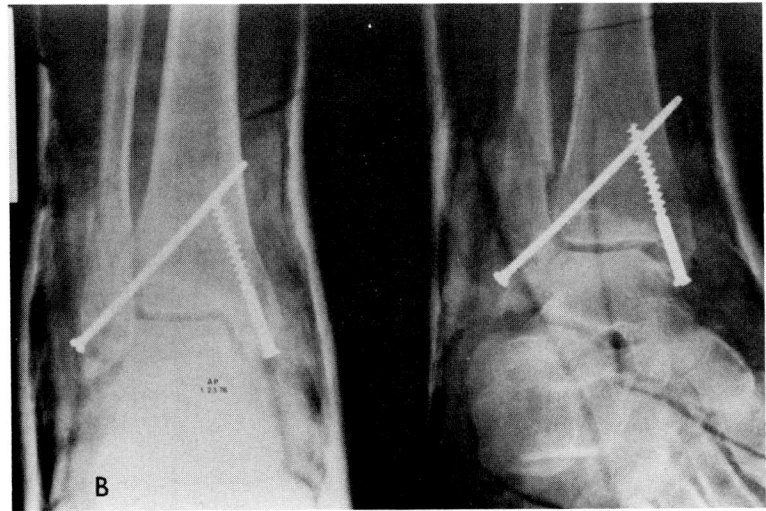

Figure 26–9 A. A stage 4 supination-external rotation injury. *B.* Treated with open reduction and internal fixation with the use of a cancellous compression screw for the medial malleolar fragment, and a transfibular screw spanning the syndesmosis for the lateral aspect.

injury. The ligament is then approximated in two separate layers, as outlined by Close.[19] The sutures are placed in position, but are not snugly secured until after the lateral aspect of the joint is exposed. The lateral portion of the ankle is exposed through a Kocher incision.[37] The fracture of the distal fibula may be internally secured by a small 4-holed compression plate.

The author prefers to reduce the fibular fracture and then to insert an oblique screw across the syndesmosis and into the opposite cortex of the tibia (Fig. 26–10). This provides for secure fixation of the syndes-

mosis. The alternative is to insert a Webb bolt, as previously outlined. Once the lateral aspect of the ankle joint has been properly secured with an internal fixation device, the sutures in the deltoid ligament are tied, with the foot in slight inversion. If there has been a fracture of the medial malleolus it is secured in position with a lag compression screw through the fragment into the distal tibia.

Partial weight bearing is permitted in a short leg cast at four weeks, with progression to full weight bearing by six weeks. If a fixation device has been placed across the

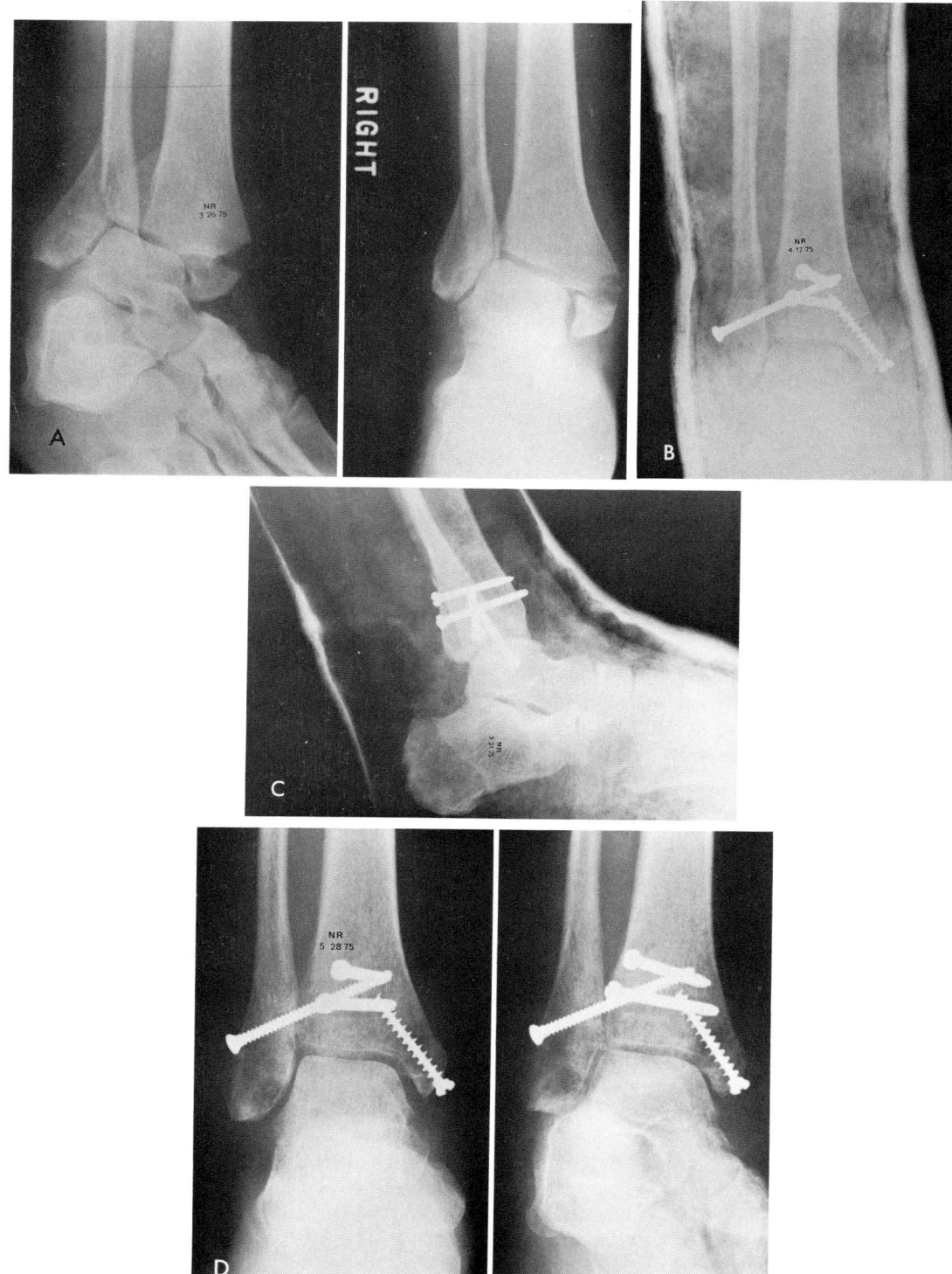

Figure 26–10   A. A severe stage 4 supination-external rotation type injury. This was indeed a trimalleolar fracture. It involved greater than 25 per cent of the posterior tibial margin portion. *B.* Postoperative anteroposterior view, demonstrating anatomical restoration of the ankle mortise. *C.* Lateral view, demonstrating satisfactory position of the posterior margin fracture. *D.* Two months postoperative, demonstrating satisfactory evidence of fracture healing and anatomical restoration of ankle.

syndesmosis, weight bearing is not allowed until six weeks later when it is removed. All plaster support may be removed by eight to ten weeks postoperatively.

SUPINATION-ADDUCTION ROTATION INJURIES

MECHANISM OF INJURY

This injury occurs with the foot in a position of supination at the time an adduction deforming force is exerted. The force produces a stage 1 injury, which includes a traction fracture of the lateral malleolus at or below the level of the ankle joint, or rupture of the talofibular ligaments. A further progression results in a stage 2 injury, which is a fracture of the medial malleolus at the level of the tibial plafond, extending in a proximal direction.

PHYSICAL EXAMINATION

The stage 1 injury presents with gross swelling over the anterolateral aspect of the ankle joint. There is acute tenderness to direct palpation along the area of the lateral malleolus owing to the fracture in this location. Any attempt at inversion of the ankle will elicit pain, particularly along the lateral aspect.

A stage 2 injury presents with tenderness and swelling along the entire ankle joint as the result of a bimalleolar fracture. Specifically, there is acute tenderness to direct palpation in the vicinity of the medial malleolar fracture, which is present at the level of the tibial plafond, and there is also tenderness over the lateral malleolar fracture. Ecchymosis may extend down into the dorsal aspect of the foot secondary to the bimalleolar fracture.

ROENTGENOGRAPHIC EXAMINATION

A stage 1 injury is evident on an anteroposterior roentgenogram as a horizontal fracture through the lateral malleolus, usually just below the ankle joint, which has the typical appearance of a traction type of fracture. The mortise view will reveal that the syndesmosis is intact.

The bimalleolar fracture of a stage 2 injury is evident on the anteroposterior view. The fracture of the medial malleolus occurs at the level of the tibial plafond and extends in a proximal direction. The traction fracture of the lateral malleolus is also seen. The mortise view fails to reveal any evidence of diastasis.

TREATMENT

Stage 1 Injury

Stage 1 injuries may be managed with the use of a below-knee weight-bearing cast for six to eight weeks. Patients are usually most comfortable with partial weight bearing for the first two weeks, followed by full weight bearing. These fractures go on to uneventful healing, usually with no restriction of joint motion.

Stage 2 Injury

Stage 2 fractures may be managed conservatively or operatively. The conservative approach may be taken if the bimalleolar fractures appear to be in satisfactory position. A long leg non–weight-bearing cast is then applied. The cast must be carefully observed for loosening caused by decreased swelling over a period of time. If this is not carefully monitored the position of the fragments may be lost in the cast. Patients presenting with a displaced bimalleolar fracture may be treated first by closed reduction, followed by application of a long leg cast. If closed reduction is not satisfactory, operative reduction and internal fixation are then performed.

The author prefers the operative approach, as the medial malleolar fracture occurs at the level of the tibial plafond and extends proximally, which tends to make this a relatively unstable injury in regard to the medial aspect. This situation is different from the one in a fracture of the medial malleolus which occurs within the body of the malleolus, but still has a proximal portion intact, to act as a buttress for the talus. In a true stage 2 fracture there is no such buttress along the medial aspect, and displacement may occur.

The medial portion of the ankle joint is exposed, and the malleolar fragment is anatomically reduced. This is followed by transfixion with a compression screw, which extends through the fragment into the distal portion of the tibia. The compression screw required for this procedure is one that has a lag effect. In other words, once the screw is inserted through the fragment the portion in the fragment is nonthreaded and smooth, while the portion in the distal aspect of the tibia has large threads, accounting for the compression effect. The danger in using a regular threaded screw is that the fracture site may be held apart by the threads of the screw. If the lateral malleolar fracture occurs at the level of the joint surface, open reduction and internal fixation of this fragment are indicated. The fragment is exposed through a lateral approach, and a Rush rod may be inserted through the tip of the distal malleolus, extending in a proximal direction to span the fracture site. A compression screw inserted in a similar fashion may also be used in the treatment of this fracture.

The postoperative management will depend upon the degree of internal fixation achieved at the time of the operative procedure. If the surgeon feels that he has obtained rigid internal fixation, a plaster cast does not necessarily have to be applied postoperatively. The alternative is to allow early range of motion of the ankle until the sutures are removed, at which time the extremity may be placed in a below-knee weight-bearing cast. If the internal fixation is not thought to be secure the patient should be placed in a below-knee cast postoperatively, and weight bearing should be postponed for three to four weeks. All plaster immobilization can usually be discontinued by 10 weeks.

PRONATION-EXTERNAL ROTATION INJURIES

MECHANISM OF INJURY

This injury occurs while the foot is in a pronated position as an external rotation deforming force is exerted. A stage 1 injury results in fracture of the medial malleolus or rupture of the deltoid ligament. If the deforming force is maintained a stage 2

injury occurs with a rupture of the anterior tibiofibular ligament or an avulsion fracture of its osseous insertion. There is a definite rupture of the interosseous ligament. Stage 3 is a fracture of the fibula above the syndesmosis. Stage 4 occurs with rupture of the posterior tibiofibular ligament or fracture of the posterior tibial margin.

PHYSICAL EXAMINATION

Stage 1 presents with swelling and tenderness over the medial malleolar area. If the medial malleolus has been fractured, tenderness is present directly over the fracture site. If there is a tear of the deltoid ligament, there will be tenderness along the course of the ligament. An abduction strain of the heel will cause severe pain at the medial aspect of the joint. In the presence of a fracture of the medial malleolus some slight toggle of the talus may be evident.

In addition to these findings, stage 2 presents with tenderness to direct palpation over the anterior tibiofibular ligament. Stage 3 includes fracture of the distal fibula together with the previously described injuries. Therefore, there is specific tenderness to direct palpation over the area of the fibular fracture. The syndesmosis is not completely disrupted, as the posterior tibiofibular ligament is still intact.

Stage 4 occurs with a complete diastasis of the syndesmosis besides the aforementioned injuries. There is gross instability of the ankle joint with an abduction and adduction strain. Marked swelling of the ankle is evident. There is tenderness over the entire anterior joint capsule as well as over the medial and lateral malleoli. Ecchymosis may well extend in a proximal and distal direction owing to the severity of the injury.

ROENTGENOGRAPHIC EXAMINATION

Stage 1 and 2 injuries will present with a fracture of the medial malleolus on the standard anteroposterior projection. There is no evidence of any diastasis on the mortise view (Fig. 26–11). Stage 3 presents with the medial malleolar fracture as well as

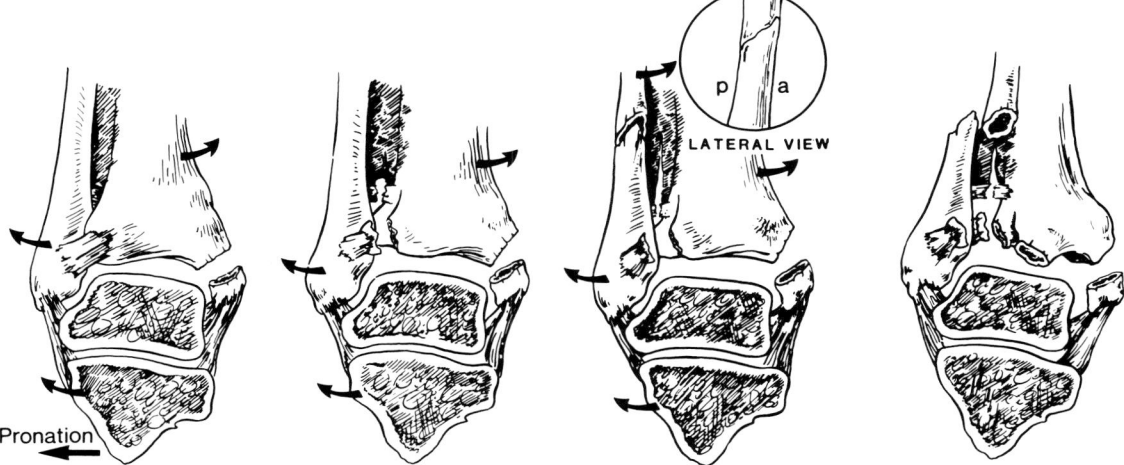

Figure 26–11 Fracture of the fibula proximal to the distal tibial fibular syndesmosis. Mechanism of injury and lesions in various stages of a pronation-external rotation fracture. (Courtesy of A. M. Pankovich and *Journal of Bone and Joint Surgery*, J. Bone Joint Surg., 60A:221–229, 1978.)

with a fracture of the distal fibula having a specific pattern, as outlined by Pankovich.[52] This includes a fracture of the fibula approximately 5 cm or more proximal to the distal portion. The fracture line is short and oblique and extends from the anterior edge in a posteroinferior direction. There is no evidence of a diastasis on the mortise view. Stage 4 presents with a similar picture, but in addition has definite diastasis demonstrable on the mortise view.

TREATMENT

Stage 1 and 2 Injury

Stage 1 and 2 injuries may be managed with the use of a plaster cast if the malleolar fracture appears to be in satisfactory position. In the presence of displacement of the malleolar fragment, an attempt at closed reduction is in order. If the closed reduction fails to obtain satisfactory alignment an open reduction and internal fixation with the use of a compression screw is probably the most appropriate treatment (Fig. 26–12). If a secure internal fixation has been obtained a plaster cast will not be required postoperatively. The patient can regain range of motion and then begin partial weight bearing, progressing to full weight bearing. If the fracture has been initially

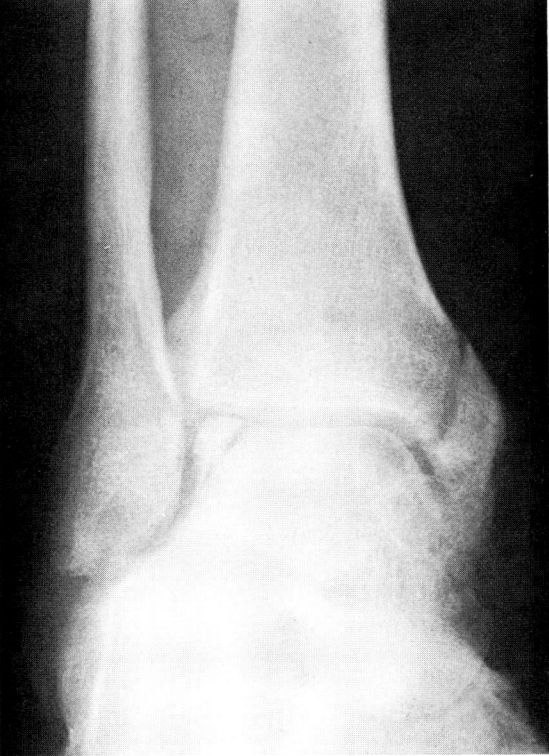

Figure 26–12 Stage 2 of a pronation-external rotation fracture with an associated lateral talar dome fracture. This was managed conservatively which resulted in eventual healing of the medial malleolar fragment. However, the lateral talar dome fragment did not heal.

managed with the conservative nonoperative approach, plaster immobilization can be discontinued at the end of 10 weeks.

Stage 3 Injury

Stage 3 injuries may be treated in a conservative fashion if the fractures are in appropriate alignment, since the syndesmosis is not completely disrupted. In the presence of malposition the injury requires an attempt at closed reduction to improve the position. If proper alignment cannot be obtained with this maneuver, appropriate open reduction and internal fixation of the medial malleolar fracture with a compression screw is the method of choice.

Stage 4 Injury

A stage 4 injury is one of significant magnitude. The author believes that all these fractures should be managed with open reduction and appropriate internal fixation (Fig. 26–13). The talus is frequently shifted to a lateral position owing to the frank diastasis as well as to the medial malleolar and distal fibular fractures. The medial malleolar fragment may be treated with the use of a compression screw, and the distal fibular fragment may be adequately secured with a semitubular compression plate. The last hole in the compression plate may be reserved for a transfixion screw extending across the syndesmosis.

The alternative is to reduce the fibular fracture and then place a Webb bolt across the syndesmosis to hold it in appropriate position. However, as Yablon and colleagues have demonstrated, the talus will follow the position of the distal fibula. Therefore, it is very important to obtain appropriate anatomical reduction and rigid internal fixation of the distal fibular fragment, as the talus will then be correctly positioned.[65] A semitubular compression plate is useful for this purpose.

It is probably no longer acceptable to obtain only internal fixation of the medial portion of the ankle with the expectation of molding the lateral aspect of the fracture with the use of plaster postoperatively. If internal fixation is selected, then appropriate secure internal fixation of *all* fragments is probably the best method of management.

Occasionally, a posterior tibial margin fracture is associated with a stage 4 injury. This produces the true trimalleolar type of fracture. If the posterior tibial margin involves one fourth to one third of the articular surface it should be managed by open reduction and internal fixation. The Gatellier approach is very versatile in this type of injury.[33] It involves reflecting the fibular fragment in a distal direction, but leaving the ligamentous attachments at the distal portion intact. This gives the surgeon excellent exposure of the posterolateral portion of the tibia and is very useful for operative reduction and internal fixation of posterior tibial fractures. The alternative is to approach the tibia through a direct posterior incision, but if the injury already involves a fracture of the distal fibula with a diastasis the Gatellier approach is probably the simplest.

PRONATION-ABDUCTION INJURIES

MECHANISM OF INJURY

This injury occurs with the foot held in a position of pronation when an abduction force is exerted. Stage 1 is a rupture of the deltoid ligament or a fracture of the medial malleolus. If the force is maintained a stage 2 injury occurs, which is a rupture of all ligaments of the syndesmosis or an avulsion fracture of one of the bone insertions. Stage 3 is a fracture of the fibula proximal to the syndesmosis.

PHYSICAL EXAMINATION

A stage 1 injury presents with swelling and tenderness along the medial aspect of the ankle. If forced pronation of the ankle is attempted there may be evidence of a valgus tilt of the talus. Stage 2 is marked by a diastasis of the syndesmosis secondary to disruption of the ligamentous structures in addition to the injury produced in stage 1.

Swelling and tenderness are present in the medial malleolar area, with similar findings along the anterolateral and posterolateral aspects of the ankle joint. Visible

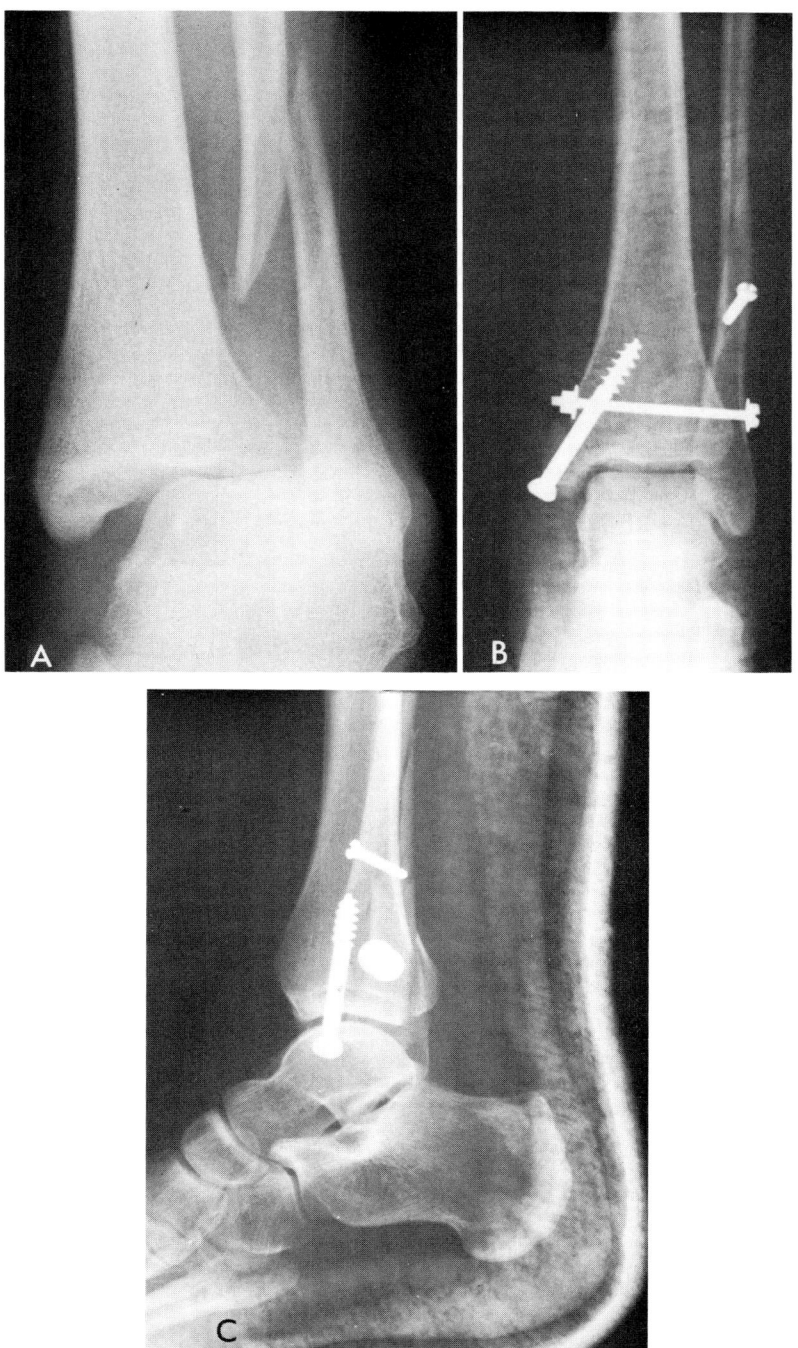

Figure 26–13 A. Severe type 4 pronation-external rotation injury. *B.* Anteroposterior view following open reduction and internal fixation. *C.* Lateral view following open reduction and internal fixation.

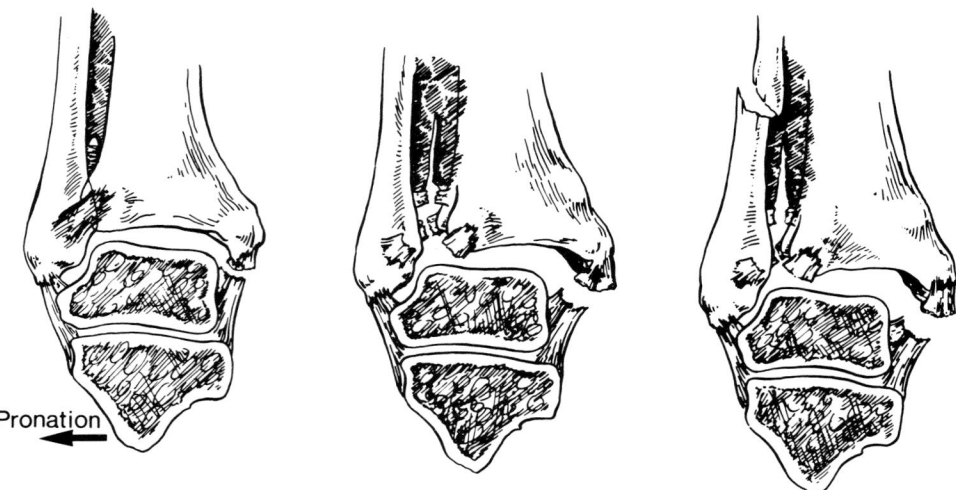

Pronation

Figure 26–14 Mechanism of injury and lesions in various stages of a pronation-abduction injury. (Courtesy of A. M. Pankovich and *Journal of Bone and Joint Surgery.* J. Bone Joint Surg., 60A:221–229, 1978.)

ecchymosis frequently extends both proximally and distally. If the heel is placed in pronation there will be a definite "give" to the ankle joint such that the talus will have definite valgus tilt and will be displaced laterally. A stage 3 includes the injuries already mentioned plus a fracture of the fibula proximal to the syndesmosis. This is an extremely unstable injury, as there is no support along the medial or lateral aspects of the ankle joint. Visible swelling and ecchymosis are present along the medial aspect as well as along the lateral aspect of the ankle. There is exquisite tenderness to direct palpation along both the medial and the lateral aspects of the ankle. The talus is noted to be very unstable in the ankle mortise. It is particularly susceptible to lateral displacement within the ankle mortise.

ROENTGENOGRAPHIC EXAMINATION

Stage 1 injuries frequently will not have any specific findings apart from a mild valgus tilt to the talus, indicative of deltoid ligament tear. If there is an avulsion fracture of the medial malleolus it will be evident on the roentgenogram. Stage 2 injuries will demonstrate a frank diastasis of the syndesmosis on the mortise view. There will be no evidence of a fibular fracture, but a rupture of the deltoid ligament with lateral dis-

placement of the talus in the ankle mortise will be shown. An avulsion fracture of the medial malleolus may be seen. A stage 3 injury has a fracture of the distal fibula, which in the presence of a frank diastasis and a rupture of the deltoid ligament predisposes the talus to a lateral position in the ankle mortise. The fracture of the fibula is located approximately 6 cm or more proximal to the distal tip of the fibula. The fracture line is oblique, extending from the lateral surface in an inferomedial direction (Fig. 26–14).

TREATMENT

Stage 1

Stage 1 injuries may be treated in a conservative manner. This usually consists of applying a below-knee weight-bearing cast. For a deltoid ligament tear the cast remains in place for six to eight weeks, when it is succeeded by aggresssive physical therapy to the ankle. The foot in the cast should be in a position of inversion to favor approximation of the separated deltoid ligament surfaces. A small avulsion fracture of the medial malleolus is treated in a similar fashion.

Stage 2

Stage 2 injuries should be treated with operative repair of the deltoid ligament and

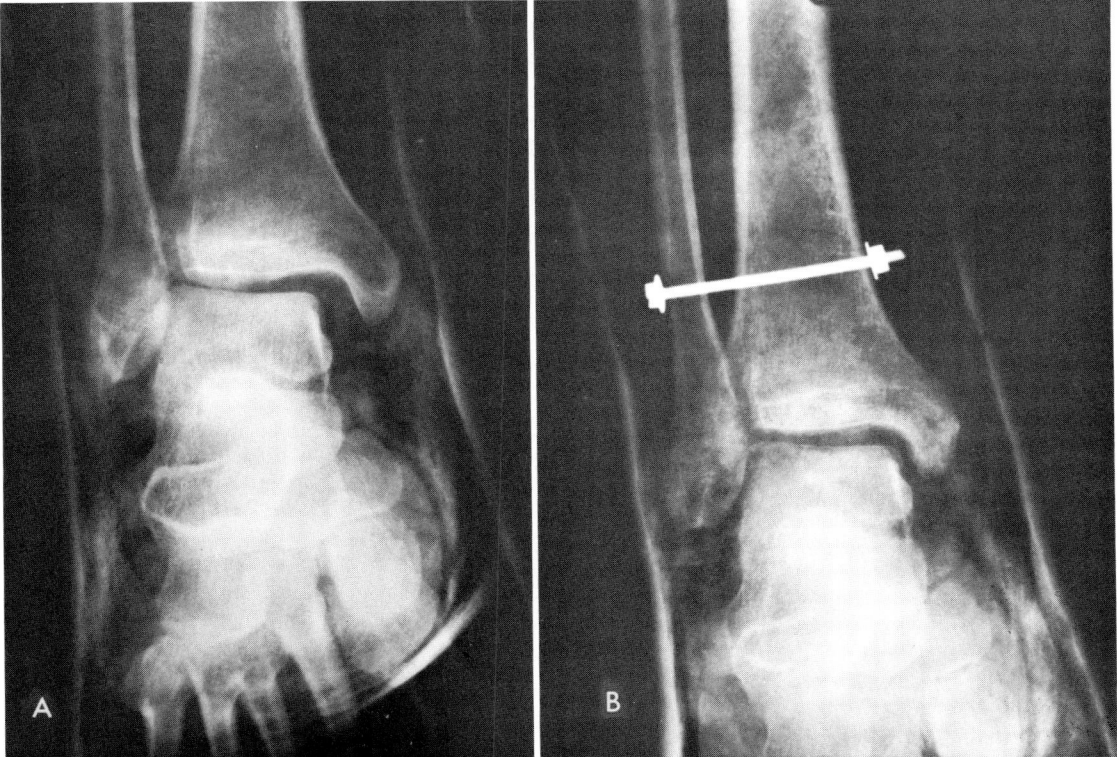

Figure 26–15 A. A stage 2 pronation-abduction injury. Note the lateral talar shift. *B.* Treated with operative repair of the deltoid ligament and transfixation of the syndesmosis with a Webb bolt.

also with a transfixion device for the distal syndesmosis (Fig. 26–15). The deltoid ligament is closed with sutures in two separate layers. The diastasis may be treated with a long oblique screw or a Webb bolt. Patients are maintained on non-weight bearing until six weeks when the transfixion device is removed. Then active weight bearing is initiated in a short leg walking cast for four weeks, at which time the plaster immobilization is discontinued. If the plaster support of the diastasis is removed earlier than 10 weeks post-injury there is a chance that the diastasis may recur.

Stage 3

Stage 3 injuries should also be managed operatively. This injury may be treated by the method outlined for a stage 2 fracture. Alternatively, the fibula may be treated with

a semitubular compression plate, and the last hole of the plate may be reserved for a transfixion screw for the syndesmosis.

If a Webb bolt is selected for internal fixation of the diastasis it is important technically not to place the bolt in too proximal a position along the distal fibular fragment, or the distal portion of the fibula will be sprung in a lateral direction. It is more appropriate to place the Webb bolt just above the tibial plafond, so that equal pressure will be exerted against the fibula, tending to hold the fibula in a neutral position rather than tilting the fibular fragment at either end. These patients are maintained in a non–weight-bearing plaster cast for six weeks, and return for removal of the internal fixation device across the syndesmosis at that time. Active weight bearing in a below-knee weight-bearing cast is then encouraged. All plaster is discontinued at 10 to 12 weeks postinjury.

PRONATION-DORSIFLEXION INJURIES

MECHANISM OF INJURY

This type of fracture is produced by a fall from a considerable height with the lower extremity striking the ground as the foot is held in a pronated position. With the force of the impact the foot and ankle are subjected to a severe dorsiflexion motion. Three distinct stages may be identified. The initial force will result in a stage 1 injury with a near-vertical fracture of the medial malleolus. The fragment is situated proximally and medially. A stage 2 injury results from a continued dorsiflexion force at the ankle, producing a fracture of the anterior articular margin of the distal tibia as well as of the medial malleolus. A stage 3 injury requires considerable force, and causes a fracture of the distal tibia extending into the articular surface of the ankle with a supramalleolar fracture of the fibula.

PHYSICAL EXAMINATION

A stage 1 fracture will produce considerable swelling and tenderness over the medial malleolar region. There will be pain associated with attempted motion at the ankle joint. Stage 2 injuries may result in instability at the ankle joint. The talus will have a tendency to glide forward out of the ankle joint owing to the fracture of the anterior articular margin of the tibia. In fact, the examiner may be able to passively move the talus in a forward direction. There is usually a great deal of swelling along the anterior and medial aspects of the ankle joint proper. A stage 3 fracture is extremely unstable. Since the fracture involves the distal tibia as well as the supramalleolar portion of the fibula, the talus may be freely mobile in all directions. Because this injury results from a significant force at the ankle joint, there is always a great deal of swelling around the entire ankle joint.

ROENTGENOGRAPHIC EXAMINATION

In a stage 1 injury of the ankle, routine roentgenograms will demonstrate a near-vertical fracture of the medial malleolus, with displacement of the fragment in a proximal and medial direction. Stage 2 presents with fractures of the medial malleolus and the anterior articular margin of the distal tibia. The fragment of the distal tibia is displaced in a proximal direction and is usually of significant size. It may involve from one half to one third of the anterior articular surface of the distal tibia. Stage 3 results in a relatively transverse fracture of the distal tibia above the tibial plafond, but the fracture extends into the articular surface with significant distortion of the articular contour. There is also an associated supramalleolar fracture of the fibula. The talus is usually located in a proximal and lateral direction in this injury.

TREATMENT

Stage 1

Stage 1 injuries may be treated with closed reduction and maintained in plaster immobilization if the fracture is anatomically reduced. The method of reduction is a plantar flexion of the foot with slight supination. Direct pressure in a distal direction may be applied to the medial malleolar fragment as this maneuver is performed. If the reduction is not anatomical, this injury should be treated with open reduction and internal fixation with the use of a cancellous compression screw to maintain the medial malleolar fragment in an anatomical position. Once again, it is essential to obtain anatomical reduction of the fracture fragment as the vertical nature of the fracture makes this an unstable injury. If secure fixation has been obtained with a cancellous compression screw, the patient may be ambulated with full weight bearing, in a below-knee weight-bearing cast. The cast is maintained for six weeks and then discarded. If closed reduction is selected as the form of treatment the patient is maintained in a below-knee non–weight-bearing cast for at least six to eight weeks. Progression to full weight bearing is undertaken for an additional four weeks in a below-knee weight-bearing cast.

Stage 2

Stage 2 injuries may be treated with a closed reduction. Direct pressure must be applied to the anterior aspect of the distal tibia at the same time as the foot is placed in plantar flexion with slight supination. Direct pressure distally is required, since the only attachment remaining between the ankle joint and the articular margin is the joint capsule. This itself may be torn secondary to the injury, necessitating forced manipulation of the fracture fragments back into anatomical location. The talus may also be subluxated in an anterior direction owing to the injury, in which case a direct posterior force must be applied to the talus in order to accomplish reduction. If an acceptable reduction is obtained, the foot is maintained in a position of slight plantar flexion in a long leg cast for four to six weeks. Non-weight bearing during this time is the rule. The foot is then brought up to a neutral position at the end of four to six weeks, but it is maintained in a plaster cast, non–weight-bearing, for an additional four to six weeks. If weight bearing is attempted prior to this time the danger is that the talus may gradually subluxate in an anterior direction, with compression of the distal articular margin portion of the fracture.

Stage 3 injuries are extremely unstable secondary to the magnitude of the fracture. These injuries are frequently best managed with a pin through the calcaneus and skeletal traction to realign the fracture fragments. Operative intervention at the fracture site is not indicated, as the fracture fragments tend to be multiple and firm fixation is almost impossible to accomplish. The alternative to skeletal traction is to insert pins above the fracture fragments as well as a pin in the calcaneus, incorporating the pins in a plaster cast following appropriate reduction. Weight bearing is generally delayed for at least 10 to 12 weeks with this type of injury because of the comminution at the articular surface.

SPECIAL TYPES OF ANKLE FRACTURES

POSTERIOR MALLEOLAR FRACTURES

Fractures of the posterior tibial margin have been referred to as posterior malleolar fractures. They may occur as isolated events, or they may be seen in association with other malleolar fractures. These injuries are frequently termed trimalleolar fractures.

Mechanism of Injury

Bonnin has stated that the isolated posterior malleolar fracture may result from striking a solid object with the ankle held in a neutral or plantar flexed position.[4] In other words, the mechanism of injury is a vertical compression force.

Trimalleolar fractures are usually caused by a combination of vertical compression and external rotation forces. This is a very complex fracture, and its severity is frequently due to the action of multiple forces.

Physical Examination

In an isolated posterior malleolar fracture there is gross swelling along the posterior aspect and acute tenderness to direct palpation along the posterior capsule. Motion of the ankle is painful. Most patients are able to bear weight on the extremity following the injury, but the pain progressively increases in intensity. The trimalleolar fracture presents with gross swelling of the entire ankle joint, with acute tenderness to palpation along the anterior capsule, posterior capsule, and all three malleolar areas. This type of injury is extremely unstable, and the talus will frequently subluxate posteriorly and laterally in the ankle mortise. The examiner is aware of the gross motion achieved with very little force exerted on the ankle.

Roentgenographic Examination

Isolated posterior malleolar fractures show no evidence of a fracture of the medial or lateral malleoli on the routine anteroposterior view. However, in the lateral roentgenographic view the fracture of the posterior malleolus is apparent. The extent of involvement of the articular surface may be judged from the lateral view. The injury appears as a near-vertical fracture through the posterior portion of the distal tibia, involving the articular surface. An oblique view is occasionally helpful in determining

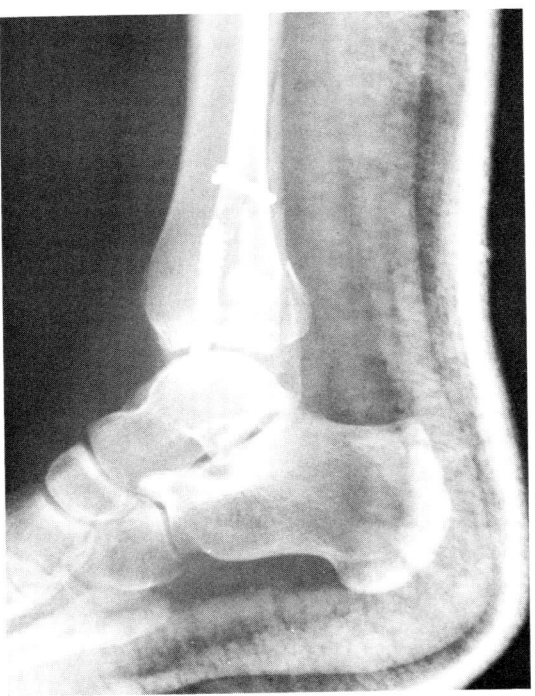

Figure 26-16 The posterior malleolar fragment is less than one fourth of the articular surface and did not require internal fixation per se.

the extent of involvement of the articular surface. A trimalleolar fracture will demonstrate a fracture of the medial malleolus and the lateral malleolus in the routine anteroposterior view. The posterior malleolar fracture will be evident in the lateral view (Fig. 26–16). The amount of displacement is determined by a combination of the mortise and lateral views. Since this is a very unstable fracture it is frequently noted that there is a subluxation of the talus in a posterolateral direction.

Treatment

The size of the posterior malleolar fragment warranting an open reduction has been the subject of a great deal of debate in the past. McLaughlin reported that all his cases in which the fragment involved greater than 25 per cent of the articular surface, developed subluxation and eventually progressed to traumatic arthritis.[49] He maintained that articular surface fractures involving greater than 25 per cent of the

surface required open reduction and internal fixation. Joy and co-workers, in a large series of bimalleolar and trimalleolar fractures, concluded that 25 per cent or more of articular surface involvement was significant.[35] They also advocated open reduction and internal fixation in these cases. Vasli stressed the importance of open reduction and internal fixation for a posterior malleolar fracture that involved greater than one third of the tibial articular surface.[63] Nelson and Jensen also recommended open reduction and internal fixation if the posterior tibial articular surface involvement was one third or greater.[50] In a follow-up study, Joy and associates were of the opinion that three specific factors influenced the end results:[35] (1) The type of fracture involved was important. The more severe trimalleolar fractures had a guarded prognosis. (2) Significant displacement of the talus was felt to be a poor prognostic factor. (3) A tear of the deltoid ligament was believed to have significant bearing on the end results.

Interestingly, all deltoid ligament tears were surgically repaired, but not all lateral malleolar fragments received internal fixation. It is possible that stricter attention to the lateral malleolar repair, as outlined by Yablon, may have led to an improvement in the overall results.[65]

The author has adopted the policy of performing open reduction and internal fixation if the posterior malleolar fragment involves 25 per cent or greater of the articular surface. The rationale is that significant instability of the talus may result otherwise. In the presence of a trimalleolar fracture two specific approaches have been useful. First, the direct posterior approach with reflection of the Achilles tendon provides excellent exposure of the posterior tibial margin and allows easy reduction and appropriate internal fixation. The use of a lag compression screw is preferred. The second approach that may be applied to the trimalleolar fracture is that of Gatellier.[33] This is particularly helpful if the lateral malleolar fracture occurs above the syndesmosis and is associated with a frank diastasis. Under these conditions the fibular fragment may be reflected in a distal direction while the integrity of the lateral ligaments is maintained, as outlined by Gatellier. This allows adequate exposure of the posterolateral aspect of the distal tibial articular surface, and operative reduction and internal fixation may be performed without difficulty. Once the posterior malleolar fragment has been secured the fibula may be repositioned. It is then held in appropriate position with a Webb bolt or a long oblique transfixion screw which is placed in a slightly anterior position to avoid the repair of the posterior malleolar fragment. Postoperatively, if the fixation is felt to be secure the patient is placed in a soft bandage and allowed early range-of-motion exercises, but is kept non-weight bearing. At the time of suture removal the patient is placed in a below-knee weight-bearing cast. If fixation is adequate, partial weight bearing is allowed and progression to full weight bearing ensues. At the end of two months the plaster immobilization is removed, and active ankle motion is initiated, with partial weight bearing progressing to full weight bearing.

Isolated nondisplaced posterior malleolar fragments may be treated with a below-knee non–weight-bearing cast, with the foot held in a neutral position or in slight dorsiflexion. The reason for this position is that the flexor hallucis longus tendon is located adjacent to the fragment, and if the foot is placed in a slightly dorsiflexed position the tendon will aid in securing fixation of the fragment and preventing displacement. At the end of one month the plaster cast is removed, and active range-of-motion exercises are initiated. However, weight bearing is not allowed for at least two months postinjury. If weight bearing is initiated earlier, there is always the danger that the fragment may displace, allowing mild posterior subluxation of the talus.

BOSWORTH FRACTURE

In 1947 Bosworth described five patients having a specific and relatively uncommon injury—a fracture-dislocation of the ankle with entrapment of the fibula behind the tibia.[5] More recently, Mayer and Evarts reported four additional cases.[48] Although this is a relatively rare injury, its presence must be recognized and appropriate treatment initiated if a functional result is to be expected.

Mechanism of Injury

This injury is produced by a severe external rotation force applied to the foot. The result is that two forces are exerted on the leg, one forward and lateral and the other rotatory. The talus is forced backward out of the mortise, resulting in a tearing of the anterior and posterior syndesmotic ligaments. The fibula is then carried in a posterior direction by the intact lateral collateral ankle ligaments. Either the inferior part of the fibula fractures at the posterior tibial border, or the shaft remains intact and is dislocated behind the tibia. The distal talofibular and calcaneofibular ligaments usually remain intact.

Physical Examination

Physical examination will reveal that the foot is severely externally rotated in relation to the tibia. Gross swelling and tenderness are evident. A frank posterolateral dislocation of the ankle is usually seen.

Roentgenographic Examination

Routine roentgenograms of the ankle demonstrate a fracture-dislocation of the ankle with the fibula entrapped behind the tibia. The lateral view will reveal that the lateral malleolus is posterior to the medial malleolus. Normally, the lateral and medial malleoli are superimposed one on the other. The anteroposterior view may demonstrate that the lateral malleolus, which has rotated outward with the talus, may be superimposed over the medial malleolus. These abnormal relationships are usually evident if the knee is included on the initial roentgenographic study.

Treatment

The majority of these fracture-dislocations have been managed with operative intervention. The fibula is explored through a lateral incision. The proximal fibular fragment must be disengaged from its posterior position; once this is performed it will reposition properly since the distal talofibular and calcaneofibular ligaments are usually intact. A Rush rod can then be inserted to provide stability of the fibular fracture.

Mayer and Evarts found that three out of four of their cases were managed appropriately by closed reduction. They recommended positioning one hand around the ankle and foot to apply axial traction and internal rotation of the foot in a medial direction. At the same time the opposite hand is placed along the posterolateral aspect of the distal fibular shaft to apply an anterolaterally directed force in an attempt to reposition the shaft of the fibula. It appears at the present time that a closed reduction should be attempted; if this fails an open reduction is indicated.

Maisonneuve Fracture

Maissonneuve was the first to postulate that an external rotation force may be a prime mechanism of injury to the ankle joint.[47] He observed that an external rotation force at the ankle produces an oblique fracture of the lateral malleolus if the anterior tibiofibular ligament is adequate to resist the stress. However, if the ligament ruptures, the force is transmitted to the proximal portion of the fibula. A fracture of the proximal third of the fibula occurs,

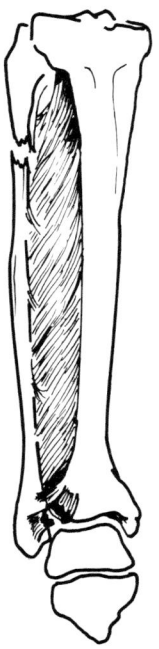

Figure 26–17   A Maisonneuve fracture.

which is known as a Maisonneuve fracture (Fig. 26–17). Ashhurst and Bromer described 3 such cases in their series of 300 ankle fractures.[1] Bonnin was able to identify 19 cases in his series of 178 fractures produced by external rotation of the foot.[3, 4]

More recently, Pankovich extensively studied 12 classic Maisonneuve fractures.[53] He was able to identify five specific stages in the classification of the Maisonneuve fracture. Stage 1 involves a rupture of the anterior tibiofibular ligament or avulsion of one of its bone insertions, either being associated with rupture of the interosseous ligament. Stage 2 is a fracture of the posterior tibial tubercle or rupture of the posterior tibiofibular ligament. In stage 3 there is a rupture of the anteromedial joint capsule or an avulsion fracture of one of its bone insertions. Stage 4 is marked by fracture of the proximal portion of the fibula, and stage 5 by rupture of the deltoid ligament or fracture of the medial malleolus.

In the Lauge-Hansen classification the interosseous ligament remains intact with a supination-external rotation fracture.[41] Cedell stated that the interosseous ligament ruptures during a supination-external rotation fracture of the fibula.[14] Bonnin observed that in a Maisonneuve fracture the interosseous ligament and membrane and the posterior tibiofibular ligament remain intact.[4] However, Pankovich noted a rupture of the interosseous membrane in three of the seven patients who received operative intervention.[53] It is not readily evident at which stage the interosseous membrane ruptures, how far proximally the rupture extends, or whether the rupture occurs only exceptionally. Pankovich believed that the interosseous membrane may be ruptured in the late stages.

Pankovich advocated conservative management of patients with advanced stages of the fracture complex, provided the deltoid ligament and the medial malleolus were intact. If these anatomical structures are damaged, early operative repair is indicated. Following repair of the injured structures along the medial aspect of the ankle, the lateral structures must be explored to rule out any instability of the syndesmosis. If there is gross motion of the fibula relative to the tibia, stabilization of the syndesmosis by fibulotibial transfixation should be performed. If there is only slight motion present, operative repair of the anterior tibiofibular ligament is all that is necessary.

The author has preferred to treat the later stages by operative repair of the medial structures with placement of a transfixion screw across the syndesmosis or insertion of a Webb bolt to treat the diastasis. Postoperatively the patient is maintained in a below-knee non–weight-bearing cast with the foot in slight inversion. At six weeks the internal fixation device for the syndesmosis is removed, and range-of-motion exercises for the ankle are initiated. Partial weight bearing is allowed, with progression to full weight bearing.

OPEN FRACTURES

The reader is referred to Chapter 30 for a discussion of the general management of open fractures. Open ankle fractures are not especially uncommon. They are usually produced by a deforming force that displaces the osseous fragment through the skin. It is relatively rare to encounter an open injury produced by an external device penetrating the skin. The one exception is gunshot wounds associated with fractures of the ankle. These are also discussed in Chapter 30.

A fall from a height or a motorcycle or vehicular accident is usually responsible for open ankle fractures. In general, these wounds are severely contaminated, and it is not good surgical practice to consider internal fixation at the time the patient is first evaluated. It is more appropriate to thoroughly cleanse and debride the wounds and then attempt to treat the ankle fracture in a conservative manner until there is some evidence of healing without signs of infection.

If there is no indication of skin loss over the heel area and no evidence of a fracture of the calcaneus, insertion of a calcaneal pin should be considered, to provide traction for the lower extremity in an attempt to realign the osseous fragments. A pin may also be inserted through the proximal tibia for countertraction to apply balanced suspension. This is also applicable to fractures in which there has been a significant amount of skin loss over the ankle. Split-thickness grafts or free pedicle grafts may then be applied to the area of skin loss, while the lower extremity is maintained in balanced skeletal traction. If at the end of seven to ten days the skin coverage appears adequate, consideration may be given to primary open reduction and internal fixation if the severity of the fracture warrants this type of operative intervention. Otherwise the leg may be placed in a plaster cast incorporating the proximal and distal traction pins in order to maintain the position of the fracture fragments.

This technique may also be useful in patients with severe peripheral arterial or venous disease of the lower extremity that precludes internal fixation, as outlined by Laskin.[40]

SWELLING IN ANKLE FRACTURES

Patients presenting 24 to 48 hours following a severe ankle fracture will frequently have gross edema accompanied by skin blebs or open blisters. These are difficult injuries to manage, as operative intervention is not ideal. For this reason the author feels that ankle fractures are a relative emergency. If they are managed by early closed reduction or early open reduction and internal fixation the swelling is definitely decreased, and skin blebs are encountered relatively seldom. This is because the sooner the deformity is corrected, the sooner the blood flow to and from the foot improves, decreasing the incidence of edema. It is not sound treatment to delay operative intervention for an ankle injury over 24 to 48 hours for the surgeon's convenience. In the presence of gross swelling and skin blebs it has been the author's practice to suspend the lower extremity in a stockinette, as outlined by Quigley.[57] This is very useful in controlling edema and also is helpful in reducing external rotation and abduction injuries (Fig. 26–18). The foot tends to assume a position of internal rotation with adduction. Frequently the fractures will be reduced spontaneously, as the ankle edema subsides in this type of suspension. If the position of the fracture fragments is satisfactory following the decrease in edema and the disap-

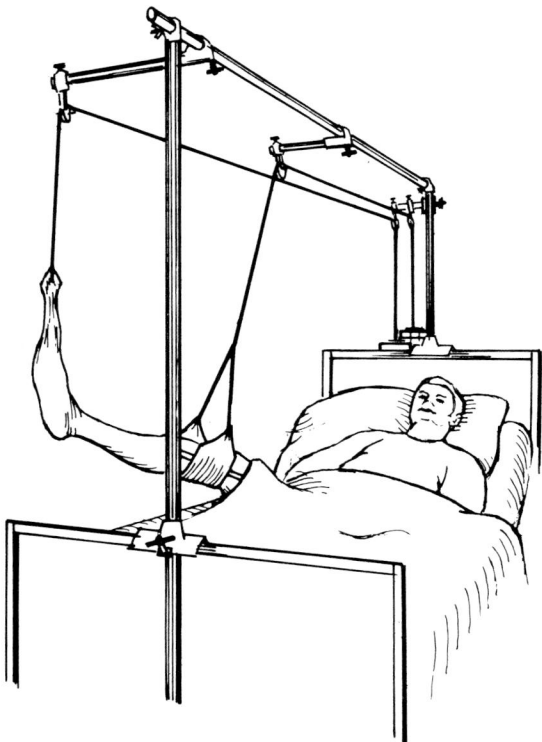

Figure 26–18   Quigley traction.

pearance of the ankle blebs, then a proper plaster cast may be applied. If it is a very unstable injury, operative reduction and internal fixation may be performed.

LIGAMENTOUS INJURIES

Many physicians fail to realize the importance of ligamentous injuries. Frequently, disruption of the ligamentous structures about the ankle can be as disabling as fractures of the ankle joint. This statement must be well digested by both the lay public and the medical profession. All too frequently, serious ligamentous ruptures about the ankle are dismissed as "ankle sprains." It is also necessary to realize that ligamentous injuries of the ankle joint are probably the most common ligamentous injuries of the body. If we bear in mind these two facts it is not difficult to understand the importance of proper diagnostic evaluation and treatment of ligamentous injuries about the ankle. A thorough knowl-

edge of wound healing in general, as outlined in Chapter 1, is required for a proper understanding of ligamentous healing. There is no doubt that ligamentous injuries require a longer time for repair than regular soft tissue injuries, such as those of the skin. An important difference is that ligaments in general do not have as abundant a blood supply as the skin. This is one of the significant factors in the length of time required for repair and for structural integrity and resistance to deformation.

CLASSIFICATION

A uniform definition of the term sprain is required in order to discuss ligamentous injuries about the ankle. Sprains may be classified into three degrees according to the standard nomenclature of athletic injuries, as outlined by the American Medical Association. A first degree sprain is mild, with evidence of slight point tenderness, minimal hemorrhage and swelling, no specific abnormal motion, and little disability. Little if any tearing of the ligamentous fibers is noted. A second degree sprain is moderate, with a greater loss of function than a first degree sprain. There is localized tenderness, more joint reaction, slight abnormal motion, and partial tearing of the ligamentous tissues. A third degree sprain is a more severe injury, evidenced by marked abnormal motion indicative of a complete tear of the ligament. This classification may be applied to the lateral ligament, deltoid ligament, and syndesmotic ligaments.

LATERAL LIGAMENT INJURIES

Injuries to the lateral collateral ligament are very common. This is probably because there is an increased susceptibility to inversion injuries of the ankle during normal walking and running, compared with eversion injuries. A thorough knowledge of the anatomical structure of the lateral collateral ligament is required. As outlined in the beginning of this chapter, the lateral collateral ligament consists of the anterior talofibular ligament, the posterior talofibular ligament, and the middle portion known as the calcaneofibular ligament. These three

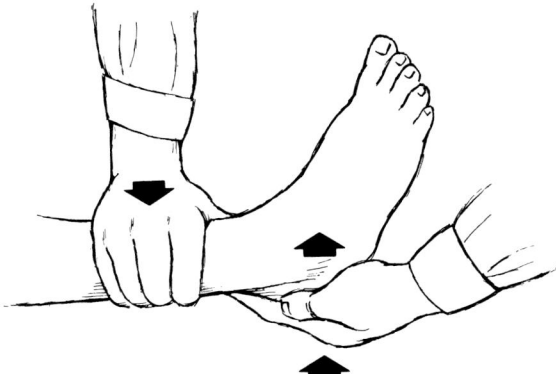

Figure 26–19   The anterior drawer sign.

separate structures constitute the lateral collateral ligament complex.

Mechanism of Injury

Adduction of the foot places increased stress on the lateral collateral ligament. Therefore, adduction or inversion injuries of the foot account for sprains of the lateral ligaments. A frequent mechanism of injury is stepping on an uneven portion of ground, throwing the foot and ankle into marked inversion. Athletic activities also place an additional stress on the lateral structures of the ankle. The anterior tibiofibular ligament is usually the first to be injured. If the deforming force continues the calcaneofibular ligament is next in order of injury. It is interesting that the posterior talofibular ligament is rarely injured owing to its larger size and to the fact that it is maximally stressed in forced dorsiflexion. The susceptibility of the anterior talofibular ligament to injury causes it to be the most common lateral ligament injury encountered in clinical practice.

Physical Examination

Most patients will volunteer the fact that they "turned over" on their ankle. There is usually obvious swelling and ecchymosis along the lateral aspect of the ankle. Cedell felt that the anterior talofibular ligament was the most important stabilizing ligament of the ankle.[15] If it is ruptured a positive anterior drawer sign may be evident (Fig. 26–19). This sign appears when the talus is placed in slight plantar flexion, and an attempt is made to displace the talus anteriorly. If there is a grade 3 sprain or tear of the anterior talofibular ligament a positive anterior drawer sign will be obtained. This is a very useful test, and in some areas has been found to be more effective in diagnosing a torn anterior talofibular ligament than stress inversion radiography. The amount of anterior drawer is increased if the calcaneofibular ligament is also torn. It must be emphasized that this test has to be performed soon after the injury. If a time lapse occurs following the injury, reflex muscle guarding about the ankle will limit the usefulness of the anterior drawer test. Under these circumstances the test should be performed under some type of anesthesia.

Roentgenographic Examination

Routine anteroposterior and lateral roentgenographic examination of the ankle usually does not reveal any abnormality with a tear of the lateral ligament. Stress films and arthrography have been used to document tears of the lateral ligament of the ankle. Stress films have produced conflicting results in the past. The author's impression has been that stress radiography is useful only if both ankles are examined with maximal stress and a comparison made of the normal and abnormal ankle (Fig. 26–20). Olson found that a talar tilt of up to 25 degrees may be noted in a relatively normal ankle without any preceding history of trauma.[51] Yablon and co-workers found in a cadaver study that if the fibular collateral ligament was sectioned a 30 degree rotatory instability with evidence of marked talar instability resulted.[65] Therefore, it appears that talar tilt is important in relation to recent injury, but it must be compared with the opposite normal extremity to be of value in determining the degree of injury present. Adequate anesthesia is also important if the study is to be meaningful.

Ankle arthrography is frequently helpful in the initial evaluation of ligament injuries. In 1965 Broström and colleagues described the arthrographic diagnosis of recent ligament injuries.[9] The study is relatively easy to perform. It involves inserting a needle along the anteromedial aspect of the ankle

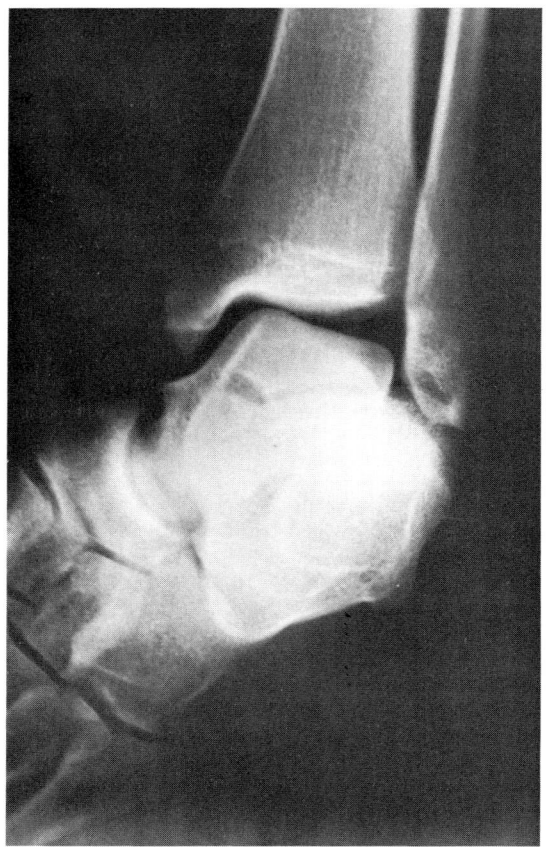

Figure 26–20 Stress inversion view. Note the tilt of the talus.

and aspirating blood from within the joint. Following this maneuver, 5 ml of contrast media is injected into the joint. Recently, Staples studied the value of arthrography in recent lateral ligament injuries in 26 patients.[62] All but one of the arthrograms revealed massive lateral extraarticular spread of the contrast media. However, only half of the patients with a tear of the talofibular and calcaneofibular ligaments demonstrated contrast material in the peroneal sheath (Fig. 26–21). This is in contrast to Broström's study, which found that filling of the peroneal sheath with contrast material indicated a rupture of the calcaneofibular ligament. However, Fordyce and Horn were unable to confirm Broström's finding of leakage of dye into the peroneal sheath with rupture of the calcaneofibular ligament.

The author believes the study is useful if it produces positive results. In other words, if there is definite filling of the peroneal sheath a tear of the calcaneofibular ligament probably is present. However, there also may be false negative results with this study, and the absence of contrast material in the peroneal sheath does not rule out a tear of the calcaneofibular ligament. Therefore, a positive study has value, but a negative study may fail to reveal the presence of a torn lateral ligament.

Treatment

The treatment of a grade 1 or 2 sprain of the lateral ligament is simple taping of the ankle for comfort and avoidance of vigorous activities. A grade 3 sprain in an older, relatively nonathletic individual should be treated with a below-knee weight-bearing cast with the foot held in neutral position for three to four weeks. The management of a grade 3 sprain in a young athletic individual is probably best managed with operative repair of the torn ligaments, if chronic instability and limitation of athletic activities are to be prevented. Staples found that conservative treatment of severe lateral ligament injuries revealed poor results in follow-up.[62] Only 58 per cent of patients were symptom-free without limitations. Also, half of the patients demonstrated instability by stress at follow-up. An anterolateral curved fibular incision is probably the most appropriate incision for operative repair. Broström found that 90 out of 95 patients who had early operative repair had stable ankles in follow-up.[11]

The author's practice is to treat a grade 3 sprain of the lateral ligament in a young athletic patient very aggressively with operative repair. This approach is taken in the expectation that it will result in a stable ankle in follow-up. In the older, occasionally athletic individual this injury is probably best managed with a below-knee weight-bearing cast for three to four weeks.

DELTOID LIGAMENT INJURIES

Isolated injuries of the deltoid ligament are rare. The deltoid ligament is a strong structure consisting of a superficial and a deep portion.

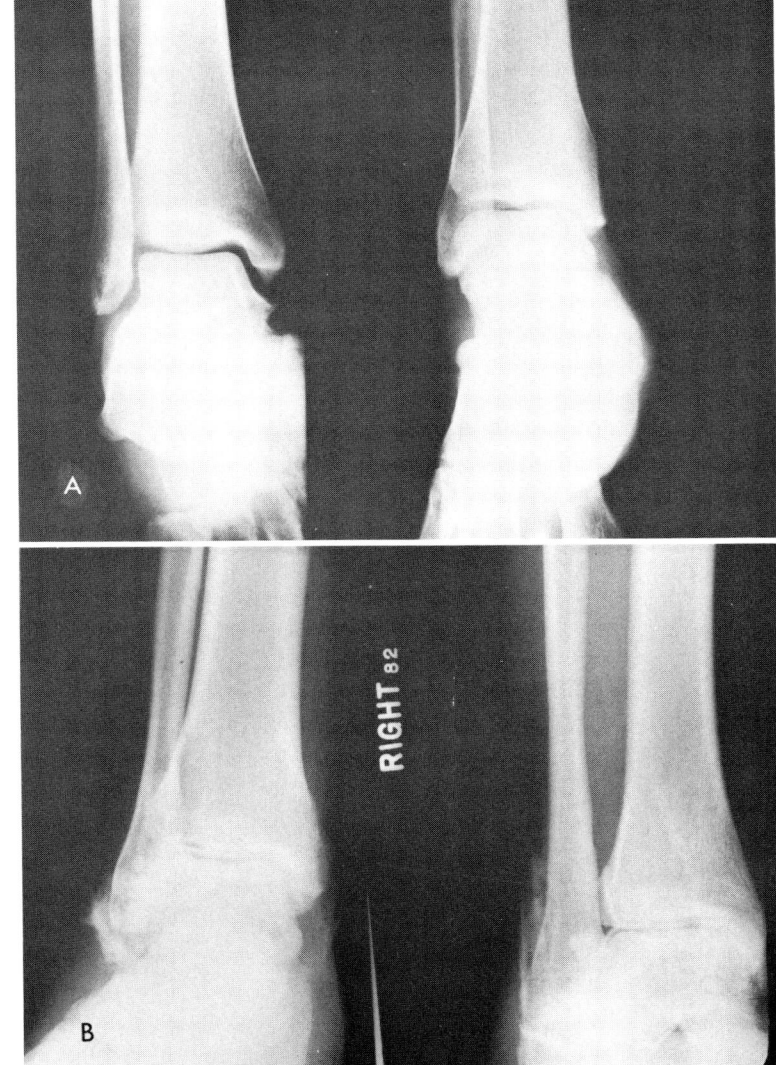

Figure 26–21 *A.* Routine roentgenograms fail to reveal lateral ligament injury. *B.* Following arthrography, contrast material is demonstrated in the peroneal sheath, indicative of a lateral ligament disruption.

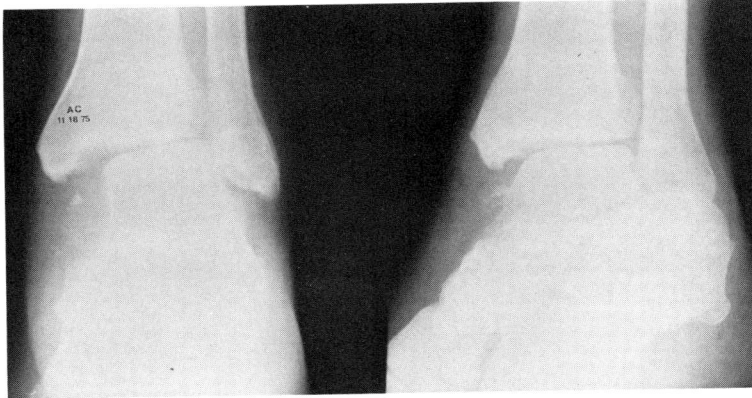

Figure 26–22   An avulsion injury of the deltoid ligament.

Mechanism of Injury

The deltoid ligament is placed under tension when the foot is subjected to an abduction or to external rotation stress. Therefore, these two mechanisms are the ones most commonly encountered with injuries to the deltoid ligament (Fig. 26–22). The force required to produce a rupture of the deltoid ligament is substantial and is usually associated with significant injuries to the fibula or syndesmosis.

Physical Examination

Since isolated tears of the deltoid ligaments are rare, examination usually reveals evidence of other associated injury. Gross swelling and ecchymosis are noted over the area of the deltoid ligament. If there is an associated fracture of the fibula or diastasis of the syndesmosis, gross swelling will also be present along the lateral aspect of the ankle. In the presence of a fracture of the fibula the examiner may be able to produce a subluxation of the talus laterally with a mild abduction strain.

Roentgenographic Examination

Since deltoid injuries are frequently associated with other injuries of the ankle, routine anteroposterior, lateral, and mortise views are indicated. The mortise view is particularly helpful, as it will enable the examiner to determine whether or not a lateral shift of the talus away from the articular surface of the medial malleolus has occurred. If there is significant lateral dis-placement of the talus a definite tear of the deltoid ligament must be present. In 1956 Close found that unless the deltoid was torn, lateral displacement of the talus in relation to the tibia would not exceed 2 mm even if all the tibiofibular ligaments were severed.[19] In 1960 Staples confirmed this observation.[62] Therefore, if there is a lateral shift of the talus of between 2 and 4 mm on the mortise view there is probably a tear of the deltoid ligament. A shift of greater than 4 mm in a lateral direction confirms a definite tear of the deltoid ligament.

Treatment

Grade 1 and grade 2 sprains may be treated with simple taping and avoidance of vigorous activities. Grade 3 sprains are usually associated with other injuries of the ankle, and the definitive form of treatment will depend on the associated injuries. If these are of significant magnitude, such as a diastasis of the ankle or a significant fracture of the distal fibula, then the deltoid ligament is openly repaired at the same time as internal fixation for the lateral aspect of the ankle is performed. If the deltoid ligament injury occurs in association with a relatively simple fracture of the fibula a closed reduction is attempted. If the talus appears to be situated in proper position in the ankle mortise and the fibular fracture appears to be appropriately aligned, the patient is placed in a plaster cast with the foot held in slight inversion in an attempt to approximate the ruptured ends of the deltoid ligament. Any tendency for lateral subluxation of the talus in the ankle mortise in follow-up requires operative repair of the deltoid ligament injury as well as fixation of the lateral aspect of the ankle.

There are two technical points in regard to operative repair of the deltoid ligament. It has been the author's experience that occasionally an attempt at closed reduction is unsatisfactory, as the talus cannot be repositioned appropriately in the ankle mortise. In other words, there appears to be a definite space of 4 mm or greater between the talus and the articular surface of the medial malleolus. Under these circumstances the deltoid ligament will occasionally be turned under the medial malleolus, blocking the proper reduction of the talus in the ankle mortise. This is a definite indication for operative repair. It is important to reflect the deltoid ligament from between the talus and medial malleolus during the procedure. Second, if operative treatment is performed the deltoid ligament should be sutured in two separate layers corresponding to the superficial and deep portion of the deltoid ligament, as outlined by Close.[19]

SYNDESMOTIC LIGAMENT INJURIES

Severe injuries of the syndesmotic ligaments are reflected by the presence of a diastasis of the ankle joint. The management of diastasis has been referred to earlier in this chapter in the evaluation of ankle injuries according to the modified Lauge-Hansen classification.

It is important to realize that under normal conditions slight motion occurs at the distal syndesmosis. This permits the fibula to ascend at the ankle mortise in a proximal and distal direction to accommodate the broad talar surface in dorsiflexion. Therefore, the syndesmosis plays an important role in normal gait. Any condition that limits motion at the syndesmosis will affect motion at the ankle joint. For example, if osseous union occurs at the distal syndesmosis this reciprocal motion cannot occur, and motion at the ankle joint is definitely altered (Fig. 26–23). This is more disabling than most physicians realize. The author's experience has been that osseous union at the syndesmosis as a result of prior injury is very difficult to treat. The osseous bridge will frequently have to be excised, but it may well recur.

Mechanism of Injury

Complete diastasis at the ankle joint occurs when the anterior and posterior tibiofibular and interosseous ligaments are completely disrupted. This may be seen in association with a Maisonneuve fracture, as

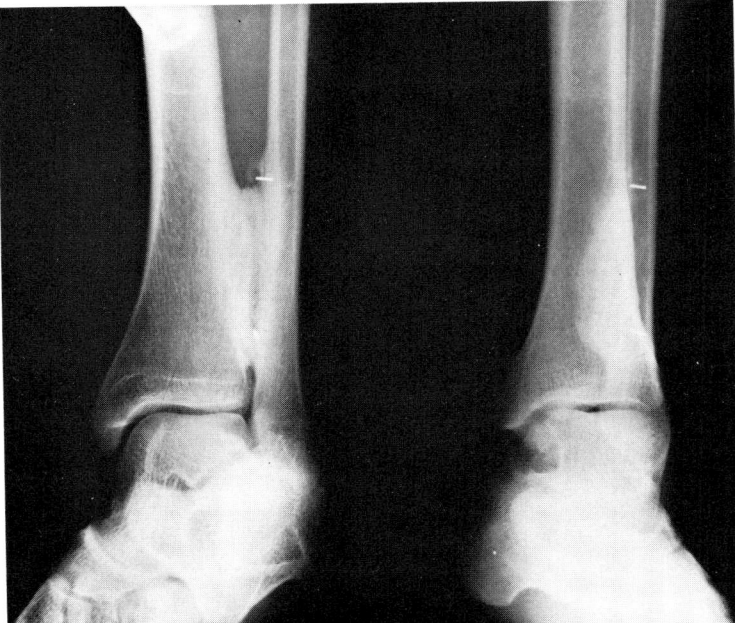

Figure 26–23 Osseous union across the syndesmosis. Severe disability which required operative removal.

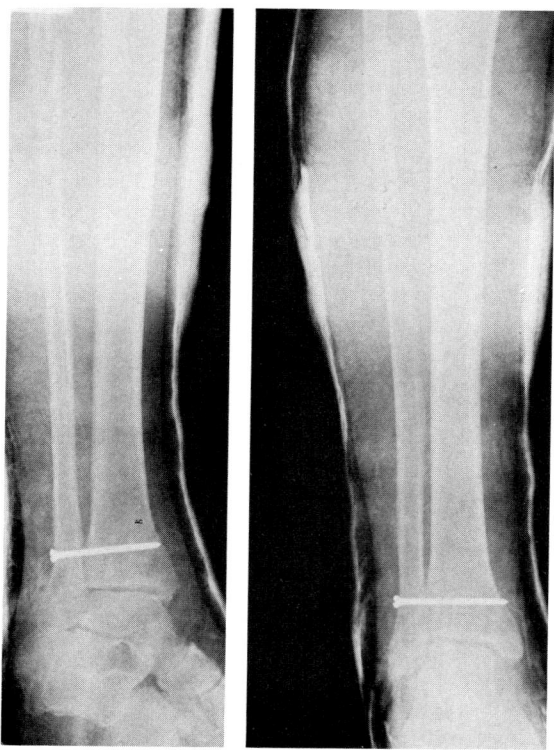

Figure 26–24 Operative fixation of a diastasis due to a Maisonneuve injury.

previously outlined (Fig. 26–24). External rotation and abduction are the two primary mechanisms involved in the production of a diastasis. The reader is referred to the modified Lauge-Hansen classification.

Physical Examination

If a diastasis has occurred in the absence of a fibular fracture there will be definite tenderness and swelling over the area of the anterior and posterior talofibular ligaments. This is an important diagnostic sign, as frequently young athletic individuals will receive a twisting injury to the ankle and present with pain and tenderness directly over the tibiofibular ligament area. The examining physician should be suspicious of a partial or complete diastasis of the ankle if this finding is present. If there has been a tear of the deltoid ligament in association with the diastasis the examiner may note a slight lateral toggle of the talus in the ankle mortise.

Roentgenographic Examination

A complete diastasis is usually evident on the mortise view. A clear space visualized between the distal tibia and the fibula is presumptive evidence of a diastasis (Fig. 26–25). Normally a distinct clear space between these two osseous structures is not possible in the presence of intact syndesmotic ligaments. If there is a space greater than 5 mm between the medial cortex of the fibula and the posterior edge of the peroneal groove in the anteroposterior view, a definite diastasis has occurred.

Treatment

The treatment of a diastasis depends on the other associated injuries. As indicated in the discussion of Maisonneuve fractures, the later stages of this fracture require internal fixation of the syndesmosis as the appropriate form of treatment. Occasionally a mild diastasis may be treated by closed methods, but careful follow-up examination

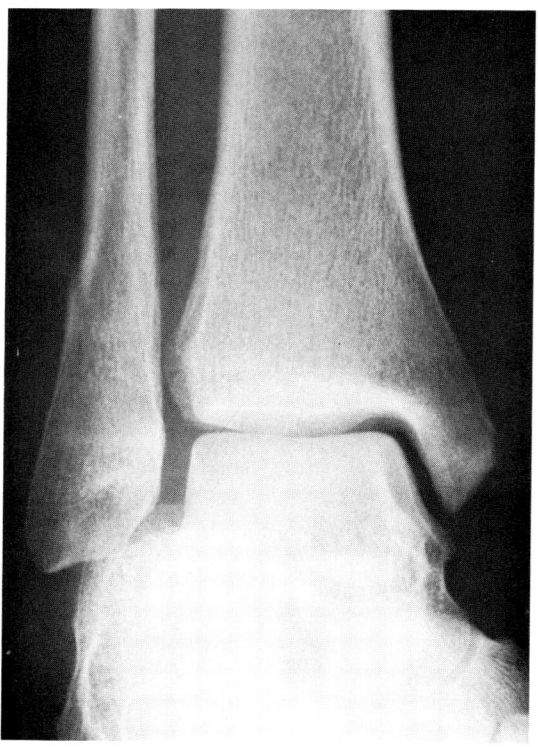

Figure 26–25 A mild diastasis evident in the mortise view.

in plaster is recommended in order to evaluate whether or not the spread between the distal tibia and fibula has recurred. If operative management is selected, a transfixion screw or a Webb bolt may be used to maintain the syndesmosis in proper alignment. As already stated, cross union between the distal tibia and fibula following treatment of an ankle injury may be a very disabling condition which is difficult to treat. Under these conditions the author has attempted to excise the area of cross union at the syndesmosis and insert a thin sheet of Silastic membrane in the hope of preventing recurrence of the cross union.

SALVAGE PROCEDURES

In the presence of disabling degenerative arthritis following ankle fractures two operative procedures are available. The first is the time-honored ankle fusion. This is an excellent method for relief of pain. It does limit the mobility of the ankle, but since significant motion occurs at the subtalar as well as at the midtarsal joints the limited motion is well tolerated by the patient. This procedure is performed with the use of the Charnley compression arthrodesis device. The joint surface is denuded of all viable cartilage down to raw bleeding bone, and then the talus is compressed against the distal tibia with the use of the Charnley device. The results of this treatment show a very high rate of success with a solid ankle fusion. This procedure is preferred by the author, as it provides a stable painless ankle in follow-up examination. It also allows patients to perform relatively heavy labor and to engage in athletic activities.

The second procedure which is still under extensive clinical trials is that of total ankle replacement. It is early in the development of this technique, and it is probable that ankle fusion will still be selected as the salvage procedure for degenerative arthritis of the ankle until improved components and methods of fixation are available for total ankle replacement. At the present time it may have a limited application in the elderly patient with severe degenerative arthritis of the ankle and relative limitation of activites.

REFERENCES

1. Ashhurst, A. P. C., and Bromer, R. S.: Classification and mechanism of fractures of the leg bone involving the ankle. Arch Surg., 4:51–129, 1922.
2. Berndt, A. L., and Harty, M.: Transchondral fractures (osteochondritis dessicans) of the talus. J. Bone Joint Surg., 41A:988, 1959.
3. Bonnin, J. G.: Injury to the ligaments of the ankle. J. Bone Joint Surg., 47B:609, 1965.
4. Bonnin, J. G.: Injuries to the Ankle. Darien, Conn., Hafner Publishing Co., 1970.
5. Bosworth, D. M.: Fracture-dislocation of the ankle with fixed displacement of the fibula behind the tibia. J. Bone Joint Surg., 29:130–135, 1947.
6. Braunstein, P. W., and Wade, P. A.: Treatment of unstable fractures of the ankle. Ann. Surg., 149:217–226, 1956.
7. Broomhead, R.: Discussion on fractures in the region of the ankle joint. Proc. R. Soc. Med., 25:1082, 1932.
8. Broström, L.: I. Anatomic lesions in recent sprains. Acta Chir. Scand., 128:483–495, 1964.
9. Broström, L., Liljeahl, S. O., and Lindvall, N.: II. Arthrographic diagnosis of recent ligament ruptures. Acta Chir. Scand., 129:485–499, 1965.
10. Broström, L., and Sundelin, P.: IV. Histologic changes in recent and "chronic" ligament ruptures. Acta Chir. Scand., 132:248–253, 1966.
11. Broström, L.: Sprained Ankles. V. Treatment and prognosis in recent ligament ruptures. Acta Chir. Scand., 132:537–550, 1966.
12. Broström, L., Liljedahl, S. O., and Lindvall, N.: Isolated fracture of the posterior tibial tubercle. Aetiologic and clinical features. Acta Chir. Scand., 128:51–56, 1964.
13. Burwell, H. N., and Charnley, A. D.: The treatment of displaced fractures at the ankle by rigid internal fixation and early joint movement. J. Bone Joint Surg., 47B:634–660, 1965.
14. Cedell, C.: Supination-outward rotation injuries of the ankle. A clinical and roentgenological study with special reference to the operative treatment. Acta Orthop. Scand. (Suppl.), 110, 1967.
15. Cedell, C.: Ankle lesions. Acta Orthop. Scand., 46:425–445, 1975.
16. Charnley, J.: The Closed Treatment of Common Fractures. Baltimore, Williams & Wilkins Co., 1963.
17. Chrisman, O. D., and Snook, G. A.: Reconstruction of lateral ligament tears of the ankle. An experimental study and clinical evaluation of 7 patients treated by a new modification of the Elmslie procedure. J. Bone Joint Surg., 51A:904–912, 1969.
18. Clayton, M. L., and Weir, G. J., Jr.: Experimental investigations of ligamentous healing. Am. J. Surg., 98:373–378, 1959.
19. Close, J. R.: Some applications of the functional anatomy of the ankle joint. J. Bone Joint Surg., 38A:761–781, 1956.
20. Colonna, P. C., and Ralston, E. L.: Operative approaches to the ankle joint. Am. J. Surg., 82:44, 1951.
21. Coltart, W. D.: Aviator's astragalus. J. Bone Joint Surg., 34B:545, 1952.

22. Coonrad, R. W.: Fracture-dislocations of the ankle joint with impaction injury to the lateral weight-bearing surface of the tibia. J. Bone Joint Surg., 52A:1337–1344, 1970.
23. Cotton, F. J.: A new type of ankle fracture. J.A.M.A., 64:318–321, 1915.
24. Davidson, A. M., Steele, H. D., MacKenzie, D. A., and Penny, J. A.: A review of twenty-one cases of transchondral fractures of the talus. J. Trauma, 7:378, 1967.
25. Denham, R. D.: Internal fixation for unstable ankle fractures. J. Bone Joint Surg., 46B:206, 1964.
26. Destot, E.: Traumatismes du Pied et Rayons. 2nd ed. Paris, Masson et Cie., 1937.
27. Dupuytren, G.: Of fractures of the lower extremity of the fibula and luxations of the foot. (reprinted in) Med. Classics, 4:151–172, 1939.
28. Dziob, J. M.: Ligamentous injuries about the ankle joint. Am. J. Surg., 91:692–698, 1956.
29. Evans, D. L.: Recurrent instability of the ankle—a method of surgical treatment. Proc. R. Soc. Med., 46:343–344, 1953.
30. Evans, D. L.: Recurrent disability of the ankle—a method of surgical treatment. J. Bone Joint Surg., 39B:795, 1957.
31. Fussel, M. E., and Godley, D. R.: Ankle arthrography in acute sprains. Clin. Orthop. Rel. Res., 93:278, 1973.
32. Gaston, S., and McLaughlin, H. L.: Complex fracture of the lateral malleolus. J. Trauma, 1:69–78, 1961.
33. Gatellier, J.: The juxtaretroperoneal route in the operative treatment of fracture of the malleolus with posterior marginal fragment. Surg. Gynecol. Obstet., 52:67–70, 1931.
34. Grath, G.: Widening of the ankle mortise. A clinical and experimental study. Acta Chir. Scand. (Suppl.), 263:1–88, 1960.
35. Joy, G., Patzakis, M. J., and Harvey, J. P.: Precise evaluation of the reduction of severe ankle fractures. J. Bone Joint Surg., 56A:979–993, 1974.
36. Klossner, O.: Late results of operative and non-operative treatment of severe ankle fractures. Acta Chir. Scand. (Suppl.), 293:1–93, 1962.
37. Kocher, T.: Textbook of Operative Surgery. 3rd ed. London, Adam and Charles Black, 1911.
38. Kristensen, T. B.: Fractures of the ankle. VI. Followup studies. Arch. Surg., 73:112–121, 1956.
39. Lane, W. A.: The operative treatment of simple fractures. Surg. Gynecol. Obstet., 8:344–354, 1909.
40. Laskin, R. S.: Steinman-Pin fixation in the treatment of unstable fractures of the ankle. J. Bone Joint Surg., 56A:549–555, 1974.
41. Lauge-Hansen, N.: Fractures of the ankle. II. Combined experimental surgical and experimental roentgenologic investigations. Arch. Surg., 60:957–985, 1950.
42. Lauge-Hansen, N.: "Ligamentous" ankle fractures; diagnosis and treatment. Acta Chir. Scand., 97:544–550, 1949.
43. Lauge-Hansen, N.: Fractures of the ankle. V. Pronation-dorsiflexion fracture. Arch. Surg., 67:813–820, 1953.
44. Laurin, C. A., Ouellet, R., and St. Jacques, R.: Talar

and subtalar tilt: An experimental investigation. Can. J. Surg., 11:270–279, 1968.
45. Leonard, M. H.: Injuries of the lateral ligaments of the ankle—a clinical and experimental study. J. Bone Joint Surg., 31A:373–377, 1949.
46. Magnusson, R.: On the late results of non-operative cases of malleolar fractures. Acta Chir. Scand. (Suppl.), 90:1–136, 1944.
47. Maisonneuve, J. G.: Recherches sur la fracture du perone. Arch. Gen. Med., 7:165–187, 433–473, 1840.
48. Mayer, P., and Evarts, C. M.: Fracture-dislocation of the ankle with posterior entrapment of the fibula behind the tibia. J. Bone Joint Surg., 60A:320–324, 1978.
49. McLaughlin, H. L.: In: Trauma. Philadelphia, W. B. Saunders, 1959.
50. Nelson, M. C., and Jensen, N. J.: The treatment of trimalleolar fractures of the ankle. Surg. Gynecol. Obstet., 71:509–514, 1942.
51. Olson, R. W.: Arthrography of the ankle; it use in the evaluation of ankle sprains. Radiology, 92:1439–1446, 1969.
52. Pankovich, A. M.: Fractures of the fibula proximal to the distal tibio-fibular syndesmosis. J. Bone Joint Surg., 60A:221–229, 1978.
53. Pankovich, A. M.: Maissonneuve fracture of the fibula. J. Bone Joint Surg., 58A:337–342, 1976.
54. Patrick, J.: A direct approach to trimalleolar fractures. J. Bone Joint Surg., 47B:236–239, 1965.
55. Pott, P.: Some few general remarks on fractures and dislocations. London, Hawes, Clarke, Collins, 1768.
56. Quigley, T. B.: Analysis and treatment of ankle injuries produced by rotatory, abduction and adduction forces. In AAOS Instructional Course Lectures, 19:172–182. St. Louis, C. V. Mosby, 1970.
57. Quigley, T. B.: Management of ankle injuries. J.A.M.A., 169:1432–1435, 1959.
58. Rubin, G., and Witten, M.: The talar-tilt angle and the fibular collateral ligament. J. Bone Joint Surg., 42A:311, 1960.
59. Ruth, C. J.: The surgical treatment of injuries of the fibular collateral ligaments of the ankle. J. Bone Joint Surg., 43A:229–239, 1961.
60. Speed, J. S., and Boyd, H. B.: Operative reconstruction of malunited fractures about the ankle joint. J. Bone Joint Surg., 43A:270–286, 1936.
61. Staples, O. S.: Injuries to the medial ligaments of the ankle. J. Bone Joint Surg., 42A:1287–1307, 1960.
62. Staples, D. S.: Ruptures of the fibular collateral ligaments of the ankle. J. Bone Joint Surg., 57A:101–107, 1975.
63. Vasli, S.: Operative treatment of ankle fractures. Acta Chir. Scand. (Suppl.), 226:1–74, 1957.
64. Wilson, F. C., and Skilbred, L. A.: Long term results in the treatment of displaced bimalleolar fractures. J. Bone Joint Surg., 48A:1065–1078, 1966.
65. Yablon, I. G., Heller, F. G., and Shouse, L.: The key role of the lateral malleolus in displaced fractures of the ankle. J. Bone Joint Surg., 59A:169–173, 1977.

R. BRUCE HEPPENSTALL, M.D.

Injuries _____ 27
of the
Foot

SURGICAL ANATOMY

Injuries to the foot occur in all age groups. Fractures are common; dislocations also occur, but are not as frequent. If improperly managed these injuries cause significant pain and disability. Therefore, a proper evaluation and treatment program, based on a thorough knowledge of the anatomy and biomechanics of the foot, is essential to their management.

SURGICAL ANATOMY

For descriptive purposes, the osseous portion of the foot may be divided into three regions. The forefoot includes the metatarsals and the phalanges (Fig. 27–1). The midfoot comprises the navicular, the cuboid, and the three cuneiforms. The hindfoot includes the calcaneus and the talus. The articulations between the tarsal bones and the metatarsals have been referred to as Lisfranc's joint (Fig. 27–2). The midtarsal joints located between the hindfoot and the midfoot are known as Chopart's joint.

On the dorsum of the foot, progressing from medial to lateral, the following structures are present. The superficial area is made up of the tibialis anterior, the extensor hallucis longus, the extensor digitorum longus, and the peroneus tertius tendons. The deep layer consists of a branch of the peroneal nerve, the dorsalis pedis artery,

and the extensor hallucis brevis and extensor digitorum brevis. The sensory supply derives from the superficial branch of the common peroneal nerve and the sural nerve.

The sole of the foot is made up of several specific layers. The plantar fascia is a dense fibrous structure that resembles the palmar aponeurosis but is thicker. It originates from the medial process of the tuber calcanei and extends distally to fan out to each toe. The underlying muscles and tendons of the foot are also separated into distinct layers. The first layer, progressing from medial to lateral, includes the abductor hallucis, the flexor digitorum brevis, and the abductor digiti minimi. The second layer of the foot, again from medial to lateral, consists of the flexor hallucis longus tendon, the flexor digitorum longus tendon, the quadratus plantae, and the lumbrical muscles. The third layer includes the flexor hallucis brevis, the adductor hallucis, and the flexor digiti minimi. The tibialis posterior tendon, the peroneus longus tendon, and the underlying interossei make up the fourth layer. The source of the nerve supply to the plantar muscles is the medial and lateral plantar branches of the posterior tibial nerve. The blood supply derives from the posterior tibial artery.

On the medial aspect of the foot the abductor hallucis extends from the calcaneus to the base of the proximal phalanx of the great toe (Fig. 27–3). From the dorsal

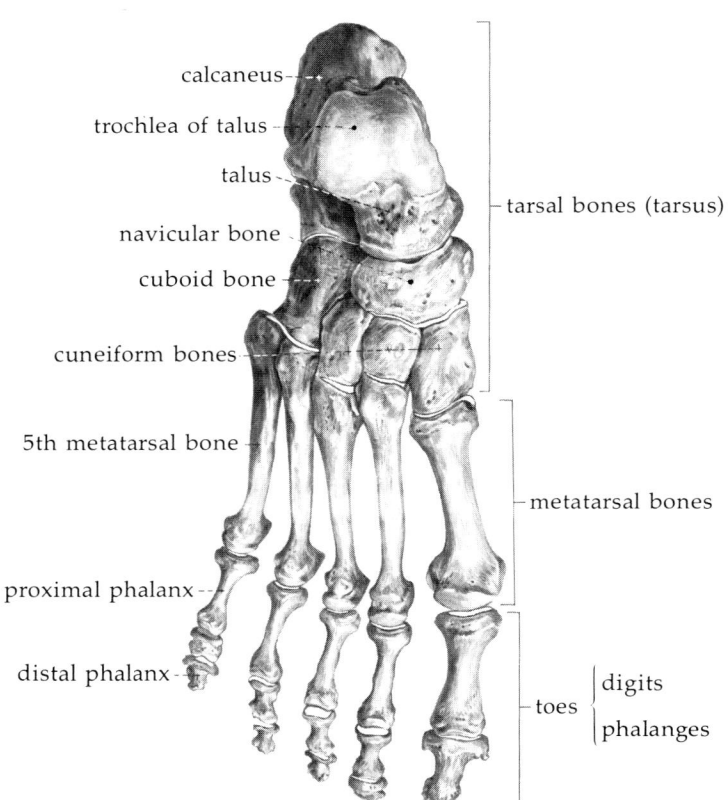

calcaneus
trochlea of talus
talus
navicular bone
cuboid bone
cuneiform bones
5th metatarsal bone
proximal phalanx
distal phalanx

tarsal bones (tarsus)

metatarsal bones

toes — digits / phalanges

Figure 27–1   Dorsal aspect of the bones of the right foot. (Courtesy of J. Langman and M. W. Woerdeman, and W. B. Saunders Co., Philadelphia. *Atlas of Medical Anatomy*, 1978.)

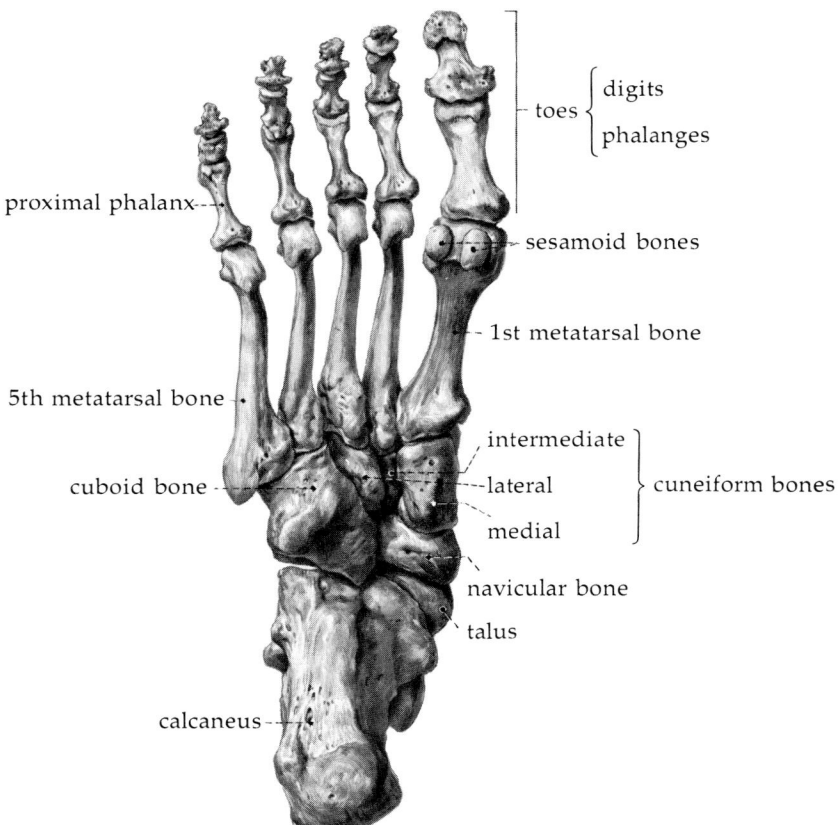

Figure 27–2 Plantar aspect of the bones of the right foot. (Courtesy of J. Langman and M. W. Woerdeman and W. B. Saunders Co., Philadelphia. *Atlas of Medical Anatomy,* 1978.)

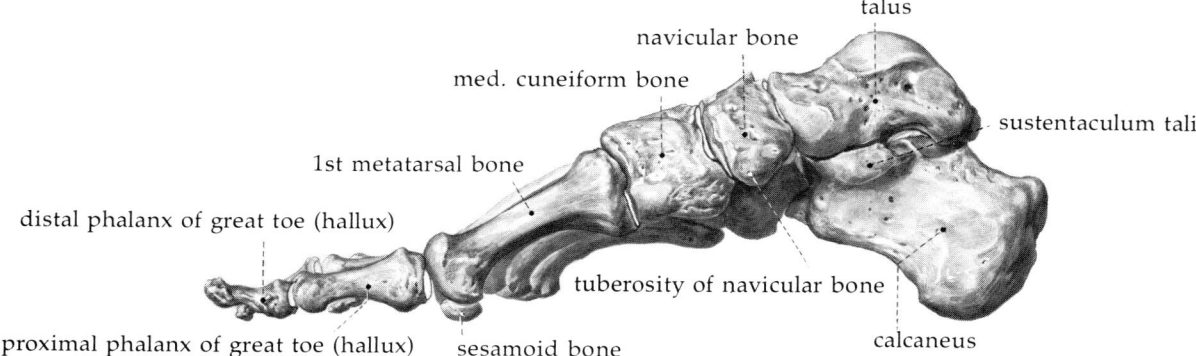

Figure 27-3 Medial aspect of the bones of the right foot. (Courtesy of J. Langman and M. W. Woerdeman and W. B. Saunders Co., Philadelphia. *Atlas of Medical Anatomy*, 1978.)

aspect, moving downward medially, the tibialis anterior tendon extends to the first cuneiform and the base of the first metatarsal. The tibialis posterior tendon extends to the navicular tubercle and the first cuneiform. The flexor hallucis longus tendon is located in a specific groove along the medial and posteromedial surface of the talus.

On the lateral aspect of the foot the peroneus brevis tendon extends to its insertion into the base of the fifth metatarsal (Fig. 27–4). The peroneus longus tendon is in a more plantar location, extending in a groove between the cuboid and the fifth metatarsal. The sural nerve is located just inferior to the peroneal tendons.

The anatomy of the talus deserves special attention (Fig. 27–5). As outlined in Chapter 26, the superior articular surface of the talus is wider anteriorly than posteriorly. There are no specific muscular or tendinous attachments to the talus. Stability is provided by the anatomical structure of the talus and by the articular capsule and synovial membrane. The os trigonum is an accessory bone, that is, an osseous mass located at the posterior aspect of the talus that fails to unite with the talus. It should not be confused with a fracture in this area.

The blood supply of the talus is complex, involving branches of all three major arteries, the anterior tibial, posterior tibial, and perforating peroneal. An important blood supply is located in the tarsal canal and the

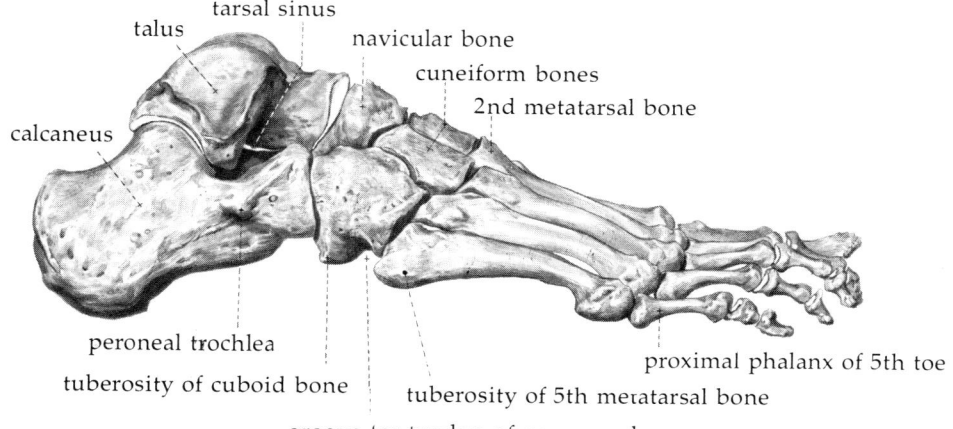

Figure 27-4 Lateral aspect of the bones of the right foot. (Courtesy of J. Langman and M. W. Woerdeman and W. B. Saunders Co., Philadelphia. *Atlas of Medical Anatomy*, 1978.)

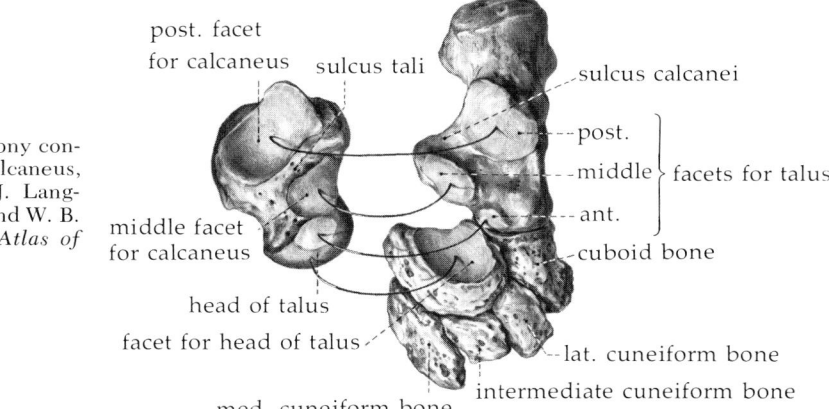

Figure 27–5 Surfaces of bony contact between the left talus, calcaneus, and navicular. (Courtesy of J. Langman and M. W. Woerdeman and W. B. Saunders Co., Philadelphia. *Atlas of Medical Anatomy*, 1978.)

sinus tarsi. The tarsal canal is situated between the talus and calcaneus, distal and posterior to the tip of the medial malleolus. A branch of the posterior tibial artery is located in the tarsal canal, and a branch of the perforating peroneal artery is located in the sinus tarsi. Both of these arteries anastomose to form a vascular channel that distributes branches to the neck of the talus. Branches of the anterior tibial artery extend into the superior aspect of the neck of the talus. The posterior tubercle also has a specific blood supply. The reader is referred to the article by Kelly and Sullivan[36] for a detailed explanation of the blood supply of the talus.

Three articular facets, anterior, middle, and posterior, are present along the superior aspect of the calcaneus. The anterior facet, the smallest structure, is located along the medial aspect of the calcaneus on the distal portion of the superior aspect. It frequently merges with the middle facet, which is located just posterior to it. The middle facet is a slightly larger structure situated over a projecting aspect of the calcaneous known as the sustentaculum tali. The posterior facet is the largest of the three structures. Between the middle and posterior facets is a sulcus for the interosseous ligament. This area opens up laterally to form, with the talar sulcus, the sinus tarsi.

On the medial aspect, slightly posterior and distal to the sustentaculum tali, is a groove for the tendon of the flexor hallucis longus. The tuber calcanei is a downward

projection at the posteroinferior aspect of the calcaneus. Two other projections, the medial and lateral tuberal processes, extend from the tuber calcanei and aid in supporting weight placed on the heel.

FRACTURES OF THE TALUS

TRANSCHONDRAL FRACTURES

In the past, there have been several misconceptions in regard to this injury. In 1888, König observed loose bodies in joints other than the ankle joint,[40] which he believed were due to a process of spontaneous necrosis. He coined the term "osteochondritis dissecans" for this type of lesion. In 1922, Kappis applied this term to the ankle joint.[35] Since that time, many authors have considered loose bodies in the joint to be due to osteochondritis dissecans.

It was not until the classic studies of Berndt and Harty in 1959 that the true nature of transchondral fractures was defined.[6] They proposed the term "transchondral fracture" as the correct name for this entity from both an anatomical and an etiological point of view. They felt that a transchondral fracture was by definition a fracture of the articular surface of the bone, produced by a force transmitted from the articular surface of a contiguous bone across the joint, and extending through the articular cartilage to the subchondral trabeculae of the fractured bone. Since the avulsed segment of bone has no attendant soft tissue attachments, there is no blood supply to the fragment and it is therefore susceptible to the development of avascular necrosis. The true incidence of this injury is difficult to determine. However, it appears that it is not as rare as was once supposed. Bosien, Staples, and Russell made a study of a series of ankle sprains in college students in 1955,[10] reporting 133 sprains in 113 patients. A careful review revealed that nine patients demonstrated cortical avulsion fractures of the talus, for an incidence of 6.75 per cent.

Mechanism of Injury

In their anatomical study, Berndt and Harty were able to produce transchondral fractures of the dome of the talus with specific deforming forces. Lesions of the lateral dome were usually found in the middle or anterior half of the lateral border, with damage limited to two sites: (1) the talar dome itself, and (2) the lateral collateral ligament (Fig. 27–6). The basic applied force was strong inversion of the dorsiflexed ankle. Anatomically, the dome of the talus is wider in the anterior portion, which provides for a snug fit in the ankle mortise with dorsiflexion of the ankle. If excessive inversion is applied to the dorsiflexed ankle, the talus is rotated laterally, impacting and compressing the lateral talar margin against the articular surface of the fibula. This produces a typical stage 1 lesion—a small area of indentation in the talar margin, with the lateral collateral ligament remaining intact.

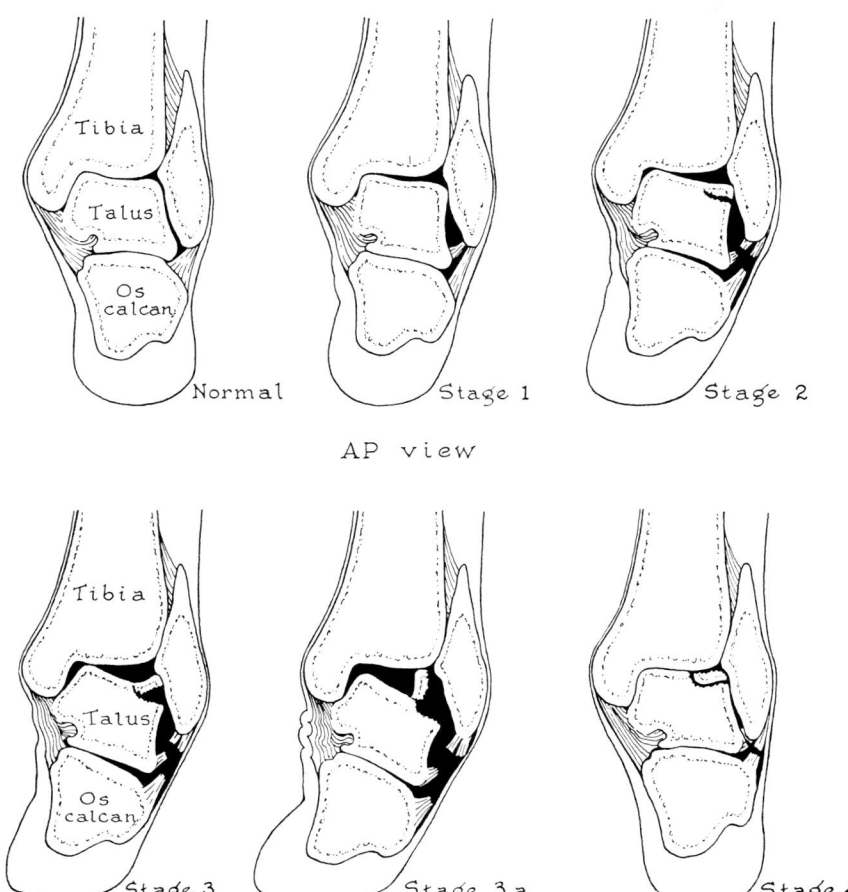

Figure 27–6 Mechanism of transchondral fractures of the lateral border of the talar dome. (Courtesy of A. L. Berndt and M. Harty and *Journal of Bone and Joint Surgery*. J. Bone Joint Surg., 41A:988–1020, 1955.)

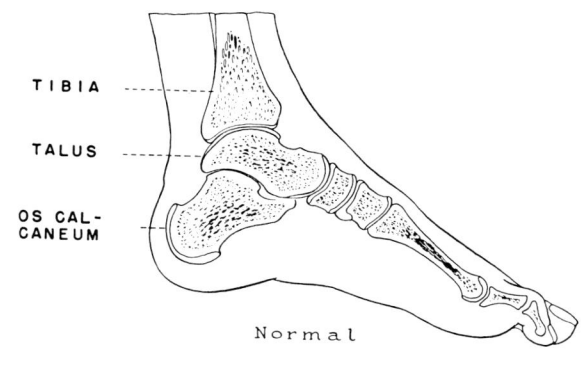

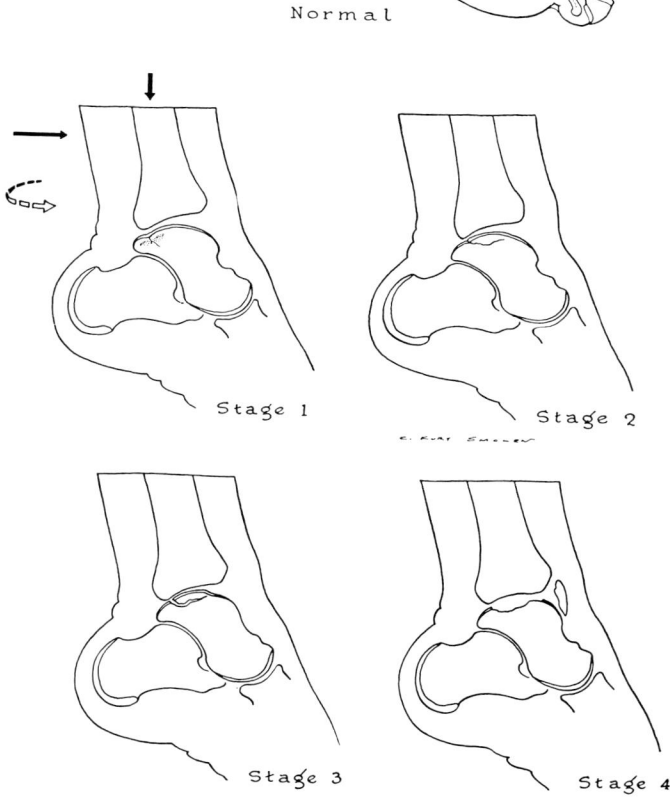

Figure 27-7 Mechanism of transchondral fractures of the medial border of the talar dome. (Courtesy of A. L. Berndt and M. Harty and *Journal of Bone and Joint Surgery.* J. Bone Joint Surg., *41A*:988–1020, 1955.)

A stage 2 lesion results when the inversion stress is continued, resulting in a shearing-off of a portion of the lateral dome of the talus. This may also be associated with a rupture of the middle and anterior fasciculi of the lateral collateral ligament. A stage 3 lesion is produced by further inversion, in which a portion of the lateral dome becomes completely detached and may be slightly displaced. A stage 4 lesion causes significant displacement or inversion of the talar dome fragment.

Medial dome lesions are produced by a combination of forces. These include (1)

plantar flexion of the ankle; (2) slight anterior displacement of the tibia upon the talus; (3) inversion of the ankle; and (4) lateral rotation of the tibia upon the talus (Fig. 27–7). A stage 1 lesion is caused by plantar flexion and inversion followed by rotation of the tibia on the talus. This produces a small area of compression of the articular surface with the collateral ligaments remaining intact. The same sequence of events occurs in a stage 2 lesion in addition to anterior displacement of the tibia on the talus. This results in the posterior inferior lip of the tibia gouging out

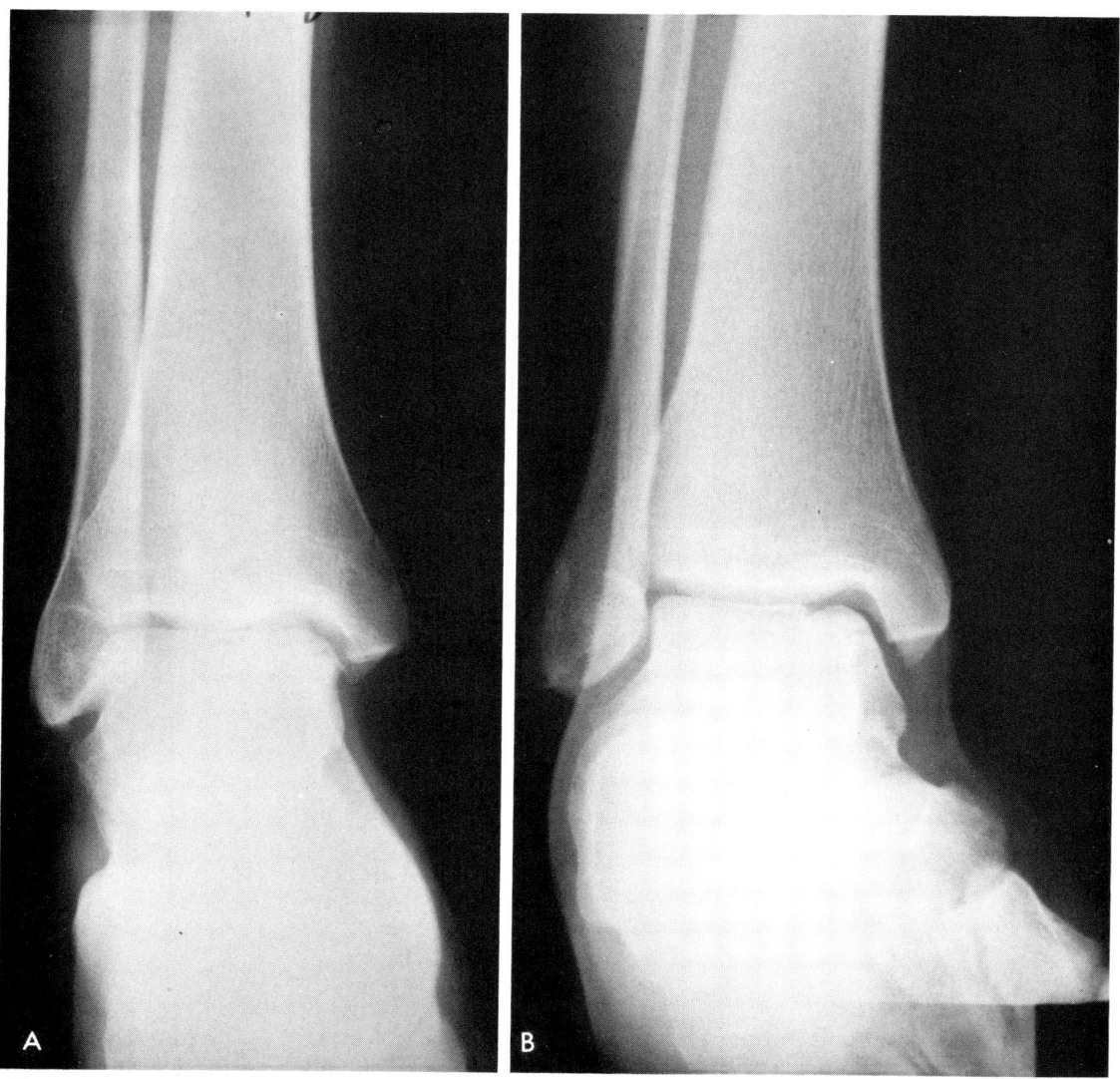

Figure 27–8   *A.* A routine anteroposterior view of the ankle demonstrating a type 2 transchondral fracture of the medial border of the talar dome. It is difficult to appreciate the lesion in this view. *B.* A mortise view providing a better demonstration of the lesion.

an osteochondral chip that is partially detached. A stage 3 lesion results from further application of the force combined with lateral rotation of the tibia upon the talus. This produces a completely detached osteochondral fragment along the medial talar dome. A stage 4 lesion is caused by still greater progression of the applied force, resulting in a displacement of the involved fragment into the anterior portion of the joint. It is interesting to note that in these anatomical studies the posterior fibers of the deltoid ligament ruptured with production of a stage 2 or greater lesion.

Physical Examination

Stage 1 lesions present with a relatively painless and free range of motion of the ankle, since the ligamentous structures remain intact and the articular cartilage lacks sensory nerve endings. Stage 2 lesions are painful because of the associated collateral ligament injury. In lateral dome lesions there is tenderness over the lateral collateral ligament, while in medial dome lesions there is tenderness over the deltoid ligament. There may be an associated traumatic synovitis, limiting range of motion of the ankle. In stage 3 and stage 4 lesions synovitis is increased, with a corresponding decrease in range of motion; the remaining motion is painful. There may also be evidence of collateral ligament instability.

Roentgenographic Examination

Standard anteroposterior mortise and lateral views of the ankle usually demonstrate the associated transchondral fracture. Because stage 1 lesions are due to compression, there is no detachment of the involved fragment. Therefore, it is difficult to appreciate this injury on routine roentgenograms (Figs. 27–8 and 27–9). Stage 2 lesions are usually clearly delineated by the fracture through the cancellous surface of the appropriate talar dome. Stage 3 and 4 injuries are more evident because the detachment and displacement are complete.

Treatment

Stage 1 lesions are not always apparent following routine physical and roentgeno-

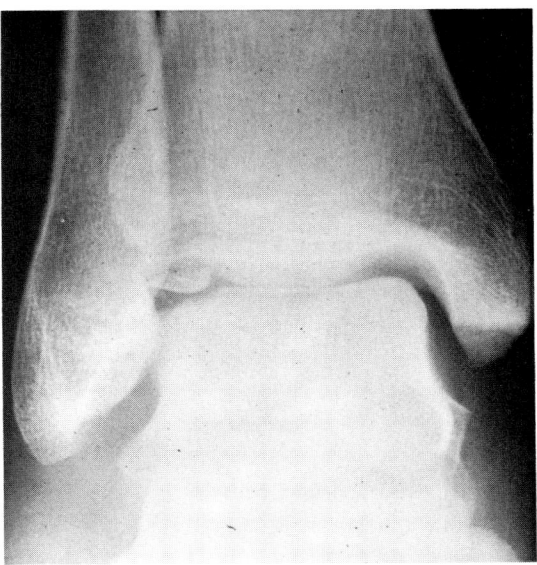

Figure 27-9 A type 4 transchondral fracture of the lateral border of the talar dome. Note that the fragment is completely displaced by inversion.

graphic examinations. Therefore, patients may present with an almost painless range of motion of the ankle. A mild decrease in physical activities for two to three weeks will resolve any residual symptoms. Stage 2, 3, and 4 lesions frequently demand more aggressive treatment. In these injuries the blood supply to the fragment has been disrupted, and the fragment itself is susceptible to changes of avascular necrosis. For this reason, stage 2 lesions often require an extended period of conservative therapy in order to completely heal. If immobilization is less than complete, disruption of the reparative process with interference of the ingrowth of the capillary structure will delay healing.

The author supports the findings of Berndt and Harty, who noted an increased percentage of good results with operative management compared with conservative treatment. At the time of surgery, it is always striking that the fragment appears larger than had been anticipated from reviewing the roentgenograms. This is because a large articular portion is involved, which is not always evident on the roentgenogram. If the fragment is relatively large, it may be replaced in its bed with some type of small pin fixation, but the majority of these injuries are best treated with excision of the fragment and curettage of the base. This allows for ingrowth of fibrous tissue, which will fill in the defect that is created by removal of the fragment. A good result can be expected from the operative approach, while only a fair or poor result may be obtained with conservative nonoperative treatment. The reader is referred to the article by Berndt and Harty for further appreciation of this subject.[6]

FRACTURES OF THE NECK OF THE TALUS

Fractures of the neck of the talus are probably the second most common talar injury, the most common being small chip or avulsion fractures. In spite of this fairly frequent occurrence, few large series are reported in the literature. In 1919, Anderson coined the term "aviator's astragalus"[2] to refer to fracture-dislocations of the talus. He was the first to recognize the primary role played by dorsiflexion in the mechanism of injury. A thorough knowledge of the anatomy and blood supply of the talus is essential if these injuries are to be managed intelligently. Avascular necrosis of the talus may result from disruption of the blood supply and is a very difficult complication to treat. An added problem in the management of patients with this injury is that 50 per cent or more have associated fractures. Hawkins noted that 64 per cent of patients in his series of fractures of the neck of the talus had associated fractures, including 21 per cent who had open fractures.[32]

Mechanism of Injury

The main deforming force in this injury is forced dorsiflexion of the foot and ankle. The neck of the talus is driven against the anterior leading edge of the distal tibia, which produces the characteristic fracture of the talar neck. The displacement of the fracture fragments depends upon the magnitude of the dorsiflexion force and also upon the presence or absence of rotatory components.

Classification

In 1970, Hawkins reviewed a series of 57 fractures of the neck of the talus and developed a very valuable working classification[32] based on the roentgenographic appearance at the time of injury. In type 1, a vertical fracture of the neck of the talus is present and is undisplaced. A fracture line enters the subtalar joint between the middle and posterior facets. The body of the talus is maintained in its normal position with respect to the ankle and subtalar joints. This injury accounted for 10.6 per cent of the total in his series. Avascular necrosis of the talus is uncommon, as only one of the three main sources of blood supply is interrupted.

Type 2 injuries are vertical fractures of the neck of the talus that are displaced. The subtalar joint is subluxated or dislocated, but the ankle joint itself is normal. The fracture line frequently enters a portion of the body and posterior facet of the talus. This injury represents 42.1 per cent of the total in the series. Two of the main sources of blood supply are interrupted in this injury. These are the supply proceeding proximally from the neck and that entering the foramina in the sinus tarsi and tarsal canal. Occasionally, the blood supply entering the foramina in the medial surface of the body may be disrupted, resulting in avascular necrosis. In Hawkin's study, 42 per cent of type 2 fracture-dislocations resulted in avascular necrosis of the talus, but union of the fracture occurred in all cases.

A type 3 injury is a displaced vertical fracture of the neck of the talus, with the body of the talus dislocated from both the ankle and the subtalar joints. The fracture line frequently enters a portion of the body of the talus. The body is often extruded posteriorly and medially, finally becoming located between the posterior surface of the tibia and the Achilles tendon. The head of the talus usually remains in normal relationship to the navicular. Since the three main routes of blood supply to the body of the talus are damaged in this injury, avascular necrosis of the talus frequently occurs. Type 3 injuries represented 47.3 per cent of cases in this series.

In 1978, Canale and Kelly published an excellent long-term evaluation of 71 cases of fractures of the neck of the talus from the Campbell Clinic.[13] They described a new type of injury that they called type 4, in which the fracture of the talar neck is associated with dislocation of the body from the ankle or subtalar joint, with an additional dislocation or subluxation of the head of the talus from the talonavicular joint. They noted a type 4 injury in 3 out of 71 cases, for an incidence of 4.2 per cent. The author recommends the use of the Hawkins classification with the addition of the type 4 injury of Canale and Kelly.

Physical Examination

Significant swelling is usually present in the forefoot and midfoot of patients presenting with fractures of the neck of the talus. There may be gross deformity of the foot, depending upon the amount of displacement of the fracture fragments. Any attempt at motion of the foot or ankle produces pain. The arterial supply to the foot is usually not significantly impaired with these injuries. However, the gross swelling and stasis that result from the deformity may compromise the blood flow to the toes. Therefore, it is advisable to assess the vascular supply to the distal foot by determining the amount of capillary return in the nailbeds. Likewise, the viability of the skin overlying the injury should be determined. If there is significant displacement of the foot owing to an associated subluxation or dislocation of the head and neck of the talus, the overlying skin may be "tented" over the injury. A delay in performing an appropriate reduction may cause

the skin to break down because of tensile pressure. This will result in an open fracture of the talus.

If the patient presents with an open fracture of the talus, sterile dressings should be applied and irrigation and debridement of the wound performed at the time of the reduction. A rule of thumb is to avoid frequent inspection of the wound by several examining physicians prior to definitive treatment. In order to decrease the risk of contaminating, the author recommends applying a sterile dressing and then taking the patient to the operating room for appropriate inspection and irrigation and debridement.

Roentgenographic Examination

Routine anteroposterior and lateral views of the foot and ankle are usually sufficient to evaluate these injuries. In type 1 lesions there is minimal displacement of the fracture of the neck of the talus (Fig. 27–10). The fracture line enters the subtalar joint between the middle and posterior facets. Frequently, a portion of the fracture line enters the body, involving the posterior facet of the subtalar joint or the most anterior portion of the articular cartilage of the talus.

A type 2 lesion is a vertical displaced fracture of the neck of the talus (Fig. 27–11). The subtalar joint is either subluxated or dislocated. The fracture line frequently

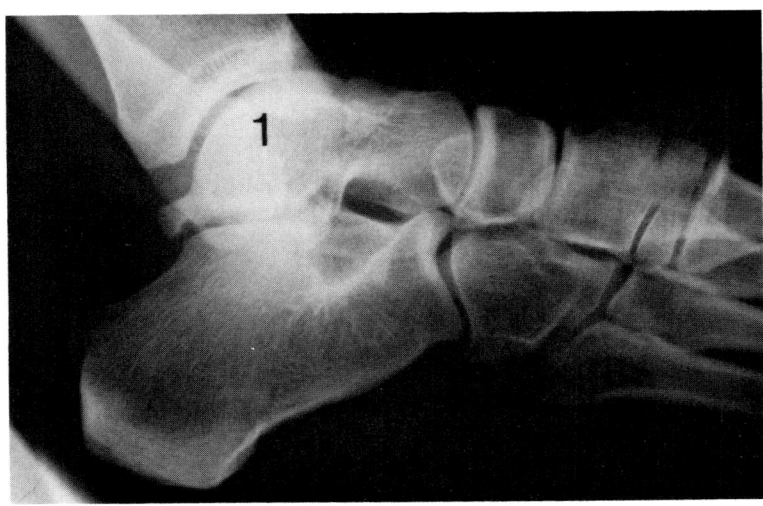

Figure 27–10 A type 1 fracture of the neck of the talus. (Courtesy of S. T. Canale.)

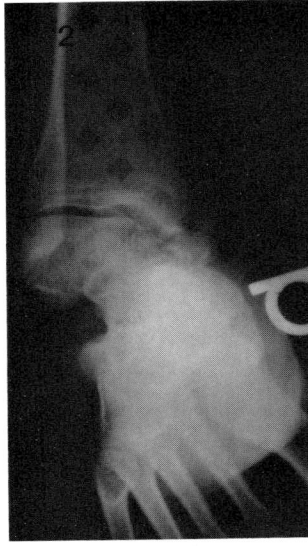 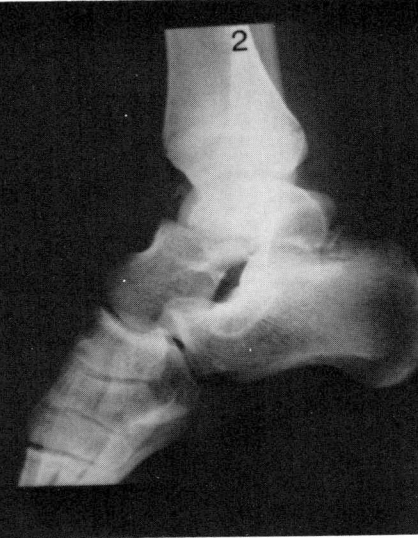

Figure 27-11 A type 2 fracture of the neck of the talus. (Courtesy of S. T. Canale.)

enters a portion of the body and posterior facet of the talus. The head of the talus usually maintains a normal relationship to the navicular and the anterior facet of the subtalar joint.

In a type 3 lesion there is displacement of the vertical fracture of the neck of the talus, and the body of the talus is dislocated from both the ankle and the subtalar joints (Fig. 27-12). The talar body is frequently displaced posteriorly and medially and is finally positioned between the posterior surface of the tibia and the Achilles tendon.

Another frequent deformity is the one that occurs when the body of the talus rotates within the ankle mortise. It may then become wedged in varying positions between the tibia and calcaneus. In this injury the head of the talus is situated normally in relationship to the navicular.

In type 4 lesions the fracture of the neck of the talus is associated both with dislocation of the body from the ankle or subtalar joint and with an additional dislocation or subluxation of the head of the talus from the talonavicular joint (Fig. 27-13).

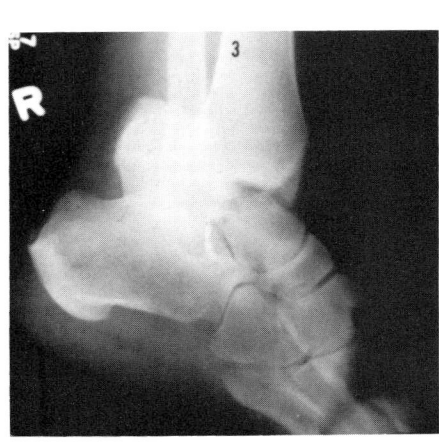 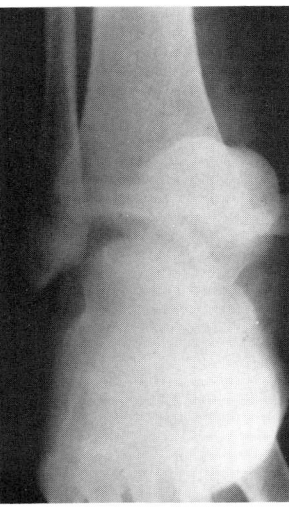

Figure 27-12 A type 3 fracture of the neck of the talus. (Courtesy of S. T. Canale.)

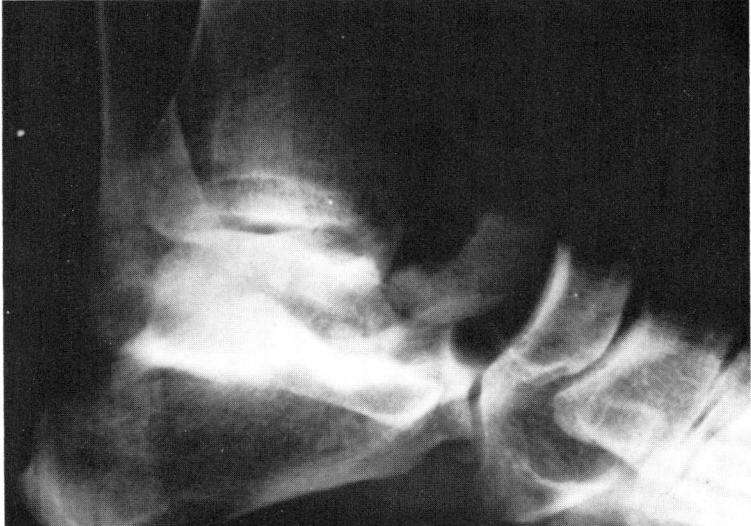

Figure 27–13 A type 4 fracture of the neck of the talus. (Courtesy of S. T. Canale and F. B. Kelly and *Journal of Bone and Joint Surgery.* J. Bone Joint Surg., *60A:*143–156, 1978.)

Treatment

Type 1 lesions are managed with the application of a non–weight-bearing, below-knee cast for 12 weeks (Fig. 27–14). The patient is then removed from the cast, but kept non–weight-bearing for an additional eight weeks. Active range-of-motion exercises for the ankle are encouraged during this time.

Type 2 lesions are treated with a closed reduction and application of a below-knee, non–weight-bearing cast. Open reduction and internal fixation are performed under two specific circumstances: (1) if an attempted closed reduction does not result in satisfactory apposition of the fracture fragments; and (2) if an initial closed reduction is satisfactory but follow-up roentgeno-

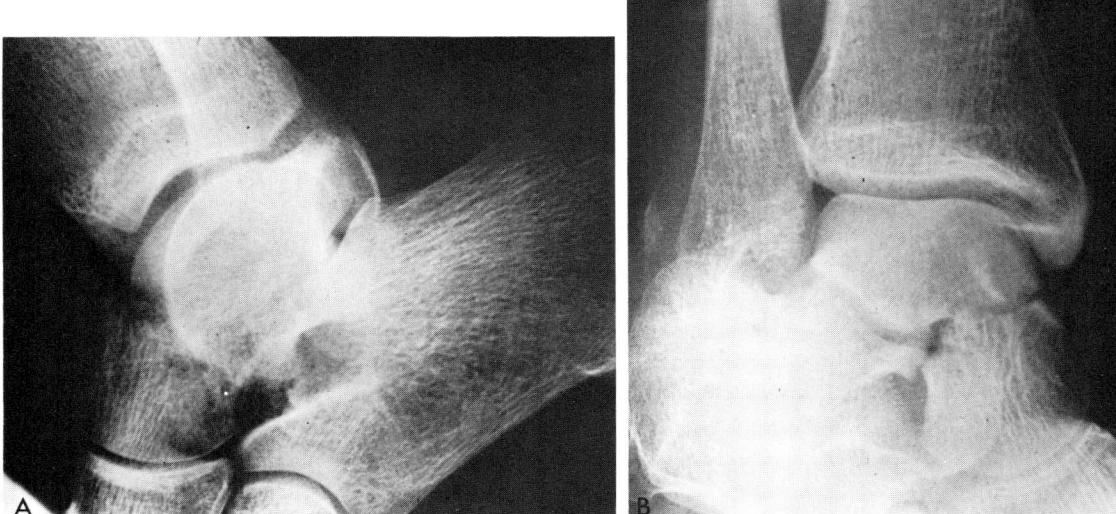

Figure 27–14 *A.* A lateral view of a type 1 fracture of the neck of the talus. *B.* An oblique view demonstrating the nondisplaced fracture of the neck of the talus. Treated with application of a non–weight-bearing cast for 12 weeks.

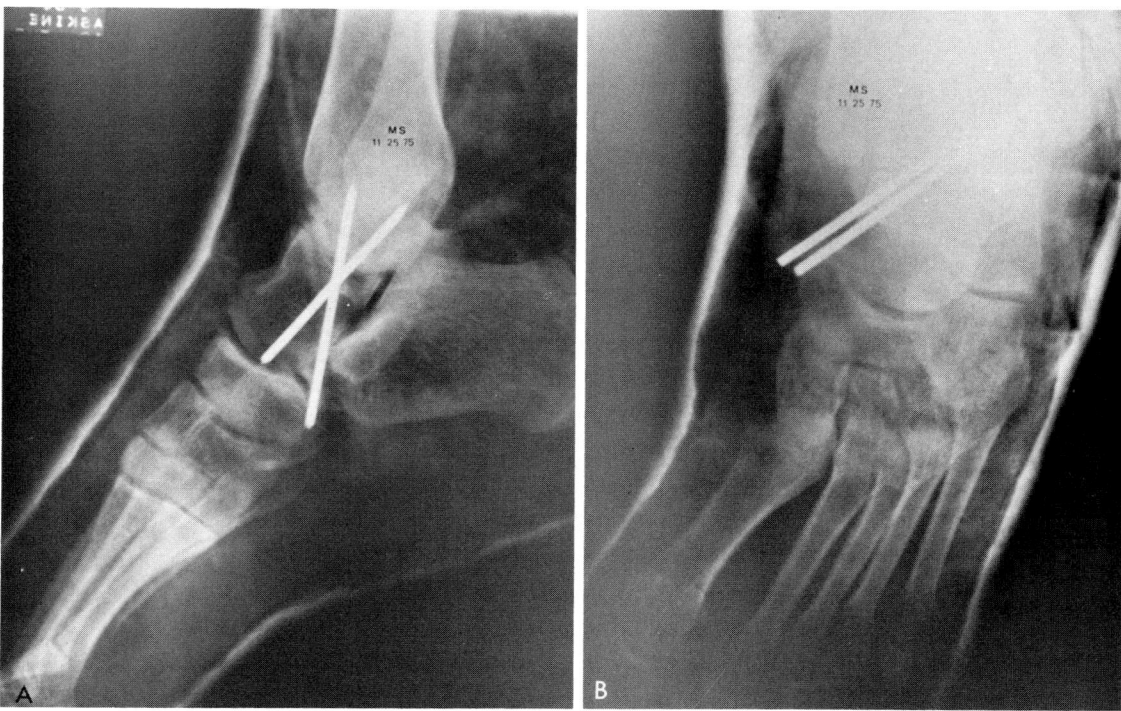

Figure 27–15   A. A type 2 fracture of the neck of the talus that required an open reduction and internal fixation with the use of two threaded pins. B. An anteroposterior view of the foot demonstrating the adequate reduction of this fracture.

graphic evaluation shows the reduction has not been maintained (Fig. 27–15). The open reduction is usually performed through an anteromedial incision, which allows excellent visualization of the medial and superior aspects of the neck of the talus. Internal fixation may be accomplished by inserting two Steinmann pins in a proximal direction across the navicular, through the head of the talus, across the fracture site, and into the body of the talus. An alternative form of fixation may be accomplished with the use of a lag compression screw. This has the added advantage of applying active compression across the fracture site proper. The internal fixation device is removed after 12 to 16 weeks, depending on roentgenographic evidence of healing.

Type 3 lesions are all managed with open reduction and internal fixation. It is important to achieve an appropriate reduction of the displaced body of the talus into the ankle mortise. If this is difficult, an osteotomy of the medial malleolus may facilitate the reduction of the body of the talus. The osteotomy may then be repaired with the

use of a lag compression screw. Internal fixation of the talar neck fracture may be accomplished with the use of Steinmann pins or a lag compression screw. A below-knee, non–weight-bearing cast is applied for 12 to 16 weeks. As will be discussed, the incidence of avascular necrosis is very high in this fracture.

The management of type 4 lesions is extremely difficult, as outlined by Canale and Kelly. All three of their type 4 lesions were open fractures. These injuries should probably be treated with aggressive irrigation and debridement of the wound followed by open reduction and internal fixation. In any event, the patient should be informed that results with this injury are not good and that secondary procedures are frequently necessary.

Open Fractures

These injuries require an aggressive course of operative management. This includes thorough irrigation and debridement, as outlined in Chapter 30. Whether or not to close the wound following irrigation and debridement is still slightly controversial. The author believes these wounds are best managed by open packing with Betadine-soaked sponges, followed by inspection of the wound in the operating room three to four days later. If there is no evidence of infection at that time, internal fixation of the fracture of the talar neck may be performed, followed by closure of the wound. However, if the wound does not appear to be viable enough for a secondary closure, packing with Betadine-soaked sponges is repeated. The patient is brought back to the operating room after three to four days for reinspection of the wound. Secondary closure is accomplished at this time if the tissue appears viable and has no evidence of infection.

Complications

The main complications of fractures of the neck of the talus are the following: (1) avascular necrosis of the talus; (2) arthritis of the ankle or subtalar joints; (3) malunion; and (4) infection.

Avascular Necrosis. This complication is uncommon in type 1 lesions. In both Hawkins'[32] and Kleiger's[39] series, there was no evidence of avascular necrosis with this injury. However, Canale and Kelly's series showed a 13 per cent incidence of avascular necrosis in type 1 lesions.[13]

Type 2 lesions have significant associated avascular necrosis (Fig. 27–16). In Hawkins' series there was a 42 per cent incidence, and in Canale and Kelly's series a 50 per cent incidence. This results from the fact that two and possibly all three sources of blood supply to the body of the talus are jeopardized.

Type 3 injuries are associated with an exceedingly high rate of avascular necrosis: In Hawkins' series it was 91 per cent, and in Canale and Kelly's series 84 per cent. All three sources of blood supply to the talus are compromised in this injury, and avascular necrosis of the talus is to be expected (Fig. 27–17).

In type 4 lesions, Canale and Kelly noted that one of their two fractures not treated by primary talectomy resulted in avascular necrosis. This is too small a series to be

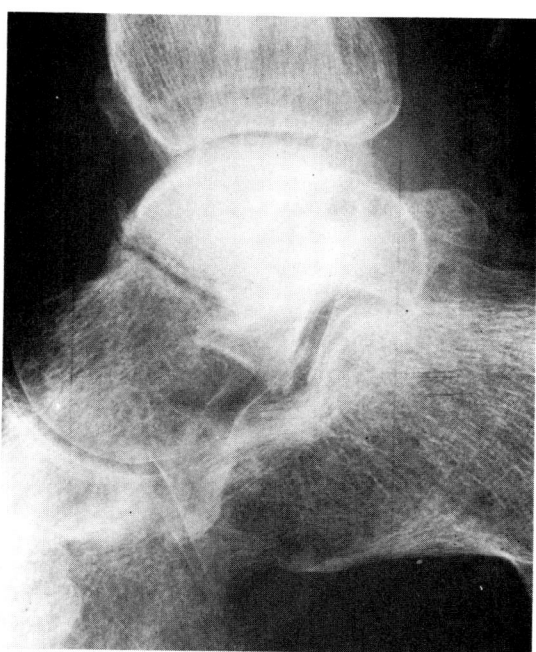

Figure 27–16 A type 2 fracture of the neck of the talus that was treated by closed reduction resulting in avascular necrosis of the body of the talus.

statistically significant, but a high incidence of avascular necrosis can be anticipated.

In an attempt to predict whether avascular necrosis of the talus would develop in the future, Hawkins described a specific diagnostic sign.[32] He stated that if a subchondral radiolucency was visible in the body of the talus six to eight weeks following fracture, the patient was unlikely to develop avascular necrosis. He claimed this finding is indicative of disuse osteopenia and vascular congestion, suggesting continuity of the blood supply and evidence of vascularity of the body of the talus. Its presence is a reliable indication that avascular necrosis will not occur in the future. If it does develop, then non-weight bearing for a prolonged period or partial weight bearing with the use of a patellar tendon-bearing device is probably the best form of initial treatment. As in other areas of the body, bone grafting procedures for avascular necrosis with collapse are probably not indicated.

If a secondary procedure is required for the management of avascular necrosis because of persistent pain, tibial calcaneal fusion or a Blair ankle fusion is probably the

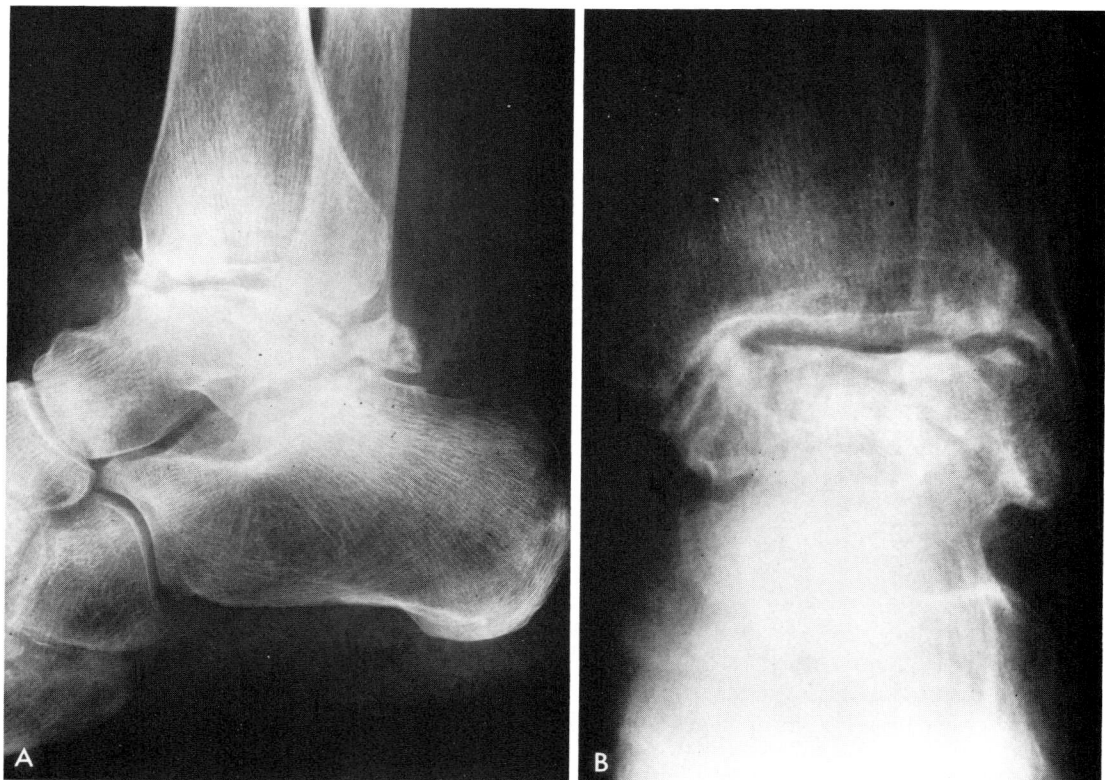

Figure 27–17   *A.* A lateral view of a type 3 fracture that was treated with appropriate reduction resulting in avascular necrosis of the body of the talus. *B.* An anteroposterior view of the same patient demonstrating avascular necrosis of the body of the talus. Note the lack of a subchondral radiolucency, as outlined by Hawkins.

most satisfactory. Talectomy is of questionable benefit.

Malunion. This complication occurs most frequently in the management of type 2 and type 3 lesions. The type of malunion that develops is usually a dorsal or varus malposition. Dorsal malunion can be managed with simple dorsal beak resection from the talar neck, which produces very satisfactory results. Varus malunion will frequently lead to degenerative changes of the subtalar joint. This condition may be appropriately managed with a triple arthrodesis.

Traumatic Arthritis of the Ankle and Subtalar Joints. The most common cause of traumatic arthritis of the ankle joint is a previous dislocation of the body of the talus with or without an associated malleolar fracture. Arthritis of the subtalar joint is frequently seen with malunion of the talar neck fracture. If there is no evidence of sig-

nificant arthritis of the subtalar joint, the appropriate treatment for traumatic arthritis of the ankle joint is an ankle fusion. Likewise, patients with traumatic arthritis of the subtalar joint without significant arthritis of the ankle joint will benefit from a subtalar or triple arthrodesis. A more difficult diagnostic problem is the patient who presents with degenerative arthritis of both the ankle and the subtalar joints. With these conditions, a fusion of one of the involved joints will place additional stress on the other joint, frequently causing great pain. If there is significant avascular necrosis of the talus, the appropriate treatment is a tibial calcaneal fusion; if not, a pantalar arthrodesis may be indicated.

Infection. An established osteomyelitis of the talus may be extremely difficult to manage, as demonstrated by McKeever.[44] This is because the talus is composed almost entirely of cancellous bone, and a fracture through the neck of the talus may interfere with the blood supply, compounding the problem. Under these conditions it is probably best to excise the involved portion of the talus and attempt an arthrodesis.

FRACTURES OF THE BODY OF THE TALUS

These fractures usually result from forced dorsiflexion of the foot associated with axial loading and are often produced by a fall from a height. As the individual strikes the ground, axial loading of the distal tibia and talus is compounded by forced dorsiflexion of the talus. Significant stress is applied to the body of the talus to produce a fracture. This injury is not as common as a fracture of the neck of the talus.

Physical Examination

The patient presents with marked swelling about the ankle. Any attempt at motion of the ankle joint elicits pain, and the patient is unable to bear any weight without considerable discomfort.

A careful examination of the lumbar spine is necessary with this injury. Since it is frequently associated with a fall from a height with axial loading, there may be an associated fracture of the thoracolumbar spine, which could be overlooked.

Roentgenographic Examination

Routine anteroposterior and lateral roentgenograms usually delineate the extent of the injury. One of three fracture patterns is likely to be seen. The first is an undisplaced linear fracture of the body of the talus; the second, a displaced linear fracture of the body of the talus; and the third, a comminuted fracture of the body of the talus.

Treatment

Simple undisplaced fractures of the body of the talus may be managed in a below-knee, non–weight-bearing cast for eight weeks. In displaced fractures, a closed reduction should be attempted initially. However, since this is usually unsuccessful,

an open reduction with internal fixation is usually necessary. Open reduction is accomplished through a medial incision. An osteotomy of the medial malleolus is frequently required to obtain adequate exposure of the body of the talus. A lag compression screw or two Steinmann pins may be used for internal fixation. The osteotomy of the medial malleolus is repaired with a lag compression screw. The extremity is then placed in a long leg, non–weight-bearing cast. The long leg cast is maintained in position for six weeks and then converted to a short leg cast. At the end of 12 weeks the patient is returned to the operating room, and the internal fixation device is removed. Roentgenograms are taken at this time. If the fracture has healed without evidence of avascular necrosis, the patient is started on partial weight bearing, gradually progressing to full weight bearing. If Hawkins' radiolucent sign is present in the talus, the patient is maintained non–weight bearing for an additional four to six weeks.

If severe avascular necrosis of the talus develops, a tibial calcaneal fusion, a Blair fusion, or a pantalar arthrodesis may be performed. Comminuted fractures of the body of the talus have a higher incidence of avascular necrosis. These patients are treated with a posterior plaster splint and elevation of the involved extremity for four to six weeks. At the end of that time, when the swelling has decreased, a pantalar arthrodesis or a tibial calcaneal fusion may be performed.

FRACTURES OF THE HEAD OF THE TALUS

Fractures of the talar head are less common than fractures of the talar body, which in turn are less common than fractures of the talar neck. These injuries are produced by a fall from a height on the hyperextended foot.

Physical Examination

There is usually swelling of the ankle joint, principally over the talonavicular joint. Motion of the ankle joint is surprisingly well preserved, but is painful at the extremes. There is tenderness to direct palpation over the head of the talus and the talonavicular joint.

Roentgenographic Examination

Routine anteroposterior and lateral roentgenograms of the foot usually demonstrate the fracture. Comminution is frequently present, but significant displacement is rare. Oblique views of the foot may further delineate the fracture if routine roentgenograms are questionable.

Treatment

A posterior plaster slab is appropriate for immobilization of the foot and ankle. The extremity is then elevated to reduce the swelling. At one week, the swelling has usually diminished enough for a long leg, non–weight-bearing cast to be applied. The patient is maintained non–weight bearing for four weeks, when the cast is converted to a weight-bearing cast for an additional four weeks. At the end of that time the fracture has usually healed.

CHIP AND AVULSION FRACTURES OF THE TALUS

These fractures tend to occur primarily in four locations—the superior surface of the neck and the lateral, medial, and posterior aspects of the body.

The mechanism of injury in fractures of the superior surface of the neck is a longitudinal compression force combined with acute plantar flexion (Fig. 27–18). If the fragment is large and displaced, the appropriate treatment is surgical excision. A small fragment can be treated conservatively.

Fractures of the lateral process of the talus are particularly important. Hawkins[31] and Mukherjee and co-workers[49] each collected a series of 13 cases.

The lateral process has both articular and nonarticular surfaces, and a fracture of the lateral process will therefore involve the posterior subtalar joint. The mechanism of injury is compression of the lateral process with the foot in inversion and dorsiflexion. A useful physical finding is local tenderness over the lateral process just below the tip of the lateral malleolus. The fracture involves the lateral aspect of the articular surface of the posteroinferior portion of the talus and is usually comminuted or displaced. The significance of this fracture is that an irregularity or a loose body in this area may predispose to arthritic changes in the subtalar joint. The large single fracture fragment should be openly reduced in order to maintain congruity of the surfaces of the subtalar joint and should be maintained in position with a small Kirschner wire. Small or comminuted fragments are best treated by operative excision.

Avulsion fractures may occur on the

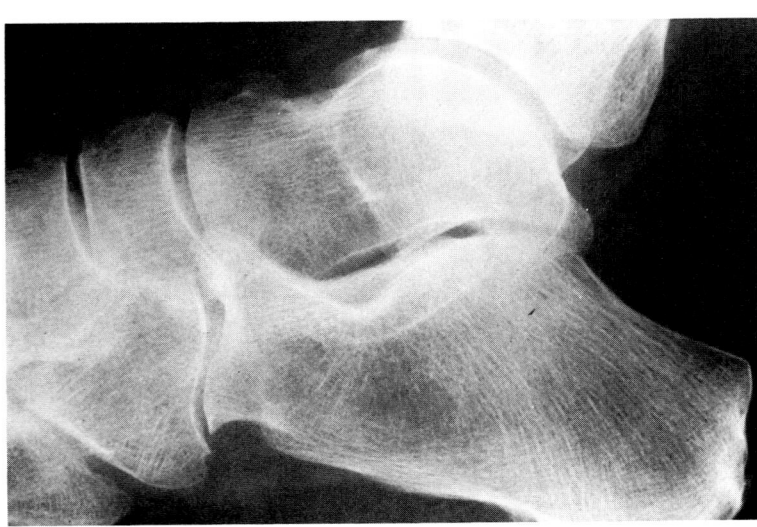

Figure 27–18 A lateral view of a chip fracture from the dorsal aspect of the talus.

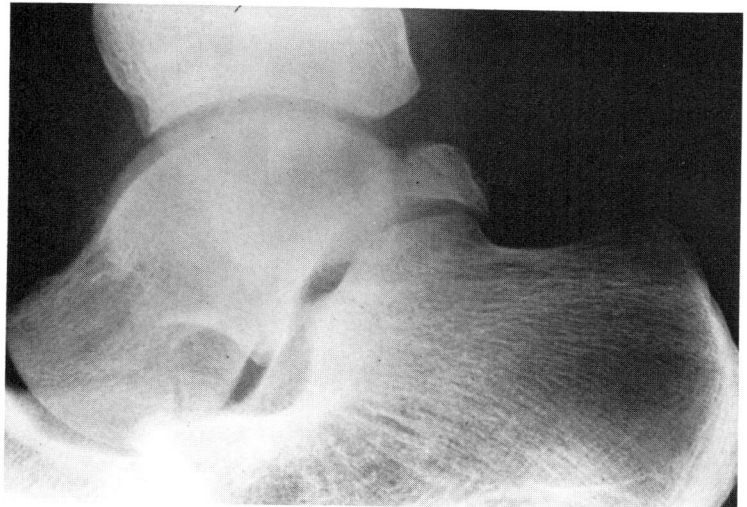

Figure 27–19 A fracture of the posterior tubercle of the talus. The patient experienced exquisite tenderness in this area following the injury.

medial aspect of the body of the talus. The deep fibers of the deltoid ligament are attached just below and behind the tip of the medial malleolus; stress on these fibers may result in an avulsion fracture. If the fragment is large, the fracture line may extend posteriorly to involve the medial portion of the groove for the flexor hallucis longus tendon. If significant displacement is present, operative excision is the treatment of choice. An important point in operative excision is to avoid injury to the small but important arteries that supply blood to the body of the talus and enter the medial surface of the talus deep to the deltoid ligament.

The posterior tubercle of the talus is also vulnerable to injury. The usual mechanism is a severe plantar flexion force, which wedges the posterior aspect of the talus between the tibia and the os calcis, fracturing the posterior tubercle. It is important to distinguish this injury from an accessory bone, the os trigonum, which also may be found in this location (Figs. 27–19 and 27–20). A fracture line is usually irregular, whereas an os trigonum has smooth outline. Significant disability may result from this

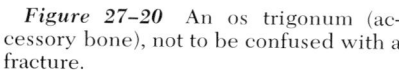

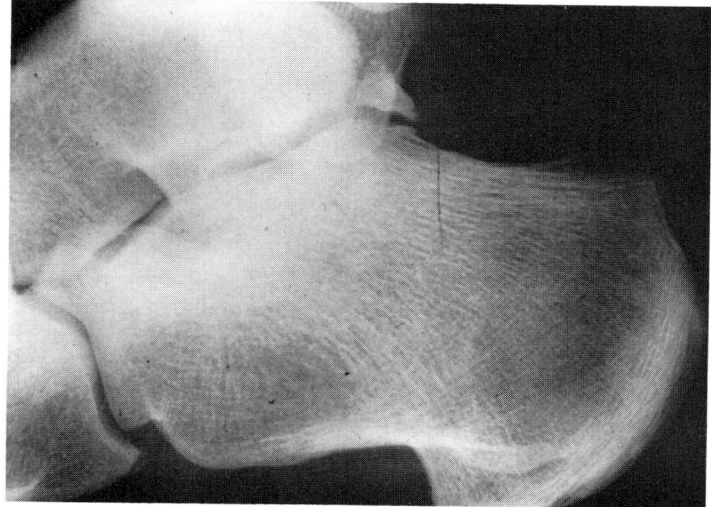

Figure 27–20 An os trigonum (accessory bone), not to be confused with a fracture.

injury, because the fracture line may involve both the subtalar joint and the groove for the flexor hallucis longus tendon. Initial treatment includes a short leg walking cast for six weeks. At the end of that time, if pain has not been relieved by conservative measures, operative excision is indicated. The fragment may be approached through a posterolateral incision which displaces the peronei forward.

DISLOCATIONS OF THE TALUS

TOTAL DISLOCATION

Fortunately, this is a relatively rare injury. The mechanism of injury is believed to be forced plantar flexion of the foot associated with a compression force, which causes the talus to be literally "popped out" of the ankle joint. There is complete disruption of the capsular and ligamentous structures. The talus assumes an anterior and lateral position out of the ankle mortise, so that it rests under the skin in front of the ankle. Since considerable force is required to produce the injury, many of these dislocations are open. Frequently the talus extrudes through the anterior wound.

Physical Examination

Examination of the foot and ankle reveals gross swelling along the anterolateral aspect of the ankle. The talus may be palpated in an anterolateral position just under the skin. The remainder of the forefoot and the midfoot lie in a medial position. As stated, many of these dislocations are open, and the talus may be frankly extruded through the wound.

Roentgenographic Examination

Routine anteroposterior and lateral views of the foot and ankle show the talus to be dislocated out of the ankle mortise in an anterolateral position and the calcaneus to have settled upward into the medial and lateral malleolar region. If the talus has been completely extruded, the superior border of the calcaneus will be seen to abut the malleoli. There may or may not be associated fractures of the malleoli.

Treatment

This is a very serious injury indeed and requires immediate treatment. If the talus is dislocated without a break in the integrity of the skin, a large Kirschner wire should be inserted through the calcaneus and a traction bow applied to this device. An effort is then made to distract the calcaneus away from the malleoli. Longitudinal traction is applied through the traction bow, while countertraction is applied to the leg with the knee in the flexed position. Once the calcaneus has been distracted away from the malleoli, the surgeon exerts direct pressure on the talus in an attempt to force it back into the ankle mortise. If reduction is not possible with this maneuver, immediate open reduction is indicated. The talus is exposed through an anterior incision, and traction is applied to the calcaneus. The talus is then pushed in backward to sit in the ankle mortise. Following reduction the extremity is placed in a long leg cast for four to six weeks. At the end of this time the cast is removed, and the patient begins range-of-motion exercises of the foot and ankle. Once satisfactory motion is obtained, usually at the end of two more weeks, the patient is allowed to begin weight bearing.

A great danger in the management of these cases is the ever-present risk of infection. Detenbeck and Kelly reported a series[21] in which eight of nine patients developed infection following open reduction. There is no apparent explanation for the high incidence of infection in this injury.

A patient presenting with an open dislocation with the talus extruded from the wound is managed in a standard fashion, as outlined in Chapter 30. Once the wound has healed without evidence of infection, a tibial calcaneal fusion should be considered.

ISOLATED SUBTALAR DISLOCATIONS

Subtalar dislocations produce a gross deformity of the foot. Medial subtalar dislocations are more common by far than lateral subtalar dislocations. Interestingly, with medial subtalar dislocations there may be no evidence of an associated fracture. However, with lateral subtalar dislocations, a fracture of the lateral malleolus is often present. Buckingham found that with medial subtalar dislocations the head of the talus is prominent laterally, appearing between the extensor hallucis longus and the extensor digitorum longus tendons.[12] In a

lateral subtalar dislocation the head of the talus is in a medial position.

Mechanism of Injury

The most common cause of subtalar dislocations is a fall from a height or an automobile accident. However, significant force is not necessary to produce this injury. Medial subtalar dislocation is produced by a combination of flexion and inversion of the

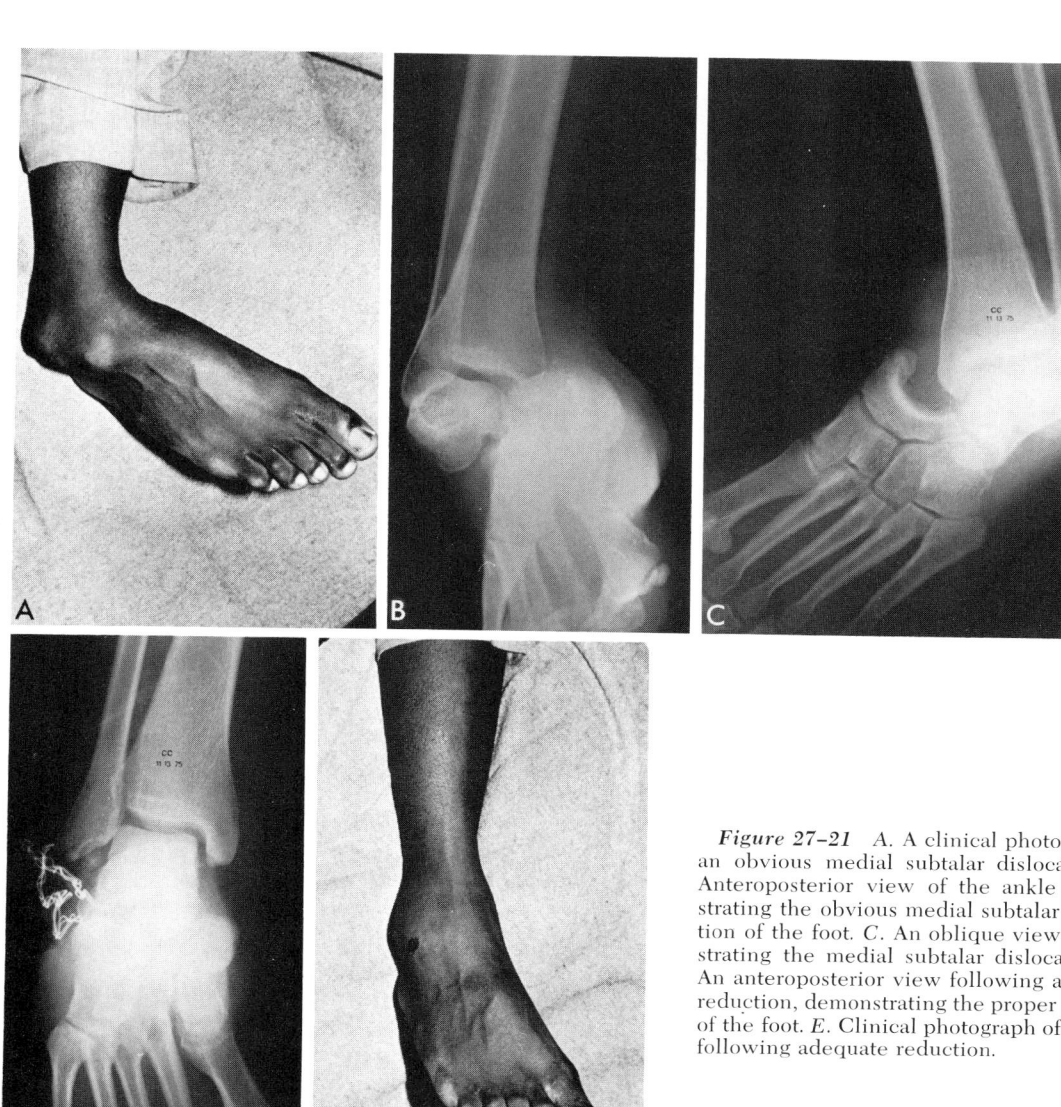

Figure 27–21   *A.* A clinical photograph of an obvious medial subtalar dislocation. *B.* Anteroposterior view of the ankle demonstrating the obvious medial subtalar dislocation of the foot. *C.* An oblique view demonstrating the medial subtalar dislocation. *D.* An anteroposterior view following adequate reduction, demonstrating the proper position of the foot. *E.* Clinical photograph of the foot following adequate reduction.

foot. Lateral subtalar dislocation is produced by a combination of flexion and eversion of the foot.

Physical Examination

The deformity produced by a subtalar dislocation is quite obvious (Fig. 27–21). With a medial subtalar dislocation, the entire forefoot is resting in a medial position and the talus is palpable laterally. Significant swelling is present, and any attempt at motion of the ankle or subtalar joints causes discomfort.

In lateral subtalar dislocation, the forefoot is in a lateral position and the talus is located medially. Considerable swelling is present, and frequently there is an associated fracture of the lateral malleolus. The majority of these injuries are closed, and the skin is noted to be tented over the talus.

Roentgenographic Examination

Standard anteroposterior and lateral views of the foot and ankle usually reveal the subtalar dislocation. Oblique views may be necessary to determine whether an associated fracture is present. As stated, medial dislocations frequently present without an associated fracture. Roentgenograms show the talus to be normally positioned within the ankle mortise. The midfoot and forefoot are situated medially in relation to the talus, and the navicular is located dorsally, behind the head of the talus.

In lateral subtalar dislocations the entire midfoot and forefoot are in a lateral position, and the talus is located normally within the ankle mortise. Frequently there is an associated fracture of the distal fibula.

Treatment

The majority of these injuries can be reduced in the emergency room under intravenous or intramuscular analgesics. The medial subtalar dislocation may be reduced by flexion and slight adduction of the foot. This is followed by gentle traction and abduction of the midfoot and forefoot to accomplish reduction of the talonavicular joint. A lateral dislocation is reduced by applying an adduction force to the midfoot

and forefoot. If there is resistance to the reduction, it should not be forced. The patient should be taken to the operating room and given a general anesthetic. Occasionally, a closed reduction is not possible. Buckingham described an osteochondral separation of both the talus and the navicular as an obstacle to reduction.[12] If open reduction is necessary in this case, a lateral incision is useful. The reduction may then be accomplished by unlocking the osteochondral separation and swinging the forefoot into appropriate position. A below-knee cast is applied postoperatively, and weight bearing is delayed for four weeks. At the end of that time, full weight bearing is allowed, but the cast is maintained for an additional two weeks. After six weeks the cast is removed, and range-of-motion exercises of the ankle and midfoot are encouraged. If there is an associated fracture of the distal fibula, particularly in a lateral subtalar dislocation, the cast may have to be maintained for six to eight weeks until there is sufficient healing of the fibular fracture to allow weight bearing without plaster.

The results are excellent in follow-up care of these injuries. The only important problem that may occur is degenerative arthritis of the subtalar joint. Avascular necrosis of the talus is rare. If significant degenerative arthritis of the subtalar joint develops in long-term follow-up, it is managed with a subtalar or triple arthrodesis.

FRACTURE OF THE CALCANEUS

This injury is frequently encountered in clinical practice. In spite of the fact that this is the most common type of tarsal bone fracture, there is considerable debate in regard to its proper management. All age groups are affected by this very difficult fracture. The pendulum of treatment appears to swing back and forth between conservative and operative management. It is probably fair to state that most fractures of the calcaneus can be managed nonoperatively. The majority of long-term follow-up for both conservative and operative treatment reveals that 30 per cent or greater of these injuries result in pain and disability. The financial impact on industry is substantial. Most discussion regarding long-term disability centers on injury to the subtalar joint. Although deformity of the subtalar joint due to intraarticular calcaneal fractures leads to disability in a high percentage of cases, damage to other important structures is equally critical.

CLASSIFICATION OF CALCANEAL FRACTURES

It is important for the physician to have a thorough understanding of the various types of calcaneal fractures in order to plan appropriate treatment. In general, these fractures are either extraarticular or intraarticular. In the intraarticular type, the fracture line extends into the subtalar joint. Extraarticular fractures do not involve the subtalar joint and therefore have a much higher percentage of good results. Most studies of fractures of the calcaneus refer to either the Essex-Lopresti[24] or the Rowe[56] classification. The author prefers the classification of Rowe and co-workers,[56] which describes five specific types of calcaneal fracture (Fig. 27–22).

Type 1 fractures are those of relatively minor consequence. They have been subdivided as follows:

    a. Fractures of the tuberosity.
    b. Fractures of the sustentaculum tali.
    c. Fractures of the anterior process.

Type 2 fractures have been grouped as follows:

    a. Fractures of the beak of the calcaneus.
    b. Avulsion fractures of the insertion of the Achilles tendon.

It is important to differentiate the specific type, as the treatment program may differ.

Type 3 fractures are oblique fractures that extend down through the body of the calcaneus but do not involve the subtalar joint or the articular facets.

Types 4 and 5 are intraarticular fractures; these account for greater than 50 per cent of all fractures of the calcaneus. Type 4

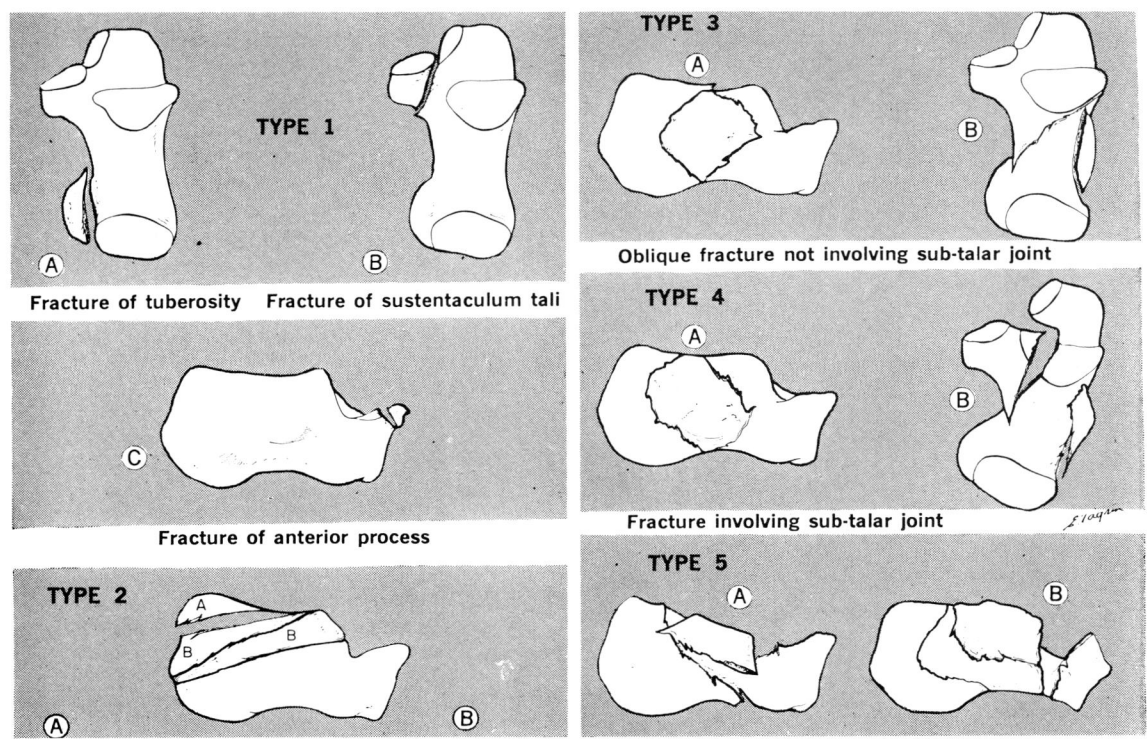

Figure 27–22 The Rowe classification of fractures of the calcaneus. (Courtesy of C. R. Rowe et al. and *Journal of the American Medical Association*. JAMA, *184*:920–923, 1963.)

involves the subtalar joint. The fracture line extends across the subtalar joint, separating the calcaneus into two or three primary portions that demonstrate various degrees of displacement. These injuries are very difficult to manage.

Type 5 intraarticular fractures involve the subtalar joint and result in a central depression fracture with comminution. These are subdivided into two specific types. In the first, the entire posterior articular surface is displaced in one piece; this is referred to as central depression. In the other, the entire articular surface may be fractured into several small fragments that may have lost their primary relationship with the talus.

MECHANISM OF INJURY

This fracture is the result of acute axial loading of the calcaneus. It is produced by falling from a height, landing directly on the heel of the foot. In fact, this has been referred to as lover's heels, as it may result from a hasty escape through a second-story window when approaching footsteps are heard.[15]

However, the majority of these injuries occur in industrial accidents when a worker falls from a height. As illustrated by Harty, the calcaneus has a very thin cortical shell enclosing a pattern of cancellous bone that reflects the static and dynamic strains to which it is repeatedly exposed (Fig. 27–23).[30] Traction trabeculae radiate from the inferior cortex, and pressure lamellae con-

verge to support the posterior and anterior articular facets, resulting in a neutral triangle of sparse trabeculae. A fine network of vessels traverses the neutral triangle approaching the medullary cavity. Therefore, the neutral triangle is a common site of fracture, as it lacks the support of a surrounding osseous structure. An intraarticular type of fracture with axial loading of the heel results.

It is the author's impression that too much emphasis has been placed on disruption of the subtalar joint as the cause of continued pain and disability with calcaneal fractures. Again, it is extremely important to realize that associated structures are also damaged owing to the amount of force required to produce this injury. The calcaneus may "spread" as a consequence, encroaching upon the peroneal tendons and possibly causing a secondary tenosynovitis.

The fat pad of the heel is very significant in this injury. The fatty elements are contained within septa, and when the injury occurs there is disruption of the septa with secondary changes in the fatty tissue and eventual scar formation. This is a very important but frequently overlooked source of pain and disability in follow-up.

Although the major impact force is absorbed by the calcaneus, with resultant fracture, there is no doubt that some force is transmitted to the ankle joint proper. It is possible that the articular surface of the ankle joint sustains compression injury which may result in arthritic symptoms. An associated fracture of the spine may also occur. Rowe and co-workers[56] and Lance and associates[41] have both demonstrated that approximately 10 per cent of these injuries have related spinal injury.

ROENTGENOGRAPHIC EXAMINATION

Lateral, oblique, and axial views are helpful in delineating calcaneal fractures. Occasionally, a special view, such as that described by Anthonsen,[3] may be useful in evaluation. In the lateral view the Böhler tuber-joint angle is demonstrated. As illustrated in Figure 27–24, this is the angle formed by drawing a line through the anterior and posterior facets. A second line is then drawn along the axis of the superior

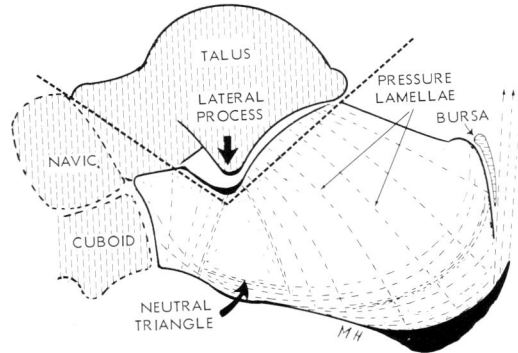

Figure 27–23 The crucial angle of the calcaneus indicated by the lateral process of the talus. Note the neutral triangle. Also note the direction of the pressure lamellae. (Courtesy of M. Harty and *Orthopedic Clinics of North America.* Orthop. Clin. North Am., 4:182, 1973.)

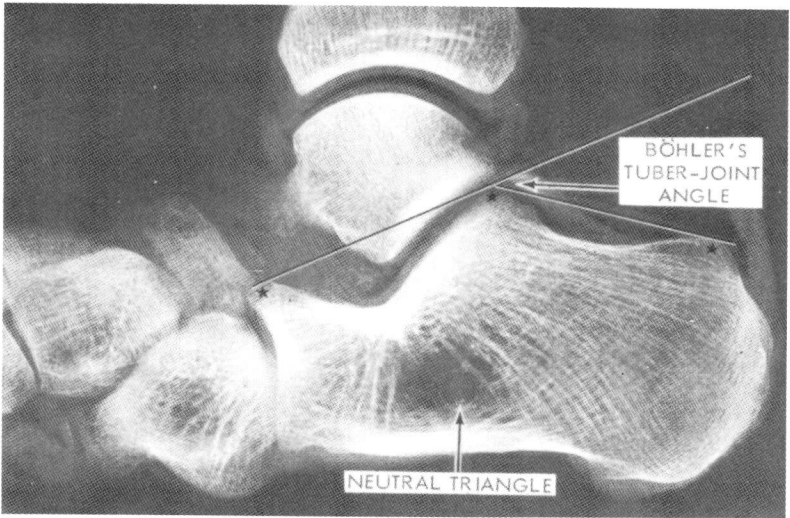

Figure 27–24 Böhler's tuber-joint angle. (Courtesy of M. Harty and *Orthopedic Clinics of North America*. Orthop. Clin. North Am., 4:180, 1973.)

cortex of the body. The angle formed by the intersection of these two lines is referred to as Böhler's angle. This normally measures between 25 and 40 degrees. If there has been significant collapse of the intraarticular portion of the subtalar joint, this angle will be decreased. In the past, great emphasis was placed on this angle. If the angle was severely decreased, it was thought that the fragments had to be operatively manipulated into position in order to reconstitute it. However, today most authors do not place as much emphasis on Böhler's angle in the management of this injury.

It is also customary to obtain anteroposterior and lateral roentgenograms of the dorsal lumbar spine in all patients with calcaneal fractures. As stated, the incidence of associated spinal fractures is approximately 10 per cent.

TREATMENT

A great deal of controversy surrounds the management of fractures of the calcaneus. The literature supports both an operative and a nonoperative approach to these injuries. However, it is fair to state that there has been a trend to conservative treatment over the past decade. As stated previously, it is not only the fracture that must be

considered but also the surrounding soft tissue injury, which plays a significant role in pain and disability in follow-up. Together with the resurgence of conservative therapy there is a trend to early functional treatment. This is in keeping with the management of other fractures, as outlined throughout this book. Functional therapy appears to return the individual to full activity at an earlier date and also appears to decrease pain and disability in follow-up.

Type 1A

The majority of tuberosity fractures are relatively nondisplaced. The initial management includes the application of a Jones soft dressing. Ice contained in a plastic bag is applied over the soft dressing for the first 48 hours. Once the swelling has subsided, usually after four to five days, either a new snug Jones dressing or a short leg, weight-bearing cast may be applied. The patient is then ambulated, with instructions to apply 25 per cent of the weight on the injured extremity. This can usually be achieved by the end of one or two weeks. Weight bearing is gradually increased within the limits of pain tolerance. If a soft Jones dressing has been applied, it is maintained in place for 6 to 7 weeks. The advantage of this form of therapy is that the patient may remove the dressing once or twice a week to soak the injured extremity in warm water and begin gradual range-of-motion exercises. If a cast is utilized it will generally have to be changed at the end of the first or second week owing to a decrease in swelling. A new cast is then applied and maintained in position for an additional five to six weeks. By the end of this time the fracture has usually united.

Type 1B

This injury is managed with the use of a Jones soft dressing together with elevation and an ice pack for the first 48 hours. At the end of this time the ice pack may be discontinued. Weight bearing is delayed with this fracture, as it involves the middle facet which is attached to the superior portion of the sustentaculum tali. Fortunately, these fractures are also relatively nondisplaced and usually heal with conservative management. The patient is ambulated with the use of a soft dressing, but is maintained non–weight-bearing and advised to keep the injured extremity elevated when not ambulatory to help reduce swelling. Partial weight bearing is initiated at six to eight weeks postinjury, progressing to

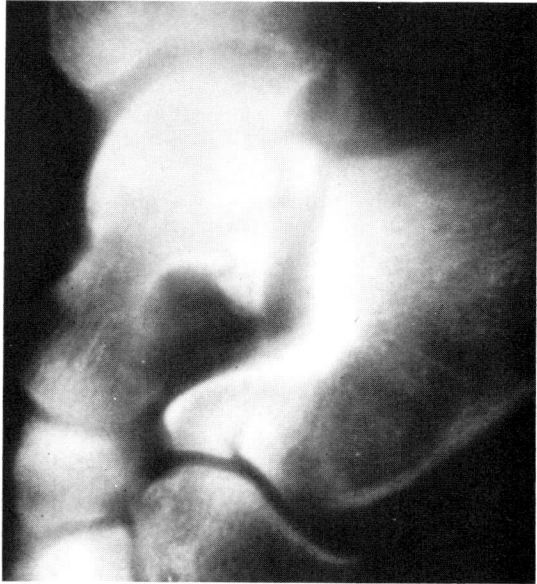

Figure 27–25 Lateral tomogram demonstrating an avulsion fracture of the anterior process of the calcaneus.

full weight bearing over the next two to three weeks. At the end of this time the fracture has usually united, and ambulatory aids may be abandoned. Vigorous activities, such as athletics, are not permitted for an additional four weeks. Nonunion is rare with this injury. If it does develop it may or may not be painful. If it is not particularly painful, no active therapy is required. If, however, a painful nonunion results, simple excision of the fragment will relieve symptoms.

Type 1C

This avulsion fracture of the anterior process may also be managed in a conservative fashion (Fig. 27–25). It is treated with a soft dressing together with elevation and ice packs. The patient is then ambulated with the use of crutches, and early weight bearing is encouraged. Results are good to excellent with this form of therapy, and even if the fracture fragment does not unite, very few symptoms are usually present.

Type 2A

This beak type of fracture can usually be managed conservatively with a closed reduction if it is displaced, followed by application of a short leg cast for six weeks. If there is significant displacement, and the reduction can be maintained only with the foot held in marked equinus, open reduction and internal fixation are indicated. During the six-week period of immobilization in a plaster cast, the patient is maintained in a non–weight-bearing status.

Type 2B

These avulsion fractures of the insertion of the Achilles tendon frequently require open reduction and internal fixation. The fragment is usually displaced in a cephalad direction by the pull of the Achilles tendon. Open reduction and internal fixation are performed through a posterior approach. Internal fixation may be secured with a compression screw or a circlage wire (Fig. 27–26). The author prefers using a compression screw for these injuries. The extremity is then placed in a below-knee, non–weight-bearing cast with the foot

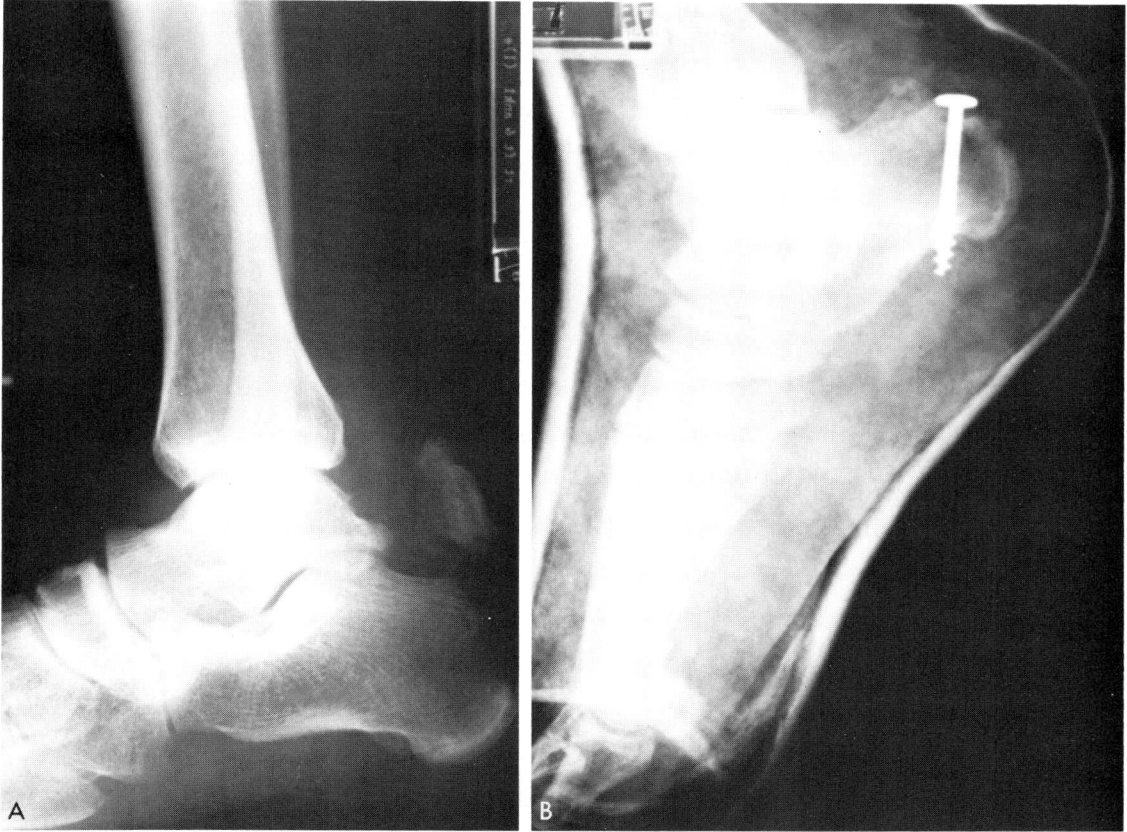

Figure 27–26   *A.* A type 2-B avulsion fracture of the insertion of the Achilles tendon. *B.* Following open reduction and internal fixation with the use of a lag compression screw.

maintained in neutral position for six weeks. At the end of this time, healing is usually sufficient to discard the cast and begin active weight bearing and range-of-motion exercises. Operative treatment of this injury usually produces good to excellent results.

Types 3A and 3B

These oblique fractures through the body of the calcaneus, but not involving the subtalar joint, can usually be managed conservatively. A soft Jones dressing is applied, and elevation and ice packs are prescribed for the first 48 hours. The patient is then encouraged to attempt active ambulation with the injured extremity maintained in a non–weight-bearing status. Weight bearing is not permitted until six to eight weeks postinjury, when healing is usually sufficient to allow partial and then full weight bearing. A short leg, non–weight-bearing plaster cast may also be used in this injury, but the author prefers the soft Jones dressing. Active ankle motion may be initiated within the soft dressing. It also can be easily removed to periodically inspect the skin for bleb formation and to soak the extremity in warm water.

Types 4A and 4B

These intraarticular fractures involve the subtalar joint. A review of the literature will find ample support for both an aggressive open approach and a conservative nonoperative approach. In fact, the results do not appear to be substantially different in the two forms of treatment. Therefore, the author has adopted the policy of managing most of these fractures in a conservative fashion, similar to that outlined by McLaughlin.[45, 46] This includes the application of a soft Jones dressing along with elevation and ice treatment for the first 24 hours. The ice is then discontinued, but the patient is maintained at bed rest with marked elevation of the involved extremity for an additional two to three days. By this time the acute discomfort has gradually decreased. The dressing is then removed, the skin is inspected for blebs, and a new soft Jones dressing is applied. The patient is then allowed to begin to dangle the legs over the side of the bed. Ambulation with the use of crutches, non–weight-bearing on the involved extremity, is usually started seven to eight days postinjury. Once the patient is comfortable on crutches he may be discharged, usually 12 to 14 days postinjury, and then seen in the office one week later. At that time the Jones dressing is removed and replaced with a fresh dressing. The patient is advised to begin partial weight bearing (approximately 25 per cent of the weight) on the involved extremity. This is increased to full weight bearing at

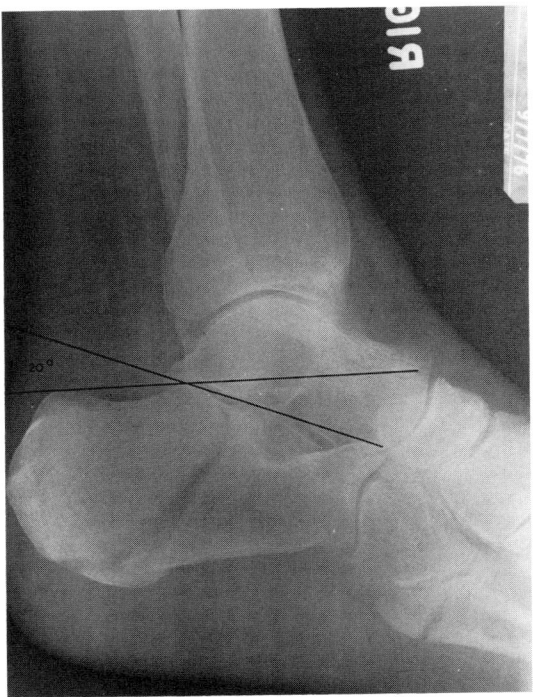

Figure 27–27   A lateral view of an intraarticular fracture involving the subtalar joint. This was managed in a conservative fashion with excellent results. Note the 20 degree tuber-joint angle.

six to eight weeks postinjury. The Jones dressing is removed at that time and replaced with an Ace bandage. The majority of patients are able to return to active employment at three to four months postinjury. It has been the author's impression that the sooner patients are ambulated and encouraged to begin weight bearing, the quicker they seem to recover from the injury (Fig. 27–27). In contrast, many patients who are placed in a non–weight-bearing cast for 12 to 16 weeks seem to end up with a painful stiff foot. Once again, the functional weight-bearing method appears to be advantageous in the management of these fractures. One interesting finding is that many patients with a distorted subtalar joint on follow-up roentgenograms are relatively pain-free at active employment. On the other hand, some patients with radiological evidence of minimal subtalar residual deformity have pain in this area. It is very difficult to predict whether a patient will experience pain on the basis of the follow-up roentgenographic examination.

Operative approaches to this injury have been advocated in the past, and these will be discussed in a separate section.

Types 5A and 5B

These are intraarticular fractures of the central depression type with comminution (Fig. 27–28). They are managed conservatively, in a fashion similar to type 4A and 4B injuries.

ALTERNATIVE TREATMENT FOR INTRAARTICULAR FRACTURES

The treatment programs outlined in the preceding sections are those recommended by the author. However, there certainly are other approaches to these problems and these will be discussed briefly.

Böhler[9] and Hermann[33] have been active enthusiasts for reconstitution of the tuber angle by closed reduction. The Böhler technique involves the insertion of two Steinmann pins, one through the calcaneal tuberosity and the other through the midportion of the tibia. The pins are placed in a transverse fashion to allow for traction and countertraction. Traction is applied through

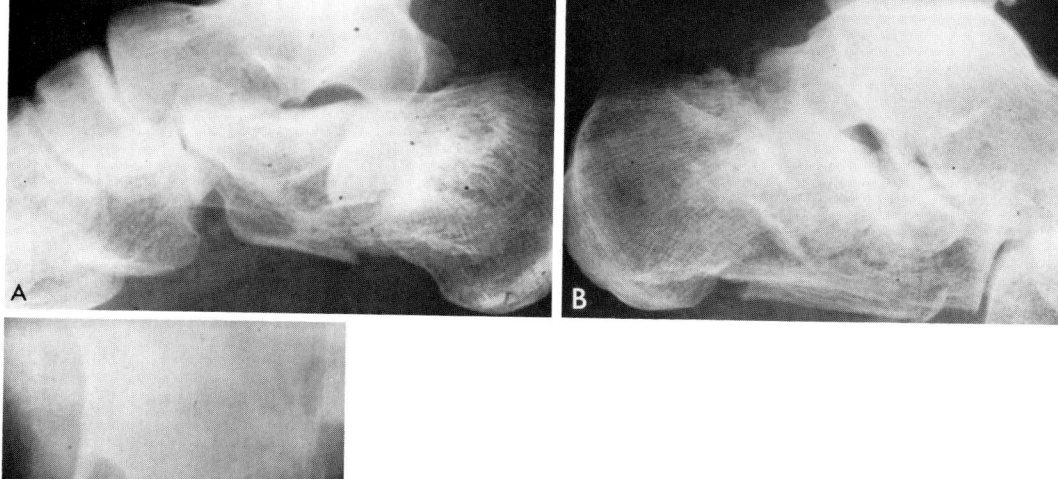

Figure 27-28 *A.* A lateral view of an intraarticular comminuted fracture that was treated in a conservative fashion with excellent results. *B.* A lateral view of the opposite calcaneus reveals a similar comminuted intraarticular fracture that also had a good result with conservative management. *C.* An axial view of one of the calcanei demonstrating the obvious fracture.

the calcaneal pin, with the Böhler clamp inserted around the calcaneus under the lateral and medial malleoli. Direct lateral compression of the calcaneus is achieved by tightening the Böhler clamp (Fig. 27-29) to produce direct lateral compression of the comminuted fragments. The clamp is then removed, and a plaster cast incorporating the pins is applied. Particular attention is given to molding the cast under the malleoli to maintain the lateral compression achieved with the use of the clamp. After four weeks the cast and pins are removed, and a well-molded short leg cast is applied for an additional six weeks. At the end of that time, weight bearing is initiated with the use of a prescribed, specially constructed shoe.

Good results have been reported with this form of therapy. However, in the author's opinion, the heel has suffered an acute injury with gross swelling and edema; to apply a rigid clamp that compresses the already damaged soft tissues in an attempt to mold the fracture fragments appears to

invite problems of skin damage or slough. Consequently, the author has had no particular experience with this form of treatment.

Essex-Lopresti advocates a method of closed reduction with the use of a longitudinally applied Steinmann pin.[24] The reduction is performed with the patient in the prone position as a heavy Steinmann pin is introduced just lateral to the insertion of the Achilles tendon. The pin is then advanced longitudinally into the tongue fragment. The correct positioning of the pin is under the depressed fragment. Manipulation is then performed by applying an upward force on the pin. This will frequently realign the facet fragment into proper position. A calcaneal spread may then be corrected by closed reduction. Once this is accomplished, the pin is placed across the fracture and into the anterior fragment of the calcaneus. This is the usual position for the tongue type of fracture. However, in the joint-depression type of fracture, the pin is inserted into the calcan-

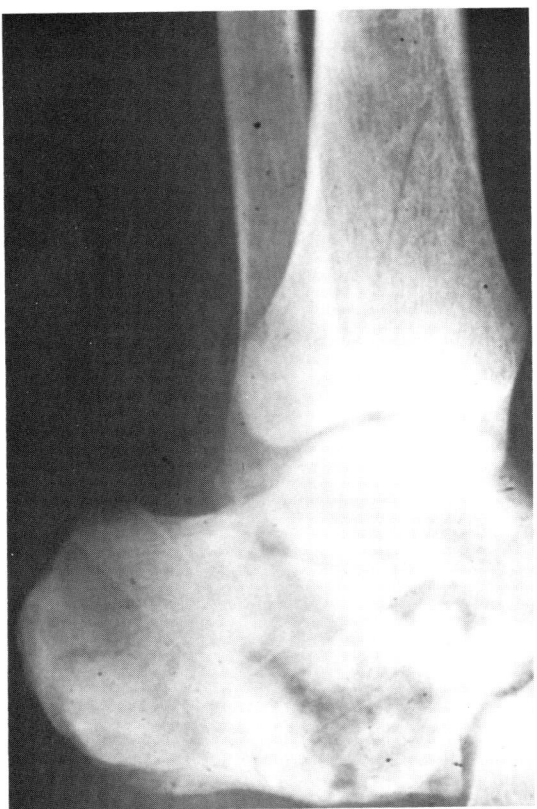

Figure 27–29   A comminuted intraarticular fracture of the calcaneus treated with a Böhler clamp, with resulting improvement in the tuber angle.

eocuboid joint. A slipper cast, which incorporates the pin, is applied for two weeks. The patient is maintained at complete bed rest during this time. The reader is referred to the original article for further details.[24]

Open reduction has also been advocated for intraarticular fractures. Palmer[51] recommended this approach, and Maxfield[47] has reported good to excellent results with his modification of Palmer's original method. This technique involves exposure through a lateral approach at the level of the sinus tarsi. The depressed articular surface is directly visualized and raised into appropriate position with the use of a small periosteal elevator. This maneuver will reveal a large cancellous defect under the elevated articular surface fragment. This defect is then filled in with cortical bone from the iliac crest. A long leg cast is applied, and immobilization is maintained for 10 to 12 weeks. Although Maxfield

reports good results with this technique, the author's impression is that they are not substantially better than the results of conservative management. In fact, Rowe and co-workers[56] reported that 50 per cent of type 5 fractures treated by the Palmer procedure had good results, while 52 per cent of the fractures treated by casts, with or without prior manipulation, achieved good to excellent results. In other words, conservative measures appeared to have a slightly higher rate of success compared with Palmer's open operative technique.

Primary subtalar arthrodesis has also been advocated for the treatment of these injuries by Hall and Pennal[27] and by Harris.[28] In the Harris procedure, the deformity of the heel is corrected first. This may be accomplished by skeletal traction with a pin through the posterior superior corner of the calcaneus and a second pin through the distal tibia. The width of the calcaneus is reduced either by hand molding or by use of the Böhler clamp. At the end of three or four weeks the plaster and pins are removed, and a Gallie posterior subtalar fusion is performed. Harris advocates the use of tibial grafts, which act as splints until solid fusion has been achieved.

The rationale for this approach is that the majority of these fractures demonstrate distortion of the subtalar joint on follow-up roentgenographic examination. Therefore, these patients are likely to develop subtalar arthritis in the future, even though their calcaneal fracture has healed. Operative treatment has been advocated in order to decrease the duration of pain and disability and to reduce time lost from work. However, as stated previously, the author has seen several cases in which the subtalar joint is distorted but the patient is back at work following the conservative functional ambulatory type of management. If a subtalar or triple arthrodesis should be required, it can always be performed at a later date.

FRACTURES OF THE NAVICULAR

Fractures of the tarsal navicular are of three basic types:

1. Chip fractures of the navicular.
2. Fractures of the navicular tuberosity.

3. Fractures of the body of the navicular.

With the exception of chip avulsion fractures of the navicular, these injuries are relatively infrequent.

CHIP AVULSION FRACTURES

Chip fractures of the navicular are fairly commonly encountered in an office orthopedic practice. They are very disabling initially and, if improperly managed, result in a painful foot.

Mechanism of Injury

These injuries are produced by a combination of forces, including both inversion and flexion. The taut talonavicular capsule is placed under acute stress, which results in an avulsion of the proximal portion of the navicular along the dorsal aspect.

Physical Examination

There is obvious acute swelling along the dorsal aspect of the midfoot and tenderness to palpation directly over the dorsal aspect of the navicular. Frequently, an abnormal osseous mass may be palpated just under the skin along the dorsal aspect and motion of the midfoot causes pain in this area. Attempts at ambulation produce pain directly over the navicular.

Roentgenographic Examination

This injury is usually evident on the lateral roentgenogram. A small portion of bone will be noted to be avulsed from the proximal and dorsal aspect of the navicular. There is usually some mild separation of the fragment. The fracture line enters the talonavicular joint.

Treatment

Chip fractures may be managed in a very conservative fashion. The customary treatment is to place the foot and ankle in an Ace bandage. The patient is advised to use crutches without weight bearing for the first one to two weeks, gradually advancing to partial and then to full weight bearing as the symptoms subside. Elevation is recommended between ambulatory periods to reduce the swelling. Crutches are usually discontinued at the end of three to four weeks, and the patient may progress to use of a cane or to walking without support.

Some patients experience exquisite pain over the area and are unable to ambulate even without weight bearing. For this individual, the best form of treatment is an Ace bandage and elevation for the first week until the gross swelling subsides. This is followed by the application of a short leg, weight-bearing cast for four to six weeks. At the end of this time the cast is removed, and the tenderness over the area is reassessed. Usually the patient can be ambulated with the use of an Ace bandage without additional support. The chip avulsion fracture is frequently encountered in young persons following vigorous athletic activity. In this group the functional Ace bandage is preferable to plaster cast treatment. In the middle-aged to elderly patient, cast treatment may be needed to provide support for ambulation.

FRACTURES OF THE NAVICULAR TUBEROSITY

This is the second most common navicular fracture.

Mechanism of Injury

This is also classified as a form of avulsion fracture, because the posterior tibial tendon inserts on the medial portion of the navicular tuberosity. Therefore, if the foot suffers a severe eversion injury, extreme tension is applied to the posterior tibial tendon, avulsing the navicular tuberosity.

Physical Examination

There is evidence of acute swelling along the medial aspect of the navicular. There is also pinpoint tenderness to direct palpation along the entire medial portion of the navicular. Any attempt at eversion of the foot elicits considerable pain along the medial border of the navicular.

Roentgenographic Examination

The injury is usually evident on a routine anteroposterior view of the foot. The fracture line extends through the tuberosity of the navicular and must not be confused with an accessory bone that occasionally occurs, known as the os tibiale externum. The accessory navicular can be distinguished by the fact that it is usually bilateral. As with other accessory bones, the separation line appears to be rounded rather than jagged and sharp, as it is in an acute fracture.

Treatment

A fracture of the navicular tuberosity may be managed either with an Ace bandage and crutch walking or with a below-knee, weight-bearing cast. The author prefers to apply a cast in the majority of cases, as many patients with this injury are young athletic individuals who wish to be ambulatory and weight-bearing as soon as possible. If a cast is applied, it should be maintained for four to six weeks and then removed for reevaluation of tenderness at the fracture site. If there is no acute tenderness, the patient is placed in an Ace bandage and allowed full weight bearing.

If a painful nonunion results from this injury, the small tibial tuberosity fragment may be carefully excised from the posterior tibial tendon. This will usually lead to increased painless function.

FRACTURES OF THE NAVICULAR BODY

This is the least common of the three types of fracture of the navicular.

Mechanism of Injury

A direct blow to the dorsal aspect of the foot, as occurs in industrial accidents, or if a horse steps on the dorsum of the foot, usually produces a comminuted fracture of the body of the navicular.

Physical Examination

Acute swelling is seen on the dorsal aspect of the midportion of the foot, and any attempt at weight bearing elicits pain. There is also acute tenderness to direct palpation over the navicular. Motion of the midfoot produces extreme pain.

Roentgenographic Examination

Routine anteroposterior views of the foot demonstrate the fracture (Fig. 27–30). If it is comminuted, multiple fracture lines will be evident within the body of the navicular. However, most of these fractures are relatively undisplaced.

Treatment

Since the majority of these fractures are relatively undisplaced, they may be man-

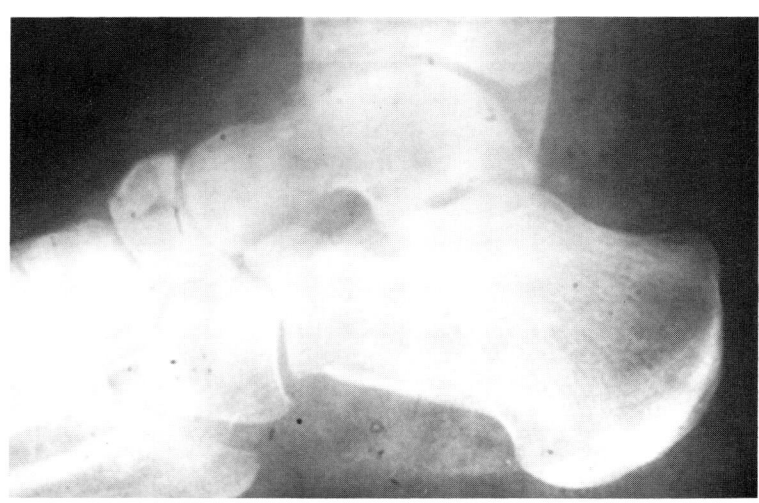

Figure 27–30 Lateral view revealing a fracture of the body of the navicular. This was managed conservatively with the use of a below-knee weight-bearing cast for eight weeks.

aged with a below-knee, weight-bearing cast for 8 to 10 weeks. At the end of that time the fracture has usually united enough so that the patient may be managed with an Ace bandage for support. If there is gross displacement of a fragment, open reduction and internal fixation are mandatory. The fragment is usually approached from the dorsomedial aspect, and fixation is accomplished with the use of small crossed Kirschner wires. The wires are cut parallel to the osseous surface. The patient is then placed in a below-knee, weight-bearing cast for six to eight weeks, when the plaster is removed for reassessment of tenderness at the fracture site. At that time an Ace bandage is usually all the support that is required for an additional two to three weeks. If there is gross comminution of the fracture fragments with separation, the author prefers to manage it with a non–weight-bearing cast for 8 to 10 weeks and then to reassess the injury. If there is continued pain and disability three to four months following the injury, an arthrodesis may be performed. However, patients may present with evidence of incongruity of the joint surface and yet still be functioning without much pain or discomfort. It is probable that they will require an arthrodesis at a later date, but this can always be performed as an elective procedure. An alternative is to perform a primary arthrodesis at the time of the accident. However, this is probably an aggressive form of therapy unless there is very gross comminution with significant distraction.

DISLOCATIONS OF THE NAVICULAR

This is not a common injury, but it is a serious one. It is extremely important to recognize it and to perform an adequate reduction in order to prevent future severe arthritis.

MECHANISM OF INJURY

The probable mechanism of injury in this unusual dislocation is severe plantar flexion combined with inversion of the foot. The dorsal ligaments are ruptured, and the navicular is forced out of its normal alignment to a more dorsal position.

PHYSICAL EXAMINATION

Physical examination reveals a grossly swollen foot along the dorsal aspect, particularly on the dorsomedial portion. There is acute tenderness to direct palpation in this area. A definite firm osseous mass is palpable along the medial portion of the dorsal aspect of the foot and reflects the abnormal position of the navicular.

ROENTGENOGRAPHIC EXAMINATION

A lateral view usually demonstrates the abnormal position of the navicular (Fig. 27–31). Oblique views are also helpful in determining the amount of rotation of the navicular.

TREATMENT

A closed reduction is attempted in the operating room with the expectation of proceeding to an open reduction if it fails. The patient is administered an appropriate anesthetic, and then the foot is placed in severe plantar flexion. Direct pressure is applied to the dorsal aspect of the navicular in a downward direction, "popping" the navicular back into correct position. Once this has been achieved, a small Kirschner wire or Steinmann pin may be inserted through the base of the first metatarsal across the navicular into the talus to hold the position. The wire may then be bent under the skin for removal at a later date, or it may be left protruding through the skin and the foot incorporated in plaster. At the end of three to four weeks the pin is removed, and the extremity is placed back in a below-knee cast. The cast is maintained in position for an additional four weeks, when it is removed and ambulation is allowed with the use of an Ace bandage.

If there is any problem in achieving appropriate reduction by closed methods, the area is approached through a dorsal incision and the navicular is wedged back into position under direct visualization.

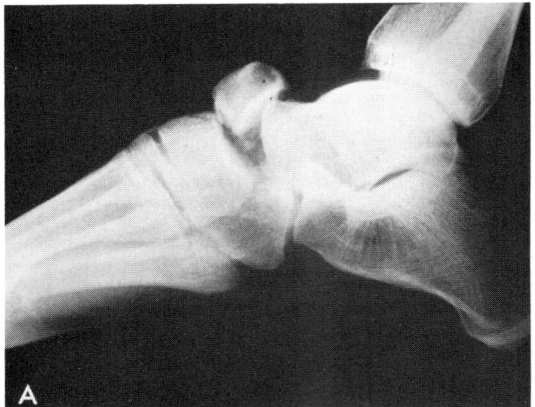
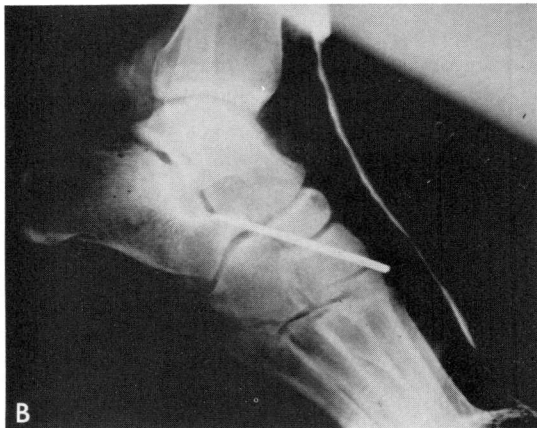
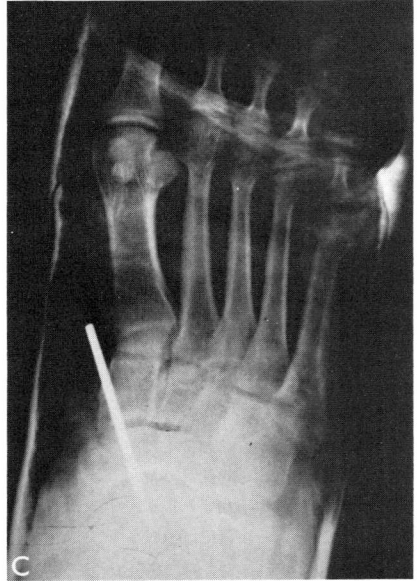

Figure 27–31 *A.* A dislocation of the navicular. *B.* Following appropriate reduction and fixation with a threaded Steinmann pin. *C.* An anteroposterior view of the foot revealing satisfactory reduction.

Once reduction is obtained it is secured with an internal fixation device, as outlined earlier.

FRACTURES OF THE CUNEIFORMS

These are not common injuries.

MECHANISM OF INJURY

The usual mechanism of injury is direct trauma along the dorsal aspect of the foot. This usually results from an industrial accident. The fractured cuneiforms may also be associated with a fracture of the cuboid.

PHYSICAL EXAMINATION

There is evidence of swelling along the medial portion and midportion of the midtarsal area. There is tenderness to direct palpation directly over the cuneiform bones, and ambulation produces pain in this vicinity.

ROENTGENOGRAPHIC EXAMINATION

Routine anteroposterior and oblique views of the midfoot usually demonstrate fractures of the cuneiform bones. A single fracture of the cuneiform is unusual; fracture of two or three of the cuneiform bones is more likely. This again is due to the amount of force required to fracture these bones. These fractures are usually relatively undisplaced.

TREATMENT

The patients are placed in a short leg, non–weight-bearing cast initially and then ambulated on crutches for two to three weeks. Partial weight bearing then progresses to full weight bearing. At the end of six to eight weeks the cast is removed, and residual tenderness over the fractured area is reassessed. There is usually sufficient healing at this time to allow mobilization with the use of an Ace bandage.

FRACTURES OF THE CUBOID

This is a relatively uncommon injury.

MECHANISM OF INJURY

This fracture is usually caused either by direct trauma to the lateral aspect of the foot, as occurs in an industrial accident, or by a severe inversion injury of the foot.

PHYSICAL EXAMINATION

There is gross swelling along the dorsolateral aspect of the midfoot and localized tenderness on direct palpation over the cuboid. Attempted inversion of the foot produces significant pain, as does attempted ambulation.

ROENTGENOGRAPHIC EXAMINATION

Anteroposterior views usually delineate this fracture, but it is best viewed on an oblique roentgenogram. As a rule, these fractures are relatively undisplaced.

TREATMENT

The patient is most comfortable in a below-knee, non–weight-bearing cast for the first two weeks. At the end of that time partial weight bearing is allowed, progressing to full weight bearing. At the end of six to eight weeks the cast is removed, and tenderness over the fracture site is reassessed. An Ace bandage is normally all that is required at this stage.

DISLOCATION OF THE CUNEIFORMS AND CUBOID

This injury is also relatively rare. However, as with navicular dislocations, prompt recognition and appropriate treatment are essential if severe arthritis is to be avoided.

MECHANISM OF INJURY

The most probable mechanism of injury is severe plantar flexion of the foot with a component of inversion.

PHYSICAL EXAMINATION

Gross examination reveals swelling and edema along the dorsolateral aspect of the foot. There is acute tenderness to direct palpation in this area. The cuboid or cuneiform bones may be noted to be in a more dorsal position than normal.

ROENTGENOGRAPHIC EXAMINATION

Routine anteroposterior, lateral, and oblique views aid in delineating this injury. Careful scrutiny of the roentgenograms may reveal an associated fracture of the cuboid or cuneiform bones.

TREATMENT

A closed reduction should be attempted with this injury. The foot is placed in severe plantar flexion, and direct pressure is applied to the cuboid or cuneiform bones to relocate them in appropriate position. Once the reduction has been obtained, Kirschner wires may be run longitudinally through the base of the metatarsal across the involved bone and into the talus. One or two

Kirschner wires may be necessary to achieve satisfactory internal fixation. The pins may be either buried or left protruding through the skin. The involved extremity is then placed in a short leg cast. At the end of six weeks the wires are removed, and the patient is placed in an Ace bandage to begin full weight bearing.

DISLOCATIONS OF THE TARSOMETATARSAL JOINTS

These injuries are being seen more frequently with the increased popularity of bicycle and motorcyle riding. The dislocations occur through the tarsometatarsal joints and have come to be known as Lisfranc dislocations. Although Jacques Lisfranc did not describe this particular dislocation, he did describe an amputation through the tarsometatarsal joints, and these joints have come to be known as Lisfranc's joints.[14]

MECHANISM OF INJURY

Several mechanisms may produce this dislocation pattern. A twisting injury that is being seen with increasing frequency occurs secondary to a fall from a high-speed bicycle with the foot strapped into the stirrup. The rider falls to the ground, and a sudden twisting force on the foot produces either a medial or a lateral dislocation of the tarsometatarsal joints.

Another mechanism of injury is seen in industrial accidents, when a worker falls from a height, landing on the foot. The force on impact may be transmitted through the tarsometatarsal joints, producing a dorsal dislocation of the metatarsals on the tarsal bones. If the individual lands more securely on the calcaneus, the calcaneus fractures and dissipates the force.

Automobile accidents also account for a significant number of these injuries. As the floor board is driven upward, the sudden force is absorbed by the sole of the foot and transmitted to the tarsometatarsal joints.

A final mechanism of injury has been reported by Wiley.[61] This occurs with the foot in maximum plantar flexion, as in the stance of a ballet dancer. Sudden force is applied to the foot in the same linear axis, producing further forced flexion of the foot and resulting in a plantar dislocation of the metatarsal heads in relationship to the tarsal bones.

PHYSICAL EXAMINATION

There is usually gross swelling and edema along the midportion of the foot. In dorsal dislocations of the tarsometatarsal joints the metatarsal shafts may be located more dorsally than normal. There may be a step-off deformity at the site of the dislocation. Any attempt at motion of the midportion of the foot elicits considerable pain. In medial and lateral dislocations the foot may be noted to be in an abnormal position owing to the associated displacement. It is important to evaluate the capillary return to the nailbeds, as a dorsal dislocation may interfere with the dorsalis pedis blood supply.

ROENTGENOGRAPHIC EXAMINATION

Routine anteroposterior, lateral, and oblique roentgenograms of the foot usually demonstrate the disruption at the tarsometatarsal joints (Fig. 27–32). Although the roentgenograms may look comparatively normal, a clue to the extent of the injury may be furnished by a fracture of the base of the second metatarsal or cuboid bone. These frequently occur with this type of dislocation and are indicative of the severity of the primary injury.

TREATMENT

Complete relaxation is required for a proper reduction, and this usually necessitates general anesthesia. The dorsal and plantar aspects of the foot around the metatarsal heads may be painted with benzoin. Once this is dry and sticky, a cloth sheet may be passed under the metatarsal heads and then crisscrossed over the dorsal aspect of the foot, providing an excellent means of traction. The surgeon's assistant then applies countertraction through the heel. A closed reduction is attempted by

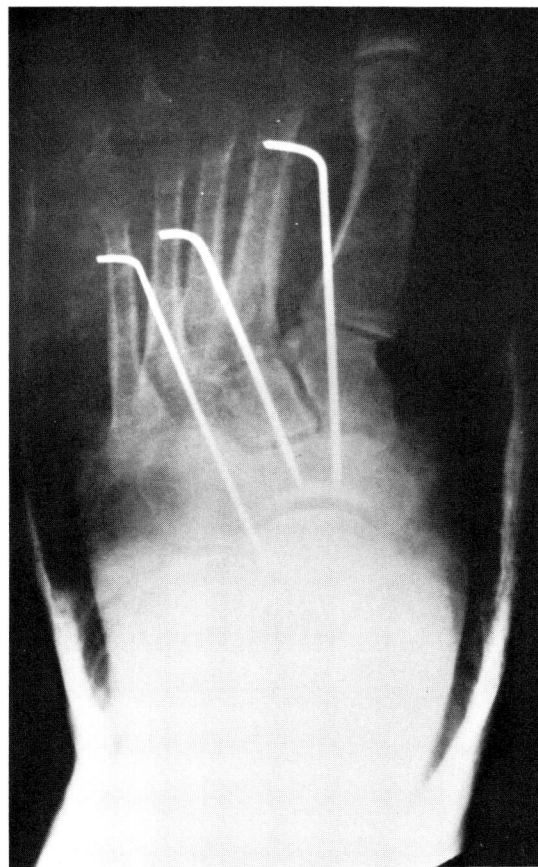

Figure 27-32 An anteroposterior view of a tarso-metatarsal dislocation treated with a reduction and internal fixation using Kirschner wires.

this maneuver, with direct pressure applied over the base of the metatarsals in an attempt to wedge them back into appropriate position. Occasionally, this method is not successful, and an open reduction is required. Following reduction the joints are usually relatively unstable, and it is best to provide internal fixation to prevent redislocation. This may be done by passing Kirschner wires longitudinally down through the metatarsal shaft and into the appropriate tarsal bone. If the injury is very unstable, it is possible to pass a small wire through each individual metatarsal shaft into the appropriate tarsal bone. The wires may be inserted percutaneously if a closed reduction has been performed, or may be inserted through the incision in an open reduction. The wires may then be buried under the skin. The extremity is placed in a below-knee, non–weight-bearing cast for six weeks. After that time the wires are removed, and the patient is placed in an Ace bandage and allowed partial weight bearing, progressing to full weight bearing. Once again, it should be stressed that these injuries require stabilization with Kirschner wires. If internal fixation has not been employed, a careful follow-up series of x-rays is required to insure that redislocation in the cast has not occurred.

If the dislocations are not perfectly reduced, these joints are susceptible to degenerative arthritis in the future.

FRACTURES OF THE METATARSALS

These are not uncommon injuries and are often seen in industrial accidents. Stress fractures are becoming increasingly frequent owing to the greater number of people running for exercise.

MECHANISM OF INJURY

The most common mechanism of injury is a direct blow to the dorsal aspect of the metatarsals, as in an industrial accident. Most patients present with a history of a very heavy weight having fallen across the dorsal aspect of the foot, producing a crush injury. The metatarsal shaft and neck absorb the energy, resulting in fracture.

PHYSICAL EXAMINATION

Physical examination usually demonstrates gross swelling and edema along the dorsal aspect of the foot. This injury is similar to a wringer injury of the forearm in that the amount of soft tissue destruction is not always appreciated on the initial evaluation. Since the majority of these injuries are due to a very heavy object falling on the dorsal aspect of the foot, there is significant soft tissue disruption in addition to the metatarsal fractures. A careful evaluation of the blood supply to the toes is essential, as there may be significant vascular compromise caused by gross swelling, direct damage to the dorsalis pedis artery, or both.

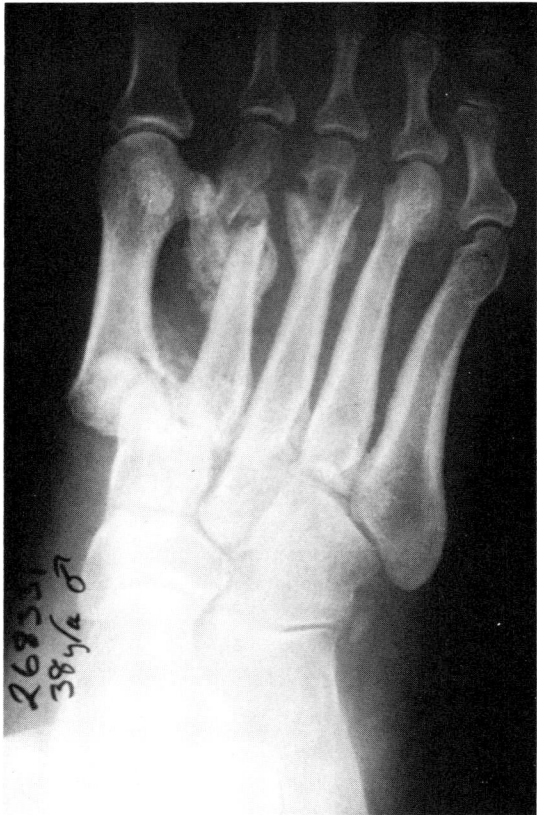

Figure 27–33 Fractures of the second and third metatarsal shafts with evidence of abundant callus formation in follow-up. Note displacement at the first tarsometatarsal joint.

ROENTGENOGRAPHIC EXAMINATION

Routine anteroposterior, lateral, and oblique views usually demonstrate these fractures. There may be evidence of multiple metatarsal fractures rather than involvement of one or two bones (Fig. 27–33). It is important to determine the amount of angulation present, particularly with fractures of the metatarsal necks, as the metatarsal heads may be rotated in a plantar direction. This produces distinct visible prominence of the metatarsal heads in the plantar surface and sets the stage for future callosities and pain.

TREATMENT

The majority of these fractures can be treated conservatively. Fractures that are relatively undisplaced may be managed with a below-knee, partial weight-bearing cast for six weeks.

Displaced fractures require an attempt at closed reduction. If this fails, open reduction and internal fixation are necessary. Closed reduction is performed under general anesthesia, with traction applied through the toes by a Chinese finger trap device. As with the wrist, countertraction may be applied by the use of a muslin bandage over the distal tibia with a weight attached to provide countertraction. Once the reduction is accomplished the patient is placed in a below-knee, non–weight-bearing cast for six weeks.

A case deserving special mention is fracture of the metatarsal necks with definite plantar rotation of the metatarsal heads. As stated previously, this injury sets the stage for plantar callosities and pain and discomfort in the future (Fig. 27–34). Therefore, it is extremely important to correct the plantar angulation at the metatarsal fracture site. This may be done by suspending the foot in a Chinese finger trap device and then applying direct pressure along the plantar aspect of the metatarsal heads by pushing in a dorsal direction. Following appropriate reduction the extremity is placed in a short leg, non–weight-bearing cast for six weeks.

If closed reduction techniques fail to correct an obvious angulation deformity at the fracture site, open reduction and internal fixation are indicated. Open reduction may be accomplished through a dorsal incision with direct manipulation at the fracture site. A smooth Kirschner wire may then be passed down the shaft of the metatarsal to maintain the reduction. The wire is removed at four weeks postinsertion, and the patient is allowed weight bearing in a below-knee, weight-bearing cast. The cast is maintained for an additional three to four weeks and then replaced with an Ace bandage.

If pain and discomfort develop under the metatarsal heads, a metatarsal bar may be inserted into the shoe for relief of symptoms.

The Jones Fracture

This fracture is commonly encountered in clinical practice. It is a fracture through the base of the fifth metatarsal and is an avulsion type of injury.

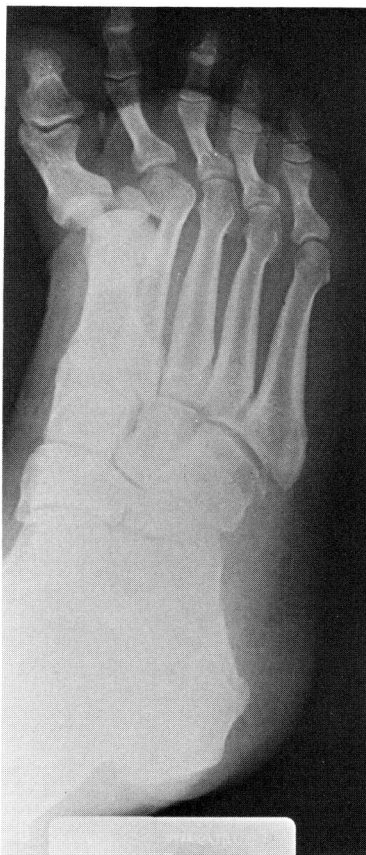
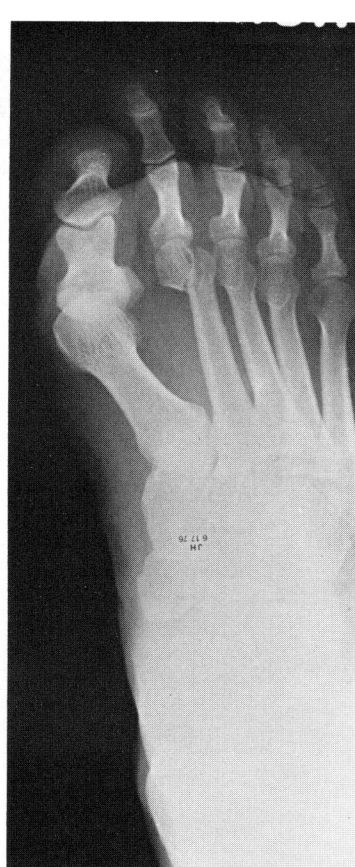

Figure 27–34 Fracture of the second metatarsal neck with angulation. The angulation must be corrected, or the patient may end up with painful callosities.

Mechanism of Injury

This injury occurs through an inversion of the foot. The peroneus brevis tendon is attached to the base of the fifth metatarsal. If the foot is suddenly subjected to severe inversion, the peroneus brevis muscle may contract in an attempt to prevent the inversion deformity and thus may avulse a segment of bone from the base of the fifth metatarsal. This produces the true Jones fracture.[34] Another type of fracture occurs at the base of the fifth metatarsal but in a more distal location. This may be a comminuted fracture and is more difficult to heal than a typical Jones avulsion fracture (Fig. 27–35). It is usually due to a direct blow along the lateral aspect of the foot.

Physical Examination

There is usually mild to moderate swelling along the lateral aspect of the involved foot and acute tenderness to direct palpation over the base of the fifth metatarsal. Any attempt at inversion of the foot elicits pain, because the peroneus brevis is still attached to the avulsed fragment and attempted inversion causes motion at the fracture site.

Roentgenographic Examination

The most useful roentgenographic views for demonstrating this fracture are the true anteroposterior and oblique views. The Jones fracture is a true avulsion fracture and involves a small segment of bone at the base of the fifth metatarsal. As stated previously, another type of fracture, which has a more guarded prognosis, occurs in a more distal location and may be comminuted.

Treatment

The typical Jones fracture may be treated in two different ways. The first method is to supply the patient with an Ace bandage for

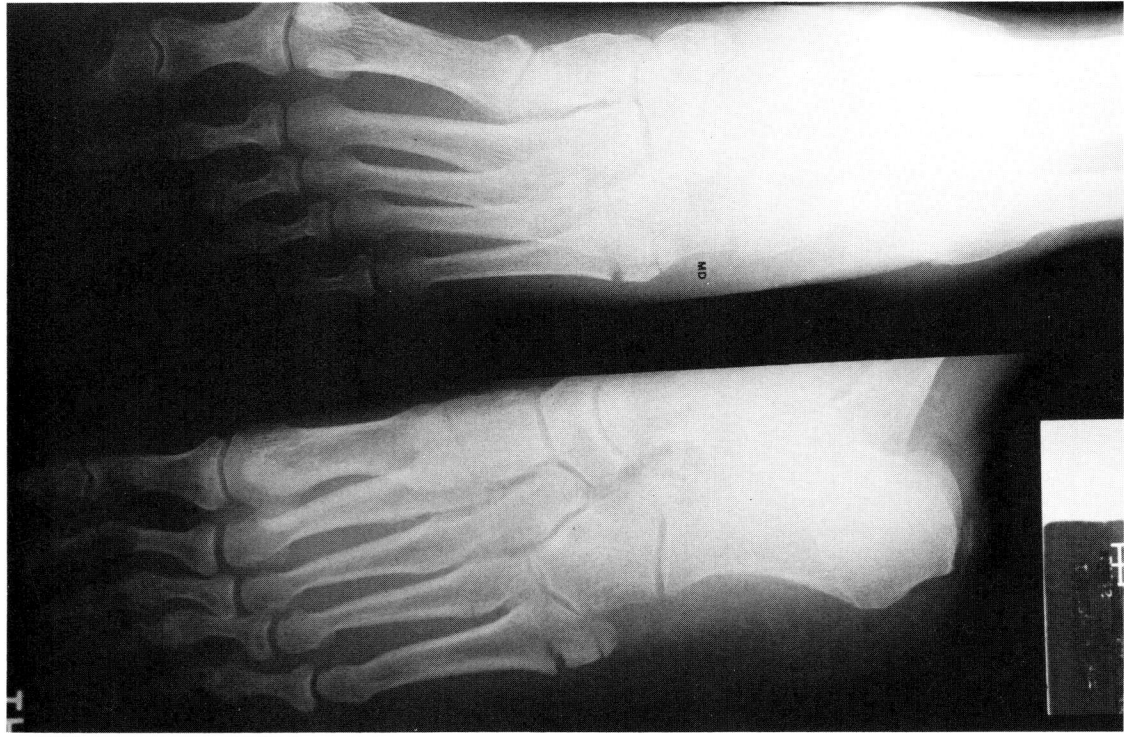

Figure 27–35   A comminuted Jones fracture at the base of the fifth metatarsal.

comfort and crutches for partial weight bearing. Progression to full weight bearing occurs over the next two to three weeks. The alternative form of treatment is to place the patient in a below-knee, weight-bearing cast initially. The advantage of cast treatment is that weight bearing can usually begin within the first three days. If an Ace bandage is utilized as definitive treatment, the patient may not be able to actively bear weight for two to three weeks. The author favors cast treatment for younger patients, who wish to return to full activity as soon as possible. Cast treatment allows them to reach this goal faster than the Ace bandage method.

At the end of six weeks the cast is removed. The patient is placed in an Ace bandage and is usually able to bear weight with minimal discomfort. Vigorous athletic activities are curtailed for an additional four weeks.

The often comminuted fracture that occurs in a more distal location than the true Jones fracture is much more difficult to

treat. As a rule, this fracture requires longer than six to eight weeks to heal. It usually results from a different mechanism of injury and involves a larger portion of bone, which is also comminuted.

STRESS FRACTURES

This fracture of the metatarsal shaft and neck area is described in Chapter 29.

FRACTURES OF THE PHALANGES

These injuries are extremely common. They occur in all age groups and are usually due to direct trauma.

MECHANISM OF INJURY

Fractures of the phalanges are produced by direct trauma and are seen frequently in industrial accidents. A heavy weight may fall and strike the toes, fracturing one or more phalanges. The injury may also result from stubbing the toe against a chair or table leg.

PHYSICAL EXAMINATION

There is usually gross swelling and edema of the involved toe. There may also be an angulatory deformity secondary to angulation at the fracture site. This is particularly evident with a fracture of the fifth toe produced by striking the toe against a table leg. Frequently the toe will be pointed in a more lateral direction than normal owing to angulation at the fracture site. There is definite tenderness to direct palpation over the fracture.

ROENTGENOGRAPHIC EXAMINATION

Routine anteroposterior views usually demonstrate the fracture as well as any angulation at the fracture site.

TREATMENT

These injuries are usually very simple to manage. A basic form of treatment is to splint the injured toe against an uninjured one, using tape with cotton padding between the toes. The patient is advised to resplint the toes if the tape becomes loose. If an angulatory deformity is present, this must be corrected prior to splinting. A local anesthetic is first injected in a ring block fashion around the metatarsal head. Direct longitudinal traction is then applied to the toe in order to pull it over into appropriate position. The involved toe is then splinted to the uninjured toe. Discomfort usually subsides after the first two weeks. The splinting may be discontinued at the end of four to six weeks. The fractures are usually completely healed by six to eight weeks.

DISLOCATION OF METATARSOPHALANGEAL JOINTS

This is a relatively uncommon injury. The big toe is the digit most often involved in this type of dislocation.

MECHANISM OF INJURY

The typical mechanism of injury is a sudden dorsiflexion force applied to the great toe, which results in tearing of the plantar capsule and dorsal displacement of the proximal phalanx on the metatarsal head. A lateral dislocation may also occur, but the dorsal dislocation is more common.

PHYSICAL EXAMINATION

Routine physical examination usually reveals the dorsal displacement of the proximal phalanx on the metatarsal head. There is gross swelling and edema secondary to the dislocation. There is also pinpoint tenderness to direct palpation at this level.

ROENTGENOGRAPHIC EXAMINATION

The lateral roentgenographic view usually demonstrates the dorsal displacement of the proximal phalanx.

TREATMENT

The majority of these injuries may be managed with a closed reduction. This is accomplished with the use of a ring block around the metatarsal head with local anesthetic. Following this the examiner grasps the great toe by one hand and applies longitudinal traction while applying countertraction on the metatarsal area with the opposite hand. Along with longitudinal traction, a definite hyperextension maneuver will usually relocate the base of the proximal phalanx into proper alignment with the metatarsal head. If there has been lateral displacement, a medial force is required in addition to longitudinal traction. The toe is protected with a simple metal splint, which is placed under the toe and bent back over the dorsal aspect. The splint is maintained in position for three weeks. Non–weight bearing is the rule during this time. Occasionally the reduction may be somewhat unstable; if this is the case, a simple corrective maneuver is to place a percutaneous Kirschner wire through the proximal phalanx and into the metatarsal head. The wire should remain in place for three weeks before being removed.

Occasionally a dorsal dislocation may be extremely difficult to reduce by closed measures. The problem associated with this type of irreducible dislocation is that the sesamoid bones and the volar capsule become interposed between the base of the proximal phalanx and the metatarsal head, blocking the reduction. Under these circumstances an open reduction is required. A simple dorsal incision is made, with removal of the sesamoid bones from the joint surfaces, followed by appropriate reduction under direct visualization.

FRACTURES OF THE SESAMOIDS OF THE FIRST TOE

This injury is frequently overlooked. There are normally two large sesamoid bones located within the flexor hallucis brevis tendon, just under the first metatarsal head. The sesamoid bones have an articular surface for active articulation with the inferior aspect of the metatarsal head.

MECHANISM OF INJURY

The most common mechanism of injury is repetitive, direct trauma to the sesamoid, such as that seen with jumping exercises or ballet dancing.

PHYSICAL EXAMINATION

There is usually mild tenderness to direct palpation directly under the first metatarsal head. There is also pain under the metatarsal head associated with attempted weight bearing.

ROENTGENOGRAPHIC EXAMINATION

The fracture of the sesamoid bone appears as a jagged line through the substance of the sesamoid itself. A bipartite sesamoid bone may be present and fool the unwary observer into thinking that this is an acute fracture. However, a bipartite sesamoid bone will usually demonstrate a smooth edge through the substance, rather than the jagged edge characteristic of acute fracture

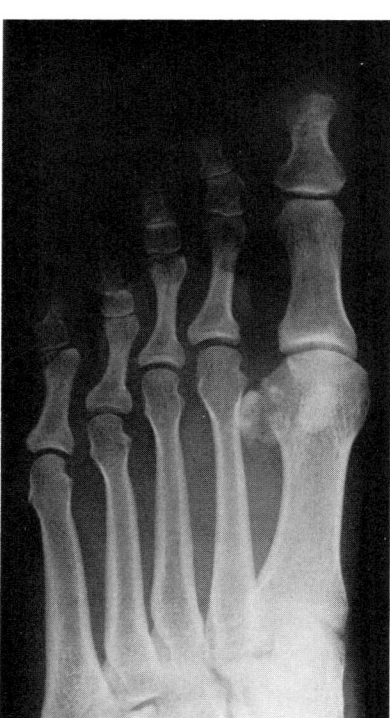
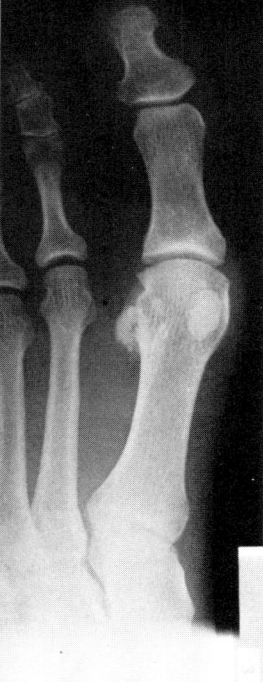

Figure 27–36 A comminuted fracture of the lateral sesamoid of the foot.

(Fig. 27–36). Because these injuries are bilateral in a high percentage of cases, it is frequently useful to x-ray both feet. A defect in the sesamoid of both great toes probably indicates a bipartite sesamoid rather than a true fracture. The medial sesamoid appears to be more frequently fractured than the lateral sesamoid.

TREATMENT

These injuries are an acute event, and it is beneficial to provide the patient with an Ace bandage and advise non–weight bearing for the first week. During this time the patient should have a metatarsal bar built into his shoe. At the end of one week he is usually able to walk with the use of the metatarsal bar, and at the end of four to five weeks he is generally asymptomatic.

If the patient still complains of pain under the metatarsal head sometime after the accident and has evidence of fracture of the sesamoid, a metatarsal bar should be advised. If the symptoms persist, however, the local area may be injected with a Xylocaine solution. If the symptoms appear to subside after Xylocaine injection, in a small percentage of cases the patient may benefit from excision of the sesamoid bone.

REFERENCES

1. Aitken, A. P., and Poulson, D.: Dislocations of the tarsometatarsal joint. J. Bone Joint Surg., *45A*:246–260, 1963.
2. Anderson, H. G.: The Medical and Surgical Aspects of Aviation. London, Oxford University Press, 1919.
3. Anthonsen, W.: An oblique projection for roentgen examination of the talocalcaneal joint particularly regarding intraarticular fracture of the calcaneus. Acta Radiol., *24*:306, 1943.
4. Ashurst, A. P. C.: Divergent dislocation of the metatarsus. Ann. Surg., *83*:132–136, 1926.
5. Bankart, A. S. B.: Fractures of the os calcis. Lancet, *2*:175, 1942.
6. Berndt, A. L., and Harty, M.: Transchondral fractures (osteochondritis dissecans) of the talus. J. Bone Joint Surg., *41A*:988–1020, 1955.
7. Bertelsen, A., and Hasner, E.: Primary results of treatment of fracture of the os calcis by "foot-free walking bandage" and early movement. Acta Orthop. Scand., *21*:140, 1951.
8. Blair, H. C.: Comminuted fractures and fracture dislocations of the body of the astragalus. Operative treatment. Am. J. Surg., *59*:37–43, 1943.
9. Böhler, L.: Diagnosis, pathology, and treatment of fracture of the os calcis. J. Bone Joint Surg., *13*:75, 1931.
10. Bosien, W. R., Staples, D. S., and Russell, S. W.: Residual disability following acute ankle sprains. J. Bone Joint Surg., *37A*:1237–1243, 1955.
11. Brindley, H. H.: Fractures of the os calcis: a review of 107 fractures in 95 patients. South. Med. J., *59*:843–847, 1966.
12. Buckingham, W. W., Jr.: Subtalar dislocation of the foot. J. Trauma, *13*:753–765, 1973.
13. Canale, S. T., and Kelly, F. B.: Fractures of the neck of the talus. Long term evaluation of 71 cases. J. Bone Joint Surg., *60A*:143–156, 1978.
14. Cassebaum, W. H.: Lisfranc fracture-dislocations. Clin. Orthop., *30*:116–129, 1963.
15. Cave, E. F.: Fracture of the os calcis: the problem in general. Clin. Orthop., *30*:64–66, 1963.
16. Charnley, J.: Compression arthrodesis of the ankle and shoulder. J. Bone Joint Surg., *33B*:180–191, 1951.
17. Coltart, W. D.: "Aviator's astragalus." J. Bone Joint Surg., *34B*:545–566, 1952.
18. Conn, H. R.: The treatment of fractures of the os calcis. J. Bone Jont Surg., *17A*:392–405, 1935.
19. Cotton, F. J., and Henderson, F. F.: Results of fracture of the os calcis. Am. J. Orthop. Surg., *14*:290–298, 1916.
20. Dameron, T. B.: Fractures and anatomical variations of the proximal portion of the fifth metatarsal. J. Bone Joint Surg., *57A*:788–792, 1976.
21. Detenbeck, L. C., and Kelly, P. J.: Total dislocation of the talus. J. Bone Joint Surg., *51A*:283–288, 1969.
22. Dimon, J. H.: Isolated displaced fracture of the posterior facet of the talus. J. Bone Joint Surg., *43A*:275–281, 1961.
23. Eftekhar, N. M., Lyddon, D. W., and Stevens, J.: An unusual fracture-dislocation of the tarsal navicular. J. Bone Joint Surg., *51A*:577–581, 1969.
24. Essex-Lopresti, P.: Results of reduction in fractures of the calcaneum. J. Bone Joint Surg., *33B*:284, 1951.
25. Gaul, J. S., Jr., and Greenberg, B. G.: Calcaneus fractures involving the subtalar joint: a clinical and statistical survey of 98 cases. South. Med. J., *59*:605–613, 1966.
26. Haliburton, R. A., Sullivan, C. R., Kelly, P. J., and Peterson, L. F. A.: The extraosseous and intraosseous blood supply of the talus. J. Bone Joint Surg., *40A*:1115–1120, 1958.
27. Hall, M. C., and Pennal, G. F.: Primary subtalar arthrodesis in the treatment of severe fractures of the calcaneum. J. Bone Joint Surg., *42B*:336–343, 1960.
28. Harris, R. I.: Fractures of the os calcis: treatment by early subtalar arthrodesis. Clin. Orthop., *30*:100–110, 1963.
29. Harris, W. R., and Bobechko, W. P.: The radiographic density of avascular bone. J. Bone Joint Surg., *42B*:626–632, 1960.
30. Harty, M.: Anatomic consideration in injuries of the calcaneus. Orthop. Clin. North Am., *4*:179–183, 1973.
31. Hawkins, L. G.: Fracture of the lateral process of the talus. J. Bone Joint Surg., *47A*:1170–1175, 1965.

32. Hawkins, L. G.: Fractures of the neck of the talus. J. Bone Joint Surg., 52A:991–1002, 1970.

33. Hermann, O. J.: Conservative therapy for fracture of the os calcis. J. Bone Joint Surg., 19:709–718, 1937.

34. Jones, R.: Fracture of the base of the fifth metatarsal bone by indirect violence. Ann. Surg., 35:697–700, 1902.

35. Kappis, M.: Weitere Beiträge jur Traumatisch-mechanischen Entstehung der "spontanen" Knorpelablösungen (sogen. Osteochondritis dissecans). Dtsch. Z. Chir., 171:13–29, 1922.

36. Kelly, P. J., and Sullivan, C. R.: Blood supply of the talus. Clin. Orthop., 30:37–44, 1963.

37. Kenwright, J., and Taylor, R. G.: Major injuries of the talus. J. Bone Joint Surg., 52B:36–48, 1970.

38. King, R. E.: Axial pin fixation of fractures of the os calcis (method of Essex-Lopresti). Orthop. Clin. North Am., 4:185–188, 1973.

39. Kleiger, B.: Fractures of the talus. J. Bone Joint Surg., 30A:735–744, 1948.

40. König, F.: Ueber freie Körper in den Gelenken. Dtsch. Z. Chir., 27:90–109, 1888.

41. Lance, E. M., Carey, E. J., and Wade, P. A.: Fractures of the os calcis: treatment by early mobilization. Clin. Orthop., 30:79–90, 1963.

42. Lindsay, W. R. N., and Dewar, F. P.: Fractures of the os calcis. Am. J. Surg., 95:555–576, 1958.

43. Lowy, M.: Avulsion fractures of the calcaneus. J. Bone Joint Surg., 51B:494–497, 1969.

44. McKeever, F. M.: Treatment and complications of fractures and dislocations of the talus. Clin. Orthop., 30:45–52, 1963.

45. McLaughlin, H. L.: Trauma. Philadelphia, W. B. Saunders, 1959.

46. McLaughlin, H. L.: Treatment of late complications after os calcis fractures. Clin. Orthop., 30:111–115, 1963.

47. Maxfield, J. E., and McDermott, F. J.: Experiences with the Palmer open reduction of fractures of the calcaneus. J. Bone Joint Surg., 37A:99–106, 1955.

48. Mindell, E. R., Cisek, E. E., Kartalian, G., and Dziob, J. M.: Late results of injuries to the talus. J. Bone Joint Surg., 45A:221–245, 1963.

49. Mukherjee, S. K., Pringle, R. M., and Baxter, A. D.: Fracture of the lateral process of the talus. J. Bone Joint Surg., 56B:263–273, 1974.

50. Mulfinger, G. L., and Trueta, J.: The blood supply of the talus. J. Bone Joint Surg., 52B:160–167, 1970.

51. Palmer, L.: The mechanism and treatment of fractures of the calcaneus. Open reduction with the use of cancellous grafts. J. Bone Joint Surg., 30A:2–6, 1948.

52. Parkes, J. C. H.: The nonreductive treatment for fractures of the os calcis. Orthop. Clin. North Am., 4:193–195, 1973.

53. Peltier, L. F.: Eponymic fractures: Robert Jones and Jones's fracture. Surgery, 71:522–526, 1972.

54. Pennal, G. F.: Fractures of the talus. Clin. Orthop., 30:53–63, 1963.

55. Pennal, G. F., and Yadev, M. P.: Operative treatment of comminuted fractures of the os calcis. Orthop. Clin. North Am., 4:197–211, 1973.

56. Rowe, C. R., Sakellarides, H. T., Freeman, P. A., and Sorgie, C.: Fractures of the os calcis: a long term follow-up study of 146 patients. J.A.M.A., 184:920–923, 1963.

57. Sammarco, G. J., Burstein, A. H., and Frankel, V. H.: Biomechanics of the ankle: a kinematic study. Orthop. Clin. North Am., 4:75–96, 1973.

58. Thompson, K. R.: Treatment of comminuted fractures of the calcaneus by triple arthrodesis. Orthop. Clin. North Am., 4:189–191, 1973.

59. Thompson, K. R., and Friesen, C. M.: Treatment of comminuted fractures of the calcaneus by primary triple arthrodesis. J. Bone Joint Surg., 41A:1423–1436, 1959.

60. Warrick, C. K., and Brenner, A. E.: Fractures of the calcaneum. With an atlas illustrating the various types of fractures. J. Bone Joint Surg., 35B:33–45, 1953.

61. Wiley, J. J.: The mechanism of tarsometatarsal joint injuries. J. Bone Joint Surg., 53B:474–482, 1971.

62. Wilson, D. W.: Injuries to the tarsometatarsal joints: etiology, classification, and results of treatment. J. Bone Joint Surg., 54B:677–686, 1972.

R. BRUCE HEPPENSTALL, M.D.

Pathological ——————————————— 28
Fractures
Secondary to
Metastatic
Disease

A simple definition of a pathological fracture is a break in the continuity of bone within an abnormal bone structure. This broad definition encompasses pathological fractures in three basic categories: (1) metabolic bone disease, (2) primary bone tumors and (3) metastatic bone tumors. The reader is referred to Chapter 32 for a discussion of fractures secondary to metabolic bone disease. The diagnosis and management of pathological fractures due to primary bone tumors involves treating the tumor per se and is beyond the scope of this book. This chapter will be limited to the diagnosis and treatment of pathological fractures secondary to metastatic disease. It is fair to state that a very aggressive approach to the management of these problems has developed in the past two decades.

SURGICAL ANATOMY

Since pathological fractures occur throughout skeletal structure it is impossible to discuss pertinent surgical anatomy. The reader is referred to the chapter dealing with the specific regional fracture for this information. Knowledge of the surgical anatomy is essential before any form of treatment for these serious problems is undertaken.

DIAGNOSIS

HISTORY

As with the general work-up of any patient with a tumor, certain questions should be asked in an attempt to determine a possible primary etiology. The presence or absence of recent weight loss should be ascertained. A change in activities resulting from a general lack of energy will frequently be found.

A recent change in bowel habit or evidence of abnormal bleeding from the GI tract may be an early sign of malignancy. Patients should be specifically questioned about the appearance of any abnormal soft tissue or osseous masses. Despite the presence of these early signs, it has been reported that in up to 24 per cent of patients with pathological fractures due to malignant disease the fracture is the initial complaint.[25] The attending physician must be aware of the relatively high incidence of a pathological fracture manifesting metastatic disease as the initial presentation. Such fractures are frequently produced by minimal trauma. This is a specific warning signal to the physician that this may indeed be a pathological fracture.

PHYSICAL EXAMINATION

A thorough and specific examination is required in the initial work-up of these patients. Each system must be examined for clues to the primary location of the malignancy. The fact that many patients do not appear to have the severe pain that is associated with a fracture through healthy bone may be a helpful sign. Also, there may be little swelling associated with the fracture, as it is frequently produced by muscle contraction rather than by direct external violence. Muscle spasm and guarding likewise may be less than that associated with a fracture through normal bone. The presence or absence of cachexia may be a clue to the diagnosis. There may be evidence of recent weight loss with redundant skin folds. Tissue turgor may be severely decreased.

The specific deformity will depend upon the exact location of the fracture, and these are discussed in appropriate sections throughout this book.

LABORATORY INVESTIGATION

Several laboratory investigations are in order during the initial evaluation of a patient with metastatic disease. That is not to say, however, that a large number of diagnostic tests must be ordered. The more realistic approach is to order a base set of laboratory investigations and then order further studies as needed. The following laboratory investigations are regarded as a baseline in the evaluation of a patient with a pathological fracture.

A serum calcium value should be determined in all patients presenting with a pathological fracture. This value is frequently elevated in patients with metastatic lesions. Another frequent cause of an elevated serum calcium value is primary hyperparathyroidism. If there is rapid destruction of bone by a metastatic lesion, this may well release an increased amount of calcium into the circulation. Since a portion of the calcium is bound to protein, the level of protein may affect the end result. This is discussed further in Chapter 32.

The serum phosphorus value should also be determined. Although the serum phosphorus is not as frequently affected by metastatic disease as the serum calcium, this test is useful to help rule out renal malfunction and metabolic bone disease.

The serum alkaline phosphatase is a very useful determination and may reflect the state of bone turnover. It has also been useful as a prognostic indicator in the management of osteogenic sarcoma. If the value of the alkaline phosphatase is very high when the patient is initially evaluated, the prognosis may not be as good as if it were normal. An important point to remember is that the alkaline phosphatase may be of bone or liver origin. Tests are now available that make this differentiation.

An acid phosphatase value is useful if the patient is suspected of having metastatic prostatic carcinoma. For accuracy the blood sample must be obtained prior to digital examination of the prostate. The reason for this is that digital examination may cause an elevation of the acid phosphatase for 24 to 48 hours. An elevation of the acid phosphatase in the absence of digital examination is highly specific as an indicator of prostatic carcinoma.

A complete blood count is usually obtained in these patients. The white cell count may or may not be elevated in the presence of metastatic disease. Frequently the hemoglobin and hematocrit will reveal a relative state of anemia in the presence of metastatic disease. This is not just academic, as patients may require an operation for the pathological fracture, and it is important to determine whether anemia is present and whether it should be corrected prior to surgery. The author has found that as long as the blood volume is maintained, the presence of a moderate anemia does not alter the fracture healing process.[23]

The sedimentation rate is a relatively nonspecific test, but an elevated value may be an indication of malignancy or infection. It is common to find an elevation of the sedimentation rate in the presence of metastatic disease. However, it is important to bear in mind that a normal sedimentation rate does not rule out metastatic disease.

Like a complete blood count, a urinalysis is a standard laboratory examination performed on all patients in the hospital. It is valuable in determining whether or not primary renal disease is present. It may also reflect the presence of a urinary tract infection and is a useful study in patients with diabetes. A careful search for Bence Jones protein in the urine is indicated in the management of a pathological fracture. This protein is present in the urine of slightly over 50 per cent of patients with multiple myeloma.

A serum electrophoresis is also useful in ruling out multiple myeloma as a cause of the pathological fracture. This test will reveal an elevation of globulin and also of the M component of the electrophoretic pattern.

ROENTGENOGRAPHIC EVALUATION

All patients admitted to the hospital with a fracture should have a routine chest examination at the time of the initial roentgenograms for the fracture. If a surgical procedure is necessary for management of the fracture, a chest roentgenogram will be required. By obtaining roentgenograms in proper sequence, additional trips to the radiology department can be avoided.

There are several specific roentgenographic findings in a patient with metastatic disease. First of all, the exact location of the lesion is established. The lesion may be anywhere within the bone. It may present in the cortex, the substantia spongiosa, the articular portion, or the shaft portion. Certain tumors have a predilection for a particular area of bone, such as the giant cell tumor which tends to develop in the secondary epiphyses.

Second, the osseous response of the lesion should be documented. This is probably the most important roentgenographic finding. The osseous response may be one of lysis, calcification, or ossification. As an example, a prostatic metastatic carcinoma may present with a lytic or a blastic area.

The third roentgenographic determination is the perilesion osseous response. There may be no obvious response, or there may be evidence of cortical thinning. Subperiosteal new bone formation may be present, and there may be an area of sclerosis or margination.

Finally, the gross character of the lesion must be ascertained. Cortical expansion or actual cortical breakthrough, such as that seen with malignant lesions, may be seen. Loculation may be present, and there may be evidence of trabeculation.

Careful evaluation of the roentgenographic findings will yield information that the physician can use to arrive at the correct diagnosis. Once again, the correct diagnosis can be reached only through a careful and systematic assessment of these findings.

MECHANISM OF INJURY

A pathological fracture may be produced by direct or indirect trauma. Patients presenting with this type of lesion frequently report having sustained a very trivial injury. Since this sort of fracture occurs through an area of structural weakness within the bone, it is not hard to comprehend why patients present with minimal trauma. In the author's experience the majority of fractures that are secondary to pathological lesions are the result of an indirect mechanism.

TREATMENT

Metastases to the skeleton are relatively common in the cancer patient. The true incidence of skeletal metastases in patients who die of cancer probably approaches 70 per cent if the sampling size is large enough. That is not to state that all patients with metastatic lesions develop pathological fractures. Only a small percentage of those with metastatic lesions incur a frank pathological fracture. Marcove and Yang have reported that approximately 40 per cent of patients with pathological fractures caused by metastatic carcinoma survive for six months after the first such injury, and 30 per cent survive for one year or longer.[28] Thus, a fair percentage of patients survive for an extended period following a pathological fracture.

For this reason a more aggressive surgical approach has been favored in the past two decades. For example, the fracture may be stabilized by open reduction and appropriate internal fixation, allowing the patient increased comfort as well as increased functional activity including active mobility. In the past, these fractures were looked on as a terminal event in the patient's downhill clinical course. This view, however, is no longer feasible. It is much more reasonable to undertake an aggressive approach to make the patient more functional and pain-free during the remaining life span. Harrington and co-workers have reviewed 375 cases of pathological fractures.[22] Of these, 139 patients had metastases from breast carcinoma, 142 had metastases from other tumors, and 42 had metastases from myeloma or lymphoma. The mean survival rate for the 210 patients who had undergone surgery two years or more before final evaluation was 15.4 months. It is interesting that 94 per cent of the patients who were ambulatory before fracture regained the ability to walk, and 85 per cent had excellent or good relief of pain. There were only four failures of fixation and six functionally poor results.

Their treatment included early operative intervention, with adequate stability obtained by internal fixation devices or prostheses supplemented with methyl methacrylate. These authors found that the addition of methyl methacrylate increased structural stability to withstand the stresses of immediate weight bearing. It has been seen over the years that fractures secondary either to metastatic malignancy from the breast or prostate or to myeloma or lymphoma tend to have a higher rate of union than those from the lung, kidney, or gastrointestinal tract.

Methyl methacrylate also does not appear to appreciably intensify ionization. Therefore, radiotherapy may be initiated shortly after the operative procedure. It is customary to allow a one to two week interval prior to initiating radiation therapy. In this manner the wound itself has a chance to begin the reparative process. A dose of 2000 roentgens is enough to prevent tumor progression in the majority of cases, and this dose may be administered over a two-week period. It has also been demonstrated by Murray and colleagues that irradiation seems to have no specific effect on the shear strength, compressibility, or durability of the acrylic cement.[33]

The specific goals of early aggressive operative management of pathological fractures are the following: (1) to afford adequate pain relief, (2) to increase functional mobility of the patient, (3) to facilitate nursing care, and (4) to improve the mental attitude of the patient for the remaining limited life span. The nonoperative conservative approach fails to attain these goals, and for this reason the author advocates surgical treatment.

With the recognition that all cases must be treated individually, the following sum-

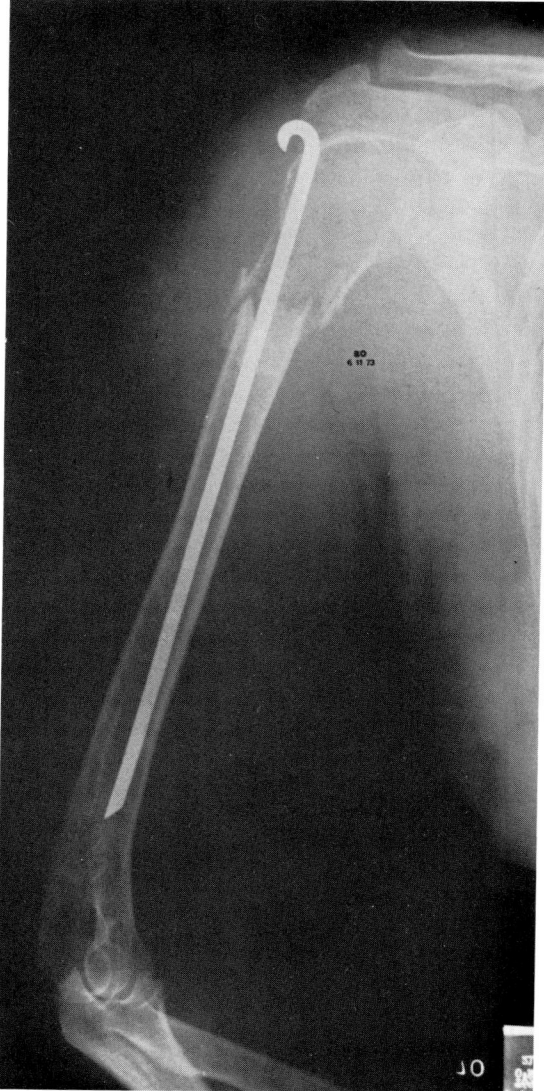

Figure 28-1 Pathological lesion of the proximal humerus managed with the use of a Rush rod.

marizes the methods available to obtain stability in pathological fractures of the long bones.

Humerus

Pathological fractures in the shaft of the humerus may be managed by conservative or operative treatment. Conservative therapy includes the use of a posterior plaster splint or a functional brace. The author prefers the operative method because it achieves relative stability at the fracture site and permits motion without the use of a splint or brace. Three internal fixation devices are effective in stabilizing this fracture. First, a Rush rod may be passed from the humeral head down the shaft of the humerus (Fig. 28–1). One or two Rush rods may be employed. Although this does provide relative stability at the fracture site to prevent angulation, it does not provide rigid immobilization, and patients still experience some pain with motion.

The second type of internal fixation involves the use of the Küntscher rod. This device does furnish adequate stability at the fracture site (Fig. 28–2). However, the author has found that in order to insert the Küntscher rod it is frequently advantageous to perform a partial acromionectomy. This provides a better exposure for passing the rod through the humeral head down the humeral shaft. If this is not done, it is often technically difficult to pass the rod down the shaft of the humerus because the tip of the rod tends to abut the medial cortex of the proximal humerus. Another technical advantage is to have the humerus in full extension and adduction, which exposes the proximal humerus sufficiently for insertion of the rod. The medullary canal of the humerus decreases in size in a distal direction. Therefore, it is extremely important to select a rod of appropriate size to fit the distal half of the shaft. If a rod is selected to provide a tight fit of the proximal portion of the shaft, it cannot be inserted into the distal portion. Since this is not a weight-bearing bone, a tight fit is not as important as it is in the lower extremity. The rod may also be passed in a retrograde manner from the fracture site. If this is performed, the biopsy of the pathological lesion can be accomplished through an open incisional area. The problem with

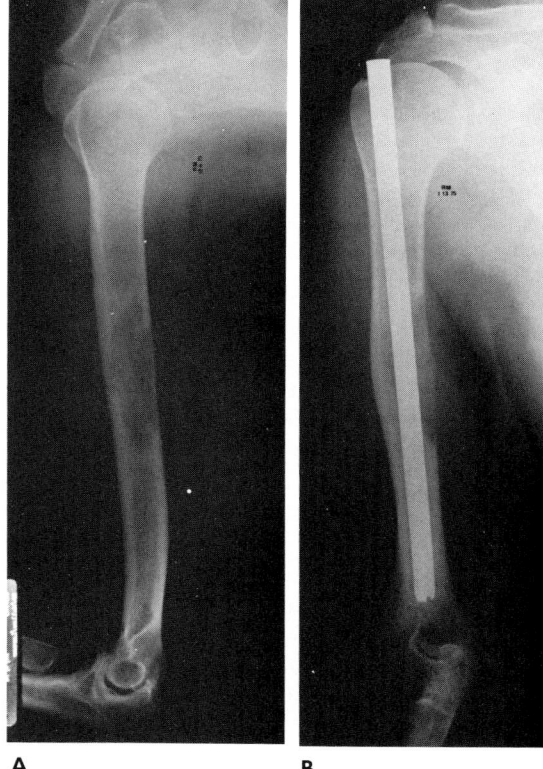

A   **B**

Figure 28–2   A. A renal carcinoma metastatic to the midshaft of the humerus. B. Managed with the use of a "blind" insertion of a Küntscher rod. An excellent result.

such exposure is that blood loss is greater than in a "blind" rodding. The biopsy can also be performed during a blind rodding by passing a curette down the shaft of the humerus and obtaining a piece of bone at the fracture site, for histological study. Image intensification is helpful in performing a closed rodding of the humerus.

The final method of fixation for the humeral shaft is the use of a Sampson fluted rod. This resembles the femoral rod in its fluted design, and it is also slightly curved to provide for tight fixation. Like the Rush rod, this device is passed through the humeral head and down the shaft. Adequate fixation of the fracture site is insured by the fluted design and the prebent shape of the rod.

The postoperative course of intramedullary rod fixation is one of increased functional ability with decreased pain. A compression plate may also be applied for fixation across the fracture site, but this involves increased surgical exposure with its attendant blood loss.

Forearm

A single forearm pathological fracture may be managed with the use of a functional brace for comfort (Fig. 28–3). If this does not provide sufficient pain relief, internal fixation may be accomplished by a compression plate with or without a bone graft, or by a Sage intramedullary nail. Patients with single fractures usually have some stability, as the rest of the forearm bone remains intact. Hence, the majority of patients may be managed with a functional brace.

Hip

Lesions involving an extensive portion of the femoral neck may be treated by a smooth-stem Austin-Moore or Thompson prosthesis supplemented by methyl methacrylate. In this manner the patient may be ambulated very early and may remain mobile for the duration of his life. The alternative is to insert a sliding hip compression screw, but if a substantial portion of the neck and proximal portion of the head is in-

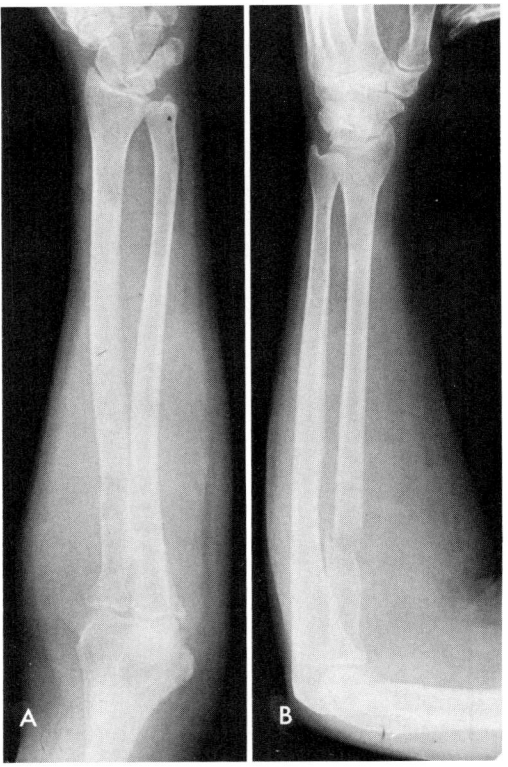

Figure 28–3 *A.* Anteroposterior view of a metastatic lesion to the proximal radius. *B.* Lateral view demonstrating the complete fracture. This was managed with a long arm cast and later by a functional brace.

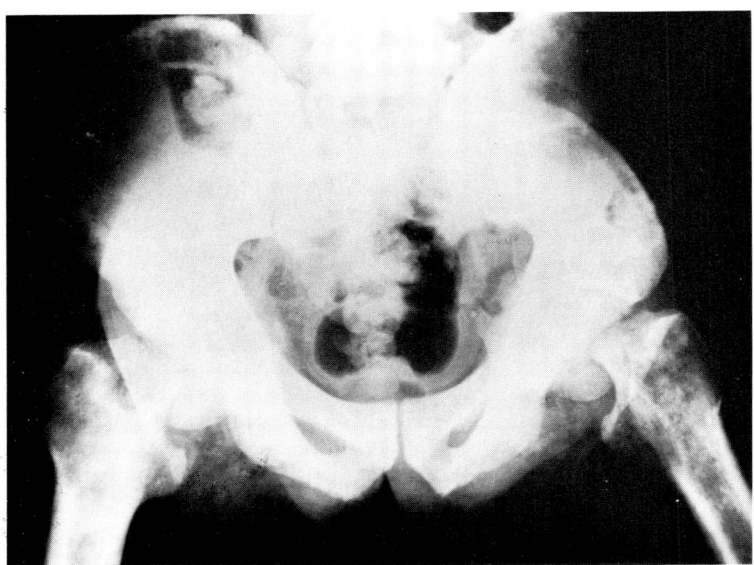

Figure 28–4 Diffuse metastatic disease with bilateral subcapital fractures. This was managed with bilateral Austin-Moore prosthesis.

volved this device will not achieve adequate purchase. For this reason, prosthetic replacement of large lesions of the femoral neck is preferred (Fig. 28–4). If the lesion extends through the femoral head and involves a portion of the acetabulum, a total hip replacement is the procedure of choice.

Lesions in the intertrochanteric area may be managed with the use of a sliding hip compression screw. This device does have one advantage. If the lesion increases in size and the fracture site collapses, the device will collapse along with it, preventing protrusion of the metallic screw through the femoral head into the acetabulum. The

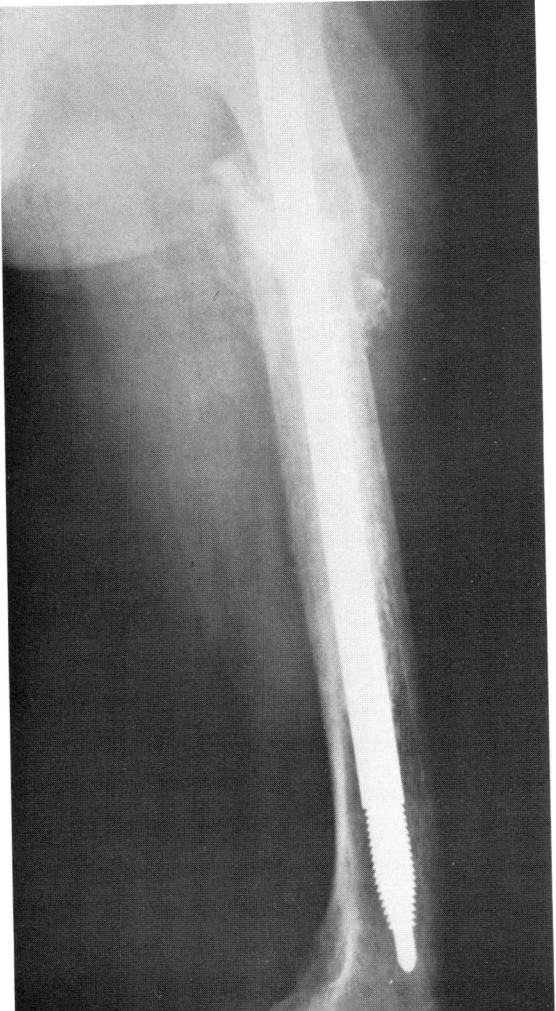

Figure 28–5 Metastatic lesion to the subtrochanteric area of the femur. Treated with insertion of a Schneider intramedullary device.

alternative is to insert a one-unit device supplemented by methyl methacrylate. This has the disadvantage of not allowing for collapse at the fracture site, but may slightly increase the structural stability of the device itself. If the lesion is large, involving a significant portion of the intertrochanteric area and extending into the femoral neck, a custom-made prosthesis may be required following resection of the large amount of tumor. Methyl methacrylate may be used in conjunction with this treatment.

Subtrochanteric lesions may be managed with the use of a Zickel nail or intramedullary device (Fig. 28–5). This type of fixation may or may not be supplemented by methyl methacrylate. Zickel and Mouradian have recently reported the use of this device for the management of pathological fractures in the subtrochanteric area in 35 patients.[43] They did not utilize methyl methacrylate with the device. Early mobilization was possible in nearly all of their cases. Of the 35 patients with fractures, 14 demonstrated union after an average of 4.5 months. In a separate study by Mickelson and Bonfiglio, the Zickel nail was employed in the management of 21 patients with neoplastic pathological fracture of impending pathological fractures in the proximal femur.[30] Twenty of their patients were able to walk following internal fixation, and failure of fixation did not occur in any of their cases. These two independent studies confirm that the Zickel nail is an excellent device for the management of pathological fractures of the proximal femur. It is especially applicable to the subtrochanteric area. In the author's experience, the Zickel nail provides strong fixation, and a failure has not occurred to date.

Femoral Shaft

The use of intramedullary rods for the management of pathological fractures is particularly applicable to lesions of the femoral shaft (Fig. 28–6). Several devices are available for the management of fractures in this area, as outlined in Chapter 23. The author prefers the fluted Sampson intramedullary device, because of its inherent strength, its fluted design which allows ingrowth of new vasculature, and its ability to achieve solid,

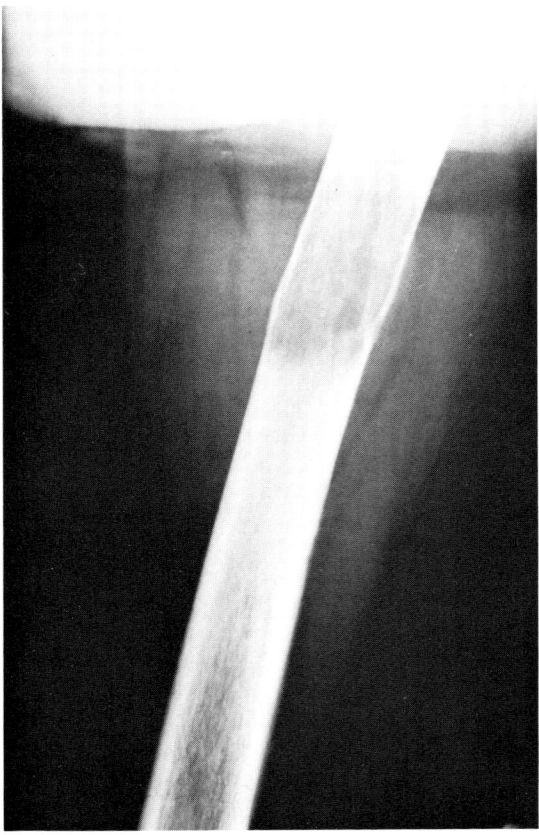

Figure 28–6 Pathological lesion of the proximal femur treated by observation. A complete fracture through the lesion was eventually sustained and was treated with the use of an intramedullary rod, supplemented with methyl methacrylate.

stable fixation. Since the Sampson rod has such inherent strength, the supplementary use of methyl methacrylate is not required as often as with internal fixation devices. If the Küntscher device is employed in the management of these fractures, methyl methacrylate may be useful as an adjunct in internal fixation (Fig. 28–7). Stubbs and co-workers have demonstrated experimentally that the injection of cooled methyl methacrylate into the distal portion of the femur through the canal of the Küntscher rod increases tortional stability at the fracture site.[41]

The method of insertion for either device is generally open exposure of the fracture site and retrograde insertion of the intramedullary device following a satisfactory bone biopsy. The fracture site is then reduced, and the rod is driven down the shaft of the femur. Bank bone may be utilized if needed to fill in any large osseous gap produced by resection of the tumor (Fig. 28–8).

Tibia

Pathological fractures of the tibia may be managed with the use of a patellar tendon-bearing cast followed by a functional brace, or with the use of an intramedullary device, such as the Lottes nail. The Lottes nail provides stability at the fracture site and may well have application in the management of pathological lesions of the tibia.

PROPHYLACTIC INTERNAL FIXATION

There appears to be almost universal acceptance of the early aggressive operative approach to the management of a complete pathological fracture. However, there is still some debate concerning the management of an impending pathological fracture. Parrish and Murray felt that pain together with involvement of half of the cortex of the osseous structure was a definite indication for prophylactic operative intervention.[36] Zickel and Mouradian described a category of patients with femoral pathological fractures that they designated the "high-risk femur."[43] They considered the following to be high-risk characteristics: (1) pure lysis as evidenced on roentgenograms; (2) development of a malignant lesion not previously demonstrable in the bone; (3) involvement of even small portions of the cortex, especially in association with the first two signs; and (4) increasing pain.

There can be no doubt that both the technical procedure of internal fixation and the condition of the patient are improved when the fracture is incomplete (Fig. 28–9). This stands in contrast to the case of a complete fracture treated by internal fixation. The author has applied the guidelines of Parrish and Murray in combining the amount of pain with the involvement of half the cortex as an indication for prophylactic internal fixation.[36] Although this is a general statement and may not apply to all pathological lesions, it is a good rule of thumb. If the lesion occurs in the midshaft

Text continued on page 894.

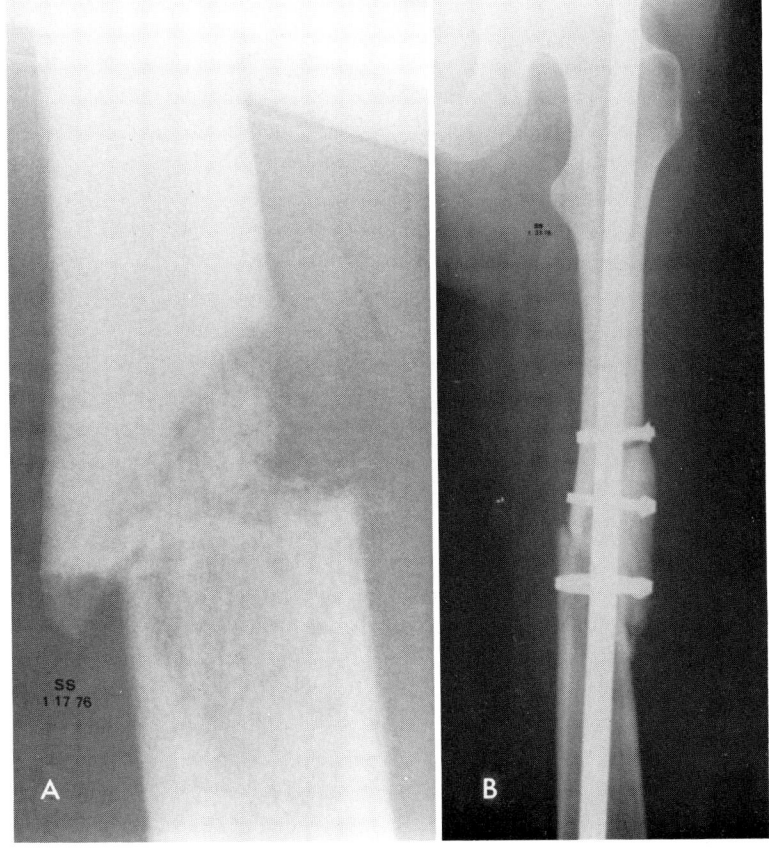

Figure 28–7 *A.* Metastatic lesion to the midfemur. *B.* Managed with open reduction and internal fixation with the use of an intramedullary rod, bone graft, and Parham bands.

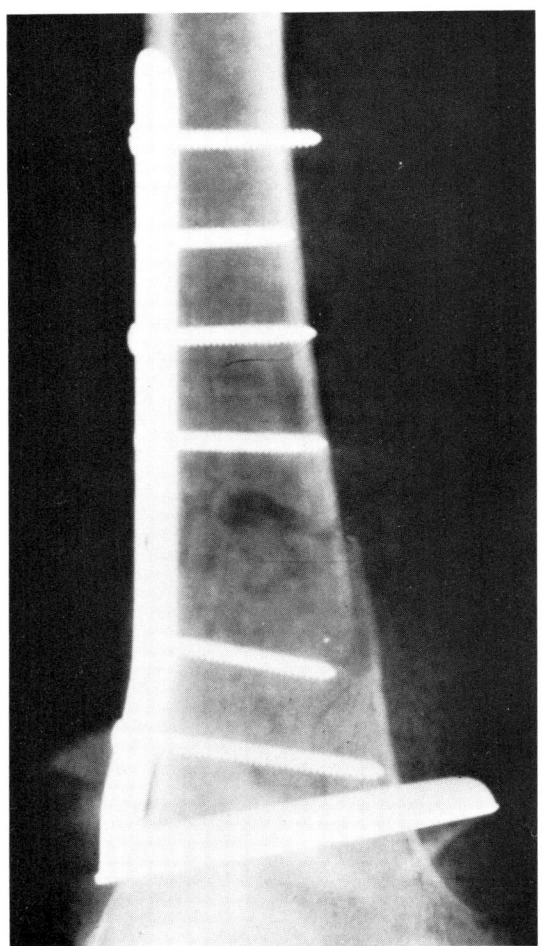

Figure 28–8   A pathological fracture through a lesion in the supracondylar area. Managed with the use of a blade plate.

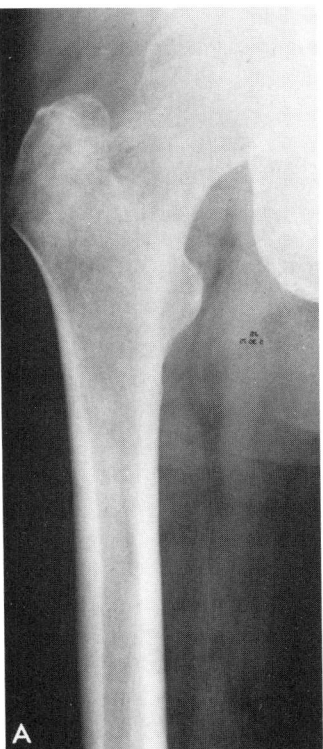

Figure 28–9 *A.* Bilateral metastatic prostatic carcinoma to the femoral neck. This is an incomplete fracture involving at least half the cortex, and the patient was having pain. *B.* Three months post-treatment with the insertion of a sliding hip compression screw along with appropriate therapy. There is evidence of beginning resolution of the femoral neck lesion. *C.* Six months following prophylactic pinning, with evidence of healing of the femoral neck lytic defect.

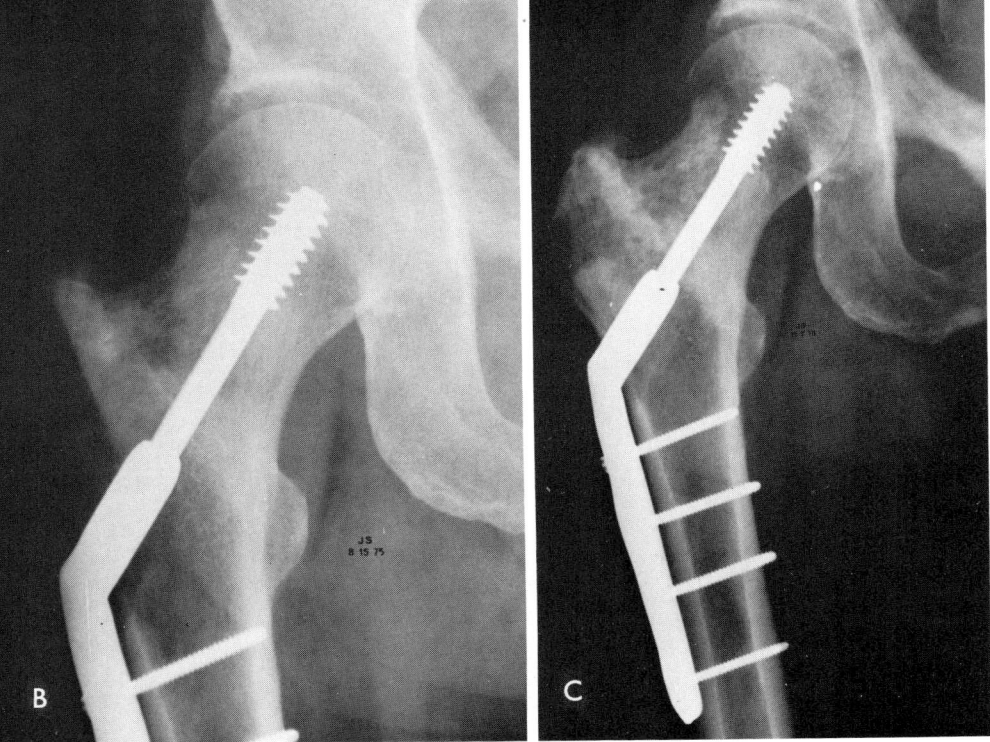

of the humerus, femur, or tibia it may be treated with a blind rodding of the involved bone with a pathological specimen from the intramedullary canal reamings. This type of operative intervention is not as major as the formal open procedure with its attendant blood loss. The author has found that occasionally an incomplete fracture will be converted to a complete fracture during the preparation of the patient for surgery. In this event, a blind rodding may still be possible with the use of an image intensifier. If this becomes too difficult, the fracture site is opened directly. In any event, the intramedullary rod has proved to be a very useful device for shaft fractures in long bones. The sliding hip compression screw is useful in the management of impending lesions in the femoral neck and intertrochanteric areas. The Zickel device is very useful for treating impending subtrochanteric pathological fractures.

REFERENCES

1. Altman, H.: Intramedullary nailing for pathological impending and actual fractures of long bones. Bull. Hosp. Joint. Dis., *13*:239–251, 1952.
2. Barry, H. C.: Paget's Disease of Bone. Edinburgh, E. & S. Livingstone, 1969.
3. Barry, H. C.: Fractures of the femur in Paget's disease of bone in Australia. J. Bone Joint Surg., *49A*:1359–1369, 1967.
4. Beals, R. K., Lawton, G. D., and Snell, W. E.: Prophylactic internal fixation of the femur in metastatic breast cancer. Cancer, *28*:1350–1354, 1971.
5. Blake, D. D.: Radiation treatment of metastatic bone disease. Clin. Orthop. Rel. Res., *73*:89–100, 1970.
6. Bonarigo, B. C., and Rubin, P.: Nonunion of pathologic fracture after radiation therapy. Radiology, *88*:889–898, 1967.
7. Bremner, R. A., and Jelliffe, A. M.: The management of pathological fracture of the major long bones from metastatic cancer. J. Bone Joint Surg., *40B*:652–659, 1958.
8. Charnley, J.: A biomechanical analysis of the use of cement to anchor the femoral head prosthesis. J. Bone Joint Surg., *47B*:354–363, 1965.
9. Coley, B. L., and Higinbotham, N. L.: Diagnosis and treatment of metastatic lesions in bone. *In*: AAOS Instructional Course Lectures. Vol. 7. Ann Arbor, J. W. Edwards, 1950, pp. 18–25.
10. Coran, A. G., Banks, H. H., Aliapoulios, M. A., and Wilson, R. E.: The management of pathologic fractures in patients with metastatic carcinoma of the breast. Surg. Gynecol. Obstet., *127*:1225–1230, 1968.
11. Devas, M. B., Dickson, J. W., and Jelliffe, A. M.: Pathological fractures: Treatment by internal fixation and irradiation. Lancet, *2*:484–487, 1956.
12. Douglass, H. D., Jr., Shukla, S. K., and Mindell, E.: Treatment of pathological fractures of long bones excluding those due to breast cancer. J. Bone Joint Surg., *58A*:1055–1060, 1976.
13. Enis, J. E., Hall, M. F., and Sarmiento, A.: Methylmethacrylate in neoplastic bone destruction. *In*: The Hip. Proceedings of the Hip Society. St. Louis, C. V. Mosby, 1973, pp. 118–138.
14. Enneking, W. F.: Local resection of malignant lesions. J. Bone Joint Surg., *48A*:991–1007, 1966.
15. Fidler, M.: Prophylactic internal fixation of secondary neoplastic deposits in long bones. Br. Med. J., *1*:341–343, 1973.
16. Fitts, W. T., Jr., Roberts, B., and Ravdin, I. S.: Fractures in metastatic carcinoma. Am. J. Surg., *85*:282–289, 1953.
17. Francis, K. C.: The role of amputation in the treatment of metastatic bone cancer. Clin. Orthop. Rel. Res., *73*:61–63, 1970.
18. Francis, K. C.: The treatment of metastatic fractures with internal fixation. Am. J. Surg., *97*:484–487, 1959.
19. Francis, K. C., Higinbotham, N. L., Carroll, R. E., et al.: The treatment of pathological fractures of the femoral neck by resection. J. Trauma, *2*:465–473, 1962.
20. Griffiths, D. L.: Orthopaedic aspects of myelomatosis. J. Bone Joint Surg., *48B*:703–728, 1966.
21. Harrington, K. D., Johnston, J. O., Turner, R. H., and Green, D. L.: The use of methylmethacrylate as an adjunct in the internal fixation of malignant neoplastic fractures. J. Bone Joint Surg., *54A*:1665–1676, 1972.
22. Harrington, K. D., Sim, F. H., Enis, J. E., et al.: Methylmethacrylate as an adjunct in internal fixation of pathological fractures. Experience with three hundred and seventy-five cases. J. Bone Joint Surg., *58A*:1047–1054, 1976.
23. Heppenstall, R. B., and Brighton, C. T.: Fracture healing in the presence of anemia. Clin. Orthop. Rel. Res., *123*:253–258, 1977.
24. Higinbotham, N. L., and Marcove, R. C.: The management of pathological fractures. J. Trauma, *5*:792–798, 1965.
25. Koskinen, E. V. S., and Nieminen, R. A.: Surgical treatment of metastatic pathological fracture of major long bones. Acta Orthop. Scand., *44*:539–549, 1973.
26. Leabhart, J. W., and Bonfiglio, M.: The treatment of irradiation fracture of the femoral neck. J. Bone Joint Surg., *43A*:1056–1067, 1961.
27. MacAusland, W. R., Jr., and Wyman, E. T., Jr.: Management of metastatic pathological fractures. Clin. Orthop. Rel. Res., *73*:39–51, 1970.
28. Marcove, R. C., and Yang, D. J.: Survival times after treatment of pathologic fractures. Cancer, *20*:2154–2158, 1967.
29. Martin, N. S., and Williamson, J.: The role of surgery in the treatment of malignant tumors of the spine. J. Bone Joint Surg., *52B*:227–237, 1970.
30. Mickelson, M. R., and Bonfiglio, M.: Pathological fractures in the proximal part of the femur

treated by Zickel-nail fixation. J. Bone Joint Surg., 58A:1067–1070, 1976.

31. Milkman, L. A.: Multiple spontaneous idiopathic symmetrical fractures. Am. J. Roentgenol., 32:622–784, 1934.

32. Murray, J. A., and Parrish, F. F.: Surgical treatment of secondary neoplastic fractures about the hip. Orthop. Clin. North Am., 5:887–901, 1974.

33. Murray, J. A., Bruels, M. C., and Lindberg, R. D.: Irradiation of polymethylmethacrylate. In vitro gamma radiation effect. J. Bone Joint Surg., 56A:311–312, 1974.

34. Nicholas, J. A., Wilson, P. D., and Frieberger, R.: Pathological fractures of the spine: etiology and diagnosis. J. Bone Joint Surg., 42A:127–137, 1960.

35. Parrish, F. F.: Treatment of bone tumors by total excision and replacement with massive autologus grafts. J. Bone Joint Surg., 48A:968–990, 1966.

36. Parrish, F. F., and Murray, J. A.: Surgical treatment for secondary neoplastic fractures. J. Bone Joint Surg., 52A:665–686, 1970.

37. Patterson, R. L., Jr., and Eichenholtz, W.: Man-agement of patients with pathological fractures. J. Bone Joint Surg., 37A:1119, 1955.

38. Poigenfurst, J., Marcove, R. C., and Miller, T. R.: Surgical treatment of fractures through metastases in the proximal femur. J. Bone Joint Surg., 50B:743–756, 1968.

39. Rose, C. A.: A critique of modern methods of diagnosis and treatment of osteoporosis. Clin. Orthop. Rel. Res., 35:17–42, 1967.

40. Sim, F. H., Daugherty, T. W., and Ivins, J. C.: The adjunctive use of methylmethacrylate in fixation of pathological fractures. J. Bone Joint Surg., 56A:40–47, 1974.

41. Stubbs, B. E., Matthews, L. S., and Sonstegard, D. A.: Experimental fixation of fractures of the femur with methyl methacrylate. J. Bone Joint Surg., 57A:317–321, 1975.

42. Takita, H., and Watne, A. L.: Operative treatment of pathologic fractures. Surg. Gynecol. Obstet., 116:683–692, 1963.

43. Zickel, R. E., and Mouradian, W. H.: Intramedullary fixation of pathological fractures and lesions of the subtrochanteric region of the femur. J. Bone Joint Surg., 58A:1061–1066, 1976.

JAMES M. MORRIS, M.D.

29 _____ *Stress*
Fractures

INTRODUCTION

Stress fractures are fractures in which no initial overt break occurs as a result of a single traumatic incident. Rather, there is a gradual alteration of the bone caused by repeated submaximal and usually unaccustomed stresses, which may or may not eventually result in a complete fracture. There is generally no audible or subjective sensation of fracture, and therefore it is not suspected. As a result of long experience with military trainees, physicians in the past used the terms "fatigue" or "march" fracture to refer to the fracture of a metatarsal associated with prolonged walking, marching, or running. Similar fractures occurring in other bones, such as the calcaneus, tibia, fibula, femur, and pelvis, were less well known and until fairly recently were often not recognized.

Although experience with stress fractures is most rapidly acquired in a basic training center, these fractures are by no means limited to military personnel. Any person engaging in an unaccustomed vigorous physical activity over a period of time is a prime subject. Thus the ballet dancer, the weekend hunter or fisherman, the eager athlete at the beginning of the season, and the young student working toward a gold medal in a physical fitness program may all develop such injuries.

Stress fractures also are not unusual in osteoporotic bone, that is, in postmenopausal females or after disuse. In these individuals, the bone is not "abnormal"; however, as Devas[1] has pointed out, there may be a discrepancy in muscle strength com-

pared with bone strength at any given time, which may result in a stress fracture. Even minor increases in exertion may lead to a stress fracture.

Painful, swollen feet in soldiers after long marches were first described in 1855 by Breithaupt, a German military surgeon.[2] He believed that this condition was a traumatic inflammatory reaction in tendon sheaths and named it *Fussgeschwulst*. Weisbach[3] believed that the lesion was in the ligaments and in 1877 coined the term "syndesmitis metatarsea." Pauzat[4] also pointed out its occurrence in soldiers and noted that there was palpable periosteal proliferation on the second, third, or fourth metatarsals, the second being most common. After these reports, other observers suggested a variety of explanations for this lesion. In 1897 Stechow,[5] of the Prussian Guard in Madrid, using the newly discovered roentgen ray, defined the nature of the disorder. He reported on the roentgen examination of 36 patients and found that metatarsal fracture was the basic lesion. Many reports then followed; some investigators held that a fracture always occurred, while others noted that in a certain number of cases no fracture developed. The descriptions of these lesions are now easily recognized to be those of stress or fatigue fractures.

It was gradually recognized that such fractures occurred in other bones. In 1905 Blecher[6] first reported on a case involving the femoral neck. Aleman[7] described a similar lesion in the tibia in 1929, and Burrows[8, 9] discussed cases of fatigue fracture in the fibula in 1940 and 1948. Hullinger[10] reported 53 cases of fracture of the calcaneus in 1944. In 1966 Blickenstaff and Morris[11] reported a series of femoral neck fractures in recruits undergoing basic training. Involvement in other areas, such as the pelvis, ulna, humerus, and ribs, has also been reported occasionally.

In the past, lack of recognition of the true nature of the causative factors led to the use of many different descriptive terms for this disorder, including swollen foot (*Fussgeschwulst*), syndesmitis metatarsea, march fracture, *Deutschländer's* disease, *pied forcé*, insufficiency fracture, overload fracture, wear-and-tear fracture, recruit's disease, periostitis ab exercitio, osteopathia itineraria, soldier's fracture, spontaneous fracture, pseudofracture, insidious fracture, and creeping fracture. The best descriptive terms for this condition are now considered to be "stress fracture" or "fatigue fracture."

ETIOLOGY

It is common knowledge that bone is remarkably sensitive to the amount of stress or use to which it is subjected and that it reflects this stress. Disuse or immobilization results in rapid osteoclastic resorption followed by a decrease in osteoblastic activity, which is only slowly revealed by roentgenograms. Less easy to explain is the fact that excessive use, as in the case of stress fracture, also leads initially to resorption of bone.

It follows from the concept of a stress fracture (which is essentially a process rather than an event) that it is extremely difficult, if not impossible, to determine the exact moment at which the process begins, or even the precise nature of the change in bone that may be considered the initial event. In all of the series reviewed, the reported time sequence was calculated as beginning with the onset of symptoms—usually pain. Yet in all true stress fractures such pain must be considered the result of a process already under way, in the course of which a stage characterized by at least some osteoporosis has already been reached.

The matter is complicated still further by the normal physiological processes in the bones of young people. In the age group most commonly affected by stress fractures (18 to 28 years), the bones are still undergoing internal remodeling of circumferential lamellar bone into adult osteonal bone. For new osteons to be laid down, some of the existing osteons and the circumferential lamellar bone must be removed. Thus osteoclastic resorption of bone and replacement by new bone are entirely normal processes at this age. When repeated submaximal stresses are applied to such bones the normal process appears to be accelerated. However, resorption occurs more rapidly than replacement, so that local osteoporosis, followed by callus reinforcement, results.

From Johnson and co-workers' studies of pathology[12] and from my own critical evaluation of many roentgenograms, it seems that the sequence of events is as follows: During the first 5 to 14 days of symptoms, the bone undergoes active osteoclastic resorption, resulting in demonstrable local osteoporosis. Periosteal and endosteal callus formation then begin. Excessive stress during the stages of osteoporosis or early callus formation may result in a cortical crack or a complete fracture. If a fracture line develops, it does so during the peak period of osteoporosis, before sufficient callus is present. If the stress is discontinued early, however, a roentgenographically visible fracture usually does not occur. Reconstitution of the osteoporotic cortex by osteon formation gradually takes place over a period of several months.

Whenever a fatigue fracture is encountered, the quality of the bone is immediately open to question. Although the affected bone may have some innate defects in crystalline structure, trabecular orientation, or ground substance, it is not possible to detect, by the gross clinical methods of evaluation now available, any abnormality of bone affected by stress fracture.

AREAS OF INVOLVEMENT

Stress or fatigue fracture of the os calcis or metatarsal in a recruit during basic military training is a relatively frequent occurrence and is generally readily recognized. However, when this type of fracture occurs in other bones, such as the tibial or femoral shafts, the femoral neck, or the ischiopubic

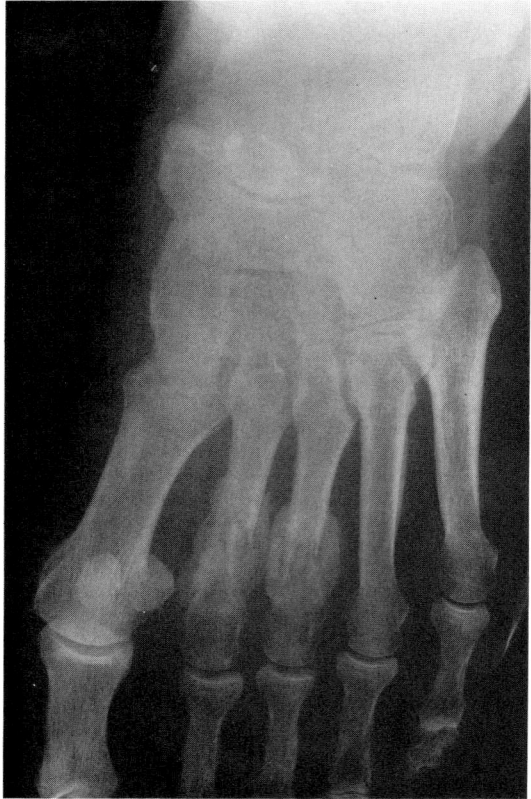

Figure 29–1 Healed stress fractures six to seven weeks after onset of symptoms in a young male training for a marathon run.

ramus, it may be difficult to make an accurate diagnosis. Stress fractures of the tibia have been mistakenly diagnosed as "tibialis anterior syndrome," shin splints, "growing" pains, and pes anserinus bursitis. Fractures of the femoral neck have been misdiagnosed as synovitis of the hip, muscle strains, gluteal bursitis, and other ailments.

In military recruits the metatarsal, os calcis, and medial tibial plateau are the most commonly encountered sites of stress fracture (Fig. 29–1); less frequently, fractures occur in the femoral neck and shaft, the tibial and fibular shafts, and the ischiopubic rami. Os calcis and medial tibial plateau fractures are bilateral in 50 per cent or more of cases.

While stress fractures are most frequently seen in men 18 to 25 years of age in basic military training, certain other very physically active groups are prone to stress

fractures, usually in specific areas (Fig. 29–2). For example, ballet dancers are subject to tibial shaft fractures; runners are especially susceptible to femoral neck and

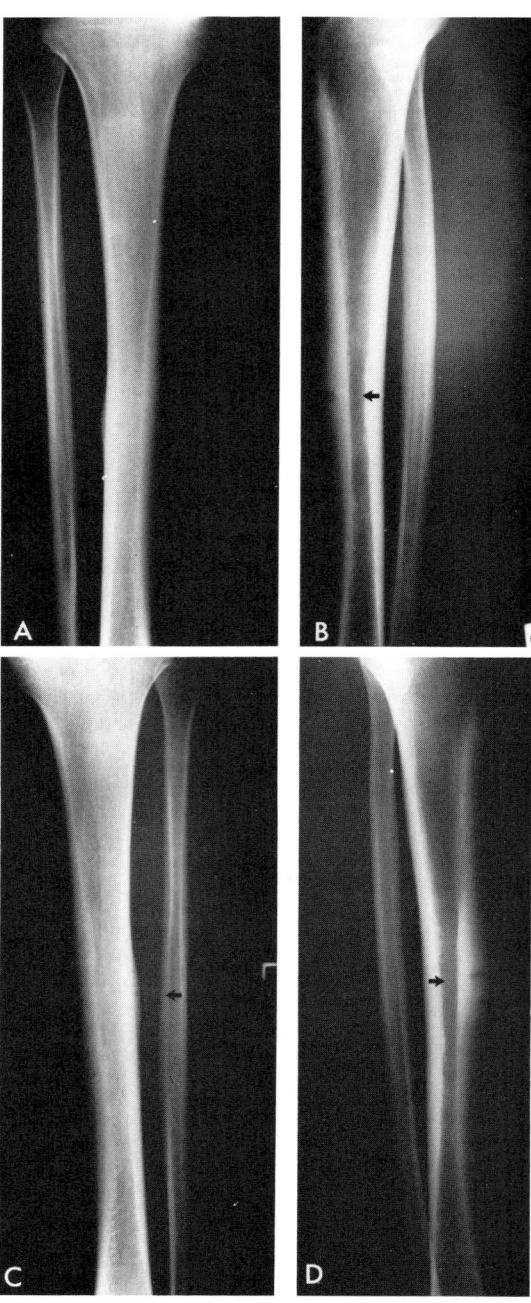

Figure 29–2 *A* and *B.* Stress fracture of the right midtibia in a ballet dancer; the roentgenograms were obtained several weeks following onset of symptoms. *C.* and *D.* Similar findings were noted on roentgenograms obtained eight months later on the opposite extremity.

proximal femoral shaft fractures; and gymnasts and down linemen have been noted to develop fractures of the pars interarticularis (spondylolysis) as a result of excessive lumbar lordotic stresses.

Stress fractures have been described in patients of all ages from 15 months to over 70 years and are being recognized and diagnosed more frequently among children and the elderly than before. In recent years a significant number of cases have been described in children, generally in those who have engaged in strenuous activity. Among these cases may be included "Little League elbow," a traction type of stress fracture. So-called growing pains in children may in reality be aborted stress fractures; in the upper part of the tibia, at the point of maximal stress, there is frequently later roentgenographic evidence of buttressing in the medial, lateral, or posterior aspect of the bone. This may be the result of slow development and healing of a stress fracture; it is similar to the reaction that is known to occur with muscle pull in certain areas over a long period of time. An increased number of fractures have also been diagnosed among the elderly, who presumably have more osteoporotic bone. The distal tibia and fibula and the ischiopubic ramus are the most frequently encountered areas of involvement in these patients.

SYMPTOMS AND PHYSICAL FINDINGS

Pain is the universal complaint of persons affected by a stress fracture. However, because of the frequently insidious onset of discomfort and pain, there may be a considerable interval between the onset of symptoms and the request for medical consultation. This period depends on the severity of the discomfort, and no doubt on the activity in which the patient is engaged (Fig. 29–3). During military training the avoidance of medical treatment is sometimes a point of honor, and the athlete, in the belief that he is simply "out of shape," may assume that such discomfort is a consequence of the early phases of athletic training. Because of the lack of specific trauma, the affected person usually fails to realize the severity of the condition and does not immediately

seek medical advice. For these reasons, it is common for a week or more to elapse between the onset of symptoms and the initial medical consultation.

In almost all instances the pain is aggravated by such activities as running and marching, when, as is usually the case, the lower limb is affected. Rest generally relieves the discomfort, though on occasion there may be aching discomfort during rest. Generally the pain is sharply localized within a specific and circumscribed area, which is tender to palpation or pressure.

Swelling, occasionally to the point of pitting edema, is the next most frequently encountered clinical finding upon physical examination. It is often rather diffuse, as in the case of a stress fracture of a metatarsal bone, when the entire dorsum of the foot may be swollen. Initially, the swelling is reduced only slightly by elevation of the extremity for short periods. Less commonly, the affected area is erythematous with an associated elevation in temperature on palpation.

When the fracture occurs near a joint, as in fractures of the femoral neck or of the distal portion of the fibula (Fig. 29–4), passive movement of the adjacent joint to the extremes of its range of motion generally causes discomfort in the region of the fracture. This, however, is not a constant finding. In addition, there may be swelling and effusion of the adjacent joint.

LABORATORY FINDINGS

With stress fractures, systemic responses, such as fever, elevated white blood cell count, and elevated sedimentation rate, are absent, and if occasionally noted are undoubtedly incidental and unrelated. Results of laboratory tests such as those for blood calcium, phosphorus, and alkaline phosphatase levels have been reported or examined on many occasions and have always been within normal limits.

ROENTGENOGRAPHIC ASPECTS

Although the diagnosis of stress fracture may be reasonably established by an appropriate history in association with the

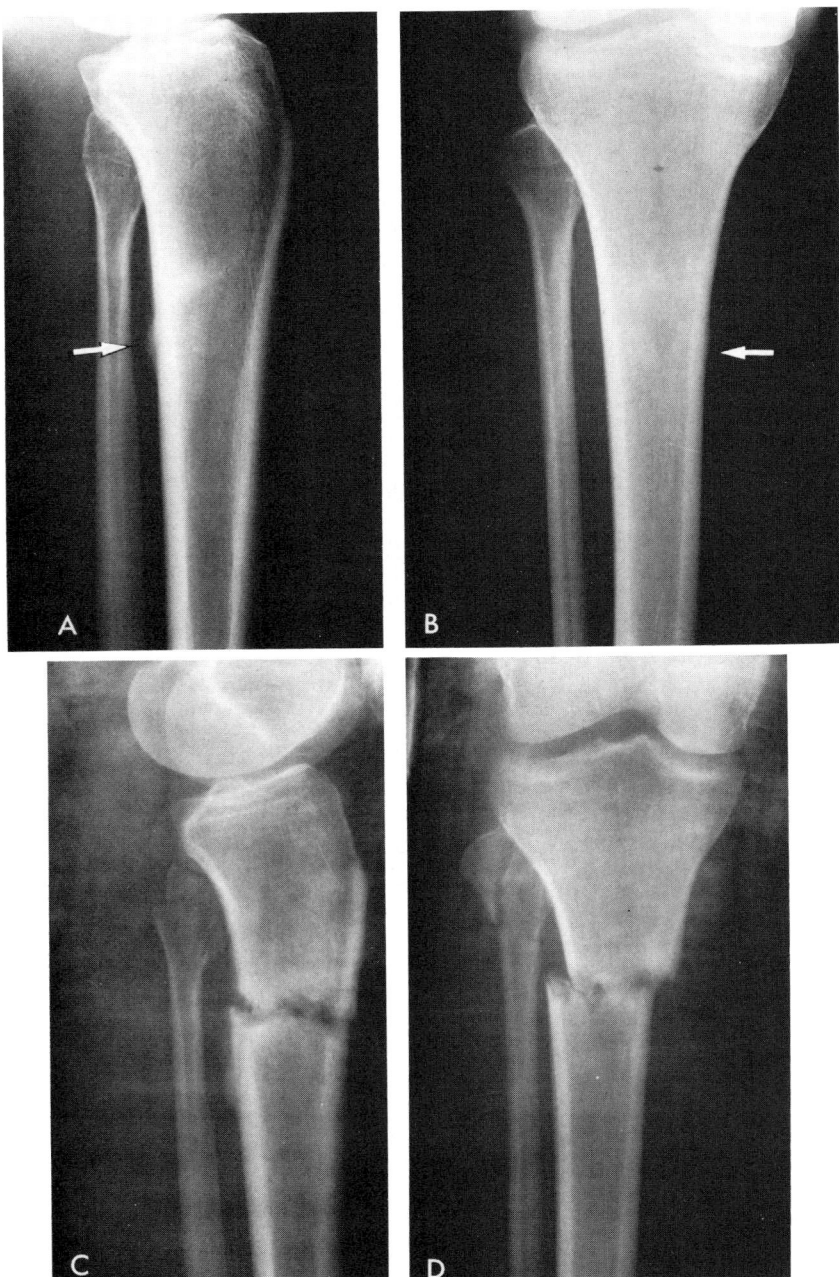

Figure 29–3 A and B. After jogging one to two weeks, a young nurse developed symptoms; she continued her activity, however, and after five weeks obtained these roentgenograms. She was placed on crutches, but after one month resumed her activities because of subsidence of symptoms. C and D. On the first day of skiing she sustained a minor twisting injury of the tibia, resulting in a complete fracture through the area of the previous stress fracture. She was subsequently placed in a long leg cast.

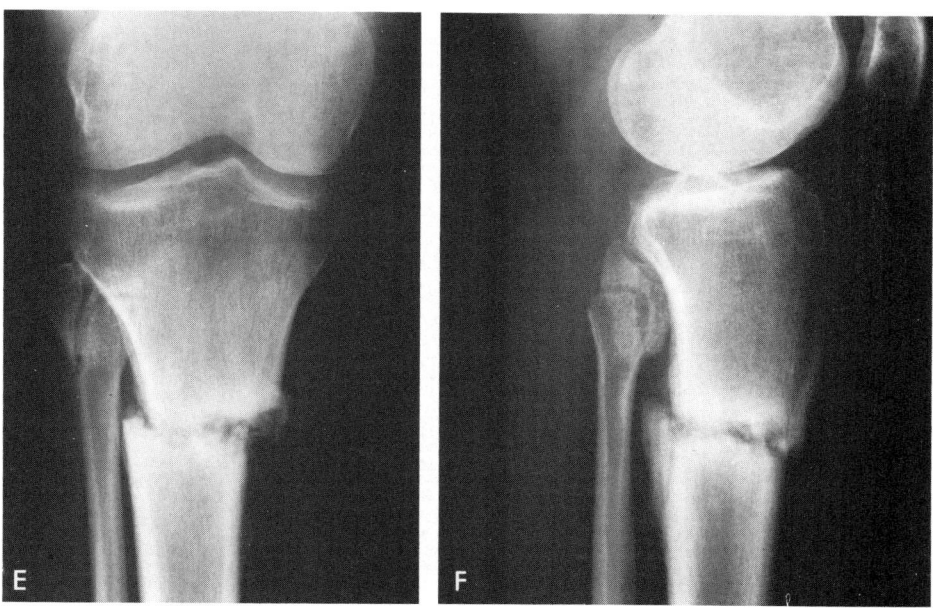

Figure 29–3 Continued. E and F. Four months later, roentgenograms demonstrate a delayed union and a potential nonunion.

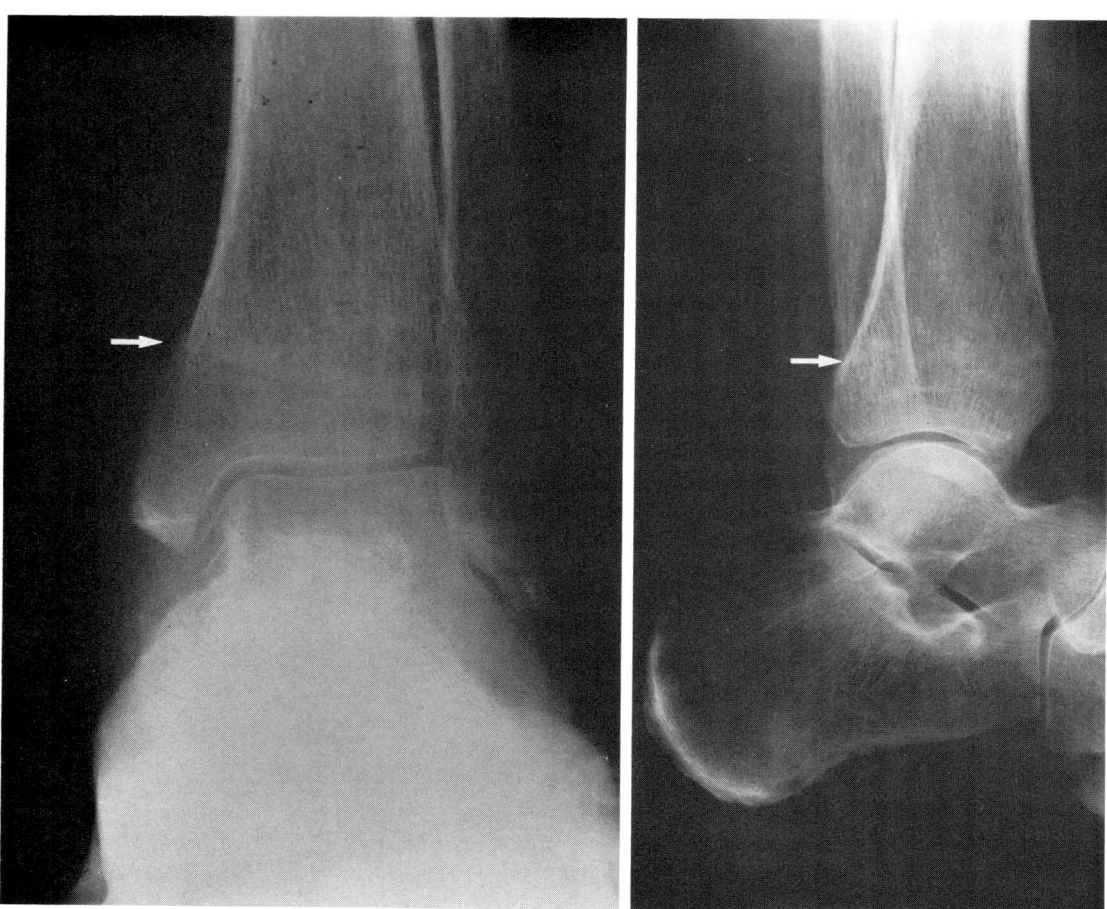

Figure 29–4 A and B. Stress fracture through distal tibia in a middle-aged female after unaccustomed activity. Roentgenograms obtained two and one-half weeks after onset of symptoms.

symptoms and findings of localized pain, tenderness, and edema over the affected bone, confirmation depends on the progressive changes of the disorder as observed roentgenographically. It should be pointed out, however, that in all probability stress reactions frequently fail to develop the diagnostic roentgenographic findings because of the subsidence of the initiating stress. This may account for the so-called, poorly explained growing pains of the child and the nonspecific "shin splints" or "ligamentous strains" seen in the athlete and weekend outdoorsman.

If roentgenograms are obtained shortly after the onset of symptoms, the bony architecture generally appears completely normal (Fig. 29–5). Quite frequently, changes are not discernible on the roentgenogram until 14 to 21 days after the first symptoms. At this point, subperiosteal or endosteal callus formation, with or without a small cortical crack, may be the first observable change. The progression of the stress fracture, however, depends on its severity as well as on the particular bone involved. In the case of the metatarsal stress fracture, the crack in the cortex may be evident at the time of onset of symptoms, whereas subperiosteal bone proliferation may become evident only after two weeks (Fig. 29–6). In the case of fractures of cancellous bone, such as the calcaneus, the tibial plateau, or the distal portion of the femur, progressive subperiosteal and endosteal callus may be the only finding. It must be emphasized that a definite fracture line or crack need not be present for the diagnosis of a stress reaction or of a fracture. The absence of a fracture line frequently leads to the confusion of this lesion with a primary sarcoma of bone. In stress fractures of the femoral neck or the shafts of the femur and tibia, the subperiosteal and endosteal callus formation may be followed by the development of a true fracture—partial or complete—through the bone two to three weeks after the onset of symptoms. Subsequently, the callus formation progresses slowly to a fusiform area of maturing callus, which leads to healing of the fracture. This may require a period of several weeks. Each bone—in fact, each area of a particular bone affected by the stress fracture—appears to have its own pattern or patterns of callus formation and repair. As a general rule, however, the cortex of the shaft of a bone heals by subperiosteal new bone, whereas the metaphyseal cancellous bone heals by proliferation of endosteal new bone (medullary sclerosis) (Fig. 29–7).

It should be pointed out again that because of the length of time between the onset of symptoms and the development of findings that are visible roentgenographi-

Text continued on page 907.

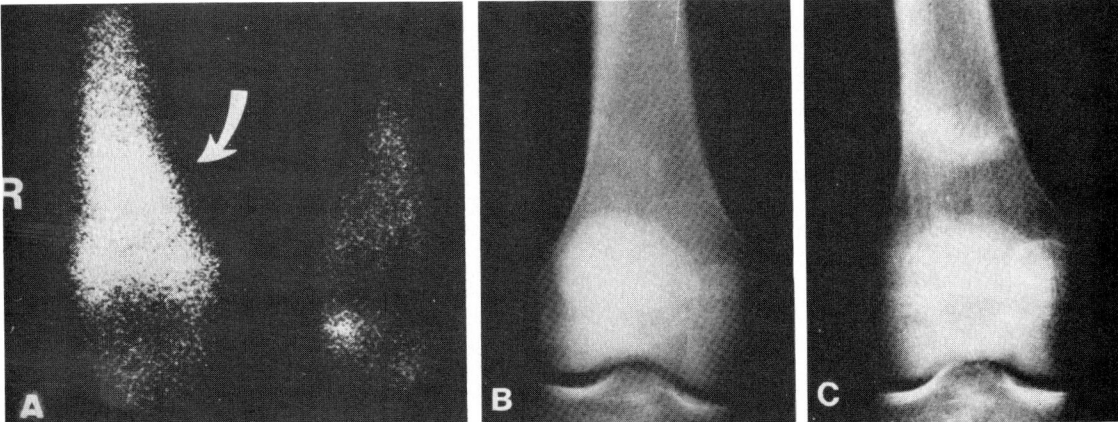

Figure 29–5   A. Stress fracture of the distal right femur. Anterior view shows increased radioactivity (*arrow*) B. Anteroposterior roentgenogram taken at the same time, interpreted to be normal. C. Two weeks later, roentgenogram demonstrates sclerosis and periosteal reaction secondary to a femoral stress fracture. (Courtesy of Geslien, G. E., Thrall, J. H., Espinosa, J. L., et al. and *Radiology*. Early detection of stress fractures using ^{99m}Tc-polyphosphate. Radiology, *121*:683–687, 1976.)

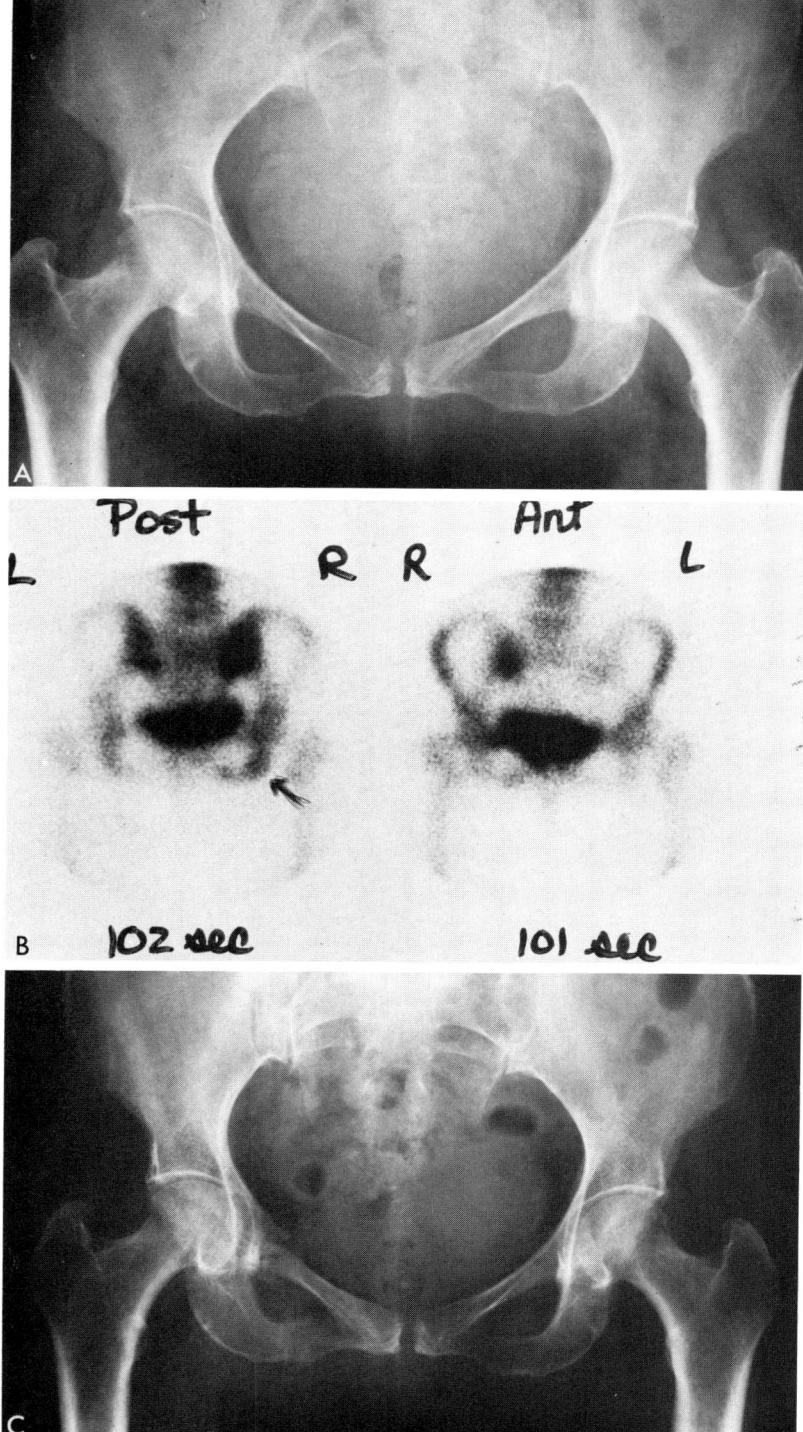

Figure 29–6   A. This patient had onset of pain in the right groin, with radiation into the right medial thigh, after prolonged repetitive stooping and bending while cleaning an attic. The initial roentgenogram was negative. *B.* Bone scan demonstrates increased activity in the ischiopubic ramus on the right. A presumptive diagnosis of stress fracture was made. *C.* A roentgenogram taken two months later demonstrates a well-developed stress fracture of the ischiopubic ramus. Delayed union occurred.

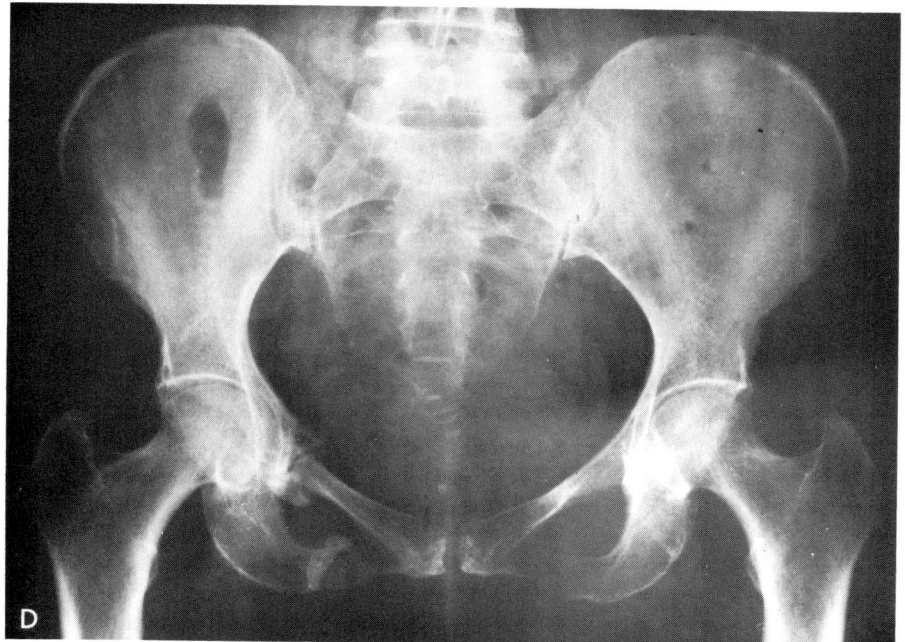

Figure 29–6 Continued.   D, Eight months after onset of symptoms.

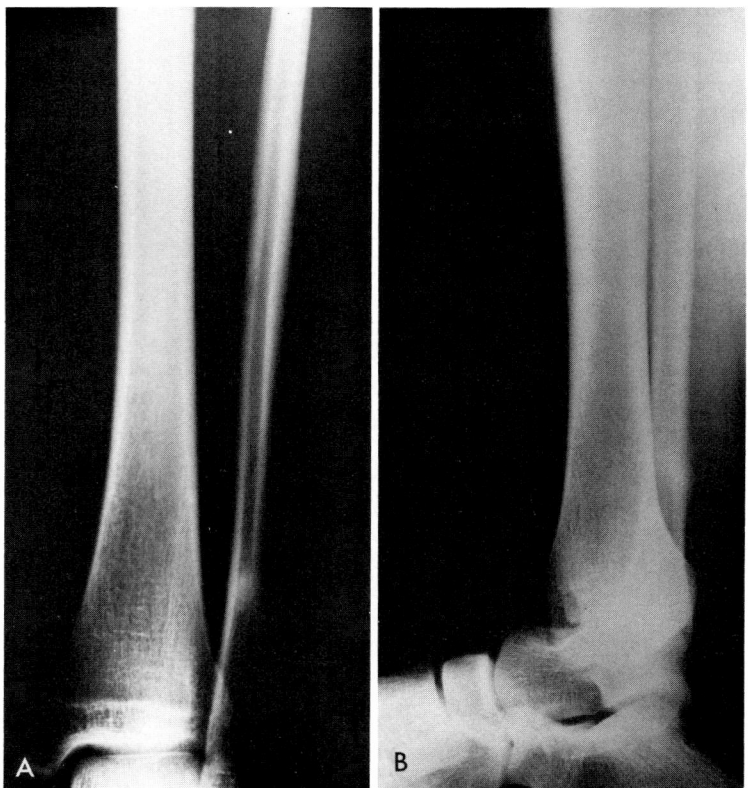

Figure 29-7   A and B. Typical stress fracture of the distal fibula, seen in runners and ice skaters especially.

cally, many cases of fatigue fracture are completely missed or misdiagnosed. This is probably particularly true in civilian practice, because the expense of roentgenograms and repeat examinations limits follow-up examination in suspected cases. Frequently, roentgenograms are taken at the time of onset of pain that may or may not be due to stress fracture. However, because subsequent rest of the involved part relieves the symptoms, no further roentgenograms are made; in many cases such x-rays might have demonstrated the true nature of the disorder. I have seen several cases in military personnel that proved to be stress fractures which would not have had serial roentgenograms in civilian practice. The diagnosis would therefore have been missed. One can only speculate about the incidence of such cases.

In recent years, the use of ^{99m}Tc-polyphosphate scintigraphy has been valuable in the early detection of stress fractures. The unique ability of these compounds to accumulate primarily in areas of high metabolic activity and blood flow in bone makes them useful in the detection of early stress fractures that cannot be demonstrated by roentgenograms.

Geslien and co-workers[13] studied 200 consecutive patients between the ages of 17 and 30 years who had clinically suspected stress fractures. Initial roentgenograms of the painful or suspected area and those taken two to three weeks later were correlated with the radionuclide images. A total of 188 stress fractures in 140 patients were initially detected by bone imaging and later confirmed by roentgenograms within two to three weeks. Sixty per cent of the roentgenograms showed no evidence of stress fracture at the time of positive bone image. In those cases that demonstrated positive roentgenograms at the time of scintigraphy, two to three weeks had elapsed between the onset of symptoms and the scan.

A small number of false-positive results were noted. These occurred mainly in the medial tibial plateau. In 10 out of 78 cases, there was intense accumulation of isotope, but the patients were asymptomatic in that area and subsequent roentgenograms were negative. Accelerated bone remodeling associated with repeated stress does not always result in a stress fracture. If the exercise or stress is reduced, osteonal bone reinforces the weakened remodeled bone enough to prevent fracture. In such cases the roentgenogram is normal and the scan is positive, because the increased blood flow and surface area produced by the remodeling process allow increased chemisorption of polyphosphate. This demonstrates the sensitivity and nonspecificity of bone scintigraphy and the need for confirmatory roentgenograms.

CLINICAL MANAGEMENT

Treatment of these fractures in general is conservative and consists simply of reduced activity or rest, and at times immobilization of the affected part. In most instances, mere limitation of activity results in complete healing of the fracture without sequelae (Fig. 29–8). This is particularly true of fractures of the metatarsals, calcaneus, fibula, and proximal portion of the tibia. These most common types of stress fracture may also require a period of partial weight bearing or non–weight bearing, or in some cases immobilization for a period of two to six weeks, depending on the severity of the symptoms. Symptoms generally disappear in two to ten weeks, and in none of these cases have serious sequelae been seen.

However, stress fractures of the tibial shaft, the femoral shaft, and particularly the femoral neck demand careful supervision and treatment. Fractures of the tibial and femoral shafts may progress and become displaced, which may then result in delayed union and prolonged incapacitation. These fractures require a sufficient period of partial weight bearing, non–weight bearing, or plaster immobilization to allow adequate healing of the fracture. Generally this takes from 10 to 16 weeks, depending on the severity of the fracture as determined by roentgenographic evidence. These findings may range from subperiosteal and endosteal callus to complete fracture of the bone.

Fractures of the femoral neck are by far the most serious and significant of all stress fractures (Fig. 29–9). Even for the simplest undisplaced fractures, with evidence of only subperiosteal and endosteal callus formation, non–weight bearing for a period

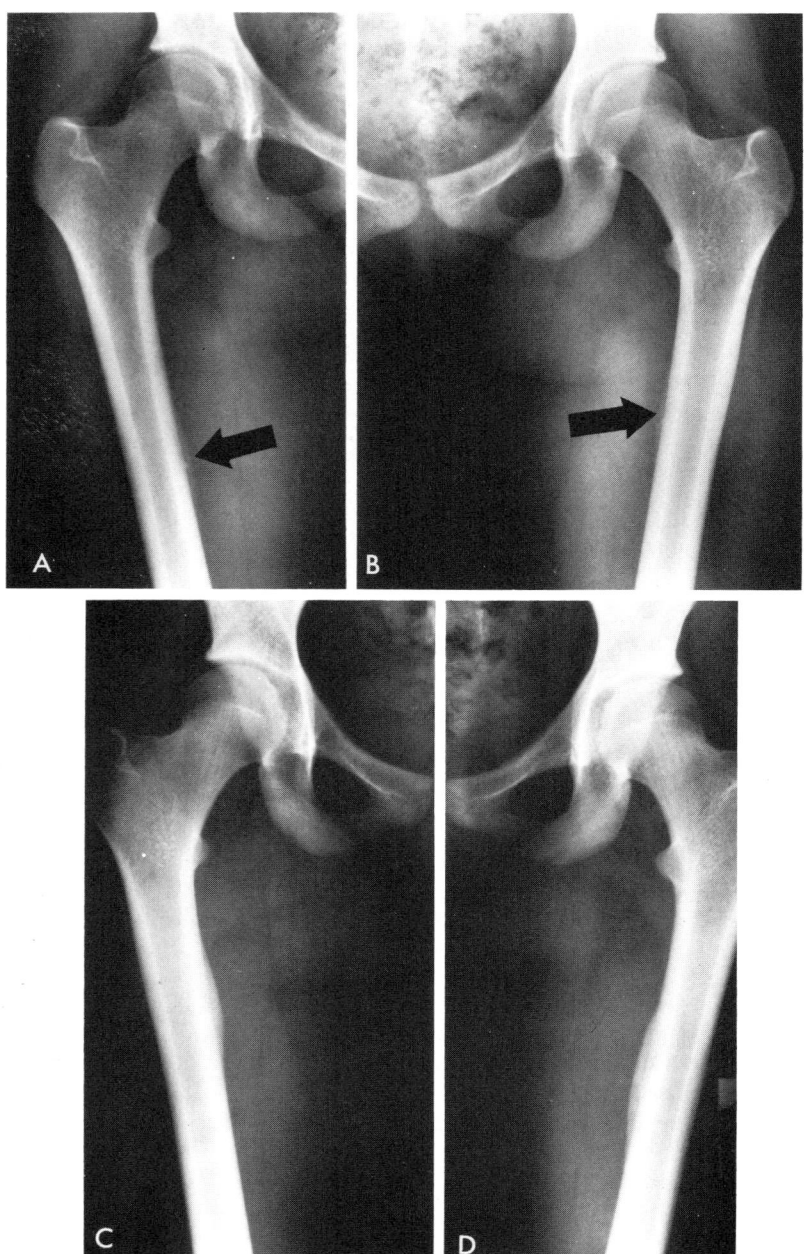

Figure 29-8   *A* and *B.* A 17-year-old female marathon runner who after seven to eight weeks of running developed increasing pain in both thighs. Roentgenograms demonstrated periosteal elevation, and the diagnosis of possible bone tumor was entertained. *C* and *D.* Subsequent films one month later demonstrated periosteal ossification, indicative of stress fracture. She had been running up to 10 to 15 miles a day, and despite her pain persisted in the exercises. Fortunately, a displaced fracture did not occur.

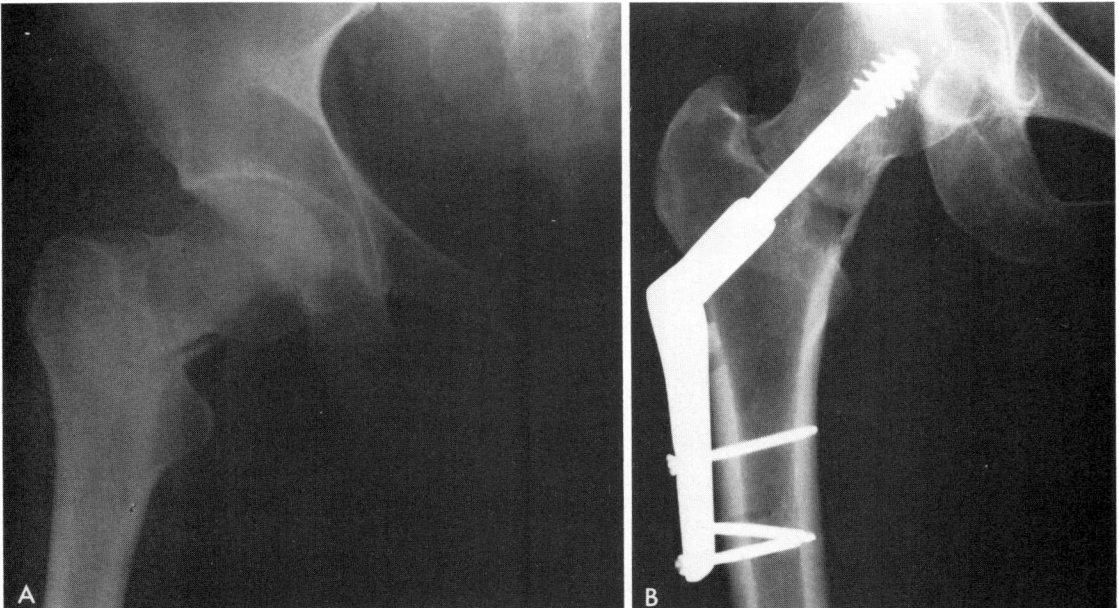

Figure 29–9   A. A 25-year-old jogger presented at the orthopedic clinic after a two-week period of jogging with increasing pain in the right groin. Diagnosis of a muscle strain was made, and she was advised to remain non–weight-bearing on crutches. She discarded the crutches, however, and in crossing a street suffered severe pain in the hip and fell to the ground. Subsequent roentgenograms demonstrated this fracture. *B*. Roentgenograms taken at the time of the internal fixation demonstrated the characteristic findings of osteoporosis at the femoral neck fracture site, indicative of a stress fracture. Prognosis in such cases, especially in younger individuals, is guarded.

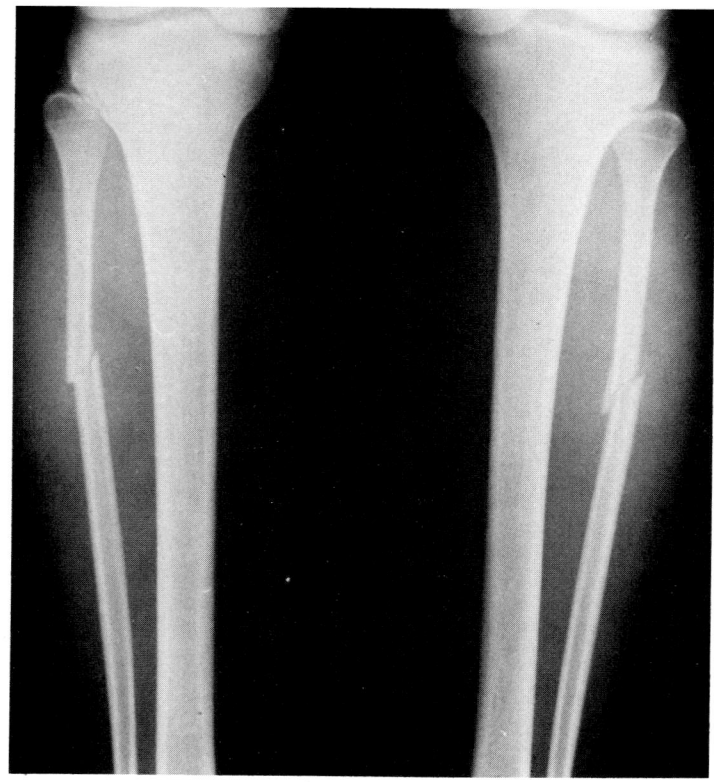

Figure 29–10   High bilateral stress fractures of the fibula, frequently associated with air troop exercises or jumping exercises. Fibular fractures are apparently associated with muscular action, since the bone is essentially non–weight-bearing.

of three to eight weeks is indicated. If the stress fracture develops to the point of displacement, operative reduction and internal fixation are necessary. The outcome of complete fracture of the femoral neck treated by reduction and internal fixation is, in the majority of cases, poor. Severe and prolonged incapacitation, nonunion, and aseptic necrosis are not uncommon. Thus extreme caution and conservatism must be exercised in the handling of this type of stress fracture. Based on my experience with displaced femoral neck fractures in young military recruits, I feel that if even a slight cortical crack occurs, or if pain is not controlled by minimizing weight bearing, internal fixation should be performed at once (Fig. 29–10).

SUMMARY

The prognosis for complete recovery from stress fractures is generally excellent. In all stress fractures, except for some of the tibial shaft, femoral shaft, and femoral neck, healing is eventually complete and uncomplicated. This is true despite the fact that the fractures may occasionally be unrecognized or inadequately treated. The period of debility of course depends on the treatment. In general, the person with a stress fracture naturally and instinctively rests the affected part, so that adequate healing takes place with time. Only in rare instances has delayed union of a fracture in a bone such as the fibula been described. Nonunion of the tibia has to my knowledge not been described, but is a possibility. Fractures of the femoral shaft and especially

of the femoral neck have led to nonunion and necessitated open reduction and internal fixation; in this one type the sequelae have occasionally been disastrous.

REFERENCES

1. Devas, M.: Stress Fractures. Edinburgh, Churchill Livingstone, 1975.
2. Breithaupt: Zur Pathologie des menschlichen Fusses. Med. Z., 24:169, 1855; 24:175, 1855.
3. Weisbach: Die sogenannte "Fussgeschwulst," Syndesmitis metatarsea, der Infanteristen in Folge von anstrengenden Märschen. Deutsch. Mil.-ärtzl. Z., 6:551, 1887.
4. Pauzat, J. E.: De la périostite ostéoplastique des métatarsiens à la suite des marches. Arch. Med. Pharm. Mil., 10:337, 1887.
5. Stechow: Fussoedem und Röntgenstrahlen. Deutsch. Mil.-ärztl. Z., 26:465, 1897.
6. Blecher, A.: Über den Einfluss des Parademarsches auf die Entstehung der Fussgeschwulst. Med. Klin., 1:305, 1905.
7. Aleman, O.: Tumors of foot from long marches (syndesmitis metatarsea). T. Mil. Hälsov., 54:191, 1929.
8. Burrows, H. J.: Spontaneous fracture of the apparently normal fibula in its lowest third. Br. J. Surg., 28:82, 1940.
9. Burrows, H. J.: Fatigue fractures of the fibula. J. Bone Joint Surg., 30B:266, 1948.
10. Hullinger, C. W.: Insufficiency fracture of the calcaneus: similar to march fracture of the metatarsal. J. Bone Joint Surg., 26:751, 1944.
11. Blickenstaff, L. D., and Morris, J. M.: Fatigue fractures of the femoral neck. J. Bone Joint Surg., 48A:1031, 1966.
12. Johnson, L. C., Stradford, H. T., Geis, R. W., Dineen, J. R., and Kerley, E. R.: Histogenesis of stress fractures. Armed Forces Institute of Pathology Annual Lectures, 1963. (Abstract in J. Bone Joint Surg., 45A:1542, 1963.)
13. Geslien, G. E., Thrall, J. H., Espinosa, J. L., and Older, R. A.: Early detection of stress fractures using ^{99m}Tc-polyphosphate. Radiology, 121:683–687, 1976.

R. BRUCE HEPPENSTALL, M.D.

30 _____ *Open Fractures and Gunshot Wounds*

Part I _____ **OPEN FRACTURES** _____

INTRODUCTION

An open fracture is by definition a break in the skin with communication of the fracture site with the outside environment. In the older literature these injuries were called compound fractures. This nomenclature should be discontinued, however, and this type of injury should be referred to as an open fracture. In this manner the simple classification of "open" versus "closed" fracture may be used. Open fractures are certainly not rare, being commonly encountered in a busy orthopedic practice. Specific management has varied over the years, but there is now a trend toward aggressive open debridement with removal of all dead tissue, and definitive treatment by delayed closure five to seven days later.

Hippocrates (460–370 B.C.) was the first to describe healing by first and second intention. It was his practice to irrigate wounds with boiled water or wine. However, he did realize the significance of an open fracture and advised expectant treatment rather than primary closure in these cases. Galen (A.D. 131–201), who is considered a disciple of

Hippocrates, taught various laboratory methods through animal experimentation. He is acknowledged to be one of the first great physiologists. Galen recognized that arteries transmit blood and that arterial blood differs from venous blood. He also believed that the purulence frequently present in open wounds is necessary for active wound repair.

It remained for Ambroise Paré (1510–1590) to demonstrate that war wounds could be treated without the use of boiling oil. He observed that certain gunshot wounds healed satisfactorily after he ran out of boiling oil. It is interesting that Paré's insight into avoiding harmful interference in surgical treatment has been epitomized by an inscription on his statue, which translates into English as follows. "I treated him, God healed him."

Joseph Lister (1827–1912) completely revolutionized surgery. In 1865 he successfully applied carbolic acid as a chemical antiseptic to an open fracture and obtained satisfactory healing. William Halsted (1852–1922) introduced the use of rubber gloves in surgery in America in 1891.

During the war years several important

912

concepts were learned, abandoned, and then relearned. It is fair to state that military experience since World War I has definitely established the importance of early active debridement and delayed closure in the management of open fractures and gunshot wounds if catastrophes are to be avoided.

MECHANISM OF INJURY

An open fracture may be produced by direct external forces or by internal forces, such as penetration of a fracture fragment through the skin. There is a marked difference between the two types of trauma. In externally applied direct trauma, there is usually significant soft tissue disruption, with gross contamination of the fracture site and the surrounding soft tissues. In general, internally applied forces do not produce as much soft tissue destruction and contamination. That is not to say that soft tissue damage and infection are absent in open injuries produced by an internal mechanism. By definition, all open fractures are contaminated. The distinction between external and internal trauma is not just academic, because the appropriate therapy may depend on which mechanism was involved in producing the injury.

PHYSICAL EXAMINATION

Since the majority of open fractures are the result of significant trauma, many patients will present with multiple-system injuries. It is extremely important to perform a complete physical examination. If a life-threatening condition exists, a quick superficial examination should be made, followed by immediate corrective measures. A patient who presents in frank shock must be treated aggressively and properly. The reader is referred to Chapter 31 for the initial evaluation and management of a multiply injured patient.

Once the life-threatening conditions have been corrected, a thorough examination of the patient should be performed. It is best to ignore the obvious open fracture at first and undertake a systematic examination, so that associated injuries will not be overlooked. It is frequently advantageous to begin with the skull and neck and progress in a distal manner.

A detailed examination of the open fracture area may be performed once the initial complete evaluation has been recorded. The state of the surrounding soft tissues at the site of the open fracture should be thoroughly assessed. It is important to specifically examine the extremity for evidence of adequate blood supply. Distal pulses should be palpated and the adequacy of the pulse pressure determined. If the pulses are not present distal to the open fracture, it is important to examine for capillary flow. The blood supply to the distal limb may still be adequate for survival despite absence of the peripheral pulses, as long as the peripheral capillary filling is sufficient. The simplest measure is to depress the nail bed and observe the capillary filling following release. Skin color and temperature are additional measures of vascular viability. A Doppler machine, if available, may be utilized to determine the adequacy of the peripheral vascular flow.

At this stage any dressing that was placed on the wound for transport should be carefully removed so that the state of the soft tissue at the open fracture site may be evaluated. In some centers it is a policy to take the patient immediately to the operating room, where under sterile conditions the dressings are removed and the wound examined. It is true that there will be less contamination with this approach. Nevertheless, it is important for the examining physician to determine the amount of soft tissue damage at the wound site in order to select the appropriate form of treatment. This is not to say that the wound should be inspected by all personnel in the emergency room, because it is common sense that the more the wound is manipulated the greater the likelihood of further contamination. Therefore, it is preferable for only one physician to remove the dressing and evaluate the wound. If there is a break in the skin in the area of bone deformity it may be assumed that this is an open fracture.

The author does not recommend palpation and exploration of the wound in the emergency room to determine whether or not the fracture communicates with the outside environment. Such exploration should be reserved for the relatively sterile conditions of the operating room. All injuries with evidence of an open fracture should receive thorough debridement in the operating room. A superficial debridement in the emergency room will frequently lead to disaster, since all the dead tissue may not be removed. The examiner should be able to determine the degree of contamination by visual inspection of the wound. The presence or absence of dirt particles and foreign matter, such as glass or lead, should be determined as well as the degree of superficial abrasion of the surrounding skin and muscle tissues. The presence of an associated burn in the surrounding area should also be recorded. The size and shape of the wound will allow the examining physician to assess the extent of soft tissue disruption.

The amount of instability at the fracture site is generally evident with any attempt at motion of the injured part. A careful examination of the joints above and below the area of open fracture should be made. In this manner an associated dislocation of the joint will not be overlooked. An example of this problem is a femoral fracture in which an associated dislocation of the hip may be missed owing to inadequate physical and roentgenographic evaluation.

ROENTGENOGRAPHIC EXAMINATION

The initial roentgenographic evaluation of the open fracture requires standard anteroposterior and lateral views of the fractured osseous segment. These views must also include the proximal and distal joints. It is important to bear this point in mind in order to decrease the incidence of "missed associated dislocations." If the proximal and distal joints are not visualized in the standard roentgenograms of the fracture, separate views of the appropriate joint structures must be obtained. Occasionally it is beneficial to take oblique roentgenograms of the fracture site in order to assess the degree of comminution present.

Since many of these patients have other associated injuries, it is extremely important to obtain sufficient roentgenographic examination of the involved structures. This may call for obtaining the following: chest film, kidney, ureter, and bladder (KUB) film, intravenous pyelogram (IVP) if necessary, roentgenograms of the cervical and thoracolumbar spine, and arteriograms of the injured limb, if indicated. Although this may require several roentgenographic studies for full evaluation, it is better to obtain all the necessary roentgenographic evidence initially than to send the patient to the radiology department for further studies at a later date.

If the hospital is equipped with adequate roentgenographic equipment and operating room personnel the patient may be transferred from the emergency room to the operating room for proper roentgenographic evaluation prior to surgical debridement. However, most hospitals are not this fully equipped, and patients must still be transported to the radiology department for evaluation prior to definitive operative treatment of their open injury. It is mandatory not to accept inadequate roentgenographic evaluation prior to operative management. Few circumstances are more detrimental to patient care than finding that a patient has a related serious injury that was not appreciated prior to management of the open fracture. If this happens, the patient may be subjected not only to another operative procedure that may not be appropriate at the time, but also to the hazard of further complications from the associated injury.

TREATMENT

Treatment of open injuries is usually initiated during the evaluation of the patient in the emergency room. An intravenous line is established with a large-bore needle and saline or Ringer's lactate solution. Standard laboratory blood determinations are drawn, and the patient is crossmatched for two or more units of blood, depending on the severity of the injury. Once the patient's condition has been stabilized in the emergency room, appropriate therapeutic measures may be taken with the open injury.

Two questions frequently arise in regard to open injuries. The first concerns emergency room management of active bleeding from the open fracture site. This is best controlled with sterile compressive dressings until the patient is transported to the operating room. If an active arterial "bleeder" is visualized on initial evaluation, and it is in the subcutaneous tissues rather than deep in the wound, it is frequently useful to apply a sterile hemostat to control this bleeding while the patient is transported to the operating room. In the majority of cases it is not advisable to explore the wound in the emergency room in an attempt to seek out an active "bleeder" and ligate the vessel. Occasionally a tourniquet may be applied to the proximal portion of the limb as an initial measure. However, this treatment is not appropriate if there is going to be a delay in transporting the patient. A properly applied tourniquet will produce ischemia of the distal tissue, and a delay will increase the risk of damage to the distal tissues. A tourniquet may also lead to further hypoxia of the tissues which may promote infection. Suffice it to state that most bleeding from an open fracture site may be controlled with direct pressure through a sterile bandage.

A second frequently asked question in regard to open fracture management is, What is the appropriate initial management of exposed bone at the fracture site? By definition, the exposed osseous structure is contaminated. It is best to apply a sterile bandage over the wound proper and also over the exposed osseous structure. Manipulating the bone in the emergency room in an effort to reduce the fracture fragments into the wound is not appropriate therapy. It is also theoretically possible that foreign objects under the exposed bone may be dragged into the wound. Physiologically, it makes more sense to apply a sterile dressing and then to perform irrigation and debridement in the operating room before placing the osseous structures back into the wound proper. In this manner, the bacterial count of the exposed bone will be decreased prior to reduction. The reader is referred to Chapter 35 for the initial management of a burn associated with an open fracture.

TETANUS IMMUNIZATION

While in the emergency room the patient should be given medication to avoid the dread complication of tetanus. Tetanus, also known as lockjaw, is produced by the gram-positive bacillus *Clostridium tetani* which is a spore-forming, strictly anaerobic organism. *C. tetani* is normally found in the soil and may also be present in the gastrointestinal tract of some domestic animals. It is the elaboration of a toxin from the organism that produces the clinical syndrome of tetanus.

Fortunately, the normal host resistance to the tetanus bacillus is relatively high, so that frank infection is infrequent. However, if the host's immune system is weakened, or if there is significant devitalized tissue present, anaerobic conditions may be favored and the threat of tetanus increased. Therefore, it is important not only to debride the wound to remove the devitalized tissues, but to insure that the patient has an adequate level of tetanus antibody present. This goal may be accomplished by active or passive immunization.

Active immunization is achieved by injecting tetanus toxoid in three separate injections of 0.5 ml each. The first injection is followed by a second four to six weeks later. The third injection is administered six months to one year following the second injection. A booster dose of absorbed tetanus toxoid may then be given six to ten years following the third injection. Passive immunization may be given by injecting 250 to 500 units of human tetanus immune globulin.

The physician in the emergency room must try to establish the patient's immunization history. If the patient is awake and cooperative and can confirm that he has been immunized within the past six to ten years, a single booster dose of adsorbed tetanus toxoid is indicated. If the patient has a grossly contaminated wound with severely devitalized tissues, it is probably advisable to administer 250 units of human tetanus immune globulin in addition to the single dose of tetanus toxoid.

If the patient states that he has not been previously immunized, then 0.5 ml of adsorbed tetanus toxoid should be injected when he is first evaluated. The full immunization regime is then followed as outlined. If the wound is relatively clean and without significant devitalization of tissue, this is probably all the therapy required. If, on the other hand, the wound is contaminated and devitalized tissue is present, 250 to 500 units of human tetanus immune globulin should be administered in addition to the initial adsorbed tetanus toxoid.

It cannot be overstated that all patients presenting with open injuries must have adequate protection against tetanus. If this dread complication does develop the clinical picture will usually be evident seven to ten days following injury. The patient will demonstrate irritability, tremor, insomnia, and rigidity or spasm of muscles, particularly of those muscles adjacent to the wound. In the presence of this syndrome it is important to insure that all devitalized tissues have been surgically excised. The patient is then administered human tetanus immune globulin on a daily basis for 10 days in an attempt to destroy the circulating tetanus toxin. Antibiotics are also given, in the form of penicillin or cephalosporin. It is important to initiate active immunization with tetanus toxoid at the same time. However, it is interesting that affliction with this syndrome does not always confer future immunity.

ANTIBIOTIC SELECTION

All patients presenting with an open fracture should receive prophylactic intravenous antibiotics. In a retrospective and prospective study of 1025 open fractures of long bones, Gustilo and Anderson reported that cephalosporin is currently the prophylatic antibiotic of choice.[29] They found that most series demonstrated an infection rate that varied from 3 to 25 per cent. Their prospective study showed that initial wound cultures revealed a bacterial growth in 70.3 per cent of cases, with an ultimate infection rate of 2.5 per cent. The single best antibiotic in their series was a cephalosporin, either cephalothin or cefalozin. The antibiotics are administered preoperatively, intraoperatively, and postoperatively. Subsequent alterations in antibiotic coverage are based on the sensitivity of the organisms isolated from the infected open fractures.

Patzakis and co-workers also demonstrated the effectiveness of antibiotics in the management of these injuries.[45, 46] They felt that the term prophylactic antibiotics was inappropriate, as all the injuries were open fractures and they were dealing primarily with contaminated wounds. Of the three different groups they studied, the first group of patients did not receive antibiotics. Those in the second group received penicillin and streptomycin; the third group received cephalothin (Keflin). The results showed that in patients treated without antibiotics the infection rate was 13.9 per cent. In the group treated with penicillin and streptomycin, the infection rate was 9.7 per cent. In the group treated with cephalothin, the infection rate was 2.3 per cent, which was significantly lower than the other two groups. These authors recommended using an antibiotic effective against both gram-positive and gram-negative organisms as well as against coagulase-positive *Staphylococcus aureus* organisms. *Staphylococcus aureus* was isolated in 50 per cent of the infected wounds in this series. The authors felt that a culture specimen of an open fracture wound obtained prior to any treatment is the one most likely to isolate an infection-causing organism. The antibiotic treatment should be altered if the bacterial sensitivity study demonstrates an organism in the wound that is resistant to the antibiotic or antibiotics that are being utilized.

Burke had previously demonstrated that the optimum period for the administration of prophylactic antibiotics in the management of contaminated wounds is within three hours postinjury.[6]

It is important to recognize that the administration of antibiotics is not a substitute for extensive surgical debridement of all devitalized tissues in the management of open fractures. Antibiotics are useful in conjunction with appropriate surgical debridement.

IRRIGATION

Irrigation in association with active debridement of all devitalized tissue allows the wound the best chance of healing without infection. The irrigation solution usually employed is normal saline or Ringer's lactate, and a large quantity is required. Gustilo reported that at least 10 liters of normal saline is needed as an irrigating solution.[28] His investigation showed that patients treated with less than 10 liters of irrigating solution demonstrated a higher incidence of infection than those treated with 10 liters or more. The irrigation not only washes superficial bacteria away from the wound, but also removes blood clots and small necrotic portions of muscles, fascia, and fat which may contain bacteria. It has always been a surgical dictum to irrigate fully with an irrigating solution, but Gustilo's series definitely proved the beneficial effect of quantities of solution greater than 10 liters. The irrigating solution is collected in a fenestrated pan under the affected extremity and is then drained off into a separate area away from the operating table.

Recently an advance in irrigation has come into use. Gross and co-workers demonstrated the effectiveness of a pulsating water jet lavage in the management of contaminated crushed wounds.[27] The pulsating effect of the irrigating solution under pressure is definitely beneficial in removing necrotic debris and also in decreasing the bacterial count. Several devices now on the market accomplish this purpose. The Water-Pik is probably the one most frequently employed to deliver a pulsating jet lavage to a wound surface. Initially it was feared that the pulsatile jet flow might itself damage cell structures. However, it has been demonstrated that it is not detrimental to cell function, and that it does aid in loosening dead tissue and flushing bacteria out of the wound. If such a device is available in the operating room, it should definitely be employed in the management of open fractures.

DEBRIDEMENT

There is no substitute for formal irrigation and debridement of all devitalized tissues in the surgical treatment of open fractures. The type of anesthesia selected depends on the degree of injury and also on the associated injuries. The reader is referred to Chapter 8 for the various techniques of anesthetization. In most medical centers the wound has been inspected by the examining physician in the emergency room and a new dressing applied. The dressing that is in place should not be removed until debridement in the operating room is performed. This will decrease the amount of contamination of the wound. Remember, all open wounds by definition are contaminated.

If the wound is present in the mid- to distal aspect of the extremity, a pneumatic tourniquet may be applied to the proximal portion of the extremity prior to preparation and draping for surgery. The pneumatic tourniquet may or may not be employed during the debridement process, but it is always better to have it in place in case it is needed to temporarily control active bleeding. If it is utilized it must be released when appropriate, and all active "bleeders" must be ligated.

Surgical preparation of the open fracture is performed in a meticulous manner. A sterile dressing is applied to the wound itself. Then the surrounding skin is cleansed with a Betadine solution. A formal 10-minute scrub is applied to this area. The preparation solutions are then discarded, and a new preparation tray is opened. The surgeon changes gloves, and the dressing is removed from the wound. Obvious foreign bodies are removed from the wound with the use of hemostats, and the wound is cleansed with a Betadine solution. It has been demonstrated that Betadine is not a harmful substance to viable cells. The wound is draped sterile in the usual fashion, allowing for extension as necessary for appropriate debridement and exploration.

It is frequently useful to apply a sterile plastic sheet under the wound prior to preparation and draping, so that if the drapes become soaked with the irrigating solution the sterile plastic sheet underneath will allow for adequately sterile technique. A fenestrated pan is placed under the extremity in order to catch all the irrigating solution and to prevent contamination of the surrounding drapes. The wound is now ready for debridement. If osseous fragments protrude from the wound these are scrubbed with a Betadine solution prior to the draping procedure. The undersurfaces of the osseous fragments are then inspected to insure that no foreign material will be dragged into the wound on reduction of the fracture fragments. There is no hurry to perform a reduction of the osseous fragments. It is more important at this time to inspect the bone for residual debris and foreign objects. The viability of the underlying muscle and soft tissue structures must then be determined.

Several measures are employed to assess the viability of muscle. The four main criteria are color, consistency, contractility, and capacity to bleed. Scully determined in a very important study that consistency and a capacity to bleed are the most important criteria for muscle viability.[53] He correlated the color, consistency, contractility, and capacity to bleed with the histological evidence of viability. Color has been found to be the least useful criterion for viability. Contractility is an important criterion and may be useful in determining viability. The author's experience has been that if the muscle actively bleeds and there is a definite tendency toward contractility, the muscle is probably viable. At this point the active resection of the injured muscle may be discontinued. However, it is best to resect all muscle that is of doubtful viability. This will insure removal of dead tissue, which is a nidus for the development of an anaerobic infection. The alternative is to leave questionable muscle in place and return the patient to the operating room two to three days later for a second look. The best overall approach is probably the surgical excision of all muscle that is of doubtful viability. This will decrease the possibility of the dread complications of tetanus or gas gangrene.

Once all the muscle has been actively debrided, attention may be shifted to the surrounding skin margins. The skin is debrided back to bleeding healthy tissue. This will frequently allow for wider exposure of the underlying muscle. At this point the fracture fragments may be reduced into proper position. One of the most difficult controversies concerns the management of a free osseous fragment that appears to be devitalized owing to lack of surrounding soft tissue structures. The author's preference is to thoroughly clean and irrigate these osseous structures and then place them back into the wound as a free bone graft. If the osseous structure is excised and removed, a large gap may be produced at the fracture site which may well lead to nonunion in the future.

WOUND MANAGEMENT FOLLOWING DEBRIDEMENT

There are three separate methods of managing a wound after an open fracture. These are primary closure, delayed closure, and open packing of the wound. Most centers encourage delayed closure or open packing of contaminated wounds. The distinct disadvantage of primary closure is that an infection may develop which could lead to loss of the extremity or loss of life.

PRIMARY CLOSURE

Conditions must be ideal for this type of wound management to produce good results. It is not an easy decision for a surgeon to make, and the author has always felt that he is unable to determine the amount of bacterial contamination still present following initial irrigation and debridement procedures. Therefore, he has elected not to perform primary closure as a definitive method of wound closure unless rigid criteria are met. These include the following:

1. The open fracture is essentially an isolated event. This type of wound management is not suitable for patients who have sustained multiple-system injuries. The author has demonstrated previously that the oxygen delivery to a standardized wound in a patient with multiple trauma is diminished for at least four to five days postinjury.[33] It is well documented that soft tissue wounds demonstrate a delay in repair and an increased susceptibility to infection under conditions of relative hypoxia. The combination of a multiply injured patient and definitive wound management by primary closure usually results in a very high incidence of infection in the management of open fractures. Under these conditions definitive wound management is usually by delayed closure or open packing.

2. The blood flow to the involved extremity should be essentially normal if primary closure is selected. This type of treatment is not appropriate for patients who demonstrate end artery disease.

3. Irrigation and debridement have, in the surgeon's opinion, essentially elimi-

nated all dead tissue and converted the wound from an open wound to one suitable for a primary surgical incision. For this procedure the amount of devitalized tissue must be small, and the degree of initial contamination of the wound must be minimal.

4. The surgeon must be able to close the wound edges without significant tension. Otherwise, the wound is exposed not only to increased risk of infection owing to the initial contamination, but also to the hazards of necrosis of the wound edges because of a lack of blood supply secondary to the tension. There is also the possibility that the wound may break open under these circumstances.

5. Finally, the surgeon must be able to close the wound without any significant dead space remaining. If the wound margins are mobilized in an effort to achieve primary closure without any provision for closure of the underlying dead space, a catastrophe may result. Not only will a hematoma form in this area, but bacterial organisms will settle in any remaining devitalized tissue. Needless to say, these conditions provide an ideal medium for bacterial growth.

The foregoing are very stringent criteria for performing primary wound closure, but serious complications will be avoided if these standards are rigidly adhered to. It should also be clear to the reader that primary closure is not often used in the management of open injuries because of the serious complications that may ensue.

If, however, all these criteria can be satisfied, it may be appropriate to attempt primary closure as a definitive method of wound management.

DELAYED CLOSURE

This type of wound management is preferred by the author, because it definitely reduces the incidence of serious wound complications and the possibility of future osteomyelitis. The patient is taken to the operating room, and the wound is primarily irrigated and debrided and packed open with Betadine-soaked sponges. The packing is loosely applied to allow for adequate drainage. Sterile dressings are then applied

to the wound, which is not disturbed until two to four days later. The patient's general condition, temperature, and white blood cell count are closely observed during this time. If the patient's condition appears to be improving he is taken back to the operating room where the packing is removed and the wound is reinspected. Any residual devitalized tissue is excised at this time. If the wound seems to be developing healthy granulation tissue and there is no evidence of frank infection, a secondary closure should be considered.

If, however, there are signs of an infection, such as visible pus, an increased amount of devitalized tissue, or poor granulation tissue, the wound is irrigated and debrided once again and managed with the insertion of new Betadine-soaked packing. Two to four days later the patient is returned to the operating room, and if inspection of the wound reveals healthy granulation tissue, and no evidence of infection, delayed closure is performed.

In the presence of a significant soft tissue deficit, several techniques may be used to obtain a delayed closure. These include split-thickness skin grafts, a pedicle or flap graft, muscle transfers and relaxing incisions.

Skin Grafts

Split-thickness skin grafts are very useful when beginning healthy granulation tissue is seen in association with a soft tissue deficit. The skin for grafting may be obtained from an adjacent area or from an uninvolved normal extremity. The viability and success of the skin graft depends on the thickness. It has been demonstrated that relatively thin split-thickness skin grafts are more likely to survive than thick split grafts. The author prefers to utilize 0.010- to 0.012-inch split-thickness skin grafts. This is a very thin skin graft which has a very high rate of survival.

The graft is placed over the area of skin loss and is seated on the underlying healthy beginning granulation tissue. The graft is then sutured to the surrounding skin margins, and a pressure stint is applied directly over the graft to insure maximal contact between the skin graft and the underlying granulation tissue. This also will decrease the amount of hematoma formation, which will threaten the survival of the skin graft. Sterile dressings are then applied to the skin graft site. The graft donor site may be managed with the application of a Vaseline gauze strip, which is allowed to eventually fall off. The alternative is to place a superficial dressing over the donor site, which is removed early, and to then apply topical thrombin. The skin graft itself is not inspected for a four to five day interval. At that time the amount of skin "take" is usually evident.

Placing the patient in an enriched-oxygen gaseous environment for four to five days to stimulate ingrowth of granulation tissue into the split-thickness skin graft has been advocated. There is no doubt that a locally elevated oxygen tension will better the survival chances of a skin graft. However, this beneficial effect must be weighed against the adverse effect on the pulmonary parenchyma of breathing an enriched oxygen mixture over a prolonged period.

Pedicle Grafts

Pedicle or flap grafts have been utilized to provide soft tissue closure in the face of soft tissue loss. There has been recent enthusiasm for the application of a vascular pedicle free soft tissue flap. This type of graft includes the skin and subcutaneous tissue with its underlying arterial and venous pedicle. It is ideal if the vascular pedicle can be connected to an artery and vein within the wound. This is in contrast to an abdominal pedicle or a cross-leg pedicle flap, in which one of the skin flaps is elevated and attached to the area of skin loss. The proximal portion of the graft remains attached to the abdomen or to the opposite extremity. A time interval is allowed for incorporation of the graft at the graft site. The proximal portion of the pedicle is then cut loose from its parent blood supply. The problem with this type of graft is that if infection develops underneath the pedicle, both the original open wound and the area where the pedicle graft originates are in jeopardy of developing a serious infection.

Muscle Transfers

Muscle transpositions have also been advocated as a means of providing soft tissue coverage over an area of open fracture. Ger has successfully managed both osteomyelitis and open fractures with this method.[24] Its best application is in open fractures of the lower extremity. In fact, the area most suited to this form of treatment is the proximal half of the tibia. In this region the soleus or deep flexor muscles may be useful for transposition. The author has found this technique to be most valuable in the management of chronic osteomyelitis in the lower extremities, but it does have application for soft tissue coverage in the management of open fractures.

Relaxing Incisions

Relaxing incisions allow the surgeon to mobilize an area of skin in order to provide coverage for the area of skin loss. The incision site may then be closed with a skin graft. This technique is appropriate for open fractures of the tibia associated with significant soft tissue loss. It is particularly applicable to the anterior subcutaneous border of the tibia, where significant skin loss, such as that seen in association with a "bumper" type of injury, may occur. A relaxing incision may be made along the lateral or medial aspects of the calf, and the skin margins may be mobilized to cover the area of skin loss and allow closure. A skin graft is then applied to the area where the relaxing incision was made. The relaxing incision does have limitations, but it is a useful method for providing soft tissue coverage.

OPEN PACKING

This is an extremely useful technique in the management of grossly contaminated open fractures. As an example, it is appropriate for injuries incurred in motorcycle accidents, in which there is a significant amount of ground-in dirt or foreign particles. The patient is taken to the operating room, and a standard irrigation and debridement procedure is performed. The wound is then loosely packed open with Betadine-soaked sponges, and sterile dressings are applied over the wound surface. The patient is returned to the operating room three to four days following the initial

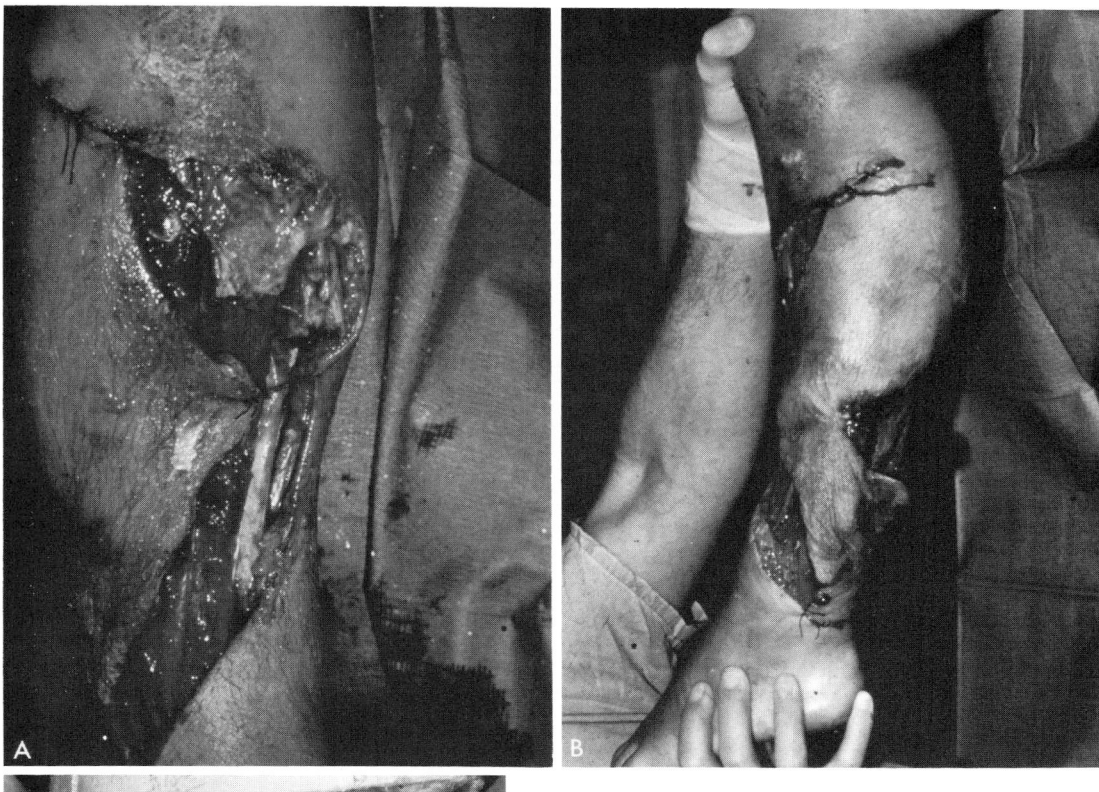

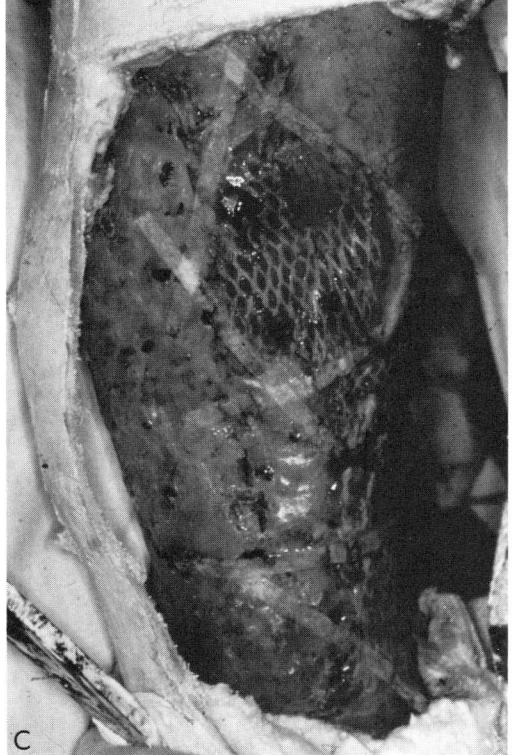

Figure 30–1 *A.* A severe open tibial fracture with obvious skin loss. This is a view of the posterior aspect of the tibia. *B.* Lateral aspect of the same open injury. *C.* Following appropriate debridement and open packing, the remainder of the open wounds were treated with open meshed split-thickness skin grafts.

treatment, and the loose packing is removed. Inspection of the wound will reveal the extent of residual devitalized tissue as well as any evidence of frank infection. The wound is irrigated and debrided again, and this is followed by insertion of loose Betadine-soaked packing. Another three to four days are allowed to pass without inspection of the wound. At the end of this time the packing can usually be removed on the ward under intravenous sedation. Sterile techniques are used for removal of the packing, and new Betadine-soaked packing is inserted. This may be repeated every two to six days as necessary.

The wound is allowed to close through the formation of granulation tissue. It is true that this is a very slow process, but it does allow for adequate drainage of the wound and it insures healthy granulation tissue. If at the end of two to three weeks there appears to be adequate healthy granulation tissue, the process may be hastened by the application of a meshed split-thickness skin graft, as outlined by Tanner (Fig. 30–1).[55] This type of graft has the advantage of being fenestrated, which allows for the escape of transudate and exudate which would normally lift up the graft and decrease the likelihood of its survival. However, with the fenestrations in place free drainage is provided, and small islands of skin will usually take and be viable. After a time these small islands of skin will rapidly coalesce and provide adequate skin coverage.

CLASSIFICATION OF OPEN FRACTURES

Gustilo and Anderson performed a retrospective and prospective analysis of the prevention of infection in the treatment of 1025 open fractures of long bones.[29] In the prospective study they were able to classify open injuries into three distinct categories. Type 1 is an open fracture with a clean wound less than 1 cm long. Type 2 is an open fracture with laceration greater than 1 cm long, but without extensive soft tissue damage, flaps, or avulsions. Type 3 is either an open segmental fracture, an open fracture with extensive soft tissue damage, or a traumatic amputation. The special categories in type 3 include gunshot injuries, open

fractures due to a farm injury, and open fractures with accompanying vascular injury requiring repair. It was their policy to perform primary closure in type 1 and type 2 fractures, but to perform delayed primary closure, including split-thickness skin grafts or appropriate flaps, for type 3 injuries. They recommended administering antibiotics before, during, and following surgery. Cephalosporins were the antibiotics of choice. If the wound was closed primarily, the antibiotics were stopped on the third postoperative day. In injuries that required secondary closure of the wound, the antibiotics were continued for an additional three days following the procedure. With this approach infection developed in 2.4 per cent of 326 open fractures studied prospectively. If the type 3 fractures were isolated, the infection rate was 9.9 per cent. These figures are very impressive in the overall management of these severe injuries; the reader is referred to the original study.[29]

GAS GANGRENE

This is a very serious life-threatening complication in the management of open injuries. Traditionally, gas gangrene has been associated with war injuries. However, it now is being seen in civilian practice and is not as rare as was once supposed.[10, 14] This dread complication is caused by the Clostridium organism. There are six species of Clostridium that are capable of producing gas gangrene. However, the most important by far is *Clostridium perfringens*. These gram-positive rods are obligate anaerobes. They thrive in an anaerobic environment and are unable to survive in the relatively high oxygen-reduction potentials that exist in healthy human tissue. Clostridium organisms are widely distributed in nature and are commonly found in soil and in the feces of most animals.

The clinical picture of gas gangrene has been described as an invasive, anaerobic infection of muscle, characterized by extensive local edema, massive tissue necrosis with variable degrees of gas production, and profound toxemia. The organisms produce a variety of highly potent toxins, 12 of which have been identified. The most important toxin by far is the alpha-toxin, a dermonecrotizing lecithinase. The importance of lecithinase is that most cell walls have a lipoprotein complex containing lecithin. The alpha-toxin produces its effect by disrupting the cell wall and eventually causing death of the cell.

It is important to realize that one of the most important requirements for clostridial infection is the presence of an area of decreased oxygen-reduction potential. Since these organisms are obligate anaerobes, they survive in areas of very low oxygen tension. For this reason it is extremely important to debride all devitalized tissues in managing open fractures. If conditions are favorable for the growth of this organism, that is, an area of hypoxia such as that in devitalized tissue, the organism will flourish. The severe muscle destruction that is seen with profound toxemia produces the clinical syndrome. Clostridial myonecrosis is the definitive term for the clinical syndrome of gas gangrene. It is interestng that more than 90 per cent of the lesions occur in the extremity. The incubation period of the organism is usually less than 24 hours and always less than 3 days.

The typical clinical presentation is heralded by the sudden onset of pain in the region of the wound which is out of proportion to the pain expected with this type of injury. Localized edema and swelling occur together with a thin hemorrhagic exudate. A distinct tachycardia is present. As the syndrome progresses, there is increasing pain, swelling, edema, fever, and toxemia. The systemic toxemia results in a profound state of shock. The odor of the wound has been described as a typical "mousy" smell. The changes in the muscle produce an increased reddened appearance with mottled areas of purple, which progresses to frank gangrenous myonecrosis. Gas is produced in the tissues, but it is the severe muscle necrosis and profound toxemia that may lead to death. It is occasionally helpful to obtain a Gram stain of the wound exudate. This will reveal an abundance of gram-positive rods and a few pus cells.

Once this syndrome is recognized, it requires immediate decompression and debridement of the involved area. Antibiotics are administered in massive doses (penicillin is still favored by many investigators).[10, 14, 21] Wide excision of the necrotic muscle is required, with fascial decompressions as necessary. Hyperbaric oxygen is useful in reducing the advancing myonecrosis, but will not alone cure the infection. Surgery is the all-important key, and high doses of penicillin and hyperbaric oxygen are supportive measures. It may be necessary to perform an immediate amputation in an attempt to save the patient's life. Most centers having access to a hyperbaric chamber find that surgery combined with hyperbaric oxygen treatments will limit the amount of muscle resection that is necessary. However, it should be emphasized that primary amputation is occasionally the method of choice. The hyperbaric oxygen treatments are usually given at three times atmospheric pressure with an exposure of 60 to 90 minutes. This is repeated every 8 to 12 hours as necessary.

In summary, it must be stated that the only definitive treatment for gas gangrene is its prevention. This can be accomplished only by adequate irrigation and debridement of open injuries. This complication is seen in civilian practice, and a recent report of five cases seen by Fee and co-workers in the management of open forearm fractures reminds us that this problem is not as rare as had been thought.[21]

Part II ———————— **GUNSHOT WOUNDS** ————————

All orthopedic surgeons must have a thorough understanding of gunshot wounds in order to manage these injuries successfully. It is true that war produces mass experience with management of gunshot wounds. However, it is also fair to state that during World Wars I and II, the Korean War, and the Vietnam War, several well-established surgical principles were learned, abandoned, and then relearned. There is certainly a marked difference between wounds produced by low-velocity missiles, such as those seen in civilian practice, and wounds produced by the high-velocity missiles of combat. War wounds lead to far more tissue destruction than civilian wounds.

WAR WOUNDS

As stated, war wounds are essentially wounds produced by high-velocity missiles. In a series of articles, DeMuth reviewed the various components of military missiles that lead to severe wound destruction.[16-18] Three theories out of a large number emerged as the most plausible in explaining the wounding mechanism. These are: (1) kinetic energy, (2) momentum, and (3) power. All three involve missile speed and weight. In simple form, the theories are as follows.

(1)   Kinetic energy $= \dfrac{\text{Mass} \times \text{Velocity}^2}{2}$

(Kinetic energy equals mass times velocity squared, divided by two.)

(2) $\text{Momentum} = \text{Mass} \times \text{Velocity}$

(3) $\text{Power} = \text{Mass} \times \text{Velocity}^3$

(Power equals mass times velocity cubed.)

It is clear that the kinetic energy theory applies best in conjunction with experimental observations. The important factor in the kinetic energy theory is that doubling the mass doubles the kinetic energy, but doubling the velocity quadruples the kinetic energy. In other words, velocity is the crucial factor in the production of kinetic energy. Armed with these facts, it is not difficult to understand why military gunshot injuries are much more destructive than civilian ones. For practical purposes, a simple classification of bullet velocity follows. Missile velocity of less than 1000 feet per second is considered low velocity. A medium-velocity missile travels between 1000 and 2000 feet per second. A high-velocity missile is one with a speed of greater than 2000 feet per second.

A bullet wound produces an obvious tract in the wake of the bullet's passage through the tissue. A less well understood type of wound tract is known as the temporary cavity, which is produced during the passage of the projectile. The temporary cavity is the direct result of the kinetic energy expended and has little relationship to the shape or composition of the bullet. DeMuth demonstrated the significance of the temporary cavity by firing bullets into premolded substances and into animals.[16, 17] It was noted that with high-velocity missiles there is an explosive cavitational effect which can lead to a fractured bone despite the fact that the bone was not actually struck by the projectile. All the cell tissues adjacent to the wound tract then become secondary missiles which move in an outward direction at tremendous speed, producing the temporary cavity effect. The actual size of the temporary cavity is directly proportional to the energy absorbed by the expanding medium. The direction of the cell excursion reverses at the point of maximum cavitation, and the cavity then collapses to the size of the permanent wound tract. At the point of maximum cavitation, a suction effect is created, so that clothing and dirt particles may be drawn into the wound. This is an important factor, since it may lead to gross contamination. It is extremely important to recognize the severe destruction caused by the temporary cavitation in order to understand the amount of cell destruction produced by the high-velocity missile.

As far as bullet composition and design are concerned, the majority of bullets are made of a lead alloy. One of the drawbacks of this composition is its low melting point. This is important because friction in the barrel increases significantly with increase in velocity. Therefore, unjacketed lead bullets cannot be propelled more than 2000 feet per second, or they will soften in the barrel and cause it to deform. For this reason, jackets composed of metals with much higher melting points are used to cover the portion of the bullet that is in direct contact with the barrel.

In general, there are two types of high-velocity bullets—jacketed and expanding. The jacketed nonexpanding bullet does not produce as much destruction as the expanding type. International law (Geneva Convention) requires all military bullets to be of the fully jacketed, nonexpanding configuration. This type of bullet maintains its caliber as it passes through the tissues. In contrast, the expanding bullet enlarges to several times the original caliber, establishing a very wide wound tract. The significance of course is that greater destruction occurs in its path secondary to this mechanism. This type of bullet is frequently used for game hunting. The significance of this sort of injury must be fully understood, as gunshot wounds from high-velocity hunting rifles are still encountered far too frequently in our society. Management of these injuries is similar to that of a high-velocity missile military wound.

In the Vietnam conflict, American soldiers were introduced to the M-16 military rifle, which represented a major advance in technical design. The M-16 bullet was much lighter than its predecessors, and a much higher missile velocity, approximately 3250 feet per second, was obtained. This is indeed a high-velocity missile. Experiments using this weapon were performed to produce both muscle wounds and bone wounds.[17] It was noted that high-velocity bullets caused very large temporary cavities which appeared to reach a maximum size in less than one millisecond. The volume of the temporary cavity was proportional to the energy transmitted by the bullet. Muscle fibers were damaged directly, but the surrounding connective tissues and blood vessels were also injured. Therefore, a significant amount of devitalized tissue existed at a distance from the obvious wound margin.

It has been demonstrated that the most appropriate form of treatment for this type of wound is to excise all devitalized tissue back to fresh bleeding muscle margins and then to pack the wound open. The patient is returned to the operating room for a second look after three to four days, and if the wound appears clean at that time a secondary closure may be performed. If it does not appear to be clean a second debridement is carried out, and the wound is repacked. After another three to four days the wound is inspected once again. Secondary closures are performed at this time if the wound is clean on direct examination. There is no doubt that this type of wound management was one of the most important concepts to come out of World War II.

Experiments were also performed to produce standard bone wounds. It was noted that bone fragments, like muscle, acted as secondary missiles at the time of the temporary cavity formation, but that the majority of bone fragments returned in close proximity to the parent bone. It was also demonstrated that if the high-velocity bullet passed in close proximity to the bone, a fracture could result from the violent force produced by the temporary cavity. In other words, the bullet did not have to strike the bone directly to cause severe disruption of the osseous structure. It should be noted that cortical bone has a much higher specific gravity than water, and therefore it is the most severely damaged of all body tissues in this type of injury. However, it is also true that in high-velocity bullet wounds the soft tissue destruction is usually severe. The attending physician must attempt to treat the severe soft tissue destruction, frequently at the expense of the mechanical aspects of treatment of the fracture. The usual procedure in this type of fracture is to perform a wide debridement of the wound area and then attempt to treat the fracture with skeletal traction or pins in plaster fixation. Recent advances in external skeletal fixation apparatus, such as the Hoffman device, can certainly improve patient care.

In summary, the management of high-velocity gunshot wounds must include an adequate debridement of all devitalized tissues and then a packing open of the wound, to be followed by a delayed closure three to four days after the initial debridement. *It is completely inappropriate to consider primary closure following debridement of these severe injuries.* If there is one lesson that has been learned in war experience, it is the benefit derived from adequate debridement and delayed closure of these wounds.

CIVILIAN GUNSHOT WOUNDS

Civilian gunshot wounds are being encountered with increasing frequency today (Fig. 30–2). It is important to have an overall appreciation of the extent of the injury produced by the civilian type of handgun. As previously stated, civilian injuries involve low-velocity missiles—usually less than 1000 feet per second. As examples, a

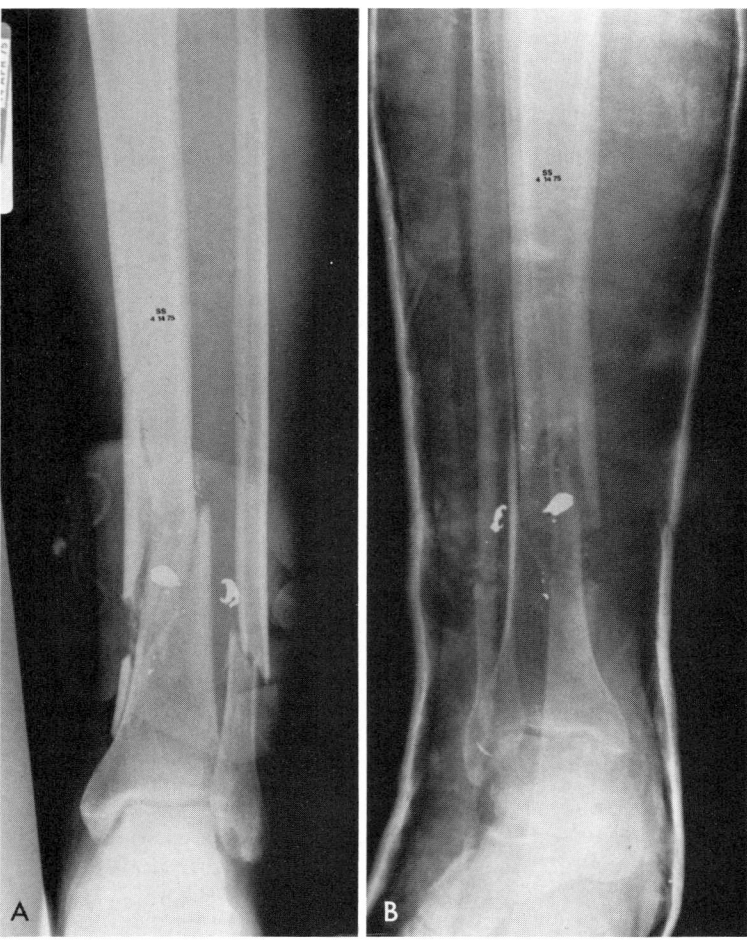

Figure 30–2   *A.* An anteroposterior view of a gunshot wound of the distal third of the tibia. This was treated with functional weight bearing in a below-knee, weight-bearing cast. *B.* An oblique view demonstrating the comminution at the fracture site. The bullet fragment was not excised, because it was buried in bone.

.45-caliber pistol bullet has been demonstrated to project at 846 feet per second. A .38-caliber revolver bullet projects at 600 feet per second, and a .22-caliber long rifle bullet at 1206 feet per second. The amount of destruction produced in the path of these bullets is much less than that caused by a high-velocity missile. This is confirmed by the fact that a low-velocity bullet will produce permanent damage only in an area bordering the bullet tract. For this reason, civilian injuries may be managed in a different fashion from war wounds.

The definite exception to this rule is the close-range shotgun wound. The significance of this injury is due not only to the destruction produced by the shotgun pellets, but to the fact that there is always the danger of a retained shell wadding (Fig. 30–3). This is a structure consisting of hair and jute which is compressed as a binding agent and placed at the base of the gunshot pellet. Its function is to drive the shot down the barrel secondary to the explosive force from the gun powder. Under normal circumstances the wadding falls behind the shot if enough distance is allowed in its projectory path. However, if a shotgun injury occurs at close range, the wadding may be found buried in the tissues. It is extremely important to surgically remove the wadding, as it is a definite foreign body which produces a severe inflammatory response in the tissues. It is not necessary to surgically remove all the shot pellets, but it is important to excise all devitalized structures.

There has been a recent trend toward conservative management of civilian handgun injuries. In 1961, Hampton reviewed

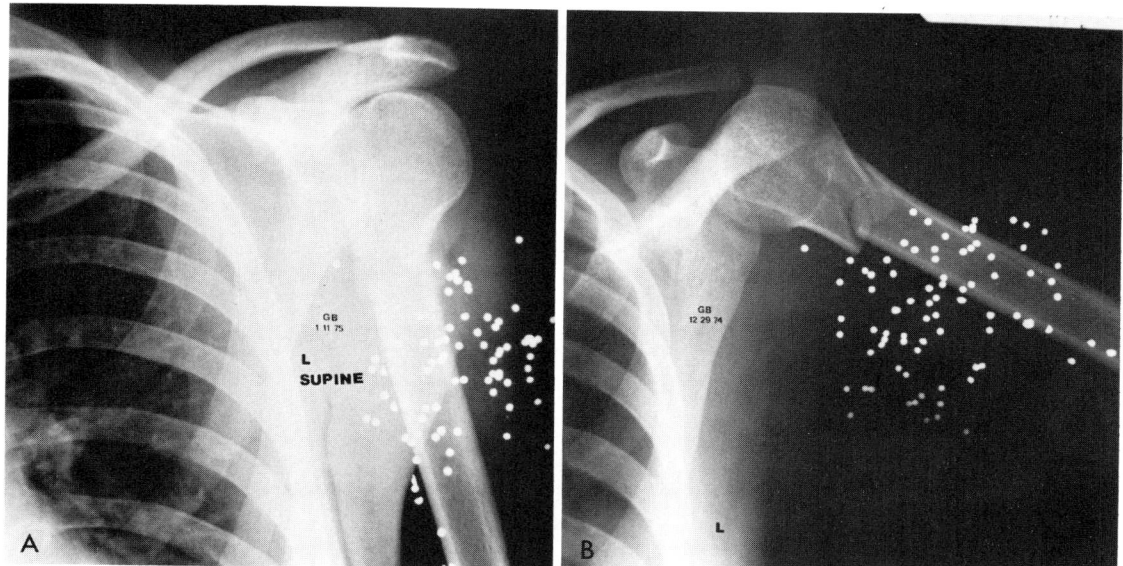

Figure 30–3 *A.* A gunshot wound of the left proximal humeral area treated with initial exploration with removal of retained wadding. *B.* One month postexcision of the wadding. No attempt was made to remove the numerous small pellets. The wound eventually went on to heal. The fracture site healed without any significant problems.

the literature and found that more than 300 of 368 bullet wounds of the extremities (approximately 50 per cent with associated fractures) were managed without wound debridement. No loss of life or limb occurred as a result of sepsis.[30] He concluded that classic surgical debridement or debridement by any definition was not necessary for the vast majority of bullet wounds of the extremities encountered in civilian practice. However, an associated injury to a major artery required a classic debridement of the wound with appropriate arterial surgical reconstruction. Hampton also cautioned that this opinion would have to be discarded in favor of an adequate and at times aggressive surgical approach when the characteristics of the wound so dictated (Fig. 30–4).

In 1961 Morgan and co-workers published a series of 105 consecutive patients with single gunshot wounds of soft tissue by single bullets with a muzzle energy of less than 400 pounds and a muzzle velocity of less than 1200 feet per second.[42] It was their policy not to operatively debride these injuries. The majority of wounds were caused by .38- and .45-caliber pistols. Their treatment consisted of placing the patient on bed rest, cleansing the surrounding skin,

and applying a dry sterile pressure dressing over the wound. The extremities were usually splinted and elevated. Antibiotics were routinely administered for at least five days. These investigators believed that debridement was unnecessary for these injuries, since they involved only brief hospitalization and disability.

An animal study was performed by Dziemian and colleagues who demonstrated that low-velocity gunshot wounds in goats healed spontaneously even when they were produced by high-velocity military bullets, provided no obvious circulatory impairment existed.[19] In the presence of obvious vascular damage, however, there was a far different prognosis in terms of progressive tissue necrosis and development of anaerobic infection.

In 1971, Howland and Ritchey reported a series of 72 patients with fractures resulting from civilian gunshot wounds.[34] They contended that the majority of these injuries could be managed by superficial debridement and immobilization with satisfactory results (Fig. 30–5). The majority of patients in their series did not receive antibiotics, and only 2 of the 72 patients developed wound infections, neither of which was serious. Bullets retained in the hand or foot

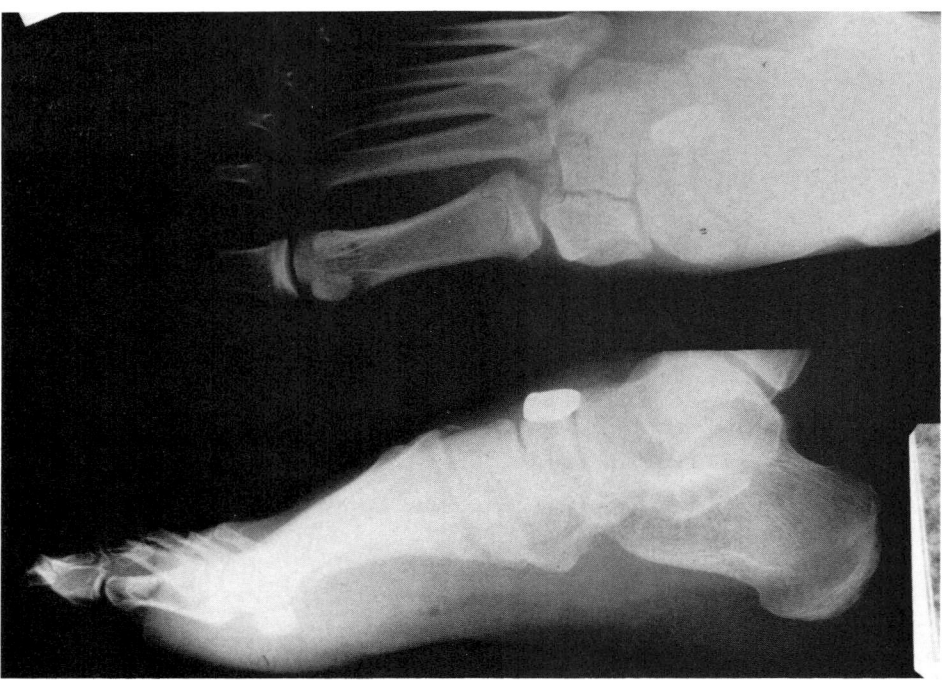

Figure 30–4   A gunshot wound to the foot. The bullet had lodged between the navicular bone and the talus. This required operative removal of the bullet owing to mechanical symptoms at the wound site.

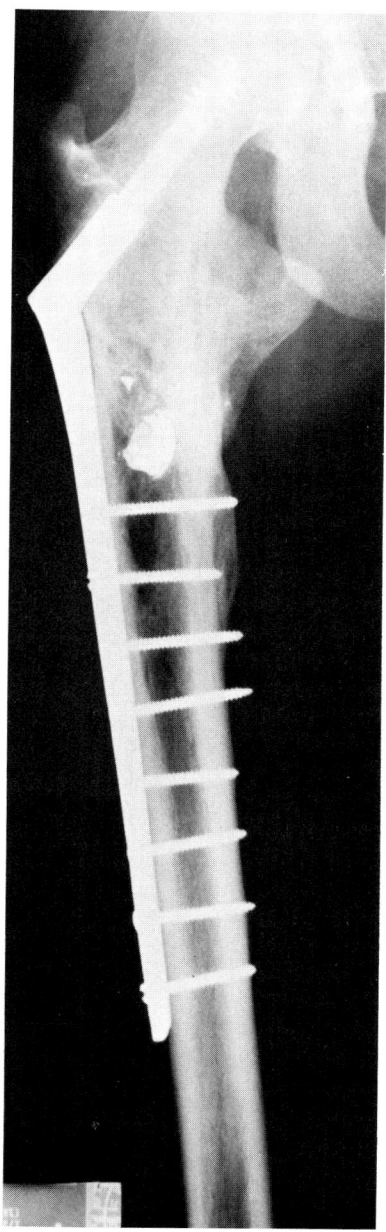

Figure 30–5 A subtrochanteric fracture due to a gunshot injury. It was treated with initial open reduction and internal fixation with a sliding compression screw device with a long side plate. This went on to uneventful healing. No attempt was made to excise the bullet which was embedded in the osseous structure.

were frequently painful and required excision at a later date.

Conversely, Ziperman advocated that all bullet wounds be explored, with the possible exceptions of obviously intradermal injuries or "crease" wounds.[63] He felt that if no foreign body or tissue devitalization was found on exploration, the wound could be sutured primarily. If, however, there was evidence of devitalized tissue, this was treated open, and the patient was taken back to the operating room on the fourth or sixth day postdebridement. At that time, secondary closure was considered if the tissues appeared viable and clean.

The author's practice has been to follow the dictum, "When in doubt, explore the wound, and if there is no evidence of devitalized tissue primary closure over a drain may be performed." Conversely, devitalized tissue should be treated with surgical excision and irrigation, followed by secondary closure four to five days postinjury. Philosophically, the small possibility of significant infection must be weighed against subjecting the patient to a negative exploration of the wound which may not be indicated. As stated, if there is any doubt it is probably better to explore the wound to rule out the presence of significant devitalized tissue and also to provide adequate irrigation of the wound.

CIVILIAN GUNSHOT WOUNDS INVOLVING JOINTS

There appears to be a different philosophy in regard to the management of gunshot wounds that enter a joint. The author feels that all these wounds should be explored and primary debridement performed, including excision of any foreign body (Fig. 30–6). This is important for two reasons. First of all, osteochondral fragments may be present in the joint and may interfere with active motion. These fragments should be surgically excised. Second, a bullet fragment retained in the joint may lead to dissolution of the lead by synovial fluid. This will produce lead deposition within the subsynovial tissues and may result in periarticular fibrosis.[39] It is also possible that the lead itself may have a toxic effect on the articular surface, producing cartilage necrosis of the articular surface.

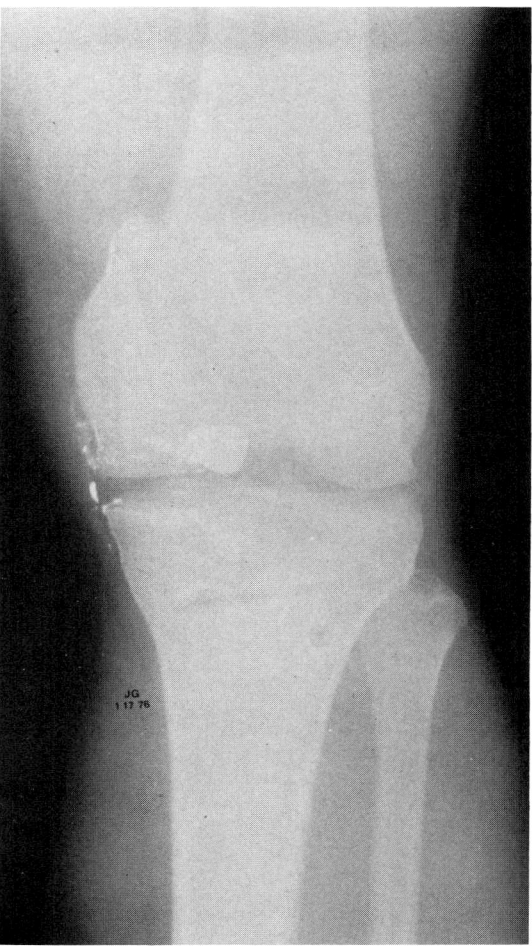

Figure 30–6   A fracture of the medial condyle in the femur produced by a gunshot wound, with the bullet remaining free in the joint cavity. This was treated with operative excision of the bullet, thorough irrigation of the knee joint, and transfixion of the femoral condyle with a Webb bolt.

Ashby reviewed seven cases of gunshot wounds to the knee, in which the bullet was retained within the joint.[1] All cases were treated by initial arthrotomy, removal of the bullet, and excision of osteochondral fragments. Four of the seven cases required numerous surgical incisions to locate the foreign body within the synovial compartment. Ashby advised obtaining roentgenograms immediately prior to the surgical procedure in order to localize the position of the bullet. Primary arthrotomy must be performed directly over the compartment in which the bullet is located. All osteochondral fragments must be excised. None of the seven wounds in this series became infected with this treatment program.

REFERENCES

1. Ashby, M. E.: Low-velocity gunshot wounds involving the knee joint: surgical management. J. Bone Joint Surg., 56A:1047–1053, 1974.
2. Bowers, W. H., Wilson, F. C., and Greene, W. B.: Antibiotic prophylaxis in experimental bone infections. J. Bone Joint Surg., 55A:795–807, 1973.
3. Braithwaite, F., and Moore, F. T.: Skin grafting by cross-leg flaps. J. Bone Joint Surg., 31B, 228, 1949.
4. Brav, E. A.: The management of open fractures of the extremities. In Instructional Course Lectures. AAOS Vol. 13, pp. 227–233. Ann Arbor, J. W. Edwards, 1956.
5. Brown, P. W., and Urban, J. G.: Early weight-bearing treatment of open fractures of the tibia. An end-result study of 63 cases. J. Bone Joint Surg., 51:59–75, 1969.
6. Brummelkamp, W. H., Hogendijk, J., and Boerema, I.: Treatment of anaerobic infections (clostridial myositis) by drenching tissues with oxygen under high atmospheric pressure. Surgery, 49:299–302, 1961.
7. Burke, J. F.: The effective period of preventive antibiotic action in experimental incisions and dermal lesions. Surgery, 50:161–168, 1961.
8. Cannon, B.: Plastic surgery skin transplantation. N. Engl. J. Med., 239:435, 1948.
9. Cleveland, M.: The emergency treatment of bone and joint casualties. J. Bone Joint Surg., 32A:235, 1950.
10. Colvill, M. R., and Mandsley, R. H.: The management of gas gangrene with hyperbaric oxygen therapy. J. Bone Joint Surg., 50B:732–742, 1968.
11. Converse, J. M.: Early skin grafting in war wounds of the extremities. Ann. Surg., 115:321, 1942.
12. Copeland, C. X., Jr., and Enneking, W. F.: Incidence of osteomyelitis in compound fractures. Ann. Surg., 31:156–158, 1965.
13. Davis, G. L.: Management of open wounds of joints—experience during the Vietnam war. A preliminary study. J. Bone Joint Surg., 51A:1032, 1969.
14. DeHaven, K. E., and Evarts, C. M.: The continuing problem of gas gangrene: a review and report of illustrative cases. J. Trauma, 11:983–991, 1971.
15. Dehne, E.: Treatment of fractures of the tibial shaft. Clin. Orthop. Rel. Res., 66:159–173, 1969.
16. DeMuth, W. E.: Bullet velocity and design as determinants of wounding capability: an experimental study. J. Trauma, 6:222–232, 1966.
17. DeMuth, W. E.: High-velocity bullet wounds of muscle and bone: the basis of rational early treatment. J. Trauma, 6:744–755, 1966.
18. DeMuth, W. E.: Bullet velocity as applied to military rifle wounding capacity. J. Trauma, 9:27–38, 1969.
19. Dziemian, A. J., Mendelson, J. A., and Lindsay, D.: Comparison of the wounding characteristics of some commonly encountered bullets. J. Trauma, 1:341–353, 1961.
20. Epps, C. H., Jr., and Adams, J. P.: Wound management in open fractures. Am. Surg., 27:766–769, 1961.
21. Fee, N. F., Dobranski, A., and Bisla, R. S.: Gas gangrene complicating open forearm fractures. Report of five cases. J. Bone Joint Surg., 59A:135–138, 1977.
22. Fogelberg, E. V., Zitzman, E. K., and Stinchfield, F. E.: Prophylactic penicillin in orthopaedic surgery. J. Bone Joint Surg., 52A:95–98, 1970.
23. Furste, W., Skudder, P. A., and Hampton, O. P.: Prophylaxis against tetanus in wound management. J. Trauma, 6:516, 1966.
24. Ger, R.: The management of open fractures of the tibia with skin loss. J. Trauma, 10:112–121, 1970.
25. Glotzer, D. J., Goodman, W. S., and Geronimus, L. H.: Topical antibiotic prophylaxis in contaminated wounds. Experimental evaluation. Arch. Surg., 100:589–593, 1970.
26. Godley, D. R., and Smith, T. K.: Some medicolegal aspects of gunshot wounds. J. Trauma, 17:866–871, 1977.
27. Gross, A., Cutright, D. E., and Bhaskar, S. N.: Effectiveness of pulsating water jet lavage in treatment of contaminated crushed wounds. Am. J. Surg., 124:373–377, 1972.
28. Gustilo, R. B., Simpson, L., Nixon, R., and Ruiz, A.: Analysis of 511 open fractures. Clin. Orthop. Rel. Res., 66:148–154, 1969.
29. Gustilo, R. B., and Anderson, J. T.: Prevention of infection in the treatment of one thousand and twenty-five open fractures of long bones. J. Bone Joint Surg., 58A:453–458, 1976.
30. Hampton, O. P., Jr.: The indications for debridement of gun shot (bullet) wounds of the extremities in civilian practice. J. Trauma, 1:368–372, 1961.
31. Hampton, O. P., Jr.: Editorial. Management of open fractures and open wounds of joints. J. Trauma, 8:475–478, 1968.
32. Harvey, E. N.: Studies on wound ballistics in service in World War II. Advances in military medicine. Vol. 1. Boston, Little, Brown & Co., 1948.
33. Heppenstall, R. B., Littooy, F. N., Fuchs, R., Sheldon, G., and Hunt, T. K.: Gas tensions in healing tissues of traumatized patients. Surgery, 75:874–880, 1974.
34. Howland, W. S., and Ritchey, S. J.: Gunshot fractures in civilian practice. An evaluation of the results of limited surgical treatment. J. Bone Joint Surg., 53A:47–55, 1971.
35. Howland, W. S., and Sterling, J. R.: Gunshot wounds in civilian practice. An evaluation of the results of limited surgical treatment. J. Bone Joint Surg., 53A:47–55, 1971.
36. Hopkinson, D. A. W., and Marshall, T. K.: Firearm injuries. Br. J. Surg., 54:344, 1967.
37. Key, J. A.: Treatment of compound fractures in the antibiotic age. J.A.M.A., 146:1091, 1951.
38. King, K. F.: Orthopaedic aspects of war wounds in South Vietnam. J. Bone Joint Surg., 51B:112, 1969.

39. Leonard, M. H.: Solution of lead by synovial fluid. Clin. Orthop. Rel. Res., 64:255–261, 1969.
40. London, P. S., and Clarke, R.: Severe accidental flaying. J. Bone Joint Surg., 41B:658, 1959.
41. Lowry, K. F., and Curtis, G. M.: Delayed suture in management of wounds. Am. J. Surg., 80:280, 1950.
42. Morgan, M. M., Spencer, A. D., and Hershey, F. B.: Debridement of civilian gunshot wounds of soft tissue. J. Trauma, 1:354–360, 1961.
43. Orr, H. W.: Compound fractures with special reference to the lower extremity. Am. J. Surg., 46:733–737, 1939.
44. Paradies, L. H., and Gregory, C. F.: Early treatment of close-range shotgun wounds to the extremities. J. Bone Joint Surg., 48A:425–432, 1966.
45. Patzakis, M., Harvey, J. I. P., and Ivler, D.: The role of antibiotics in the management of open fractures. J. Bone Joint Surg., 56A:532–541, 1974.
46. Patzakis, M. J., Dorr, L. D., Ivler, D., Moore, T. M., and Harvey, J. P.: The early management of open joint injuries. A prospective study of one hundred and forty patients. J. Bone Joint Surg., 57A:1065–1071, 1975.
47. Peebles, T. C., Levine, L., Eldred, M. C., and Edsall, G.: Tetanus-toxoid emergency boosters. A reappraisal. N. Engl. J. Med., 280:575–581, 1969.
48. Pollock, W. J., and Parkes, J. C.: Open skin grafting of war wounds. J. Bone Joint Surg., 51A:926, 1969.
49. Pool, E. H.: War wounds: primary and secondary suture. J.A.M.A., 73:383, 1919.
50. Pulaski, E. J., Meleney, F. L., and Spaeth, W. L. C.: Bacterial flora of acute traumatic wounds. Surg. Gynecol. Obstet., 72:982, 1941.
51. Rustigan, R., and Cipriani, A.: Bacteriology of open wounds. J.A.M.A., 33:224, 1947.
52. Salisbury, R.: Biological dressings for skin graft donor sites. Arch. Surg., 106:705–706, 1973.
53. Scully, R. E., Artz, C. P., and Sako, Y.: An evaluation of the surgeon's criteria for determining muscle viability during debridement. Arch. Surg., 73:1031–1035, 1956.
54. Smith-Petersen, M. N., Larson, C. B., and Cochran, W.: Local chemotherapy with primary closure of septic wounds by means of drainage and irrigation cannulae. J. Bone Joint Surg., 27:562–571, 1945.
55. Tanner, J. C., Vanderput, J., and Alley, J. F.: The mesh skin graft. Plast. Reconstr. Surg., 34:287–292, 1964.
56. Thompson, J. E., and Berry, F. B.: Penetrating wounds of major joints. Ann. Surg., 126:947, 1947.
57. Thuresby, F. P., and Darlow, H. M.: The mechanisms of primary infection of bullet wounds. Br. J. Surg., 54:359, 1967.
58. Trueta, J.: Principles and Practice of War Surgery. St. Louis, C. V. Mosby, 1943.
59. Trueta, J., and Barnes, J. M.: Immobilization in treatment of infected wounds. Br. Med. J., 2:46, 1940.
60. Waterman, N. A., Howell, R. S., and Babich, M.: The effect of a prophylactic antibiotic (cephalothin) on the incidence of wound infection. Arch. Surg., 97:365–370, 1968.
61. Wilson, F. C., Worcester, J. N., Coleman, P. D., and Byrd, W. E.: Antibiotic penetration of experimental bone hematomas. J. Bone Joint Surg., 53A:1622–28, 1971.
62. Wilson, J. N.: The management of infection after Küntscher nailing of the femur. J. Bone Joint Surg., 48B:112, 1966.
63. Ziperman, H. H.: The management of soft tissue missile wounds in war and peace. J. Trauma, 1:361–367, 1961.

WILLIAM T. FITTS JR., M.D.

Early Care of the Patient with Multiple Injuries*

31

INTRODUCTION

Patients with fractures often have multiple injuries, and management of the fracture must never prevent the physician from discovering other life-threatening conditions. Such injuries are often occult and easily overlooked. The term multiple injuries describes an injury producing two or more sites of major trauma. Every injured patient must be considered to have multiple injuries until proved otherwise. Often the most important injury—the one that may kill or maim the patient—is overlooked because the most obvious injury receives all the attention.

An immediate and thorough examination of the entire body must be made to discover all of the patient's injuries. Remember always that the saving of life comes first; treat asphyxia, hemorrhage, shock, and other life-endangering conditions before treating the fracture, or at least *while* treating the fracture. In making an immediate assessment of the injured patient's condition, primary emphasis must be placed on the functions of respiration and circulation and on the possibility of injury to the spinal cord, especially the cervical spine. Deaths that occur within a few hours of injury are usually the result of severe brain damage, asphyxia, hemorrhage, or a combination of these. Many patients with severe intracranial injuries probably could not be saved even by the most expert medical care, although recent work in neurosurgical intensive care units indicates that some of these patients can be saved by prompt attention to the respiratory damage that is associated with brain injury.

The treatment of patients with multiple injuries should be a team effort, but there must be a team captain—one person who assumes primary responsibility and who coordinates the studies and management of the patient from the beginning. Often the captain may change as more experienced personnel arrive on the scene.

---

*In the preparation of this chapter the author has drawn freely from *Early Care of the Injured Patient*, by the Committee on Trauma of the American College of Surgeons. This book should be readily available to all those taking care of the injured patient.

HISTORY AND PHYSICAL EXAMINATION

Often a complete history is impossible, but every effort should be made to establish the time and cause of the accident, and these data should be noted on the patient's record. The how, when, where of the accident must be determined and recorded. Any onlookers should be carefully questioned, and the patient, if able to answer questions, should be thoroughly interrogated. It is important to determine the presence of chronic disease and especially the history of prescribed medication, drug sensitivity, and allergy. The underlying illness may well be the cause of the accident, and proper treatment may not be possible until this is known. Such a patient, recently seen in our emergency department, had been receiving steroid therapy but had neglected to take his medication. He developed shock from hypotension due to steroid withdrawal and lost control of his automobile, causing the accident.

A complete, rapid, and thorough physical examination must be made at the same time as lifesaving measures are undertaken. Often lives are lost because occult injuries go undiagnosed as the most obvious injury is being treated. Not infrequently this is because the patient is not completely disrobed. In all severely injured patients, all the clothing should be removed and the entire body inspected and examined. In fractures, especially those of the cervical spine, great care must be taken in turning the patient. The operator must insure that there is stabilization of fractures, especially those of the neck. A rectal examination must always be performed. This examination may reveal an unsuspected pelvic fracture or injury to the urinary or gastrointestinal tract.

MANAGEMENT OF THE AIRWAY

ENDOTRACHEAL INTUBATION

Of first priority in the management of the patient with multiple injuries are evaluating the airway and insuring its continued patency. Upper airway obstruction can often be relieved by clearing the mouth and pharynx of foreign material and then tilting the head backward and elevating the lower jaw. However, patients who are unconscious as a result of head injury may have associated damage to the cervical spine. To prevent further spinal cord damage as the upper airway is cleared, the patient's head should be held immobile by one person while at least two others roll him to the side for clearing the mouth and pharynx. When the patient is returned to the supine position, extension of the neck should be restricted only to that degree required to open the airway. Proper positioning of the head, removal of foreign bodies, and endotracheal intubation, each supplemented by aspiration of the upper airway, all may be lifesaving when airway obstruction poses a threat of asphyxia.

Tracheostomy is occasionally indicated when an endotracheal tube cannot be passed. By keeping the patient's head down until an endotracheal tube can be put in place, inhalation of vomitus can be minimized. If there is any question about the adequacy of an airway, an endotracheal tube should be inserted and the tube replaced by a tracheostomy when it is obvious that the patient will require ventilatory assistance for a long period of time.

Patients who have severe respiratory stress, who are cyanotic, who are agitated owing to hypoxia, or who show evidence of face, neck, or chest injury need to have oxygen delivered directly into the trachea. The method employed will depend upon the following considerations: (1) the likelihood of an injury to the cervical spine which might be worsened by the manipulations necessary for insertion of an endotracheal tube, (2) the skill and experience of the treating physician, and (3) the probability of the need for prolonged ventilatory assistance.

Alternative Methods

Alternatives to endotracheal intubation include a number of measures. One is cricothyroidotomy, in which a tracheal catheter, consisting of a 14-gauge needle or a Teflon catheter, is inserted percutaneously through the cricothyroid membrane. It is used to insufflate oxygen by connecting the hub to an oxygen source and a self-inflating bag resuscitator. This technique is a temporary expedient that may reverse a toxic chain of events. A cricothyroidotomy consists of a transverse incision just beneath the larynx, which severs the cricothyroid membrane. It permits insertion of an instrument or tube between the thyroid and cricoid cartilages to provide an ample airway below the vocal cords. The procedure is safe and comparatively easy to perform.

Nasotracheal intubation involves insertion of an endotracheal tube through the nose and into the larynx and trachea. It avoids manipulation of the neck but requires a cooperative or an unconscious patient and an experienced and skilled operator. Since it may cause vomiting, skilled personnel and an aspirator must be available.

Orotracheal intubation is performed by inserting an endotracheal tube through the mouth by a laryngoscope. Adequate suction and prior nasogastric decompression are advisable to reduce the risk of vomiting. Since hyperextension of the neck is usually required, it is important to check first for cervical spine injury.

Tracheostomy consists of the surgical insertion of a tube, preferably through the second and third tracheal cartilages. Since this can be a difficult surgical procedure, it should rarely be performed in the emergency department or without prior tracheal intubation. Immediate intubation is seldom necessary or desirable. Of first priority are clearing the airway of obstructing objects, including the tongue, and ventilating the patient. After the patient has been oxygenated, intubation can be carried out if necessary.

If possible, patients with head and neck injuries should have x-rays to detect cervical spine fractures or dislocations. If these are present, further injury to the cord must be avoided in subsequent management. A trained anesthesiologist would know how to accomplish an "awake intubation" after the neck is splinted and the head is being supported. If the patient is assumed to have a full stomach, he should have only atropine for premedication. If available, an electrocardiographic monitor may be helpful. Much more important, in fact mandatory, is continuous pulse monitoring with a precordial or esophageal stethoscope.

It is possible that the obstructed airway should be managed by a cuffed endotracheal tube. There are times, of course, when personnel skilled in the placement of an endotracheal tube are not available. Paramedical workers are now being trained in this procedure. The esophageal airway is not, strictly speaking, an esophageal airway. It is a large-bore tube with a large balloon that almost mimics the radiologist's barium enema cuffed tube. The tube is passed blindly into the esophagus, and the balloon is then inflated to obstruct the esophagus. Proximal to the balloon are side vents—openings in the tube which with inflation of the balloon will force the air to pass into the trachea and bronchi. The device is really more of a blind pharyngeal tube or pharyngeal airway.

Tracheostomy. Tracheostomy is seldom indicated in the care of the multiply injured patient. There are perhaps two clear-cut situations in which it is advisable. One is in the patient with multiple facial injuries and a mandibular fracture or a floating mandible, in whom it is otherwise impossible to stabilize the airway. One can provide temporary stabilization with a suture or towel clip through the tongue to bring it forward while a tracheostomy is carried out. The other indication is in the patient with potential or real cervical spine fracture-dislocation, in whom movement (flexion, or extension, or lateral rotation) of the neck is contraindicated. One method is to thread an endotracheal tube over a flexible bronchoscope and then pass it through the larynx into the trachea.

Initial Treatment and Follow-up

It is likely that the patient who reaches the emergency department alive following a vehicular accident some distance away either had no immediate upper airway obstruction or was properly treated at the accident scene and during transport. Therefore, the airway management at the hospital by the trauma surgeon, anesthesiologist, and allied personnel is directed toward supplementing the initial field therapy or elaborating upon it.

The solution of the immediate airway management problem can be contained in the answers to the simple questions *who* and *how*. It is now recognized that the initial rescuer, whether a physician or a paramedic, must bear the responsibility of initiating airway management. On many occasions, initiating the airway care and providing a definite life support system are synonymous. How the initial attendant is to provide this care is not easy to solve.

Most physicians and paramedical ambulance personnel are familiar with the use of an oropharyngeal airway, located in the equipment package of emergency vehicles. This will prevent the tongue from occluding the laryngeal aperture, but it is useless in many cases of severe head and neck trauma. When edema, bleeding, aspiration, and direct laryngeal and tracheal injury occur, more complicated methods of treatment are demanded.

In the hospital, endotracheal intubation by trained personnel is the preferred method of initial airway control when it is required. However, at the scene of the accident, endotracheal intubation is often difficult for those with limited experience in intubation. It is evident, therefore, that emergency medical personnel must be trained to manage an airway immediately in prompt and efficient manner. The most direct and easiest route to the airway is through the cricothyroid membrane, creating a temporary airway stoma which can be converted to a tracheostomy if necessary in a less hectic moment after hospital admission.

The technique of cricothyroidotomy is not complicated and can be demonstrated to ambulance personnel. Indications for its use can be carefully presented to these responsible individuals, who already are beginning to play a much greater role in initial resuscitation and therapy.

ESTABLISHMENT OF AN EFFECTIVE RESPIRATORY EXCHANGE

Pneumothorax

Cardiothoracic injuries may be either penetrating or blunt. Before a dyspneic patient is intubated and placed on a mechanical ventilator, it must be ascertained that he has no pneumothorax. Tension pneumothorax develops when an opening in the lung, chest wall, or bronchus acts as a valve that allows air to enter the pleural cavity on inspiration but prevents its escape during expiration. As a result, pressure builds up in the pleural space. This elevated intrathoracic pressure collapses the ipsilateral lung, displaces the mediastinum to the opposite side, and significantly compresses the contralateral lung. Air hunger, hypertension, and cyanosis dominate the clinical picture; tracheal shift and diminished or absent breath sounds also suggest the diagnosis. Chest x-rays will confirm the diagnosis, but if doubt still exists an 18-gauge needle may be inserted into the chest and aspiration done to determine the presence of air. The necessary treatment if the lesion is present is immediate tube thoracostomy.

Hemothorax

Injuries that present with massive or moderate hemothorax are generally lacerations or other trauma to the chest wall, resulting in intercostal or internal mammary vessel damage. Other sources of hemothorax include bleeding from injuries to the lungs, heart, or mediastinal vessels. Treatment of moderate or massive hemothorax is tube thoracostomy connected to a closed-seal underwater system. All patients with minimal hemothorax should be closely watched, because bleeding may continue and progress to a more severe stage of hemothorax in only a few hours.

Massive hemothorax is generally the result of a penetrating injury to a major vessel. Open chest wounds usually require operative intervention, but as a preliminary measure an occlusive dressing should be applied, followed by a tube thoracostomy. This will prevent further shift of the mediastinum and allow ventilation of the opposite lung.

Flail Chest

Flail chest occurs when a segment of the bony thorax is fractured in more than one area, allowing the mobilized segment to move on breathing in a direction opposite to that of the remainder of the thorax (paradoxical respiration). Diagnosis is made by palpation of the flail segment or by observing the paradoxical respiration. The minimal flail chest with no severe respiratory embarrassment may be managed without operation by improving the evacuations of secretions and by administering intercostal nerve blocks for relief of pain. The patient with a more severe flail chest is probably best managed by endotracheal intubation and support by mechanical ventilation on a respirator.

Pulmonary and Myocardial Contusion

The physician should be on the alert for the more subtle injury of pulmonary contusion. Pulmonary contusion may not be obvious immediately on admission, but may become apparent only some 24 hours after injury. One of the first signs is a diminution in the P_{O_2}.

Myocardial contusion is also a subtle injury that must always be considered in injuries to the chest. Certain types of injuries should make one suspect myocardial contusion—for example, injuries in which the patient was thrown from a vehicle, struck the steering wheel, or for any other reason has an area of contusion over the anterior chest wall. Myocardial contusion *may* occur without evident chest wall injury, but it is more often found with signs of sternal contusion and rib fractures. Damage to the heart may range from minor subepicardial or subendocardial hemorrhage to rupture of the myocardium. Most injury will become evident within 48 to 72 hours with electrocardiographic alterations, particularly inverted T waves. There may also be arrhythmias, myocardial failure, cardiac tamponade, or hemothorax. The immediate management of myocardial contusion parallels the care of acute myocardial infarction.

Pericardial Tamponade

Any patient who has sustained a blunt chest injury, a gunshot wound of the chest, or a precordial or epigastric stab wound should be suspected of having pericardial tamponade unless examination definitely rules it out. The classic signs of tamponade are the triad of arterial hypotension, venous hypertension, and narrow pulse pressure. This is probably the one situation in which a static intravenous pressure reading can be meaningful, yet in the patient with cardiac tamponade it is almost redundant to establish a central venous pressure. If pericardial tamponade is suspected, one should immediately decompress the pericardial cavity by pericardial aspiration.

ESTABLISHMENT OF AN EFFECTIVE CIRCULATING BLOOD VOLUME

Once the airway has been established and oxygen has been provided to the cells, a circulating blood volume is needed to transport the oxygen to the cellular level. External hemorrhage is best controlled by direct pressure. There are exceptions, such as a massive injury to an extremity necessitating a tourniquet, but almost always the application of direct pressure will control hemorrhage. Blood loss must be evaluated and prevented from contributing to further deterioration of the patient. To provide for adequate fluid and blood replacement, insert at least two 16-gauge catheters into two different sites, one in the upper extremity and one in the lower extremity. In suspected injuries to the pelvis or extremities, avoid the lower extremities as a site for giving blood in order to prevent further loss of blood in the area of the injury.

Blood should immediately be drawn for typing, cross matching, and determination of hematocrit, electrolytes, and level of blood gases. The best fluid for immediate resuscitation is lactated Ringer's solution, since it closely resembles the extracellular fluid. The lactic acid of Ringer's lactate is metabolized into carbon dioxide and water and provides free water, so there is no need to worry about providing water in addition to the resuscitation fluid. Often there may be a need to monitor the central venous pressure of the multiply injured patient, or in the most critically ill the pulmonary wedge pressure. The sites for insertion of the central venous catheter may vary. We prefer a subclavian approach. Careful monitoring of the central venous pressure is helpful in determining the volume and type of resuscitation fluids to give. Caution is needed in monitoring the central venous pressure. It cannot be used as a static measure, because a single central venous pressure reading may offer nothing in monitoring a given patient, except to suggest cardiac tamponade. The *trend* of central venous pressure readings is helpful in all critically injured patients, especially those with heart disease, those who are digitalized, and those with incipient pulmonary edema. Determinations of central venous pressure levels can be useful indicators of how effective the fluids used for resuscitation are.

BLOOD LOSS

A proper estimation of blood loss is important in assessing the patient with multiple injuries. Usually one tends to minimize blood loss. Severe fractures of the pelvis may result in a blood loss of 3 to 4 liters, and at times as much as 15 liters may be lost. This blood will extend into the retroperitoneal area as well as throughout the pelvic region. Fracture of the pelvis is one of the most underestimated sources of blood loss in the multiply injured patient. Another injury in which blood loss is not appreciated is fracture of femur, which can result in the loss of 1 to 2 liters, which are trapped in the tight fascial compartments of the thigh. In these instances it is useful to measure the circumference of the involved thigh, which will help to estimate the increase in bleeding into the thigh.

Shock

In the unconscious patient, shock is often caused by blood loss. Blood loss may be from severe scalp lacerations, from associated facial injuries, or from injuries from closed spaces, either the thoracic or the peritoneal cavity. The unconscious patient in shock should be considered to be in shock as a result of blood loss until another cause is proved.

Whenever an injured patient is seen in profound shock out of proportion to the injury present and with massive hemothorax, a major vessel injury should be immediately suspected. These injuries often result from penetration by a bullet or knife.

Immediate thoracotomy offers the patient the only opportunity for survival. We believe that all bullet or missile wounds of the abdomen need exploration, even if shock or signs of peritonitis are absent. Diagnostic studies other than physical examination should be limited, and x-ray studies obtained only if the patient appears febrile after initial resuscitative care.

BLUNT TRAUMA

Stab sounds of the abdomen, however, can be carefully observed, and an operation can be performed if signs of peritoneal irritation are present. It is blunt abdominal injuries that pose the major problems. These commonly present with evidence of contusion of the lower chest wall, splinting of the abdominal wall, absent or diminished bowel sounds, guarding of the abdominal wall, and localized tenderness. The physician should be on the lookout for fractures of the lower third of the chest accompanied by pain in the shoulder or absence of peristalsis along with nausea, vomiting, and distention of the abdomen. Blood in the vomitus, stool, or urine is significant; it frequently indicates intraperitoneal injury.

Paradoxical respiration within the abdomen may signify injury to the diaphragm, while a ruptured diaphragm may be indicated by peristaltic sounds within the chest from the abdominal viscera in the pleural cavity. Occasionally a multiply injured patient must be turned over. This makes a point for resuscitation of the patient in the supine position.

Injuries of the thoracic cavity were considered earlier in the chapter. Abdominal injuries are often life-threatening in the patient with multiple injuries. Liver injuries are becoming more common and are difficult to manage. The clinical features of injuries to the liver are localized pain in the right upper quadrant with radiation to the shoulder, shock, and absent bowel sounds. Since the liver is a solid fixed organ, lacerations of the liver are common in deceleration injuries.

Pancreatic injury, usually the result of blunt upper abdominal trauma, is often associated with trauma to other organs, such as the stomach, duodenum, and liver. Occasionally, injury to the pancreas may be accompanied by damage to major blood vessels, including the vena cava. Determinations of serum amylase are helpful in the diagnosis of pancreatic injury.

The spleen is very frequently injured by blunt trauma; such injuries are often associated with fractures of the left rib cage. The clinical features of splenic injury include signs of blood loss, abdominal pain localized to the left upper quadrant, and pain radiating to the left scapula and the tip of the left shoulder (Kehr's sign).

Blunt abdominal injuries call for special diagnostic studies. The four-quadrant peritoneal tap is very simple, but potentially most helpful. The aspiration should be performed with a short 18-gauge needle attached to a 10-ml syringe. As little as 1 ml of blood or fluid is diagnostic of intraperitoneal injury. However, a negative tap is totally meaningless; it certainly does not rule out intraperitoneal injury.

Peritoneal Lavage

When such injuries are suspected in an unconscious or multiply injured patient and the four-quadrant tap is negative, peritoneal lavage should be performed. The urinary bladder should be catheterized first, but this should be done quite early along with other resuscitative measures in any case—both to appraise the status of the urinary tract in general and to monitor the effectiveness of fluid resuscitation.

The technique of peritoneal lavage is no different from that of inserting a peritoneal dialysis tube, which is the recommended procedure. The tube is inserted through the lower midline of the abdomen. If aspiration reveals no gross blood or fluid, 1000 ml of lactated Ringer's solution is infused into the abdomen of an adult (300 to 500 ml in a child). The bottle is then lowered to create a siphon effect, and the fluid is recovered. An obviously bloody return will of course dictate the need for abdominal exploration, but in any case the color of the return is significant; as little as 75 or 100 ml within the peritoneal cavity will tint the fluid a salmon or straw color. The fluid should be examined for white blood cells, bacteria, and fecal content. An elevated fluid amylase determination suggests pancreatic injury or perforation of the duodenum or upper small intestine.

Roentgenographic Examination

X-ray studies are important, but a negative study does *not* rule out an intraabdominal injury; a positive one may be extremely helpful. For maximal usefulness, flat-plate studies of the abdomen should include the diaphragm and the chest. X-rays may disclose free air or fluid, immobility of the diaphragm on the affected side, displacement of viscera, or obliteration of the psoas shadows. Retroperitoneal emphysema may be found in injuries of the duodenum or of the extraperitoneal rectum.

Urography. Any patient who receives blunt trauma to the perineum, genitalia, abdomen, back, or flank should be suspected of having a urinary tract injury. The urinary bladder should be catheterized in every injured patient. Blood in the urine may indicate laceration or contusion of the kidney. A word of caution: When the catheter doesn't readily enter the urinary bladder, obtain a urethrogram immediately to determine the status of the patient's urethra.

The kidney is most often injured by blunt trauma to the upper abdomen or posterior chest. Kidney injury should be suspected in blunt abdominal trauma with any degree of hematuria and in any patient with unexplained ileus or abdominal pain. The possibility of a kidney injury must be considered in the presence of any penetrating abdominal wound. It should also be considered if there is fracture of the lower rib cage or the transverse processes of the lumbar vertebrae, or if there is a flank mass or costovertebral angle tenderness.

What will an intravenous urogram show in the presence of kidney injury? One may see a negative shadow within the kidney, or there may be extravasation of the contrast medium. There may also be obliteration of the psoas shadow.

The distended bladder is easily ruptured. This occurs most commonly during deceleration in automobile accidents. Injury to the prostatic urethra is almost always caused by the shearing effect on the prostatic urethra in association with a fracture of the bony pelvis. The diagnostic signs of a ruptured bladder include rigidity of the abdomen, associated hypotension, and inability to urinate. Injuries to the prostatic urethra are accompanied by the signs of ruptured bladder plus fluctuation in the area of the prostate on rectal examination. The two most important x-ray studies are the retrograde urethrogram and the retrograde cystogram. Once more: Attempts to catheterize the urinary bladder should be abandoned if they are not immediately successful or a rupture may result.

Fractures

We should direct our attention to the life-threatening injuries that present in association with fractures. Many of these are related to the blood loss that comes with lacerations of major vessels. Arteriography has been extremely helpful in some instances, particularly when there has been vascular embarrassment below the site of fracture. One must obtain arteriograms to assess the status of the blood supply, but these should be combined with careful and repeated checking of the pulses below the fracture site.

In summary, there is a serious need for all of us involved in the care of the injured to accept responsibility for overseeing and guiding a patient after a multiple-injury accident. There is a need for one individual to direct the care of that patient and to insure that priorities are established and maintained. Without that, we are jeopardizing the patient and are not going to do the job necessary to reduce the morbidity and mortality of the injured patient.

CARDIOPULMONARY RESUSCITATION (CPR)

Cardiopulmonary resuscitation (CPR) is the first method used to restore an effective ventilation and circulation in persons who have lost these functions. At the 1973 National Conference of Standards for CPR and Emergency Cardiac Care Standards, methods were developed and published (J.A.M.A. (Suppl.), 227:7, 1974). All those caring for the injured patient should be familiar with these recommendations.

The common denominator in all instances of sudden death is anoxia. Causes include drowning, electrocution, stroke, gas inhalation, drug or chemical intoxication, injuries involving the head, neck, or chest, myocardial infarction, convulsions, and unconsciousness from other causes. Clinical death occurs when peripheral pulses, heartbeat, effective circulation and ventilation are absent, and pupils are dilated and unresponsive to light. Biological death is a progression of clinical death to the point at which irreversible anoxic damage has occurred. This varies from organ to organ (three to five minutes for the brain to several hours for the muscles).

BASIC LIFE SUPPORT

This is an emergency set of first-aid procedures. It consists of recognizing respiratory and cardiac arrest and instituting CPR immediately until the victim has recovered sufficiently to be transported to a facility where advanced life support measures are available. Basic life support includes the ABC's of CPR: (a) airway management, (b) breathing, and (c) circulation. To accomplish this, artificial ventilation and artificial circulation must be established.

The advantage of CPR is that it may be instituted immediately, anywhere, by adequately trained personnel, with no elaborate equipment required. Delay in starting CPR may lead to irreversible atoxic cerebral damage. In unconscious or collapsed persons, inadequacy of effective ventilation and circulation must be determined immediately. If ventilation alone is absent or ineffective, airway management and artificial ventilation may be all that is required. If in addition circulation is ineffective or absent, artificial circulation may be started in combination with artificial ventilation. The basic steps are opening the airway and restoring ventilation.

Ventilatory inadequacy may result from a mechanical obstruction to the airway (for example, the tongue), from foreign bodies (vomitus, food, blood), or from respiratory failure. A partially obstructed airway is recognized by

1. Noisy and labored breathing (stridor).

2. Use of the accessory muscles of breathing (e.g., sternocleidomastoids).

3. Soft tissue retractions of the intercostal, supraclavicular, and suprasternal areas.

4. Paradoxical or "seesaw" breathing. Normally, in the unobstructed airway the chest and abdomen rise and fall together. If the airway is partially or completely obstructed and cardiac arrest has not occurred, the chest is sucked in as the abdomen rises.

5. Cyanosis. For cyanosis to occur, a circulating reduced hemoglobin level of about 5 gm per 100 ml is needed; this is a late sign of hypoxia, especially if the patient is anemic.

Airway Management

The most important step for successful resuscitation is immediate opening of the airway. A head tilt is performed by placing one hand under the victim's neck, the other on the forehead. The neck is lifted with one hand, and the head is tilted back with the other. This extends the neck and lifts the tongue from the posterior pharyngeal wall. By observing the chest wall and listening at the victim's mouth, it can be rapidly determined whether or not breathing is present. If breathing has not begun, the rescuer performs four rapid mouth-to-mouth ventilations. The rescuer inhales deeply and applies his wide-open mouth to the victim's mouth, inflating the lung. The nose must be occluded by pinching. Adequate inflation can be recognized by seeing the chest rise, feeling the resistance or compliance of the victim's lungs as they expand, and hearing the escape of air during exhalation. The normal rate for ventilation is one insufflation every five seconds.

Mouth-to-nose ventilation may be used if the mouth is impossible to open, if serious injuries to the mouth are present, or if there is difficulty in obtaining a good seal with mouth-to-mouth breathing. The rescuer keeps the head tilted back with one hand on the forehead, using the other hand to lift the victim's lower jaw, which seals the lips. The rescuer inflates the lungs by sealing his lips around the victim's nose and blowing.

Infants and Children. Airway management is similar to that in adults. The larynx in infants or small children lies more anteriorly, so that overextension of the neck may obstruct the airway; consequently, the neck should be held in midposition. The rescuer covers both the mouth and the nose with this mouth, uses small puffs of air with less volume, and inflates the lungs once every three seconds.

Trauma Victims. If there is a possibility of neck fracture, caution must be taken to avoid neck extension and all neck movements. The victim's head and neck should be kept in a neutral position. Evidence of upper airway obstruction can be overcome by appropriate measures, such as the following: (1) insertion of an oropharyngeal or nasopharyngeal tube; (2) protraction of the mandible (jaw thrust); and (3) a triple airway maneuver if mouth-to-mouth respiration is necessary. This consists of protracting the jaw and sealing the nose with the rescuer's cheek while giving mouth-to-mouth ventilation.

Foreign Bodies. The rescuer should not look for foreign bodies in the airway as an initial step prior to mouth-to-mouth ventilation. Inability to ventilate with proper neck extension will determine the presence of foreign bodies. In such instances, the victim should be rolled onto the side away from the rescuer and the jaw opened with the thumb and index finger. The index finger of the other hand is used to explore the victim's oropharynx; this will identify and permit removal of large foreign bodies. If skilled personnel are available, direct laryngoscopy is indicated to remove the foreign body with forceps, followed by rapid endotracheal intubation after the victim has been ventilated with a high-oxygen concentration from a bag–valve–mask unit. If a laryngoscope is not available, three or four sharp blows with the heel of the hand should be delivered between the victim's shoulder blades, the pharynx reexplored, and attempts made to ventilate the victim.

HEIMLICH MANEUVER. This method is effective in relieving acute upper airway obstruction caused by food or foreign bodies lodged in the posterior pharynx or glottis. The victim cannot speak or breathe, may become panic-stricken, and frequently runs from the room. Pallor may develop, followed by increasing cyanosis, anoxia, and death. The maneuver may be carried out with the patient in a standing or lying position.

The Rescuer Standing. The rescuer stands behind the victim and wraps his arms around the victim's waist, with the fist of one hand grasped by the other. The thumb side of the rescuer's fist is held against the victim's abdomen between the umbilicus and the rib cage. The rescuer's fist is pressed into the victim's abdomen with a quick upward thrust. This may have to be repeated several times. Sudden elevation of the diaphragm compresses the lung within the confines of the thoracic cage, increasing intrathoracic pressure, and forcing air and the foreign object from the airway.

The Rescuer Kneeling. The victim lies supine; the rescuer kneels astride the victim's hips. The rescuer lays his hands on top of each other, places the heel of the dependent hand on the abdomen of the victim between the xiphoid and the umbilicus, and carries out the same procedure.

Tracheostomy in an obstructed patient as an emergency procedure is fraught with hazards. The opening in the cricothyroid membrane may be held open with a clamp, or a small number 2 tracheostomy tube, if available, may be inserted.

Gastric Distention and Aspiration. The most common cause of gastric distention is an inadequate airway. Vomiting is an active reflex act, while regurgitation of stomach contents is a passive phenomenon based on a pressure difference between the intragastric contents and the oropharynx. The latter occurs in cardiopulmonary arrest. Significant aspiration of gastric contents with a pH of 2.5 or less is associated with a mortality rate of close to 50 to 60 per cent, and is a common occurrence in cardiopulmonary arrest. Gross distention can be relieved by applying moderate pressure to the epigastrium. This should be done with the victim turned on his side, so that any gastric contents will drain out of the mouth by gravity.

Artificial Circulation

When sudden cessation of effective circulation occurs, the ABC's of basic life support must be instituted. The recognition of cardiac arrest should take no longer than 10 seconds. Cardiac arrest is assumed in these conditions: (1) absent large vessel pulses, (2) absent ventilation, (3) unconsciousness with a deathlike appearance and fixed dilated pupils.

The carotid pulse should be checked following four lung ventilations. Maintaining the head tilt with one hand, the index finger of the other hand locates the victim's larynx and slides into the groove between the trachea and the sternomastoid muscle. The reasons for the selection of the carotid pulse over other arterial pulses include (1) its proximity (since the rescuer is at the victim's head), and (2) the ready accessibility of the neck (no clothing has to be removed). Furthermore, (3) since the carotids are large arteries, their pulsation may still occur in low cardiac-output states when other peripheral pulses have disappeared. Femoral arterial palpation is an acceptable alternative in the hospitalized patient.

External Cardiac Compression (ECC)

Questionable absence of the carotid pulse is an indication for starting external cardiac compression (ECC). As the heart is compressed between the sternum and the vertebral column, blood is ejected from the left ventricle; during relaxation, cardiac filling occurs. Properly performed, ECC produces a cardiac output from 20 to 33 per cent of normal. It must always be accompanied by artificial ventilation.

METHOD

1. The patient must be in a horizontal position.

2. Elevation of the lower extremities may augment venous return and cardiac output.

3. A firm surface is mandatory. A board or tray placed under the victim's shoulders and thorax will suffice, although if it is not immediately available ECC should not be delayed. Placing the patient on the floor may be the best alternative.

4. The rescuer places himself close to the victim's side and locates the tip of the xiphoid process. The heel of the hand is placed three finger-breadths cephalad to this in the long axis of the sternum. The other hand is placed over the first one. The rescuer brings his shoulders directly over the victim's sternum, and with his arms and shoulders straight exerts pressure vertically downward to depress the sternum 1 1/2 to 2 inches in the adult. Compression must be

smooth, regular, and uninterrupted. Relaxation immediately follows compression, but the heel of the rescuer's hand should not be removed from the sternum.

The rate of ECC for two rescuers is 60 per minute, and a ventilation is interposed after each fifth chest compression, that is, in a ratio of 5 to 1. To maintain proper rate, the person compressing the chest must count loudly, "1-1000, 2-1000 . . ." to 5-1000. This method of counting assures the proper rate. Switching positions between rescuers is important, since properly performed CPR is tiring. This is accomplished by the ventilating rescuer's moving to the side of the victim immediately following lung inflation. The pneumonic switch is a means of switching two rescuers without missing a compression. The "chest rescuer" removes his hands, usually after the third compression, and the "heart rescuer" finishes the sequence. The "ex–chest rescuer" is now at the victim's head, has it properly extended, and is ready to inflate the lungs at the completion of the count of "5-1000."

The rate of compression for the single rescuer is 80 per minute. This rate is necessary to maintain a cardiac compression rate of 60 per minute and a respiratory rate of 2, that is, a 30 to 1 ratio. The proper rate can be maintained by the single rescuer by counting, "1 and 2 and 3" to a count of 15.

Infants and Small Children. In small children the heel of one hand is used; in infants the tips of the middle and index fingers are used. The pressure should be exerted at the midsternal area, as the heart lies higher in the chest and the danger of liver laceration is highest in this group. Infants require 1/2 to 3/4 inches of sternal compression; children require 3/4 to 1 1/2 inches. Compression rate is faster (80 to 120 per minute), and breaths are delivered as rapidly as possible at the completion of every fifth compression. A firm support can be provided by the chest compressor's using the other hand under the thorax; a folded blanket serves the same purpose. In small infants the alternative method is to include the chest with both hands and compress the midsternum with both thumbs.

Effectiveness of CPR

Pulse. The carotid pulse should be checked periodically to gauge the adequacy of chest compression. It should always be checked when rescuers change positions.

Pupils. The reactivity of pupils is the best gauge of the effectiveness of CPR. Pupils that constrict to light and remain small indicate that the cerebral circulation is probably adequate. Largely dilated pupils that are unresponsive to light indicate that serious atoxic brain damage is imminent or has already occurred.

Color. Peripheral circulation may be evaluated by squeezing the ear lobes periodically and noting capillary refill time.

Consciousness. The victim may make respiratory or other movements; these suggest adequacy of CPR, but do not necessarily mean CPR should be discontinued. On the contrary, efforts should be continued if a definite pulse cannot be detected without ECC.

Precordial Thump. In cases in which the primary cause of cardiac arrest is not hypoxia, as in witnessed arrest or in the monitored patient in the coronary care unit or intensive care unit, a single precordial thump may be effective in reversing arrhythmias or in restoring normal cardiac action. This maneuver consists of the delivery of a single sharp blow over the midsternum. The fleshy part of the rescuer's fist is used, and the blow is struck from a height of 8 to 12 inches. It should be delivered within a minute of the cardiopulmonary arrest. If there is not an immediate response, basic life support should be started.

The blow generates a small electric stimulus in a reactive myocardium. In addition, it may be effective in reversing ventricular tachycardia or ventricular fibrillation and in restoring a beat in ventricular asystole.

The following situations indicate an initial precordial thump: witnessed cardiac arrest, arrest in the monitored patient, and pacing of a known atrioventricular block.

Pitfalls in CPR Performance

1. Do not interrupt CPR for longer than five seconds, because effective circulation

falls to zero. The single exception to this rule is to allow endotracheal intubation. This is an advanced life support measure and should be performed by none but experienced personnel, and only when expert initial airway management and proper equipment are available. It should not take longer than 5 to 10 seconds to intubate the patient.

2. In penetrating wounds about the heart or when there is evidence of recent cardiothoracic surgery, closed chest massage is usually contraindicated and open thoracotomy is generally advisable.

3. Compression of the lower sternum may result in costochondral separation or lacerations of the abdominal viscera.

4. Malposition of the hands on the ribs, or lateral instead of vertical compression increases the likelihood of fracturing ribs or producing a flail chest.

5. Quick compression and relaxation should be smooth, regular, and uninterrupted. Quick jabs increase the possibility of injury to the victim and do not improve cardiac output.

6. In order to perform effective compression, to obtain a sufficient cardiac output, and to prevent rescuer fatigue, the position of the rescuer must be high enough above the victim so that vertical pressure on the sternum is assured.

7. Ventilation must be interposed between compressions, but the chest compressor should not break the compression relaxation rhythm to wait for the lungs to be inflated by the second rescuer.

8. Other complications include fractured sternum, costochondral separation, pneumothorax, hemothorax, liver lacerations, and fat embolism. These can occur with properly conducted CPR, but are far more likely to occur with improper techniques.

MISDIAGNOSES IN PATIENTS WITH MULTIPLE INJURIES

In an injured patient the most obvious injury is often not the most serious injury. Some examples of misdiagnoses in the injured patient follow.

When a patient suffers an accident, both a local injury and a series of reactions in the body as a whole are induced. Thromboembolic complications and other blood coagulation problems may be induced by a relatively minor injury as well as by multiple injuries. A freshman in the College of the University of Pennsylvania died of pulmonary fat embolism following a closed fracture of the tibia shaft with no displacement, which was treated expertly from the moment of injury. The first sign of trouble was cerebral anoxia from pulmonary fat embolism, which occurred within 12 hours after injury and which was not recognized until it became far advanced. The first indication of pulmonary fat embolism may be cerebral signs due to anoxia. One of the earliest laboratory signs is a diminution in the PO_2. The physician may not recognize such a pulmonary complication and make a mistaken diagnosis of head injury. Blood gas determination will show a depressed oxygen pressure, and proper ventilatory support may save the patient's life.

A patient with a head injury who is in coma and shock may be dying from a ruptured spleen or other abdominal viscus. Head injuries rarely produce shock. When shock is present in such a patient, its cause must be searched for elsewhere. Since intraabdominal and intrathoracic lesions may produce minimal signs in an unconscious patient, peritoneal paracentesis or lavage of a chest tap may be diagnostic.

Patients with a fractured pelvis may die because blood loss into the retroperitoneal tissues is not compensated. At times as much as 20 or 30 units of blood may be needed for replacement. Patients with such injuries must be treated in hospitals with a good blood bank. The bleeding may be stopped by precise angiographic placement of catheters and the insertion of blood clots or other material to plug the bleeding vessel. Patients with a fractured pelvis may also have injuries to intraperitoneal organs that go unrecognized, for example, a fractured liver or a ruptured diaphragm. These must be diagnosed by appropriate tests.

Patients injured by the steering wheel of an automobile may have a cardiac contusion that an electrocardiogram will not show until several days after the injury. A widened mediastinum in a patient with a chest injury may indicate a ruptured aorta, and this finding demands arteriography.

If the patient sustains blunt trauma to the

thorax and abdomen and is not disrobed in the emergency department, a flail chest may not be recognized. When a patient arrives in the emergency department in shock without evidence of blood loss, cardiac tamponade due to bleeding into the pericardial sac should be suspected. Signs include a high central venous pressure, a slow pulse, and a subsequent decline in blood pressure.

In a patient with multiple injuries, preexisting disease may be the cause of an accident as well as the cause of death. A good history is helpful here. As an example, we cite a patient who suffered a fractured femur and humerus which were correctly diagnosed. However, the physician failed to recognize that she had been taking large doses of cortisone for arthritis. The patient died in shock 16 hours after admission to the hospital; failure to administer steroids probably accounted for her death.

REFERENCES

1. Baker, R.: Emergency Cardiac Care Systems. Panel in 1973 Conference of Standards for CPR and Emergency Cardiac Care. J.A.M.A. (Suppl.), 227:7, 860–863, 1974.
2. Blakemore, W. S., and Fitts, W. T., Jr. (eds.): Management of the Injured Patient. New York, Harper & Row, 1969.
3. Bouzarth, W., Green, R., Naclerio, E. A., et al.: Picking up the pieces: Talking it over. Panel in Do's and Don'ts in the Emergency Room Care of the Patient with Multiple Trauma. Presented at the Philadelphia Sectional Meeting of the American College of Surgeons, March 1972. Emergency Med., 4:119–128, 1972.
4. American College of Surgeons Committee on Trauma: Early Care of the Injured Patient. 2nd ed. Philadelphia, W. B. Saunders, 1976.
5. Dudrick, S. J., Wilmore, D. W., Steiger, E., et al.: Spontaneous closure of traumatic pancreatoduodenal fistulas with total intravenous nutrition. J. Trauma, 10:542–553, 1970.
6. Fitts, W. T., Jr., Lehr, H. B., Bitner, R. L., et al.: An analysis of 950 fatal injuries in Philadelphia. Surgery, 56:663–668, 1964.
7. Fitts, W. T., Jr.: The assaulted abdomen. Presented at the American Medical Association Annual Meeting, Atlantic City, N. J., June, 1975. Emergency Med., September 1975, pp. 61–66.
8. Fitts, W. T., Jr., Fifty years' progress in abdominal injuries. Bull. Am. Coll. Surg., 47:17–20, 1972.
9. Fitts, W. T., Jr.: Multiple injuries. In Hawthorne, H. R. (ed.): The Acute Abdomen and Emergent Lesions of the Gastrointestinal Tract. Springfield, Charles C Thomas, 1967, pp. 364–376.
10. Fitts, W. T., Jr.: The patient with multiple traumatic injuries. In: Oaks, W. W., Moyer, J. H., and Spitzer, S. (eds.): Emergency Room Care. New York, Grune & Stratton, 1972, pp. 205–212.
11. Fitts, W. T., Jr.: Shock and hemorrhage: electric injury. In: Cole, W. H., and Puestow, C. B. (eds.): Emergency Care. 7th ed. New York, Appleton-Century-Crofts, 1972, pp. 103–114.
12. Hampton, O. P., Jr.: Keeping Them Alive—A Course on Multiple Injuries. Presented at the American Medical Association Annual Meeting, Atlantic City, N. J., June 1975. Emergency Med., September 1975.
13. Jacobs, B.: 70-second procedure may eliminate emergency endotracheal intubations. Clin Trends Ophthalmol. Otol. A1, II:6, 1974.
14. Kennedy, R. H., Fitts, W. T., Jr., Kelly, R. P., et al.: Emergency Treatment in Major Disaster: Fractures, Immobilization and Preparation for Transportation. National Research Council, September 1950.
15. Oppenheimer, R. P.: Airway ... Instantly. In: Special communication. J.A.M.A., 230:1, 76, 1974.
16. Shires, G. T. (ed.): Care of the Trauma Patient. New York, McGraw-Hill, 1966.

JOSEPH M. LANE, M.D.

32 _____ *Metabolic*
Bone
Disease
and Fracture
Healing

BONE AS A METABOLIC ORGAN

The interrelationship of metabolic bone disease and fracture healing is dependent on the skeleton's role as a metabolic resource.[51] Bone contains a mineral fraction, hydroxyapatite, and an organic fraction of which 90 per cent is in the form of collagen. The mineral fraction of bone, in the form of calcium phosphohydroxyapatite, constitutes from 65 to 75 per cent of the dry weight. The hydroxyapatite crystal is imperfect, and substitutions are found frequently in the form of carbonates. Ninety-nine per cent of the bodily calcium and eighty-five per cent of the bodily phosphorus are found in the skeleton. The hydroxyapatite is intimately related to the collagen molecule, the bulk of the crystal being found in the hole zones within the quarter-staggered collagen array and the microfibrilar structure. Only 10 per cent of the mineral is located outside the domain of the macromolecular arrangement of the collagen. The mineral provides the compressive strength of bone, and in experimental diseases in which the mineral content is increased, the compressive strength of the bone is augmented. Bone is characterized as a composite material in which the collagen provides the tensile strength and the hydroxyapatite the compressive strength. The bone itself is constantly turn-

ing over, its half-life being variable and dependent on the location within the bony structure. The phases of bone remodeling, as characterized by Frost, include a state of reabsorption initially, followed by one of formation. This reabsorption-formation modulation constitutes metabolic bone units, and specific time courses for the process have been established by using tetracycline labeling among other techniques.[17, 18, 26] The remodeling and turnover of bone appear to be under a series of influences including local humeral factors, biophysical considerations (most notably Wolff's—"form follows function"), and systemic demands. The net turnover of bone appears to represent a response to both structural and metabolic demands.[26] The large supplies of calcium and phosphorus within bone are called upon to meet the metabolic requirements of the body.

Actual formation and deposition of bone appear to be directly under the control of the cells, although the exact mechanism of cellular control has not been established. Light microscopy and electron microscopy have failed to show cellular continuity along the surface of bone. It has been suggested that the mineral surface is isolated from the extracellular fluid by a chemoabsorptive lining of pyrophosphate. Osteoblasts arising from osteoprogenitor

946

cells within the marrow line the bone-forming surfaces. They synthesize osteoid, which is essentially a collagen.

After the osteoblasts have formed collagen osteoid, it is mineralized initially in the hole zone and then later throughout the osteoid. Alkaline phosphatase is secreted by the osteoblasts at the mineralizing front of osteoid and may interact with the pyrophosphate to facilitate nucleation. Calcium phosphate concentrations are supersaturated. Once nucleation occurs within the holes in the quarter-staggered collagen, the calcium and phosphate rapidly form hydroxyapatite crystals.

The resorption of bone is under the control of osteoclasts. These are multinucleated cells arising from the consolidation of previously formed mononuclear scavenger cells. They have been postulated to originate both from a vascular source and from osteogenic precursor cells. The osteoclasts effectively isolate a limited surface of the bone and bound this area with a transitional zone. In the isolated surface bordered by the osteoclasts, a ruffled membrane forms within the osteoblast and the secretion of acid phosphatase occurs. This enzyme presumably permits access of the osteoclast to the mineral phase of bone. The osteoclast lowers the pH by secreting citrate and other acids so that the calcium phosphate concentration ceases to be supersaturated and the mineral phase will begin to dissolve. Lysosomal enzymes are released to degrade the noncollagenous organic matrix, and collagenase is secreted by the osteoclast to initiate the degradation of the collagen organic matrix.

Under normal conditions, from 60 to 90 per cent of mineral turnover occurs in and about the area of the osteocytes and their lacunae. In states of disease, growth, and bone repair, the osteoclasts and osteoblasts assume the major role in the pathological bone turnover. Bone is not a homogenous material but consists of osteons oriented so as to afford the greatest strength against tension and compression. During bone turnover, the matrix that is least essential to structural demands and contains the oldest osteons is preferentially removed first, and the trabecular and cortical osteons most essential to structural demands are retained. This phenomenon is best illustrated in the vertebrae of osteoporotic individuals in which the nonessential horizontal trabeculae are preferentially removed, leaving the vertical trabeculae to the end.

SYSTEMIC CONTROL OF BONE METABOLISM

The osteoblasts, osteocytes, and osteoclasts within bone respond to the hormonal nutritional environment of the animal. Calcium is a crucial ion and has most recently been identified with an intimate control of cellular activity throughout the animal.[54, 55, 56] There are three calcium pools within the body: extracellular, cytosol, and

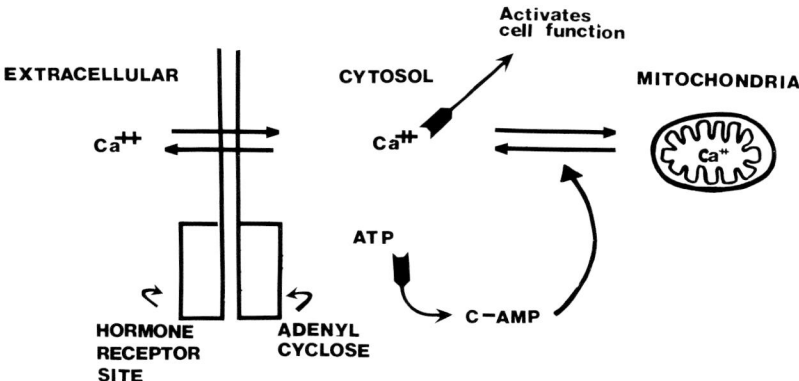

Figure 32–1   Calcium pools and cellular function. The cytosol pool is maintained by a calcium pump from the cytoplasm to the extracellular and the mitochondrial pools. Hormones alter the target cell membrane and activate adenylcyclase. Adenylcyclase, in turn, converts intracellular ATP to cyclic-AMP, which activates target cell function, in part by altering cytosol calcium concentrations.

mitrochondrial (Fig. 32–1). The extracellular calcium pool has a concentration of 10^{-3}, the mitochondrial pool one of 10^{-4}, and the cytosol calcium pool one of 10^{-6} to 10^{-7} molar. The low-level cytosol calcium pool is maintained by a calcium pump from the cytoplasm to the extracellular and the mitochondrial pools. Sutherland demonstrated that most hormones function by altering the target cell membrane and activating adenylcyclase within the cell membrane.[73] The adenylcyclase, in turn, converts intracellular adenosine triphosphate to cyclic adenosine monophosphate. The cyclic-AMP functions as a secondary messenger to activate target cell function. Most recently, Rasmussen has shown that the cyclic-AMP functions in part by altering cytosol calcium concentrations.[52, 53] There also appears to be an alternate route for calcium flux in the cell. Prostaglandins permit a direct ingress of calcium from the extracellular pool into the cytosol calcium pool to activate cell function. Cyclic-AMP augments the cytosol calcium by inhibiting the mitochondrial gradient and permitting the calcium to go from the mitochondrial to the cytosol calcium pool. The resultant increase in cytosol calcium activates the cell functions. From this schema it can be seen that calcium is crucial for cellular activity and that the body has developed a complex system to insure the proper calcium concentrations within these three pools.

Three hormones have been identified that have the primary responsibility of controlling calcium metabolism within the organism.[54] These are parathyroid hormone, thyrocalcitonin, and vitamin D.[1, 12, 13, 47] These hormones act primarily upon calcium absorption across the gut, calcium resorption in the renal tubules, and bone turnover. Parathyroid hormone is produced within the parathyroid gland and is a hypercalcemic agent. It increases the calcium reabsorption from the renal tubules, it increases calcium reabsorption from the bone by activating osteoclastic and osteocytic osteolysis as well as increasing the number of osteoclasts, and indirectly it increases calcium absorption across the gut by stimulating the production of the active vitamin D metabolite, $1,25(OH)_2$ vitamin D.

Thyrocalcitonin is produced in the thyroid gland and is an effective hypocalcemic agent. It decreases calcium reabsorption in the renal tubules, it decreases bone reabsorption by decreasing the activity of osteoclasts both in number and in activity, and it indirectly decreases calcium absorption across the gut by inhibiting the production of the active vitamin D metabolite, $1,25(OH)_2$ vitamin D.

Vitamin D has recently been shown by DeLuca and co-workers to be, in fact, a hormone.[12, 13] It is ingested in food or produced in the skin in the presence of ultraviolet light, and is converted to $25(OH)$ vitamin D in the liver and further converted to the active vitamin D metabolite $1,25(OH)_2$ vitamin D in the kidneys.[4, 7] This synthetic step is under the control of parathyroid hormone, which can increase its production. The $1,25(OH)_2$ vitamin D stimulates calcium absorption across the gut and augments parathyroid-stimulated reabsorption of bone.

Other hormones affect bone metabolism and are discussed later in the context of fracture healing.

Nutritional factors are important in bone turnover. Calcium and phosphate are the main components of the hydroxyapatite within bone, and in states of calcium and phosphate deficiency, bone is reabsorbed to provide these metabolites for the body. Mild calcium deficiency causes osteoporosis, the loss of bone mass per unit volume; phosphate deficiency causes osteomalacia, a failure of mineralization of osteoid organic matrix. Marked calcium deficiency, however, causes both osteoporosis and osteomalacia. The specific alterations that are responsible for the interplay of secondary hyperparathyroidism and mineralization are beyond the scope of this chapter.

HORMONES IN FRACTURE HEALING

Fracture healing is influenced by multiple factors including the mode of injury, the degree of tissue damage, and the method of fracture therapy. Besides the local events, there are significant systemic events that can augment or retard fracture repair. A valid generalization is that normal amounts of all hormones contribute toward fracture healing and that significant hormonal deficiencies or excesses frequently contribute to delayed bone repair. Within this generalization, certain hormones have been identified as being crucial in facilitating adequate bone repair and these include growth hormone, thyroxin, calcitonin, and vitamin D, all to various degrees of significance.[15, 28, 35, 36, 45, 72] Cortisone, uncontrolled diabetes, castration, and vitamin D excess have been identified with retardation of bone healing.[11, 14, 27, 35, 36, 65]

Conclusions drawn regarding the relative importance of hormones in fracture repair have been gathered from animal studies and observation of clinical disease states. Experimental data are incomplete, however, and further studies are currently under way in many centers to determine the exact role of various hormones in bone healing.

Growth hormone has been shown to play an important role in the fracture repair, probably through its altered form somatomedin.[36] In patients with decreased growth hormone levels, Misol and co-workers were able to show delayed bone healing.[45] In studies on the healing of long-bone fractures in hereditary pituitary insufficient mice, Hsu and Robinson demonstrated that diaphyseal tibial fractures failed to heal after 13 weeks in the pituitary dwarf mice, while fracture healing usually occurred within that time in unaffected siblings.[28]

Cortisone has been shown to be an effective catabolic agent. Many studies have been performed to evaluate the effect on fracture healing. Duthie and Barker, in a histochemical study of the preosseous stage of bone repair, demonstrated that in cortisone-treated animals the formation of the preosseous cartilaginous callus and the subsequent process of endochondral ossification were delayed.[14] Kowalewski and Gort observed delayed fracture healing in cortisone-treated rats, both when the cortisone was given prior to fracture and when it was administered during the three-week healing period.[37]

Castration has been shown by Koskinen to retard bone fracture repair.[35] Metabolic agents, particularly 17-ethyl-19-nortestosterone, as demonstrated by Kowalewski and Gort, stimulate bone healing and reverse the deleterious effects in part caused by cortisone in a rat fracture model.[37]

The three crucial hormones controlling bone metabolism, vitamin D, parathyroid hormone, and thyrocalcitonin, have been shown to have significant effects on bone metabolism and bone repair following injury.[1] Thyrocalcitonin was studied by Ewald and Tachdjian, who demonstrated a 17 per cent increase in dry bone weight in treated animals compared to untreated control animals.[15] No histological difference, however, was noted in hematoxylin and eosin and trichrome micrographs of the two groups. Parathyroid hormone is a known initiator of bone reabsorption and, in fact, can cause pathological fractures. Fracture healing may be delayed but not prevented in marked parathyroid hormone excess.

Vitamin D has been studied in both clinical and experimental animal models. Rickets resulting from a deficiency of vitamin D is associated with pathological fractures and delayed fracture healing. Steier and co-workers have shown that vitamin D enhances the initial mineralization, as evidenced by an increase in ash content and calcium percentage in human fracture and by a rise in serum alkaline phosphatase in rat fracture models.[72] Vitamin D, however, in high dosages, has been shown by Copp and Greenberg to retard bone growth and repair.[11]

Diabetes can exert a deleterious effect on fracture healing.[27, 65] Herbsman and co-workers, utilizing an alloxan diabetes model, demonstrated that fracture healing in growing rats was significantly decreased in the presence of poorly controlled diabetes and deficient diet, as determined by breaking strength measurements of healing femoral shaft fractures.[27] Well-controlled diabetic rats exhibited a lag phase of callus strength between the first and fourth week postfracture, at which time breaking strength approached normal values. Despite the differences in callus strength, there was no discernable histological or radiographic alteration in healing among the groups.

The experimental data just quoted represent histological, biochemical, and biomechanical studies in part. These data are not all-inclusive, and some of the effects of hormones may be more significant in one facet of fracture healing than the others. It has been shown, however, that certain hormones do contribute significantly to fracture repair and that aberrations in hormonal levels, either excesses or deficiencies, can delay bone repair.

METABOLIC BONE DISEASE

Pathological fractures frequently call attention to an underlying metabolic bone abnormality.[46, 51, 54] Most diseases that alter the bone matrix will lead to a certain degree of weakness in the biomechanical strength of the bone and facilitate fracture, but certain metabolic bone diseases are characterized by frequent pathological fractures (Table 32–1). These conditions represent a broad spectrum of metabolic disease and have various causes, age ranges, and bone distributions. Metabolic bone disease is frequently present but not recognized—particularly the osteomalacia of the elderly that is often discovered during treatment of hip fractures.[8]

The ease of the pathological fractures does not connote, necessarily, a significant inhibition of repair. Particularly, osteogenesis imperfecta is noted for extensive callus production and the rarity of pseudarthrosis; osteogenesis imperfecta, osteopetrosis, and hypophosphatasia are congenital diseases and are relatively rare; and Paget's disease involves one or a few bones.* The other diseases are generalized.

---

*See references: for osteogenesis imperfecta, 5, 16, 33, 69, 75; for osteopetrosis, 31, 34; for hypophosphatasia, 38; for Paget's disease, 4, 10, 23.

TABLE 32–1 Pathological Fractures and Metabolic Bone Disease*

Osteoporosis[2, 17, 18, 56, 60, 76]

Osteomalacia[8, 9, 30, 39, 47, 49, 50, 61, 67, 70, 71]

Paget's disease[3, 4, 23]

Hyperparathyroidism[1, 29, 74, 77]

Osteopetrosis[31, 34]

Osteogenesis imperfecta[5, 16, 33, 40, 69, 75]

Hypophosphatasia[38]

*For an overview of the subject, see reference 46.

Although treatment of pathological fractures associated with metabolic bone disease requires a clear understanding of the basic underlying disease, the general principles of fracture care remain valid in these conditions. The underlying condition may, however, necessitate a specific mode of therapy to prevent delayed healing even while the principles of immobilization, apposition, and alignment are followed.

The diagnosis of the primary metabolic bone disease requires a careful history, meticulous physical examination, and appropriate laboratory tests.[6, 22] By utilizing this approach, 95 per cent of the underlying conditions can be quickly diagnosed, and appropriate therapy for the metabolic disorder can be initiated while the fracture is healing. It must be remembered, however, that in very mild forms of metabolic bone disease the body has a great ability to retain normal laboratory values. In the common disorder of osteoporosis, for example, there are no routine laboratory abnormalities.[18, 56, 60, 76]

Metastatic tumors can easily mimic the osteopenia of metabolic bone disease. The most frequent tumor of this type is multiple myeloma, but other tumors on occasion may present a similar pattern. A bone scan will frequently be of great value in eliminating these possibilities, and a bone biopsy may be indicated.

Osteopenia

In the course of evaluation of patients with fractures, roentgenographic studies may indicate the presence of osteopenia.[55] In contradistinction to the metabolic disorder of osteoporosis, osteopenia is only a radiographic description of decreased radiodensity on x-ray. Although osteopenia is synonymous with osteoporosis in common parlance, there are other causes of osteopenia that have important effects on fracture healing. Osteoporosis is a loss of bone mass per unit volume.[32] Osteomalacia, while similar to osteoporosis roentgenographically, represents a failure of mineralization of osteoid, and in certain situations the bone, in fact, may have more than a normal amount of organic matrix per unit vol-

Text continued on page 955.

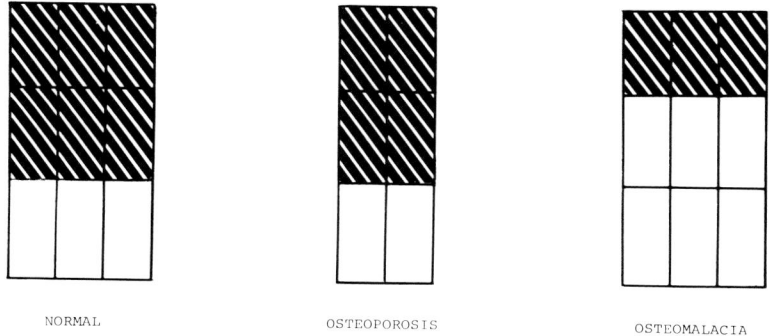

NORMAL OSTEOPOROSIS OSTEOMALACIA

Figure 32–2 Normal bone, osteoporosis, and osteomalacia. Osteoporosis is less mass per unit volume, and osteomalacia is failure of mineralization of osteoid.

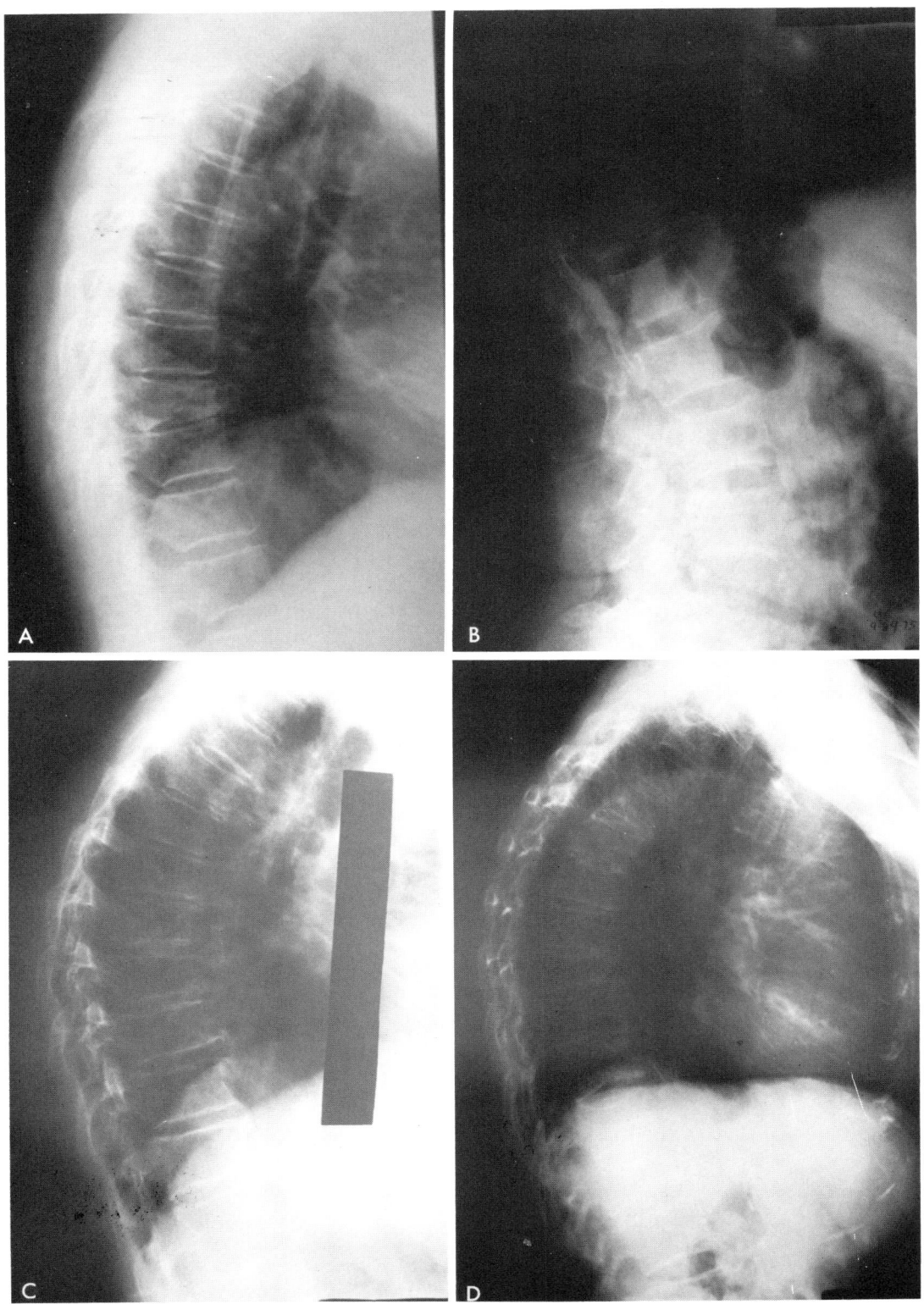

Figure 32–3 Differential diagnosis of osteopenia. *A.* Postmenopausal osteoporosis. *B.* Osteomalacia. *C.* Hyperparathyroidism. *D.* Steroid osteoporosis.

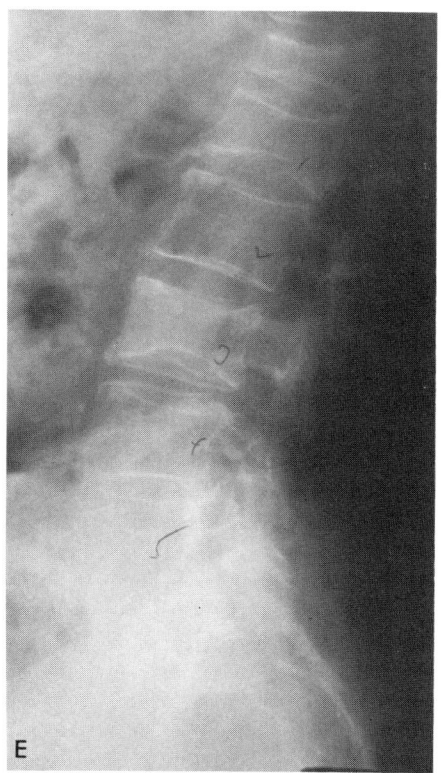

Figure 32–3 Continued.   E. Alcoholic osteoporosis.

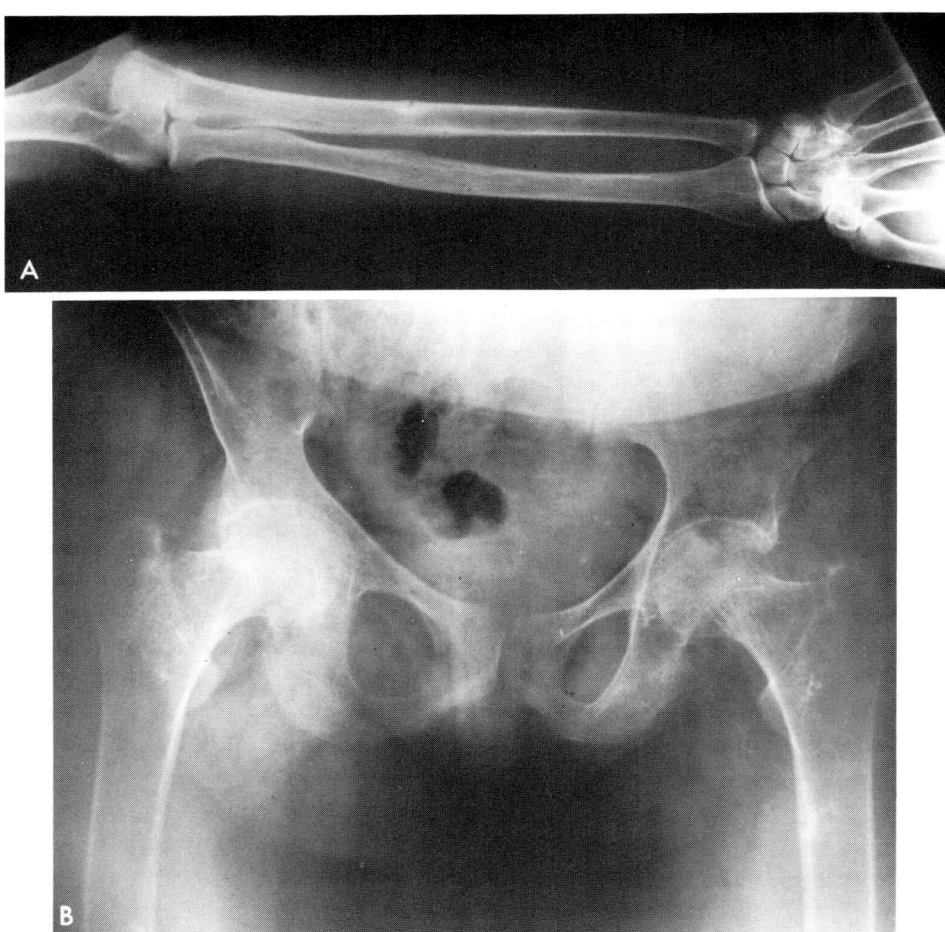

Figure 32-4 Osteomalacia with Looser lines. *A.* Ulna. *B.* Both femoral shafts and right femoral neck.

ume.[30, 34, 67] The difference between these two entities is best illustrated by Figure 32–2.[18, 56, 60]

The differential diagnosis of osteopenia includes osteoporosis; osteomalacia; hyperparathyroidism; hyperthyroidism; metastatic tumors; particularly multiple myeloma; and steroid excess whether endogenous or iatrogenic.* These disorders represent broad categories (Fig. 32–3). They are not all-inclusive, but form the framework for the subsequent discussion. Fracture healing is little affected in osteoporosis; the body will utilize the nutrient and mineral requirements from the unfractured skeletal system to provide an adequate metabolic source for fracture healing at the site of injury. Osteomalacia, however, is associated with delayed fracture healing.[30, 39, 49, 50, 67, 70, 71] In fact, one of the hallmarks of this disorder is the presence of Looser lines, which can go on to transverse pathological fractures following minimal trauma (Fig. 32–4). Pathological fractures secondary to cancer require special modes of therapy and are discussed in their entirety in Chapter 28. Hormonal excess contributes to delayed fracture healing, and the primary defect should be rectified in conjunction with fracture healing if possible.

A diagnosis of the underlying metabolic bone disease requires the combination of a detailed history, specific radiographic examination, and appropriate laboratory testing. The historical facts that are important include those that pertain to genetic and family background, nutrition, menarche or menopause, lactation, renal status, drug ingestion (particularly steroids), and gastrointestinal symptoms or surgery.[18, 20, 21, 40, 41, 47] Radiographic studies, in addition to appropriate views for careful evaluation of the site of fracture, should include x-rays of the skull, spine, pelvis, and hand. Classic findings that help in the diagnosis include the salt and pepper skull and subperiosteal erosions of hyperparathyroidism, the codfished vertebrae associated with osteoporosis, the rugger jersey spine and Looser lines of osteomalacia, the

epiphyseal widening and slipped capital epiphyses of rickets, and the lytic changes of metastatic bone disease.* First-line laboratory studies have included determinations of serum calcium, phosphorus, alkaline phosphatase, blood urea nitrogen, creatinine, electrolytes, thyroid function, serum protein electrophoresis, complete blood count, urinary pH, 24-hour urine hydroxyproline, calcium, and creatinine, and, when appropriate, liver enzymes.[6, 22] Examination of these values will often narrow the diagnosis to one or a few entities, and second-line studies can complete the diagnosis (Table 32–2). A schema for this approach is illustrated in Table 32–3. It must be noted, however, that several entities may lead to completely normal initial studies and this group is illustrated in Table 32–4.[6] The importance of diagnosing the underlying metabolic bone disease lies in the prevention of further fractures as well as the improvement of fracture healing, particularly in osteomalacia.[8, 9, 30, 39] In a series of 13 consecutive patients presenting with wedge fractures of the dorsal spine and a tentative diagnosis of osteoporosis at the metabolic bone disease clinic at the Hospital for Special Surgery, this diagnostic approach resulted in major alteration in diagnosis in 30 per cent and alteration in therapy in 70 per cent (cf. Fig. 32–3). In this series the incidence of primary hyperparathyroidism was 8 per cent, that of primary hyperthyroidism was 8 per cent, and that of multiple myeloma was 8 per cent. One patient, having been treated for prostatic carcinoma metastatic to the spine, proved to have alcoholic osteoporosis and not metastatic disease as was originally suspected.

The purpose of this chapter is primarily to emphasize the importance of recognizing the underlying entities. This is crucial if proper fracture care is to be provided. Appropriate history, x-rays, and laboratory studies will frequently be sufficient to provide the answer in very short order. Occasionally, bone biopsy and an evaluation of undecalcified specimens will be necessary for the ultimate diagnosis.

---

*See references: for osteopenia, 55; for osteoporosis, 2, 17, 18, 20, 56, 60; for osteomalacia, 8, 9, 30, 39, 67, 70, 71; for hyperparathyroidism, 1, 29, 74; for hyperthyroidism, 43, 59, 66; and for steroid excess, 19.

*See references: for osteomalacia, 30, 39, 49, 50; for rickets, 7, 39, 42, 61.

TABLE 32–2 Diagnoses Suggested by Initial Laboratory Results

Laboratory Study	Values	
	Increased	Decreased

Serum calcium	1° Hyperparathyroidism
	Multiple myeloma (60%)
	Immobilization (10%)
	Neoplasm
	  Metastases
	  Ectopic parathyroid hormone
	Hyperthyroidism (15%)
		Vitamin D deficient states
		  Malabsorption
		  Dietary deficiency
		  Vitamin D dependent rickets
		  Anticonvulsants
		Calcium deficiency
		  Lactose intolerance
		  Dietary
		  Utilization (growth, pregnancy, lactation)
		Renal osteodystrophy

Serum phosphate	Renal osteodystrophy
	Immobilization
	Widespread metastases
		Hypophosphatemic rickets
		Vitamin D deficient states
		  Malabsorption
		  Dietary
		  Vitamin D dependent rickets
		  Anticonvulsants
		1° Hyperparathyroidism
		Neoplasm
		Phosphate deficiency

Alkaline phosphatase	Paget's disease
	Renal osteodystrophy
	Vitamin D deficient states
	  Malabsorption
	  Dietary
	  Vitamin D dependent rickets
	  Anticonvulsants
	1° Hyperparathyroidism
	Hypophosphatemic rickets
	Widespread metastases
		Hypophosphatasia

Test		

24 hour urinary calcium	Hypercalcemia
	1° Hyperparathyroidism
	Neoplasm/Myeloma
	Hyperthyroidism
	Cushing's disease/steroids
	Immobilization
	Hypophosphatasia
	Renal tubular acidosis (loop diuretics)
	Phosphate deficiency
		Renal osteodystrophy
		Hypophosphatemic rickets
		Vitamin D deficient states
		  Malabsorption
		  Dietary
		Vitamin D dependent rickets
		Anticonvulsants
		Calcium deficiency
		  Lactose intolerance
		  Dietary
		  Utilization

Creatinine	Renal osteodystrophy Multiple myeloma	
Creatinine clearance		Renal osteodystrophy Poor urine collection
Hemoglobin		Neoplasm/myeloma
WBC (differential)	Leukemia (abnormal differential) Cushing's disease (↓ lymphocytes)	Thyrotoxicosis Graves' disease (↑ lymphocytes)
Electrolytes		
Chloride	Neoplasm without bone metastasis Renal tubular acidosis	Multiple myeloma Metastatic neoplasm
Potassium		Renal tubular acidosis
Carbon dioxide		Renal osteodystrophy Renal tubular acidosis

Urinalysis
  pH
  Glucose
	Renal tubular acidosis
	Cushing's disease
	Fanconi syndrome	

Protein	Multiple myeloma Renal osteodystrophy	
T₄	Thyrotoxicosis	Dilantin

Serum protein electrophoresis
  Para-protein
  Albumin
	Multiple myeloma	Hypocalcemia

TABLE 32–3   Laboratory Findings and Confirmatory Studies for the Diagnosis of Generalized Osteopenia[*]

Etiology	Initial Laboratory Results									Confirmatory Studies
	Calcium	Phosphate	Alkaline Phosphatase	Creatinine	T_4/T_3RU	Complete Blood Count	Electrolytes	U/A	24 hour Calcium	
Nutritional										
Calcium deficiency	N↓	N	N	N	N	N	N	N	→	N↑ PTH
Vitamin D deficiency	↓	→	↑	N	N	N	N	N	→	↑↑ PTH, ↓ Vit. D, Bone biopsy: ↑ Osteoid
Phosphate deficiency	N	→	↑	N	N	N	N	N	N↑	Bone biopsy: ↑ Osteoid, ↓ Urinary PO_4
Gynecological (senile)										
Post Menopausal Osteoporosis	N	N↑	N	N	N	N	N	N	N	
Calcium utilization										
Gastrointestinal										
Malabsorption	→	N	↑	N	N	N	N	N	→	↓ Serum carotene, ↓ Vit. D, ↑ Fecal fat ↑ PT, ↑↑ PTH
Lactose intolerance	N↓	N	N	N	N	N	N	N	→	Lactose tolerance test ↑↑ PTH NH_4Cl loading test
Renal										
Renal tubular acidosis	N↓	N↓	N	N	N	N	↓ CO_2	pH > 5.3+	N↑	Nephrocalcinosis on IVP
Osteodystrophy	N↓	↑↓	↑	↑↑	N	N	↓ CO_2	Prot. Casts	↓↑	↑ PTH
Hypophosphatemic rickets	N	N↓	↑	N↑	N	N	N ↓ CO_2	N	→	↑ Urinary glucose, PO_4, Urinary amino acids in Fanconi's syndrome, N PTH (sex-linked)
Vitamin D dependent rickets	→	↓↑	↑	N	N	N	N	N	↓↑	(Autosomal recessive)
Endocrine										
Cushing's syndrome/ corticosteroids	N	N	N	N	N	↑ Hb ↑ WBC ↓ Lymphs	N	↑ Glu	N↑	24° Urinary cortisol Dexamethasone suppression
Thyrotoxicosis	N↑	N	N↑	N	↑↑	↓ WBC ↑ Lymphs in Graves' disease	N	N	↑	↑ T_4, ↑ T_3RU, ↑ T_3RIA
1° Hyperparathyroidism	↑	→	N↑	N↑	N	N	N	N	N↑	↑ PTH, Phalangeal subperiosteal resorption
1° Skeletal										
Paget's disease	N	N	↑°	N	N	N	N	N	N↑	Bone scan, Bone biopsy ↑ Urinary hydroxyproline
Osteogenesis imperfecta	N	N	N	N	N	N	N	N	N	Blue sclera, deafness
Hypophosphatasia	N↑	N	↓↑	N	N	N	N	N	N↑	↑ Urinary and serum phosphoethanolamine, Renal failure
Neoplasm										
without bony metastases	↑↓	N↓	N↑	N	N	N↓ Hb	↑ Cl	N	N↑	N↑ PTH ectopic or PGE
Myeloma	N↑	N	N↑	↑	N	↓ Hb↑	N↓ Cl	↑ Prot.	N↑	Bone scan, Bone marrow biopsy Bence Jones prot. SPEP. Uric A
Metastatic	↑	N	N↑	N	N	N	N↓ Cl	N	↑	Bone scan, Bone biopsy
Other										
Immobilization	N↑	N	N	N	N	N	N	N	↑↑	
Drugs										
Dilantin/P.B.	N↓	N↓	↑	N	(↓ T_4-Dil)	N	N	N	↓↑	↑ PTH, ↓ 25OH–Vit. D, Bone biopsy: ↑ Osteoid
Heparin	N	N	N	N	↑ T_3 RU	N	N	N	N	

[*]Normal findings do not exclude a diagnosis.
†Always found.
N, Normal.

TABLE 32-4 Diseases in Which All Initial Laboratory Studies and History May Be Normal

Osteoporosis
        Postmenopausal
        Senile
Cushing's disease
Osteogenesis imperfecta tarda
Calcium deficiency
        Dietary
        Lactose intolerance
        Utilization (growth, pregnancy, lactation)
Vitamin D deficiency
        Dietary
        Malabsorption
        Anticonvulsants
Phosphate deficiency–antacid abuse
Early primary hyperparathyroidism
Occult malignant disease

Paget's Disease

Since the initial description of Paget's disease by Sir James Paget in 1871, Paget's disease has been identified as a syndrome seen in one or several bones in elderly individuals and associated with pathological fractures.[4, 48] Paget's disease (osteitis deformans) affects 3 per cent of the population over the age of 50 and is slightly more common in males than in females. One third of patients never know they have the syndrome during life, one third recognize their syndrome but are asymptomatic, and one third have symptomatic problems.[10]

The etiology of Paget's disease remains obscure; however, recent studies by Mills and Singer have suggested that nuclear inclusions are present in pagetoid osteoclasts.[44] These inclusions have been described as consisting of numerous microfilaments and having a bearded appearance. They appear to be similar to viral particles found in the cells of patients with subacute sclerosing panencephalitis. Further studies by this group and others are under way in an effort to confirm this finding.

Paget's disease repesents a three-staged bone disorder in which the first phase appears to be an abnormal destruction of bone by an excessive number of osteoclasts and is represented radiographically as a wave of osteolysis.[4] The second phase is represented by new bone formation of primarily coarse-fibered bone and the development of a vascular fibrous marrow. The third phase represents cyclical bone reabsorption and formation producing a mosaic patterned bone matrix classic for Paget's disease. The syndrome affects the single bones in entirety. It is most commonly found in descending order of frequency in the lumbosacral vertebrae, skull, pelvic bones, femur, tibia, clavicle, sternum, and fibula; rarely it is found in the scapula, humerus, radius, phalanx, mandible, ribs, and patella. Clinical problems related to Paget's disease include disabling bone pain, progressive skeletal deformity (including vertebral compression), acetabular protrusion and pathological fractures, neurological complications (paraplegia), deafness, high-output congestive heart failure, and bone enlargement.[3, 4, 24] Neoplastic changes within pagetic bone are rare but when present have an extremely poor prognosis.[4]

Pathological fractures associated with Paget's disease occur both during the early stages of Paget osteolysis and in well-established disease.[3, 4] There may initially be pseudofractures in pagetoid bone or frank transverse fractures (Fig. 32–5). These result from minimal trauma, and the most common sites are the femur and tibia. In a series of pagetoid femoral fractures the most common sites in descending order of frequency were the subtrochanteric area, the middle third of the shaft, the upper third of the shaft, the lower third of the shaft, the femoral neck, and lastly, the trochanteric region.[3, 4, 23] Fractures are frequently transverse, form a good callus, and heal well. Difficulty in the management of femoral fractures may be related in part to the problems of intramedullary fixation caused by severe bowing and difficulty of reaming.[3, 23] Fractures of the shaft can be treated conservatively with immobilization. Healing has been reported to occur in anything from 8 to 22 weeks. Nonunion is common with femoral neck fractures, and the use of an endoprosthesis is indicated.

Recent advances in pharmacological intervention have shown that Paget's disease responds favorably to treatment with salmon calcitonin therapy.[25, 62-64, 78, 79] On this regimen, alkaline phosphatase and urinary hydroxyproline values can be brought close to, if not into, normal range within six months.[25] Ninety per cent of patients show a favorable response in a limit-

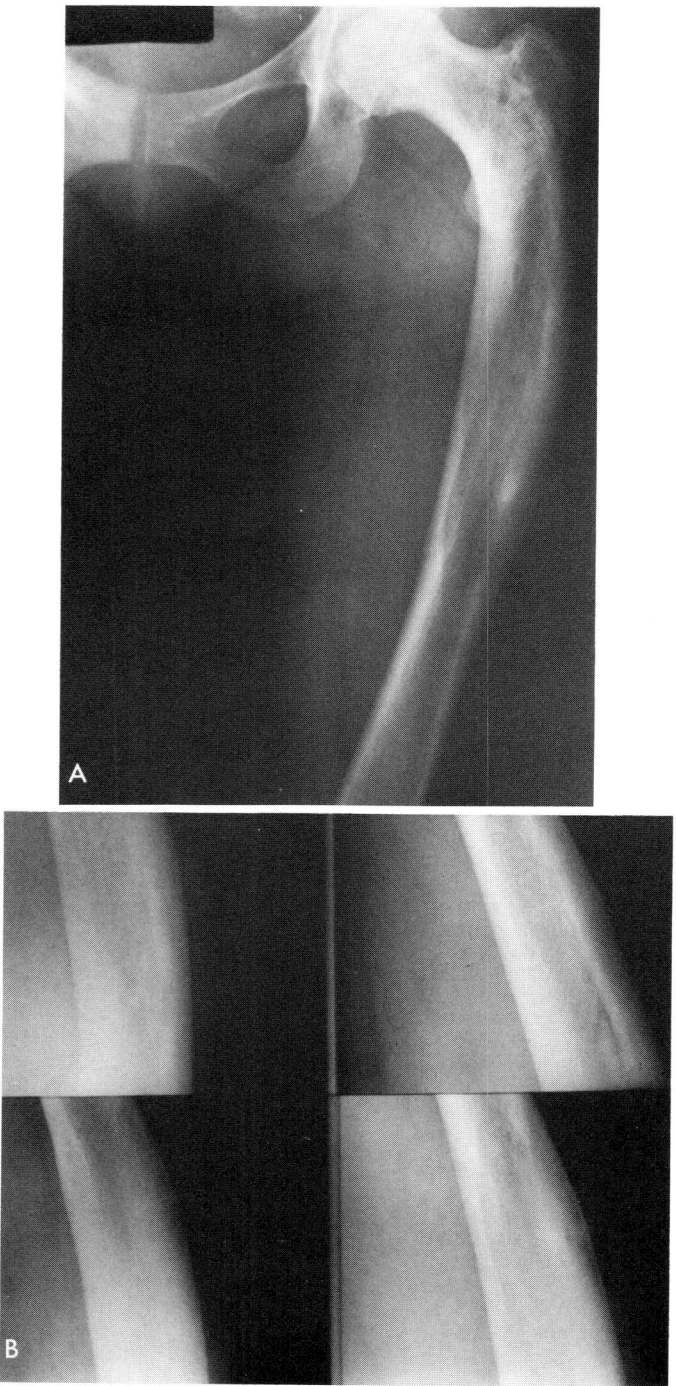

Figure 32–5 Paget's disease with pseudofracture. *A.* Anterolateral femur. *B.* Tomograms of the fracture.

ation of pain, and calcitonin has effectively healed Looser lines and partial fractures quite rapidly. Partial weight bearing and bracing may be required during the initial course of therapy to augment skeletal support until the callus is well formed. Additional modes of therapy have included intravenous Mithramycin in low dosages and oral diphosphonate, EHDP.[5, 8, 57, 68] Remodeling of the pagetoid bone toward a more normal architecture, however, occurs only with calcitonin therapy; no significant degree of remodeling has been found with the other two forms of therapy.

REFERENCES

1. Albright, F., and Reifenstein, E. C., Jr.: The Parathyroid Glands and Metabolic Bone Disease, Selected Studies. Baltimore, Williams & Wilkins Co., 1948.
2. Arnold, J. S.: Amount and quality of trabecular bone in osteoporotic vertebral fractures. Clin. Endocrinol. Metab., 2:221–238, 1973.
3. Barry, H. C.: Fractures of the femur in Paget's disease of bone in Australia. J. Bone Joint Surg., 49A:1359–1370, 1967.
4. Barry, H. C.: Paget's Disease of Bone. Edinburgh, Livingstone, 1969.
5. Bauze, R. J., Smith, R., and Francis, M. J. O.: A new look at osteogenesis imperfecta. J. Bone Joint Surg., 57B:2–12, 1975.
6. Bijvoet, O. L. M., and Van der Sluys Veer, J.: The interpretations of laboratory tests in bone disease. Clin. Endocrinol. Metab., 1:217–238, 1972.
7. Cattell, H. S., Levin, S., Kopits, S., and Lyne, D.: Reconstructive surgery in children with azotemic osteodystrophy. J. Bone Joint Surg., 53A:216–228, 1971.
8. Chalmers, J., Conacher, W. D. H., Gardner, D. L., and Scott, P. J.: Osteomalacia—a common disease in elderly women. J. Bone Joint Surg., 49B:403–423, 1967.
9. Chalmers, J.: Subtrochanteric fractures in osteomalacia. J. Bone Joint Surg., 52B:509–513, 1970.
10. Collins, D. H.: Paget's disease of bone: Incidence and subclinical forms. Lancet, 2:51–57, 1956.
11. Copp, D. H., and Greenberg, D. M.: Studies on bone fracture healing. I Effect of vitamins A and D. J. Nutr., 29:261–267, 1945.
12. DeLuca, H. F., and Steenboch, H.: 1,25 Dihydroxycholecalciferol: Isolation, identification, regulation and mechanism of action. In S. Taylor, Endocrinology. London, Heinemann, 1971, pp. 452–467.
13. DeLuca, H. F.: The kidney as an endocrine organ involved in the function of vitamin D. Am. J. Med., 58:39–47, 1975.
14. Duthie, R. B., and Barker, A. N.: Histochemistry of the preosseous stage of bone repair studied by autoradiography. J. Bone Joint Surg., 37B:691–710, 1955.
15. Ewald, F., and Tachdjian, M. D.: The effect of thyrocalcitonin on fractured humeri. Surg. Gynecol. Obstet., 125:1075–1080, 1967.
16. Falvo, K. A., and Bullough, P. G.: Osteogenesis imperfecta: a histometric analysis. J. Bone Joint Surg., 55A:275–286, 1973.
17. Frost, H. M.: Managing the skeletal pain and disability of osteoporosis. Orthop. Clin. North Am., 3:561–570, 1972.
18. Frost, H. M.: The spinal osteoporosis. Clin. Endocrinol. Metab., 2:257–276, 1973.
19. Gallagher, J. C., Aaron, J., Horsman, A., Wilkinson, R., and Nordin, B. E. C.: Corticoid steroid. Clin. Endocrinol. Metab., 2:355–368, 1973.
20. Gallagher, J. C., Aaron, J., Horsman, A., Marshall, D. H., Wilkinson, R., and Nordin, B. E. C.: The crush fracture syndrome in postmenopausal women. Clin. Endocrinol. Metab., 2:293–316, 1973.
21. Goldsmith, N. F., and Johnston, J. D.: Bone mineral: Effects of oral contraceptives, pregnancy and lactation. J. Bone Joint Surg., 57A:657–668, 1975.
22. Goldsmith, R. S.: Laboratory aids in the diagnosis of metabolic bone disease. Orthop. Clin. North Am., 3:545–560, 1972.
23. Grundy, M.: Fractures of the femur in Paget's disease of bone. J. Bone Joint Surg., 52B:252–263, 1970.
24. Haddad, J. G., Jr.: Paget's disease of bone: Problems and management. Orthop. Clin. North Am., 3:775–786, 1972.
25. Haddad, J. G., Berge, S. J., and Avioli, L. V.: Effects of prolingiacalcitonin administration on Paget's disease of bone. N. Engl. J. Med., 283:549–555, 1970.
26. Harris, W. H., and Heaney, R. P.: Skeletal renewal and metabolic bone disease. N. Engl. J. Med., 280:193–202, 253–259, 303–311, 1969.
27. Herbsman, H., Powers, J. C., Hirschman, A., and Shaftan, G. W.: Retardation of fracture healing in experimental diabetes. J. Surg. Res., 8:424–431, 1968.
28. Hsu, J. D., and Robinson, R. A.: Studies on the healing of long bone fractures in hereditary pituitary insufficient mice. J. Surg. Res., 9:535–536, 1969.
29. Jackson, C. E., and Frame, B.: Diagnosis and management of parathyroid disorders. Orthop. Clin. North Am., 3:699–712, 1972.
30. Jaworski, Z. F. G.: Pathophysiology: Diagnosis and treatment of osteomalacia. Orthop. Clin. North Am., 3:623–652, 1972.
31. Johnston, C. C., Lavy, N., Lora, T., Vellios, F., Merritt, A. D., and Deiss, W. P.: Osteopetrosis: A clinical, genetic, metabolic and morphologic study of the dominantly inherited benign form. Medicine, 47:149–167, 1968.
32. Jowsey, J., Riggs, B. L., Kelly, P. J., and Hoffman, D. L.: Effect of combined therapy with sodium fluoride, vitamin D and calcium in osteoporosis. Am. J. Med., 53:43–49, 1972.
33. King, J. D., and Bobechko, W. P.: Osteogenesis imperfecta. J. Bone Joint Surg., 53B:72–89, 1971.
34. King, R. E., and Lovejoy, J. F.: Familial osteopetrosis with coxa vara. J. Bone Joint Surg., 55A:382–385, 1973.
35. Koskinen, E. V. S.: Effect of endocrine factors in

callus development in experimental fractures. Symp. Biol. Hung., *1*:315–322, 1967.

36. Koskinen, E. V. S., Ryoppy, I., and Lindholm, T. S.: Bone formation by induction under the influence of growth hormone and cortisone. Isr. J. Med. Sci., *1*:378–380, 1971.

37. Kowalewski, K., and Gort, J.: An anabolic androgen as a stimulant of bone healing in rats treated with cortisone. Acta Endocrinol., *30*:273–276, 1959.

38. MacPherson, R. I., Kroeka, M., and Houston, C. S.: Hypophosphatasia. J. Can. Assoc. Radiol., *23*:16–26, 1972.

39. Mankin, H. J.: Rickets, osteomalacia, and renal osteodystrophy. J. Bone Joint Surg., *56A*:101–128, 352–386, 1974.

40. McKusick, V. A.: Heritable Disorders of Connective Tissue. 4th Ed. St. Louis, C. V. Mosby, 1972.

41. Meema, H. E., Bunker, M. L., and Meema, S.: Loss of compact bone due to menopause. Obstet. Gynecol., *26*:333–343, 1965.

42. Mehls, O., Ritz, E., Krempien, B., Gilli, G., Link, K., et al.: Slipped epiphyses in renal osteodystrophy. Arch. Dis. Child., *50*:545–554, 1975.

43. Meunier, P. J., Bianchi, G. G., Edonard, C. M., et al.: Bony manifestations of thyrotoxicosis. Orthop. Clin. North Am., *3*:745–774, 1972.

44. Mills, B. G., and Singer, F. R.: Nuclear inclusions in Paget's disease of bone. Science, *194*:201, 1976.

45. Misol, S., Samaan, N., and Ponsetti, I. V.: Growth hormone in delayed fracture healing. Clin. Orthop., *74*:206–208, 1971.

46. Mitchell, D. C.: Fractures in brittle bone diseases. Orthop. Clin. North Am., *3*:787–792, 1972.

47. Norman, A. W., Schaefer, K., Grigoleit, H. G., von Herroth, D., and Ritz, E.: Vitamin D and Problems Related to Uremic Bone Disease. Berlin, Walter de Gruyth, 1975.

48. Paget, J.: On a form of chronic inflammation of bones (osteitis deformans). Med. Chir. Trans., London, *60*:37, 1877.

49. Parfitt, A. M.: Hypophosphatemic vitamin D refractory rickets and osteomalacia. Orthop. Clin. North Am., *3*:653–680, 1972.

50. Parfitt, A. M.: Renal osteodystrophy. Orthop. Clin. North Am., *3*:681–698, 1972.

51. Paterson, C. R.: Metabolic Disorders of Bone. Oxford, Blackwell Scientific Publications, 1974.

52. Rasmussen, H.: Cell communication, calcium ion, and cyclic adenosine monophosphate. Science, *170*:404–412, 1970.

53. Rasmussen, H.: The cellular basis of mammalian calcium homeostasis. Clin. Endocrinol. Metab., *1*:3–20, 1972.

54. Rasmussen, H., and Bordier, P. J.: The Physiological and Cellular Basis of Metabolic Bone Disease. Baltimore, Williams & Wilkins Co., 1974.

55. Reynolds, W. A., and Karo, J. J.: Radiologic diagnosis of metabolic bone disease. Orthop. Clin. North Am., *3*:521–543, 1972.

56. Riggs, B. L., Jowsey, J., Kelly, P., Hoffman, D. L., and Arnaud, C. D.: Studies on pathogenesis and treatment in postmenopausal and senile osteoporosis. Clin. Endocrinol. Metab., *2*:317–332, 1973.

57. Russell, R. G. G., and Smith, R.: Diphosphonates. J. Bone Joint Surg., *55B*:66–86, 1973.

58. Ryan, W. G., Schwartz, T. B., and Perlia, C. P.: Effects of mithramycin on Paget's disease of bone. Ann. Int. Med., *70*:549–557, 1969.

59. Ryckewaett, A., Bordier, P., Miravet, L., and Antonini, A.: L'ostéose. Thyröidienne. Sem. Hôp. Paris, *4*:222–228, 1968.

60. Saville, P. D.: The syndrome of spinal osteoporosis. Clin. Endocrinol. Metab., *2*:177–186, 1973.

61. Shea, D., and Mankin, H. J.: Slipped capital femoral epiphysis in renal rickets. J. Bone Joint Surg., *48A*:349–355, 1966.

62. Singer, F., and Bloch, K. J.: Antibodies and clinical resistance to salmon calcitonin. Clin. Res., *20*:220, 1972.

63. Singer, F., Neer, R. M., Parsons, J. A., et al.: Treatment of Paget's disease with salmon calcitonin. J. Clin. Invest., *49*:89a, 1970.

64. Singer, F. R., Neer, R., Golzman, D., Krane, S. M., and Potts, J. T.: Treatment of Paget's disease of bone with salmon calcitonin. *In* S. Taylor: Endocrinology. London, Heinemann, 1973.

65. Singh, R. H., and Udupa, K. N.: Some investigations on the effect of insulin in healing of fractures. Ind. J. Med. Res., *54*:1071–1082, 1966.

66. Smith, D. A., Fraser, S. A., and Wilson, G. M.: Hyperthyroidism and calcium metabolism. Clin. Endocrinol. Metab., *2*:333–354, 1973.

67. Smith, R.: The pathophysiology and management of rickets. Orthop. Clin. North Am., *3*:601–621, 1972.

68. Smith, R., Russell, R. G. G., Bishop, M. C., Woods, C. G., and Bishop, M.: Paget's disease of bone: Experience with a diphosphonate (disodium etidronate) in treatment. Q. J. Med., *42*:235–256, 1973.

69. Sofield, H. A., and Millar, E. A.: Fragmentation, realignment and intramedullary rod fixation of deformities of the long bones in children: A ten year appraisal. J. Bone Joint Surg., *41A*:1371–1391, 1959.

70. Stanbury, S. W.: Azotaemic renal osteodystrophy. Clin. Endocrinol. Metab., *1*:267–304, 1972.

71. Stanbury, S. W.: Osteomalacia. Clin. Endocrinol. Metab., *1*:239–266, 1972.

72. Steier, A., Gedalia, I., Schwarz, A., and Rodan, A.: Effect of vitamin D_2 and fluoride on experimental bone fracture healing in rats. J. Dent. Res., *46*:675–680, 1967.

73. Sutherland, E. W.: On the biological role of cyclic AMP. J.A.M.A., *214*:1281–1288, 1970.

74. Taylor, S.: Hyperparathyroidism. Clin. Endocrinol. Metab., *1*:79–92, 1972.

75. Tilly, F., and Albright, J. A.: Osteogenesis imperfecta: Treatment of multiple osteotomy and intramedullary rod insertion. J. Bone Joint Surg., *55A*:701–713, 1973.

76. Urist, M. R.: Orthopaedic management of osteoporosis in postmenopausal women. Clin. Endocrinol. Metab., *21*:159–176, 1973.

77. Von Recklinghausen, F. D.: De Fibröse oder deformierende Ostitis, die Osteomalazie und die osteoplastische Carcinose in ihren gegenseitigen Beziehungen. Festschr. R. Virchow, Berlin, Reimer, 1891.

78. Woodhouse, N. J. Y.: Paget's disease of bone. Clin. Endocrinol. Metab., *1*:125–142, 1972.

79. Woodhouse, N. J. Y., Reiner, M., Bordier, P., Kalu, D. N., Fisher, M., et al.: Human calcitonin in the treatment of Paget's bone disease. Lancet, *1*:1139–1143, 1971.

PETER R. McCOMBS, M.D.
and
D. A. DeLAURENTIS, M.D.

Vascular ──────────────────────────── 33
Injuries
Associated
with
Fractures
and
Dislocations

Vascular injuries associated with fractures and dislocations frequently produce complex clinical problems. These injuries are often multifactorial, with arterial, venous, lymphatic, and microvascular components. Skeletal trauma can easily conceal vascular injuries because attention is given only to the obvious bone deformity. Consequently, arterial and venous defects are often recognized too late, when the likelihood of a successful repair is greatly decreased. Sophistication in the diagnosis and treatment of vascular injuries, coupled with better triage and faster evacuation, has improved the rate of limb salvage. Nevertheless, the incidence of functional impairment and major disability following these injuries still remains too high.

PRINCIPLES OF MANAGEMENT

Three principles should govern the management of patients with vascular damage.

First, a high index of suspicion of vascular injury must prevail during the initial evaluation and treatment of any major fracture or dislocation. Second, time lost prior to the recognition of vascular injury can never be regained. Third, prompt and appropriate definitive therapy according to established surgical principles produces the best results. Szilagyi and co-workers have written that the two greatest errors in managing these patients are delay in recognition of the arterial injury and improper orthopedic management of the fracture. Most unsatisfactory results can ultimately be traced to these basic errors.

This chapter will present a review of the current concepts concerning etiology, diagnosis, and management of vascular injuries associated with fractures and dislocations in the extremities, shoulder girdle, and pelvis. Injuries to the great vessels of the head and neck, thorax, and abdomen are beyond the limits of this discussion and are not included.

963

Much of the data and opinion concerning vascular injuries are based on reports of military experience. Several large series of vascular injuries are available from the United States Armed Forces Vascular Registries, documenting progress in surgical techniques and results in management. Strict correlation between military and civilian trauma must be made with caution. Combat injuries generally are produced by high-velocity missiles or fragments and are accompanied by extensive blast injury and soft tissue destruction, resulting in open and grossly contaminated wounds and fractures. Civilian vascular trauma more often arises from nonpenetrating injury. In these cases, the vessels are damaged by internal traction, entrapment, torsion, or laceration by fracture fragments, and although an open wound may be present the amount of contamination and devitalized soft tissue is frequently far less.

THE MILITARY EXPERIENCE

In 1946, DeBakey and Simeone summarized the results of 2471 cases of arterial injury sustained during World War II.[5] These injuries were largely to the extremities and often were associated with major skeletal trauma. They constituted only 1.4 per cent of all extremity wounds treated, but carried a high incidence of amputation: 75 per cent for popliteal, 73 per cent for femoral, 43 per cent for axillary, and 30 per cent for brachial artery injuries. In this large series, only 81 arteries were repaired by lateral suture and only 3 by end-to-end anastomosis. Most of the remainder were treated by ligation. In the context of these complex wounds, the authors concluded ". . . it is clear that no procedure other than ligation is applicable to the majority of vascular injuries which come under the military surgeon's observation."

Following the Korean War, Hughes documented the beginning of the trend away from empirical ligation for arterial injury.[11] He noted that those wounds treated by ligation had results similar to those in the DeBakey and Simeone series. However, in a group of 269 cases treated by reparative surgery, the incidence of early amputation was far lower: 9 per cent following direct anastomosis, 12 per cent following interposition vein graft, and 3 per cent following lateral suture. Nevertheless, the incidence of late amputation due to ischemia remained as high as 32 per cent following popliteal artery trauma.

The Vietnam War proved the effectiveness of improvements in evacuation, transport, resuscitation, and evaluation of wounded victims. According to Fisher, evacuation time from the combat area to a hospital averaged 45 minutes, and three quarters of those patients requiring surgery were operated on within six hours of injury.[9] Repair or reconstruction was attempted in nearly all arterial injuries, and in one series of 154 such wounds the overall amputation rate was 8.3 per cent. Popliteal artery trauma continued to produce the highest rate of limb loss (31 per cent), largely because of associated soft tissue damage, infection, instability of the fracture, associated venous injury, and delay in recognition of arterial disruption.

INCIDENCE AND ETIOLOGY

Disruption of the integrity of the arteries and veins is an uncommon complication of long bone fractures. According to Connolly, 0.6 to 3 per cent of fractures of the extremities have associated arterial injuries.[4] The incidence of venous injuries is probably somewhat lower. However, up to 40 per cent of arterial injuries occurring as a result of closed trauma are associated with a fracture.

ARTERIAL INJURIES

Vascular injuries tend to occur with fractures in areas where the vessels pass close to bone or are held in a fixed position by muscles, ligaments, or adjacent bones. So the subclavian artery, for example, is vulnerable to injury at its points of greatest fixation—at the thoracic outlet and as it passes between the clavicle and the first rib. The brachial artery may be injured at any point of its close proximity to the humerus. At the elbow it is particularly vulnerable to laceration or entrapment by dislocation or by fragments of a supracondylar fracture.

In the upper extremity the collateral circulation is normally more extensive than in the lower, so that damage to the brachial artery is less likely to lead to gangrene and amputation. However, we strongly advocate early diagnosis and surgical treatment of these injuries because, as Morton points out, Volkmann's ischemic contracture can be almost as disabling as amputation.[17] While numerous reports of successful ligation of the brachial artery are recorded in the earlier literature, most authors currently advocate vascular repair, whenever possible, for injuries at this level.

The superficial femoral artery is most commonly injured in the adductor canal, its point of tightest fixation, but the entire femoral system is vulnerable to injury when the femur is fractured. The popliteal artery and veins traverse the posterior surface of the knee joint capsule and are tethered in position by the tendinous hiatus of the adductor magnus superiorly and the soleus tendon insertion inferiorly. For this reason, posterior dislocation of the knee and fractures involving the femoral condyles or tibial plateau carry a high risk of vascular injury and distal ischemia, particularly if there is posterior displacement of the fragments (Figs. 33–1 and 33–2). The collateral geniculate branches are not well protected by soft tissue, and frequently are also injured or unable to compensate for sudden interruption of flow through the main channel. In Hoover's series of popliteal artery injuries accompanying closed trauma to the knee, 75 per cent went on to amputation despite surgical intervention, and only one patient's foot regained full viability and usefulness.[10]

Injuries to numerous other arteries, including the thyrocervical trunk, subscapular, radial, ulnar, obturator, hypogastric, posterior tibial, and dorsalis pedis have been reported sporadically in conjunction with skeletal trauma. Their complications tend to be hemorrhagic rather than ischemic, since parallel patent collateral arteries usually are present. They are frequently recognized and treated early, and results are often excellent.

The nature of the arterial injury is variable and may occur as an immediate or late complication of bone or joint injury. Disruption of the full thickness of an artery results in laceration or avulsion of small branches and generally is first appreciated by the presence of an expanding hematoma,

which may be significant enough to produce systemic hypotension or distal ischemia (Fig. 33–3). Injuries of this type are almost invariably associated with comminuted fractures and are produced by bony spicules or penetrating missiles.

Arterial injuries occurring as the result of sudden forces that produce traction or torsion account for the majority of civilian injuries. These injuries generally produce elevated flaps of intima or intramural hematomas. Flow past these injured areas may be present initially but diminishes as the lumen narrows. Thrombosis may occur within minutes or hours of injury or may be a later manifestation, depending on such factors as the degree of underlying atherosclerosis or associated venous injury. The major late complications include arteriovenous fistula, false aneurysm, and even true aneurysm formation (Figs. 33–4 to 33–6).

Distal ischemia may occur in the absence of arterial disruption because of extensive compression by hematoma formation or entrapment by soft tissue or bone fragments. Restoration of normal flow is usually the rule following treatment of fasciotomy (Fig. 33–7). If untreated, however, these injuries may progress to thrombosis and gangrene of the affected part. The only hard-and-fast rule about arterial trauma is that its presentation may be delayed or concealed. Thus, the absence of classic signs of acute ischemia, and even the presence of palpable pulses distal to the site of injury, in no way rule out the possibility of impending vascular compromise. Patients with major fractures and dislocations should be evaluated frequently for signs of ischemia. Aggressive work-up, followed by appropriate intervention, must be undertaken if signs of circulatory insufficiency develop.

VENOUS INJURIES

Isolated venous injuries associated with osseous trauma are rare except in the pelvis. However, the combination of venous and arterial disruption following skeletal trauma is common and occurs more frequently than is appreciated. The incidence varies with the anatomical relationships of artery and vein. In Rich's series of 1000 major arterial

Text continued on page 974.

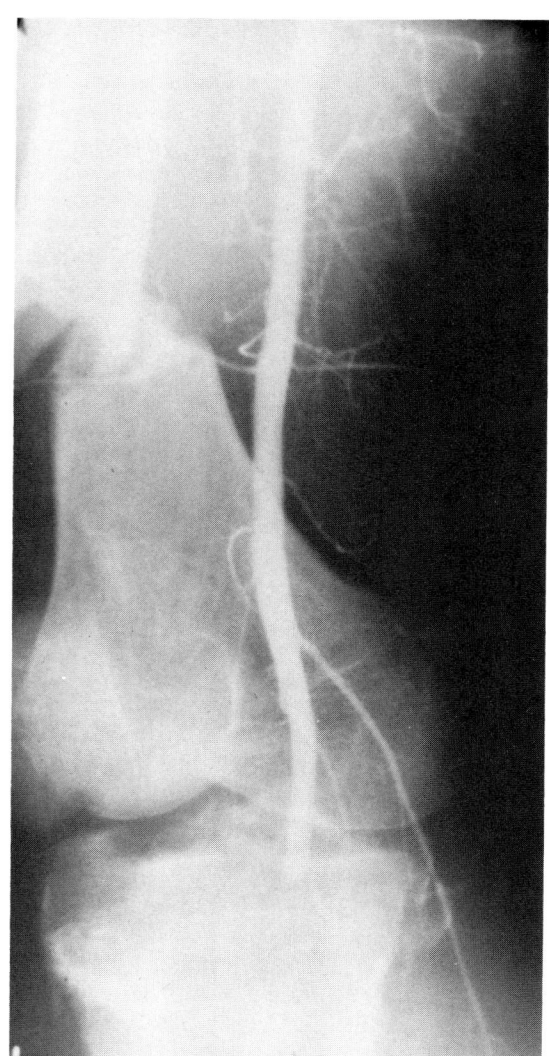

Figure 33–1   This man was struck by an automobile and sustained a supracondylar fracture of the femur and a T fracture of the tibial plateau. No distal pulses were palpable, and the foot was ischemic. Arteriogram revealed thrombosis of the popliteal artery with poor runoff. His foot has remained marginally viable following lumbar sympathectomy.

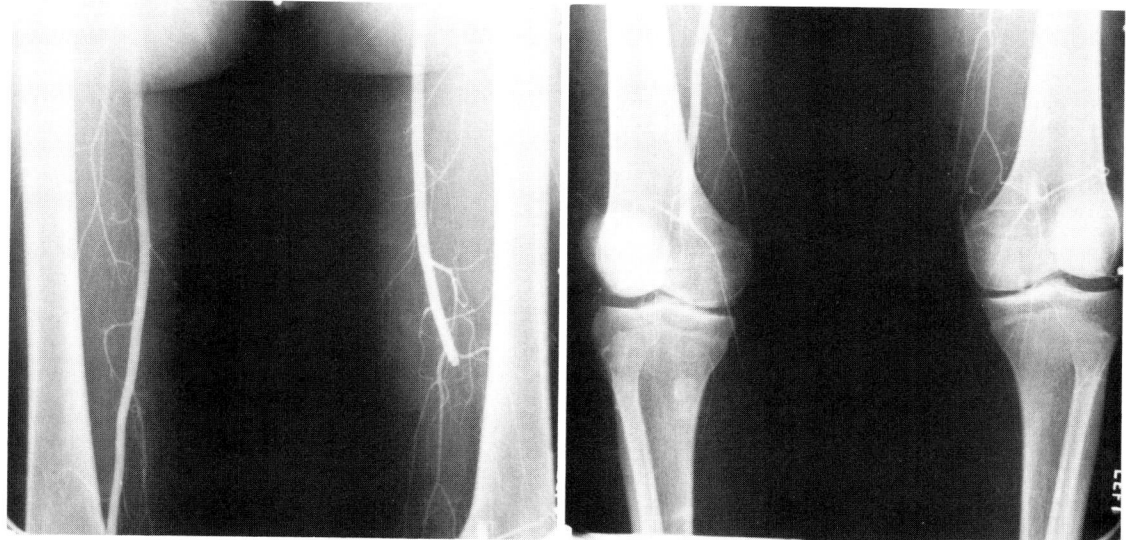

Figure 33–2 This girl developed posterior dislocation of the knees bilaterally when struck by an automobile and presented with pulseless, ischemic legs. Thrombectomy with a Fogarty catheter via the femoral arteries was attempted at a rural hospital. Arteriography, done one week later because of persistent ischemia, revealed bilateral popliteal artery thrombosis. Despite operative attempts at limb salvage, she eventually lost both legs below the knee.

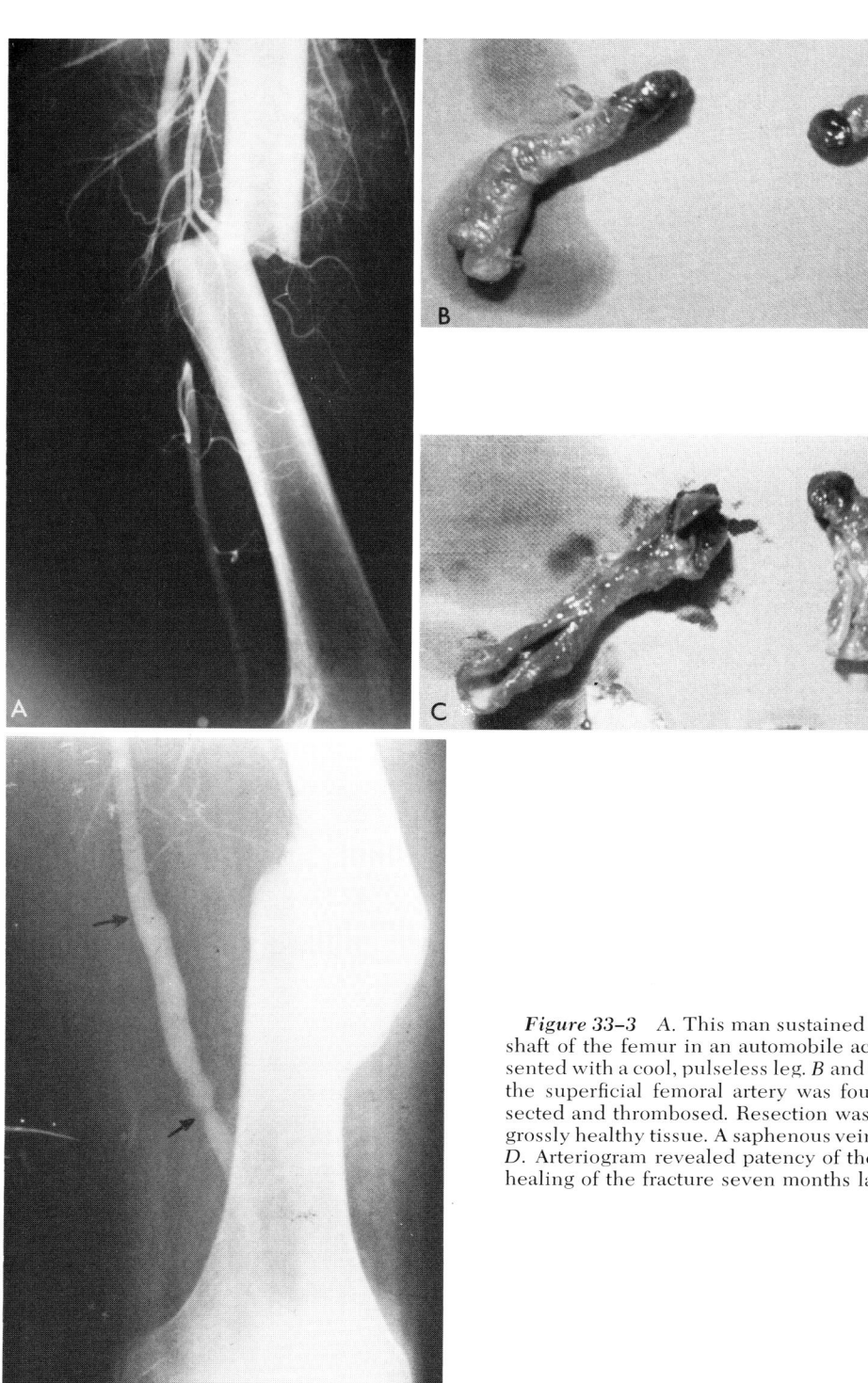

Figure 33–3 A. This man sustained a fracture of the shaft of the femur in an automobile accident and presented with a cool, pulseless leg. B and C. At operation, the superficial femoral artery was found to be transsected and thrombosed. Resection was carried back to grossly healthy tissue. A saphenous vein graft was used. D. Arteriogram revealed patency of the vein graft and healing of the fracture seven months later.

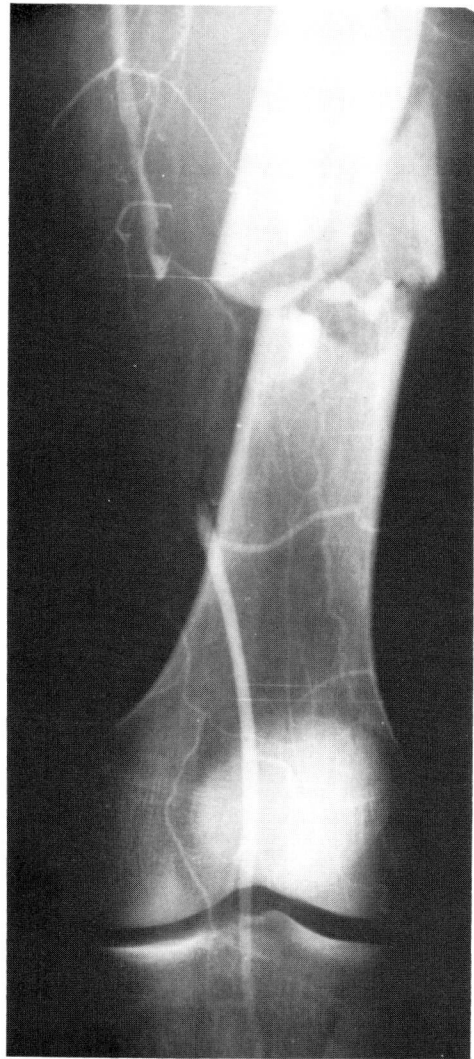

Figure 33–4   This man sustained a comminuted fracture of the femoral shaft in a fall and presented with no distal pulses. Arteriogram revealed occlusion of the superficial femoral artery at the adductor canal with prominent collaterals. This occlusion was due to underlying chronic atherosclerosis, probably was present prior to the fracture, and was not repaired. Except for mild claudication, the patient now has no evidence of ischemia.

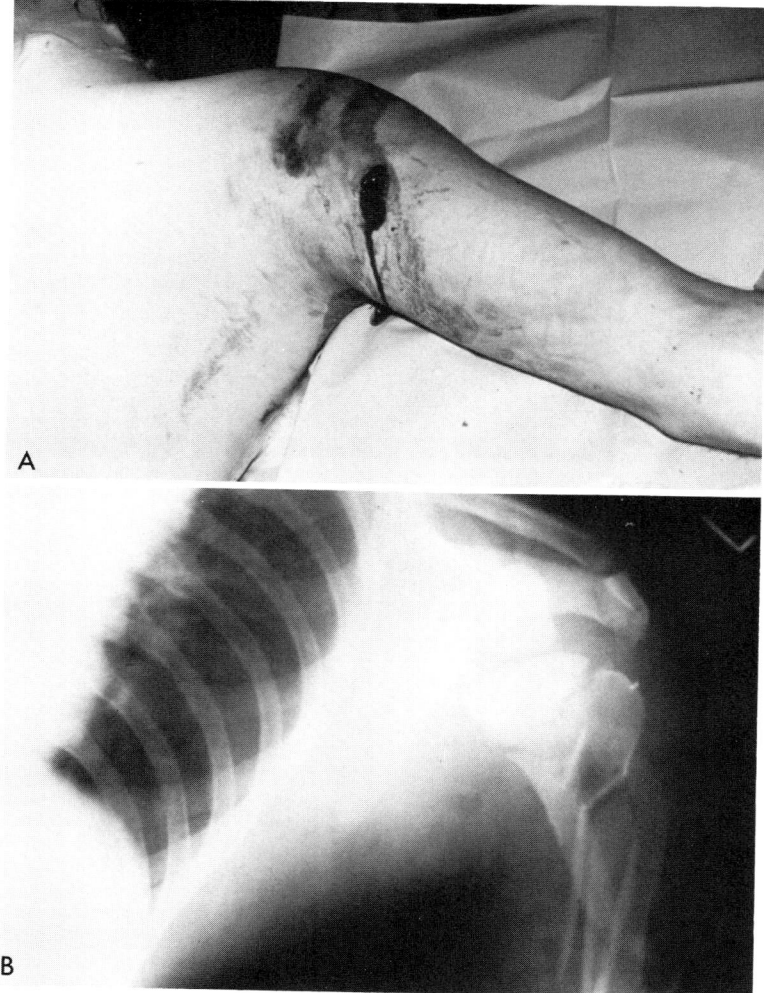

Figure 33-5 *A* and *B*. This boy sustained an open, comminuted fracture–dislocation of the proximal humerus and scapula in a motorcycle accident. Distal pulses were absent and the hand was ischemic.

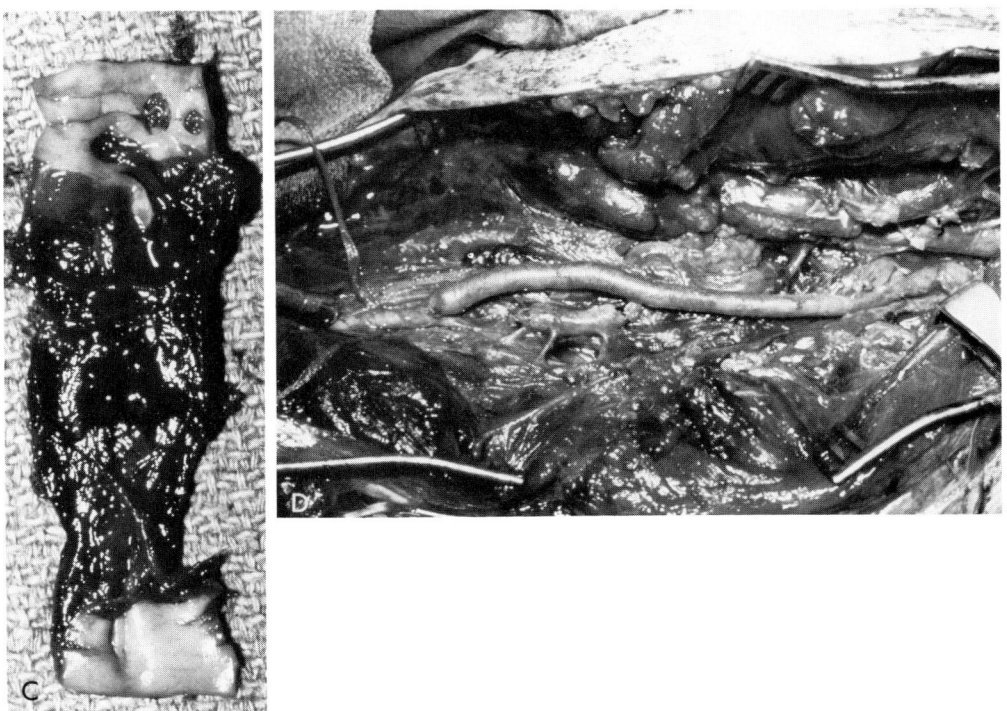

Figure 33–5 Continued.   C. The resected segment of axillary artery revealed contusion and thrombosis. *D*. It was replaced with a saphenous vein graft. Pulses were restored, and the arm regained full function.

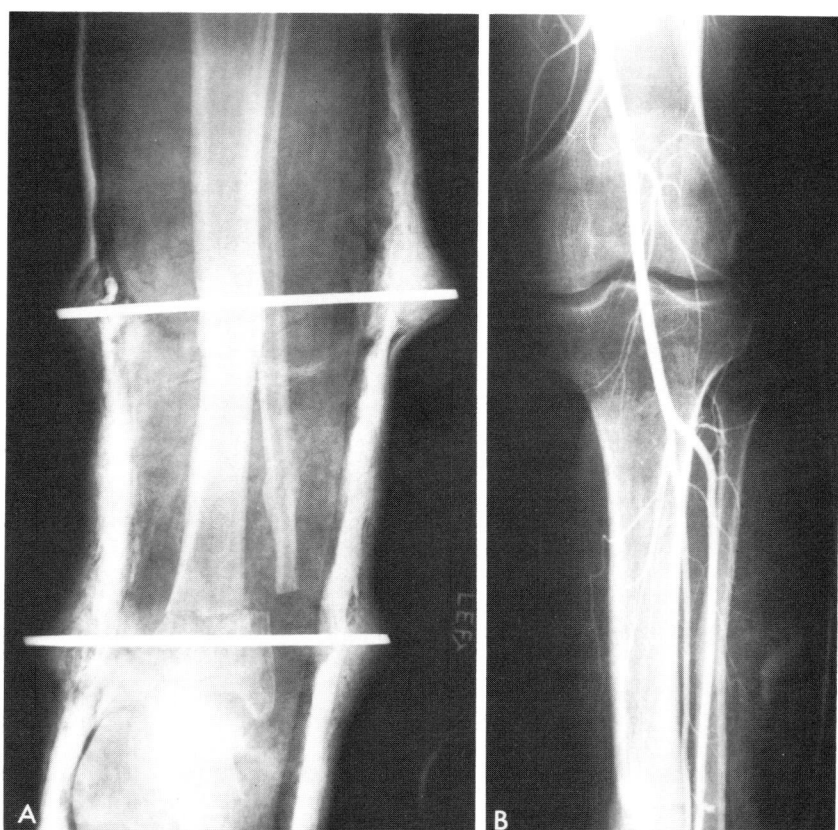

Figure 33–6   A. This young man had nonunion of an old fracture of the distal tibia and fibula, treated with pins and plaster. After insertion of the pins, the dorsalis pedis pulse was lost temporarily but returned spontaneously. On removal of the pins six weeks later, a jet of pulsatile blood occurred. *B.* Arteriogram revealed a small false aneurysm of the anterior tibial artery in the upper pin tract. Despite old damage to the posterior tibial artery, the foot remained viable with no further treatment to this iatrogenic injury.

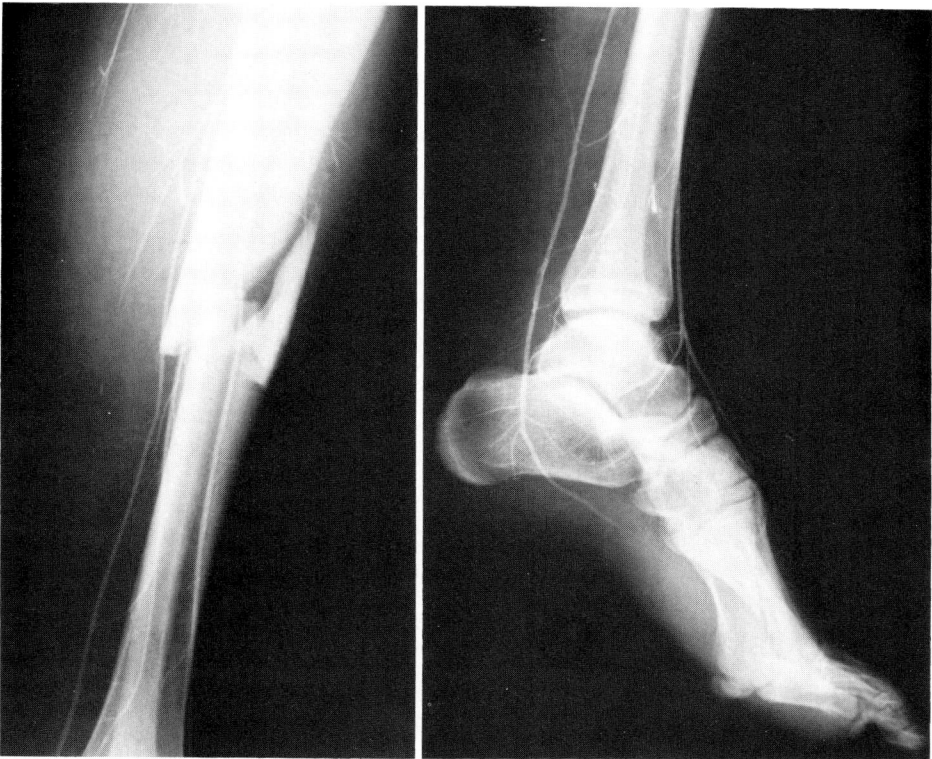

Figure 33-7   This patient developed a comminuted fracture of the midshaft of the tibia and fibula in a bicycle accident. Distal pulses were absent. Arteriogram showed diffuse narrowing of tibial vessels secondary to marked compartmental tension. Pulses were restored following three-compartment fasciotomy.

injuries incurred in Vietnam, the overall incidence of concomitant venous injuries was 37.7 per cent; with popliteal artery injuries, the incidence was 58.7 per cent.[20, 21] In general, these injuries are lacerations, often multiple, producing hematomas. Thrombosis may follow as a delayed event. When this occurs, the hemodynamic and hydrostatic effects may be significant, particularly after attempted arterial repair, since improved arterial inflow may then only contribute to hematoma formation, distal edema, and progressive tissue destruction.

DIAGNOSIS

The first and most important step in the diagnosis of vascular injury following skeletal trauma is awareness of the possibility. The absence of distal pulses, a gradient in temperature, pallor, mottling, paralysis of distal musculature, paresthesias, anesthesia, and even rapidly progressive edema or hematoma formation are classic indications for immediate and aggressive evaluation and treatment. These signs may be initially absent if the vascular injury is occult. In Drapanas's series of 128 patients with injuries to the major arteries of the extremities, 27 per cent had palpable pulses distally when first examined.[7] The diagnosis may be difficult in marginal cases in which the signs of ischemia are not clear, leading some authors in earlier references to recommend temporizing measures, such as transfusions, administration of dextran, sympathetic blockade, or intraarterial injection of vasodilators. However, this is a risky course of action. Many more extremities have been lost by erroneously ascribing early signs of ischemia to "spasm" than have ever been saved by delaying operation until classic signs are present.

The modern approach to patients in this category calls for frequent examinations and immediate diagnostic intervention, including both noninvasive and invasive techniques. The Doppler ultrasound device can be useful in localizing patent arteries and veins that are not palpable distal to a fracture or dislocation. In combination with a sphygmomanometer cuff placed between the fracture and the sensing probe, the systolic pressure can be taken accurately in the distal vasculature and compared with pressure measurements made in nontraumatized extremities. In this way, gradients of pressure across fracture or dislocation sites can be established. Serial measurements of this type may provide clues to underlying arterial injury, if the pressures obtained demonstrate a steady downward course.

Pulse volume recording is another noninvasive means of collecting information about arterial flow past a traumatized area. These instruments reproduce pulse wave contours through sensing pneumatic cuffs placed sequentially down an extremity, which detect volume changes in arterial inflow and thus yield a qualitative image of the pulsatile nature of arterial flow. By measuring the area under the pulse waves, a rough quantification of arterial flow per unit of time may be obtained. Serial pulse volume measurements and contrasting measurements between extremities may likewise be helpful in assessing the extent and progress of arterial insufficiency.

Other noninvasive methods of measuring flow, including various radionuclide scanning techniques, phonoangiography, and measurements of arteriovenous differences of oxygen saturation and the products of anaerobic metabolism, have not lent themselves well to the rapid evaluation of patients with vascular trauma.

The sine qua non in the diagnosis of arterial injury is arteriography, an invasive procedure that in good hands carries a low morbidity. Several recent reviews of this technique have emphasized the high diagnostic yield and low complication rate and have advocated that angiography be performed early in the evaluation of patients with skeletal trauma who demonstrate any sign of arterial insufficiency. The limits of confidence in the procedure match the competence and experience of the arteriographer. There is no disgrace in subjecting a patient to angiography that proves to be normal, if one's best judgment suggests that early arterial compromise may be present. The risk of lost time when unrecognized arterial disruption exists far outweighs the risk of morbidity from a negative ateriogram. The procedure will reward good clinical judgment with a positive finding in over 50 per cent of cases.

Similarly, venography should be performed when there is suspicion of either isolated or concomitant venous injury. No noninvasive venous test is as definitive about the patency or level of occlusion of major venous channels, location of venous collaterals, and point of extravasation from the lumen as venography.

TREATMENT

INITIAL MANAGEMENT

Early resuscitation and transportation of the patient from the scene of the accident to the hospital may be critical events in the evolution of vascular injury. Obviously, priority should be given to the establishment and maintenance of a good airway. If necessary, support of the circulation should be instituted according to the principles of cardiopulmonary resuscitation. If hypovolemia exists, it should be corrected, first by infusion of crystalloid and colloid solutions as soon as these are available, and later by transfusion of compatible whole blood.

The traumatized limbs should be immobilized, using the best means at hand, and protected. The patient should be kept warm and recumbent, with the affected parts not elevated. Local applications of heat or cold may be harmful if vascular injury is present. Bleeding from open wounds should be controlled by direct pressure and not by the application of clamps or a tourniquet (Fig. 33–8). The use of external counterpressure using a G-suit has been proposed for control of hemorrhage, particularly in the retroperitoneum, but experience with this technique is limited. One should resist the temptation to attempt to reduce the obvious bone deformities until sufficient assistance, light, instruments, and sedation are available. Heparin should not be given, and dextran is probably not of much value in altering the course of evolving arterial or venous trauma.

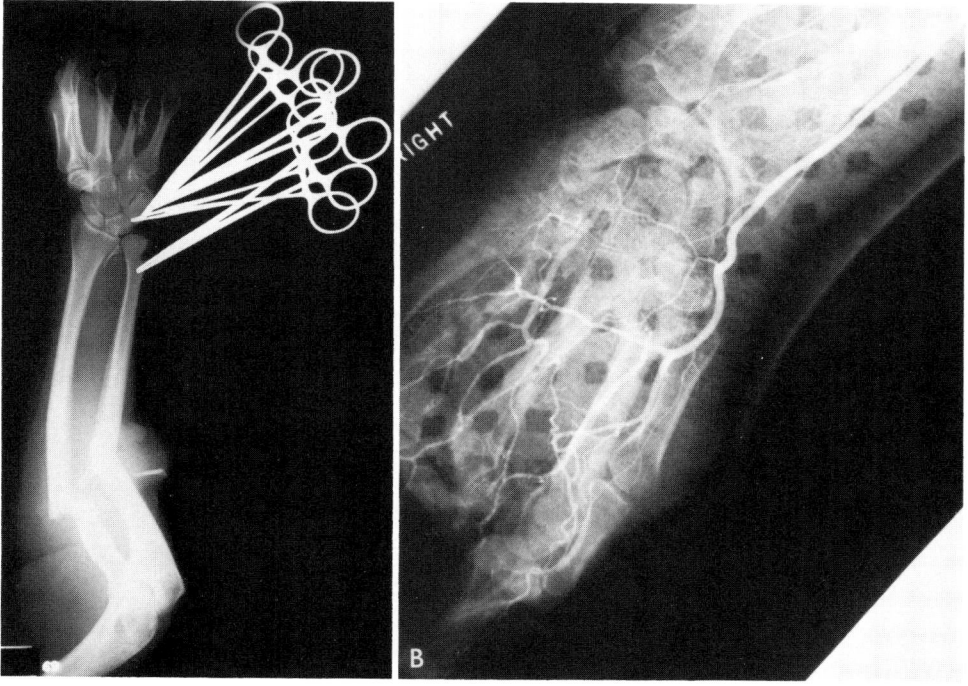

Figure 33–8   *A.* This young woman was the victim of an assault with an ax. She sustained open fractures of the proximal radius and ulna, distal radius, and fourth metacarpal. Copious bleeding from the wrist was controlled by application of clamps and ligatures. *B.* Arteriogram revealed occlusion of the distal ulnar artery. At operation, the ulnar artery was found to be ligated. The patient's hand remained viable.

PREOPERATIVE PREPARATION

Once the patient reaches the hospital, emphasis should be placed on treating the whole individual, establishing an accurate and complete diagnosis of all obvious and concealed injuries, and preparing for appropriate surgical intervention. If arterial disruption is present, this activity should proceed rapidly since, as Miller and Welch demonstrated experimentally, the longer the period of ischemia, the greater the incidence of wound complications, and later, of contractures, atrophy, and gangrene. They considered the optimal period for restorative surgery in traumatic ischemia to be the first six to eight hours. During this period, the patient should be carefully examined and stabilized hemodynamically. Acidosis should be corrected, appropriate monitoring lines should be placed, and routine venous and arterial blood and urine studies together with needed plain and angiographic x-rays, should be obtained.

If an open wound is present it should be cultured for aerobic and anaerobic organisms and irrigated copiously. Debridement should be delayed until the patient is anesthetized and optimal operating conditions are present. Tetanus prophylaxis is indicated, using hyperimmune human globulin if the details of prior immunization are vague or if gross contamination is present. Substantial intravenous doses of antibiotics, effective against gram-positive, gram-negative, and anaerobic organisms, should be given preoperatively and continued into the postoperative period, the spectrum being modified as indicated by sensitivity reports. Antibiotic prophylaxis should not be abused, since it is not a substitute for adequate debridement. Furthermore, broad-spectrum antibiotic infusions given over extended periods only favor the selective growth of resistant bacterial strains. Steroids and hyperbaric oxygen therapy generally do not have a place in the preoperative preparation of these patients.

THERAPEUTIC ARTERIOGRAPHY

In certain injuries, particularly pelvic fractures associated with expanding retroperitoneal hematomas, open operation may

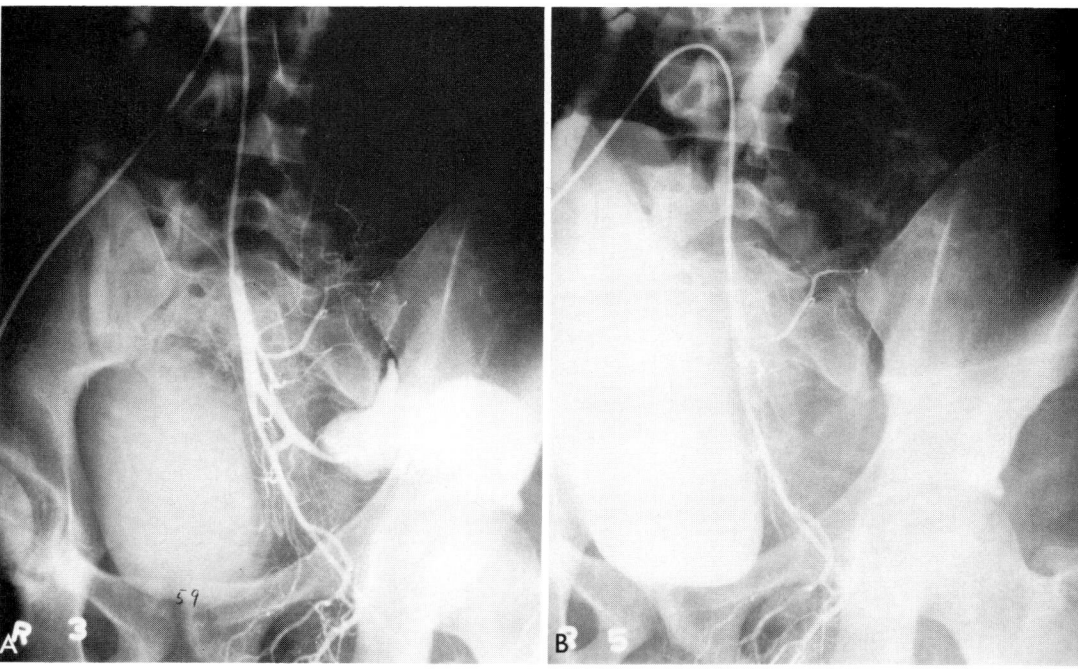

Figure 33–9 This woman developed hypotension following pelvic fracture and sacroiliac diastasis. A. Arteriogram revealed hemorrhage from the hypogastric system. B. Selective embolization with Gelfoam controlled the hemorrhage, and the patient recovered without requiring operation.

be hazardous or ineffective. Exposure and identification of the bleeding vessel may be difficult even if it is arterial. Incision into the retroperitoneum of the pelvis may destroy an effective tamponading force. Even ligation of the hypogastric artery may fail to give control because of back bleeding through the rich collateral network fed from the opposite side or from the lumbar system.

These problems led Ravitch to advocate closed management with massive whole blood replacement. Recently, Ring and co-workers demonstrated that posttraumatic arterial bleeding into the pelvis can be controlled by embolization of autologous

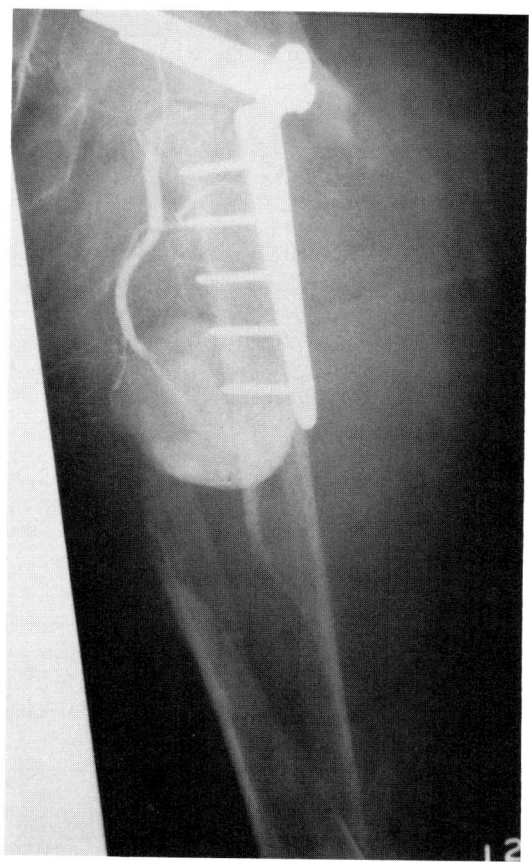

Figure 33–10 This woman had undergone pinning of an intertrochanteric fracture of the hip one year previously. She fell, fracturing the shaft of her femur and developing a large hematoma in the thigh. Distal pulses were palpable. Arteriogram revealed disruption of the profunda femoris artery with free extravasation of contrast material. Hemorrhage was controlled by selective embolization of Gelfoam.

clot or Gelfoam into the injured artery through an angiographic catheter selectively placed via the hypogastric artery.[22] Their patients had fractures of one or more rami. Contrast material was seen to extravasate from the obturator or internal pudendal arteries prior to embolization in all cases (Figs. 33–9 and 33–10). No morbidity was described, and no deaths were attributable to continued bleeding. Since their original paper, numerous case reports have appeared substantiating the effectiveness of this procedure. However, Trunkey and colleagues, in reviewing this topic, classified pelvic fractures on the basis of degrees of comminution and instability.[27] They emphasized that most pelvic hematomas accompanying severe fractures have a venous component and implied that in their hands, the operative approach was superior.

OPERATIVE MANAGEMENT

In the operating room, the patient should be widely prepared and draped to permit access to a segment of saphenous or cephalic veins, should this be necessary for patching or grafting. Closed reduction of bony deformities may restore distal pulses, particularly in injuries about the elbow, knee, or ankle. However, if preoperative studies raised the question of underlying vascular trauma, or if a change in the quality of the pulse occurs later, exploration and arteriotomy may be indicated to rule out the presence of an intimal flap.

The question of internal versus external fixation of the fracture is best resolved by the extent and contamination of the associated wound. Rich reported 21 patients treated by internal fixation, the majority presenting with large open wounds inflicted by high-velocity missiles.[21] Sixteen of the devices required removal, usually because of infection, and only five remained in place and asymptomatic at the time of his report. However, external immobilization, using bivalved casts, Steinmann pins, and balanced suspension was ultimately a superior method for the military and prevented the introduction of foreign material into the wound. Connolly's experimental work supports the contention that with a reasonable amount of immobilization arterial repairs are not jeopardized.[4] In this regard, external immobilization is as effective as internal immobilization and carries less risk of infection. For these reasons external fixation is the procedure of choice in combat surgery.

However, many civilian surgeons are satisfied with internal fixation. Separate reviews by Sher, Cole, Doty, and Morton each concluded that in clean open trauma or in closed trauma, rapid internal stabilization of the fracture prior to vascular repair produced a rigid support for arterial or venous reconstruction, permitted earlier mobilization and ambulation, and was associated with a qualitatively reduced incidence of postoperative complications.[3, 6, 17, 24] These authors, therefore, preferred their approach for patients in whom wound contamination and tissue necrosis were limited or absent. One may conclude that external fixation is an acceptable technique, which is most appropriate when any risk of infection is present, while internal fixation is probably desirable for closed injuries and those cases in which the amount of tissue trauma and contamination seems negligible. No difference in long-term patency rates of vascular repairs between the two modalities has been documented.

The keys to successful arterial repair are good arteriography, ample exposure, and strict attention to detail. The incision should be placed so that it can be extended in either direction and can pass longitudinally over a joint, if necessary. After satisfactory debridement, an assessment of the nature of the field and the nature of the injury should be made. If arterial disruption lies in a contaminated area, it should be ligated proximally and distally and then bypassed, using reversed autogenous vein through a subcutaneous or subfascial tunnel that avoids the dirty area. One such alternative for wounds in the groin is to bring an iliac-to-superficial femoral graft through the obturator foramen, as described by Mahoney and Whalen.[15]

Clean arterial injuries may be treated by direct lateral suture, venous patch grafting, resection with primary anastomosis, or resection with interposition of a reversed venous graft, depending on the extent of the injury. One should not hesitate to resect a damaged artery and resort to an interposition graft; otherwise, the traumatized portion of artery or an anastomosis that is under tension will lead to thrombosis. Prosthetic material should be avoided if at all possible, especially in contaminated cases. Suitable proximal and distal control must be achieved, and satisfactory forward and backward flow should be demonstrated. A Fogarty catheter should be used to retrieve proximal or distal clots. Systemic heparinization is preferable to regional heparinization prior to the application of clamps, but intraarterial injection of thrombolysin may be effective in improving run-off. Suture technique should be precise, and fine cardiovascular instruments and material should be used to create a hemostatic approximation of intima to intima.

Postoperative edema can be severe following arterial reconstruction and may cause thrombosis in a well-constructed arterial repair. Rich has emphasized the value of identification and repair of major venous injuries occurring concomitantly with arterial trauma.[20] Venous reconstruction decreases hydrostatic pressure and resistance across the arterial repair. Most venous lacerations can be repaired by lateral suture. More severe venous disruption may require excision and primary anastomosis or interposition venous grafting. These venous repairs are vulnerable to thrombosis, but Rich maintains that even if they remain open for only 24 to 72 hours, relaxation of vasospasm and development of venous collaterals may occur. Furthermore, thrombosed venous grafts may later recanalize. In his series of 64 venous repairs from Vietnam, most remained clinically patent, and the incidence of thromboembolic complications was not significant.

Most authors advocate fasciotomy, particularly in the lower extremities, as an adjunctive measure to reduce pressure within closed compartments postoperatively. Ernst has aptly stated that judicious fasciotomy can prevent the tragedy of gross muscle atrophy or equinovarus deformity in the presence of a palpable pedal pulse and a well-perfused foot.[8] He points out that classic fasciotomy does not decompress all four osteofascial compartments in the leg, especially the deep posterior compartment, and advocates excising the shaft of the fibula, preserving the distal portion to maintain stability of the ankle. While unanimous accord does not exist on the need for fibulectomy, most clinicians agree on the value of prophylactic or therapeutic compartmental decompression by fasciotomy, particularly in the presence of prolonged ischemia, venous interruption, or significant soft tissue damage.

Other adjunctive procedures, notably regional sympathectomy, are probably of little therapeutic value, since no measurable improvement in perfusion of traumatized muscle occurs and effects on "spasm" are generally negligible. Vasospasm itself is more often imagined than real in this clinical setting. When failure of the circulation persists following attempted surgical reconstruction, an anatomical explanation can usually be identified on close inspection and should be corrected.

AMPUTATION

Early or primary amputation is indicated for extremities that are beyond hope of salvage because of massive soft tissue loss and bone destruction. These are almost always open injuries, generally sustained in combat or in industrial, farm, or vehicular accidents. Amputation and reconstruction may require several operations, and proper bone length and viable muscle should be preserved.

Late amputation indicates failure of orthopedic, vascular, or peripheral nerve reconstruction, and may be necessary when persistent ischemia, chronic infection, or denervation with marked sensory and motor loss is apparent. According to Waddell, most clinical indications for delayed amputation are present within two to ten days following injury.[28] However, since the patient is entitled to major input into the decision, many amputations are performed long after this interval. This frustrating conclusion to complicated civilian injuries probably occurs in less than 20 per cent of cases. The nature and location of the vascular injury are the principal determinants, and disruption of the popliteal artery and vein continue to take the heaviest toll. In the military experience, the incidence of amputation is somewhat higher, for reasons that have been discussed.

COMPLICATIONS

The metabolic, renal, pulmonary, and embolic complications of these injuries are essentially those of all peripheral skeletal trauma and are discussed in Chapter 35. One complication specific to vascular trauma that deserves mention is the anterior tibial compartment syndrome. According to Bradley, this is characterized by pain in the anterolateral aspect of the lower leg, progressing to a variable amount of foot drop.[2] It is preceded by signs of inflammation in the compartment and later by weakness on dorsiflexion, especially of the great toe, and hypoesthesia in the first digital cleft. As pressure in the compartment rises, perfusion is further impaired and edema increases, leading to a vicious cycle based on microcirculatory ischemia. The increasing tension does not seem to affect all muscles equally; the extensor hallucis longus is more sensitive than the tibialis anterior or extensor digitorum longus. Treatment consists of rest and early fasciotomy prior to the onset of peroneal nerve palsy. The value of ancillary measures, such as anticoagulants, fibrinolysins, and chemical or surgical sympathectomy, is unsubstantiated. Tendon transplantation may be indicated in the management of end-stage deformities.

SUMMARY

1. The combination of skeletal and vascular trauma produces complex injuries that are best treated by a collaborative approach.

2. Evidence of arterial insufficiency may be absent or incomplete at first. Accurate diagnosis requires a high index of suspicion, knowledge of the common sites of vascular injury, and aggressive use of noninvasive modalities and arteriography.

3. Initial treatment should focus on resuscitation of the whole patient, but delay in proceeding to operation should be minimized.

4. Arteriography may be therapeutic,

particularly in pelvic retroperitoneal hemorrhage.

5. Open fractures should be immobilized after vascular repair by external fixation; closed fractures generally may be stabilized internally prior to vascular repair.

6. Good arteriography, adequate exposure, and scrupulous attention to detail are vital to successful vascular reconstruction.

7. Venous repair, fasciotomy, and fibulectomy are important adjuncts to restoration of arterial flow in selected cases and may help to reduce the severity of postoperative swelling, deformity, and disability.

8. Indications for delayed amputation are usually present within several days following injury. Popliteal arterial and venous injuries carry the greatest risk. The amputation stump should be functional.

9. Judicious use of intravenous fluids, whole blood replacement, antibiotics, and tetanus prophylaxis are important pre- and postoperatively. Indiscriminate use of antibiotics, heparin, dextran, steroids, and other temporizing measures may be counterproductive.

10. These patients are vulnerable to a multitude of postoperative complications. Good hydration, careful surgery, close postoperative attention, and aggressive rehabilitation are fundamental to a favorable result.

REFERENCES

1. Bassett, F. H., III, and Silver, D.: Arterial injuries associated with fractures. Arch. Surg., 92:13, 1966.
2. Bradley, E. L.: The anterior tibial compartment syndrome. Surg. Gynecol. Obstet., 136:289, 1973.
3. Cole, W. G.: Fractures and dislocations compounded by distal ischemia. Med. J. Aust., 1:98, 1975.
4. Connolly, J.: Management of fractures associated with arterial injuries (Editorial). Am. J. Surg., 120:331, 1970.
5. DeBakey, M. E., and Simeone, F. A.: Battle injuries of the arteries in World War II. Ann. Surg., 123:534, 1946.
6. Doty, D. B., Treiman, R. L., Rothschild, P. D., and Gaspar, M. R.: Prevention of gangrene due to fractures. Surg. Gynecol. Obstet., 125:284, 1967.
7. Drapanas, T., Hewitt, R. L., Weichert, R. F., III, and Smith, A. D.: Civilian vascular injuries: a critical appraisal of three decades of management. Ann. Surg., 170:351, 1970.
8. Ernst, C. B., and Kaufer, H.: Fibulectomy–fascio-

tomy: an important adjunct in the management of lower extremity arterial trauma. J. Trauma, 11:365, 1971.
9. Fisher, G. W.: Acute arterial injuries treated by the United States Army Medical Service in Vietnam 1965–1966. J. Trauma, 7:844, 1967.
10. Hoover, N. W.: Injuries of the popliteal artery associated with fractures and dislocations. Surg. Clin. North Am., 41:1099, 1961.
11. Hughes, C. W.: Arterial repair during the Korean War. Ann. Surg., 147:555, 1958.
12. Jahnke, E. J. and Seeley, S. F.: Acute vascular injuries in the Korean War: an analysis of 77 consecutive cases. Ann. Surg., 138:158, 1953.
13. Klingensmith, W., Oles, P., and Martinez, H.: Fractures associated with blood vessel injury. Am. J. Surg., 110:849, 1965.
14. Kurin, R.: Elbow dislocation and its association with vascular disruption. J. Bone Joint Surg., 51A:756, 1969.
15. Mahoney, W. D., and Whelan, T. J.: Use of the obturator foramen in iliofemoral artery grafting: case reports. Ann. Surg., 163:215, 1966.
16. Miller, H. H., and Welch, C. S.: Quantitative studies on the time factor in arterial injuries. Ann. Surg., 130:428, 1949.
17. Morton, J. H., Southgate, W. A., and DeWeese, J. A.: Arterial injuries of the extremities. Surg. Gynecol. Obstet., 123:611, 1966.
18. Natali, J., Maraval, M., Kieffer, E., and Petrovic, P.: Fractures of the clavicle and injuries of the subclavian artery. J. Cardiovasc. Surg., 16:541, 1975.
19. Pradham, D. J., Junteguy, J. M., Wilder, R. W., and Michelson, E.: Arterial injuries of the extremities associated with fractures. Arch. Surg., 105:582, 1972.
20. Rich, N. M., Hughes, C. W., and Baugh, J. H.: Management of venous injuries. Ann. Surg., 171:724, 1970.
21. Rich, N. M., Metz, C. W., Hutton, J. E., et al.: Internal versus external fixation of fractures with concomitant vascular injuries in Vietnam. J. Trauma, 11:463, 1971.
22. Ring, E. J., Anthanasoulis, C., Waltman, A. C., et al.: Arteriographic management of hemorrhage following pelvic trauma. Radiology, 109:65, 1973.
23. Schramek, A., Hashmonai, M., Farbstein, J., and Adler, O.: Reconstruction surgery in major vein injuries in the extremities. J. Trauma, 15:816, 1975.
24. Sher, M. H.: Principles in the management of arterial injuries associated with fractures/dislocations. Ann. Surg., 182:630, 1975.
25. Singh, I., and Gorman, J. F.: Vascular injuries in closed fractures near junction of middle and lower thirds of the tibia. J. Trauma, 12:592, 1972.
26. Smith, R. F., Szilagyi, E., and Elliott, J. P.: Fracture of long bones with arterial injury due to blunt trauma. Arch. Surg., 99:315, 1969.
27. Trunkey, D. D., Chapman, M. W., Lim, R. C., Jr., and Dunphy, J. E.: Management of pelvic fractures in blunt trauma injury. J. Trauma, 14:912, 1974.
28. Waddell, J. P., and Lenczner, E. M.: Arterial injury associated with skeletal trauma. Injury, 6:28, 1974.

FREDERICK A. SIMEONE, M.D.

Nerve _____ *34*
Injuries
Complicating
Fractures
and
Dislocations

CLASSIFICATION OF NERVE INJURY ASSOCIATED WITH FRACTURE

Accurate statistics on the incidence of peripheral nerve injuries associated with fractures in civilian life are unavailable. The Veterans' Administration and the National Research Council[13] followed 3656 peripheral nerve injuries, 40 per cent of which were associated with bone injury. Lyons and Woodhall[11] examined a smaller series of noncombat peripheral nerve injuries 21 per cent of which were associated with sufficient bone and joint damage to make combined orthopedic and neurosurgical care necessary.

Nerve injuries can be associated with fractures in a variety of ways.

1. Direct injury by the displaced fragments
   a. stretching
   b. laceration
2. Delayed injury resulting from
   a. callus and scar tissue
   b. infection
   c. ischemia from injury to vessels

Direct injury from the displaced fragments is by far the most common type. The nerve may be morphologically intact, in which case recovery of function in a matter of minutes to years may be expected. If the nerve ends are lacerated, recovery is less likely to occur, and then only after successful reapproximation.

The orthopedic literature has classified nerve injuries in terms less commonly used in neurological and neurosurgical parlance. The following classification was popularized by Seddon,[15] but is seldom used in practice today. It is included here for historical purposes.

1. *Neurapraxia:* This term has been used to describe injury in which the nerve is contused, compressed, or stretched, without disruption of the axons. This situation is presumably associated with early recovery.

2. *Axonotmesis:* The nerve has been contused or compressed. However, ". . . there has been no physical division of the axons, but the injury has been severe enough that wallerian degeneration has taken place or will take place."[15]

3. *Neurotmesis:* The nerve has been completely or partially divided, and repair is required before regeneration can take place.

In 1951, Sunderland[16] devised a more complicated classification in which injuries were rated in order of degree of anatomical

981

disruption. He identified five levels of severity.

First degree injury is a physiological disorder of conduction without anatomical disruption of even the smallest neural components. There is no wallerian degeneration, and recovery follows without treatment within a few days or weeks. A longer recovery time indicates that a more severe injury has occurred. A fracture-dislocation that compresses or stretches a nerve for an instant might produce such a phenomenon. Recovery of motor function is seen simultaneously in all muscles innervated by the nerve, as opposed to the proximal to distal sequence associated with injuries requiring nerve regeneration.

In *second degree* injury, the axon has been disrupted, with progressive proximal to distal degeneration for one or more nodal segments. All of the nerve investments, that is, the Schwann cell sheath surrounding each axon as well as the endoneural tube covering a group of axons, remain intact. Functional recovery is often satisfactory, particularly in peripheral injuries, but it is delayed for months while regeneration takes place.

In *third degree* injury, the internal components of the nerve, that is, the axons, their Schwann cell sheath, and the endoneural tubes, are damaged. The thicker perineurium is preserved. The nerve architecture is disrupted, and nerve regeneration is often hampered by intraneural fibrosis or a neuroma that develops from regenerating components unable to find their way through the area of injury. Recovery is therefore very slow or nonexistent.

The *fourth degree* injury simply describes more severe and permanent neural disruption with preservation of the epineurium and possibly some of the perineurium, so that the nerve is not entirely severed. There may be a gap in nerve contents bridged by portions of perineurium. With the regenerating axons and a few available endoneural tubes that can carry them distal to the injury, recovery cannot be expected without resection of the most severely damaged portions and accurate approximation of the remaining stumps.

In *fifth degree* injury, the nerve and all its components are transected with a variable gap between their ends. This is commonly seen in open fractures of long bones. Here, the only chance of recovery is reapproximation of the severed nerve stumps. Assessment of the precise intraneural damage is quite difficult even with the most sophisticated electrodiagnostic studies, but the severity of the nerve injury can be suggested by the nature of the fracture.

Seddon[14] reported 83.5 per cent spontaneous recovery in 109 cases of closed fracture of the upper extremity with nerve injury. Spontaneous recovery was seen in only 65 per cent of 37 open fractures.

The effect of persistent compression on nerve regeneration remains unclear. There is some evidence that a nerve might cease to function in the face of bony compression, only to return promptly when the compression is removed. There is no doubt, however, that if the nerve demonstrates third or fourth degree injury, spontaneous regeneration cannot occur in the presence of severe compression. A nerve may be trapped between the ends of a bony fragment or even within the joint itself. Occasionally, a long bone is fractured in such a way that the nerves in the limb undergo damaging traction from gravitational forces. These forces may impede regeneration.

CHARACTERISTIC FRACTURE-NERVE INJURY COMBINATIONS

The variability of the forces that can lead to a fracture and subsequent nerve injury defies a stereotyped classification. Nevertheless, anatomical relationships between nerves and bony structures are uniform, and the clinician might routinely test for certain nerve injuries when faced with a particular fracture.

What follows, therefore, is a description of the nerve injuries that may be seen in fractures and dislocations, as well as brief comments about diagnosis and treatment when appropriate. The injuries are arranged in a distal to proximal order, beginning with the upper extremity. Treatment invariably involves bony reduction and immobilization, so this point will not be repeated. Similarly, the often frustrating decision as to whether or not to explore, based on the supposition of a complete transection, will be excluded, unless useful criteria for a decision can be established.

FRACTURES OF THE UPPER EXTREMITIES

THE DIGITS

Since the nerve supply to the muscles controlling the digits is not found distal to the metacarpophalangeal joints, one is concerned only with sensory function in digital fractures. For years these injuries were overlooked, but the annoyance of insensitive fingertips can mar a worker's effectiveness, and may be more disabling to an individual who performs precision handiwork. Later studies by Seddon[15] reported reasonably good results with primary digital nerve repair without the aid of an operating microscope. Primary repair was strongly advised, and results have been significantly better than in secondary delayed repair.

Among Seddon's 22 operated digital nerve injuries, 13 underwent primary suture, and of these 7 had a good result and 5 had a fair result. Of eight secondary repairs, only two demonstrated good results, and four were considered fair. The explanation for this difference was the difficulty in retrieval and preparation of the distal nerve stump. Autogenous grafting was considered preferable to secondary suture.

More recently, Buncke[5] and others have described use of the operating microscope in such repairs. With direct visualization there is better alignment of nerve fiber bundles, and up to 10 sutures of 9–0 monofilament nylon may be used to approximate the ends. These techniques have greatly reduced the incidence of neuroma formation and have led to almost uniformly good recovery.

Digital nerves are easily stretched, rather than severed. Exploration for the repair of nerve, therefore, follows a long waiting period. Instances of open fracture of the digits, however, may warrant early exploration for the repair of digital nerves.

THE CARPAL AND METACARPAL BONES

Serious nerve damage is uncommon with carpal injuries. Fracture-dislocation of the carpus is sometimes associated with transient median nerve symptoms, which usually subside promptly. These may develop slowly with increasing signs of median neuropathy in the first week after injury, but may be secondary to preexisting carpal tunnel stenosis aggravated by the injury. The ulnar nerve may be injured by fractures of the os hamatum and os pisiforme, both of which are near the course of the nerve in the hand. Dislocation of the os lunatum may damage the median nerve, but like all other injuries of the carpal and metacarpal bones, the nerve is rarely transected, and surgical exploration is not required except under unusual circumstances.

THE RADIUS AND ULNA

At the Wrist

Nerves that enter the hand may be injured at the wrist because of their peculiar anatomical location. The trunk of the ulnar nerve runs deep to the flexor carpi ulnaris tendon and into Guyon's canal. The median nerve runs between the flexor carpi radialis and the palmaris longus, under the carpal ligament. The anterior interosseous branch of the median nerve lies on the interosseous membrane between the ulna and the radius. The posterior interosseous branch of the radial nerve lies on the posterior surface of the radioulnar interosseous membrane. Through a special sensory branch the radial nerve emerges dorsally from beneath the brachioradialis tendon 5 cm proximal to the styloid process of the radius. The dorsal cutaneous branch of the ulnar nerve lies subcutaneously on the medial surface of the ulna and emerges about 5 cm proximal to the ulnar styloid. The palmar cutaneous sensory branch of the median nerve arises from the main trunk of the nerve 4 cm proximal to the wrist crease.

In his series of 133 fractures of the lower end of the radius, Frykman[8] found 2 cases of median nerve injury and 4 cases of ulnar nerve injury. In no case were both nerves involved.

The median nerve may be injured in the following manner:[1]
1. Primary injuries.
2. Secondary injuries due to pressure by

an incompletely reduced fragment. This may develop soon after movement of the wrist is resumed.

3. Nerve involvement developing much later as the result of bony abnormalities in the nerve and alteration in the carpal ligament.

4. Injuries associated with treatment (especially in acute palmar flexion with ulnar deviation). This is caused by narrowing of the anatomical boundaries of the carpal tunnel.

Fractures of the midradius and ulnar shaft are not often associated with median nerve injury. Damage to the anterior and posterior interosseous nerves may occur, since they pass through the interosseous ligaments, but these generally heal without specific treatment.

At the Distal End Near the Wrist

Nerve injuries are uncommon despite the frequency of fractures to the distal radius or ulna. In many instances, the median or ulnar nerve is stretched. At the time of surgical restoration for other reasons, contusion and ecchymosis may be visible. Radial or ulnar nerves may be involved in callus that forms around the injury site. Surgical exploration is seldom necessary even in open comminuted fractures.

Nerve injuries are rarely associated with closed fractures involving the midportion of the radius and ulna. Nerves are injured at this site only in association with open fractures with extensive soft tissue loss, at which time the nerve injury may be identified and approximated according to the principles outlined.

THE ELBOW

The median, radial, or ulnar nerves may be injured at the time of elbow joint fracture or dislocation. The median nerve is rarely involved except in supracondylar fractures. The radial nerve and its posterior interosseous branch, however, can be injured as a result of fractures associated with anterior dislocation of the radial end. The ulnar nerve is most frequently injured in elbow fractures. It is vulnerable to fracture-dislocations, supracondylar fractures, and avulsion fractures of the medial epicondyle.

The treatment for most of these fractures is watchful waiting. If open reduction of the medial epicondyle fracture is necessary, and there is preoperative evidence of ulnar involvement, an elective ulnar nerve transposition anterior to the medial epicondyle should be performed simultaneously.

Delayed or tardy ulnar nerve palsy results from associated soft tissue and bony scar in the region of elbow fracture which ultimately restricts the normal movement of the ulnar nerve. Because of its location posterior to the medial epicondyle, the nerve is subjected to trauma if it cannot slide freely in its groove. With repeated flexion and extension of the elbow over the years, a highly localized ulnar neuropathy develops which may progress to a severe disability of the hand if it is not corrected.

Transposition of the ulnar nerve must be performed with great care. Elective removal of the medial epicondyle is favored by some, although this maneuver is not necessary. Some experienced surgeons feel that section of the branches most proximal to the flexor carpi ulnaris is necessary to immobilize the nerve above the medial epicondyle. At the time of surgery a fascial sling, which loosely directs the nerve in its new location, must be fashioned. While the nerve is still exposed, the extremity should be flexed and extended to ascertain the free course of the nerve through its new sling. If the patient awakens from surgery with greater pain or disability, immediate exploration for the cause of these symptoms is suggested. Electromyography, particularly with conduction velocity of the ulnar nerve across the elbow, has proved most useful in the diagnosis and follow-up care of these patients.

The median nerve is rarely injured, though Mannerfelt[12] has described cases in which it was trapped in the elbow joint at the time of fracture-dislocation. The medial aspect of the elbow joint was laid open and the nerve slipped inside of the joint, thereby causing complete median paralysis.

THE MIDHUMERUS

Only the radial nerve, which runs in the spiral groove around the midshaft of the humerus, is vulnerable to closed injuries at the midhumeral level. Radial palsy may result from stretching or disruption of the nerve at the fracture site. This mechanism should be considered in closed injuries associated with wrist drop and numbness of the dorsum of the hand. Radiographic evidence of fracture is usually seen, but it is not possible to discern if the nerve ends are severed or simply stretched and contused. Ordinarily, a waiting period of six months is required before exploration of the radial nerve near the fracture site should be considered. Serial electromyographic studies may be of help. Occasionally, a "tardy radial palsy" develops as a result of involvement of the nerve in scar or callus.

THE GLENOHUMERAL JOINT

The axillary nerve is most frequently injured in glenohumeral dislocations. The musculocutaneous nerve is occasionally involved, but the other peripheral nerves of the upper extremity are sufficiently remote from the joint to escape injury. Occasionally the medial cord and, very rarely, the posterior cord of the brachial plexus are involved in medial dislocations of the humeral head.

Axillary nerve injury is easily identified by palpable inability to contract the deltoid muscle and by weakness on abduction of the arm beyond 30 degrees from the chest wall. Shoulder pain may prevent the early assessment of deltoid weakness, and the sensory examination may be of help. An area of reduced sensation directly overlying the deltoid muscle (on the lateral aspect of the upper arm from the humeral head halfway down toward the elbow) is diagnostic. Musculocutaneous nerve injury is associated with weakness of flexion and supination of the forearm, palpable failure of biceps muscle contraction, and occasionally hypesthesia in the distribution of the lateral antebrachial cutaneous nerve (along the lateral aspect of the forearm from the base of the thumb to the lateral epicondylar area).

Treatment of these injuries consists primarily of reduction of the dislocation and physical therapy in anticipation of spontaneous recovery. Only rarely is the nerve actually severed, and surgical exploration should be delayed for at least six months.

INJURIES OF THE BRACHIAL PLEXUS

Throughout its course between the clavicle and the rib cage, from the conjunction of its nerve roots to the glenohumeral joint, the brachial plexus is rarely involved in closed injuries of the shoulder. The clavicle can be forcefully compressed against the first rib, with resultant brachial plexus injury. Displaced fractures of the clavicle occasionally lacerate the brachial plexus. Stretch injuries are much more likely to affect the contributing nerve roots than the brachial plexus trunks themselves. An accurate examination can identify the site of neurological injury. Roentgenograms are rarely of help unless they demonstrate a displaced clavicular fracture.

Most brachial plexus injuries caused by stretch or contusion will recover spontaneously within six months. Such injuries rarely require surgical treatment, though rest and relief of tension on the brachial plexus are of help during initial treatment. Reduction of a fractured clavicle may be required. Failure to improve over a period of several months may indicate laceration of one or more brachial plexus components, the repair of which may be complex or may require autografting. Dense cicatrix may impede regeneration, though the results of surgery for this complication are uncertain.

The neurosurgical treatment of brachial plexus lacerations requires particular expertise and careful planning. In order to gain adequate exposure, it may be necessary to extend the incision from the root of the neck across the clavicle (a portion of which must be resected) into the arm. The peripheral branches of the plexus are identified, and the disrupted nerve ends are isolated and approximated. Section of the clavicular portion of the sternocleidomastoid, the scalenus anticus, the pectoralis major and minor, and the subclavius muscles is required.

NERVE ROOT INJURIES

Injuries to the cervical nerve roots are seen with dislocations of the spine and a variety of mechanisms that produce extreme distortion of the relationship between the shoulder girdle and the cervical spine. The five nerve roots that join shortly after their exit from the cervical spine to form the trunks of the brachial plexus are normally angulated acutely in a caudal direction as they pass into the arm.

The most common mechanism of injury is traction caused by forceful straightening of the angle of the shoulder and neck. In rare instances, injury follows a forceful pull on the abducted arm. Adson[2] and others demonstrated that if the arm is abducted at the time of injury, greater stress is transmitted to the lower roots. If the arm is held adducted, the upper brachial plexus roots are most subject to traction injury. The roots may be stretched, torn, or avulsed from the spinal cord. Nerve roots are not invested with the neurilemmal sheath required for regeneration. Therefore, unlike injuries of nerve trunks or peripheral nerves, root injuries associated with disruption of anatomical continuity of the neural components are permanent and refractory to surgical therapy.

Clues to the location of the injury are available from certain facts of the history and examination. The shoulder-neck relationship at the time of injury is important. The distribution of weakness is also helpful. A nerve root injury is almost certain if there is paralysis of the diaphragm, rhomboid, or serratus muscles, because innervation of these derives directly from the root and does not pass through the trunks of the brachial plexus. Electromyographic analysis of motor potentials may suggest a nerve root, rather than a trunk or peripheral nerve, pattern. On myelography, one might see dilatations (traumatic meningoceles) of the nerve root dural sheath which are diagnostic of rupture of the nerve root sleeve. Clinical assessment of autonomic nerve function in the upper extremity devised by Bonney[3] may be helpful.

The "triple response" of the skin to an intradermal injection of 1 per cent histamine requires that the nerves innervating the site of injection be anatomically intact from the ganglion cell. If a triple response is present following upper extremity nerve injuries, this suggests that the brachial plexus and peripheral nerves are intact, and the nerve root (portion of the nerve before the ganglion cell) is the site of interruption. This signals a poor prognosis in the presence of significant paralysis. The test is

used by specialized laboratories and is not at present an important part of neurological evaluation.

Clinical Features of Nerve Root Lesions

*Upper Root (C5 to C6) or Erb-Duchenne Palsy.** With this lesion, the patient presents with an adducted, medially rotated humerus. There is paralysis of the deltoid, lateral rotators of the humerus, and the clavicular portion of the pectoralis major, as well as partial involvement of the biceps muscle. The forearm and hand are otherwise unaffected, except for an inconstant sensory deficit which proceeds along the radial aspect of the arm from the thumb and index finger to the apex of the shoulder. Paralysis of the extensors at the elbow, wrist, and fingers implies involvement of the C7 root as well.

Lower Root (C8 to T1) or Dejerine-Klumpke Palsy. This injury is far more common at birth than in adults. The arm is normal proximally, but there is weakness of intrinsic hand muscle function and loss of sensation on the palm. This syndrome is seen in so-called postoperative brachial plexus palsy and is apparently caused by prolonged hyperabduction during surgery.

Dhúner[7] estimates that this complication occurs 11 times in every 30,000 instances of use of general anesthesia. It is more frequently seen in association with abdominal surgery. To avoid this, the arm should not be abducted more than 90 degrees from the chest wall, nor should the elbows be allowed to fall below 15 cm from the tabletop. Fortunately, most postoperative brachial plexus palsies resolve spontaneously and without specific treatment in two to three months. Occasionally they are permanent, but there is no evidence that surgical exploration at any time is of help.

Rehabilitation of the Upper Extremity With Brachial Plexus Injuries

Although beyond the scope of this discussion, brief mention should be made of

---

*The eponyms refer to original clinical description of cervical nerve root injuries, most of which are associated with birth trauma.

specialized attempts to restore function in the paralyzed arm.

Leffert[10] has emphasized the importance of physical therapy in the acute and chronic phases of brachial plexus injuries. Exercises may be carried on with periodic reexamination. In the chronic phase, adjustments to persistent deficit are made. Care of the vulnerable insensate arm is emphasized. Occasional tendon transfers and fusions at the shoulder and elbow are of help. These procedures may be tailored to the patient's occupation. In rare instances, arthrodesis of the shoulder associated with amputation of the arm above the elbow and application of a prosthesis may be involved.

If shoulder flaccidity prevents useful function of the remaining muscles of the arm, stability can be achieved by surgical fusion of the glenohumeral joint. Subsequently, the humerus will move with the scapula, and this will improve proximal limb control.

FRACTURES OF THE SKULL

All of the cranial nerves are subject to injury by skull fracture. Injury to the olfactory nerve, the auditory, facial, and vestibular nerve complex, and the branches of the trigeminal nerve is relatively common. The nature of such injuries and their symptoms will be described briefly. Since many of these injuries are not treated, management will be discussed only when appropriate.

Olfactory Nerve

The olfactory nerve is the most common cranial nerve to be injured in skull fracture. Through its long course across the base of the anterior fossa of the skull, it lies relatively free. At the olfactory bulb, however, the nerve is fixed as its terminals penetrate the cribriform plate to enter the nasal mucosa. Although avulsion injuries are more common than involvement by disrupted bone ends, fractures of the cribriform plate are frequently associated with anosmia. Loss of spinal fluid from the nose is often concurrent. Because of the peculiarities in the myelinization and composition of its coverings, this nerve, like the optic

nerve, resembles more closely an extension of brain tissue than a peripheral nerve. Consequently, regeneration after transection is not possible.

Optic Nerve

Complete or partial visual loss in one eye can follow a fracture of the orbital roof which extends into the optic foramen. The fracture can be demonstrated on specialized radiographic views of the skull complemented by tomography when indicated. The patient will complain of visual loss immediately after the injury. Vision should be checked in each eye independently. Funduscopy is often of little help, though to a trained observer ischemia of the optic nerve head and occasionally retinal hemorrhages may be visible. The pupillary light reflex will be lost on the side of a severe injury, but the pupil will respond consensually to light in the other eye.

The treatment of this injury is the subject of considerable controversy in ophthalmological and neurosurgical literature. Some favor immediate surgery to widen the optic foramen and decompress the optic nerve. Others feel that since regeneration of a severed nerve is unlikely, surgery has nothing to offer. As with any injury to a cranial nerve that is surrounded by a bony opening, posttraumatic swelling of the nerve with delayed loss of function is reported. In theory, the nerve swells and becomes sufficiently confined in its bony canal so that secondary ischemia leads to disordered function. Large doses of corticosteroids may reduce the swelling. This form of treatment is favored by most clinicians. Bilateral involvement of the optic nerves in skull fractures is rare, and this devastating injury is confined to the most serious head trauma.

Oculomotor Nerve

The oculomotor nerve contains many functional components that supply the extraocular muscles, the elevator of the eyelid, and the constrictor of the pupil. It is injured by fractures that extend into the orbital apex, and it is occasionally involved in so-called orbital blowout fractures. Partial third nerve lesions may be difficult to detect because some of the muscles supplied by the nerve may be involved at the fracture site. If *all* of the muscles supplied by the third nerve are involved, the diagnosis is simpler. There is no specific treatment for fractures that injure the third nerve.

An interesting sequela of third nerve injuries is aberrant regeneration of the various fibers in the nerve, and this can produce peculiar disorders of ocular motility. For instance, the pupil may dilate pathologically, causing the individual to look toward his nose. On other occasions the eye may fall downward, though the patient has attempted to look upward. Patients can usually adapt to these anomalies.

Trochlear Nerve

The trochlear nerve, which innervates only the superior oblique muscle, is rarely involved in injury. Furthermore, minimal disability results from a trochlear nerve injury, and therefore no treatment is recommended.

Trigeminal Nerve

The trigeminal nerve sends sensory branches to the structures of the head and face. A small motor division supplies some of the muscles of mastication. Each branch leaves the skull through its foramen (superior orbital fissure, mandibular foramen, maxillary foramen), and subsequently passes through other foramina in the bones of the face to innervate the skin. These include the supraorbital foramen, the infraorbital foramen, and the mental foramen, all of which may be involved in facial fractures. Most frequently seen is infraorbital nerve damage secondary to orbital and maxillary fractures, in which the patient experiences peculiar numbness in the cheek and along the side of the nose. None of these injuries is worthy of treatment.

Abducens Nerve

The abducens nerve is rarely involved in fractures along the base of the skull or orbit. Various head injuries may be associated with avulsion of the nerve as it enters the cavernous sinus.

Facial Nerve

The facial nerve is subjected to injury in basal skull fractures that extend through the petrous bone. The nerve runs a somewhat circuitous course in this bone, and facial palsies may follow fractures through several mechanisms: (1) complete transection at the fracture site, and (2) facial nerve injury with swelling and secondary ischemia because of the tight confines of the bony facial canal.

These mechanisms are presumed, because a large percentage of postbasal skull fracture facial palsies will clear spontaneously, whereas others are permanent. Electromyographic studies can help with this differentiation.

Some otolaryngologists recommend prompt surgical decompression of the facial nerve through a translabyrinthine approach. With this operation the facial canal is opened, presumably allowing more room for the "swollen" nerve. Because of the tendency for the facial palsy to clear without treatment, there is little convincing evidence that this operation is beneficial.

Auditory-Vestibular Nerve

These nerves, which also run in the petrous bone, are similarly involved in basal skull fractures. Immediate loss of hearing, vertigo (particularly if associated with spinal fluid otorrhea), and a hematoma over the mastoid process (Battle's sign) are diagnostic of a basal skull fracture with injury to these nerves. Again, surgical decompression has been advised by some, without convincing results. Occasionally, a delayed facial nerve or auditory nerve palsy may follow the injury by several days. Some believe that the prognosis after surgical decompression is better than if these injuries are left untreated. Again, large controlled series are required to make this differentiation.

Glossopharyngeal, Vagus, Spinal Accessory, and Hypoglossal Nerves

Injury to these lower cranial nerves is most unusual. Fractures rarely occur on the ventral surface of the skull near the clivus. With the exception of the hypoglossal nerve, these nerves bear a close bony relationship to the jugular foramen, which is rarely involved in injury. They should be considered to be involved only when specific neurological deficit follows basal skull fractures.

FRACTURES OF THE PELVIS

Neurological deficit complicating pelvic fracture is often associated with injury to the sacrum or with sacroiliac disruption. The peripheral nerve most affected is the sciatic, which may be damaged anywhere along its course through the pelvic outlet. Carruthers and Logue[6] reported 3 cases of obturator nerve paralysis among 72 pelvic fractures. This injury is probably more common, in that particularly careful testing is required to assess the function of this peripheral nerve.

The nerves of greatest concern in association with these fractures are the upper sacral roots. The sacral foramina are extremely wide compared with the nerve roots exiting from them. Bonnin[4] has postulated that the pelvic nerves are injured in association with hemorrhage, fibrous tissue formation, and pressure against bone when there is significant displacement. The first and second sacral nerves are most commonly affected, so that plantar flexion and ankle jerk must be tested. These injuries are apparently not painful, a point that may distinguish them from associated herniation of a lumbar disk. Bowel and bladder function usually remain intact, because pelvic fractures are commonly unilateral and seldom involve the third sacral nerve root or below.

In some crush injuries of the pelvis, neurological findings may be scattered. Surgical exploration, either posteriorly or transabdominally, is likely to be fruitless, and therefore is rarely done. A good example is transverse comminuted fracture of the sacrum which can produce weakness in the gluteal, hamstring, and foot flexors, as well as numbness of the buttocks and posterolateral aspect of the leg. Even if the nerve roots could be identified at the fracture site, surgical repair at the root level is not effective.

FRACTURES OF THE LOWER EXTREMITIES

THE HIP

The sciatic nerve is frequently injured in dislocations or fractures about the hip. The mechanism of injury can be focal contusion, laceration, or stretch. Prompt recognition and emergency treatment are essential, since many patients will have persistent pressure from the dislocated bone which, because of secondary local ischemia, can produce permanent paralysis. Recovery has been reported in over 60 per cent of cases.[9, 17] A direct relationship between early recognition and treatment has been observed in association with a good recovery.

Fractures through the shaft of the femur are not commonly associated with nerve injury because of the interposition of a mass of muscle between the bone and the nerve. Worthy of mention, however, is the association of peroneal nerve injury with poorly managed femur traction. If the leg is maintained in external rotation during traction to align fractures of the femoral shaft, the peroneal nerve at the head of the fibula may be compressed. Flexion at the knee may not correspond to flexion in the suspension system, and this can lead to abnormal pressure on the knee. Padding over the head of the fibula can help to obviate this problem.

THE KNEE

Nerve involvement has been reported in over 25 per cent of cases of dislocation of the knee.[19] Because arterial injury is frequent in this location, some nerve damage may be secondary to ischemia. The injuries are usually of the traction type in which recovery may occur spontaneously, although late repair has been advised since the nerve may be stretched or actually torn.

Towne and co-workers[18] have described the "lateral compartment syndrome of the knee." The peroneal nerve and the lateral knee ligamentous structures are involved, and the nerve may be injured slightly or totally disrupted. This should be suspected in any adduction injury to the knee with signs of damage to the lateral ligament and capsular structures. The authors recommend early exploration of the peroneal nerve with definitive repair as soon as possible. Others suggest that exploration should be delayed for at least three months.

Surgical repair of fracture-dislocations of the knee is common, but there are a variety of neurological problems associated with such surgery. Temporary peroneal palsy may occur when excessive traction in the soft tissues of the popliteal space is necessary. Pressure on the fibular head by such traction or by casting must be recognized early and the cast windowed and padded, particularly in the area of the fibular head.

The saphenous nerve, which supplies superficial sensation to the anteromedial aspect of the foreleg, can be damaged by surgical incisions at the knee. Injury to its infrapatellar branch is associated with numbness or neuroma formation. Damage to the sartorial branch produces a numb area over the anteromedial aspect of the calf. This sensation is usually tolerated unless there is a neuroma at the site of the scar.

Fractures of the shaft of the tibia or fibula rarely cause nerve injury. The peroneal nerve may be injured in proximal fractures near the lateral aspect of the knee, but the shaft of these long bones is not otherwise contiguous with major nerve structures. The peroneal nerve may be injured in association with a midshaft tibia or fibula fracture. This is usually from direct trauma, such as that caused by the bumper of an automobile. Secondary swelling of soft tissues in the leg and cast pressure are probably more common causes of nerve injury in the leg than involvement at the fracture site.

As the peroneal nerve crosses into the anterior compartment of the leg, it is particularly susceptible to compression by swelling and hematoma. Repeated neurological examination during the first two days after this fracture is important, because secondary swelling can compress the nerve and produce gradual loss of dorsal or plantar flexion. Furthermore, an improperly applied cast is a not uncommon cause of late neurological deficit. If this pressure is not relieved within a few hours, permanent nerve damage may follow. Examination of the cast or decompression of the anterior tibial compartment must be considered.

When the paralysis immediately follows the injury, one must suspect involvement of the peroneal nerve at the fracture site, though exploration may be delayed for three to four months in anticipation of spontaneous recovery. Electromyography is helpful in making this decision.

THE FOOT

Nerve injuries associated with fractures of the foot are rare. Neural supply to the muscles of the plantar aspect of the foot comes mainly from the posterior tibial nerve which splits into medial and lateral plantar branches. The superficial branch of the common peroneal nerve supplies the dorsal aspect of the foot. Any of these nerves may be involved in crushing injuries to the foot and ankle, but they are rarely lacerated by a fracture. The medial and lateral branches of the posterior tibial nerve can become entrapped in scar tissue after fractures (particularly those involving the calcaneus), and decompression of these nerves may be required in order to relieve chronic discomfort.

REFERENCES

1. Abbott, L. C., Saunders, J. B., Hagey, N., et al.: Surgical approaches to the shoulder joints. J. Bone Joint Surg., *31A*:235–255, 1949.
2. Adson, A. W.: The gross pathology of brachial plexus injuries. Surg. Gynecol. Obstet., *34*:351–357, 1922.
3. Bonney, G.: The value of axon responses in determining the site of the lesion in traction injuries of the brachial plexus. Brain, 77:588–609, 1954.
4. Bonnin, J. G.: Sacral fractures and injuries to the cauda equina. J. Bone Joint Surg., *27*:113–127, 1945.
5. Buncke, H.: Digital nerve repairs. Surg. Clin. North Am., *52*:1267–1286, 1972.
6. Carruthers, F. W., and Logue, R. M.: Treatment of fractures of the pelvis and their complications. Am. Acad. Orthop. Surg. Lect., *10*:50–56, 1953.
7. Dhúner, K. G.: Nerve injuries following operations: A survey of cases occurring during a six year period. Anesthesiology, *11*:289–293, 1950.
8. Frykman, G.: Fracture of the distal radius including sequelae—shoulder, hand, finger syndrome, disturbance in the distal radial-ulnar joint, and impairment of nerve function: A clinical and

experimental study. Acta. Orthop. Scand. (Suppl.), *108*:1–155, 1967.

9. Hunter, G. A.: Posterior dislocation and fracture/dislocation of the hip. J. Bone Joint Surg., *51B*:38–44, 1969.

10. Leffert, R. D.: Brachial plexus injuries. N. Engl. J. Med., *291*:1059–1067, 1974.

11. Lyons, W. R., and Woodhall, B.: Atlas of Peripheral Nerve Injuries. Philadelphia, W. B. Saunders, 1949.

12. Mannerfelt, L.: Median nerve entrapment after dislocation of the elbow (report of a case). J. Bone Joint Surg., *50B*:152–155, 1968.

13. Neurosurgery in World War II. Washington, D.C., Department of the Army, 1959, p. 230.

14. Seddon, H. J.: Nerve lesions complicating certain closed bone injuries. J.A.M.A., *135*:691, 1947.

15. Seddon, H. J.: Peripheral Nerve Injuries. London, Her Majesty's Printing Office, 1954.

16. Sunderland, S.: Factors influencing the course of regeneration and the quality of recovery after nerve suture. Brain, 75:19, 1952.

17. Thompson, V. P., and Epstein, H. C.: Traumatic dislocations of the hip. J. Bone Joint Surg., *33A*:746–778, 1951.

18. Towne, L. C., Blazinia, M. D., Marmor, L., and Lawrence, J. F.: Lateral compartment syndrome of the knee. Clin. Orthop., 76:160–168, 1971.

19. White, J.: The results of traction injuries of the common peroneal nerve. J. Bone Joint Surg., *50B*:346–350, 1968.

JEROLD Z. KAPLAN, M.D.,
and
BASIL A. PRUITT, JR., M.D.

35 _____ Burns and Fractures

Optimal care of the burn patient requires a multidisciplinary approach involving specialists in many areas. Although the basic care of the patient is usually managed by a general or plastic surgeon, the orthopedist, trained in the preservation and restoration of function, should be a member of the burn care team and contribute significantly to the patient's overall recovery from the severe injury that he has suffered. Survival is obviously the prime goal, but a burned patient who survives but has lost the ability to function cannot be considered a success.

The United States Army Institute of Surgical Research admitted 3221 patients in the period 1962 through 1975 (Tables 35–1, 35–2, and 35–3). One hundred ninety-seven (6.1 per cent) of these patients sustained a total of 273 associated acute orthopedic injuries excluding fractures of the skull, facial bones, ribs, and phalanges. Seventy-one of the injuries were open, and 202 were closed.

Thermal trauma is one of the most severe forms of injury affecting man. An extensive and prolonged hospital course is the rule rather than the exception for the severely burned patient. The following brief outline and summary of burn management are presented to acquaint the orthopedist with the general care these patients require. The care of the burned patient may be subdivided into four overlapping periods of time: (1) the resuscitative phase, which lasts approximately 72 hours from the time of injury, (2) the acute phase of wound care from the time resuscitation is completed

until the patient begins to undergo his grafting procedures, (3) the subacute phase of wound closure from grafting to the patient's first discharge, and (4) the long-term convalescence and reconstructive phase.

The initial emergency evaluation and treatment of the burn patient is similar to that of any patient who has sustained massive trauma. A brief but thorough examination should be performed to ascertain whether there are any associated injuries, which there frequently are in the patient injured in an explosion or crash of an automobile or airplane. Adequacy and patency of the airway must be assured, and any hemorrhage controlled.

The burned patient, even without associated injuries, has a fluid requirement that may be massive and is directly related to

TABLE 35–1 Incidence of Upper Extremity Injuries in 3221 Patients Treated at U.S. Army Institute of Surgical Research 1962 to 1975

Injury	Open	Closed
Fracture		
Clavicle	0	17
Scapula	0	3
Humerus	4	7
Radius-ulna	9	28
Dislocation		
Shoulder	0	5
Acromioclavicular joint	0	2
Sternoclavicular joint	0	3
Elbow	0	1
Wrist	0	3
Metacarpophalangeal joint	0	7

TABLE 35–2   Incidence of Lower Extremity Injuries in 3221 Patients Treated at U.S. Army Institute of Surgical Research 1962 to 1975

Injury	Open	Closed
Fracture		
Femur	10	30
Tibia-fibula	31	32
Patella	1	4
Dislocation		
Hip	0	1
Knee	1	0
Tear		
Medial meniscus	0	1
Rupture		
Achilles tendon	1	0

burn size. Various fluid resuscitation formulas have been proposed and are used. The two most commonly used today are the Brooke formula and the more recent Ringer's lactate resuscitation advocated by Baxter.[2a] In the first 24 hours, the Brooke formula provides 1.5 ml of electrolyte-containing solution per kilogram of body weight per per cent of body surface burned and 0.5 ml colloid per kilogram of body weight per per cent of surface burned. In addition, 2 liters of 5 per cent dextrose in water is provided to cover insensible water loss. Parkland formula resuscitation provides 4 ml of Ringer's lactate per kilogram of body weight per per cent of surface burned without providing colloid-containing fluid in the first 24 hours postburn. Half the estimated fluid is given in the first 8 hours and the remainder during the next 16 hours. Both these formulas, of course, are only guidelines and should be modified as indicated by the individual patient's clinical response. If a patient has associated major fractures or soft-tissue injury, fluid

TABLE 35–3   Incidence of Injuries of Axial Skeleton* in 3221 Patients Treated at U.S. Army Institute of Surgical Research 1962 to 1975

	Open	Closed
Cervical spine	0	4
Thoracic spine	0	13
Lumbar spine	1	10
"Vertebra"—site not specified	0	8
Pelvis	13	18
Acetabulum	0	5

*Excluding ribs and skull.

resuscitation requirements may increase significantly, particularly in the case of pelvic or femoral fractures. Whole blood or components are indicated only for blood loss due to associated injuries. It should be emphasized that clinical response is the best guide to the exact volume needed for resuscitation. Blood pressure and central venous pressure should be maintained in a normal range, and a urine output of 30 to 50 ml per hour in the adult and 1 ml per kilogram of body weight per hour in children should be maintained. Tetanus prophylaxis should be given with toxoid or hyperimmune globulin as needed. Prophylactic antibiotics, unless there is an associated injury that necessitates their use, are generally no longer given in the initial postburn period.

Several methods of burn wound care can be used and each possesses certain advantages and disadvantages. Exposure therapy without a topical agent is frequently used for a small second-degree burn. The wound is merely left exposed to the air to form a clean dry crust beneath which healing occurs. Instead of leaving the wound exposed to air, several topical antibacterial agents may be used. These include mafenide acetate (Sulfamylon) burn cream, silver sulfadiazine burn cream, and 0.5 per cent silver nitrate soaks. Sulfamylon and silver sulfadiazine are supplied in a water-soluble cream emulsion that is spread on the wound after daily cleaning of the wound and reapplied as necessary, usually 12 or 24 hours later. One-half per cent silver nitrate is applied in the form of continuous soaks that are kept moist with the solution and changed twice daily. Occlusive dressings may be used for outpatients with small burns but are no longer indicated for hospitalized patients with extensive burns. Other techniques of wound management include early excision of the burn wounds and immediate or delayed grafting with autograft skin or biological dressings including human cutaneous allograft or porcine cutaneous xenograft. Definitive grafting may be done with either "meshed" autograft or sheets of autograft.

Once the wounds have been completely covered with autografts, a variable period of time, approximately 6 to 18 months, is allowed for the grafts and hypertrophic

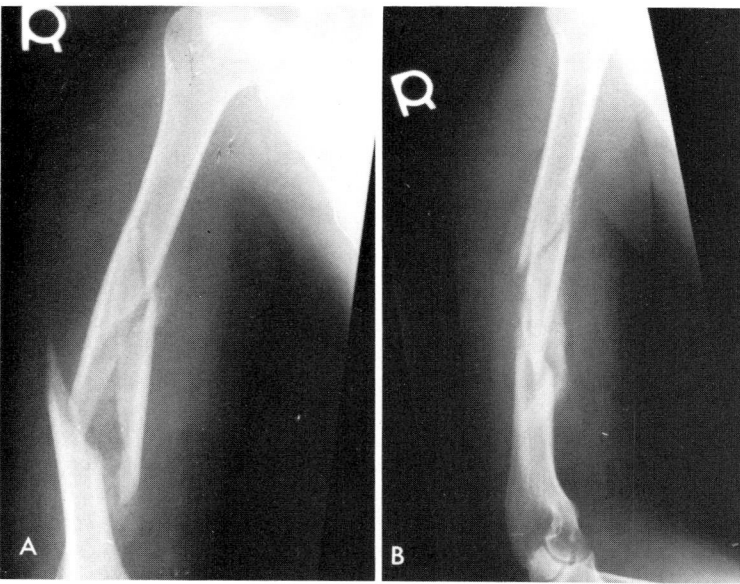

Figure 35–1 *A.* A 46-year-old woman sustained this comminuted fracture of the distal humerus in an airplane accident. Complete radial palsy was present at the time of admission to the hospital. Because of burns of the brachium, the fracture was treated with a modified sling and splint. *B.* Healing of the fracture was good, although there is some angulation of the distal fragment. The burns required grafting but healed uneventfully. Three months postinjury and following complete skin healing, reexploration of the fracture site was performed, a trapped radial nerve was released, and osteotomy was performed. Healing of the osteotomy was satisfactory, and radial nerve function has returned.

scars to mature prior to the performance of elective cosmetic or reconstructive surgery. If scar contractures result in skeletal deformity or significant functional limitation, early release should be performed. Ectropion with corneal exposure and acute neck or lip contractures that leave the mouth less than water-tight require early operative intervention, as do contractures across joints that cause subluxation or that would result in permanent loss of joint movement if not released in timely fashion. Ideally, active exercise and splinting begun on the day of the burn prevent or minimize these deformities. In some instances, however, early splinting and physical therapy may not have been utilized and the patient may not have been seen by the orthopedist until after contractures have occurred. Wide release of the contracture with onlay grafting and early physical therapy are then necessary for optimal results.

Early surgical intervention may also be necessary to release an entrapped nerve or excise heterotopic ossification (Fig. 35–1).

ORTHOPEDIC MANAGEMENT AND TECHNIQUES

Resuscitative Phase

During the resuscitative phase of burn care, orthopedic management of the patient consists of treating those fractures and dislocations that may be concomitantly present, and initiating and supervising a program of physical therapy and use of splints or positioning devices to prevent contractures or loss of motion or both.

Dislocations. Acute dislocations should be reduced by means of the same techniques that would be used for that joint in an unburned patient. Every possible effort should be made to reduce the dislocation in a closed manner. Intravenous narcotics or Valium are the most useful agents for relaxation and analgesia. Intraarticular lidocaine (Xylocaine) may also be used if muscle spasm is minimal and overlying skin is unburned. If closed reduction is not successful and open reduction is necessary, close cooperation between the primary physician managing the patient, the anesthesiologist, and the orthopedist is necessary to select the best time and technique for anesthesia and reduction. If there are no burns in the area of dislocation, standard operative techniques may be used and the wound may be primarily closed. If the involved joint underlies the burn wound, the operative techniques may be the same; however, the burn wound must be considered contaminated. In this case the wound is closed to the fascia but the skin is left open to be closed secondarily. Drainage of the joint should not be performed, as the

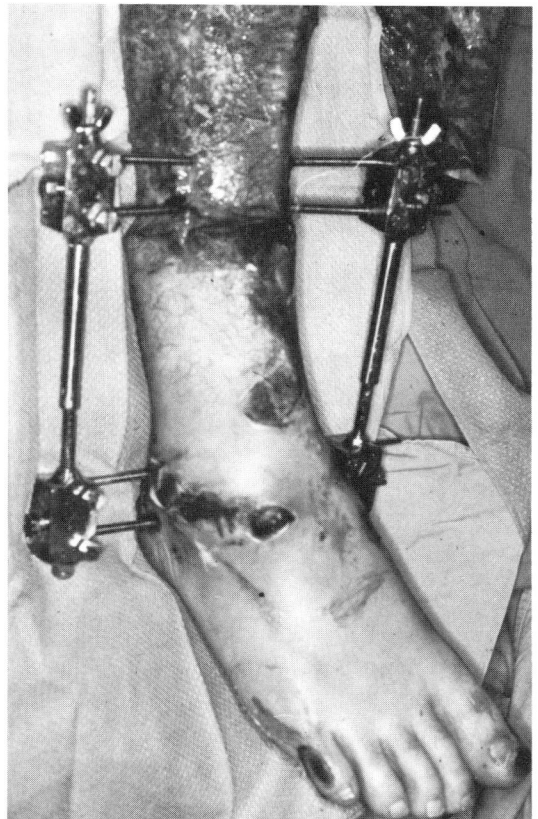

Figure 35–2 A 46-year-old man sustained a fracture-dislocation of his ankle in an airplane accident. A Charnley device was used to stabilize the foot and lower leg, facilitating nursing care.

tance will greatly simplify nursing care. Similarly, an open fracture in an unburned extremity should be treated by using standard orthopedic techniques, but reduction should preferably be held with traction or suspension rather than with a closed cast, since the patient must be bathed frequently (Fig. 35–3). Internal fixation is generally not recommended because of the theoretical risk of infection. Close attention should be paid to the wound and the fracture site. Studies at this Institute have shown that seeding of the bloodstream with organisms often follows any manipulation of the burn wound, and the possibility of an infected hematoma with resulting acute osteomyelitis is theoretically greater in these patients than in an unburned patient.

A closed fracture beneath burned skin should be reduced in a conventional manner and then held immobilized with skeletal suspension or an isoprene splint that can be removed to permit examination of the burn wound (Figs. 35–4 and 35–5). In general, open reduction should be avoided, as the probability of complications, particularly infection, is very great. Acceptance of a less than ideal position is preferable to the risk of attempting to attain anatomical alignment by an open reduction. An open fracture through a burn wound presents the greatest challenge to proper management. The patient should be taken to the operating room as soon as possible; the wounds should be cleaned and the fracture reduced. Skeletal suspension through a remote site is preferable, and internal fixation should be utilized only when nonoperative means are inadequate to reduce or stabilize the fracture. If open reduction with internal fixation is employed, the minimal amount of metal necessary to stabilize the fracture should be used (Fig. 35–6). All burn wounds are contaminated, and the risk of an infected burn wound seeding a fracture site is great if an open reduction with internal fixation is performed after the first 24 hours postburn. Vanden Bussche reported successful open reduction and rigid internal fixation of fractures but recommends this procedure only if the patient is suitable for surgery on the day of burn. The wound should be closed only to the fascial layer and then loosely packed open to await subsequent secondary closure. Close attention to the wound and

Text continued on page 999.

drainage catheter is more likely to provide ingress for bacteria than egress for fluid. Postoperatively, the reduction should be held with appropriate traction or splinting. If closed reduction cannot be performed and open reduction is contraindicated by the general condition of the patient, stabilization of the joint should be effected by splinting or pin fixation through an external device (Fig. 35–2).

Fractures. In the burned patient, fractures may be beneath burned or unburned skin and may, of course, be open or closed. A closed fracture in an unburned extremity should be handled by using standard orthopedic management. If close molding of a cast is not necessary to hold the fracture, a fiber-glass cast is preferable because, owing to the need for frequent bathing or showering of the burned patient, its water resis-

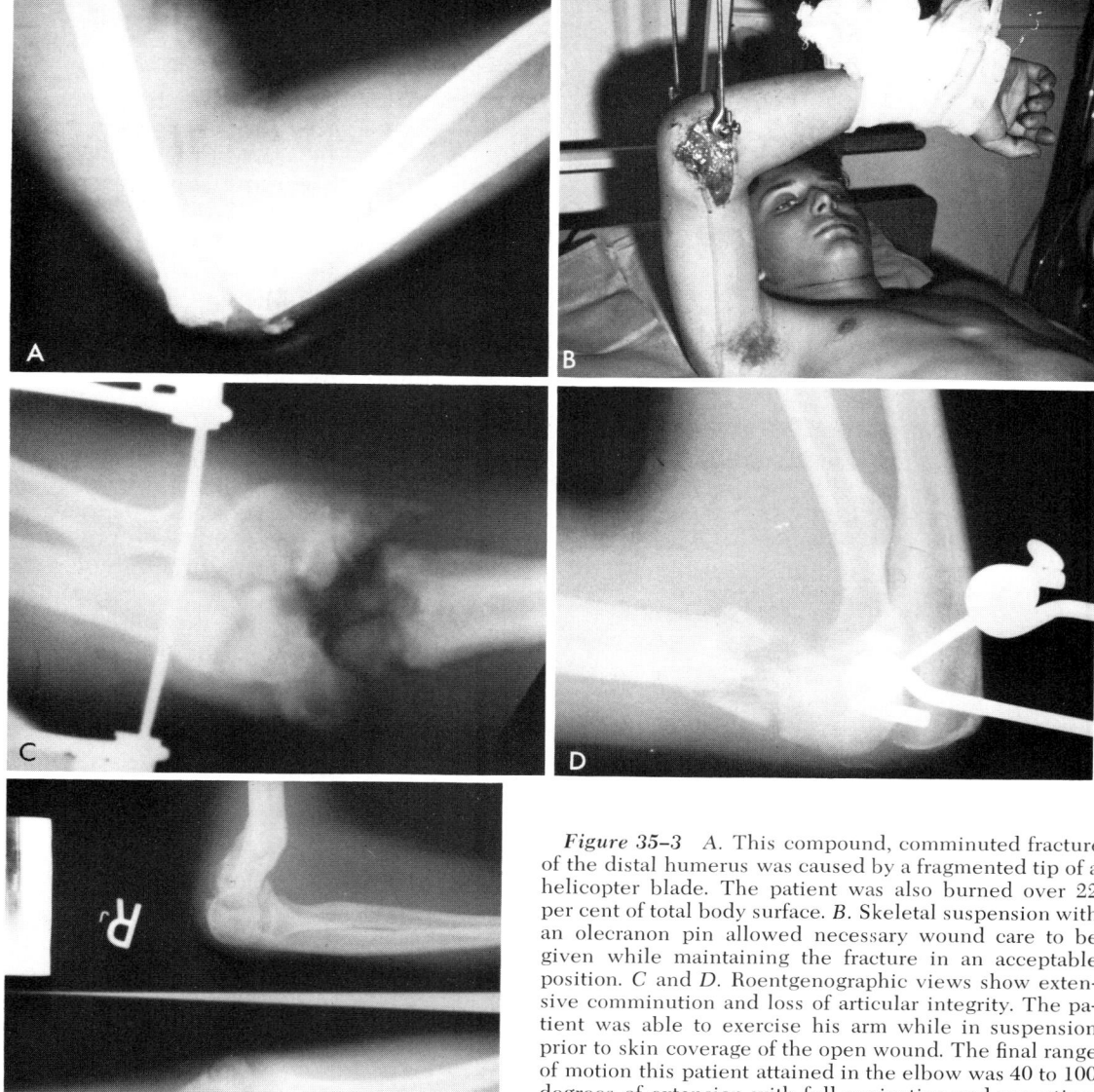

Figure 35–3 *A.* This compound, comminuted fracture of the distal humerus was caused by a fragmented tip of a helicopter blade. The patient was also burned over 22 per cent of total body surface. *B.* Skeletal suspension with an olecranon pin allowed necessary wound care to be given while maintaining the fracture in an acceptable position. *C* and *D.* Roentgenographic views show extensive comminution and loss of articular integrity. The patient was able to exercise his arm while in suspension prior to skin coverage of the open wound. The final range of motion this patient attained in the elbow was 40 to 100 degrees of extension with full supination and pronation. *E.* Roentgenographs show excellent healing despite the severe nature of this injury.

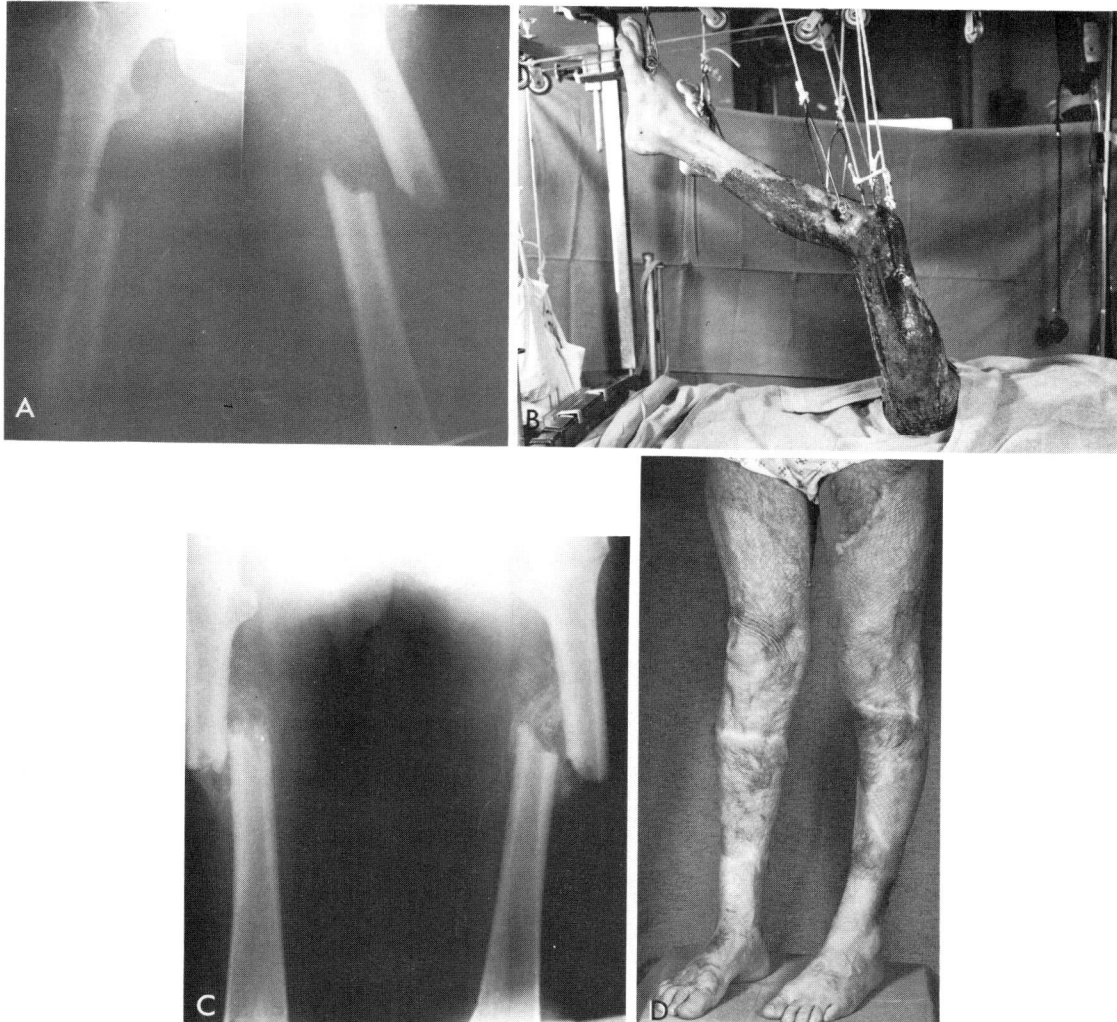

Figure 35–4   *A*. This 28-year-old man sustained burns of 50 per cent of the total body surface and these bilateral femoral fractures beneath full-thickness burns of the thighs. *B*. Skeletal pin traction provided excellent exposure of the wounds as well as maintenance of fracture position. *C*. Roentgenogram shows satisfactory position of both femoral fractures 16 weeks postinjury. There is 1 inch shortening bilaterally. *D*. The fractures healed uneventfully, and following grafting and healing of the burn wounds, the patient was fully ambulatory with excellent function of the legs.

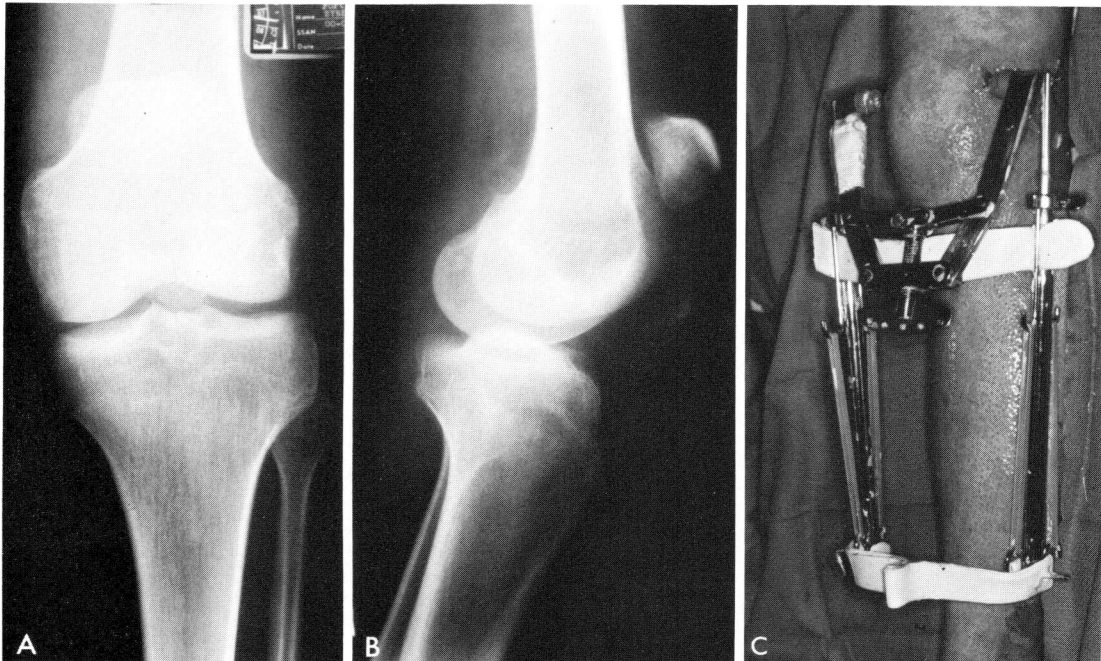

Figure 35–5 *A* and *B*. Rupture of the patellar tendon with a fracture through the distal pole of the patella occurred when this 25-year-old man leaped approximately 15 feet to escape a fire. *C*. A Kirschner wire placed through the proximal pole of the patella was fixed through a compression device to a Steinmann pin placed in the distal tibia. Although the leg was totally and circumferentially burned, optimal wound care allowed the burns to heal spontaneously. Four weeks postinjury the pins were removed and the patient was placed in a posterior splint. Healing of the tendon allowed a satisfactory range of motion of the knee with good strength and stability.

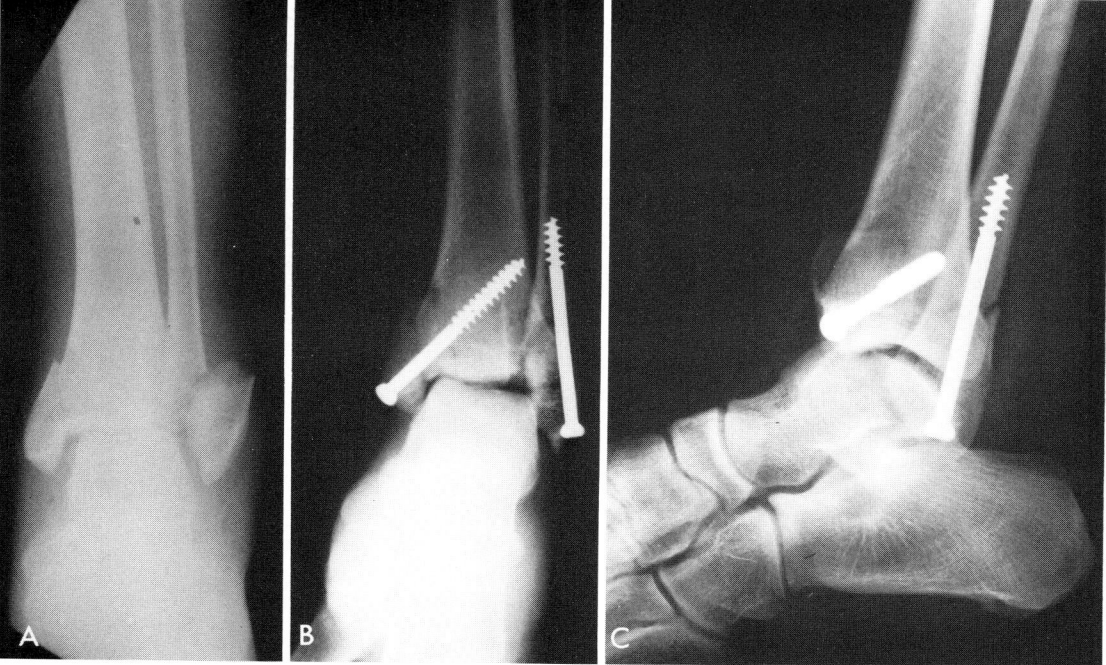

Figure 35–6 *A*. This comminuted bimalleolar fracture-dislocation of the ankle was sustained by a 26-year-old man in an airplane accident. *B* and *C*. Stabilization of the fractures with lag screws allowed adequate burn wound care to be performed.

frequent radiographic examination are necessary. The usual signs of osteomyelitis, including fever and leukocytosis, are difficult to interpret because of their prevalence in severely burned patients even without such a complication.

Amputation. Amputations may be necessitated, during the resuscitative or acute phases of burn care, by nonviability of an extremity. Associated severe compound fractures, irreparable vascular injury, extremely deep thermal injury, or electrical injuries may all lead to an early amputation. Invasive sepsis may occasionally require amputation as a lifesaving measure.

Open guillotine amputation should be performed in all cases in which surgical intervention is necessitated by sepsis. Short

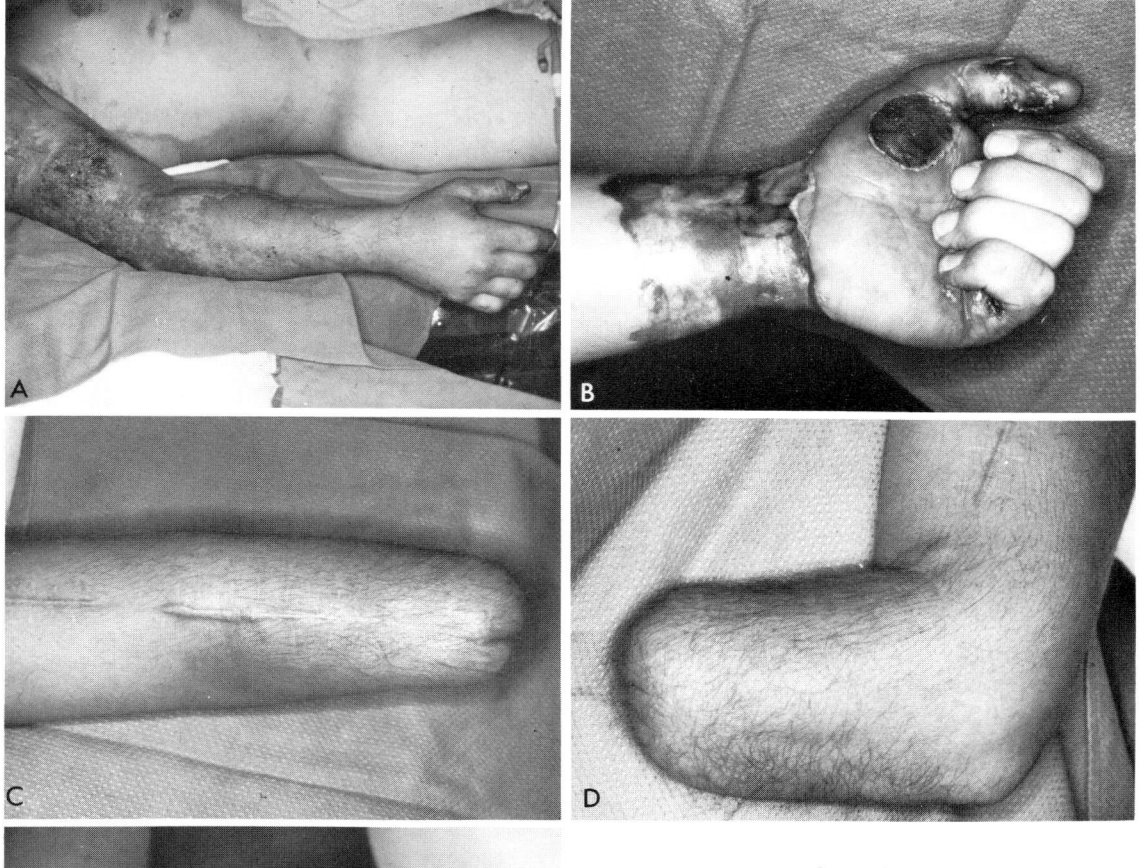

Figure 35–7 A and B. This 26-year-old man sustained a 12,500 volt electrical injury. There were severe burns over the thenar eminence and wrist and second-degree burns of the brachium. The skin on the dorsum of the hand was uninjured. Despite second-degree burns of the brachium, exploration revealed viable musculature and good vascularity. C, D, and E. Exploration revealed the distal forearm to be nonviable; a below-elbow amputation was necessary and was performed in guillotine fashion. Skin traction was not applicable because of second-degree burns of the forearm, so a subcuticular purse-string suture of 0 nylon was placed. The stump healed in "sausage" fashion, and the patient is able to use a standard below-elbow prosthesis without difficulty.

flaps should be fashioned only in the first few days postburn prior to colonization of the burn wound. If flaps are fashioned, a drain should be inserted for 24 to 48 hours and only the fascia approximated. The skin may be secondarily closed or grafted. Skin traction is generally not useful in these patients because the skin is burned. A subcutaneous suture of heavy monofilament nylon or other synthetic may be placed in a purse-string fashion in the open stump after a guillotine amputation. The suture should be pulled snugly enough that the skin will not retract proximal to the end of the stump. As healing occurs, the opening will contract, and only a small graft, if any, will be needed for closure (Fig. 35–7). Although revision is frequently performed in order to improve suitability for a prosthesis, the initial surgery should be performed as though it were the definitive procedure. Nerves should be gently placed on traction and sharply sectioned. Bone ends should be appropriately beveled, and in the leg, the fibula cut shorter than the tibia. Disarticulation rather than amputation through a bone should be performed in children in order to preserve maximum growth potential.

Acute Phase

It is during the acute phase of burn wound care, extending from the completion of the resuscitative phase through initial cutaneous autograft coverage that the orthopedist may contribute most to the care of the burned patient. Less obvious fractures or dislocations may have been missed during the initial resuscitation and be first identified only when the patient's condition has been stabilized and a more thorough examination is performed. Dislocations, if present, should be reduced under adequate analgesia or anesthesia and stabilized by splinting or skeletal traction. Succinylcholine is *not* recommended as a muscle relaxant because the burn patient is very sensitive to this agent and may develop acute and lethal hyperkalemia. Fractures should be reduced by manipulation or skeletal traction. Once the fracture is reduced, the reduction should be maintained by suspension or splinting. If the fractured extremity is not burned, standard orthope-

dic techniques may be used, but again a fiber-glass cast is preferable to plaster because of the probability that the cast will become wet during care of the burned patient.

If it is necessary to place a circumferential cast on a burned extremity, the cast should be changed frequently to allow inspection and treatment of the wound. This may be accomplished by bivalving the cast or by applying a new cast as frequently as necessary. If it is necessary to cut a window in the cast, the window should be a large one and it should be replaced at each dressing change to decrease or eliminate the possibility of window edema.

Suspension of Burned Extremities. Medical and nursing care of the circumferentially burned extremity can be quite difficult. Skeletal suspension of the burned extremity can be a valuable adjunct in the care of the burn wound, since it minimizes contracture formation by maintaining proper position of extremities and permits the burn wound to be fully exposed. Both anterior and posterior aspects of the extremity are easily accessible for application of topical antibacterial agents or grafting. Although skeletal traction pins pass through burned tissue, significant pin tract infection and osteomyelitis have been only rarely reported. Evans and co-workers have reported on the placement of several hundred pins, with only two cases of osteomyelitis.[8]

Skeletal suspension of the arm may be performed with a pin through the metacarpals or through the distal radius. If a metacarpal pin is used, it should be a .045 or .062 threaded Kirschner wire placed through the index and middle metacarpals. It should be placed approximately 1 to 2 cm proximal to the flare of the metacarpal head. A Kirschner tractor should always be used; a Steinmann bow will allow the flexible light pin to form a catenary that is likely to cut through the metacarpals. Placement of the pin must be done carefully to avoid fracturing the metacarpals, and the use of the metacarpal pin is not suggested in small children because of the difficulty in accurate placement. Suspension of the upper extremity can also be achieved by using an appropriate-sized Kirschner wire or Steinmann pin placed through the radius only, well proximal to the distal radial epiphysis to avoid impairment of growth if the epiphysis is not yet fused. Care should be taken not to spear either the radial artery or the superficial radial nerve. The pin should not transfix both radius and ulna, as this will eliminate or severely hinder radioulnar motion and may result in a permanent loss of supination or pronation of the forearm. If abduction of the arm with traction is necessary, this may be accomplished with the distal pin alone, or an olecranon pin may be used. If an ulnar pin is used, it should be a Kirschner wire of appropriate size to which a Kirschner tractor is applied, and should be placed in the olecranon well away from the joint.

Balanced skeletal suspension should always be used with any pin. Merely suspending an extremity from an overhead frame will inevitably result in complications from the pin, including osteomyelitis or the pin's cutting out through the bone and burn, or both. Local wound care, debridement, grafting, and physical therapy may all be performed with the pins in place (Figure 35–8). The pin should not be removed until one is certain that it will no longer be needed. Pin care is extremely important. No dressing should be applied to a pin site in burned skin. On each nursing shift, the pin site should be cleansed with saline, dilute peroxide, or a detergent disinfectant solution. If a topical agent is being applied to the wound, this agent will be sufficient to control bacterial growth at the pin site and no other antibiotic agent should be added. The physician should inspect the pin site frequently. Drainage from the pin site is not infrequent but should not be considered a conclusive sign of osteomyelitis. If the drainage becomes excessive or the pin loosens significantly, however, an x-ray of the pin site should be taken, and the pin should be removed if clinically significant infection is present. Another pin inserted in a more proximal site or another technique of immobilization should then be used.

Suspension without the use of skeletal pins is frequently a valuable technique in the care of burned patients. Well-padded slings or boots allow circumferential harvesting of donor sites on the legs (Fig. 35–9). This is of particular value in children. Slings may be fashioned of isoprene and lined with antibacterial-impregnated synthetic foam (Fig. 35–10). Angulation of a fracture may thus be corrected while topical chemotherapy of the burn wound is maintained.

Proper positioning of the burned patient is critical if deformities are to be avoided. As for any patient subject to contracture, the preferable position is with the knees at 0 to 10 degrees, the hips slightly abducted, and the ankles neutral. The shoulders should be abducted to 90 degrees, the elbows extended, and the wrists in neutral position or slightly dorsiflexed. The interphalangeal joints should be in full extension or 10

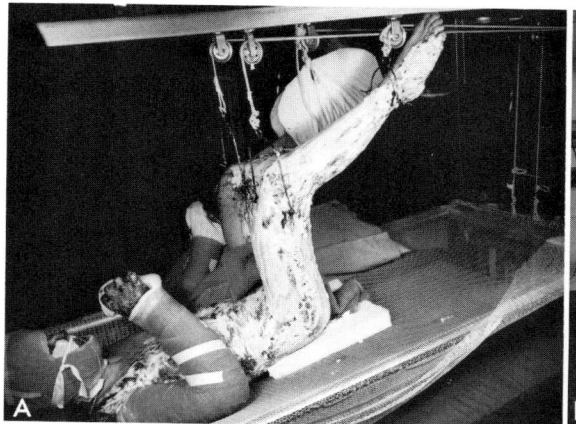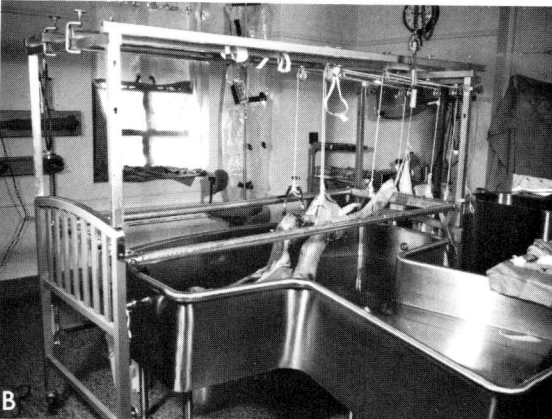

Figure 35–8 A. Suspension may be performed on a mesh bed. The open nylon mesh prevents maceration of a burned back if the patient cannot be turned frequently because of fractures. *B*. The bed frame may be placed over a Hubbard tank, the mesh can be removed, and the patient can be lowered into the tank for necessary wound care while traction and position are maintained.

degrees of flexion. The metacarpohalangeal joints should be flexed from 75 to 90 degrees in the adult or older child. In the young child, in whom it is difficult to maintain a satisfactory position in a splint, it is preferable to immobilize the hand with the wrist in neutral position and the metacarpophalangeal joints in full extension. This position is easily held on a flat hand splint, and children nearly always recover any motion lost from being splinted in this position. In all instances, the thumbs should be slightly abducted and rotated in opposition.

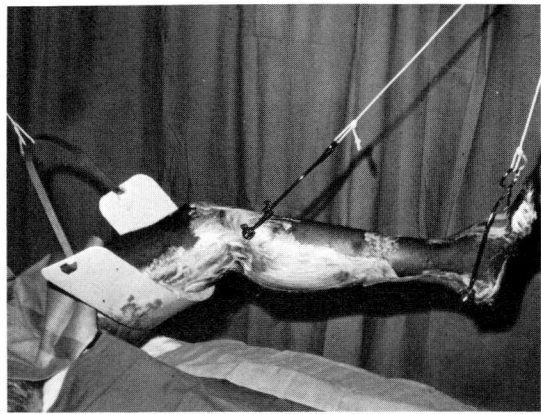

Figure 35–10   A thigh sling may be fashioned of isoprene (Orthoplast) and lined with synthetic foam (Reston). The foam may be impregnated with a topical antibacterial agent to allow correction of angulation while maintaining antibacterial therapy to the burn wound.

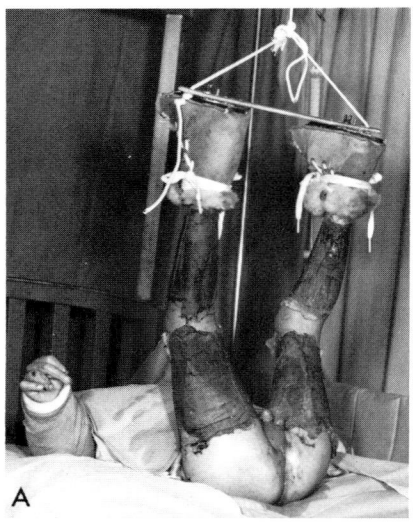

A

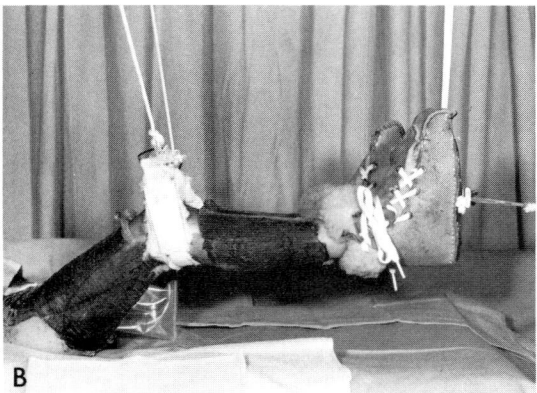

B

Figure 35–9   *A.* In a young child, well-padded boots fixed to a bar maintain full exposure of the lower limbs, thereby preventing maceration of circumferential donor sites. *B.* With the use of padded knee slings, modified split Russell traction can be utilized to allow motion of the hips and knees while maintaining exposure of the donor sites.

Internal splinting and fixation of interphalangeal and metacarpophalangeal joints with the use of smooth Kirschner wires has also been reported by Achauer and associates. They have reported prevention of deformity with good postburn function. A single or crossed .035 Kirschner wires are spun across the proximal interphalangeal joints in the first 24 hours postburn, using the smallest diameter wire sufficient to maintain the joint position. The metacarpophalangeal joint is held in position with a heavier .045 Kirschner wire at the time of grafting. All pins are removed by two weeks postgrafting.[1] Various forms of external splinting suspension devices have been devised, and many others are undergoing testing at the present time. These include banjos and hayrake-type devices for the hand and dynamic spring splinting for the ankles. Finger traction can be accomplished with small hooks cemented to fingernails with cyanoacrylate adhesive. If nails are not present, .028 or .035 Kirschner wires may be placed through the distal phalanges and used for traction (Fig. 35–11).

Active or active-assistive exercise is preferable to immobilization in most instances. During those periods in which physical therapy is not being performed, however, splinting is preferable to allowing the patient to rest a limb in a less than ideal position. In a well-staffed burn unit or

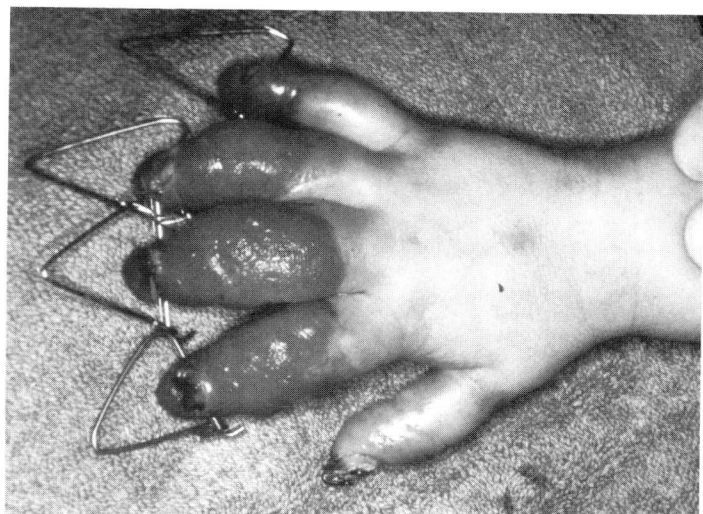

Figure 35-11 Kirschner wires inserted into the distal phalanges and bent on themselves allow traction to be applied to an infant's digits.

hospital, the occupational therapy department can make splints for the patients, and this is best done under the supervision of the orthopedist.

The most useful splinting material for the burned patient is isoprene, commonly in the form of ⅛ inch thick sheets This is easily molded after being softened with hot water and may be cut with ordinary scissors. Several basic patterns and shapes for splinting hands, elbows, and knees may be cut and then custom-molded to the individual patient. The cost is very reasonable, and splint adjustments can be made daily as indicated. In addition, the splints can be gas sterilized and remolded for use on other patients. The addition of Velcro straps to hold the splints in place makes them easy for the nursing staff to apply and remove.

Management of Exposed Bone, Joints, and Tendons. A bone either may be exposed by the initial thermal trauma destroying all overlying structures or may become exposed during the treatment of the burn by removal of overlying structures that have become necrotic and require debridement. In general, no treatment should be applied to the bone itself during the early portion of the acute phase. When exposed to air, even if beneath dressings, the superficial portion of the cortex will become desiccated and nonviable. It rarely becomes infected, however, nor does it lose its ability to act as a barrier to infection spreading deep into the marrow cavity. It is best to observe but not treat the bone and allow the surrounding burn wound to form granulation tissue. Split-thickness skin grafts may then be applied to the soft tissues surrounding the nonviable bone, and following healing of those grafts, the superficial layer of bone may be removed with an osteotome or a high-speed burr or both, going just deep enough to identify bleeding bone. At this point, the surgery should be stopped and continuous moist soaks or biological dressings kept over the bone. Granulation tissue will gradually form over the bone. Once healthy granulation tissue has covered the bone, skin grafting by standard techniques should be performed. Drilling of the cortical bone, which has been proposed in the past, is generally of little value unless intervening bridges of cortex are removed. Although multiple holes drilled through the outer table of exposed calvarium may allow sufficient formation of granulation tissue, the intervening cortex must be either resorbed or sloughed as a sequestrum; complete removal of the outer table with the high speed burr is preferable.

Subacute Phase

During this phase of recovery, orthopedic intervention continues to be important. Preservation of all possible range of motion and function must be insured during this phase of burn care or the patient will inevitably lose function permanently. It is

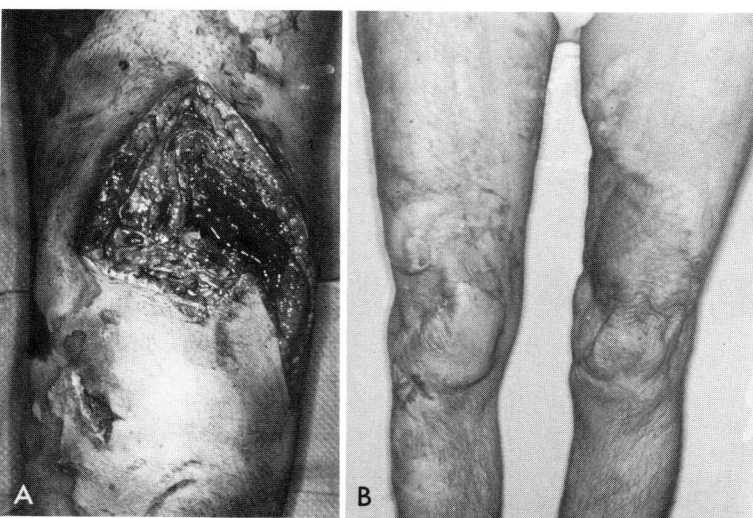

Figure 35–12 A. A 16-year-old white man sustained bilateral deep lacerations into the knees in addition to full-thickness burns. The wounds were loosely approximated and allowed to granulate and heal. Closed suction irrigation was used in the management of the open joints. *B.* Six months postinjury the patient had a full, normal range of motion in both knees and the roentgenograms were normal.

at this time that the patient may undergo repeated skin grafting procedures, and many physicians erroneously feel that all motion must be prevented in order to have a graft take. Since the only motion that must be prevented is that between the graft and its bed, a splint should not immobilize an ungrafted joint. All joints should be moved as soon as possible. In general, at 48 hours postgrafting, gentle motion may be begun under close supervision of the physician and physical therapist. Unsupervised motion cannot yet be allowed. All joints must be put through as full a range of motion as possible, preferably with active motion or, if necessary, with carefully supervised active-assisted or passive motion. A contracture allowed to develop at this point is difficult to relieve at a later date.

It is also during this phase of burn care that coverage of exposed bone and tendon is performed. Exposed bone, if previously decorticated, should by this time have developed an adequate layer of granulation tissue. If tendon is exposed but has been preserved with continuous wet dressings or biological dressings, grafting should also be undertaken at this time. If the tendon sheath is intact, it would be anticipated that motion of the tendon would be normal following grafting and healing. Generally, if the tendon is exposed and without a tendon sheath but still viable, a skin flap will be necessary for definitive closure of the wound and preservation of tendon motion.

In many patients with extensive burns, this may not be a feasible method of initial treatment; if such is the case, split-thickness skin grafting over tendons covered by granulation tissue should be done even though motion of the tendon may not be preserved.

If a joint is open because the skin and capsular structures have been destroyed, it will generally require fusion. Fusion is not inevitable, however, and if the opening into the joint is small and adequate drainage has been maintained, the wound may heal spontaneously and joint function be surprisingly well preserved (Fig. 35–12). If septic arthritis does develop in an open joint, fusion will either occur spontaneously or have to be effected surgically. It is important that such a joint be positioned so that ankylosis will occur in a functional position. A Charnley device is frequently useful in obtaining fusion, and nothing more may be necessary than placement of pins and removal of loose, necrotic articular cartilage (Fig. 35–13). Surgical closure of such joints would predispose them to the development of a septic joint or osteomyelitis and should be avoided.

Heterotopic periarticular calcification and ossification may occur during this phase.[6, 7] Calcification may increase in size as long as there is an open burn wound. In children, this extraarticular bone will often resolve completely, and in adults it may become smaller and even asymptomatic. Local signs, such as swelling and tenderness, are not reliable indicators of developing periarticular calcification, but loss of active range of motion, although frequently due to other causes, should be considered as the prime harbinger of this problem. Serum calcium, phosphorus, and alkaline phosphatase levels have not been found to be of diagnostic or prognostic usefulness in this condition. Detailed roentgenological examination including appropriate techniques to detect early soft-tissue calcification should be used as early as the problem may be clinically suspected. Xeroradiography or cardboard cassette technique may facilitate early diagnosis. Treatment of the ossification is dependent upon what functional limitation, if any, it imposes. Complete closure and primary healing of the burn wound should be effected prior to any consideration of surgical intervention for the heterotopic calcification. Unlike myositis ossificans following other injuries, this problem does not usually recur if the burn wounds are healed. If an attempt is made to remove calcification prior to complete healing of the burn wound, however, recurrence is usual. If heterotopic bone has bridged a joint, surgical removal is necessary. The most common sites for heterotopic bone formation in children are the hip and the anterior aspect of the elbow; in adults the most usual site is the posterior aspect of the elbow. Surgical excision should be complete, as the only reported recurrences have occurred when incomplete excision was performed. If neuropathy, particularly ulnar neuropathy, has developed because of entrapment, complete neurolysis should be performed at the time of operation, and anterior transposition of the ulnar nerve may be indicated. Preoperatively, the patient should be instructed in isometric exercises, and postoperatively, physical therapy should begin as soon as possible to recover any and all lost motion.

Reconstructive Phase

The reconstructive phase of burn care may extend for many years from the time of burn wound closure. It is important that the patient have a planned, logical, and consistent course of care during this period. While most of the surgery required following

complete healing of the burn wound is plastic in nature, orthopedic problems must often be considered. If contractures have been allowed to develop and are fixed, release is necessary. An initial attempt should be made to release any contracture by external splinting, and if that is unsuccessful, skeletal traction should be utilized as described by Larson and Evans and their associates, who have reported significant success in using that technique to release burn contractures in children.[8, 18] If this too is unsuccessful, surgical release should be performed. It is important that sufficient soft tissue be available for full release of a fixed contracture. If necessary, a flap should be fashioned or transferred prior to performing the release. Flap choices include pedicle, myocutaneous and free anastomosed flaps. If the joint is in an unsatisfactory functional position and adequate motion cannot be obtained by the release procedure, fusion must be performed. The position of fusion should be individualized for each patient, depending on the presence of other abnormalities or contractures. Techniques of fusion are the same as those used at any other time, and adequate soft-tissue coverage must be provided.

If amputation has been carried out during the acute phase, close cooperation between the orthopedist and the prosthetist is necessary. If a prosthesis cannot be properly fitted to the existing stump, revision will be necessary. If splinting was not adequate following amputation, flexion deformities are common, and these must be corrected by traction, splinting, or surgery as necessary. Shortening of a previously amputated bone or bones may be necessary, particularly in those instances in which the fibula has been amputated at the same or a longer length than the tibia. In the young patient, split-thickness skin graft stump coverage is adequate for prosthetic fitting; however, great care must be taken by the prosthetist to construct a very well-molded custom-fitted socket.

The patient with heterotopic bone formation may first be seen by the orthopedist at this time when he has ankylosis of the involved joints. Surgical excision is necessary and must be complete. Isometric exercises should be instituted prior to surgery so that following excision of the bone, imme-

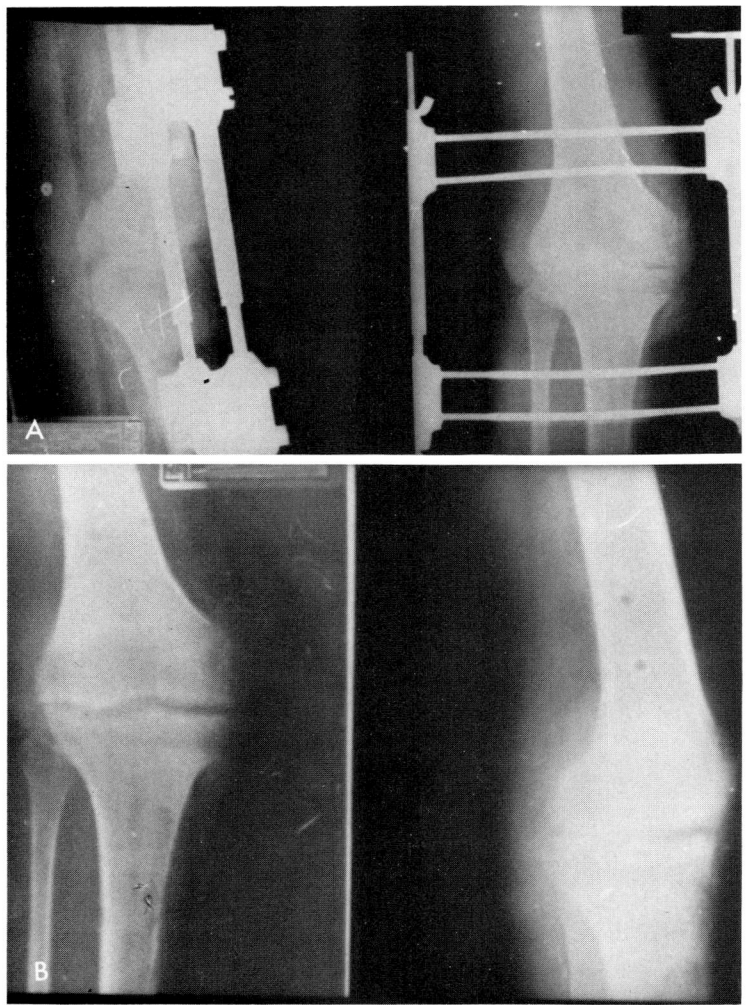

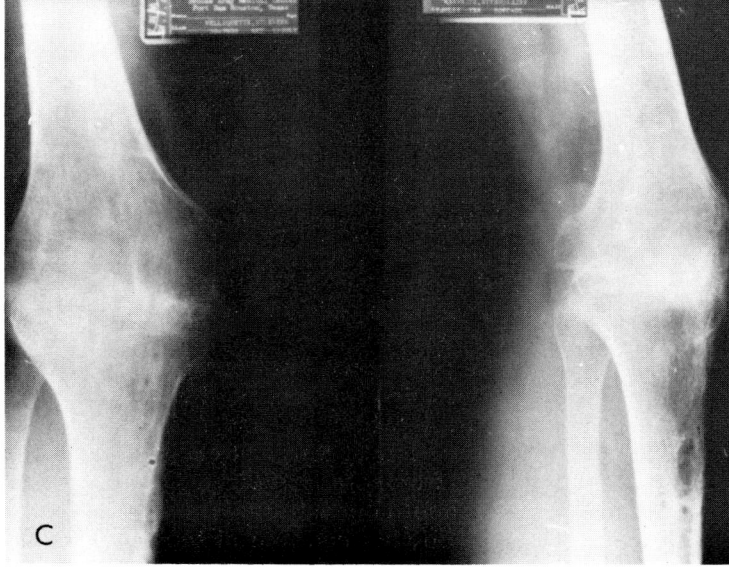

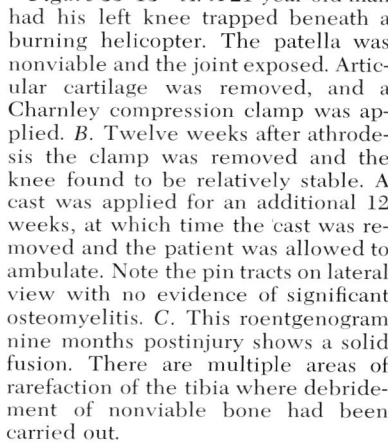

Figure 35–13 A. A 21-year-old man had his left knee trapped beneath a burning helicopter. The patella was nonviable and the joint exposed. Articular cartilage was removed, and a Charnley compression clamp was applied. *B.* Twelve weeks after athrodesis the clamp was removed and the knee found to be relatively stable. A cast was applied for an additional 12 weeks, at which time the cast was removed and the patient was allowed to ambulate. Note the pin tracts on lateral view with no evidence of significant osteomyelitis. *C.* This roentgenogram nine months postinjury shows a solid fusion. There are multiple areas of rarefaction of the tibia where debridement of nonviable bone had been carried out.

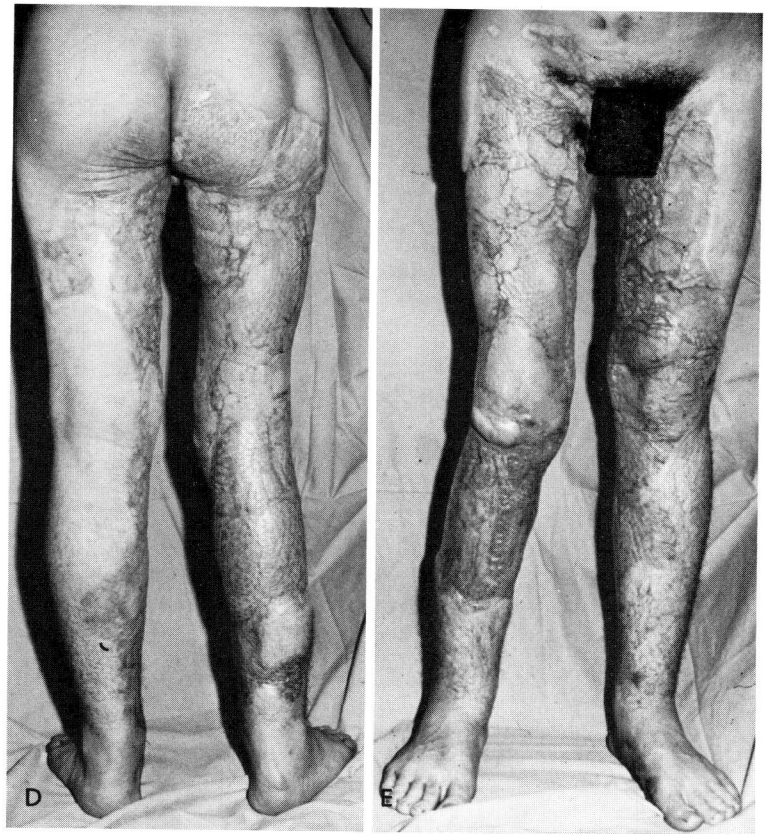

Figure 35–13 *Continued.*   *D* and *E.* The postoperative appearance of the grafted and healed legs. The patient's functional capacities are excellent.

diate and vigorous physical therapy may continue. Unlike the situation with other forms of myositis ossificans, physical therapy is not contraindicated and, in fact, is necessary to regain full range of motion.

If a tendon has been totally destroyed or ligamentous stability of a joint is lost, particularly in the hands and feet, reconstruction and stabilization of that joint must be accomplished. This is frequently difficult because overlying skin has been lost and standard procedures may not be applicable. Skin flap transfers may be necessary before tendon transfers can be considered, and in some instances even these may not be feasible. If reconstruction of an active joint is not possible, arthrodesis should be performed. Close attention must be given to the patient's overall functional capacities and long-term desires in order to select the position that is most suitable for arthrodesis in that particular patient. Boutonniere deformities of the fingers are very frequent, and Larson and co-workers have emphasized the necessity of early treatment of these deformities in burn patients.[19] If malunion of a fracture occurred during the acute phase because of wound care priorities, osteotomy may be necessary to improve alignment. In some instances, an osteotomy may serve to increase the function of a hand or foot that has been severely damaged by burn injury. Since healed burned skin does not have normal elasticity and can be damaged with very minimal pressure, great care must be taken to plan incisions so that they are long enough to allow exposure without placing undue traction on the skin edges.

Growth abnormalities following a burn may be due to direct damage of the epiphyses or due to scar contracture, and both leg length inequality and tibia vara have been reported. If an incomplete epiphyseal injury has occurred, epiphyseodesis of the entire affected epiphyses must be performed, and frequently epiphyseodesis of the opposite leg will also be necessary in order to balance growth. Although contractures initially involve only the soft tissue, once they are fixed and established in a growing child, bony abnormalities may result. Scoliosis has occurred and so has kyphosis. Soft-tissue release and suitable bracing will generally allow the bony de-

formity to be corrected by activity and further growth.

REFERENCES

1. Achauer B. M., Bartlett, R. H., Furnas, D. W., Ailyn, Z. A., and Wingerson, E.: Internal fixation in the management of the burned hand. Arch. Surg., *108*:814–820, 1974.
2. Asch, M. J., Curreri, P. W., and Pruitt, B. A., Jr.: Thermal injury involving bone: Report of 32 cases. J. Trauma, *12*:135–139, 1972.
2a. Baxter, C. R.: Fluid volume and electrolyte changes of the early post-burn period. Clin. Plastic Surg., *1*:693–703, 1974.
3. Dobbs, E. R., and Curreri, P. W.: Burns: Analysis of results of physical therapy in 681 patients. J. Trauma, *12*:242–248, 1972.
4. Dowling, J. A., Kirksey, T. D., and Moncrief, J. A.: Preservation of the burned thumb. J. Trauma, *8*:3–8, 1968.
5. Dowling, J. A., Omer, G. E., and Moncrief, J. A.: Treatment of fractures in burn patients. J. Trauma, *8*:465–474, 1968.
6. Evans, E. B., and Blumel, J.: Bone and joint changes following burns., In C. P. Artz (ed.): Research in Burns, pp. 26–52. Philadelphia, F. A. Davis Co., 1962.
7. Evans, E. B., and Smith, J. R.: Bone and joint changes following burns. A roentgenographic study—preliminary report. J. Bone Joint Surg., *41A*:785–799, 1959.
8. Evans, E. B., Larson, D. L., and Yates, S.: Preservation and restoration of joint function in patients with severe burns. J.A.M.A., *204*:843–848, 1968.
9. Fitts, W. T., Roberts, B., Grippe, W. J., Muir, M. W., and Allan, W. A.: The treatment of fractures complicated by contiguous burns: An experimental study in dogs. Surg. Gynecol. Obstet., *97*:551–564, 1953.
10. Frantz, C. H., and Delgado, S.: Limb length discrepancy after third degree burns about the foot and ankle. J. Bone Joint Surg., *48A*:443–450, 1966.
11. Grisolia, A., Forrest, W. J., and Peltier, L. F.: The treatment of fractures complicated by burns: An experimental study. J. Trauma, *3*:259–267, 1963.
12. Gronley, J. K., Yeakel, M. H., and Grant, A. E.: Rehabilitation of the burned hand. Arch. Phys. Med., *43*:508–513, 1962.
13. Jackson, D. M.: Burns into joints. Burns, *2*:90–106, 1976.
14. Koepke, G. H., and Feller, I.: Physical measures for the prevention and treatment of deformities following burns J.A.M.A., *199*:791–793, 1967.
15. Kolar, J., and Vrabec, R.: Periarticular soft tissue changes as a late consequence of burns. J. Bone Joint Surg., *41A*:103–111, 1959.
16. Kolar, J., Babicky, A., Bibr, B., and Vrabec, R.: Systemic effects of burns on bone: Mineral metabolism. Acta Chir. Plast., *13*:133–140, 1971.
17. Krizek, T. D., Flagg, S. V., Wolfort, F. G., and Jabaley, M. E.: Delayed primary excision and

skin grafting of the burned hand. Plast. Reconstr. Surg., *51*:524–529, 1973.

18. Larson, D. L., Evans, E. B., Abston, S., and Lewis, S. R.: Skeletal suspension and traction in the treatment of burns. Ann. Surg., *168*:981–985, 1968.

19. Larson, D. L., Wofford, B. H., Evans, E. B., and Lewis, S. R.: Repair of the boutonniere deformity of the burned hand. J. Trauma, *10*:481–487, 1970.

20. Marquardt, E., and Neff, G.: The angulation osteotomy of above-elbow stumps. Clin. Orthop., *104*:232–238, 1974.

21. Munster, A. M., Bruck, H. M., Johns, L. A., Von Prince, K., Kirkman, E. M., and Remig, R. L.: Heterotopic calcification following burns: A prospective study. J. Trauma, *12*:1071–1074, 1973.

22. Owens, N.: Osteoporosis following burns. Br. J. Plast. Surg., *1*:245–256, 1949.

23. Salisbury, R. E., and Palm, L.: Dynamic splinting for dorsal burns of the hand. Plast. Reconstr. Surg., *51*:226–228, 1973.

24. Salisbury, R. E., Hunt, J. L., Warden, G. D., and Pruitt, B. A., Jr.: Management of electrical burns of the upper extremity. Plast. Reconstr. Surg., *51*:648–652, 1973.

25. Schiele, H. P., Hubbard, R. B., and Bruck, H. M.: Radiographic changes in burns of the upper extremity. Radiology, *104*:13–17, 1972.

26. Tanigawa, M. C., O'Donnell, O. K., and Graham, P. L.: The burned hand: A physical therapy protocol. Phys. Ther., *54*:953–957, 1974.

27. Trapnell D. H., Jackson D: Bone and joint changes following burns. Clinical Radiology *16*:180–186, 1965.

28. Von Prince, K. M. P., Curreri, P. W., and Pruitt, B. A., Jr.: Application of fingernail hooks in splinting of burned hands. Am. J. Occup. Ther., *24*:556–559, 1970.

29. Wexler, M. R., Yeschna, R., and Newman, Z.: Early treatment of burns of the dorsum of the hand by tangential excision and skin grafting. Plast. Reconstr. Surg., *54*:268–273, 1974.

RAE R. JACOBS, M.D.

36 —————————————————————Complications of Musculoskeletal Trauma

This chapter does not purport to present a comprehensive treatment of all the possible effects of trauma and complications of fractures. An entire text could be written on each, and in fact has been written on several. Also, the details of specific diagnostic approaches and treatment regimens are omitted since these soon become out of date. For this information a continuous review of the literature is essential. A personal approach to fracture care is presented, stressing the prevention of complications and aggressive treatment once they develop. Undoubtedly much will be omitted, and some of what is said may be personal inclination. But perhaps the reader will better understand the primary role of the physician in the treatment of musculoskeletal injury: to facilitate the healing process with a minimum of added risk.

PREVENTION

Avoiding the complications of fractures is preferable by far to treating them once they have occurred. The orthopedic surgeon is the usual primary care physician for the patient with musculoskeletal injury. Therefore, he must be alert both to the multiple problems that complicate the care of the injured patient and to the complications that may result from the injuries. The orthopedist must remember that he is first a physician, second a surgeon, and only third a specialist in the musculoskeletal system. A patient entering the emergency room

1010

following an automobile accident requires a *complete* evaluation. Traffic accidents often follow a stroke or a myocardial infarction. A superficial examination that considers only evidence for a traumatic diagnosis will not suffice. The practice of "clearing" a patient on the basis of a general surgeon's evaluation may well lead to a false sense of security. Not uncommonly, intraabdominal hemorrhage due to splenic or hepatic injury is not apparent initially, particularly if the patient has not been fully resuscitated. Delayed ruptures of the spleen must be detected by the surgeon who is rendering continuing care. Although the surgeon may limit his actual practice to a small area of medicine, he must be an alert diagnostician, fully aware of those symptoms and signs that indicate further consultation. Whoever is identified as the primary physician must accept the full responsibility of a "compleat physician."

Prehospital care by properly trained emergency medical technicians is particularly important in preventing complications of musculoskeletal trauma. Certainly ventilation and circulation are the most essential functions and should be assessed and treated first. However, the spine and limbs should not be ignored. A little additional time spent determining whether there is a spinal injury may prevent lifelong confinement to a wheelchair as a result of paraplegia. Adequate splinting of the limbs helps avert further tissue trauma and possible fat embolism syndrome. Any area that appears to have a possible fracture should be splinted. Repeated manipulation in an attempt to elicit crepitus should be avoided. Gross deformities should be aligned to allow more effective splinting and to prevent neurovascular injury. Wounds should be protected with bulky dressings, applied with moderate pressure to control hemorrhage. Tourniquets are rarely, if ever, indicated. Intravenous fluid resuscitation begun in the field may help prevent the complications of hypotension. Patients with musculoskeletal injury alone should never develop shock of such a degree that it cannot be easily reversed with prompt and adequate volume replacement.

On arrival in the emergency room, a rapid initial assessment is performed with appropriate diagnostic and therapeutic measures. Later, a more complete evaluation should be made. Particularly to be condemned is the common practice of removing all the splints, so carefully applied by the emergency medical technician, in order to examine the extremities and then failing to reapply them when the patient is sent to the radiology department. Another practice to be avoided is the removal of dressings in order to evaluate wounds in the area of possible fracture. A better policy is to keep the wounds completely covered, isolating them from bacteria. Once the suspicion of an open fracture has been confirmed by the presence of a wound and a fracture in proximity to each other, the wound should be evaluated under sterile conditions with mask, gloves, and gown.

The question of whether to close a wound or to leave it open is answered by the

Of the edge of the skin
Take a piece very thin.

The tenser the fascia
The more you should slash-er.

Of muscle much more
'Til you see fresh gore,

And bundles contract
To the least impact.

Hardly any of bone
Only bits quite alone.

Sir James Learmonth
Edinburgh

completeness of the debridement rather than by an arbitrary rule.

Shotgun wounds are difficult to debride, because the areas of injury are mixed with normal-appearing tissue and surround nerves and arteries that are sufficiently viable to retain. However, fibrosis and chronic infection usually can be prevented by removal of all ischemic tissue and foreign material, followed by coverage of the wound. The use of split-thickness skin grafts, muscle pedicles, local flaps, and relaxing incisions is frequently necessary to cover exposed arteries, tendons, nerves, and cortical bone. The practice of repeated inadequate debridement using dressing changes and allowing the wound to "granulate in" all too often results in an immobile joint, contracted muscle, and unstable scars —in short, a useless extremity that frequently requires eventual amputation.

The guide to *Initial Therapy of Shock* by the Committee on Trauma of the American College of Surgeons should be prominently displayed and practiced in every emergency room (Fig. 36–1). The degree of hypovolemia can be assessed by the expected amount of blood loss based on the extent of injuries as well as by the patient's response to intravenous infusion. Very rapid infusions of crystalloid solutions should be followed by appropriate quantities of blood. Adequate volume expansion should be obtained in a matter of minutes and the infusion then decreased. The patient who presents in shock has lost a minimum of 1500 cc of blood and needs this volume replaced immediately, not slowly over a period of hours. This cannot be done without large-size needles or cannulas. One thousand cc of volume should be infused in not more than 10 minutes. A patient in profound shock needs volume replacement almost instantaneously. This frequently requires a catheter, such as a nasogastric tube, to be inserted into the vena cava through the saphenous vein. In short, hypovolemia can never be treated too rapidly. On the other hand, it is just as important to recognize when volume replacement is complete and to slow the infusion rate to maintenance levels.

Central venous pressure is the only quantitative index of the relationship of the vascular fluid volume to the capacity of the vascular space. Isotopic dilution volume

A guide to
the initial therapy of
SHOCK

Prepared by
Committee on Trauma
American College of Surgeons   April, 1976

DO

Start flow sheet and record vital signs (sample flow chart, facing page)

Use a pressure dressing on major bleeding

Maintain an adequate airway

Obtain venous sample for hematocrit, type, and crossmatch

Aid venous return and prevent air embolism during subclavian catheterization by placing patient in the Trendelenburg position

Insert large bore (15–18) central venous catheter and start infusion of electrolyte solution or plasma expander

Record CVP on flow sheet Q 30–60 minutes

Obtain arterial blood sample for pH, pO_2, and pCO_2 in all patients with severe chest trauma, respiratory distress, or profound shock

Splint fractures as soon as possible

Treat the underlying disorder resulting from the injury

Get a chest X-ray

Consider cardiac contusion with chest injury

Get an IVP with hematuria

Get a systematic history and physical examination

Obtain information regarding accident

DO NOT

Use vasopressors

Move patient until vital signs are stable

Use uncrossmatched blood

Move patient until spine has been evaluated

Fail to obtain a history of associated diseases and drugs

Forget tetanus prophylaxis

Use a tourniquet except in traumatic amputations

Blame head injury as a cause of shock

NOTE: this is one in a series of guides prepared by, and available from, the Committee on Trauma of the American College of Surgeons. Other available titles include guides to the initial management of burns, initial therapy of soft tissue wounds, the evaluation of serious head injuries, and tetanus prophylaxis. Reprints of these five titles are available, as are posters, from: *Committee on Trauma; American College of Surgeons; 55 East Erie Street; Chicago, Illinois 60611.*

Figure 36–1 A and B. These principles for the treatment of shock should be conspicuously displayed in every emergency room and practiced by all who work there. (Courtesy of The American College of Surgeons.)

FLOW SHEET

Patient name

Hospital No.

Time of injury _____ am _____ pm

History:

Month Day Year

VITAL SIGNS

Time	B/P	P	R	T	CVP

INTAKE

IV#1	IV#2	Acc. Total

OUTPUT

Urine	Acc. Total

Acc. total

_____ RN

Resident

Intern

Attdg. MD

Major Problems or Parameters

Problem #	Problem #	Problem #	Minor Problems, Notes, and Medications

Summary:

studies require comparison with arbitrary norms, which all too often are inappropriate to the status of the individual patient. Central venous pressure lines, such as those inserted through the arm or by subclavian stick, should not be used for rapid fluid infusions. In fact, the subclavian vein is frequently completely collapsed in hypovolemic patients, leading to failure of percutaneous puncture. The external jugular vein is a far more reliable route for insertion of a central venous pressure line in this case.

The matter of the appropriate fluid for initial resuscitation remains controversial. Gaisford demonstrated in monkeys that resuscitation from hemorrhagic shock with lactated Ringer's solution led to pulmonary edema but with 5 per cent albumin did not.[20] In contrast, Siegel[57] and Holcroft[31] have demonstrated precisely the opposite in baboons. The possible immunological significance of evaluating *human* albumin in subhuman primates was ignored by both. Skillman[59] evaluated concentrated salt-poor albumin and ethacrynic acid in a group of patients. He found that although a combination of both was most effective in producing diuresis and improvement in the alveolar-arterial gradient, the albumin acted chiefly to maintain plasma volume and was relatively ineffective alone. Both Walker[65] and Fulton[19] demonstrated that early post-traumatic pulmonary insufficiency responds to fluid restriction and diuresis. In contrast, the late variety is associated with sepsis and remains lethal.

Therefore, resuscitation of the patient in hemorrhagic shock must remain for the present a vigorous attempt to promote homeostasis. Central venous pressure (CVP) is maintained with crystalloid solutions which can be easily excreted when the blood is transfused. Colloid solutions should be used only when the CVP cannot be maintained or for the hypoproteinemia of sepsis.

The question of priorities in the management of the patient with multiple trauma, although essential for the prevention of complications, lies beyond the scope of this chapter. The reader is referred to Chapter 31 and to the comprehensive discussion by Border,[10] which should be read by all surgeons involved in trauma care.

Two points deserve emphasis. First, the order of *importance*, that is, establishing ventilation, replacing blood and controlling blood loss, followed by treating injuries of the extremity, does not imply a *chronological* sequence. All can frequently be accomplished simultaneously. Possible fractures should have been splinted in the field. Antibiotics and tetanus prophylaxis should be started immediately in open fractures. If a period of observation is necessary for a head injury, initial debridement of musculoskeletal injuries should be performed under local anesthesia. Avoid the temptation to accept a less than optimal result in the seriously injured patient, because the risks are usually not as high as was once assumed. For example, open reduction and internal fixation is the treatment of choice in the spastic head injury patient whose fractures cannot be controlled with traction.[24] The patient with brain damage frequently cannot adapt to the amount of shortening or limitation of motion that would be tolerable for a normal patient. Second, continued observation and repeated assessment of the patient are the responsibility of the primary care physician. Sophisticated care of the seriously ill trauma patient requires accurate and precise quantitative information. To quote Lord Kelvin:

When you can measure what you are speaking about and express it in numbers you know something about it. When you cannot express it in numbers your knowledge is of a meagre kind.

Blood pressure, temperature, heart and respiratory rates, urinary output, central venous pressure, and arterial oxygen tension should be measured frequently. Calculation of the arterial-alveolar oxygen tension ratio (normally > 0.75) will demonstrate pulmonary insufficiency. The alveolar oxygen tension is calculated from the alveolar gas equation:

$$PAO_2 = F_I O_2 \times \text{barometric pressure} - 1.25 \times PACO_2$$

In patients with multiple injuries or delayed resuscitation, who are candidates for posttraumatic pulmonary insufficiency, the central venous catheter should be replaced with a Swan-Ganz pulmonary artery catheter, inserted to monitor both pressure and mixed central venous oxygen tension.[22] An increase in pulmonary artery pressure indicates impending pulmonary insufficiency.[18] An increase in capillary wedge pressure indicates left heart failure and the need for cardiotonic drugs.

The per cent pulmonary shunt can be determined by calculating the oxygen content of the arterial and mixed venous blood from their respective oxygen tensions, pH, and hemoglobin concentration. The theoretical value for the blood equilibrating with the alveolar gas is calculated from the alveolar oxygen tension. The per cent shunt is equal to this value less the arterial content divided by the same value less

the mixed venous content: $\% \; Q = \dfrac{C_A - C_a}{C_A - C_{\bar{v}}}.$

The peripheral arteriovenous shunting of sepsis and the increased arteriovenous oxygen tension difference of shock can also be detected. Although these calculations may seem difficult, pocket programmable computers are now available to calculate them quite simply.[39] Even without sophisticated equipment, a great deal of information can be gained from the simple bedside observation described by Border: Estimate arterial hypoxia by comparing the patient's arterial blood with a second sample equilibrated with your own end-expiratory air, and approximate cardiac output by measuring the arteriovenous oxygen difference, using a tuberculin syringe system.[9]

Bedside contact with the patient is equally important. The phrase "Your patient is doing well" may be full of meaning or worthless, depending on the experience of the observer. The restlessness of hypoxia, the mental deterioration of cerebral epidural hematoma, the peripheral manifestations of sepsis, the sacral edema of slowly progressive heart failure, and the petechiae of fat embolism may be missed without astute bedside observation. The increased use of monitoring equipment to record *quantitative* data should allow better patient observation by the health care team to detect these equally important *qualitative* changes.

MANAGEMENT OF LOCAL COMPLICATIONS

PROBLEMS OF UNION

This subject has been dealt with extensively in previous chapters, but a few comments are in order. First, fractures in animals, such as those of the femur in the dog, will eventually heal with no treatment whatsoever. The normal process of fracture healing is a progressive immobilization of the fracture fragments, initially by replacement of the hematoma with fibrous tissue, followed by conversion to cartilage and eventually to bone. Not uncommonly, the result will be an angulated, shortened bone. When the trauma surgeon chooses to intervene in the process of fracture healing, he must have distinct goals in mind. If one's only goal is to obtain union, no therapy whatever is indicated because nonunion of untreated fractures is rare. On the other hand, the musculoskeletal surgeon does have the opportunity to return the limb to a more normal state with anatomical length and shape without stiffness of the distal and proximal joints, and possibly to increase the speed of "functional" union.

The major alteration in the natural healing process that the orthopedist can offer is control of the fracture fragments. This can be accomplished by either external immobilization with plaster, external skeletal fixation with pins, or internal skeletal fixation with plates or intramedullary rods. The first carries the least risk of infection, but the greatest likelihood of loss of joint motion. The second technique allows control of the fracture without covering the limb, and is specifically indicated for fractures associated with severe soft tissue injury. The last method is essential for anatomical reduction of intraarticular fractures. If properly executed it offers the opportunity for early return to full function of the injured limb. Accurate reduction, atraumatic technique, rigid fixation, and early joint motion are essential.[43]

The days of brute force in orthopedics are over. Strong force on the retractors is never indicated; it is always better to extend the incision. Self-retaining retractors must be applied lightly and released frequently to insure adequate vascularity of the soft tissues. The fracture must be anatomically reduced and fixed with absolutely rigid technique. A resultant fixation that requires the addition of external plaster immobilization has the disadvantages of both open and closed treatment, that is, possible infection plus joint stiffness. Supplemental plaster fixation following an open reduction is an indication of failure of the open reduction. This is not to say that full weight bearing would be allowed immediately following open reduction and internal fixation. On the contrary, progressively increasing weight bearing in an intelligent, cooperative patient is the ideal.

Cast brace treatment frequently achieves the goal of joint motion without the risks of internal fixation. It is also a more appropriate supplement for the comminuted shaft fracture which may not be adequately treated by internal fixation. Although not everyone may agree with the specific indications for internal fixation, once the decision has been made, it is imperative to obtain the most rigid fixation possible in order to avoid the complications of external plaster immobilization. The reader is encouraged to learn the principles of fracture management of the Association for the Study of Internal Fixation. If we exercise the same degree of care, precision, and sterility in the treatment of fractures as we insist on for total joint replacement, the infection rate should be comparably low.

The timing of operative treatment of fractures is particularly important to avoid complications. If surgical treatment is carried out within the first 24 to 48 hours following injury, infection is much less likely. After this time, bacteremia due to bladder catheterization, atelectasis with

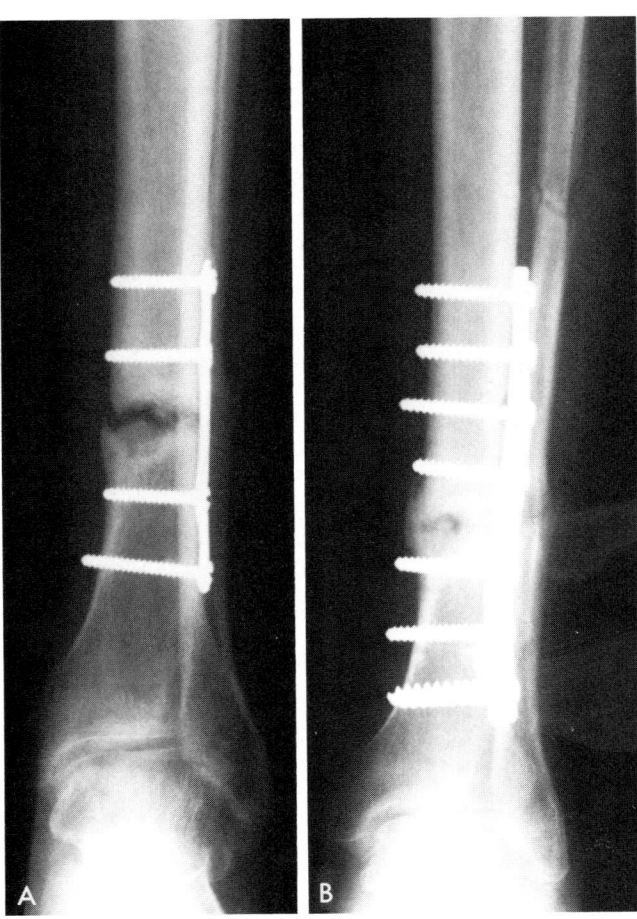

Figure 36–2 Inadequate internal splintage with this implant resulted in non-union of this distal tibia fracture. Replacement with adequate internal fixation by a dynamic compression plate resulted in prompt union.

pneumonia, and fecal contamination of the skin are more common. In addition, wound edema in the area of the injury increases.

If closed treatment is selected the fracture should be reevaluated at about four to six weeks to determine whether treatment is progressing satisfactorily. Eventual malunion, delayed union, and nonunion are often apparent at this time from the amount of angulation or shortening or the lack of ossification in the fracture callus. Gross motion at six to eight weeks should arouse suspicion of delayed union. The adequacy of reduction of intraarticular fractures is reevaluated at one week; open treatment by internal fixation or bone grafting should be considered at that time. At the completion of closed fracture treatment in four to six months, a malunion, delayed union, or nonunion necessitates open treatment. If initial management with plaster immobilization led to one of these complications, it is unreasonable to assume that repeating or continuing that treatment is likely to resolve the problem.

Malunions require osteotomy and correction of the deformity and use of more rigid fixation to prevent a second malunion. A delay in union generally requires more rigid fixation (Fig. 36–2). This usually indicates internal fixation, but in a case such as a fracture of the tibia and fibula a "physiological plating" can be obtained by performing a posterolateral bone graft (Fig. 36–3).[30] In cases of nonunion that are "hypertrophic" more rigid fixation is required, and internal fixation is usually indicated. Delayed union and nonunion may also be caused by devascularization of the fracture, resulting in a more atrophic appearance. These fractures require stimulation of osteogenesis by bone grafting.

An investigation of dynamic bone scanning to detect impending union problems is currently in progress. The net increase in isotope at the fracture site corrected for the normal portion of the bone, from 7.5 to 15 minutes after injection, is measured and plotted against time postfracture. In normally healing fractures treated with plaster immobilization, the uptake is 3 per cent per month; in delayed union 1.5 per cent per month; and in cases requiring operative intervention, grafting, or internal fixation, 0 to 1 per cent per month. The usual two-hour

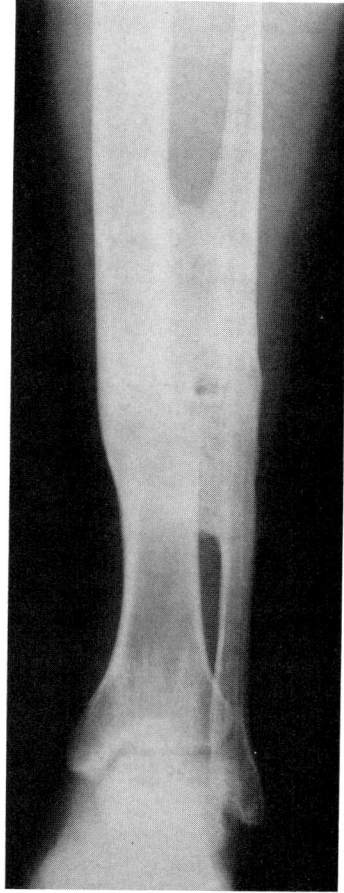

Figure 36–3 "Physiological plating" of a tibial nonunion by posterolateral grafting of the tibia to the fibula at a distance from the nonunion site where there is less motion progressively immobilized the fracture, resulting in complete union.

bone scan image interpretation correlates with clinical outcome in only 10 per cent of the studies. Only the rate of uptake of isotope after the rapid vascular phase correlates with "fracture healing." The two-hour image is the sum of these two phases, and therefore may be misleading in a case of adequate vascularity without active bone formation.[32]

INFECTION

The definition of infection varies greatly in different reports. To some, only persistent osteomyelitis is considered infection, and acute soft tissue infections that resolve with conservative treatment are ignored. At the other extreme, some report positive cultures of serous drainage without abscess formation or cellulitis.

Basically there are two types of infections: those that are acute, but resolve with local treatment and antibiotics in a few days or weeks, and those that do not resolve with this treatment, but become chronic and require more aggressive therapy. The former are chiefly soft tissue problems, whereas the latter develop established bone infection. The acute infection rate in an orthopedic facility should be less than 1 per cent in elective procedures. For operatively treated closed fractures the rate has been less than 2 per cent, and for open fractures about 10 per cent.[11]

In a recent prospective series of 352 open fractures the infection rate was 2.5 per cent in the 81 per cent of fractures treated by debridement and primary closure. In the remaining 19 per cent (segmental fractures, extensive soft tissue damage, and traumatic amputations), closure was delayed and the infection rate was 9 per cent. All cases received prophylactic treatment with antibiotics effective against penicillin-resistant organisms. No cases had primary internal fixation, but external skeletal fixation was frequently indicated.[27] The degree of tissue injury contributes to the variation in the infection rate in these groups. In addition, elective procedures frequently allow better patient preparation, both local and systemic, as well as a smoother operative procedure. Obviously, open injuries allow the entrance of bacteria.

The surgeon's goal is to convert an open, contaminated, ischemic injury to as sterile and vital a wound as possible. This requires both liberal debridement of all ischemic tissue and irrigation. The use of antibiotic irrigating solutions has been demonstrated to reduce wound infection. The fixation attained should be as rigid as possible, because the persistence of motion at the fracture site produces a void in which tissue fluid turnover and cellular invasion are minimal, allowing bacterial colonization. Any remaining dead space should be eliminated by suction catheters to close the soft tissues and prevent hematoma formation. Muscle pedicle transfers will allow covering of vital structures, such as bone, nerve,

and artery. The skin should be closed primarily, but only if this can be done with no tension whatever and if the surgeon is confident that the remaining tissues are viable and bacterial contamination minimal.

Frequently, primary closure can be obtained without tension by using relaxing incisions or local flaps, and covering the resultant defects with a split-thickness skin graft. In addition, a split-thickness skin graft frequently can be used to close the primary wound if there is a bed of muscle. The application of split-thickness skin to tendon and bone is not advised, as this usually results in high shear stress and resultant breakdown, although the initial graft may appear to be successful. When one is not confident of the success of the debridement, homograft can be valuable. This technique allows coverage of the wound and prevention of bacterial invasion, but also allows escape of possible infection under the homograft without loss of the patient's valuable skin. At two to four days following homografting the wound is reinspected. If the homograft appears to be taking, it is replaced with split-thickness skin; otherwise, the homograft is repeated.

Similarly, if after debridement internal fixation does not seem advisable owing to the extent of the open wound or the degree of contamination, the advantages of both closed and open treatment can often be obtained by use of external skeletal fixation. Figure 36–4 illustrates an open unstable distal tibia fracture in which the wound was debrided, the bone covered with a muscle pedicle transfer, the skin closed with a 1:1.5 meshed split-thickness graft, and the fracture immobilized with external skeletal fixation. Rigid internal fixation of the fracture fragments was achieved without placing large metallic implants within the wound.[33]

Environmental factors are also important in wound infection. Charnley has demonstrated that the infection rate will decrease as the bacterial flora in the operating room is reduced. The surgeon's scrub technique, gowning, and hair covering are also significant factors. The value of "prophylactic systemic antibiotics" remains controversial. Perhaps a better term is "preventive antibiotics." If bacteria enter the patient's inter-

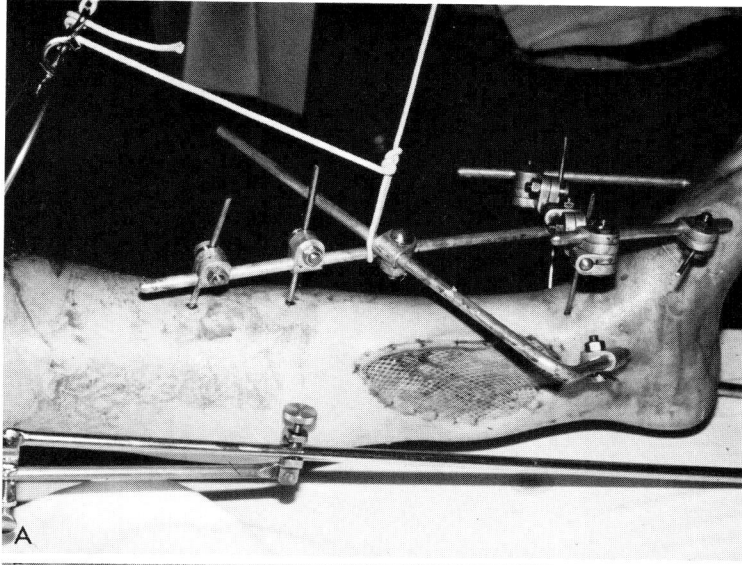

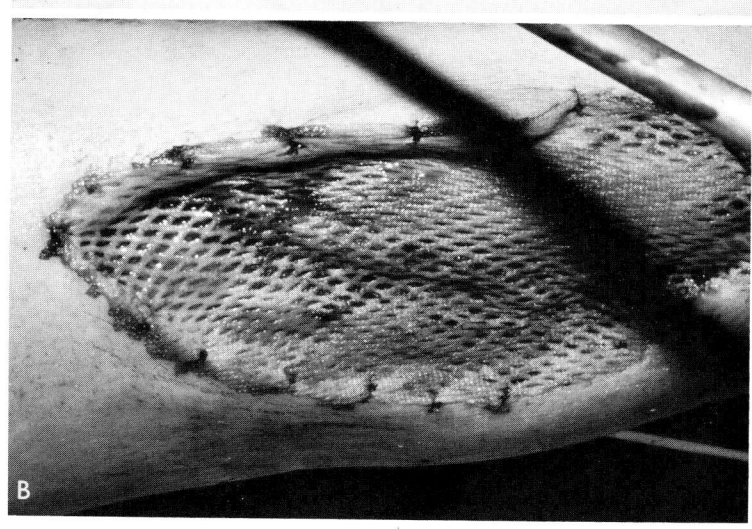

Figure 36–4 External skeletal fixation, complete debridement, and primary closure with skin graft gave an excellent result in this case of a severe, contaminated, comminuted, unstable open tibia fracture. The temptation to leave the wound open and allow it to granulate is often an excuse for inadequate debridement and failure to stabilize the fracture. The result all too often is a barely usable extremity, even if union without osteomyelitis is achieved.

nal environment through an open wound, it is rational to attempt to prevent colonization by administration of systemic antibiotics.

Proper antibiotic selection requires a study of the hospital's bacterial culture and antibiotic sensitivity spectrum. Adequate pharmacological doses must be administered as soon as possible after recognition of an open wound. They should be continued until such time as debridement is complete, vascularity has returned, and the wound is closed, allowing the initial phase of wound healing to be completed. Burke has demonstrated that three to four days is the maximum time during which these antibiotics can be expected to be effective.[2] If treat-

ment has been aggressive and debridement adequate, the wound should be closed by this time and organisms will not be able to colonize it. An attempt to prevent infection by use of antibiotics without adequate debridement inevitably leads to colonization by resistant organisms.

Acute infection may develop in spite of all efforts to prevent it. Alertness and diligence to the signs of infection are important for its early recognition. Any tachycardia, fever, or wound pain demands inspection of the area of injury. If local signs of infection are present, the wound should be opened immediately and the pus evacuated. Specimens of tissue should be obtained not only

A guide to
prophylaxis against Tetanus in wound management
<u>1972 Revision</u>

General principles

I. The attending physician must determine for each patient with a wound, individually, what is required for adequate prophylaxis against tetanus.

II. Regardless of the active immunization status of the patient, meticulous surgical care, including removal of all devitalized tissue and foreign bodies, should be provided immediately for all wounds. Such care is essential as part of the prophylaxis against tetanus.

III. Each patient with a wound should receive adsorbed tetanus toxoid[1] intramuscularly at the time of injury, either as an initial immunizing dose, or as a booster for previous immunization, unless he has received a booster or has completed his initial immunization series within the past five (5) years. As the antigen concentration varies in different products, specific information on the volume of a single dose is provided on the label of the package.

IV. Whether or not to provide passive immunization with tetanus immune globulin (human) must be decided individually for each patient. The characteristics of the wound, conditions under which it was incurred, its treatment, its age, and the previous active immunization status of the patient must be considered.

V. To every wounded patient, give a written record of the immunization provided, instructing him to carry the record at all times, and, if indicated, to complete active immunization. For precise tetanus prophylaxis, an accurate and immediately available history regarding previous active immunization against tetanus is required.

VI. Basic immunization with adsorbed tetanus toxoid requires three injections. A booster of adsorbed tetanus toxoid is indicated ten[2] years after the third injection or ten[2] years after an *intervening* wound booster. All individuals, including pregnant women, should have basic immunization and indicated booster injections.

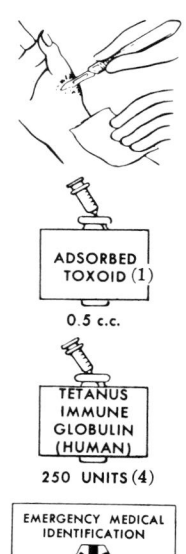

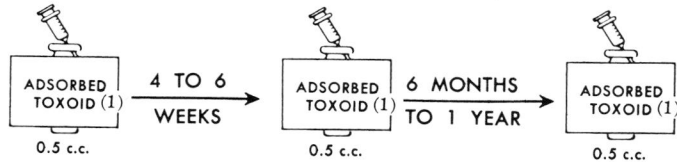

This guide from the Committee on Trauma of the American College of Surgeons is the work of the ad hoc subcommittee on prophylaxis against tetanus: Roger T. Sherman, MD, FACS, Tampa, Florida, Chairman; Wesley Furste, MD, FACS, Columbus, Ohio; Paul A. Skudder, MD, FACS, New York; and Oscar P. Hampton, Jr., MD, FACS, St. Louis.

Posters and reprints may be obtained from the Committee on Trauma, American College of Surgeons, 55 East Erie Street, Chicago, Illinois 60611.

Figure 36–5 Active tetanus prophylaxis must be maintained and passive immunization considered in tetanus-prone wounds and when the history of prior active immunization is questionable. (Courtesy of The American College of Surgeons.)

from the Committee on Trauma of the American College of Surgeons

Specific measures for patients with wounds

I. Previously immunized individuals

A. When the patient has been actively immunized within the past ten[2] years:
   1. To the great majority, give 0.5 cc of adsorbed tetanus toxoid[1] as a booster unless it is certain that the patient has received a booster within the previous five years.
   2. To those with severe, neglected, or old (more than 24 hours) tetanus-prone wounds, give 0.5 cc of adsorbed tetanus toxoid[1] unless it is certain that the patient has received a booster within the previous year.

B. When the patient has been actively immunized more than ten[2] years previously:
   1. To the great majority, give 0.5 cc of adsorbed tetanus toxoid[1].
   2. To those with severe, neglected, or old (more than 24 hours) tetanus-prone wounds:
      a) Give 0.5 cc of adsorbed tetanus toxoid[1] [3],
      b) Give 250 units[4] of tetanus immune globulin (human)[3],
      c) Consider providing oxytetracycline or penicillin.

II. Individuals NOT previously immunized

A. With clean minor wounds in which tetanus is most unlikely, give 0.5 cc of adsorbed tetanus toxoid[1] (initial immunizing dose).

B. With all other wounds:
   1. Give 0.5 cc of adsorbed tetanus toxoid[1] (initial immunizing dose)[3],
   2. Give 250 units[4] of tetanus immune globulin (human)[3],
   3. Consider providing oxytetracycline or penicillin.

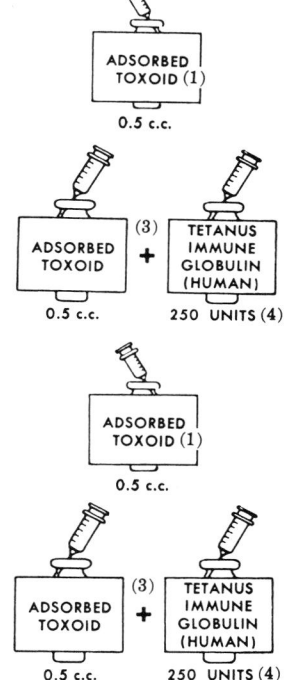

NOTE: With different preparations of toxoid, the volume of a single booster dose should be modified as stated on the package label.

(1) The Public Health Service Advisory Committee on Immunization Practices in 1972 recommended DTP (diphtheria and tetanus toxoids combined with pertussis vaccine) for basic immunization in infants and children from two months through the sixth year of age, and Td (combined tetanus and diphtheria toxoids: adult type) for basic immunization of those over six years of age. For the latter group, Td toxoid was recommended for routine or wound boosters; but, if there is any reason to suspect hypersensitivity to the diphtheria component, tetanus toxoid (T) should be substituted for Td.
(*Morbidity and Mortality Weekly Report, Vol. 21, No. 25, National Communicable Disease Center*)

(2) Some authorities advise six rather than 10 years, particularly for patients with severe, neglected, or old (more than 24 hours) tetanus-prone wounds.

(3) Use different syringes, needles, and sites of injection.

(4) In severe, neglected, or old (more than 24 hours) tetanus-prone wounds, 500 units of tetanus immune globulin (human) are advisable.

PRECAUTIONS regarding passive immunization with tetanus antitoxin (equine):

If the patient is not sensitive to tetanus antitoxin (equine), and if the decision is made to administer it for passive immunization, give at least 3000 units.

Do not administer tetanus antitoxin (equine) except when tetanus immune globulin (human) is not available within 24 hours, and only if the possibility of tetanus outweighs the danger of reaction to heterologous tetanus antitoxin.

Before using tetanus antitoxin (equine), question the patient for a history of allergy and test for sensitivity. If the patient is sensitive to tetanus antitoxin (equine), do not use it, as the danger of anaphylaxis probably outweighs the danger of tetanus; rely on penicillin or oxytetracycline. Do not attempt desensitization, as it is not worthwhile.

for culture and sensitivity testing, but also for inspection for bacteria. To delay the recognition and treatment of an acute infection invites development of the far more difficult problem of a chronic infection.

Occasionally one is faced with the dilemma of a wound hematoma versus an infection. The problem frequently presents as serous wound drainage with a positive culture. In the operating room, under sterile conditions and adequate anesthesia, the wound is opened and its contents evacuated. This is followed by closure over irrigation catheters and the usual laboratory procedures to determine if infection is present. Allowing a wound hematoma to spontaneously open and drain is to invite retrograde infection. In early infection of a hematoma, evacuation and administration of local antibiotics through a suction irrigation system and systemically usually resolves the problem promptly. The tube system requires meticulous care and early removal to prevent retrograde infection.

In addition, at the time of treatment of an acute infection the stability of the bone fragments should be reevaluated and improved if necessary. Under no circumstances should the stability of the fracture fragments be decreased by removing the internal fixation equipment. However, if the internal fixation is loose, it should be removed and stabilization obtained with external skeletal fixation. This allows treatment of the wound itself, and achieves stability by immobilizing the bone at a distance from the area of injury.

The treatment of chronic osteomyelitis is similar. The principles are the same and easily stated, but success is difficult to obtain. Debridement of all poorly vascularized tissue is primary. This may include bone and tendon as well as fibrotic scar tissue. Stabilization of the fracture fragments is essential and may be achieved by either internal or external fixation. Plaster rarely provides adequate stabilization. Control of infection usually requires systemic antibiotics based on current cultures and sensitivities.

These problems usually present as one of three types. The first is that of a healed fracture with infection manifest by recurrent and chronic drainage. Treatment consists of current cultures and appropriate antibiotic administration, debridement of all nonviable tissue, and drainage of the infection.

The second type has the same signs in addition to a pseudarthrosis. For a more complete discussion of this problem, the reader is referred to the text by B. G. Weber.[67] The essential principle is that with infection stability must be obtained first, which leads to union of the fracture; the infection will then resolve with removal of the metal. If internal fixation is removed and no stabilization is provided, the result will be a persistent infected nonunion, because infection cannot be eliminated with mobile fracture fragments.

The third type is chronic osteomyelitis in the presence of a bone defect, usually the result of sequestrectomy. This first requires treatment of the infection by debridement and then bone grafting. Acute infection is better treated with an early course of antibiotics and drainage, possibly with closure over irrigation catheters and a delayed bone graft. If the bone defect is large, cortical, and cancellous, bone grafting is required. If only a portion of the cortex is missing, a cancellous bone graft will usually suffice.

In summary, the treatment of osteomyelitis involves (1) debridement of all abnormal tissues; (2) stabilization of the bone fragments, primarily with either short plates or external skeletal fixation (usually the latter); and (3) improvement of bone strength, by grafting either in the area of deficiency or at a distance, such as the posterolateral bone graft technique used for tibial fractures.

The specific infections deserve special mention. Tetanus is an inexcusable disease.[16] Immunization levels must be maintained (Fig. 36–5). Even in minor wounds, active immunization is indicated. Gas gangrene also is a consequence of inadequate local treatment of the wound, but there is no active immunization. Gas gangrene almost always results from an open fracture that was inadequately debrided and usually closed. To resolve this problem, the emergency room physician must be better trained to consider all fractures with wounds in the same limb segment as open fractures, requiring surgical exploration and debridement.

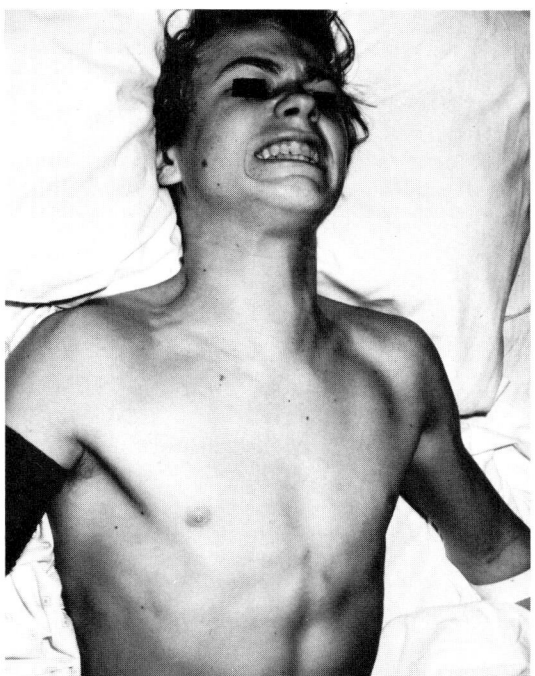

Figure 36–6   Patient with tetanus in opisthotonus.

Diagnosis of both tetanus and gas gangrene depends on familiarity with the clinical picture and not on identification of bacteria on smear or culture. The patient with tetanus typically presents with a history of a minor subcutaneous wound, such as a splinter or a laceration incurred outdoors, which has not been treated. The patient complains of trismus, difficulty in swallowing, or opisthotonus (Fig. 36–6). In contrast, gas gangrene usually results from a deep injury involving muscle and is characterized by pain in the area of injury with distention and crepitus. Systemically, the patient appears quite septic. On exploration of the wound, the amount of gas found is quite small, but the degree of muscle necrosis is extensive.

Treatment of both conditions involves debridement and appropriate antibiotic therapy, specifically with penicillin.[14, 23] Antitoxin appears to be of no value for gas gangrene, but active immunization for tetanus is highly effective in patients with previous immunization. In those without it, passive immunization with human antitetanus globulin is indicated. In addition,

tetanus patients require sedation and muscle relaxants to prevent muscle spasms. With gas gangrene, treatment with hyperbaric oxygenation appears to reduce the degree of debridement required.[48] Evidently, hyperbaric oxygenation also has the specific effect of neutralizing the toxin.

NEUROVASCULAR COMPLICATIONS

Direct injury of arteries and nerves should be detected in the emergency room by an adequate physical examination. A detailed knowledge of the motor and sensory distribution of the various peripheral nerves, including the brachial plexus, is necessary. Knowledge of the vascular anatomy is also required. The autonomous radial sensory distribution is to the dorsum of the hand between the thumb and index finger. The corresponding area for the median nerve is the palmar surface of the index finger, and for the ulnar nerve the palmar surface of the little finger. The radial nerve supplies the wrist extensors; the median supplies the flexors of the digits of the radial side of the hand; and the ulnar supplies the flexors of the digits of the ulnar side of the hand. There is frequently a crossover between the motor distribution of the median and ulnar nerves, including the innervation of the interosseous muscles. The level of injury can usually be detected by the location of the wound and the distribution of the deficit.

Common peripheral nerve injuries include the following: (1) brachial plexus stretch with motorcycle injuries involving landing on the shoulder; (2) injury to the radial nerve with fractures of the humerus; (3) injuries of all three nerves of the upper extremity with elbow injuries or gunshot wounds; (4) injury of the sciatic nerve, particularly its peroneal branch, associated with posterior dislocation of the hip; and (5) injuries of the peroneal nerve associated with injuries about the knee, particularly the head of the fibula. Common associated vascular injuries are involvement of the brachial artery with supracondylar humeral fractures, the superficial femoral artery with femoral shaft fractures, and the popliteal artery with knee dislocations. Diagnosis of these injuries requires diligence during the physical examination in eliciting all appropriate pulses as well as in making a general evaluation of the vascularity of the limbs.

Two more obscure vascular and neurologic problems of the extremities deserve special attention. The first is the compartment syndromes. These syndromes can appear in any closed space containing muscle. They typically occur in the anterior compartment of the leg, but may involve any or all of the four compartments of the leg. Frequently, the deep posterior compartment syndrome is missed and presents late with clawing of the toes. In the upper extremity, the flexor compartment of the forearm is typically involved.

The development of this syndrome requires a transitory period of relative ischemia followed by cellular swelling and progressive impairment of the circulation due to the closed space. Permanent total arterial occlusion does not result in the compartment syndrome. Also venous occlusion results in generalized enlargement of the entire extremity distal to the occlusion. Thus the unique characteristic of the syndrome is a period of muscle ischemia followed by swelling of the muscle within a closed compartment.

The classic four "P's" of Volkmann's contracture—pain, pallor, paralysis, and pulselessness—can be misleading. In the upper extremity, pulselessness is usually sought in the radial artery. This artery does *not* traverse the compartment involved, and therefore a pulse may be present. On the other hand, the radial pulse is frequently absent because the brachial artery injury precedes the development of the compartment syndrome. Similarly, the pallor in the hand is also due to the radial artery involvement which precedes the development of the syndrome. The anterior interosseous artery, which *is* occluded with the syndrome, comes off the *ulnar* recurrent. Thus the presence of a radial pulse is *not* relevant to the diagnosis of a possible flexor compartment syndrome. In fact, the presence of a good radial pulse after a period of ischemia, such as occurs prior to reduction of a supracondylar humeral fracture, should arouse one's suspicion of a developing compartment syndrome.

Inordinate pain in the area of the compartment—particularly pain produced by stretching the involved muscles, such as extending the fingers—and paralysis of these muscles are much more reliable signs of the syndrome. A clear-cut case of a compartment syndrome may be missed because of the apparent normal vascularity of the hand or foot distal to the compartment and the presence of a distal pulse in an artery that actually bypasses the compartment. Again, the best treatment is prevention. Thus in any injury involving the femoral or brachial artery a release of the distal compartment should be performed at the completion of the procedure. This is particularly important when revascularization has been delayed.

Cases of compartment syndrome should never result from the use of casts, because all acute injuries are more appropriately treated with elevation of the part and either splints or a bivalved cast to prevent this problem. Treatment of compartment syndromes obviously includes release of the compartment itself by dividing the fascia and frequently the skin in addition to repair of the arterial lesion. Any muscle that is necrotic should be removed. Any peripheral nerves traversing the compartment should be released, and if partially ischemic muscle remains which can be expected to fibrose, the nerve should be transferred subcutaneously.[1] An unusual variant of this syndrome is seen in the drug abusers, apparently owing to long periods of pressure on muscle while sleeping off an overdose.

Another condition of somewhat obscure etiology has been variously named Sudeck's osteodystrophy, reflex sympathetic dystrophy, and causalgia. Many authors take great pains to distinguish between these syndromes, but for no apparent significant reason. The diagnosis is based on the clinical findings of pain, hypersensitivity, swelling, coldness, increased sweating, and later joint stiffness. The original injury frequently includes a large component of tissue crushing and associated partial ischemia. Also, there is commonly a prolonged period of immobilization. Roentgenograms demonstrate marked osteopenia, typically spotty in appearance (Fig. 36–7). Early return of the injured part to normal function by elevation to prevent edema and active motion of the extremity is primary in the prevention of this syndrome. When it

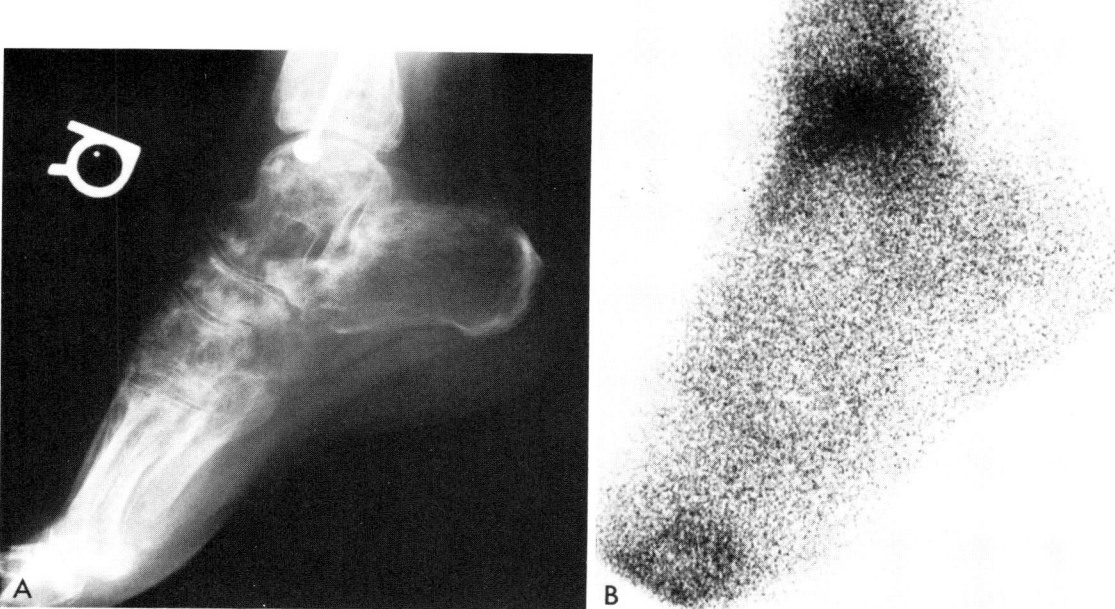

Figure 36–7   The typical appearance of Sudeck's osteodystrophy in an ankle fracture. Note the concentration of 99-MTC pyrophosphatate at the ankle joint, suggesting articular damage.

appears the syndrome is developing in the first four to six weeks following trauma, an aggressive active physical therapy program is important. Sympathetic blockade also seems to be of value. The program includes slowly progressive active motion and physical contact with the skin to overcome the abnormal sensations and to avoid increasing the symptoms.[45]

MANAGEMENT OF SYSTEMIC COMPLICATIONS

EXPERIMENTAL INVESTIGATION OF THE EFFECTS OF INJURY

To understand the possible complications of musculoskeletal trauma we must first investigate its systemic effects. Some degree of pulmonary insufficiency is a nearly constant effect of musculoskeletal injury. Musculoskeletal trauma in dogs has been demonstrated to produce intravascular fibrin deposition, alveolar membrane thickening, septal invasion by inflammatory

cells, and frequent intravascular fat emboli.[34] Ultrastructural studies of the lung of the traumatized dogs are very revealing. The type II pneumocytes showed an increase in activity to the point of exhaustion. Within 24 hours postinjury their lamellar bodies had emptied themselves into the alveolar spaces (Fig. 36–8). These structures are responsible for surfactant production. Even the lattice structure of surfactant was identified in the alveolar space (Fig. 36–9). This represents the lungs' attempt to prevent the progressive atelectasis of quiet breathing seen in the trauma patient in acute pain with decreased consciousness from the cerebral effects of injury or narcotics.

Another change is the dissolution of collagen, the skeleton of the lung, which allows the atelectasis and "blister" formation in its place as well as throughout the space between the alveolar and endothelial components of the pulmonary membrane (Fig. 36–10). The distance oxygen must diffuse from the alveolus to the capillary is increased five to ten fold. The lung attempts to restore its skeleton by abundant formation of new collagen (Fig. 36–11). Unfortu-

Text continued on page 1030.

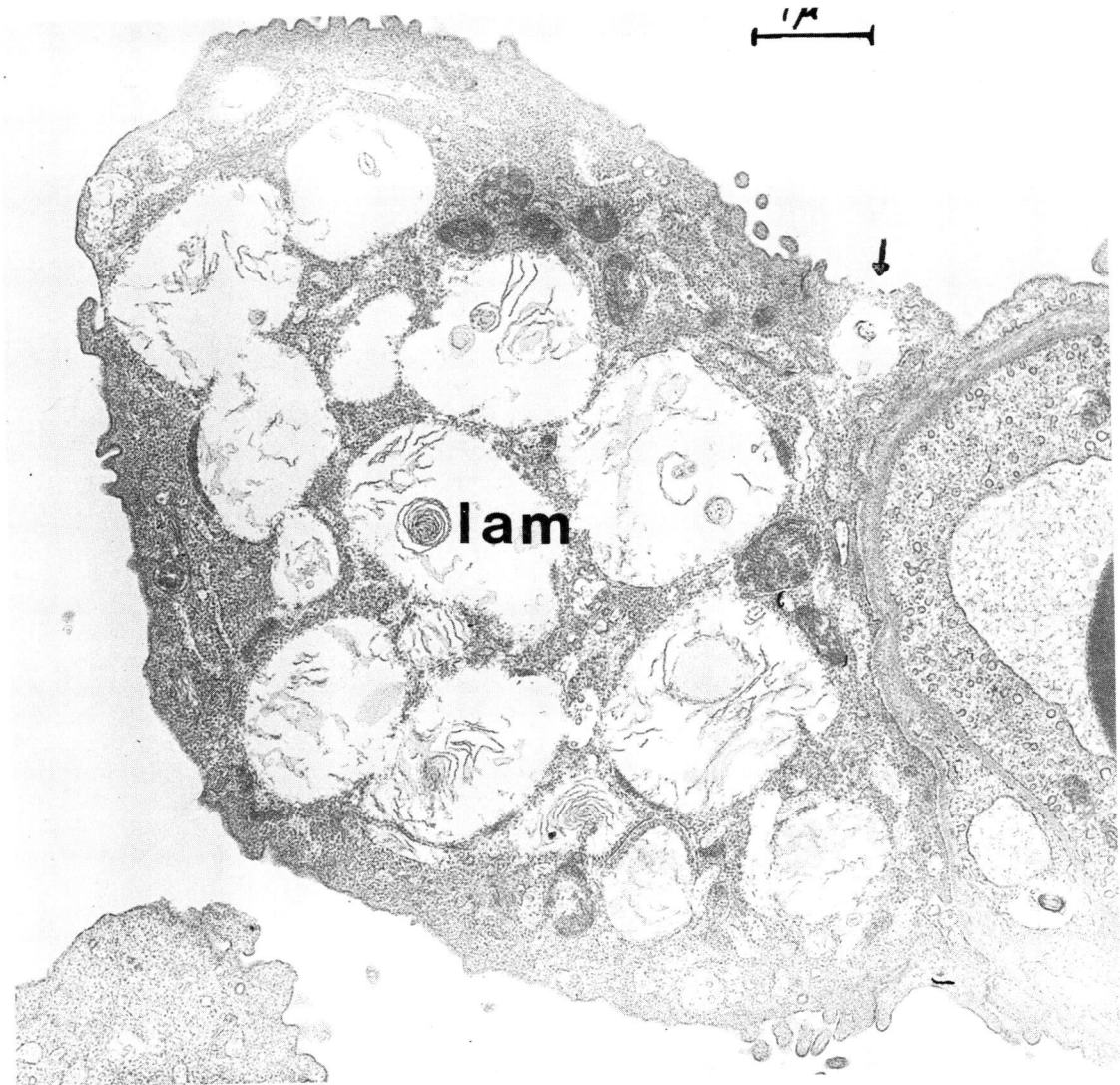

Figure 36–8 Type II pneumocytes contain lamellar bodies that are responsible for surfactant production. Following trauma the lamellar bodies empty their contents into the alveolar space.

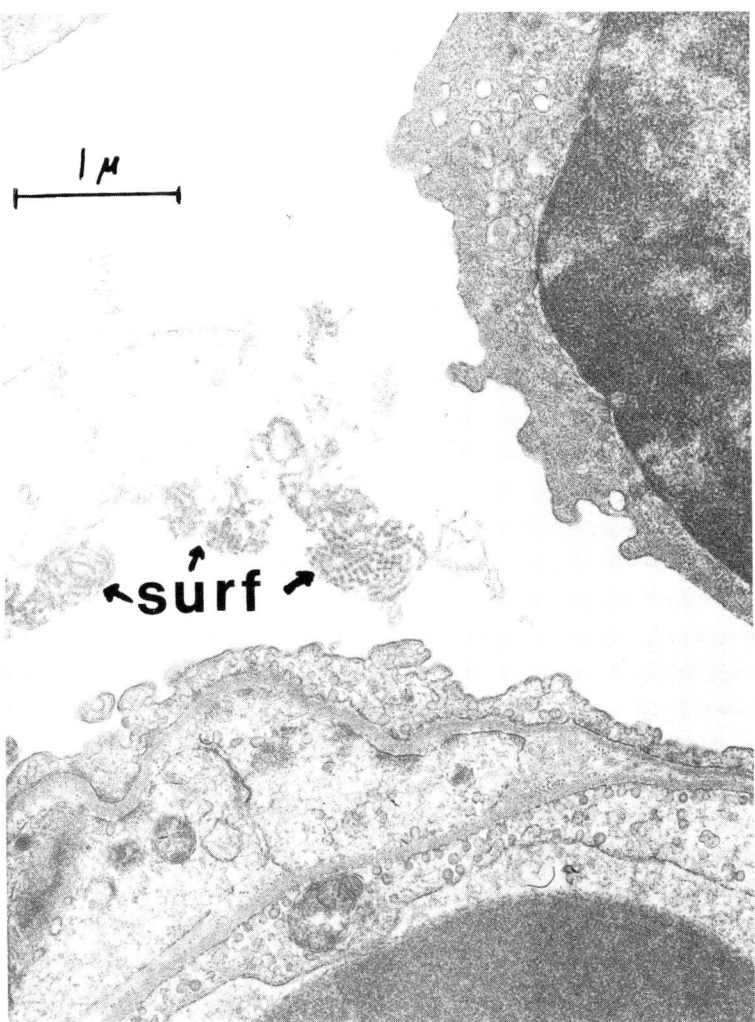

Figure 36–9   Surfactant is identified in the alveolar space by its specific lattice-type structure.

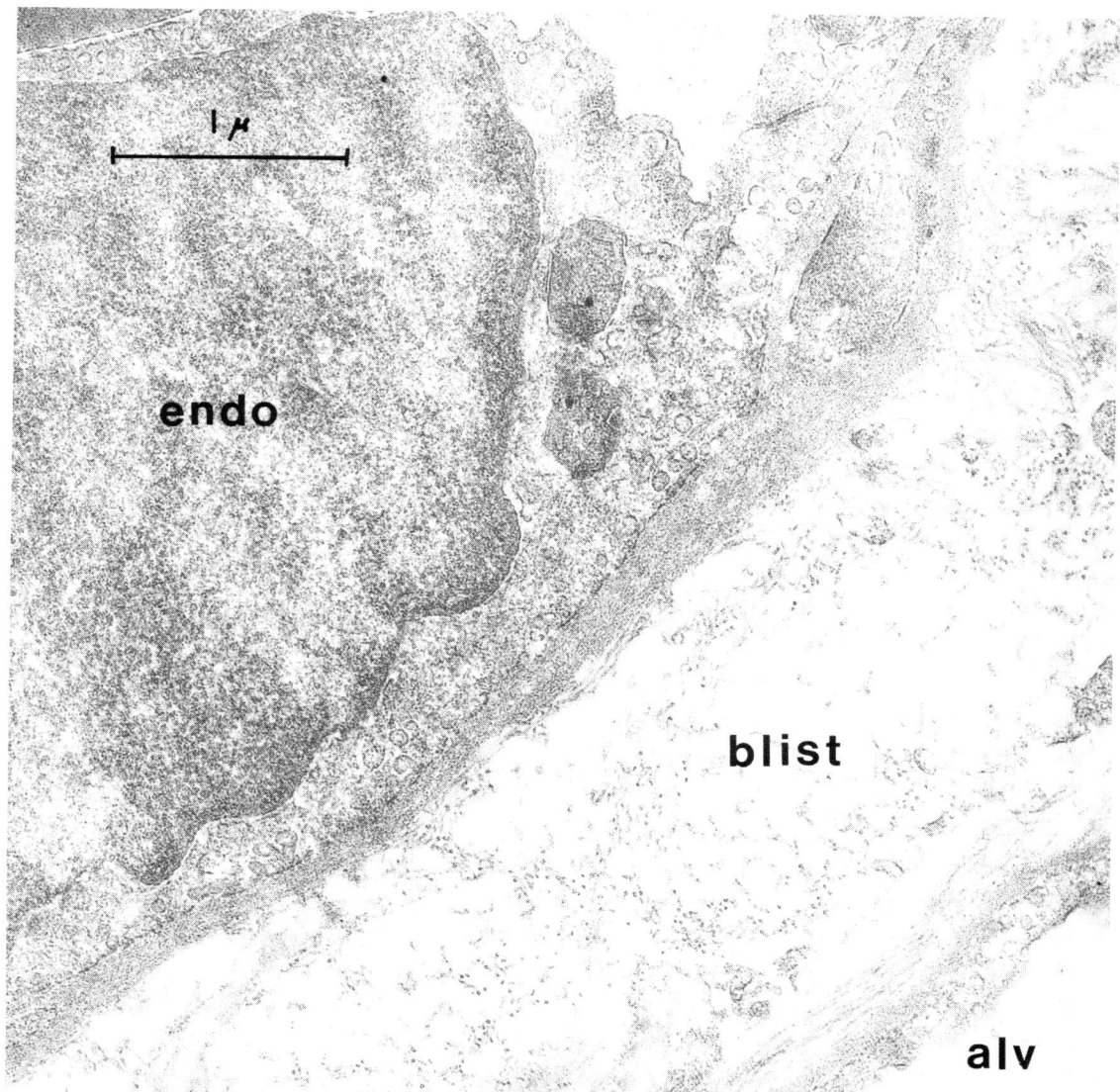

Figure 36-10   Dissolution of the collagen between the two component layers of the alveolar membrane leads to loss of the skeletal support of the alveolus and resultant atelectasis. In addition, the space between these two layers swells, forming "blisters" that impede oxygen transfer by a 5 to 10-fold increase in distance.

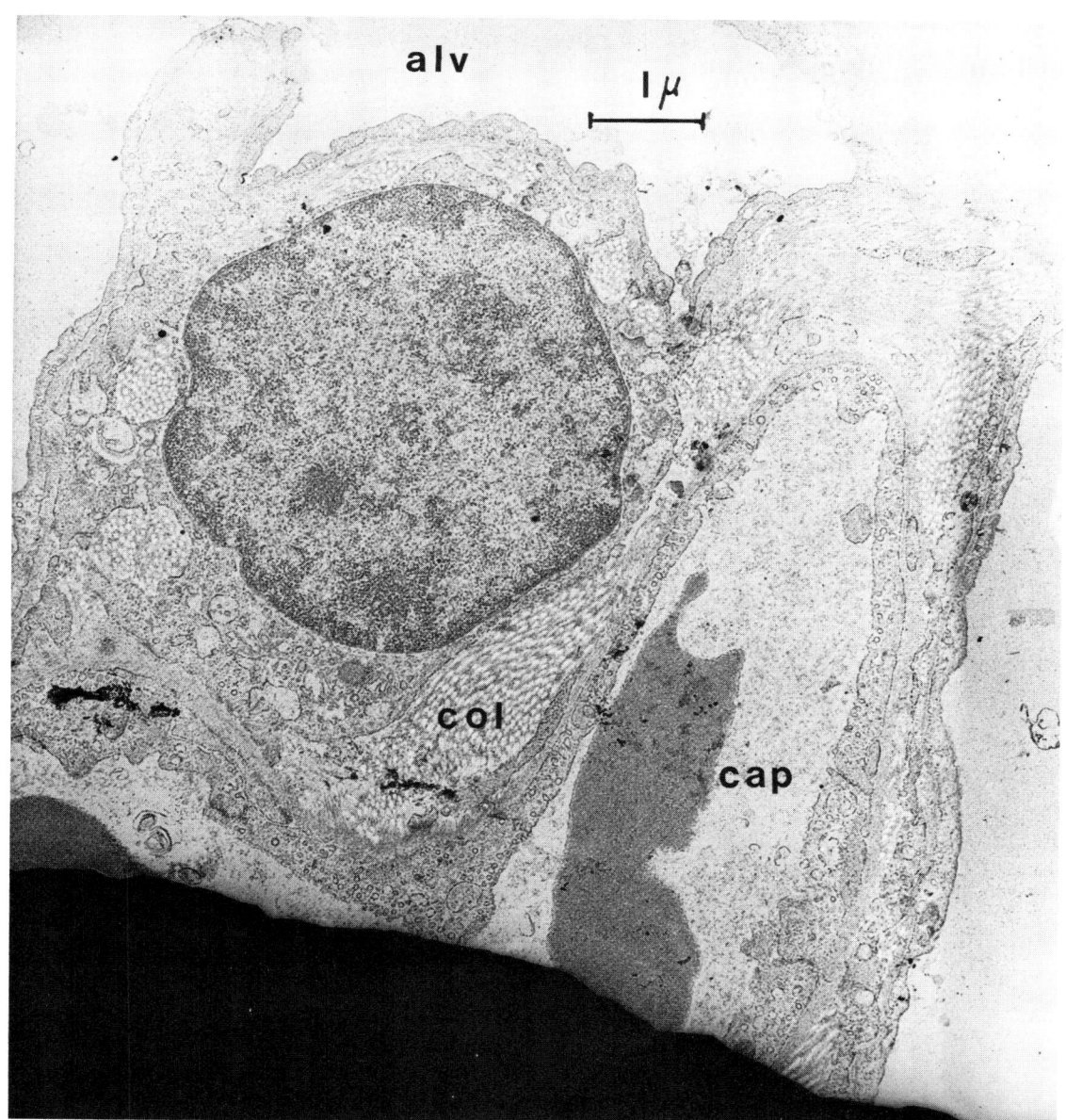

Figure 36–11   The collagen is rapidly replaced, but forms in areas where gas exchange normally occurs. This capillary is almost completely surrounded by collagen.

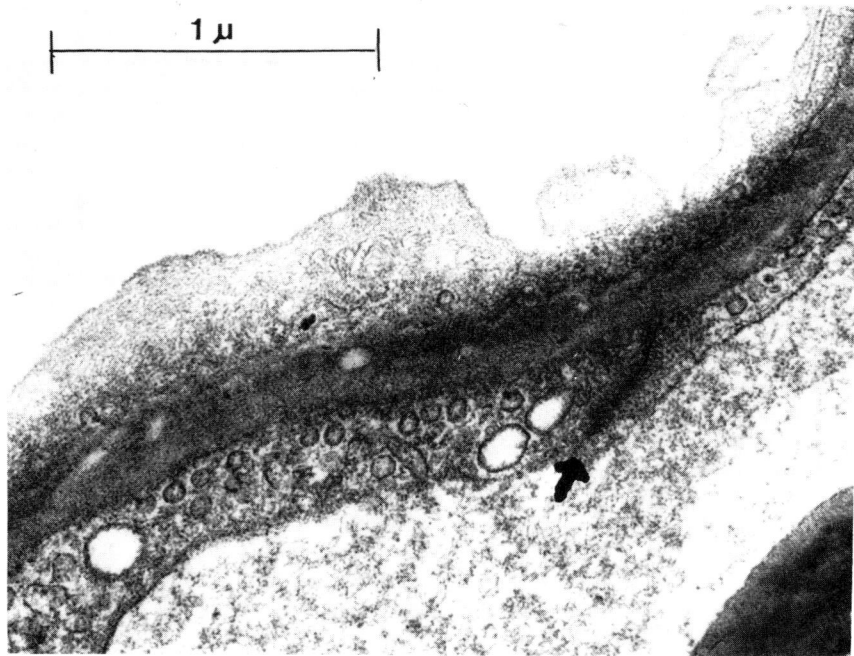

Figure 36–12   Opposite the nucleus of the endothelial cell the two thinned-out layers of cytoplasm abut each other in a characteristic junction, which identifies this as the thinnest area of the alveolar membrane. The extensive deposition of collagen between the layers in this area inhibits gas exchange.

nately, this collagen is not deposited in the proper position under the endothelial cell nucleus and the end of the septa. In fact, it frequently appears precisely where gas exchange normally occurs — opposite the nucleus of the endothelial cell where the cytoplasm of the two sides of the cell touch each other (Fig. 36–12). At the site of their junction the cytoplasm is normally very thin, and there is no space between the alveolar and endothelial layers. In the traumatized animals, the potential space was filled with collagen. The final result is a breakdown of alveolar membrane, cellular disorganization, and even free collagen both in the alveolar space, impeding gas exchange, and in the capillary, contributing to intravascular coagulation (Fig. 36–13).[36]

Hematological studies showed the commonly observed decrease in hemoglobin concentration of 29 per cent, an increase in the white cell count of 36 per cent, and a fourfold increase in the corrected sedimentation rate. Coagulation studies showed a 33 per cent decrease in platelet concentration and a 59 per cent increase in the partial thromboplastin time (Fig. 36–14). Triglycerides increased nearly twofold. Cholesterol showed only a slight increase, with phospholipids demonstrating a slight decrease. The ratio of cholesterol to phospholipids, which is inversely related to the suspension stability of the blood, increased 68 per cent (Fig. 36–15). Lipoprotein electrophoresis showed an increase in the cholesterol containing pre-beta fraction of from 15 to 35 per cent at the expense of the alpha portion.[35] The combination of these two changes contributes to agglomeration of fat particles which forms a nidus for platelet aggregation.

Hemodynamic studies demonstrated an initial increase in pulmonary artery pressure of 16 per cent associated with a 22 per cent decrease in pulmonary flow, resulting from a 25 per cent increase in pulmonary vascular resistance. Arterial oxygen tension decreased 11 per cent, and pulmonary shunting increased from 11 per cent prior to injury to 30 per cent the day following injury (Fig. 36–16). The large increase in the pulmonary shunt with only a moderate

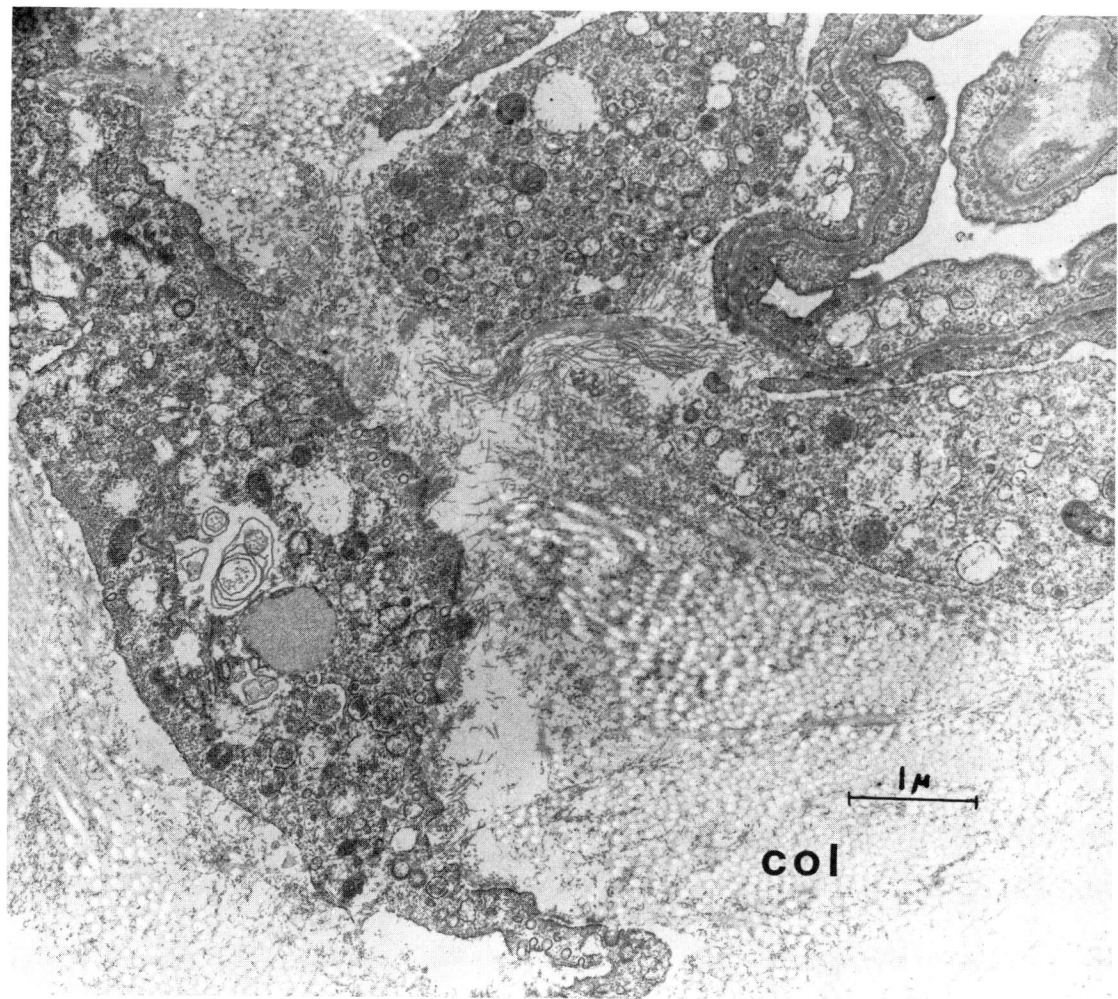

Figure 36–13 Cellular disorganization and membrane breakdown result in free collagen in both the alveolar space, preventing gas exchange, and the capillary, contributing to intravascular coagulation.

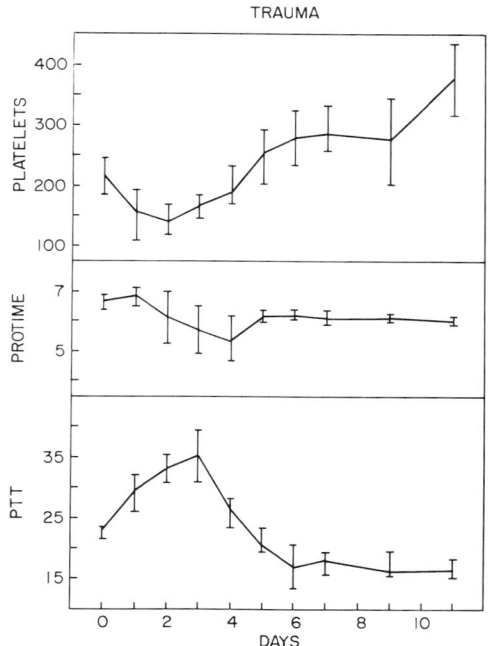

Figure 36–14 Musculoskeletal trauma produces a consumptive coagulopathy characterized by a decrease in platelets and an increase in partial thromboplastin time. The over-response of replacement at 7 to 10 days produces a hypercoagulable condition contributing to thromboembolism.

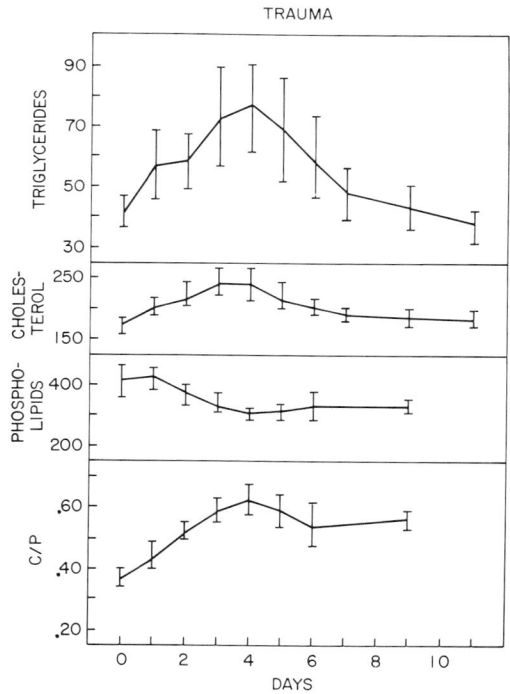

Figure 36–15 The mobilization of depot fat results in a marked increase in the serum triglyceride level. The cholesterol to phospholipid ratio increases, resulting in a decrease in the suspension stability of the blood. This contributes to agglomeration of fat particles, which may become centers of platelet aggregation.

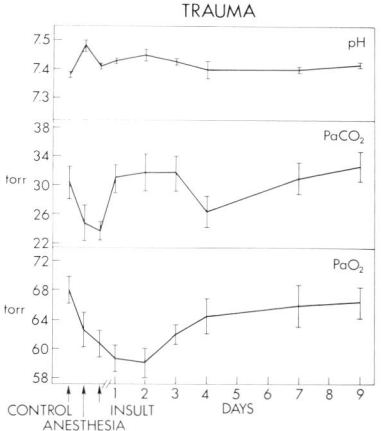

Figure 36–16 Arterial hypoxia consistently follows musculoskeletal injury and is the result of pulmonary insufficiency, not hypoventilation.

decrease in arterial oxygen is explained by the decrease in mixed venous oxygen resulting from the initial decrease in cardiac output. Oxygen content of the arterial blood was decreased even more owing to the loss

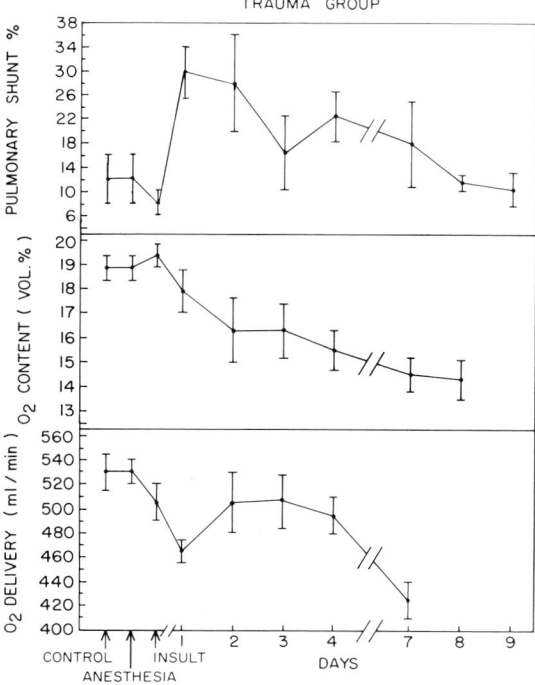

Figure 36–17 The pulmonary shunt increased to 30 per cent, the oxygen content decreased, and the cardiac output decreased, resulting in a fall in the systemic delivery of oxygen immediately following injury. After a temporary period of compensation the fall was 20 per cent.

of blood and subsequent anemia. The final physiological parameter, the systemic delivery of oxygen, decreased 13 per cent (Fig. 36–17).

In summary, these studies show that musculoskeletal injury produces a mild pulmonary insufficiency, as quantitated by the increase in pulmonary shunt. Associated with this is evidence of a decrease in platelet count and an increase in partial thromboplastin time, suggesting a consumptive coagulopathy picture. The lipid studies demonstrate a possible contribution to the fat emboli in the lung from the cholesterol-containing lipoprotein fraction. The histological studies confirm the presence of pulmonary microemboli and demonstrate an anatomical basis for the pulmonary insufficiency. Combined with hypovolemic shock, the result is a fall in the systemic delivery of oxygen (Fig. 36–18).

Other investigators have demonstrated similar relevant findings. Saggau found the same coagulation and pulmonary hemodynamic changes, and also suggested a vasoactive rather than a mechanical cause for the pulmonary blockade.[51] Berman demonstrated that the source of the platelets was the injured limb and showed concentration of radioactively labeled serotonin in the lung.[8] Ljungqvist,[37] using experimental trauma as his model and radioactive labeling techniques, proved that the platelets were sequestered in the lung initially, followed by fibrin.

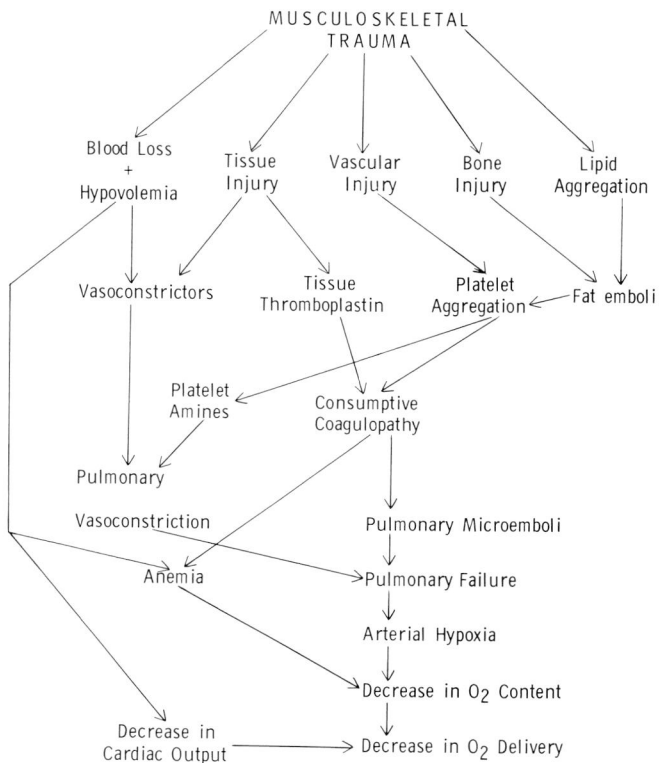

Figure 36–18   Musculoskeletal trauma produces many local and systemic effects, all culminating in failure of the cardiopulmonary system to provide adequate systemic delivery of oxygen during a period of marked increase in need.

Modig demonstrated in patients undergoing total hip replacement a sequestration of labeled platelets during the phase of broaching and impaction. During impaction, labeled fibrinogen was also concentrated in the lung and was associated with a decrease in arterial oxygen tension.[40] Vaage has demonstrated the release of prostaglandinlike substances during platelet aggregation and pulmonary microembolism.[63] Saldeen has detected in posttraumatic autopsy material the association of embolic fat and intravascular coagulation.[52] He demonstrated in an experimental preparation with embolic fat that intravascular coagulation results.[53] Unfortunately, his experimental model used homogenized adipose tissue, which is now recognized to contain large amounts of free fatty acids and is therefore quite toxic.

In our previously cited experimental investigation we also evaluated chromatographically pure neutral triolein, which is known to be released from injured bone. We found this material, when injected in doses equal to those seen in patients dying of fat embolism,[3] did not produce pulmonary insufficiency and had only a very mild effect on the platelet count. The histological studies showed a rather benign appearance of the lung, although a moderate amount of embolic fat, over three times that seen in the trauma model, was present. None of the inflammatory changes seen in the traumatized animals was noted. The hemodynamic studies failed to demonstrate the changes seen in the trauma preparation. Many investigations using various forms of fat have reported significant amounts of pulmonary insufficiency and pulmonary changes. Unfortunately, none of these studies has verified that the material injected was truly neutral lipid. It is well recognized that presumably neutral lipid is rapidly broken down into highly toxic free fatty acids. This is particularly true of any model using homogenized adipose tissue that contains the enzymes necessary for this conversion.[13] Furthermore, the doses required are nearly 10 times that seen in patients dying of the "fat embolism syndrome."

Our studies also demonstrated a second phase of changes. At about five days following injury there was a marked reversal of the coagulation picture with an outpouring of

platelets and replacement of the thromboplastin, thus producing a hypercoagulable state. This phenomenon may well contribute to the most common and serious unresolved problem of the injured patient, that is, thromboembolism.

THROMBOEMBOLIC PHENOMENON

The literature is filled with studies demonstrating the high incidence of deep vein thrombosis following elective surgery in general, total hip surgery, and trauma, more specifically hip fractures. This is particularly a problem in the elderly.[41, 60] Clinical signs are apparent in only about half of the cases of deep vein thrombosis.[70] Laboratory verification by isotopic studies at bedside are now possible for venous thrombosis with I-131-labeled fibrinogen and for pulmonary embolism with the ventilation-perfusion scan using a mobile gamma camera.* The entire dynamic scan is tape recorded for playback analysis (Fig. 36–19). Young women on contraceptive estrogens are also at high risk, as are paraplegics.[58]

Studies of patients with total hip replacements have shown an increase in platelet coagulant activity.[66] Atik demonstrated in trauma patients a 30 per cent increase in platelet count and a 13 per cent increase in platelet adhesiveness. These changes were prevented by dextran 70.[4] Peer found that dextran 40, dextran 70, and methylprednisolone would prevent the sequestration of platelets in the lung following soft tissue trauma in animals.[46] In elective hip surgery patients, Evarts demonstrated that deep vein thrombosis detected by venography decreased from 50 to 26 per cent with dextran 40 administration begun at the end of surgery. When dextran 40 was started at the beginning of surgery, the decrease was from 56 to 6 per cent.[17]

In 1959, using oral anticoagulants, Sevitt found the incidence of pulmonary embolism in 150 patients with hip fractures was reduced from 15 to only 2.[55] With oral anticoagulants, Hamilton reduced the incidence of venous thrombosis in hip frac-

*Sigma 420 Mobile Gamma Camera, Ohio-Nuclear, Inc., Solon, Ohio.

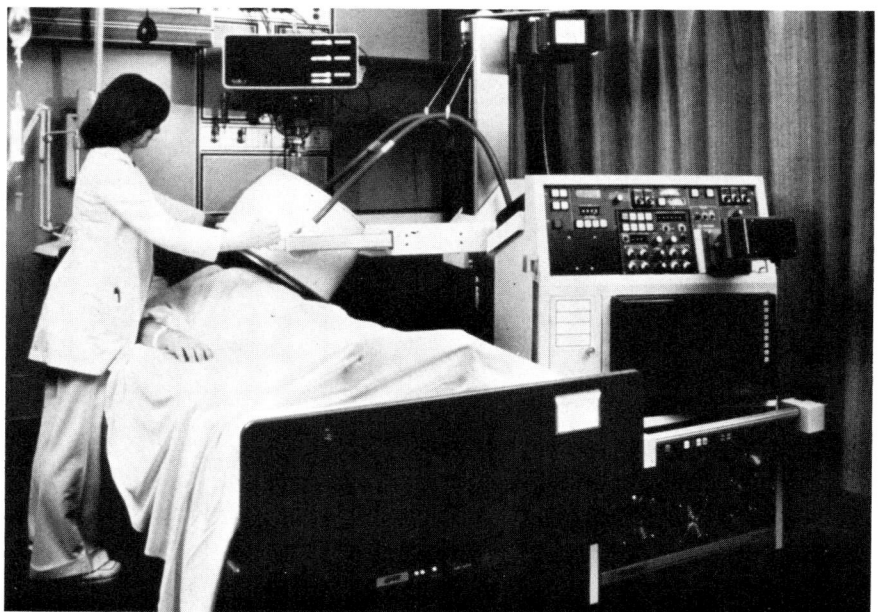

Figure 36–19   Mobile gamma cameras now allow verification of venous thrombosis and pulmonary embolism at the bedside.

tures from 48 to 19 per cent.[28] Results of prophylaxis with low-dose heparin are inconsistent. Gallus reported in 820 patients a decrease of deep vein thrombosis from 16 to only 14.2 per cent.[21] Sagar reported 8 fatal pulmonary emboli in the untreated group of 236 patients and none in the 252 treated patients.[50]

Some authors have found heparin superior to oral anticoagulants[64] and to dextran,[38] while others have found it not effective in fractures[12] or in total hip replacement.[29] When patients are treated prophylactically with anticoagulants, careful observation is required to detect complications.[61] Although the specific drug for anticoagulation in trauma remains controversial, the value of venous support and elevation of the foot of the bed should not be overlooked,[15] and some form of anticoagulation should be used in the majority of patients.

PULMONARY INSUFFICIENCY

Fat embolism syndrome is the orthopedist's usual diagnosis upon observation of fever, tachypnea, tachycardia, pulmonary distress, and cerebral disorientation within the first few days of musculoskeletal injury. The presence of petechiae seems to be a highly specific sign of this syndrome. The importance of hypoxia was first stressed by Wertzberger[68] and reemphasized by Benoit.[5] Ross,[49] Gruner,[26] and Whitson[69] are so impressed with the importance of hypoxia they seem convinced that the syndrome is simply the result of hypoxia regardless of cause, and not the result of embolic fat.

Sevitt, in his classic monograph, emphasized the relative benignity of embolization of fat to the lungs, but was convinced that if hypoxia does develop it is due to the presence of fat emboli in the brain.[56] Moss has also demonstrated that hypoxia in the brain produces a lesion in the lung which in turn produces arterial hypoxia.[42] In our previously cited experimental work, we also demonstrated the rather benign result of injection of *pure neutral* triolein. Several other works previously cited also question the role of embolic fat in posttraumatic pulmonary insufficiency. It is the opinion of Armin and Grant,[3] Grant and Reeve,[25] and Scully[54] that pulmonary embolic fat plays

little role in the syndrome. Bergentz was one of the first to demonstrate the contribution of platelet abnormalities and tissue thromboplastin to this syndrome.[6, 7]

In any event, it should be remembered that treatment of "fat embolism" must be based on increasing the delivery of oxygen to the tissues by maintaining adequate levels of oxygen tension, hemoglobin concentration, and cardiac output. Oxygen enrichment may even be prophylactic in preventing progression of the syndrome.[62] Treatments directed specifically toward fat, such as the "operative embolectomy" performed by Nelson,[44] seem ill conceived at best.

To conclude, following musculoskeletal trauma the patient is subject to three major pulmonary problems. First, pulmonary microembolism occurs early and is associated with pulmonary insufficiency. Second, the possibility of embolization of deep vein thrombi to the lungs requires prophylactic attention. Prophylaxis of pulmonary thromboembolism with anticoagulants is difficult in a trauma patient because of the changing degree of coagulation and the numerous sites that are likely to form large hematomas. A third clinically distinct entity is the pulmonary insufficiency associated with sepsis, frequently the result of atelectasis and pneumonia. This condition remains a very difficult problem and does not respond well to the usual measures for treatment of early posttraumatic pulmonary insufficiency, namely, fluid restriction and diuretics.

An aggressive approach to avoid the pulmonary problems of trauma is currently being evaluated in twelve major trauma centers.

The management of the musculoskeletal trauma patient in such a way that the chest can be upright in association with freely moving painless extremities is important in preventing the prolonged cardiopulmonary failure that leads to death.

The results of this approach have been recently reported by Riska[47] and will soon be reported by the group from Basel. Although the data cannot be considered incontestable, the results with this aggressive approach to date seem far superior to the "do nothing" attitude that relies on the homeostatic mechanisms of the human or-

THE GOAL OF THE TRAUMA SURGEON IS COMPLETE REHABILITATION OF THE INJURED PATIENT AS RAPIDLY AND SAFELY AS POSSIBLE BY:

1. Prompt and adequate resuscitation of the cardiorespiratory system.

2. Closure of all wounds after complete debridement.

3. Stabilization of fractures and mobilization of the joints.

4. Prevention of complications.

5. Evaluation of management by the risk-benefit ratio.

Figure 36-20 The trauma surgeon must keep in mind his goal when designing a plan of management and evaluating various treatments and their effects.

ganism to correct all of its deficiencies, with studious neglect on the part of the trauma surgeon. Posttraumatic pulmonary insufficiency—in particular, "fat embolism syndrome"—has nearly disappeared.

SUMMARY

The surgeon dealing with fractures must first become completely familiar with his patient and organize a total plan of care (Fig. 36-20). To be effective, resuscitation must be rapid and aggressive. The fractures must be stabilized by whatever method is appropriate. Open fractures should be debrided, converted to closed fractures, and stabilized as necessary. The patient should be rapidly mobilized to an upright position and begin moving all the joints. This will avoid the problems of pulmonary thromboembolism and pulmonary insufficiency. Most important, avoid sepsis, which will lead to lethal pulmonary insufficiency. And last, avoid delayed wound treatment and fracture immobilization. This approach all too often leads to eventual union, but with a dystrophic limb because of stiff contracted joints, shortened bones, weakened muscles, and grotesque skin scars requiring plastic surgery revision. The risk-benefit ratio of both active direct surgical intervention and passive "conservative" forms of treatment must be determined and a plan of management selected.

REFERENCES

1. Ahstrom, J. P.: Treatment of established Volkmann's ischemic contracture of the forearm and hand. Curr. Pract. Orthop. Surg., 6:213, 1975.
2. American College of Surgeons. Manual on Control of Infection in Surgical Patients, p. 175. Philadelphia, J. B. Lippincott, 1976.
3. Armin, J., and Grant, R. T.: Observation on gross pulmonary fat embolism in man and the rabbit. Clin. Sci., 10:441, 1951.
4. Atik, M.: Platelet adhesiveness and thromboembolism. 5th European Conference on Microcirculation, Gothenburg, 1968. Bibl. Anat., 10:494, 1969.
5. Benoit, P. R., Hampson, L. G., and Burgess, J. H.: Value of arterial hypoxemia in the diagnosis of pulmonary fat embolism. Ann. Surg., 175:128, 1972.
6. Bergentz, S.-E.: Studies on the genesis of posttraumatic fat embolism. Acta Chir. Scand. (Suppl.), 282, 1961.
7. Bergentz, S.-E.: Fat embolism. Prog. Surg., 6:85, 1968.
8. Berman, I. R., Smulson, M. E., Pattengale, P., and Schoenbach, S. F.: Pulmonary microembolism after soft tissue injury in primates. Surgery, 70:246, 1971.
9. Border, J. R.: Bedside study of the surgical patient. J. Surg. Res., 7:591–601, 1967.
10. Border, J. R., LaDuca, J., and Seibel, R.: Priorities in the management of the patient with polytrauma. *In* Allgower, M., Bergentz, S. E., Calne, R. Y., and Gruber, U. F. (eds.) Progress in Surgery. Vol. 14, pp. 84–120. Basil, S. Karger, 1975.
11. Burri, C.: Post-traumatic Osteomyelitis, pp. 19–27. Bern, Hans Huber, 1975.
12. Checketts, R. G., and Bradley, J. G.: Low-dose heparin in femoral neck fractures. Injury, 6:42, 1974.
13. Collins, J. A., and Caldwell, M. C.: Relationship of depot fat embolism to pulmonary structure and function in rabbits. Am. J. Surg., 119:581, 1970.
14. DeHaven, K. E., and Evarts, C. M.: The continuing problem of gas gangrene: A review and report of illustrative cases. J. Trauma, 11(12):983, 1971.
15. Doran, F. S. A., White, M., and Drury, M.: A clinical trial designed to test the relative value of two simple methods of reducing the risk of venous stasis in the lower limbs during surgical operations, the danger of thrombosis, and a subsequent pulmonary embolus, with a survey of the problem. Br. J. Surg., 57:20, 1970.
16. Edsall, G.: The inexcusable disease. J.A.M.A., 235(1):62, 1976.
17. Evarts, C. M., and Feil, E. J.: Prevention of thromboembolic disease after elective surgery of the hip. J. Bone Joint Surg., 53A:1271, 1971.
18. Fishman, A. P.: Hypoxia on the pulmonary cir-

culation. How and where it acts. Circ. Res., 38:221, 1976.

19. Fulton, R. L., and Jones, C. E.: The cause of post-traumatic pulmonary insufficiency in man. Surg. Gynecol. Obstet., 140:179, 1975.

20. Gaisford, W. D., Pandey, N., and Jensen, C. G.: Pulmonary changes in treated hemorrhagic shock. II. Ringer's lactate solution versus colloid infusion. Am. J. Surg., 124:738, 1972.

21. Gallus, A. S., Hirsh, J., O'Brien, S. E., McBride, J. A., Tuttle, R. J., and Gent, M.: Prevention of venous thrombosis with small, subcutaneous doses of heparin. J.A.M.A., 235:1980, 1976.

22. Ganz, W., and Swan, H. J. C.: Balloon flotation cathether in the management of critically ill patients. *In* Shoemaker, W. C., and Tavares, B. M. (eds.): Current Topics in Critical Care Medicine. Vol. pp. 2–22. Basel, S. Karger, 1977.

23. Garnier, M. J.: Tetanus in patients three years of age and up. A personal series of 230 consecutive patients. Am. J. Surg., 129:459, 1975.

24. Glenn, J. N., Miner, M. E., and Peltier, L. F.: The treatment of fractures of the femur in patients with head injuries. J. Trauma, 13:958–961, 1973.

25. Grant, R. T., and Reeve, E. B.: Observations on the general effects of injury in man. Special report. Med. Res. Coun. (London), 277:99, 1951.

26. Gruner, O. P. N.: Post traumatic syndrome ascribed conventionally to fat embolism. J. Oslo City Hosp., 21:81, 1971.

27. Gustilo, R. B., and Anderson, J. T.: Prevention of infection in the treatment of one thousand and twenty-five open fractures of long bones. J. Bone Joint Surg., 58A:453, 1976.

28. Hamilton, H. W., Crawford, J. S., Gardiner, J. H., and Wiley, A. M.: Venous thrombosis in patients with fracture of the upper end of the femur. J. Bone Joint Surg., 52B:268, 1970.

29. Hampson, W. G. J., Harris, F. C., Lucas, H. K., Roberts, P. H., McCall, I. W., Jackson, P. C., Powell, N. L., and Staddon, G. E.: Failure of low-dose heparin to prevent deep-vein thrombosis after hip-replacement arthroplasty. Lancet, 2:795, 1974.

30. Harris, L. W., and Reckling, F. W.: Cancellous bone grafting. Posterolateral approach to union problems of the tibia. J. Kans. Med. Soc., 75:82–86, 1974.

31. Holcroft, J. W., and Trunkey, D. D.: Pulmonary extravasation of albumin during and after hemorrhagic shock in baboons. J. Surg. Res., 18:91, 1975.

32. Jackson, R. P., Jacobs, R. R., Preston, D. F., Williamson, J. A., and Gallagher, J.: Dynamic bone scanning in fractures. American Academy of Orthopedic Surgeons, San Francisco, 1979.

33. Jackson, R., Jacobs, R. R., and Neff, J. R.: External skeletal fixation in severe limb trauma. J. Trauma, 18:201, 1978.

34. Jacobs, R. R., Wheeler, E. J., Jelenko, C., III, McDonald, T. F., and Bliven, F. E.: Fat embolism: A microscopic and ultrastructure evaluation of two animal models. J. Trauma, 13:980, 1973.

35. Jacobs, R. R.: Fat embolism syndrome: A comparison of hematologic coagulation and lipid changes in two animal models. Clin. Orthop., 116:240, 1976.

36. Jacobs, R. R., McClain, O. M., and Neff, J. R.: Pulmonary microscopic and ultrastructural effects of femur fracture and 15% hemorrhage in dogs. Surg. Forum, 28:492, 1977.

37. Ljungqvist, U., Bergentz, S. E., and Lewis, D. H.: The distribution of platelets, fibrin and erythrocytes in various organs following experimental trauma. Eur. Surg. Res., 3:293, 1971.

38. MacIntyre, I. M. C., Vasilescu, C., Jones, D. R. B., et al.: Heparin versus dextran in the prevention of deep-vein thrombosis. Multi-unit controlled trial. Lancet, 2:118, 1974.

39. Mattar, J. A., Esgaib, A. S., Tavares, B., Velasco, I. T., and Factore, L. A.: Measurements of hemodynamic and oxygen transport in critically ill patients. *In* Shoemaker, W. C., and Tavares, B. M. (eds.): Current Topics in Critical Medicine. Vol. 3, pp. 43–51. Basel, S. Karger, 1977.

40. Modig, J., Busch, C., Olerud, S., and Saldeen, T.: Pulmonary microembolism during intramedullary orthopaedic trauma. Acta Anaesthesiol. Scand., 18:133, 1974.

41. Morrell, M. T.: The incidence of pulmonary embolism in the elderly. Geriatrics, 25:138, 1970.

42. Moss, G., Staunton, C., and Stein, A. A.: Cerebral hypoxia as the primary event in the pathogenesis of the "shock lung syndrome." Surg. Forum, 22:211, 1971.

43. Muller, M. E., Allgower, M., and Willenegger, H.: Manual of Internal Fixation, p. 2. New York, Springer-Verlag, 1970.

44. Nelson, C. S.: Cardiac and pulmonary fat embolectomy for suspected fat embolus. Thorax, 29:1, 1974.

45. Pak, T. J., Martin, G. M., Magness, J. L., and Kavanaugh, G. J.: Reflex sympathetic dystrophy. Minn. Med., 53:507, 1970.

46. Peer, R. M., and Schwarts, S. I.: Development of treatment of post-traumatic pulmonary platelet trapping. Ann. Surg., 181:447, 1975.

47. Riska, E. B., von Bonsdorff, H., Hakkinen, S., Jaroma, H., Kiviluoto, O., and Paavilainen, T.: Prevention of fat embolism by early internal fixation of fractures in patients with multiple injuries. Injury, 8:110, 1976.

48. Roding, B., Groeneveld, P. H. A., and Boerema, I.: Ten years of experience in the treatment of gas gangrene with hyperbaric oxygen. Surg. Gynecol. Obstet., 134:579, 1972.

49. Ross, A. P. J.: The fat embolism syndrome: with special reference to the importance of hypoxia in the syndrome. Ann. R. Coll. Surg., Engl., 46:159, 1970.

50. Sagar, S., Massey, J., and Sanderson, J. M.: Low-dose heparin prophylaxis against fatal pulmonary embolism. Br. Med. J., 4:257, 1975.

51. Saggau, W. W., Ulmer, H. E., and Bleyl, U.: Changes of coagulation and fat-metabolism following pulmonary microembolism after trauma and hemorrhage. Thromb. Diath. Haemorrh., 33:477, 1975.

52. Saldeen, T.: Fat embolism and signs of intravascular coagulation in a posttraumatic autopsy material. J. Trauma, 10:273, 1970.

53. Saldeen, T.: The importance of intravascular coag-

ulation and inhibition of the fibrinolytic system in experimental fat embolism. J. Trauma, *10*:287, 1970.

54. Scully, R. E.: Fat embolism in Korean battle casualties. Its incidence, clinical significance, and pathologic aspects. Am. J. Pathol., *32*:379, 1956.
55. Sevitt, S., and Gallagher, N. G.: Prevention of venous thrombosis and pulmonary embolism in injured patients. Lancet, *2*:981, 1959.
56. Sevitt, S.: Fat Embolism. London, Butterworth, 1962.
57. Siegel, D. C., Moss, G. S., Cochin, A., and Tapas, K. D. G.: Pulmonary changes following treatment for hemorrhagic shock: Saline versus colloid infusion. Surg. Forum, *21*:17, 1970.
58. Silver, J. R., and Moulton, A.: Prophylactic anticoagulant therapy against pulmonary emboli in acute paraplegia. Br. Med. J., *2*:338, 1970.
59. Skillman, J. J., Parikh, B. M., and Tanenbaum, B. J.: Pulmonary arteriovenous admixture. Improvement with albumin and diuresis. Am. J. Surg., *119*:440, 1970.
60. Sternlieb, C. M.: Incidence of silent postoperative pulmonary emboli in geriatric patients. J. Am. Geriatr. Soc., *18*:242, 1970.
61. String, S. T., and Barcia, P. J.: Complications of small dose prophylactic heparinization. Am. J. Surg., *130*:570, 1975.
62. Szabo, G.: The syndrome of fat embolism and its

origin. J. Clin. Pathol., *23*. (Suppl.) (R. Coll. Pathol.) *4*:123, 1931.
63. Vaage, J., and Piper, P. J.: The release of prostaglandin-like substances during platelet aggregation and pulmonary microembolism. Acta Physiol. Scand., *94*:8, 1975.
64. van Vroonhoven, T. J. M. V., van Ziji, J., and Muller, H.: Low-dose subcutaneous heparin versus oral anticoagulants in the prevention of postoperative deep-venous thrombosis. A controlled clinical trial. Lancet, *1*:375, 1974.
65. Walker, L., and Eiseman, B.: The changing pattern of post-traumatic respiratory distress syndrome. Am. J. Surg., *181*:693, 1975.
66. Walsh, P. N., Rogers, P. H., Marder, V. J., Gagnatelli, G., Escovitz, E. S., and Sherry, S.: The relationship of platelet coagulant activities to venous thrombosis following hip surgery. Br. J. Haematol., *32*:421, 1976.
67. Weber, B. G., and Cech, O.: Pseudarthrosis. New York, Grune & Stratton, 1976.
68. Wertzberger, J. J., and Peltier, L. F.: Fat embolism: importance of arterial hypoxia. Surgery, *63*:626, 1968.
69. Whitson, R. O.: A critique of fat embolism. J. Bone Joint Surg., *33A*:447, 1971.
70. Wright, I. S.: Pulmonary embolism: A most underdiagnosed and untreated disorder. J. Am. Geriatr. Soc., *22*:433, 1974.

ROBERT M. GLAZER, M.D.

Rehabilitation _____ 37

Musculoskeletal injury causes loss of function. The goal of rehabilitation is to return the damaged part and the injured person to the maximum possible *function* in the minimum possible *time*. The relationship of time to recovery is a key point. The sooner joints move, the faster they recover motion. The earlier active exercises begin, the faster functional strength returns. The quicker the patient is mobilized, the lower the risk of complications from immobilization. Early return to function minimizes hospitalization costs, loss of wages, and related insurance expenses. Prompt institution of rehabilitation helps overcome the psychological damage of injury, inactivity during recovery, dependence on others, and lack of productivity. The emphasis on early return to function may improve the chances for the patient with a "compensation injury" (job-related and vehicular accidents, disability insurance cases) to return to productive activity. Rehabilitation aims to treat the aftermath of injury that has caused:

Pain
Loss of joint motion
Loss of muscle strength
Loss of endurance
Loss of coordinated muscle activity
Loss of mobility (ambulation)
Paralysis
Bowel and bladder dysfunction
Skin breakdown
Damage to the psyche
Damage to the family structure
Inability to care for self (activities of daily living)
Inability to care for family (homemaking)
Inability to participate in recreational activities
Inability to earn a living

Although many patients will not need formal rehabilitation, others will benefit from some participation in an organized program. The team concept is a useful foundation on which to construct an effective program, bringing in appropriate team members and techniques according to the demands of the individual case.

THE REHABILITATION TEAM

The patient must play an active role in his own rehabilitation. He must not only cooperate passively, but more important, work actively in spite of pain, fatigue, and inconvenience. His motivation will be the most important element in the speed of his recovery as well as in the ultimate success of his rehabilitation program.

The physician directs the overall program. He recommends and may teach the necessary techniques. He may request support from other specialists to provide more frequent and intensive treatments demanding more time or skill than he can provide.

Physical and occupational therapists furnish training and supervision in all the techniques of rehabilitation. These include exercise techniques and equipment, ambulation training and equipment, training in coordination and functional activities, and therapeutic application of different forms of energy. They may also fabricate and apply slings and splints and may provide essential information for brace prescription. They have the time to work closely with the patient as often as every day and even twice a day. A well-trained therapist should be expected to function with significant independence in designing and executing the specifics of an individual rehabilitation program, under the general direction of the physician.

The patient's family and friends can be taught to apply various therapeutic techniques. They will often do so with much more care and concern than anyone else. Their help is especially valuable in outpatient treatment, since they may be with the patient regularly and can assist in treatment several times a day.

Nursing personnel can do much to carry on details of rehabilitation for the inpatient. They too will be in contact with the patient several times a day and can suggest various exercises, encourage their use, and give emotional support. They are the first line of defense against the development of pressure sores (decubitus ulcers, bed sores).

The social worker organizes the use of community resources. Both the more severely injured hospitalized patient and the ambulatory injured one may benefit. This team member may help in arranging for nursing home placement, evaluating home facilities, including possible architectural barriers, mobilizing family resources, arranging for transportation to and from outpatient treatment, bringing therapists or home-health aides to the patient, and directing patients to agencies that can be helpful in one way or another.

The psychiatrist or psychologist can provide support for the patient with an emotional disturbance that impedes participation in the rehabilitation program. Depression and anxiety are common problems, especially in the patient with major injuries, loss of limb, or paralysis, as well as the one with major financial problems, or persistent pain. The psychotherapist may provide relief with psychotrophic drugs and individual therapy sessions, and by counseling the other members of the team in the best approach for dealing with the patient's emotional problems.

The vocational rehabilitation counselor should enter the picture as soon as it becomes apparent that the patient will not be able to return to his usual occupation as a result of his injuries. This team member may arrange for vocational testing, retraining programs, or contact with the local bureau of vocational rehabilitation for further help.

The rehabilitation center concentrates the skills of all the team members to provide the optimal environment and the most efficient service to the more severely injured patient. It is the best arrangement for the patient with major deficit from brain or spinal cord injury, for the patient with multiple major extremity injuries, and for the elderly, who need intensive therapy to enable return to function. The physical facilities are arranged for efficient delivery of all rehabilitation services. The staff is oriented toward the problems of the more severely disabled and is better able to function in the team approach setting.

THERAPEUTIC EXERCISE

Injuries to the spine and extremities may cause any combination of restricted joint motion, muscle weakness, loss of endurance, and impaired coordination. Restriction of joint motion results from prolonged cast immobilization of the joint, adhesions within an injured joint, scar formation in the healing of adjacent and distant soft tissue injuries, edema, muscle spasm from painful motion, or spasticity from injury to the brain or spinal cord. Bony ankylosis from heterotopic bone will produce the same effect. Muscle weakness comes from direct injury to the muscle or to its innervation, and from disuse. Inactivity also causes loss of endurance. A loss of neuromuscular coordination may result from central nervous system injury or may occur for unidentified reasons following certain major injuries. Therapeutic exercise is basic in the prevention and treatment of these problems.

Exercise ought to start at the outset—as an integral part of the overall treatment. The patient should exercise all parts of the body that do not have to be immobilized, whether he is ambulatory or confined to bed. The treatment program should direct special attention to the joints of the injured extremity, since pain or fear of causing damage may discourage the patient from moving the joints that are left free to move. The patient must learn that such motion may produce some pain but won't cause damage or, impair healing. He needs to understand that controlled exercise is essential to optimum recovery.

RANGE-OF-MOTION

Range-of-motion (ROM) exercise can maintain the normal extent of joint motion. *A joint taken through its full range of motion at least once a day is not apt to develop a contracture.* If joint motion becomes restricted it is essential to identify the cause of the limitation in order to apply the correct treatment. Soft tissue shortening frequently responds to exercise, sometimes with the help of a cast, splint, or brace. Edema is treated with heat, elevation, exercise, and massage.[19] Spasm requires analgesics, muscle relaxants, and various forms of heat. Spasticity that doesn't respond to exercise, icing, heating, splinting, or medication will require surgical alleviation by myotomy, tenotomy, or neurectomy. Bony ankylosis will require surgical excision of the ectopic bone when roentgenograms indicate maturity and when alkaline phosphatase level and bone scan indicate inactivity.[16]

Passive Exercise

Passive exercises carry the joint through its range of motion without the active use of the muscles crossing that joint. The patient can do this himself, or another person, such as a physical therapist, can administer the exercise. Passive exercise is needed when the muscles are paralyzed or significantly weak, when the patient is unconscious, severely debilitated, or can't cooperate or when it is necessary to avoid activating muscles, as in the early period following tendon surgery. This type of exercise is usually done without much force.

Stretching Exercise

Stretching exercises do involve the use of force—as much as the patient can tolerate within pain limits, or as much as is felt safe at that stage of fracture or soft tissue healing. Stretching is needed when contractures have developed. In addition to stretching by the patient and the therapist, this maneuver can be executed by positioning the contracted joint with weights applied to use the constant pull of gravity. Relatively small weights pulling constantly for long periods of time can be very effective. The prone position may help to stretch out hip flexion contractures. At the same time, weights hung from the ankles work on knee flexion contractures. Heat, ice, or massage may help if applied prior to stretching. Splints, casts, or braces can help to gain motion or to preserve motion gained by stretching.

Manipulation under Anesthesia. This is the extreme degree of stretching. For restricted motion owing to intraarticular adhesions or to other soft tissue limitations, manipulation can be quite effective. It is almost always used for restricted shoulder motion[39] or for the knee that lacks sufficient flexion. It should be considered when an excellent trial of exercise has failed, and not before fracture or soft tissue healing are secure. Manipulation is performed under anesthesia with profound drug-induced muscle relaxation or paralysis—using considerable force. It is important to remember that bones may be osteoporotic from disuse and are at some risk of fracture. Therefore, roentgenograms of the involved part should be taken routinely before and after manipulation.

The safest way to manipulate a joint is by firm, steady, unremitting pressure, using a short lever arm. Sudden jerks or snaps are not only unhelpful but dangerous. After several minutes of steady pressure, adhesions will stretch and then tear, producing audible and palpable snapping and cracking. Motion may at first be imperceptible but will gradually and noticeably increase as pressure is maintained. Local anesthetic and steroids may be instilled into the joint, but the most important postmanipulation treatment is a vigorous exercise program, begun the same day or the next day and continued without letup, lest the gains from the manipulation be lost. Adequate analgesics given 30 to 60 minutes prior to the exercise session will be helpful. An elastic bandage helps to control knee swelling. The shoulder needs constant positioning in abduction and external rotation when not undergoing exercises. Skin traction and suspension in bed can achieve this positioning.

Active Exercise

Active exercises use voluntary contraction of the muscles to provide range of motion to the joints. The muscle contraction can apply as much force as available strength and tolerance to pain permit. The average patient should use pain tolerance as a guideline to the safe amount of force for the muscles to apply. Vigorous patients or those with a high pain threshold may overdo the exercises and need supervision to prevent damage. At the other extreme are patients with a low pain threshhold and those who are fearful of causing damage. They need reassurance and encouragement to tolerate some degree of pain in order to get any benefit from the exercise.

Active Assisted Exercises. These are helpful for the patient who needs encouragement or close supervision, or whose muscles are too weak to provide sufficient power to move the joint. With this type of exercise, as with passive exercises, another person can assist the patient in motion of the joint while the muscles are actively contracted.

EXERCISES TO INCREASE STRENGTH AND ENDURANCE

These exercises prevent disuse atrophy, restore lost strength and endurance, and help to restore lost joint motion. To increase strength, muscles must work against increasing resistance. To increase endurance, muscles must contract an increasing number of times against a relatively low resistance to the point of fatigue.[19]

Isometric Exercise

Isometric or "muscle-setting" exercises are those in which the muscles contract without producing any motion of the joint. They may be used for any muscle group. Isometrics are most useful when the joint is immobilized, as in traction, splint, or cast, or when motion would be detrimental, as in chondromalacia patellae or incompletely healed fractures. Quadriceps setting is the most common type of isometric exercise. The patient tightens the thigh muscles and pushes the back of the knee against the bed, or straightens the knee, lifting the heel off the bed. To roughly quantitate this exercise, the patient should count both the number of seconds the contraction is held and the number of repetitions in a given exercise period. For example, he should do three sets of ten repetitions three times a day, holding each contraction for five seconds. Used in this form, isometrics would be expected at least to maintain muscle tone.

To increase strength, it is necessary to make the muscle work against increasing resistance. This is done by increasing the weight attached to the end of the extremity. The muscles must contract with enough force so that the joint does not bend from the selected fixed position. Taking the knee as an example again, the patient raises the leg with the knee fully extended, bringing the foot 12 to 18 inches off the bed. Two or three sets of ten repetitions done once or twice a day would be sufficient. Once the patient is accustomed to the exercise, he suspends weights from the ankle (Fig. 37–1). Starting with 5 lb, he increases the amount of weight lifted by 1 or 2 lb every one or two days. Rather than arbitrarily starting at 5 lb, the DeLorme method[8] can be used to identify a starting point that challenges the muscles to the point of fatigue. This is done by determining the

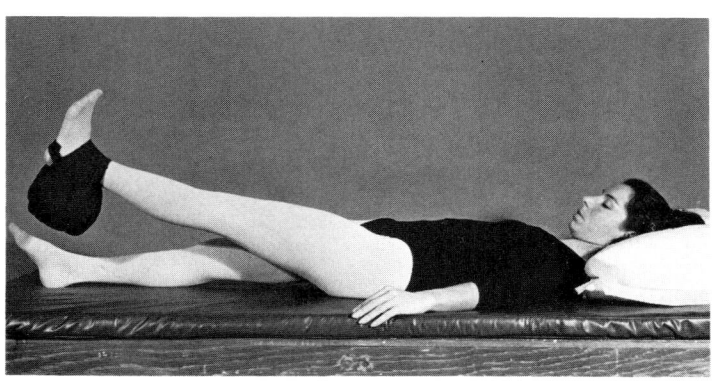

Figure 37–1 Muscle setting exercises against resistance. The patient lies supine, raises leg with knee extended, weights on ankle.

maximum weight that can be lifted for 10 repetitions by adding additional weights after each series of 10 lifts during the testing session.

This type of progressive resistance isometric quadriceps exercise may demand more of the hip flexors than is needed and may limit the amount of stress that can be applied to the knee extensors. A variation that avoids this problem has the patient sitting on a table with a sandbag under the knee which is locked in full extension or 45 degrees of flexion. The therapist applies a given amount of weight to the foot, starting from the 10-repetition maximum weight.[20] The amount of weight may be increased at intervals to build strength, or the same weight may be held for an increasing number of seconds to build endurance. The end point is arbitrary and depends on the individual, the functional recovery achieved, and the demands of leisure, sport, and work activities.

Isotonic Exercise

Isotonic exercises move the joint through an arc of motion against a constant resistance which is increased at regular intervals. As developed and refined by DeLorme, these became known as Progressive Resistance Exercises (PRE). Although originally designed to strengthen the knee extensors, PRE may be used to strengthen any muscle group.[8-10]

As in quadriceps strengthening, the patient sits on a table with a pad under the knee, which is flexed to 90 degrees. A weighted boot is strapped to the foot. Quadriceps contraction extends the knee smoothly and steadily for as far as available joint motion allows (Fig. 37–2). A controlled relaxation of the quadriceps allows the knee to flex slowly. There should be a momentary pause between repetitions. At the beginning of the exercise program, the quadriceps strength is tested to determine the initial amount of weight to use. By gradually adding weight to the boot, the maximum amount of weight that can be lifted 10 times is determined. This is the 10-repetitions maximum (10 RM), which is the weight to be lifted once a day over the next four days. On the fifth day, the maximum weight to be lifted for only one repetition is determined

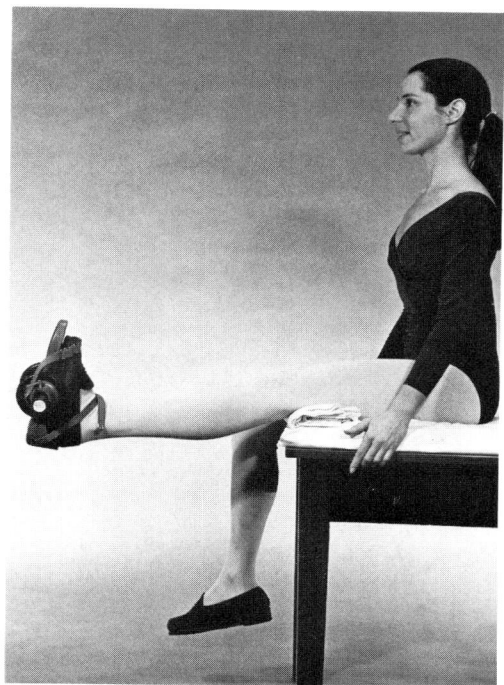

Figure 37–2 Progressive resistance exercises. The patient is seated on a table, weight boot attached to foot, knee maximally extended.

(1 RM), and a new 10 RM is established for the next week. No exercises are done in the next two days. DeLorme's original program was complicated and time-consuming. It has subsequently been modified and condensed by DeLorme and by others. A sample routine is:

First set of 10 repetitions—use 1/2 of 10 RM weight.

Second set of 10 repetitions—use 3/4 of 10 RM weight.

Third set of 10 repetitions—use full 10 RM weight.[37]

In order to achieve optimum results with various types of resistance exercises, the muscles must work to the point of fatigue.[7] As muscles become stronger, they must be regularly challenged by increasing the demands upon them.

A variation of the DeLorme technique uses a bolster or an adjustable wedge under the knee, with the patient in the supine position (Fig. 37–3). This method prevents discomfort from the pull on the knee ligaments by heavy weights suspended from the foot. It also utilizes that part of the

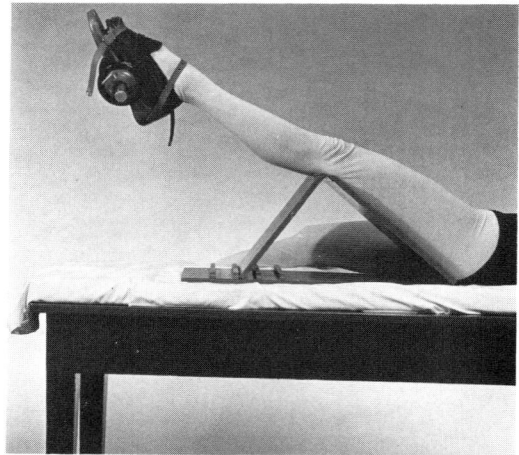

Figure 37-3 Variation of the DeLorme technique. The patient lies supine with an adjustable wedge under the knee, weight boot attached to foot, knee maximally extended.

arc of knee motion that derives the maximum resistance from gravity.

The patient can exercise the hamstrings using the same type of weights. In the prone position, the patient flexes the knee about 30 degrees, holds, and slowly lets the leg down (Fig. 37-4). In the standing position, the weighted boot is lifted, held, and slowly let down (Fig. 37-5). The same techniques of progressive resistance are applicable to the hamstrings, and for that matter to any muscle group. These exercises are intended to be suitable for a home exercise program. In the physical therapy gymnasium, more sophisticated equipment is available, but the techniques are basically the same.

Whether isometric or isotonic exercises

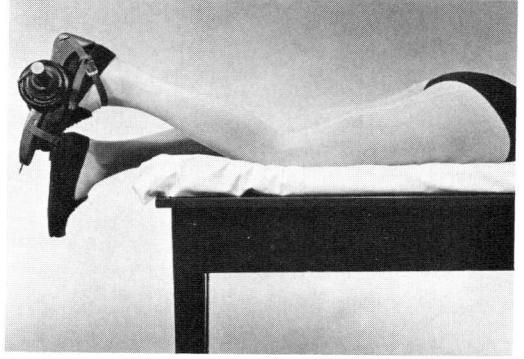

Figure 37-4 Hamstring exercises. The patient lies prone, weight boot attached to foot, knee flexed about 30 degrees.

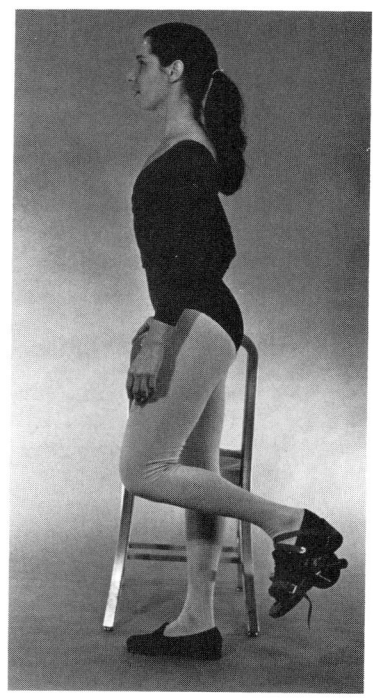

Figure 37-5 Hamstring exercises. The patient stands erect, holding chair for balance, weight boot attached to foot, knee flexed.

are superior is open to question. There is some evidence that the isometric type may be more efficient and more effective.[7, 21, 40]

Brief Maximal Exercise. This is a variety of strengthening exercise that combines features of isometric and progressive resistance exercise. This method was described by Rose and his associates who also worked with the quadriceps and positioned the patient according to DeLorme's method. Their program starts with the determination of a one-repetition maximum, with the knee moving from 90 degrees of flexion to full extension against resistance, and held in that position for a timed five seconds. Once the maximum value is obtained, the exercise session ends. At the next session an additional 1 1/2 lb is added. If the knee won't fully extend, that weight is removed. If it still won't fully extend, 1 1/4 lb more is removed for a third and last attempt at that session.[32]

Proprioceptive Neuromuscular Facilitation

This technique of neuromuscular reeducation is useful for weak or paretic muscles. A specially trained therapist administers exercises to achieve increased muscle strength and joint motion. The method aims to elicit a maximal activation of motor units of the affected muscles with each effort, through strong facilitation and summation of central stimuli. The therapist applies proprioceptive sensory input in the form of deep pressure (stretching the joint prior to muscle contraction) and manual resistance to the patient's muscle activity.

Rather than working on isolated muscle groups, the therapist encourages diagonal patterns of mass muscle movements of limbs and trunk, similar to the patterns of daily use of the involved part. The therapist has close control of all stages of the exercise and does not use any apparatus. Although good results are claimed for this method, it is time-consuming, requiring the therapist's full attention to only one patient during the entire therapy session. It is probably best reserved for problem cases.[18, 27]

Isokinetic Exercise

Isokinetic exercise requires the use of an apparatus that holds joint motion to a constant speed. The machine (Cybex, Kinetron) offers resistance to muscle activity that matches the degree of that activity. The device assures ". . . optimal exercise under maximum muscle tension at a constant speed. . ."[42] This has given rise to the term *accommodating resistance exercise*. "By allowing the exercise motion to start and stop in any position, the mechanism is able to accommodate to a patient's limited range of motion, and yet give maximal resistance within that range."[42] The machine is versatile and adjustable, allowing a variety of exercise patterns. It also provides a graphic means of recording progress. Exercising on this machine can also improve coordination and increase endurance.[19, 30]

CONDITIONING PROGRAMS

Other programs to increase coordination are based on regular repetition of complex groups of muscle activity with reinforcement of good performance. The muscles must act together in correct sequence at the appropriate speed and tension. Functional activities, such as those used in activities of daily living, crafts, gait training, and calisthenics, are beneficial. The more productive and useful the activities, the more likely that the patient will maintain interest and continue working at them. While trying to improve coordination, the patient will also be making gains in endurance.[19, 27]

More detailed conditioning programs are needed to achieve maximum recovery and performance, especially in sports. Team trainers provide the detailed reconditioning program for the athlete, in cooperation with the team physician. Athletic training must be intensive in order to bring the participant back to a level of physical development both to compete successfully and to protect against reinjury.

The average person does not need this extreme degree of conditioning to return to normal function. However, if an active conditioning program is contemplated, especially in the older patient, it may be wise to pursue a thorough medical evaluation, including an exercise stress test with monitoring of electrocardiogram, heart rate, and blood pressure. This may reveal underlying cardiac abnormalities as well as give a baseline value of the patient's capacity for endurance exercise.[1, 44]

It is possible to follow one of several available programs or to have a detailed individualized prescription. In *The New Aerobics*, Cooper outlines a program of exercises using walking, running, swimming, or handball-basketball-squash activities. These consist of a carefully graded increase in activity according to many variables, including age, type and intensity of exercise, frequency of participation, and duration of training session. Points are assigned according to the level of activity, and the participant aims to increase the number of points earned per week up to at least 30.[6]

Another "do it yourself" exercise program is the Royal Canadian Air Force Exercise Plans For Physical Fitness. This book describes a graded progression of a series of calisthenic exercises. Those for men (5BX) use variations of toe touch, sit-up, back extension, push-up, and running, in increasing degrees of difficulty. Those for women (XBX) include other calisthenics and are somewhat less demanding. These exercises specify a fixed (11-minute) duration of training session and a daily frequency of participation until the maximum recommended level is reached, after which the program should be followed three times per week. The intensity (number of repetitions of a given exercise in the allotted time) of the exercise should be regularly increased. It may take several months before a maximum level of conditioning is reached.[33]

The American College of Sports Medicine suggests, "The frequency of exercise will depend in part on the duration and intensity of the exercise session. The optimal frequency of sessions may vary from several daily sessions of only a few minutes during early rehabilitation of a severely limited patient, to three to five 20- to 45-minute periods per week."[1] Wilmore agrees with these suggestions and points out that many types of activity are suitable as long as they test endurance. Therefore, the permanently disabled can also participate in conditioning exercises, using, ". . . wheelchair propulsion, wheelchair sports, or various endurance activities in physical and occupational therapy departments."[44]

THERAPEUTIC HEAT

A useful adjunct to the exercise program is the application of local heat—to treat inflammation, relieve pain, and relax muscles. To heat large areas the patient can take a hot shower or tub bath. A sink basin or bucket can be used to immerse hands or feet, and fingers will fit conveniently into a glass or cup of hot water. Hot compresses, using hot wet towels, are a traditional way to apply heat. The hydrocollator pack, a canvas-enclosed pack of silica gel, can be used for a more sustained release of wet heat. It must be heated in a hot water bath at 140° to 160° F and then wrapped in towels to avoid burning the skin.[19]

Whether wet heat is better than dry heat is uncertain. Dry heat is available in the form of a hot water bottle or a heating pad. The latter is much more convenient, since it can be wrapped around the extremity. Its temperature is easily adjusted, and it maintains its heat as long as electricity is available. For all of these methods the temperature should be warm to comfortably hot—not "as hot as you can stand it." Burns and scalds are not uncommon if heat is misused, and can inflict severe damage. Great care must be taken with the use of heat in anyone with sensory impairment. Also more susceptible to heat damage is any part lying on a heat-producing device in a way that the pressure diminishes local circulation.

More sophisticated methods of applying heat require special equipment. Paraffin dips use a bath of melted paraffin into which the hand is dipped and then removed with a coating of paraffin. This is a useful adjunct for exercise of interphalangeal and metacarpophalangeal joints. Heating of deeper structures by diathermy or ultrasound may be helpful in decreasing pain related to exercising. There is some evidence that ultrasound can assist in treating joint contractures resulting from capsular tightness and scarring, especially in joints covered by a thick layer of soft tissue.[19]

Whirlpool has some advantage in providing controlled application of heat along with the gentle massage of water in motion. Temperature guidelines are 90° to 100° F for the whole body, 100 to 102° F for the legs, and 105° F for the upper extremities.[19] A treatment session may last about 20 minutes; active or passive exercise of the immersed part can be carried on during the treatment.

The other commonly used apparatus for hydrotherapy is the Hubbard tank, in which as much of the body as desired can be immersed. The water functions as an antigravity assist by buoying the extremities. This makes it easier for the patient with weak muscles to carry out active exercises. At the same time, the heat of the water helps to relax tight muscles. Water can be used to provide resistance exercises by increasing the speed of motion of the extremity through the liquid. Water also serves an antigravity function for the entire body if a "walk-in" tank is available. The patient with bilateral lower extremity injuries can ambulate in water, with the water level controlling the amount of stress applied to the lower extremities. As the water level is lowered, more weight is carried by the lower extremities.

AIDS TO AMBULATION

THE TILT TABLE

The tilt table is convenient to use with the patient who has been recumbent for a period of time. It is relatively easy to transfer the patient from bed to litter and then to the tilt table to which he is secured by straps. A crank-operated mechanism allows the table to tilt gradually toward the vertical. In this manner, the patient can slowly become adjusted to an increasingly upright position. This decreases the problem of syncopal episodes from postural hypotension caused by abrupt assumption of the vertical position. At the same time, weight bearing on one leg can be prevented by placing blocks under the other foot against the foot rest of the table. The tilt table also provides a convenient way of taking the patient from the recumbent to the standing position, avoiding flexion of the hip.[16] This is desirable in the immediate postoperative period for the patient who has a femoral head replacement for a femoral neck fracture.

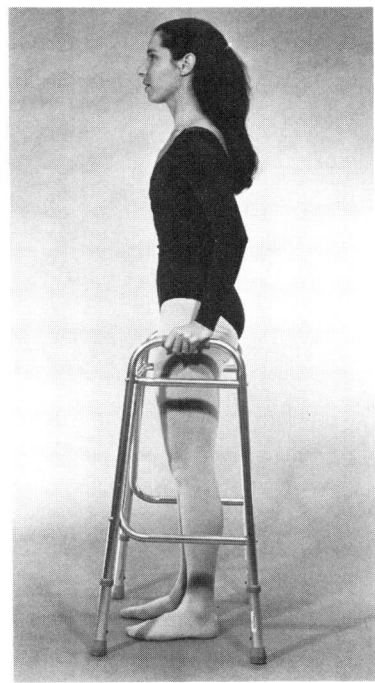

Figure 37-6 The pick-up walker.

PARALLEL BARS

Parallel bars are adjustable for height and are anchored securely to a platform. Electrically adjustable models change the distance between the bars as well as their elevation from the floor. Parallel bars provide a stable support for the patient while he is learning any of the various types of gait. After becoming competent in the parallel bars, the patient can progress to a device that allows more mobility.

WALKERS

The pick-up walker or walkerette is a lightweight, four-footed device constructed of tubular aluminum. It gives maximum stability to a device that still allows the patient to be mobile. The hand grips should be adjusted to a height that produces a 20 degree angle of elbow flexion (Fig. 37–6).[3] Technique modification in a recently introduced model allows the walker to be used to ascend and descend stairs. The

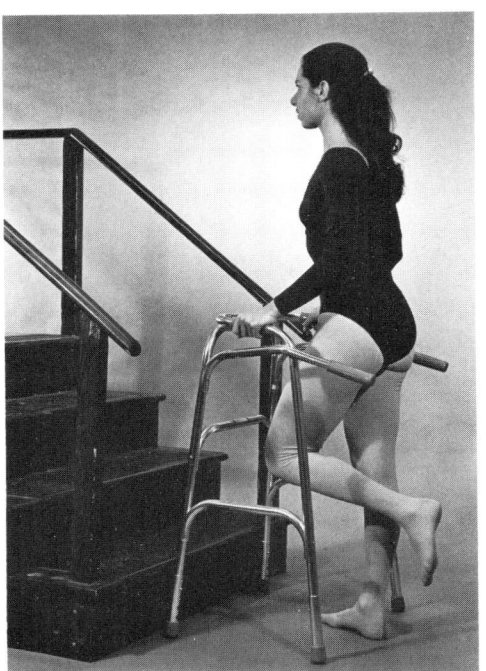

Figure 37-7 Stair climbing with a "stair walker," start position.

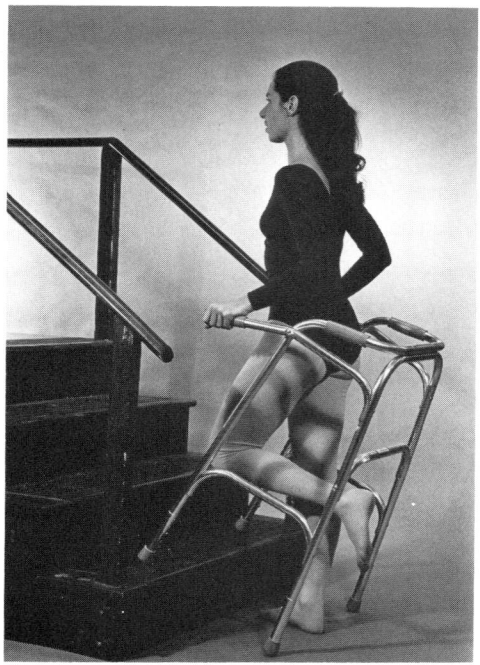

Figure 37–8 The "stair walker" is turned around, leading legs on first step, patient's hands on handle extensions.

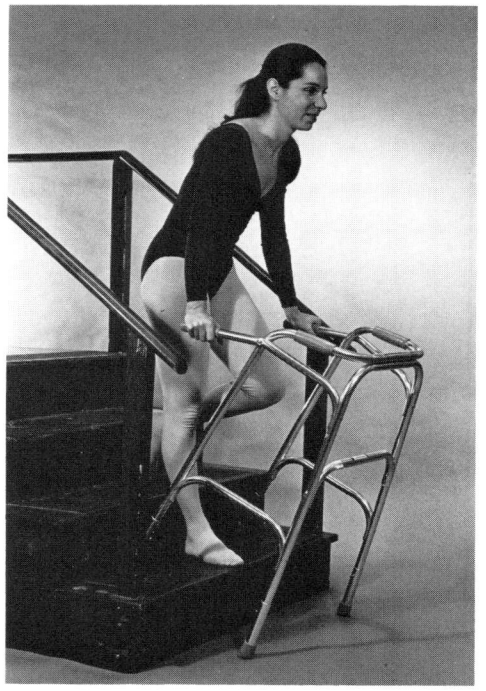

Figure 37–10 Descending stairs with "stair walker," leading legs placed on next step down, hands on extensions.

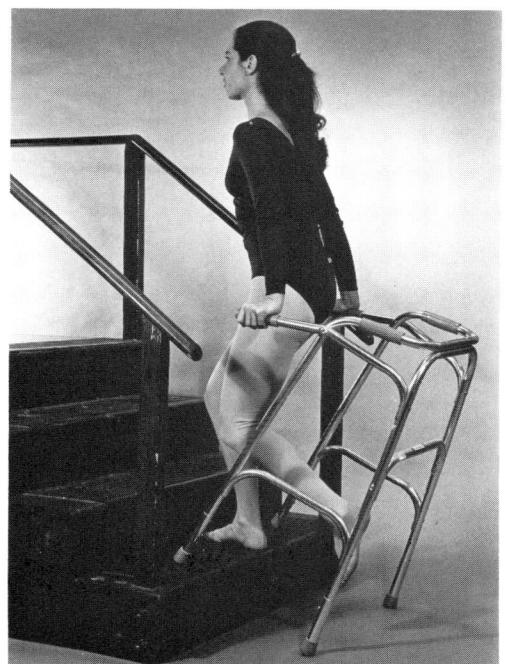

Figure 37–9 Patient advances well leg up to next step.

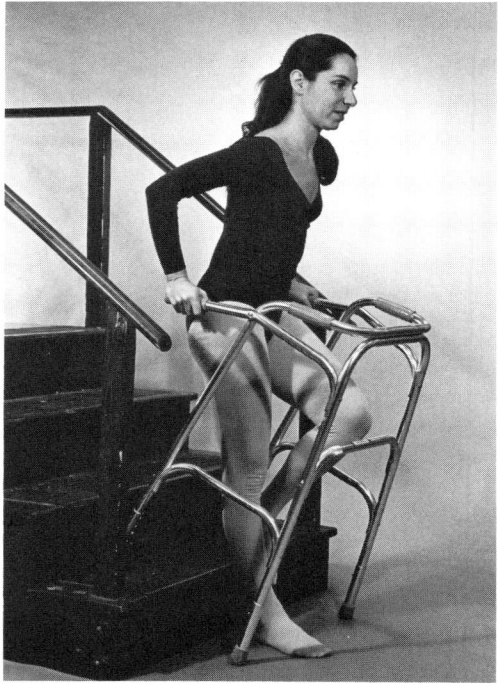

Figure 37–11 Patient advances well leg down to next step.

patient approaches the stairs using the "stair-walker" in the conventional fashion (Fig. 37–7). To ascend stairs, he turns the walker around 180 degrees, places the leading legs on the first step, and moves his hands to the grips of the extension handles (Fig. 37–8). Taking weight on both hands, he advances his feet to the first step up (Fig. 39–9). After achieving his balance, he advances the walker up one step and repeats the cycle. To descend stairs, the patient uses the walker in the conventional orientation. He places the walker's leading legs on the first step down and transfers his hand position to the grips of the extension handles (Fig. 37–10). Taking weight on both hands, he advances his feet to the first step down (Fig. 37–11). After achieving his balance, he advances the walker down one step and repeats the cycle.

CRUTCHES

Crutches allow more mobility and versatility but are less stable than other aids

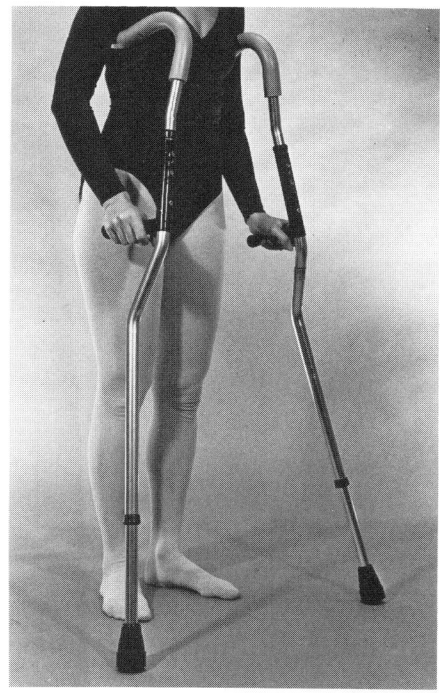

Figure 37–13 Patient using adjustable aluminum axillary crutches.

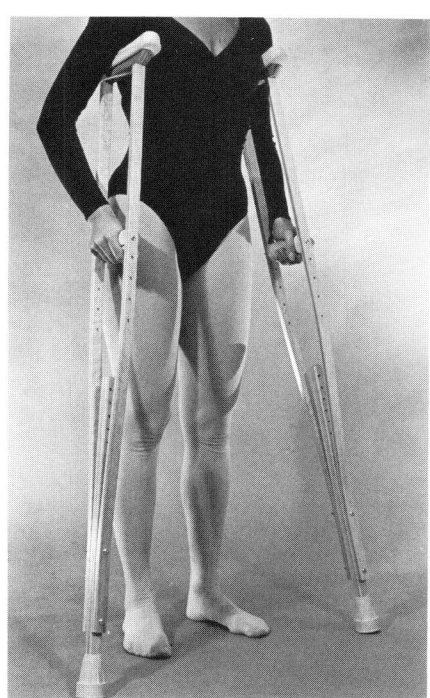

Figure 37–12 Patient using adjustable wood axillary crutches. Note proper height with flexion of the elbows.

to ambulation. Axillary crutches are so called because they have an upper transverse component contoured to fit under the axillae. The most commonly used axillary crutches are made of wood and come in fixed sizes to cover a wide range of patient height. There are adjustable wood crutches in child and adult sizes, permitting a much smaller inventory to be kept on hand (Fig. 37–12). There are different styles of adjustable tubular aluminum crutches as well (Fig. 37–13). The crutches may be fitted with sponge rubber axillary and hand grip pads for comfort. The most important attachment is a nonskid, flexible, moderately large rubber crutch tip.

To size crutches properly, with the patient standing erect and the crutch tips 6 inches away from the lateral side of the foot, the top of the crutch should come from 2 to 3 finger-breadths below the axilla. The hand grip should provide an angle of flexion of the elbow of about 20 degrees. It is most important to instruct the patient to carry his weight on his hands, not in the axillae, lest he develop neurovascular compression in the axillae. The axillary portion is used only

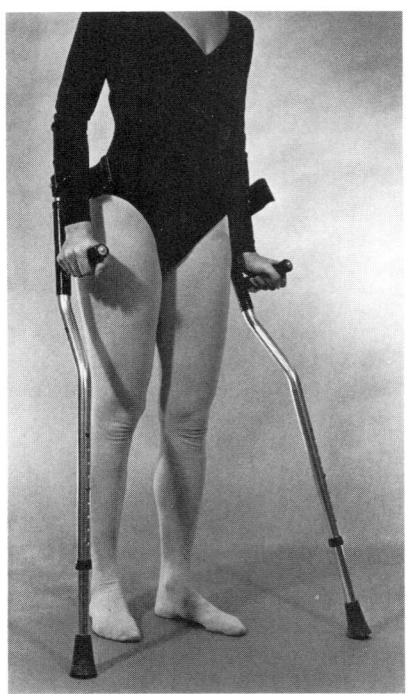

Figure 37–14   Patient using Lofstrand crutches.

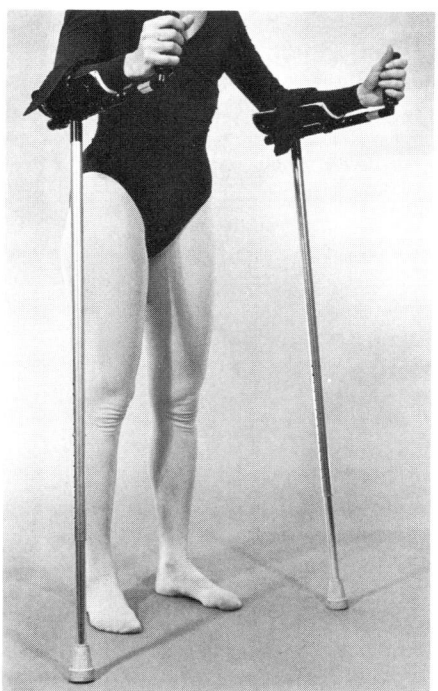

Figure 37–15   Patient using platform crutches.

to provide control, except in patients with preexisting upper extremity weakness who have no choice but to bear weight in the axillae.

Other types of crutches may be used for various special circumstances. Lofstrand or Canadian crutches are made of aluminum tubing with an open, oval, pivoting, metal band that partially encircles the upper forearm for proximal control while weight is borne on a hand grip (Fig. 37–14). The metal band allows the crutch to hang from the forearm while the hand is performing some other activity. A similar function is served by shortened wooden crutches with a proximal leather cuff. For patients with upper extremity weakness, various leather cuffs can be attached to increase stability in weight bearing. The forearm or platform crutch is most useful for patients with triceps weakness, significant elbow contractures, or impaired ability to grip with or bear weight on the hands. With the elbow flexed 90 degrees, the forearm rests in a trough or cradle. Weight is borne on the elbow and forearm while the hand holds a vertical grip for control (Fig. 37–15).

CANES

The quad-cane or four-foot cane is made of tubular metal and is adjustable in height. The feet are covered with nonskid rubber tips and may be broad- or narrow-based (Fig. 37–16). Its purpose is to provide more stability than a traditional one-point cane. It is most useful for the injured person who has one upper extremity tied up or otherwise nonfunctional.

The conventional cane, like crutches, should have an excellent nonskid tip, and should be long enough to provide about 20 degrees of elbow flexion, with the tip about 6 inches lateral to the midfoot. An alternate guide to cane length is for the handle to reach the level of the greater trochanter. In general, when one cane is used, it should be held in the hand on the side opposite the injured side. Weight should be borne on the cane and injured leg simultaneously if the cane is to do more than simply provide an additional balance point (Fig. 37–17). This arrangement does allow some unloading of the injured leg, and it is especially useful in

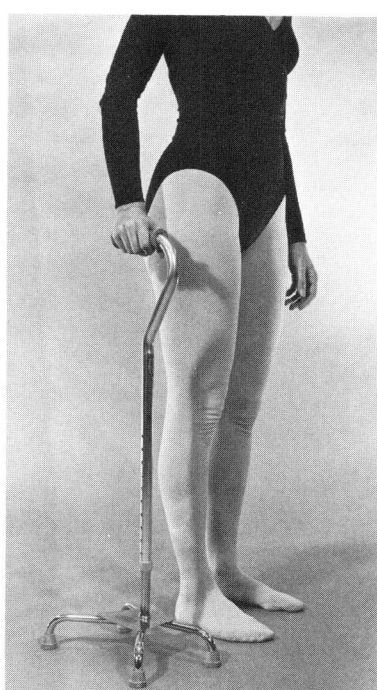

Figure 37–16 Patient using quad-cane.

protecting a hip that is painful or has weak abductors. The use of a cane in the hand on the uninjured side produces a smoother gait and averts the development of an awkward gait, which may turn into a troublesome habit pattern.

Crutch Gaits

A patient with a fracture of the lower extremity needs crutches to take all or part of his weight off the injured extremity while allowing him to get about.

The *swing-to gait* allows non–weight-bearing ambulation. The patient places both crutches evenly ahead of the weight-bearing foot by 12 to 24 inches, transfers his weight to the crutches through his hands, and hops up toward the crutches (Figs. 37–18 and 37–19).

The *swing-through gait* works the same way, except that instead of the weight-bearing leg hopping up to the crutches it is advanced 12 to 24 inches beyond the crutches. This gait can allow a rapid means of locomotion for the vigorous, coordinated patient (Figs. 37–20 and 37–21). If the hip

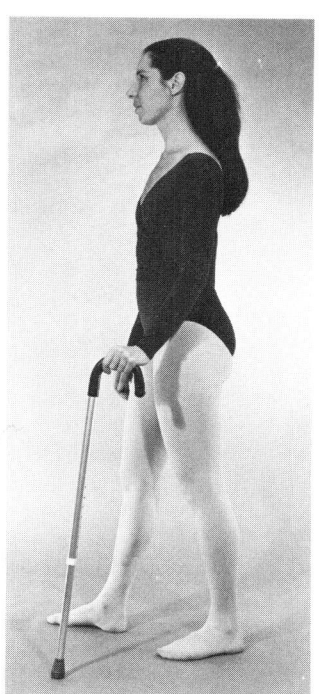

Figure 37–17 Patient advances cane and injured leg simultaneously.

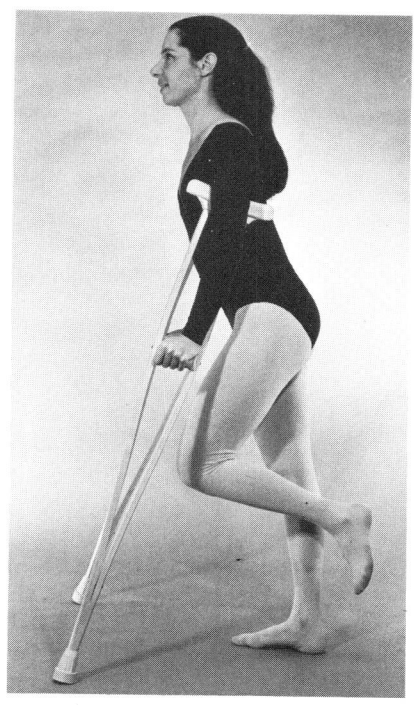

Figure 37–18 Swing-to crutch gait, starting position.

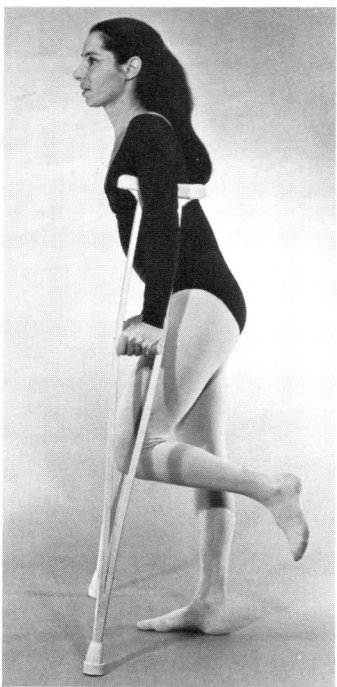

Figure 37–19 Swing-to crutch gait, finish position.

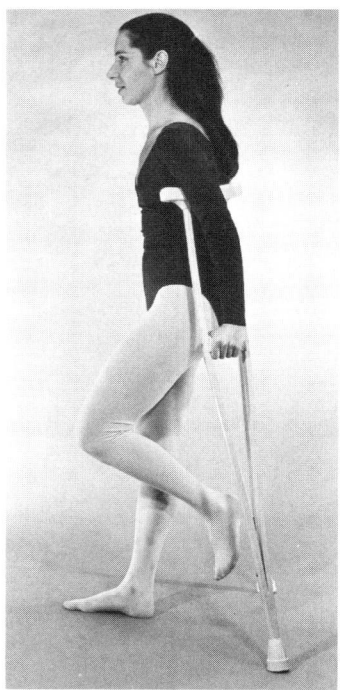

Figure 37–21 Swing-through gait, finish position.

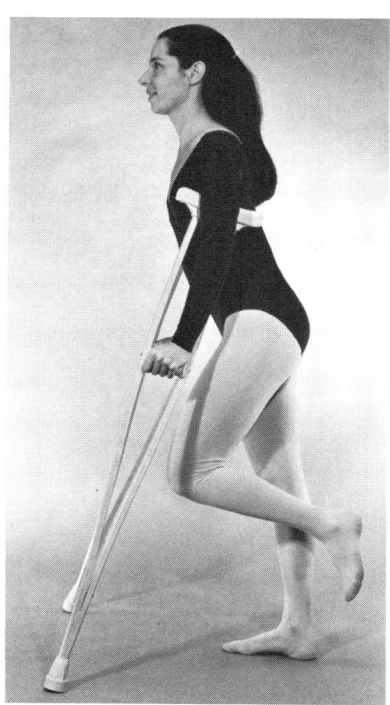

Figure 37–20 Swing-through gait, start position.

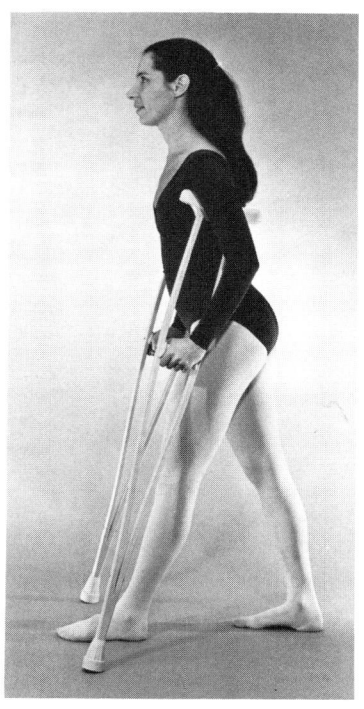

Figure 37–22 Three point gait, weight on foot controlled by amount of weight taken on hands.

and knee of the injured side are flexed, progression can be quite smooth. If the knee must be kept fully extended, it is helpful to attach a 1½- or 2-inch lift to the shoe on the uninjured leg.

The *three-point gait* is used when the patient is ready to progress to weight bearing. The foot on the injured side is placed just to "touch down" simultaneously with the crutches (Fig. 37–22). This provides additional balance and starts the progression to increasing weight bearing as symptoms and stage of healing allow. The amount of weight borne by the injured extremity can be closely controlled by carrying more or less weight on the hands. A gross quantitation of the weight carried on the foot may be obtained by stepping on a bathroom scale and correlating the feel of a given pressure with the weight registered on the scale. A more accurate and practical way to quantitate the weight is to use a limb load monitor that is set to give an audible signal each time a given weight is exceeded.

The *four-point gait* is suitable when full weight bearing is allowed but crutches are still needed for balance or for more protection than canes provide. The gait cycle starts by advancing the right crutch followed by the left foot and then the left crutch followed by the right foot.

A *walk-to gait* offers maximum stability with crutches or a walker. It is a full weight-bearing gait commonly used by elderly individuals who are unsteady. The walker or crutches are advanced, and the patient takes one step (often shuffling) with each foot, walking up to the support.

The *two-point gait* allows more rapid ambulation. The patient advances the right crutch and left foot simultaneously, then the left crutch and the right foot together. This is the same gait that is used with bilateral canes.

A *drag-to gait* is used by paraplegics who lack hip control. This patient advances one crutch, then the other, and then shifts his weight forward, dragging his feet toward the crutches. The paraplegic who has sufficient strength, control, and balance can advance both crutches simultaneously, then bring both feet together up to (swing-to gait) or past the crutches (swing-through gait).

Crutch Training

In addition to the appropriate crutch-gait training, many patients need to learn how to use crutches to assist in other activities. To arise from a bed or chair using crutches for support, the patient must grasp both crutch handles together with one hand. That hand pushes down on the crutches while the other pushes down on the bed or chair (Fig. 37–23). When he has stood erect and gained his balance, the patient arranges the crutches in the usual fashion for walking.

For stair climbing, if there is a secure railing, one hand grasps the railing while the other holds both crutches together (Fig. 37–24). With weight supported evenly by the crutches in the one hand and by the railing with the other, the well leg is raised to the next step (Fig. 37–25). As this leg accepts body weight and its knee is extended, the hand on the railing is advanced, and the crutches are brought to the same step as the well leg (Fig. 37–26). If there is no railing, the crutches are used as in normal ambulation, one on each side (Fig. 37–27). The well leg is brought up to the next step (Fig. 37–28). As it accepts weight and its knee extends, the crutches are

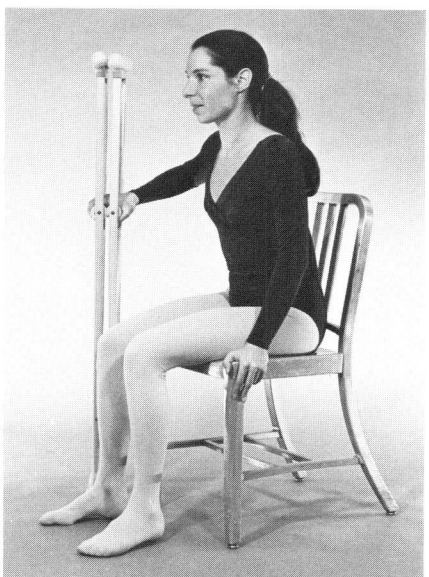

Figure 37–23 Arising from chair with crutches, patient pushes down on crutch handles and on chair.

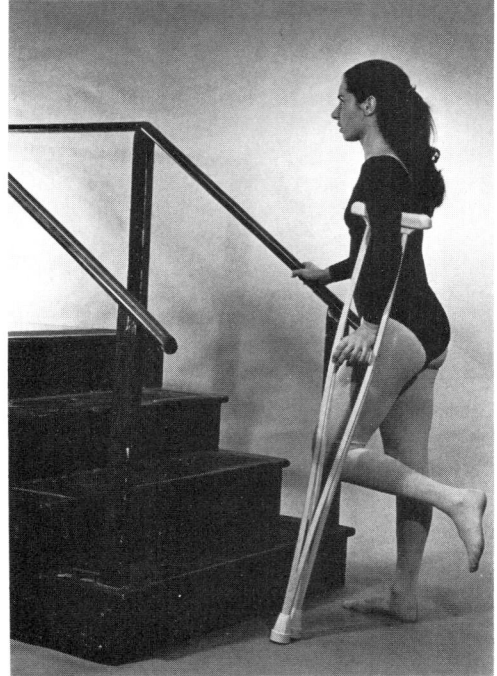

Figure 37–24 Stair climbing with crutches and railing, start position.

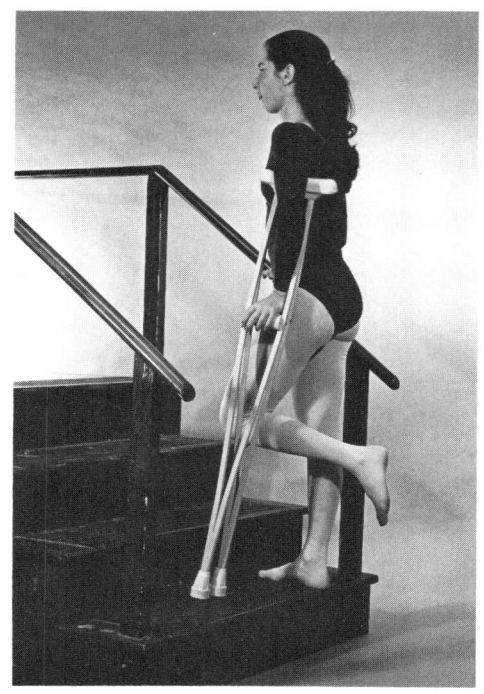

Figure 37–26 Stair climbing with crutches and railing, railing hand advanced as crutches are placed on step with well leg.

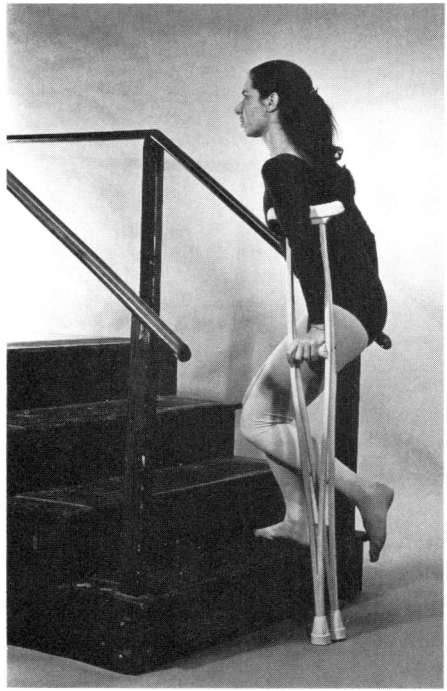

Figure 37–25 Stair climbing with crutches and railing, well leg raised to next step.

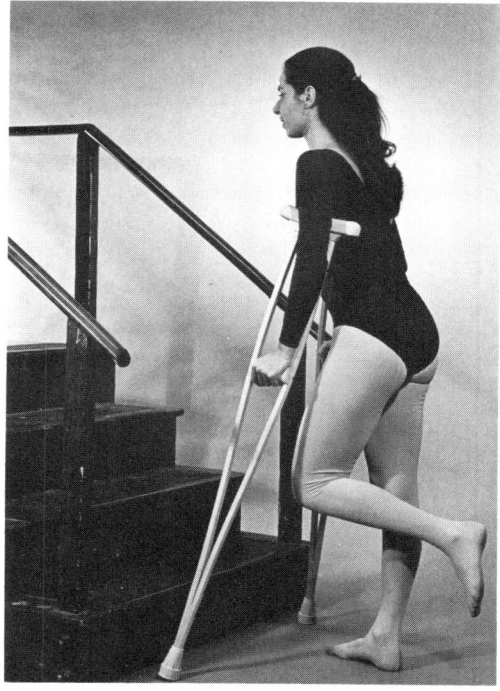

Figure 37–27 Stair climbing with crutches, start position.

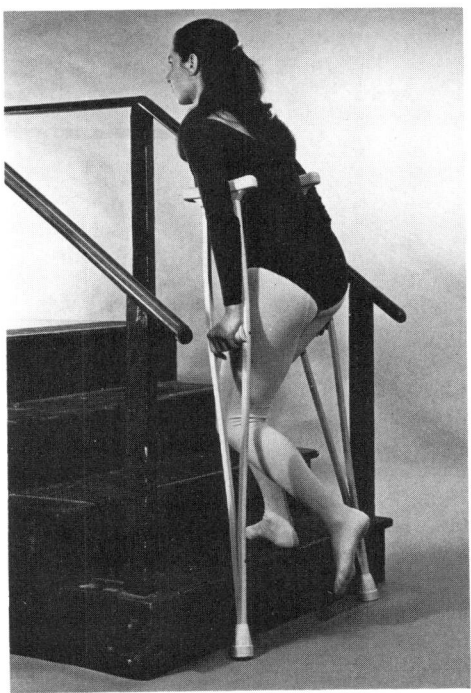

Figure 37–28 Stair climbing with crutches, well leg raised to next step.

brought up to the same step as the well leg.

To descend stairs that have a secure railing, one hand grasps the railing while the other holds the two crutches together. The railing hand and the injured leg are advanced as the crutches are brought to the next step down (Fig. 37–29). As balance is achieved and weight is accepted on both hands, the well leg is brought down to the same step as the crutches. If there is no railing, the crutches are used as in normal ambulation. Both crutches and the injured leg are advanced forward, and the crutches are brought to rest on the next step down (Fig. 37–30). As balance is achieved and weight is accepted on both hands, the well leg is brought down to the same step as the crutches. Ascending and descending a curb is carried out in a similar manner.

These techniques may be taught by a therapist or other trained person until the patient is as secure as possible. Patients who have impaired balance or inadequate muscle strength or coordination should not be allowed to do these maneuvers until it is

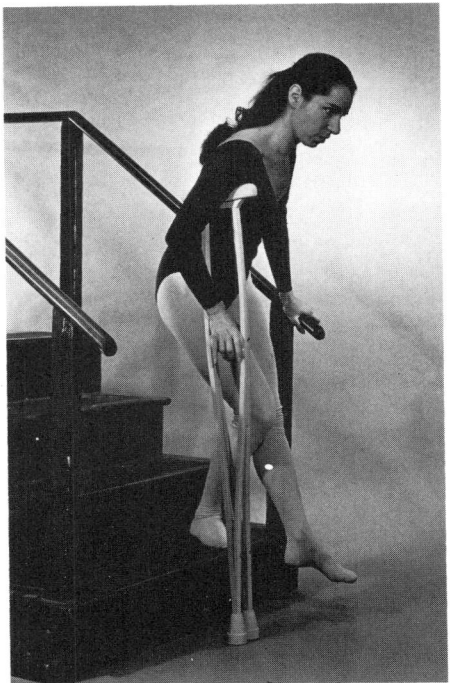

Figure 37–29 Descending stairs with crutches and railing; railing hand, crutches, and injured leg advanced simultaneously.

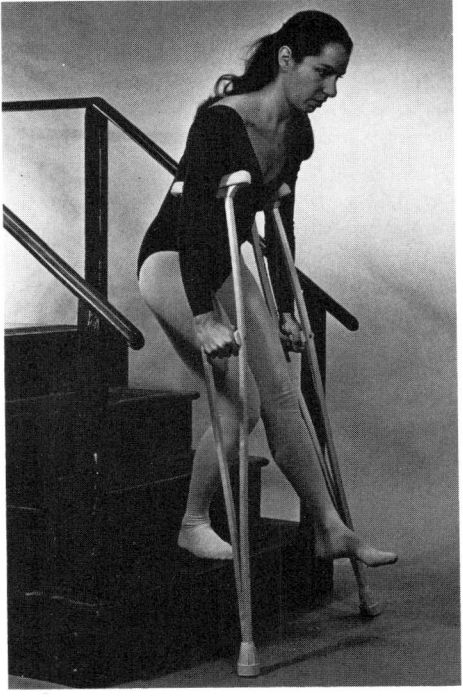

Figure 37–30 Descending stairs with crutches, crutches and injured leg advanced simultaneously.

certain they are ready. One cautious guideline, especially useful with children and the elderly, is to allow them to do one level of activity less than their estimated level of capability—anticipating that they will do at least one level of activity beyond what is permitted.

REHABILITATION OF THE BED-CONFINED PATIENT

From the outset, bed confinement should not be equivalent to solitary confinement. The patient needs to avoid sensory deprivation and to remain in touch with the outside world. Television, radio, reading material, and visitors should be encouraged. Students who are bed-confined, as in traction for femur fractures, can continue their studies. Often arrangements can be made for examinations to be taken while the student is bedridden. Seminars can be held in the hospital room, or the bed can be moved to a nearby conference room for more space and privacy. The self-propelled litter or "prone gurney" allows continued recumbency and, at the same time, mobility around the hospital.

Care of the Skin

It is essential to prevent skin breakdown, also known as pressure sores, bed sores, and decubitus ulcers. The skin of patients with sensory loss is most susceptible to breakdown, but sores commonly occur in spite of normal sensation. The stuporous or comatose patient is at high risk, as is the multiply injured patient. These people require a great deal of time and attention for their primary problems, but the skin must not go unattended, especially when pain or fracture instability makes one reluctant to change the patient's position. The underlying principles are:

1. Be ever vigilant! Look at the skin in all areas at risk. This also serves a therapeutic function, because in order to look at all areas it is necessary to turn the patient.

2. Do not allow unremitting pressure over bony prominences for longer than two to four hours. This may vary with the patient's own padding and the efficacy of what he's lying on to distribute pressure. Sacrum (supine lying) and trochanters (side lying) are the most common areas of breakdown. Ischial sores usually result from uninterrupted pressure in the sitting position. Sores also occur over the heels, malleoli, scapulae, occipital area, and elbow.

3. Avoid skin maceration. Prevent constant wetness from lying in bed clothes soaked with urine, wound drainage, faulty irrigation set-ups, or leaking intravenous tubes.

4. Avoid friction and rubbing. Foam heel and elbow protectors should be used.

Air or water mattresses, alternating pressure mattresses, foam pads, or sheepskins are helpful, but will not eliminate the need for excellent nursing care. Air rings or rubber doughnuts should not be used, since they may hinder circulation.

The prone position, although uncomfortable, should be used for one or two hours two or three times a day if at all possible. Not only does this help avert or treat pressure sores, but it helps prevent hip flexion contractures. The prone position is not without its own problems, and one must pay attention to anterior bony prominences, such as the patellar areas.

At the first sign of persistent redness over a bony prominence, the patient must be kept off that area until the redness clears. At this stage, damage is minor and should heal without much problem. Once the skin turns black, there has been irreversible damage to the epidermis and deeper layers. As long as this area is clean and closed it can be left alone until it sloughs out. As soon as there is a demarcation of necrotic tissue, it may be sharply debrided to bleeding tissue. Cellulitis and abscess formation demand appropriate *systemic* antibiotic therapy and local surgical incision, drainage, and debridement. Topical care is based on the same program that it should have been followed to prevent the sore—keep the pressure off it! Local cleansing with antibacterial soap is helpful, together with regular (one to three times a day) dressing changes for superficial debridement. Large deep sores are often extensively undermined, exposing a large area of raw tissue which is a source of much serum protein loss. A high-calorie, high-protein diet should be encouraged.

When the sore is large and long established, shows no sign of healing, and has underlying osteomyelitis, it needs extensive surgical debridement. At that time, areas of protruding and infected bone can be removed, and a smooth, broad surface of clean, bleeding bone should be fashioned. In general, it is not wise to try to close the wound at this stage. It is better to wait about a week until the area is covered with pink, clean granulation tissue. At this stage the wound is suitable for closure with large flaps of skin and subcutaneous tissue. Occasionally smaller wounds, especially in the ischial area, can be closed directly. Split-thickness skin is not suitable over bony prominences, since it is not mobile and tends to break down easily. For the same reason, it may be better to swing a flap of mobile skin and subcutaneous tissue rather than to have the immobile scar that results when the sore heals by itself.

CARE OF THE JOINTS

In the debilitated, weak, or paralyzed patient, gravity tends to produce equinus deformity of the ankles. The neatly made bed, with sheets tightly tucked in at the foot, exaggerates that deformity. Instead, the sheets ought to be draped over a foot cradle or a footboard. The footboard has the added advantage of providing a prop to support the feet in a neutral position. However, once the patient moves out of position, the support is lost. It is more efficient then to use heavily padded (foam, sheepskin) commercially available splints (Fig. 37–31), or splints made of plaster with a heavy layer of cast padding.

All joints that don't have to be immobilized can be exercised in bed. Range-of-motion exercises can be carried out by the patient and supervised or assisted by nursing personnel, therapists, medical staff, or regularly visiting friends and family. It helps for the physical or occupational therapist to set up a detailed exercise program. For paralyzed and comatose patients, it is essential for the nursing staff to carry on a regular program of passive range-of-motion exercises to all joints. The alert and cooperative patient can also do muscle-building exercises to maintain or improve muscle tone. He can do pull-ups on the overhead trapeze, push-ups with hand-held weights (to prepare for crutch walking), and hand strengthening with grip exercisers. He can work to strengthen various muscle groups of upper and lower extremities by using weights, ropes, and pulleys attached to the overhead frame of the bed.

In the lower extremities, the muscle groups to exercise to prepare for future ambulation are the knee extensors, the hip abductors, and the hip extensors. Isometric or "setting" exercises are useful to start with, especially in casted extremities. Straight leg-raising, using one or two sets of ten repetitions several times a day, should be started as soon as possible. This can be advanced to progressive resistance exer-

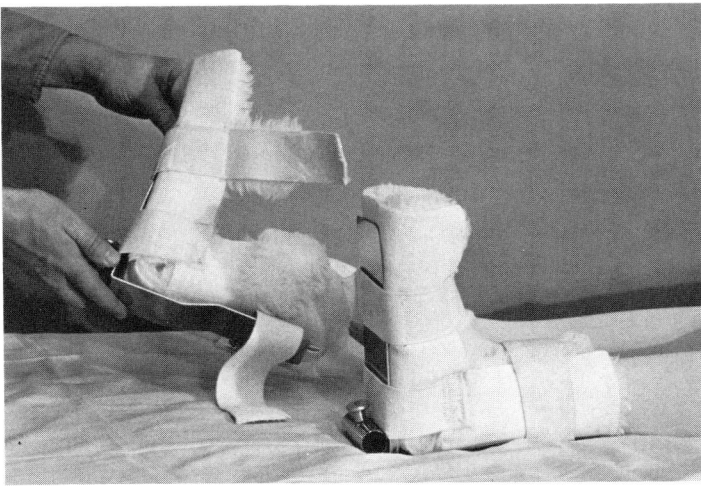

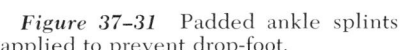
Figure 37–31 Padded ankle splints applied to prevent drop-foot.

cises by regularly adding weights to the ankle. Hip extensors can be exercised in the supine position by pushing the leg against the bed (isometric), or in the prone position by lifting the extremity up off the bed against gravity or even against resistance.

More important are the abductors, which often are weak when exercise is first begun. Wide slings used to support the calf and thigh are attached to weights by ropes and pulleys suspended from the overhead frame of the bed. They counterbalance as much of the weight of the leg as desired, according to how much weight is attached. Slings facilitate hip flexion and abduction. The same result is achieved by using a powder board or skate board. This is a very smooth board placed across the lower third of the bed. Talcum powder is liberally applied to the surface, and the patient's foot is covered by a sock. This arrangement greatly decreases friction in moving the extremity in all directions. Friction can be decreased even more by using a universal ball-bearing skate on which the heel rests. The disadvantage of this method is that it is quite noisy and may be irritating to those nearby.

REHABILITATION FOLLOWING UPPER EXTREMITY INJURY

When immobilization is in place, all unrestricted joints must be taken through as complete a range of motion as the immobilizing device allows. Shoulders and fingers get stiff quickly. Dependent edema can become a major problem, prolonging restriction of finger motion. Slings may help to decrease edema, but at the same time tend to promote shoulder stiffness. When immobilization can be discontinued the exercise program should be expanded to include the joints now liberated. Just how vigorous the exercises should be will depend on the state of healing and the judgment of the orthopedist in charge of the case. Since there is no practical accurate way to measure the strength of a healing fracture, one's enthusiasm for rapid progress must be tempered by fear of an inadvertent return to the starting point. In making this judgment, there is no substitute for clinical experience.

Shoulder motions to be emphasized in an exercise program include full upward motion in forward flexion and abduction. Functionally, this motion must be combined with external rotation, so the hand can be brought to the back of the head to tend the hair and scratch the upper back. Internal rotation must be preserved or restored for scratching the lower and middle back, hooking the bra strap, and reaching into the back pocket for a wallet. Abduction and external rotation are important for ball-throwing and racket-swinging. Adduction and internal rotation are necessary to wash the opposite side of the body.

A preliminary exercise to restore shoulder motion is the Codman or pendulum exercise. This is predominantly a means of eliminating gravity as a force to be overcome. Instead, gravity is used as a force to bring the arm into forward flexion and abduction. The patient stands, bending over forward so the trunk is parallel to the floor. The arm is allowed to fall away from the body as much as pain and stiffness permit. This can be done with the extremity hanging free or supported in a sling. The extremity is then made to swing forward and backward, side to side, and around in circles in one direction and then the other. A weight grasped in the hand or secured to the wrist will increase the range of the arm swing (Fig. 37–32). The key point is to encourage *glenohumeral* joint motion. The patient must not substitute trunk motion for shoulder joint motion, or the exercise will be of little value. Shoulder exercises in the supine position also decrease the resistance from gravity and facilitate motion in various directions.

In the wall-climbing exercise, the fingers "walk" up the wall or the hand slides up the wall. To work on forward flexion, the patient faces the wall; for abduction, his side is to the wall. In either case, maximum motion comes from moving the body progressively closer to the wall as the hand slides higher up the wall. A pulley in the ceiling with a thin rope through it provides a means for the uninjured extremity to assist the injured one in upward motion. Stretching should be carried to the point of discomfort, but not severe pain.

To maintain or restore internal rotation, the patient places his hand behind his back

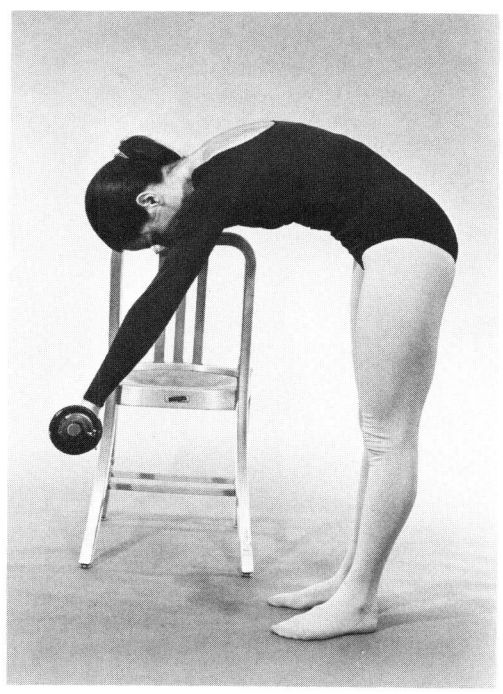

Figure 37–32 Shoulder pendulum exercises with hand-held weights, arm swings forward.

and tries to reach as far up toward the midback as possible. He may use his other hand to assist.

Shoulder muscle-building exercises usually concentrate on deltoid strengthening, but any of the muscle groups can be strengthened if needed for special activities. The progressive resistance formula can be used with hand-held weights or with rope–pulley–weight arrangements as found in a physical therapy gymnasium or as set up at home. Swimming is an excellent exercise to restore motion, strength, and endurance.

Restoration of elbow motion requires active and active assisted range-of-motion exercises. In general, passive stretching exercises of this joint have been discouraged, owing to their possible relation to the formation of ectopic bone. Muscle-building exercises for elbow flexors and extensors use the PRE technique, with hand-held weights or rope–pulley–weight setups. Proprioceptive neuromuscular facilitation is a good technique for patients with much muscle weakness or a great deal of muscle spasm.

Restoration of pronation and supination requires vigorous exercise, when healing permits, for injuries from the elbow down to and including the wrist. Active and active assisted exercises are done with the elbow at 90 degrees of flexion and the arm stabilized against the chest so as to avoid misleading rotation at the shoulder. For muscle strengthening, functional activities, such as driving in and removing wood screws or wringing out a wet towel, provide resistance exercises.

The patient will regain hand function most rapidly if active motion is started at the time the cast or splint is applied. The trim lines on long and short arm casts and splints (for fractures of the wrist and above) should allow full extension and 90 degrees of flexion at the metacarpophalangeal joints. They should also allow opposition of the thumb sufficient for it to pinch against each finger.

The traditional rubber ball squeezing has value only as an isometric exercise unless very small balls are used. Waving or wiggling the fingers is fine as a greeting, but useless as a range-of-motion exercise. Instead, the patient must concentrate on moving each joint to its maximum extent, and then a bit further. He should make a concentrated, continuous, sustained active pull of the flexors and then of the extensors. He can assist this motion with his other hand, or a therapist can assist. Functional activities are of particular value. About the only activities to avoid with the usual plaster cast are those that wet the plaster. Even that restriction is surmountable if a fiber-glass cast is used. The fracture brace made of Orthoplast or other plastic is also waterproof. Moreover, it allows great freedom of joint motion and is believed to shorten fracture healing time by the early introduction of functional activity to the entire extremity.[34, 36]

Edema is the enemy of hand motion, and motion is the best weapon to combat edema. It is helpful to elevate any extremity that has a tendency to swell. Even more important is the avoidance of excessively tight, constricting casts or bandages. For difficult cases, massage may help to milk edema out of the extremity. One technique of massage is effleurage, a deep stroking motion in a centripetal direction. Another method is compression or pétirssage, which uses kneading, squeezing, and friction to mobilize tissue fluid and to stretch adhesions.[19]

REHABILITATION FOLLOWING LOWER EXTREMITY INJURY

Fractures of the pelvis may be unstable and require bed rest until healing is sufficient and pain has abated enough to allow mobilization. Patients with stable fractures also need bed rest until pain subsides. During this period the patient should carry on a regular program of passive and active exercises of all joints not restricted by pain or fracture instability. Early upright position is possible on a tilt table or in the walk-in tank with a high water level. As healing progresses and pain subsides, the patient can progress to crutch-supported ambulation. The type of gait will depend on the limitations imposed by the individual fracture and its state of healing.

Rehabilitation after femoral neck fractures treated by prosthetic replacement is designed to be rapid. Unless there are other medical problems, these patients should progress rapidly from tilt table to parallel bars to walker or crutches. These activities can start as soon as three to five days after surgery and progress as rapidly as the patient's pain, vigor, and coordination allow. The femoral head replacement is generally quite stable since the capsule, trochanteric attachments, and muscles remain intact. Whether the prosthesis is inserted with a force fit or secured with methacrylate cement, the hip mechanism can safely bear full weight immediately. The use of crutch or walker support is preferable, however, to allow stretched muscles to recover function and to provide stability and safety in gait.

These patients should be able to sit up in a few days, but they must keep their hips abducted and avoid hip flexion beyond 70 or 80 degrees until healing is secure. The patient should sit on a chair with an elevated seat or an additional firm cushion. An armchair is best, since it provides a platform for the hands to push against on arising. If chair arms are not present, the patient tends to lean forward to shift the center of gravity over the feet. This maneu-

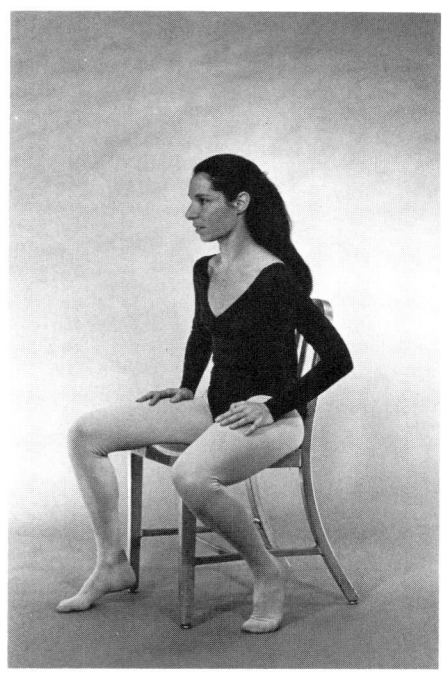

Figure 37–33   Arising from chair, foot placed below hip.

ver acutely flexes the hips and may lead to dislocation. If he inadvertently sits down in a low chair or in one without arms, the patient can arise without excessive hip flexion by abducting the hip on the uninjured side to bring the leg alongside the chair and the foot as far back as convenient. This places the foot more nearly under the center of gravity, so the patient doesn't have to lean over to get up (Figs. 37–33 and 37–34). The hands can push down on the thighs to assist. A similar technique may be used to safely arise from a toilet if an elevated toilet seat is not available.

Exercises for range of motion should stress abduction, external rotation, and extension. These motions are the ones most subject to the development of contractures. These exercises are appropriate if the posterolateral approach to the hip has been used to insert the prosthesis. Muscle strengthening for the abductors is most important for regaining normal gait without an abductor lurch. Next most important are the extensors and last the flexors.

The treatment of femoral fractures by open reduction and internal fixation is designed to minimize the complications of

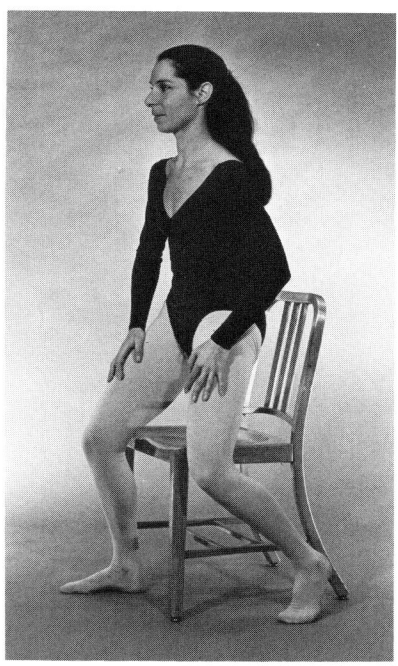

Figure 37–34 Arising from chair, hands push on thighs to assist.

subsides and the fracture achieves some internal stability, muscle-setting exercises for the muscles across the fracture can commence. This of course is only a part of the overall exercise program for all parts not immobilized.

When healing has advanced enough to discontinue traction and suspension, it has been traditional to apply a one-and-a-half hip spica. This precludes upright ambulation, but the patient can be mobile on a self-propelled gurney. Muscle-setting exercises should continue during cast immobilization. In cases in which a single hip spica provides sufficient immobilization, independent ambulation with crutches is a realistic goal except for the weak, debilitated, or otherwise impaired patient. Although cumbersome, the single hip spica does permit independent sitting, standing, walking, and change of position.

It is also possible to start early knee motion by applying hinges at the knee after removing an adequate cylinder of plaster. The location and state of fracture healing will dictate whether and when this is feasible. If the knee can be hinged, it greatly facilitates the restoration of strength and motion. The cast brace and the fracture brace for appropriate femoral shaft fractures permit early hip motion as well as knee motion. If early weight bearing is allowed, there are the added benefits of faster fracture healing and faster return to all types of activities.[24, 35] When immobilization can be discontinued, range-of-motion and strengthening exercises for hip, knee, and ankle should begin.

Patients with fractures of the tibia usually don't need to be confined to bed after the initial swelling has subsided unless there are concomitant injuries. If a long leg cast with flexed knee is the immobilizing device, the patient has to learn a non–weight-bearing, crutch-walking gait (swing-to, swing-through). Exercises of the injured extremity are appropriate and can include muscle setting, leg lifts, and leg lifts with increasing weights (PRE). Active toe motion should be encouraged to minimize edema in the foot. If the knee can be extended in a long leg cast and weight bearing is allowed, a three-point gait is appropriate, the amount of weight borne on the foot increasing as pain allows. If a

bed confinement and to allow a much more rapid rehabilitation of the injured extremity. Once the fracture fragments are securely fixed and postoperative pain has subsided, range-of-motion and muscle strengthening exercises for the hip and knee can commence. The orthopedic surgeon must specify any restrictions in stress applied during exercise, depending on the security of the fixation. As early as the day following surgery, it may be suitable and even desirable to have the patient sitting in a chair and starting physical therapy in the gymnasium. The patient must learn crutch walking, transfers, and activities of daily living within the constraints of limited weight bearing until the fracture heals.

For fractures treated by traction and suspension, the principles described in the treatment of the bed-confined patient apply. A common problem to watch out for is the development of an equinus contracture at the ankle. It may be very resistant to correction and will impair walking. A posterior splint or other foot support along with active and stretching dorsiflexion exercises will prevent this complication. As pain non–weight-bearing, swing-through gait is required, a lift on the other shoe will help the cast to clear the ground in the swing phase.

If the PTB (patellar tendon–bearing) cast or fracture brace for tibial fractures can be used, early motion of the knee can be started, as it can in the ankle if a hinge is used.[35] The same benefits of early return to unsupported ambulation with faster fracture healing are available with this technique. Early in the course of treatment, the patient uses a three-point gait, progressing gradually from touch-down to full weight bearing as pain allows. He should switch to a cane which can be discarded altogether as healing progresses.

In any method of immobilization, the longer the limb is immobilized, the more likely the patient is to develop a "habit limp" unrelated to joint motion or return of muscle strength. Therefore, when the cast comes off the patient may need gait retraining along with exercises and activities to restore joint motion, muscle strength, endurance, and coordination.[29]

For injuries about the ankle and foot, the same principles apply as for tibial fractures. Once the cast comes off, range-of-motion exercises of the active and active assisted type are needed to restore dorsiflexion, plantar flexion (ankle joint), and pronation-supination (subtalar and midfoot joints). Gentle stretching, especially of contracted toes, may be needed.[26] For the common problem of post-cast edema an elastic stocking or anklet is best. The rolled-on elastic bandage is less desirable, since its bulk makes it difficult to wear a shoe. It often wrinkles and causes areas of constriction if it is not very well applied and regularly rewrapped. Local heat, especially whirlpool, and sometimes massage will help reduce edema. The most effective treatments for edema remain elevation, active exercise, and functional use.

REHABILITATION FOLLOWING INJURY TO THE SPINE

The major determinant of the outcome of injury to the vertebral column is the integrity of the spinal cord and its nerve roots.

INJURIES WITHOUT NERVE DAMAGE

In the absence of cord or root damage, rehabilitation aims to keep the patient as mobile as possible and to preserve joint motion and muscle strength while the fracture is healing. The stability of the fracture together with the method of immobilization will determine the level of function permissible and the timetable for safe return to function. For stable fractures of the cervical spine, as little as a plastic cervical collar for pain control may be sufficient. For less stable fractures, a more effective orthosis, such as the Plastazote (Philadelphia) collar, the four-poster orthosis, or a more secure cervicothoracic orthosis, is needed.[17] The most secure external immobilization device is the halo-body jacket which relies on solid skeletal fixation to the skull, with attachment by an outrigger to a plaster or plastic body jacket.[11, 17, 31] The most unstable fractures may require open reduction and internal fixation to provide enough security for ambulation in anything less than the halo-body jacket. When circumstances require traction and recumbency, an active, in-bed exercise program is in order.

For fractures of the thoracic and lumbar spine the same principles apply. A plaster body jacket provides satisfactory immobilization for relief of pain in many stable fractures. When healing has progressed, the patient can use an orthosis, such as the Knight, Taylor, or hyperextension (Jewett) thoraco-lumbosacral orthoses.[2] For less stable fractures, internal fixation and spine fusion, supplemented by orthotic or cast support, may be needed to allow early ambulation. When circumstances delay early assumption of the upright position, the active, in-bed exercise program should start at the outset.

INJURIES WITH NERVE DAMAGE

Cord or root damage resulting from spinal injury presents the major problem, the complexity of which depends on the level of the injury, on the degree of "completeness" of the injury, and on whether any recovery takes place. Whether there is any potential for recovery of nerve function or not, the rehabilitation program aims to prevent the occurrence of many major complications. It also tries to maximize return to function within the limits of the patient's physical abilities and with the support of modern technology. In any case, rehabilitation should start with the earliest treatment of the acute injury and should be continued in a rehabilitation center or spinal cord injury center as soon as medical stability permits.

Urinary Complications

The urinary tract needs careful attention to eliminate or minimize the problem of infection. If there is a lower motor neuron lesion (cauda equina) and a continent sphincter, emptying the bladder can be controlled by strain (Valsalva) and Credé (manual pressure on the bladder) at intervals, as long as the residual urine in the bladder is minimal. The male patient who has no sphincter control needs a condom catheter. There is no equivalent device for the female, who must use diapers or an indwelling catheter.

If there is an upper motor neuron (spinal cord) lesion, there will be sphincter tone and reflex contraction of the detrusor. If the sphincter tone is not excessive and the detrusor can be stimulated to contract by some form of sensory input in the perineal area, the patient can develop a predictable and controllable reflex bladder emptying and may not need any other device.[4] If this method is unsuccessful or if there is too much residual urine in the bladder, a program of intermittent catheterization is the next best long-term treatment. A nurse or technician catheterizes the patient at frequent intervals until either he or a family member can take over this function. If this fails or if the patient has too high a cord lesion to catheterize himself, an indwelling catheter is necessary. This device must be irrigated once or twice a day and be changed at one- to three-week intervals. The patient should force fluids, take regular doses of ascorbic acid to acidify the urine, and use an appropriate urinary tract antiseptic.

When recurrent urinary tract infections resist control, the best solution may be the construction of a ureteroileostomy. In any case, it is important to assess the integrity of the urinary tract with an intravenous urogram at regular intervals as determined by the urologist, who ought to be in close consultation regarding this aspect of the patient's care.

Pressure Sores

The prevention and management of pressure sores is most important in the sensory-impaired patient.[38] The principles of management for the bed-confined patient have been outlined earlier. The cord-injured patient remains at risk when he leaves his bed to sit in a wheelchair. The paraplegic with sufficient upper extremity strength must protect himself by doing push-ups in his wheelchair at hourly intervals to preserve circulation over the ischial tuberosities. He should also use a cushion made of thick foam or gel material to distribute pressure. Patients at high risk might do well to use a cut-out seat board under the cushion to further minimize ischial pressure. Paraplegics and quadriplegics and their attendants must understand that this is a lifelong problem requiring daily attention. The paraplegic who is on his own should inspect his skin twice a day, using a mirror to see all areas. The quadriplegic's attendant should do the same. If a developing pressure sore is noted and treated early, it will save a great deal of grief, morbidity, and expense.

Heterotopic Bone

Heterotopic bone, ectopic bone, or paraarticular ossification develops in as many as 20 per cent of patients with spinal cord injury, for unknown reasons. It starts within the first few weeks or months of injury and involves predominantly hips and knees, although elbows, shoulders, and occasionally other joints may be affected. Local warmth, swelling, and stiffness precede roentgenographic evidence. At first, a lacy, ill-defined calcification appears, which gradually matures to trabecular bone. Alkaline phosphatase values will be elevated, and technetium diphosphonate bone scan will show increased activity in the involved area.[13, 16]

The early treatment is range-of-motion and stretching exercises. This will often maintain adequate motion for functional activities. If restricted motion impairs function, one can attempt to excise sufficient bone to allow motion, but not before roentgenograms show mature bone with no further progression on serial studies (usually many months after onset). A normal alkaline phosphatase level and a normal bone scan would be reassuring before embarking on this often difficult surgical adventure.[13, 16, 43]

Spasticity

Spasticity occurs to some degree in most patients with spinal cord injury and usually involves the lower extremities. It requires an intact reflex arc and cannot be present in lower motor neuron (root, peripheral nerve) injuries. It is caused by loss of inhibitory input from higher centers in the central nervous system. It can be increased by local noxious stimuli (which would be painful if pain perception were intact), such as pressure sores, urinary tract infections, fractures, and local surgery. Tension and emotional upset can increase spasticity; sleep, tranquilizers, and muscle relaxants (such as diazepam) can decrease it.

Spasticity can be beneficial and is thought to help maintain mineralization of bone by constant muscle pull. Lower extremity extensor spasticity can occasionally substitute for bracing in ambulation with crutches. Mild spasticity is not a problem unless range-of-motion exercises are not carried out and contractures develop. Moderate spasticity can usually be controlled by range-of-motion exercises, including stretching when necessary. Muscle relaxants, local heat, or local ice may be helpful prior to and during the exercise program. Occasionally, splints for positioning are useful.

Severe spasticity can present difficult management problems. The dose of diazepam needed to control the spasms will often be so high as to produce excessive sedation. Stretching and splinting trigger strong stretch reflex muscle contraction. Little by little, contractures develop and may produce extreme degrees of deformity of the extremities. As deformity worsens, the patient loses the ability to don orthoses, transfer, and even sit in a chair. Nursing care becomes increasingly difficult in terms of cleansing and positioning, and the patient becomes more susceptible to pressure sores. The usual deformity is flexed, adducted hips, flexed knees, and plantarflexed feet.

Treatment depends on static and dynamic assessment of deformity forces. It should be instituted when it becomes obvious that the deformities are worsening and are interfering with the rehabilitation program. Hip flexion deformity responds well to iliopsoas myotomy, in which a cutting cautery is used to transect the muscle as it dips over the pelvic brim.[15, 23, 25, 41] An obturator neurectomy, performed via the intrapelvic or extrapelvic route, will abolish adductor spasticity. It is occasionally necessary to perform a percutaneous or open adductor tenotomy. Posteromedial and posterolateral knee incisions provide access to the hamstring insertions which can be transected. In severe cases the medial and lateral heads of the gastrocnemius should also be transected. It is important to avoid making the incisions too far back and thus close together, since that will produce a narrow skin bridge that might slough.

Full knee extension is not possible at first, being limited by tight skin, vessels, and nerves. Serial, very well padded casts or splints will gradually stretch the knees out over the next two to four weeks. As the hips and knees straighten, the patient should lie prone for several hours each day. Splints must protect the newly gained position part of each day for several months. The joints will also need a routine range-of-motion program.

If ambulation or brace-wearing is a goal that is being frustrated by equinus deformity, percutaneous tendo Achillis lengthening, combined with tenotomy of other deforming-force muscles is appropriate.[15, 25, 41]

Fracture

Fractures in the paraplegic and quadriplegic occur more readily from minor trauma to osteoporotic bone. It is not uncommon to hear the story of a paralytic whose joints were being exercised by a therapist or family member when a snap was heard and felt. This often indicates a fracture of the femur or other long bone. If the extremity is sensate and functional, the fracture should receive the treatment customary for its particular characteristics. Where there is no skin sensation, cast immobilization is apt to cause pressure sores. If there is no pain, the only immobilization necessary may be a pillow wrapped longitudinally around the fractured area. This can be changed at regular intervals for observation and care of the skin. These fractures usually heal rapidly, with abundant callus. Especially with the nonambulatory patient, no more vigorous treatment of a lower extremity fracture is indicated. On the other hand, if there is pain, or if a malunion would impair ambulation or other function, open reduction and internal fixation may be indicated, especially if it is necessary to avoid casts over insensate skin.[22]

Autonomic Dysreflexia

Autonomic dysreflexia is a complication of injury to the upper thoracic and cervical cord segments. Uncontrolled activity of the sympathetic nervous system produces a severe hypertension with symptoms of severe headache and sweating about the face. It is commonly triggered by stimulation of the rectum or bladder or by pain-producing skin stimuli. Therefore, the initial treatment includes clearing a blocked catheter to allow the bladder to empty, bringing the patient to a sitting posture, or using dibucaine ointments prior to rectal care. If the hypertension is not controlled by these measures, it may be necessary to use intravenous hydralazine or even to proceed to spinal anesthesia.[5]

Physical Therapy

Physical therapy concentrates on two major groups of activities. The first aims to maintain or restore joint motion and to build muscle strength in order to maximize function with the remaining muscles. The second aims to train the patient in the use of techniques and equipment that allow the greatest function in spite of physical restrictions.

PARAPLEGIA

The paraplegic needs to learn how to transfer from bed to wheelchair to commode and back. He must learn dressing and undressing, bathing, bowel and bladder

care, and other activities of daily living. He can learn to drive a car with hand controls and must learn independent transfer of himself and his wheelchair into and out of the car. If his level of cord damage will allow ambulation he must be fitted with the appropriate (hip) knee-ankle-foot orthoses, and he must learn to use crutches. He will have to learn how to apply and remove his orthoses and how to get up from the floor if he falls. He will need the proper size wheelchair with removable arms to allow transfers and swing-away foot rests for mobility and flexibility. Edberg has outlined a realistic projection of goals of function to be expected, depending on weight, sex, age, and level of injury.

Patients with a complete cord injury between T1 and T12 would be expected to ". . . wheel their wheelchairs up over curbs, transfer to and from a tub, get themselves from a wheelchair to the floor and return, and take care of their own catheters."[12] Most paraplegics with this level of injury will not be functional ambulators with crutches and braces, because the energy expenditure is too great. A few young, vigorous patients may achieve this function.

If the cord injury is at the L1 to L2 level, some ambulation will be possible, based on the presence of pelvic muscle control.

With an injury level at L3 to L4, the patient is likely to ambulate well with bilateral ankle-foot orthoses and crutches or canes. Some may need orthotic control of the knee as well.[12]

QUADRIPLEGIA

The quadriplegic faces problems of even greater magnitude, increasingly so with higher levels of injury. He must rely more on the help of another person and on special devices, such as an electric-powered wheelchair and even electric-powered upper extremity orthoses. Stauffer has summarized the functional expectations of the quadriplegic, depending on the level of injury.

Above the C4 level, the patient needs permanent assisted respiration.

At the C4 level, the patient can drive an electric wheelchair with a tongue or chin control switch. With a mouth-held stick he can manipulate small objects, such as the keys of an electric typewriter. He is dependent on others for all activities of daily living.

The C5 quadriplegic still requires an electric wheelchair with chin or tongue switch control and can use a powered hand splint for manipulation of small objects.

At the C6 level, the patient should be independent in some functions, since he has active wrist extensors. He may be able to transfer from bed to wheelchair and into a car. He should do much of his own dressing, and he can push a standard wheelchair. The flexor-hinge hand splint allows function in other activities of daily living, including writing, personal hygiene, and a number of daily self-care activities.

Patients with a C7 level should be independent in most activities of daily living, including dressing, personal hygiene, and transfers. Their major upper extremity lack is functional activity of finger flexors for grasp. If necessary, a flexor-hinge hand splint will permit grasping small and large objects.[14, 41]

Spinal–cord-injured patients need strong support at the outset from the entire rehabilitation staff. The injuries may have produced the most severe physical deficits while sparing the intellectual process. This usually leads to depression, which may be profound enough to thwart all efforts at rehabilitation. Support from the psychiatrist may be especially helpful.

The patient with significant deficit from spinal cord injury presents a major challenge that can best be handled by a team of specialists who are skilled and interested in handling this type of problem.

REFERENCES

1. American College of Sports Medicine. Guidelines for Graded Exercises Testing and Exercise Prescription, p. 46. Philadelphia, Lea & Febiger, 1975.
2. Berger, N., and Lussken, R.: Orthotic components of systems. In Atlas of Orthotics: Biomechanical Principles and Application, pp. 351–357. St. Louis, C. V. Mosby, 1975.
3. Burgess, E. M., and Alexander, A. G.: Canes, crutches and walkers. In Atlas of Orthotics. Biomechanical Principles and Application, p. 423. St. Louis, C V. Mosby, 1975.
4. Comarr, A. E.: Urological management of the traumatic cord bladder. Clin. Orthop. Rel. Res., 112:53–59, 1975.
5. Comarr, A. E.: Autonomic dysreflexia. In Pierce, D. S., and Nickel, V. L. (eds.): The Total Care of Spinal Cord Injuries, pp. 181–185. Boston, Little, Brown, 1977.
6. Cooper, K. H.: The New Aerobics, pp. 22–23. New York, Evans, 1970.
7. Delateur, B., Lehmann, J., Stonebridge, J., and Warren, C. G.: Isotonic versus isometric exercise: a double-shift transfer-of-training study. Arch. Phys. Med. Rehab., 53:216, 1972.
8. DeLorme, T. L.: Restoration of muscle power by heavy-resistance exercises. J. Bone Joint Surg., 27:645–667, 1945.
9. DeLorme, T. L., West, F. E., and Shriber, W. J.: Influence of progressive-resistance exercises on knee function following femoral fractures. J. Bone Joint Surg., 32A:910–924, 1950.
10. DeLorme, T. L.: Recent Developments in Progressive-Resistance Exercises. AAOS Instructional Course Lectures, Vol. X, pp. 225–232. Ann Arbor, Edwards, 1953.
11. DeWald, R. L.: Halo traction systems. In Atlas of Orthotics; Biochemical Principles and Application, pp. 407–417. St. Louis, C. V. Mosby, 1975.
12. Edberg, E.: Physical therapy for thoracic and lumbar paraplegia. In Pierce, D. S., and Nickel, V. L. (eds.): The Total Care of Spinal Cord Injuries, p. 230. Boston, Little, Brown, 1977.
13. Freehafer, A. A.: Long term management of lumbar paraplegia. In Pierce, D. S., and Nickel, V. L. (eds.): The Total Care of Spinal Cord Injuries, pp. 135–163. Boston, Little, Brown, 1977.
14. Garrett, A.: Functional potential of patients with spinal cord injury. Clin. Orthop. Rel. Res., 112:60–65, 1975.
15. Glazer, R. M., and Mooney, V.: Surgery of the extremities in patients with multiple sclerosis. Arch. Phys. Med. Rehab., 51:494, 1970.
16. Hsu, J. D., Sakimura, I., and Stauffer, E. S.: Heterotopic ossification around the hip joint in spinal cord injured patients. Clin. Orthop. Rel. Res., 112:165–169, 1975.
17. Johnson, R. M.: Cervical orthoses. J. Bone Joint Surg., 59A:332–339, 1977.
18. Kabat, J.: Studies on neuromuscular dysfunction. XV. The role of central facilitation in restoration of motor function in paralysis. Arch. Phys. Med., 33:521–533, 1952.
19. Krusen, F. H., Kottke, F. J., and Ellwood, P. M.: Handbook of Physical Medicine and Rehabilitation. Philadelphia, W. B. Saunders, 1971.
20. Leach, R. E., Stryker, W. S., and Zohn, D.: A comparative study of isometric and isotonic quadriceps exercise programs. J. Bone Joint Surg., 47A:1422, 1965.
21. Leach, R. E., Stryker, W. S., and Zohn, D.: A comparative study of isometric and isotonic quadriceps exercise programs. J. Bone Joint Surg., 47A:1425, 1965.
22. McMaster, W. C., and Stauffer, E. W.: The management of long bone fractures in the spinal cord injured patient. Clin. Orthop. Rel. Res., 112:44–52, 1975.
23. Michaelis, L. S.: Orthopaedic Surgery of the Limbs in Paraplegia, pp. 1–51. Berlin, Springer, 1964.
24. Mooney, V.: Cast bracing. Clin. Orthop. Rel. Res., 102:159–166, 1974.
25. Mooney, V., and Goodman, F.: Surgical approaches to lower-extremity disability secondary to stroke. Clin. Orthop. Rel. Res., 63:151, 1969.

26. Moskowitz, E.: Rehabilitation in extremity fractures, p. 130. Springfield, Charles C Thomas, 1968.

27. Nicholas, P. J. R., and Hamilton, E. A.: Rehabilitation Medicine: The Management of Physical Disabilities, pp. 25–26. London, Butterworth, 1976.

28. Nicholas, P. J. R.: Rehabilitation after fractures of the shaft of the femur. J. Bone Joint Surg., *45B*:96–102, 1963.

29. Nicholas, P. J. R., and Parish, J. G.: Rehabilitation of fracture of the shafts of the tibia and fibula. Ann. Phys. Med., 5:73–87, 1959.

30. Perrine, J. J.: Isokinetic Pre-ambulation Weight-bearing Therapy with the Kinetron. New York, Cybex Division of Lumex, Inc., 1971.

31. Pierce, D. S.: Acute treatment of spinal cord injuries. *In* Pierice, D. S., and Nickel, V. L. (eds.): Total Care of Spinal Cord Injuries, pp. 10–16. Boston, Little, Brown, 1977.

32. Rose, D. L., Radzyminski, S. F., and Beatty, R. R.: Effect of brief maximal exercise on the strength of the quadriceps femoris. Arch. Phys. Med. Rehab., 38:157–164, 1957.

33. Royal Canadian Air Force Exercise Plans for Physical Fitness. New York, Pocket Books, 1972.

34. Sarmiento, A., Kinman, P. B., Murphy, R. B., and Phillips, J. G.: Treatment of ulnar fractures by functional bracing. J. Bone Joint Surg., 58A: 1104–1107, 1976.

35. Sarmiento, A.: Fracture bracing. Clin. Orthop. Rel. Res., *102*:152–158, 1974.

36. Sarmiento, A., Kinman, P. B., Galvin, E. G., Schmitt, R. H., and Phillips, J. G.: Functional bracing of fractures of the shaft of the humerus. J. Bone Joint Surg., *59A*:596–601, 1977.

37. Schram, D. A.: Resistance exercises. *In* Licht, S. L. (ed.): Therapeutic Exercise, p. 298. New Haven, Elizabeth Licht, 1961.

38. Shea, J. D.: Pressure sores. Classification and management. Clin. Orthop. Rel. Res., *112*:89–100, 1975.

39. Simon, W. H.: Soft tissue disorders of the shoulder. Orthop. Clin. North Am., 6:534–537, 1975.

40. Smodlaka, V.: Rehabilitating the injured athlete. Phys. Sports Med., 5:50, 1977.

41. Stauffer, E. S.: Long-term management of traumatic quadriplegia. *In* Pierce, D. S., and Nickel, V. L. (eds.): The Total Care of Spinal Cord Injuries, pp. 81–102. Boston, Little, Brown, 1977.

42. Thistle, H. G., Hislop, H. J., Moffroid, M., and Lowman, E. W.: Isokinetic contraction: a new concept of resistive exercise. Arch. Phys. Med. Rehab., 48:280, 1967.

43. Wharton, G. W., and Morgan, T. H.: Ankylosis in the paralyzed patient. J. Bone Joint Surg., *52A*:105–112, 1970.

44. Wilmore, J. H.: Exercise prescription: role of the physiatrist and allied health professional. Arch. Phys. Med. Rehab., 57:315, 1976.

Index

Note: Page numbers in *italics* indicate illustrations; page references to tables include the designation (t).

Bone graft(s) (*Continued*)
   tibial, 104
   vascular pedicle, survival of, 102
Bone metabolism, hormones in, 58–60
   systemic control of, 947–948, *947*
   vitamins and, 60
Bosworth fracture, 827
Bosworth technique, for surgical repair of
      acromioclavicular dislocation, 414, *415*
Boutonnière deformity, 568, *568*
Boxer's fracture, 589, *589, 590*
Brachial plexus, injury of, in fractures and
      dislocations, 985–987
Brachial plexus block, 175–178
   axillary approach, 176, *177, 178*
   interscalene approach, 175, *175*
   supraclavicular approach, 175, *176, 177*
Bracing, functional, biomechanics of, 148
   of humeral shaft fracture, 427
Bristow method, of coracoid process transfer,
      398, *399*
Buckle fracture, of distal radius and ulna,
      202, *202*
Burns, fractures and, 992–1009
   orthopedic management and techniques
         for, 994–1008
      acute phase, 1000–1003, *1001–1003*
      reconstructive phase, 1005
      resuscitative phase, 994–1000, *995–999*
      subacute phase, 1003–1005, *1004, 1006*

Calcaneus
   anatomy of, 843, *843*
   fracture of, 860–868
      classification of, 861, *861*
      mechanism of injury of, 862
      roentgenographic examination of, 862
      treatment of, 863–868, *864–868*
Calcar femorale, 632, *633*
Calcification, theories of, 55–58, *57, 58*
Calcitonin, in bone metabolism, 59
Calcium, metabolism of, calcitonin and, 59
      parathyroid hormone and, 58, 948
Callus, hard, 43, *43*
   soft, 42, *43*
Cancellous bone graft, histological sequence
      of repair in, 98
   with internal fixation, 109
Canes, as aid to ambulation, 1052, *1053*
Capitate bone, fracture of, 546
Capitellum, fracture of, 455, *455, 456*
Caput succedaneum, 238
Cardiopulmonary resuscitation, of multiply
      injured patient, 940–944
Cardiothoracic injury, management of, in
      multiply injured patient, 936–937
Carpal bone(s)
   dislocation of, 547–551
      lunate, 549, *549, 550*
         with navicular fracture, *549, 550*
      lunate-navicular, *549, 550*
      perilunar, 547, *548*
         with navicular fracture, 548, *548*
      perilunar-navicular, *548, 549*
   fracture of, 536–547
      capitate, 546

Carpal bone(s) (*Continued*)
   fracture of, distribution of, 536(t)
      incidence of, 536(t)
      lunate, Kienböck's disease and, 544, *545*
      navicular, 536–543. See also *Navicular
         bone, of wrist, fracture of.*
      nerve injuries complicating, 983
      of hook of hamate, 546, *546*
      of trapezium, 546
      of triquetrum, 543, *544*
      pediatric, 201
   fracture-dislocation of, 547–551
   gross anatomy of, *505*
   subluxation of, 551–553
Carpal mechanism, 505, 533–536, *534–536*
Carpometacarpal joint, 505
   fracture-dislocation of, 591, *592, 593*
   of thumb, dislocation of, 580, *581*
Cast
   for humeral shaft fracture, hanging, 428,
      430, 431
      shoulder spica, 431
   for supracondylar femoral fracture, 714
   for tibial fracture, 782–784
   orthopedic walking, stresses in, 149
Cast brace, for femoral fracture, 700–703, *701,
      718, 719*
Cast wedging, of tibial fracture, 784
Cellular interactions, in wound, 28–32, *30, 31*
Cephalhematoma, 238
Chest
   injury of, 286–291
      cartilaginous, 289
      flail, 289–290
         management of, in multiply injured
            patient, 936
      of rib, 288–289, *288*
      of sternum, 286–288, *287*
   surgical anatomy of, 286
Child abuse, 232–233, *232, 233*
Chronic granulomatous disease, infection in,
      25, *26*
Clavicle
   fracture of, 360–365, *361*
      birth, 199
      classification of, 361, *361*
      mechanism of injury of, 360
      of distal third, 365
         classification of, 361, *361*
      of inner third, 364, *364*
      of middle third, 364
      pediatric, 216, *216, 217*
      physical examination of, 362
      roentgenographic evaluation of, 362, *363*
      treatment of, 362
   pseudarthrosis of, congenital, *91, 92*
Clothespin(H) graft, 109
Coccyx, fracture of, 622
Collagen, 9–18
   extracellular assembly of, 12, *13*
   fiber formation of, role of proteoglycans in,
      19
   lysis of, 14
      balance of, with synthesis, 15, *15, 17*
      factors increasing, 18(t)
   of bone, 11, 37
   orientation of, by electric current, 78
   registration peptides of, 12